8TH EDITION

ESSENTIALS OF
HUMAN DISEASES AND CONDITIONS

8TH EDITION

ESSENTIALS OF
HUMAN DISEASES
AND CONDITIONS

TRACIE FUQUA BS, CMA (AAMA) (*Retired*)

Former Program Director and Instructor
Medical Assisting Program Chair
Wallace State Community College
Hanceville, Alabama

ELSEVIER

Elsevier
3251 Riverport Lane
St. Louis, Missouri 63043

ESSENTIALS OF HUMAN DISEASES AND CONDITIONS, EIGHTH EDITION   ISBN: 978-0- 443-11452-6

Senior Content Strategist: Yvonne Alexopoulos
Senior Content Development Specialist: Rebecca M. Leenhouts
Publishing Services Manager: Deepthi Unni
Senior Project Manager: Manchu Mohan
Design Direction: Brian Salisbury

Printed in Canada.

Last digit is the print number: 9 8 7 6 5 4 3 2 1

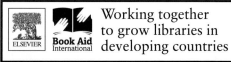

To my husband of 30 years, Michael David, and our children, Ethan and Kaitlynn, for supporting me throughout the revision of the book.
To my father John Wesley Griffin and in memory of my mother Ann Griffin, for teaching me to appreciate my blessings and to be thankful for each day. To my sister Lisa for continuing to be my rock as we care for our father. And to all my other family members and friends who are an important part of my life.
In memory of Margie Schell Frazier for showing her faith in me.
Love you always,

Tracie

Contributors and Reviewers

CONTRIBUTORS

Brandon Brooks, M.Ed., CPhT
Director of Distance Learning
Calhoun Community College
Decatur, Alabama

REVIEWERS

Brandon Brooks, M.Ed., CPhT
Director of Distance Learning
Calhoun Community College
Decatur, Alabama

Tiffany Brown, CMA (AAMA), AAS-MA, BSEd
State of AZ Teaching License; American Heart Association
   BLS, HeartSaver, and First Aid Certified Instructor;
   Certified Community Nutrition Counselor
Teacher
Central AZ Community College
Coolidge, Arizona

Michelle Buchman, MA, BSN, RN
Assistant Professor
Cox College
Springfield, Missouri

Artis Ann Howard, MHA, RHIA, CCS, CCS-P
Program Director, Health Information Technology and
   Management
Laramie County Community College (LCCC)
Cheyenne, Wyoming

LaToya Mason, MHA, MBA, CMA(AAMA)
Director, Health Sciences
Lake Michigan College
Benton Harbor, Michigan

Preface

Essentials of Human Diseases and Conditions, Eighth Edition, is a user-friendly reference intended to serve as an informative, stimulating, and practical textbook for students. This book is also an invaluable tool as a handbook for health care providers in any type of health care setting. Instructors of anatomy and physiology, disease conditions, medical insurance coding, pharmacology, massage therapy, and medical transcription may appreciate the value of this edition as a required text. This encyclopedic, but simplified, handbook includes comprehensive information on hundreds of diseases and conditions. Students in the field of medical assisting, medical transcription, medical insurance coding, pharmacy technology, massage therapy, or other allied health programs with prior introduction to basic anatomy and physiology of the human body and medical terminology will find the text format orderly, concise, and easy to comprehend. Approximately 100 new or replacement images have been added to this edition of the textbook throughout the chapters. Credentialing examination questions have been added in every chapter of the text.

Distinctive Features of Our Approach

Content and topics new to this edition include the following, in addition to updated existing content:
- In Chapter 1, a case study of a patient who was diagnosed with methicillin-resistant *Staphylococcus aureus* after a trimalleolar fracture has been added. Full-color images are presented, which follow a 2.5-year progression. Stem cell research information has been expanded. Cupping therapy with an image has been added. Magnetic therapy (transcranial magnetic stimulation) has been updated to include US Department of Food and Drug Administration (FDA) approval.
- Chapter 2 includes an explanation of amniotic band syndrome. Genetic influence has been included.
- Chapter 3 includes new information regarding preexposure prophylaxis for reducing the risk of contracting the human immunodeficiency virus. Gene therapy has been expanded to include updated information.
- Chapter 4 includes updated information on bioidentical hormone replacements and types, which are now approved by the FDA for use. Changes regarding options for continual glucose monitoring have been updated.
- In Chapter 5, macular degeneration has been expanded to include geographic atrophy. Proton therapy for ocular tumors has been included.

- Chapter 6 includes updated information for preventing herpes zoster (shingles). Newer, current treatment methods for keloid scars are included too.
- Chapter 7 updates include the most recent diagnostic criteria for fibromyalgia. Scoliosis section has been updated to include treatment using nonfusion surgery called posterior dynamic distraction for patients who do not respond to bracing.
- Revolutionary "Jaw in a Day Surgery" has been included in Chapter 8. Information about head and neck cancers and the link to specific genes is covered. Nissen fundoplication, an updated treatment for gastroesophageal reflux disease, is included. An explanation of the procedure of fecal microbiota transplantation is new to this edition.
- In Chapter 9, a section on the coronovirus disease (COVID-19) has been added. Olfactory training is explained.
- Chapter 10 includes expanded information and a new treatment option for broken heart syndrome, which includes LifeVest. Updated information for the genetic cause or etiology of polycythemia vera is included.
- In Chapter 11, en bloc kidney transplant is explained. Updated information is included in the current recommended treatment plan for pyelonephritis.
- Chapter 12 updates include the condition of HELLP (hemolysis, elevated liver enzymes, and low platelets) syndrome, which has been identified in the preeclampsia and eclampsia information. Guidelines for age groups who need to be screened for prostate-specific antigen levels have been updated in this chapter, and information regarding the etiology of uterine cancer has been updated.
- In Chapter 13, the information regarding migraine headaches and genetic links has been updated. The section covering epilepsy has been expanded and updated to include the three identified types of epilepsy and specific signs and symptoms for the identified types. The identification of specific genes involved in Huntington disease has been updated and explained. Amyotrophic lateral sclerosis has been updated to include genetic influences. Botox injections, in some cases, are updated as a treatment for trigeminal neuralgia (tic douloureux).
- The information in the Enrichment section that covers poliomyelitis and postpolio syndrome has been expanded.
- Chapter 14 includes updated information regarding applied behavior analysis as one of the methods for treating autism. Oppositional defiant disorder section

includes updated criteria which providers use to diagnose this condition. Diagnostic criteria for the determination of whether or not a person has schizophrenia have been updated. The patient teaching information has been expanded for those patients' taking risperidone. A new enrichment, neuroleptic malignant syndrome which is a unique life-threatening reaction to antipsychotic drugs, has been added. Sleep disorders has been expanded to include six major categories, as identified in the *text revision of the third edition of International Classification of Sleep Disorders (ICSD-3-TR)*.

- In Chapter 15, a new enrichment section has been added on trauma and compassion, which includes courtesy images of a patient who was in an automobile accident. Information regarding required employer forms for crushing injuries which occur on the job is included. Synthetic and biological skin substitutes in the use of burn treatment are included. Information on different types of lightning injuries has been updated. Methods identified to prevent heat stroke are expanded in this chapter. Treatment for lateral humeral epicondylitis or tennis elbow has been expanded. The information on bioterrorism, including the new term **biodefense**, has been updated and expanded. The suicide prevention number has been updated in Chapter 15.

General concepts of diseases are presented in Chapter 1 as a basis for the discussion of conditions. Chapter 1 introduces the reader to the general principles of pathophysiology. In conjunction with a breakdown of the mechanisms of disease, the subject matter flows through integrant aspects important for the student to consider in the study of human diseases, such as genetics, immune disorders, preventive health care, nontraditional medicine, and patient teaching. Additionally, the topic of cancer is introduced in Chapter 1 with foundational information about the pathology, pathogenesis, and prognostic indicators of the disease (*staging* and *grading* of malignant tumors). Specific sites and types of cancers are then comprehensively addressed in subsequent chapters. This is followed by a discussion of pediatric situations in Chapter 2. After these general discussions, the text progresses through body systems from Chapters 3 to 12. Chapter 3 introduces the student to the immune system, including discussions of immunodeficiency disorders and autoimmune disorders. Chapter 4 deals with the endocrine system and its disorders resulting from both deficiency and overactivity. This is followed by the special senses of sight and hearing in Chapter 5. Chapter 6 progresses to the largest sensory organ, the skin, or the integumentary system and its disorders. Chapter 7 describes the upright structure of the human body, its movement, and the disorders that disrupt the normal functioning of the musculoskeletal system. Chapter 8 addresses the body's nourishment system: the gastrointestinal system and its accessory organs. Chapter 9 presents discussions on the oxygen-carbon dioxide exchange and the respiratory system. The cardiovascular system (including the heart, blood, and blood vessels) is the topic of Chapter 10. Chapter 11 follows with a discussion of the urinary system, which maintains homeostasis and is a major factor in excretion of urinary

waste products. Chapter 12 discusses both male and female reproductive systems, pregnancy, and disorders of the breast. Chapter 13 covers the diseases and conditions of the neurologic system. Chapter 14 provides a discussion of mental disorders, including phobias, grief response, posttraumatic stress disorders, alcohol abuse, sleep disorders, and other conditions covered by the *Diagnostic and Statistical Manual of Mental Disorders (DSM-5-TR)*. This chapter also includes a comprehensive chart on drugs of abuse, their street names, and their effects on the abuser. Chapter 15 includes information to help health care providers with practical knowledge to deal with a variety of traumatic injuries. This material includes trauma; lightning injuries; insect, animal, and snake bites; child abuse; psychological abuse; elder abuse; sexual abuse; intimate partner violence; rape; and suicide.

Organization of Material

Each chapter is introduced with a brief review of the normal function of the specific body system discussed in the chapter, and this review is reinforced with clear illustrations. Important pathologic mechanisms are explained and illustrated as well. A disease entity is presented with a description and discussion of the symptoms experienced by the patient and the signs detected by the physician. The chapter continues with sections devoted to etiologic factors, diagnosis, treatment options, prognosis, prevention, and patient teaching related to the disease entity. A diagnostic code is assigned to each disease entity. (See important notes at the end of the preface.) **ICD-10-CM codes are included to aid in locating appropriate insurance codes**. This format also follows the inherent progression of a patient's experience: (1) the individual reports symptoms to a health care provider, usually in a clinical setting; (2) abnormal signs of a clinical disorder may be elicited during the physical examination and/or subsequent diagnostic testing; (3) an appropriate treatment option is initiated and monitored for results; (4) the patient is given appropriate teaching to encourage compliance and thus to ensure an optimal outcome. The usual prognosis for the condition and the possible preventive measures are discussed.

Italicized words found in the chapters are defined in the Glossary for purposes of review or clarification of meaning. The advantages to the student and health care worker in better understanding clinical terminology include (1) great professional gain when one comprehends the effects that a disease has on a person, (2) increased communication skills with the entire health care team, and (3) personal education that has many practical applications.

I believe it is important to define the role of *patient screening* in each discussion. Therefore the discussion of each disease entity begins with a feature called Patient Screening; the remarks therein are usually tailored to the disease entity being discussed. Because the vast majority of patients first seek access to health care services over the telephone, many health care facilities have a written, standardized protocol for medical personnel who take incoming calls. The comments offered in the *Patient Screening* feature of this text are not intended to help diagnose the caller's medical condition or give curative advice. The feature typically offers *general clues* to recognizing the urgency for an appointment, identifying emergencies, and discerning the kind of calls that require referral to the physician for action. This feature is not to be confused with the skill of medical triage, which state practice acts generally reserve for certain licensed or registered professionals. Careful listening to the patient who is calling often identifies information that helps the telephone screener select the appropriate action required by the caller. Ideally the outcome of telephone communication between the caller and the screener will benefit the patient and avoid potential medical-legal problems. Maintaining sensitivity to human suffering, keeping strict confidentiality, and upholding the priority of meeting the needs of patients cannot be overemphasized as skills necessary in a medical telephone screener.

In this regard, we also would like to add a list of serious and life-threatening conditions that require immediate assessment and intervention. These include, but are not limited to:

- Sudden onset of unexplained shortness of breath
- Crushing pain across the center of the chest
- Difficult breathing occurring suddenly and rapidly worsening, often in the middle of the night
- Vomiting of blood that is bright red or has a very dark "coffee grounds" appearance
- Sudden onset of weakness and unsteadiness or severe dizziness
- Sudden loss of consciousness or paralysis
- Flashes of light in field of vision
- Sudden and progressively worsening abdominal, flank, or pelvic pain
- Sudden onset of blurred vision accompanied by severe throbbing in the eye

A report of any of these symptoms must be immediately relayed to the physician. The physician will then offer additional instructions to give to the individual calling for help.

The appendices offer valuable information about diagnostic testing, pharmacology, and resource agencies. The appendix "Common Laboratory and Diagnostic Tests" discusses tests often ordered by the physician. Reference values for laboratory tests are listed, followed by possible causes of each variation above or below normal. Reference values or expected normal results are discussed for imaging and other studies. Again, causes of variations from normal are provided. It is imperative that the reader using this information recognize that reference values may vary, depending on the laboratory in which the test is performed and reported. Another appendix contains pharmacology information, which has been updated and revised. Representative drugs are listed by group and include the name of the drug, the usual intended therapeutic objective, possible side effects, and general comments. The presentation of this appendix follows the chapters in the text. Once again, the reader must recognize that drugs and drug substances may be continually changing and that any specific material must be confirmed by referencing a current drug reference or pharmacology reference source.

Chapter Features

Key features of each chapter include:

Each chapter begins with a set of **Learning Objectives** that list important actions the student will be able to perform after reading the chapter content.

The **Key Terms** list provides pronunciations for important words related to chapter content. Boldfaced words found in the text are listed in the Key Terms at the beginning of each chapter and in the Glossary unless the term has been adequately defined within the text of the chapter.

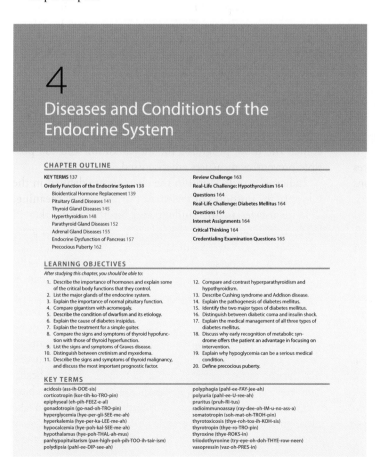

4

Diseases and Conditions of the Endocrine System

LEARNING OBJECTIVES

After studying this chapter, you should be able to:

1. Describe the importance of hormones and explain some of the critical body functions that they control.
2. List the major glands of the endocrine system.
3. Explain the importance of normal pituitary function.
4. Compare gigantism with acromegaly.
5. Describe the condition of dwarfism and its etiology.
6. Explain the cause of diabetes insipidus.
7. Explain the treatment for a simple goiter.
8. Compare the signs and symptoms of thyroid hypofunction with those of thyroid hyperfunction.
9. List the signs and symptoms of Graves disease.
10. Distinguish between cretinism and myxedema.
11. Describe the signs and symptoms of thyroid malignancy, and discuss the most important prognostic factor.
12. Compare and contrast hyperparathyroidism and hypothyroidism.
13. Describe Cushing syndrome and Addison disease.
14. Explain the pathogenesis of diabetes mellitus.
15. Identify the two major types of diabetes mellitus.
16. Distinguish between diabetic coma and insulin shock.
17. Explain the medical management of all three types of diabetes mellitus.
18. Discuss why early recognition of metabolic syndrome offers the patient an advantage in focusing on intervention.
19. Explain why hypoglycemia can be a serious medical condition.
20. Define precocious puberty.

KEY TERMS

acidosis (ass-ih-DOE-sis)
corticotropin (kor-tih-ko-TRO-pin)
epiphyseal (eh-pih-FEEZ-e-al)
gonadotropin (go-nad-oh-TRO-pin)
hyperglycemia (hye-per-gli-SEE-me-ah)
hyperkalemia (hye-per-ka-LEE-me-ah)
hypocalcemia (hye-poh-kal-SEE-me-ah)
hypothalamus (hye-poh-THAL-ah-mus)
panhypopituitarism (pan-high-poh-pih-TOO-ih-tair-ism)
polydipsia (pahl-ee-DIP-see-ah)

polyphagia (pahl-ee-FAY-jee-ah)
polyuria (pahl-ee-U-ree-ah)
pruritus (pruh-RI-tus)
radioimmunoassay (ray-dee-oh-IM-u-no-ass-a)
somatotropin (soh-mat-oh-TROH-pin)
thyrotoxicosis (thye-roh-tox-ih-KOH-sis)
thyrotropin (thye-ro-TRO-pin)
thyroxine (thye-ROKS-in)
triiodothyronine (try-eye-oh-doh-THYE-row-neen)
vasopressin (vaz-oh-PRES-in)

Enrichment boxes give the reader pertinent or relevant information that enhances knowledge of a discussion topic in the text.

◆ ENRICHMENT

Cochlear Implants

Individuals who experience severe sensorineural hearing loss that is not helped by hearing aids may have partial hearing restored by means of cochlear implants. Cochlear implants are electronic devices that use minute electrical currents to stimulate the auditory nerve and help the currents travel to the auditory cortex to be perceived as sound.

Cochlear implant systems are complex and include an electrode array, a receiver, a speech processor, a transmitting coil, and a microphone. The electrode array is placed surgically in the cochlea, and the receiver is implanted and fixed to the skull behind the mastoid bone. The surgical incision is allowed to heal for 4 to 6 weeks, after which the external components (the microphone, transmitting coil, and speech processor) are fitted to the patient. Fitting includes calibration of the transmitting coil and programming of the speech processor. Auditory and speech training are provided to the implant recipient.

Cochlear implants do not restore normal hearing; however, they can improve a deaf person's functioning in a hearing world. Candidates for the implants are selected carefully and should have severe to profound bilateral sensorineural hearing loss and be older than 2 years of age. Many still employ lip reading and American Sign Language as adjunct therapies to communicate.

An alternative implant device uses the principle of bone conduction to conduct sound waves to the inner ear. The bone conduction system is for individuals who experience conductive hearing loss, mixed, or single-sided hearing loss. Sound waves are transmitted to the inner ear by bone conduction bypassing outer or middle ear problems. A bone conduction system has an internal bone conduction implant (BCI) that is placed entirely subcutaneously. It contains a magnet to hold the externally placed audio processor above the BCI. The audio processor consists of a battery, microphones, and a digital processor. Fig. 5.23 shows cochlear implans.

• **Fig. 5.23** Cochlear implant. (From Patton KT, Thibodeau GA: *The human body in health & disease*, ed 6, St Louis, 2014, Elsevier.)

❶ ALERT!

Ototoxicity

Ototoxicity occurs when a drug or chemical causes damage to CN VIII (acoustic nerve) or to the inner ear, resulting in temporary or permanent hearing loss or disturbances in balance. Symptoms and signs of ototoxicity usually have an insidious onset and include tinnitus, a feeling of fullness or pressure in the ears, hearing loss, vertigo, and occasionally nausea.

Drugs that can cause ototoxicity include salicylates (aspirin and aspirin-containing products); NSAIDs; certain antibiotics (aminoglycosides, erythromycin, and vancomycin); loop diuretics (furosemide [Lasix], bumetanide [Bumex], and ethacrynic acid [Edecrin]); chemotherapeutic agents (cisplatin, vincristine, and vinblastine); quinines (quinidine and quinine); and heavy metals, including mercury and lead.

The physician should be notified of any of the aforementioned symptoms when the individual is taking or going to receive any of the previously mentioned medications.

Discontinuing aspirin, aspirin-containing products, and NSAIDs often reverses the ototoxic effects of these drugs. None of the other drugs should be discontinued unless so ordered by the physician. Quinine ototoxicity, like aspirin-induced ototoxicity, can usually be reversed when the medication is stopped. Large dosages of antibiotics that may be ototoxic usually are administered in life-threatening situations.

Chemotherapeutic agents are monitored for any ototoxic side effects. In normal dosages, loop diuretics usually have very few ototoxic side effects; it is when they are given in massive doses for treatment of acute kidney failure or acute hypertension that ototoxicity may occur.

Environmental chemicals include butyl nitrite, carbon disulfide, hexane, styrene, toluene, trichloroethylene, and xylene, but they are not limited to these.

Once damage has occurred, it cannot be reversed. Hearing loss may be helped somewhat by hearing aids or cochlear implants. When the patient experiences loss of balance, physical therapy may be needed to help the patient regain the ability to balance.

Alert boxes provide essential warnings (cautions and precautions) that require discussion or may require special treatment.

A **diagnostic code** used in the health care setting has been assigned to each disease entity in this publication to help students and workers in the health care setting understand the ICD-10-CM coding process when reporting clinical information.

Patient Teaching

Emphasize the importance of hydration to the parents. Care of the anal area may be required as a result of the irritation caused by the loose and irritating stools. Good hand washing is necessary after handling soiled diapers or any other clothing that may contain stool. Teach the parents to observe urinary output for volume and color. When the child is in diapers, have the parents count the number of soiled or wet diapers within a set time and report this to the physician's office.

Vomiting

Description

Vomiting, or ejection of stomach contents through the mouth, is a common symptom in infants and children.

ICD-10-CM Code	R11.10 *(Vomiting, unspecified)*
	(R11.0–R11.2 = 6 codes of specificity)
	R11.11 *(Vomiting without nausea)*
	R11.12 *(Projectile vomiting)*

Symptoms and Signs

Vomiting can range from a mild regurgitation to projectile expulsion. The infant has a distended abdomen, is irritable, and often has a fever. Aspiration of vomitus into the lungs can result in pneumonia.

Patient Screening

Chronic or severe vomiting deserves special attention as a warning sign of disease or possible dehydration. Assessment is essential. Projectile vomiting requires prompt assessment.

Etiology

Vomiting, which is more common in infants than in children, usually results from trivial or temporary factors. However, it has a host of possible causes, including overfeeding, food allergy, gastric irritation, infection, drug poisoning, elevated intracranial pressure, defects (e.g., pyloric stenosis), and habitual voluntary vomiting.

indicated, it depends on the cause, severity, and nature of the vomiting. Infant feeding problems require changes in technique or intake. Other more serious causes, such as infection, poisoning, and congenital anomalies of the GI tract, may require direct medical or surgical intervention.

Prognosis

The prognosis varies depending on the cause. Most vomiting subsides in a few hours. Longer periods of vomiting requiring medical or surgical intervention may or may not be corrected. Hydration, nutrition, and electrolyte balance are important factors in resolving the condition.

Prevention

Prevention varies depending on causative factors. Avoiding overfeeding, known food allergens, and substances that cause gastric irritation is often all that is necessary to prevent recurrence. Infection, drug poisoning, elevated intracranial pressure, defects (e.g., pyloric stenosis), and habitual voluntary vomiting may not be preventable.

Patient Teaching

Emphasize the importance of hydration and nutrition along with thorough hand washing after handling emesis.

Blood Disorders

Anemia

Description

Anemia is an abnormal reduction in the concentration of RBCs or in the hemoglobin content of circulating blood. It is not a disease, but a symptom of various diseases. Anemia can lead to tissue hypoxia. See Chapter 10 for additional information on anemias.

ICD-10-CM Code	D64.9 *(Anemia, unspecified)*
	(D64.0–D64.9 = 9 codes of specificity)

Refer to the physician's diagnosis and then to the current edition of the ICD-10-CM coding manual to ensure the greatest specificity of pathology.

Multiple-choice format **credentialing examination questions** are included in each chapter.

---

3. Explain how autoantibodies cause diseases.
4. What is the relationship between pernicious anemia, shortage of intrinsic factors, and the impairment of vitamin B_{12} adsorption?
5. How does the immune system malfunction in connective tissue diseases?
6. Why is scleroderma difficult to diagnose?
7. Which gene is known to be associated with autoimmune disorders, such as AS?
8. A patient who has undergone heart transplantation shows immediate signs of organ rejection despite an accurate tissue match prior to the transplantation. What are some of the reasons for this type of rejection?

Prepare to discuss Critical Thinking case study exercises for this chapter that are posted on the Evolve website.

Credentialing Examination Questions

1. Which class of drugs must patients who have received an organ transplant take to help ensure they do not have a rejection of their new organ?
   A. Antibiotic
   B. Antihypertensive
   C. Immunosuppressive
   D. ACE Inhibitor
2. Which method is not included in ways that HIV can be transmitted?
   A. Sexual intercourse
   B. Blood products
   C. Shared needles
   D. Casual contact
3. Which disease has been referred to as Bubble Boy disease?
   A. Severe combined immunodeficiency disease
   B. X-linked agammaglobulinemia
   C. DiGeorge anomaly
   D. Wiskott-Aldrich syndrome
4. Which condition refers to persistent and recurrent candidal (fungal) infections of the skin, nails, and mucous membranes?
   A. Selective immunoglobulin A deficiency
   B. Chronic mucocutaneous candidiasis
   C. Systemic *Candida* infection
   D. Autoimmune hemolytic anemia
5. Which condition is included in hematopoietic disorders?
   A. Autoimmune hemolytic anemia
   B. Selective immunoglobulin A deficiency
   C. Human immunodeficiency virus
   D. X-linked agammaglobulinemia
6. Which deficiency causes recurrent otitis media, eye, skin, and bronchial infections, including pneumonia?
   A. IgA
   B. IgM
   C. IgG
   D. CVID
7. Which type of counseling is beneficial when a child has a diagnosis of DiGeorge syndrome?
   A. Psychological
   B. Genetic
   C. Pediatric
   D. Behavioral
8. Which person is typically the best match for a patient who needs a bone marrow transplant?
   A. Mother
   B. Father
   C. Child
   D. Sibling
9. Which option most accurately describes connective tissue diseases?
   A. Acute conditions that resolve with treatment.
   B. Caused as a result of an untreated bacterial infection.
   C. The immune system malfunctions and works against itself.
   D. Results from a viral infection.
10. Which condition has symptoms of inflammation of the joints, nervous system, kidneys, lungs, and organs in addition to a characteristic butterfly rash on the face?
    A. Goodpasture syndrome
    B. Scleroderma
    C. Sjögren syndrome
    D. Systemic lupus erythematosus

Extensive Supplemental Resources

Student Workbook

The workbook features comprehensive additional review exercises and practice activities in a variety of formats to reinforce chapter topics. The workbook has been updated to include information added to this edition.

- **Word Definitions** and **Glossary Terms** review important key terms covered in each chapter.
- **Short Answer** and **Fill in the Blanks** questions review key chapter concepts.
- An **Anatomical Structures** section in select chapters presents diagrams representing key body structures to be labeled by the student.
- A **Patient Screening** section guides students in the practice of appointment scheduling or specialist referral based on a patient's described signs and symptoms.
- A **Patient Teaching** section guides students in the practice of providing patient education regarding various diseases and disorders.
- **Essay** questions invite students to further investigate key chapter topics.
- A **Certification Examination Review** helps students prepare for the certification examination with questions focused on chapter content in multiple-choice format.

Evolve

The specially designed complementary Evolve website provides important assets to students and instructors. For students, critical thinking case study exercises linked to each chapter can be found on the Evolve website, available at http://evolve.elsevier.com/Fuqua/essentials/.

Test Bank

The Test Bank located on the Evolve site in the ExamView format gives instructors the option of evaluating students' retained knowledge by chapter in a comprehensive format. This tool is capable of assessing retention of essential information necessary for excellence in functioning in the workplace. The seventh edition's Test Bank has been updated and revised to now include answer rationales. Also, the questions have been updated to include more stem-type questions as seen on credentialing examinations, rather than statement questions, which conclude with the answer options.

TEACH Instructor Resources

The TEACH lesson plans help instructors prepare for class and make full use of the rich array of ancillaries and resources that come with the textbook. The content covered in each textbook chapter is divided across one or more lesson plans, each designed to occupy 50 minutes of class time. Lesson plans are organized into easily understandable sections that are each tied to the chapter learning objectives:

- Instructor Preparation—This section provides a checklist of all the things you need to do to prepare for class, including a list of all the items that you need to bring to class to perform any activity or demonstration included in the lesson plan and all pertinent key terms covered in that lesson.
- Student Preparation—Textbook readings, study guide exercises, online activities, and other applicable homework assignments for each lesson are provided here, along with the overall estimated completion time.
- The 50-Minute Lesson Plan—A lecture outline that reflects the chapter lecture slides that come as part of TEACH is included, as well as classroom activities and online activities, one or more critical thinking questions, and time estimates for the classroom lecture and activities. Corresponding PowerPoint slides are provided to help the instructor save valuable preparation time and create a learning environment that fully engages the student.
- Assessment Plan—To ensure that your students have mastered all the objectives, the new TEACH includes a separate "Assessment Plan" section. An easy-to-use table maps each assessment tool to the lesson plans and chapter objectives so that you can see all your assessment options—by chapter, by lesson, and by objective—and choose accordingly.
- Answer Keys to the text and the workbook.

All the above features are available to the instructor for easy download from the Evolve site, allowing the instructor to apply his or her creativity; all of these features may be revised to accommodate any instructor's lesson plan.

Important Information

The information presented in this book represents research into the mainstream of medical knowledge and its application in clinical practice. In the actual practice of the dynamic art and science of medicine, great variations and opposing views result in either more conservative or more aggressive concepts. The material presented in this text should not take the place of individualized consultation with medical experts.

Regarding the *diagnostic codes* included in this publication, it is imperative to consider the following: Medical coding is an intricate and intense process requiring study and understanding to ensure maximum reimbursement from insurance companies, for participation in Medicare and Medicaid programs, and for statistical tabulation. Diagnostic codes are subject to changes, revisions, and additions; therefore it is imperative that you always refer to the *current* listing of ICD-10-CM codes. It is understood that the financial reimbursement directly correlates with the reporting of current valid codes, which may require modification to ensure the greatest specificity found in the most current coding manual and guidelines. Therefore I recommend that you refer to the current edition of a coding manual or to digital coding tools.

With regard to *patient teaching*, I am mindful of the legal parameters addressed in state acts governing the practice of medical assistants. *Readers, please consult your state code for licensing with regard to the rules and regulations applying to medical assistant practice.* State practice laws vary; they identify the tasks a properly prepared medical assistant can perform. With regard to the responsibility issue, the medical assistant in a medical office must know who their supervisor is should a question arise about scope of practice. Medical assistants should ask about a written office policy regarding delegation of tasks by the health care providers they work for, whether it be a physician, physician assistant, or nurse practitioner.

It is very important, and in the patient's best interests, that all health care workers, as members of a clinical team, understand the principles, goals, and specifics of patient teaching. Health care workers should learn to complement each other to provide the best care possible to each and every patient/client. *Licensing regulations and state practice acts generally permit only nurses, nurse practitioners, physician assistants, and physicians to perform patient teaching and make triage judgments. Medical assistants in some states do perform some patient teaching if directed by the health care provider.*

Students completing education in medical assisting will find this book an invaluable tool as they move into the professional arena. The text has been designed to provide information relevant in the medical office environment and will remain a handy reference during employment. The website updates will offer a resource that covers current changes in the health care field to help keep graduates current.

The established health care provider, whether a medical assistant, nurse, transcriber, coder, scribe, respiratory therapist, massage therapist, receptionist, emergency medical technician, paramedic, pharmacy technician, or other, will find this reference material a valuable resource in their work with the patient. Knowledge of diseases and related factors is essential in the provision of quality care.

Tracie Fuqua, BS, CMA (AAMA)

Acknowledgments

Special thanks go to the Elsevier experts involved in the publication of this text. I gratefully acknowledge Kristin Wilhelm, Director, Private Sector Education, and Laura Klein, Content Strategist, for guidance and suggestions during the rewriting of this book. I would also like to thank Rebecca Leenhouts, Senior Content Development Specialist, for her assistance while I was learning to navigate the digital tools Elsevier provides for authors. She is patient and kind. Her role as a mentor throughout this process was invaluable. We are grateful to Manchu Mohan, Senior Project Manager, for her expert diligence as she prepared our words and illustrations as final pages for print.

A special acknowledgment goes to Brandon Brooks, M.Ed., for his expertise in updating the medications and drug appendix throughout the text and workbook. His contribution was essential and ensured the information is accurate.

Special thanks to my family, who supported me while working on this edition of the text. Their understanding of the time commitment to see such a project from beginning to end truly helped in completion of this edition of the book and workbook.

I would also like to acknowledge and thank all the physicians and health care workers who cared for thousands of patients with COVID-19. Their journey through this pandemic was not an easy one. Their contributions to health care will not be forgotten as they navigated caring for so many patients when resources were limited.

Contents

1

Mechanisms of Disease, Diagnosis, and Treatment

CHAPTER OUTLINE

LEARNING OBJECTIVES

After studying this chapter, you should be able to:

1. Explain how a pathologic condition affects the homeostasis of the body.
2. Describe the difference between:
   - Signs and symptoms of disease
   - Acute and chronic diseases
3. Identify the predisposing factors of disease.
4. Explain the body's natural defense system against infection.
5. Explain the terms *superbugs* and *super strains* as they relate to infection.
6. Describe the ways in which pathogens may cause disease.
7. Describe the difference between benign and malignant neoplasms.
8. Explain the relationship between mutations in the genetic code in cancer and other diseases.
9. List the prevention guidelines for cancer.
10. Recall the two systems used to stage and grade cancer tumor cells.
11. Describe how chemotherapy treatment fights cancer.
12. Describe the hospice concept of care.
13. Recall three classes of immune disorders that result in the breakdown of the body's defense system.
14. Explain how mild to very severe symptoms of an allergic response can be triggered in the body.
15. Explain the inappropriate response of the body in an autoimmune disease.

16. Track the essential steps in the diagnosis of a disease.
17. Define a *holistic approach to medical care*.
18. Explain why recognition of cultural diversity is important in clinical practice.
19. Describe (1) the physiology of pain, (2) how pain may be treated, and (3) what is meant by *referred pain*.
20. Name two ways an individual can practice positive health behavior.
21. Describe examples of nontraditional medical therapies.
22. Define *integrative medicine*.
23. Discuss the principles and goals of patient teaching.

KEY TERMS

allergen (AL-ler-jen)
anaphylaxis (an-ah-fih-LAK-sis)
antigen (AN-tih-jen)
asymptomatic (a-sim-toh-MAH-tik)
auscultation (aws-kel-TAY-shun)
biologic (bi-o-lo-JIK)
biosimilar (bi-o-SI-mi-lar)
cachexia (kah-KEX-e-ah)
carcinogenic (kar-sih-no-JEN-ik)
chromosome (KRO-mo-sohm)
genotype (JEN-o-type)
homeostasis (ho-me-o-STA-sis)

hospice (HAUS-pis)
ischemia (is-KEY-me-ah)
karyotype (KARE-ee-o-type)
metastasis (meh-TAS-tah-sis)
mutation (meu-TAY-shun)
nociceptor (no-see-SEHP-tor)
oncogene (AHN-ko-jeen)
pathogenesis (path-o-JEN-eh-sis)
phagocytic (fag-o-SIT-ik)
probiotic (pro-bi-ah-TIC)
somatoform (so-MAT-o-form)

Pathology at First Glance

Pathology, the scientific study of disease, is the objective description of the traits, causes, and effects of abnormal conditions. Pathologic conditions involve measurable changes in normal structure and function that threaten the internal stability, or homeostasis, of the body.

In human disease, the negative characteristics or deviations from normal status are described subjectively by patients as symptoms. Signs, or abnormal objective findings, are the evidence of disease found by physical examination and diagnostic testing. Signs of disease often correlate with the symptoms. In other instances, the signs of disease may be noted in an asymptomatic patient, as in the discovery of a painless tumor or the finding of an abnormal blood pressure reading in a person with undiagnosed essential hypertension. A defined collection of signs and symptoms that characterize a disorder or condition is termed a *syndrome*.

The development of disease occurs in stages, described as the pathogenesis. In the course of infection, for instance, the pathogenesis may include an incubation period, a period of full-blown symptoms, and then remission or convalescence. The pathogenesis of a disease varies with the individual patient, the causative factors, and the medical intervention.

Diseases often are described as acute or chronic. *Acute* refers to an abrupt onset of more or less severe symptoms that run a brief course (usually <6 months) and then resolve or, in some cases, result in death. When a disease develops slowly, is intermittent, or lasts longer than 6 months, it is described as *chronic*. Persons who have continuous pain as part of chronic syndromes often experience depression.

Mechanisms of Disease

Human disease has varied manifestations, any of which threaten a person's ability to adapt to internal and external stressors and to maintain a state of well-being. Systemic health, or internal equilibrium, is preserved by numerous body organs and structures that work in concert to meet specific cellular needs. Any disruption of the body's equilibrium produces degenerative changes at the cellular level that may produce signs and symptoms of disease. For example, if a patient experiences kidney failure, other organ systems will begin to fail. Major disruptions in the body's cellular equilibrium that threaten homeostasis include fluid and electrolyte imbalance and excessive acidity (acidosis) or alkalinity (alkalosis).

Elements involved either directly or indirectly in pathogenesis include predisposing factors, access to preventive health care, genetic diseases, infection, inflammation and repair, neoplasms, physical trauma, chemical agents, malnutrition, immune disorders, aging, psychological factors, and mental disorders.

Predisposing Factors

Predisposing factors, also called *risk factors*, make a person or group more vulnerable to disease. The recognition of risk factors may be significant in prevention, diagnosis, and prognosis but does not precisely predict the occurrence of disease. The absence of predisposing factors does not ensure a person will never develop a disease or condition. Predisposing factors include age, sex, lifestyle, environment, heredity, and *immunodeficiency*.

- Age: Some increased risks of diseases are simply intrinsic to one's stage in the human life cycle beginning.

- Sex: Certain diseases are more common in females, and others are more common in males (sex assigned at birth).
- Lifestyle: Occupation, habits, or one's usual manner of living can have negative cumulative effects that can threaten a person's health. It is possible to alter some known risk factors associated with lifestyle. Examples include smoking, excessive drinking of alcohol, risky sexual behavior, poor nutrition, lack of exercise, and certain psychological stressors. Vaping, or the use of electronic cigarettes or smoking devices, is another risk factor. Along with nicotine, the user is exposed to chemicals that can contribute to health problems.
- Environment: Air and water pollution are the most common environmental risk factors for health problems. Pesticides, radiation, toxic waste, heavy metals, disease-causing microorganisms, and chemicals in products used by consumers may pose a threat to homeostasis. The places a person lives, works, visits or participates in recreation are also areas of the environment that can play a positive or negative role on health.
- Heredity: Genetic predisposition (inheritance) is currently considered a major risk factor. Family histories of coronary disease, cancer, certain arthritic conditions, and renal disease are known hereditary risk factors. Other genetic links to diseases are rapidly being discovered. Hereditary factors in disease that appear regularly in successive generations are likely to affect males and females equally. Examples are mental illness, cancer, hypertension, heart disease, and diabetes. Some evidence shows that smoking, a sedentary lifestyle, and a diet high in saturated fat, combined with a positive family history, compound a person's risk for heart disease and cancer. Extended sitting at work, at home, or behind the wheel or screen can also lead to health problems similar to those of cardiovascular disease and cancer. Research shows people who sit for 8 or more hours a day can counteract the effects of sitting too much by performing moderate exercise of an hour or more each day.
- Immunodeficiency: An inadequate or absent immune system makes an individual susceptible to infections, diseases, and harmful substances. The degree of risk depends on which components of the immune system are inadequate or absent and are the cause of the immunodeficiency. In cases of autoimmune disease, the immune response is misdirected at one's own body tissue, potentially causing damage.

Inflammation and Repair

Injury and disease add stress to the body's equilibrium and disrupt or destroy cellular function. Acute inflammation, a normal protective physiologic response to tissue injury and disease, is accompanied by redness, heat, swelling, pain, and loss of function. Widespread inflammation is marked by systemic symptoms, such as fever, malaise, and loss of appetite. An inflammatory response is considered a nonspecific immune response. Infection with pathogens, the effects of toxins, physical trauma, ischemia, and *necrosis* are some conditions that induce the inflammatory response.

Acute inflammation, an *exudative* response, attempts to wall off, destroy, and digest bacteria and dead or foreign tissue. Vascular changes allow fluid to leak into the site; this fluid contains chemicals that permit phagocytic activity by white blood cells. The process prevents the spread of infection through antibody action and other chemicals released by cells with more specific immune activity. After the mechanisms of inflammation have contained the insult and "cleaned up" the damaged area, repair and replacement of tissue can begin (Fig. 1.1). A normal inflammatory response can be inhibited by immune disorders, chronic illnesses, or the use of certain medications such as biologics, biosimilars, and long-term steroid therapy.

A chronic or too intense inflammatory response causes damage to the affected tissue, thereby inhibiting the healing process.

Infection

Infectious diseases are caused by pathogens. The cardinal signs of local infection are redness, swelling, heat, pain, fever, pus, enlarged lymph glands, and red streaks. Symptoms of widespread infection are fever, headache, body aches, weakness, fatigue, loss of appetite, and delirium.

When disease-causing organisms find ideal conditions to grow and multiply in the body, they cause disease by (1) invasion and local destruction of living tissue and (2) intoxication or production of substances that are poisonous to the body. The result is tissue damage that has the potential to produce systemic involvement.

The sources of infection can be endogenous (originating within the body) or exogenous (originating outside the body). Modes of transmission of pathogenic organisms are direct or indirect physical contact, inhalation or droplet nuclei, ingestion of contaminated food or water, or inoculation by an insect or animal. Pathogenic agents include bacteria, viruses, fungi, and protozoa (Table 1.1).

A communicable or contagious disease can be transmitted directly from one person to another. Carriers are asymptomatic persons or animals that harbor in their bodies pathogens that can be transferred to others.

The body's natural defense systems against infection include (1) natural mechanical and chemical barriers, such as the skin, cilia, body pH, and normal body flora; (2) the inflammatory response; and (3) the immune response. When these mechanisms of defense fail to contain or eliminate infection, appropriate and prompt medical intervention is required to treat the host and control the transmission of the infectious disease. This is accomplished by first isolating and identifying the organism through laboratory testing. Subsequently, appropriate antimicrobial therapy using antibiotic (antibacterial), antifungal, antiparasitic, or antiviral agents can begin. Analgesics for pain, antipyretic agents for fever, and other comfort measures, are dispensed. Adequate fluid intake, infection control measures, and rest are important for management.

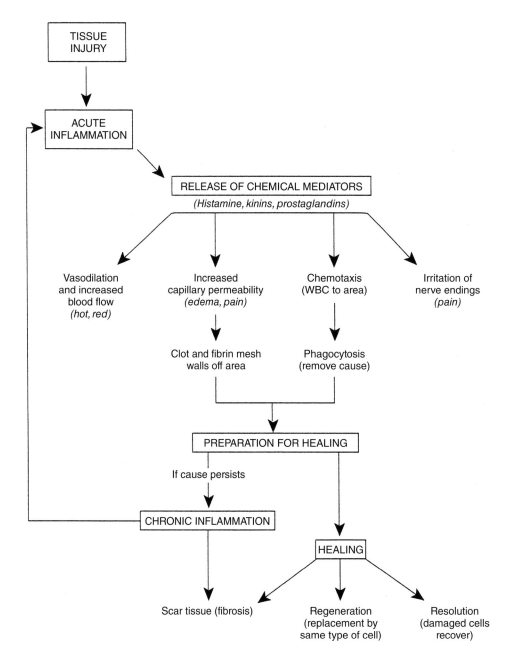

• **Fig. 1.1** The course of inflammation and healing. *WBC,* White blood cell. (From Gould BE: *Pathophysiology for the health professions,* ed 4, St. Louis, 2011, Saunders.)

Fundamental to preventing the spread of certain infections are the isolation of the infected individual when necessary, the implementation of immunization programs, and rudimentary public health teaching. To facilitate early intervention and infection control measures, many infectious diseases (e.g., encephalitis, syphilis, and tuberculosis) must be reported to the local health department. The Centers for Disease Control and Prevention (CDC) publishes a list of notifiable diseases in the United States. In hospitals, the control of postsurgical bacterial wound infections relies on breaking the chain of transmission by killing the pathogen, isolating infected persons, and using precautions, such as hand sanitization and sterilization, to prevent cross-contamination. Specific bacteria can now be isolated and identified by deoxyribonucleic acid (DNA) testing, which leads to better identification, treatment, and improved outcomes.

Virulent antibiotic-resistant strains of bacteria (commonly referred to as *superbugs* or *super strains*) present a danger even to the young and healthy. Just a few of these are *Staphylococcus, Streptococcus,* and *Pseudomonas.* Specifically, methicillin-resistant strains of *Staphylococcus aureus* (MRSA) are to blame for aggressive skin and soft tissue infections. Sometimes mistaken for spider bites, these lesions quickly develop into abscesses and cellulitis. In addition to skin infections, MRSA can cause fatal pneumonia, bone infections such as osteomyelitis, and septicemia.

TABLE 1.1 **Common Pathogens and Some Infections or Diseases They Produce**

Organism	Reservoir	Infection or Disease
Bacteria		
Escherichia coli	Colon, manure	Enteritis, mild to severe
Staphylococcus aureus Note: See section on Infection for discussion on methicillin-resistant strains of *S. aureus* ("superbugs")	Skin, hair, anterior nares	Wound infection, pneumonia, food poisoning, cellulitis
Streptococcus (β-hemolytic group A) organisms	Oropharynx, skin, perianal area	"Strep throat," rheumatic fever, scarlet fever, impetigo
Streptococcus (β-hemolytic group B) organisms	Adult genitalia	Urinary tract infection, wound infection, endometritis
Clostridium difficile	Contaminated surfaces or spores transferred to unclean hands of others	Serious intestinal conditions such as colitis
Mycobacterium tuberculosis	Lungs	Tuberculosis
Neisseria gonorrhoeae	Genitourinary tract, rectum, mouth, eye	Gonorrhea, pelvic inflammatory disease, infectious arthritis, conjunctivitis
Rickettsia rickettsii	Wood tick	Rocky Mountain spotted fever
Staphylococcus epidermidis	Skin	Wound infection, bacteremia
Pseudomonas aeruginosa	Skin, water, soil	Pneumonia, urinary tract infection, meningitis
Viruses		
Hepatitis A virus	Feces, blood, urine	Hepatitis A (infectious hepatitis)
Hepatitis B virus	Feces, blood, all body fluids and excretions	Hepatitis B (serum hepatitis)
Hepatitis C virus	Blood and body fluids	Liver disease may become chronic
Herpes simplex virus	Lesions of mouth, skin, blood, excretions	Cold sores, aseptic meningitis, sexually transmitted disease
HIV	Blood, semen, vaginal secretions (also isolated in saliva, tears, urine, breast milk but not proven to be sources of transmission)	AIDS
Hantavirus	Deer mouse urine, feces, saliva	URI to LRI to ARDS
Ebola HF	Contaminated blood or body fluid, fruit bat	Hemorrhagic fever, vascular permeability, shock, and death; potential bioterrorism threat
West Nile virus	Mosquito borne	Fever, rash, hepatitis, encephalitis
Fungi		
Aspergillus organisms	Soil, dust	Aspergillosis, allergic bronchopulmonary
Candida albicans	Mouth, skin, colon, genital tract	Thrush, dermatitis
Protozoa		
Plasmodium falciparum	Mosquito	Malaria

Modified from Potter P, Perry A: *Fundamentals of nursing: concepts, process, and practice*, ed 6, St. Louis, 2006, Mosby.
AIDS, Acquired immunodeficiency syndrome; *ARDS*, adult respiratory distress syndrome; *HF*, hemorrhagic fever; *HIV*, human immunodeficiency virus; *LRI*, lower respiratory infection; *URI*, upper respiratory infection.

❖ **ENRICHMENT**

MRSA Progression

Day 1 A patient with diabetes is 7 weeks post–trimalleolar fracture and in a boot when he starts complaining of severe pain in the foot after a shower that night. A topical anesthetic was placed by his daughter on the foot. This image is a medial view.

Day 2 The daughter calls the orthopedic surgeon and is instructed to bring the patient to the office the next day.

Day 3 The foot begins to look red and swollen. The surgeon confirms cellulitis, and the patient is placed on an oral antibiotic. On **days 4 and 5**, the patient continues the oral antibiotic.

Day 6 The patient is still in pain, and the daughter calls the surgeon to report that the foot looks "much worse" today than the past 2 days. This image is e-mailed to the orthopedic surgeon's office. The medical assistant sends the image to the physician, and the patient is "worked into" the schedule the next day to be seen. This image is taken on day 6 in the afternoon.

Day 7
The patient sees the surgeon and is immediately admitted to the hospital for an MRI and infectious disease referral. This image was taken at the doctor's office. Notice the skin is beginning to weep and the black area of necrotic tissue (gangrene). **This image was taken in the morning of day 7, less than 20 hours from the image taken in the afternoon of day 6**. The MRI was obtained after the patient was admitted, which revealed a 10-cm abscess on the tendon in the foot. Surgery was performed to open the abcess, hardware from fracture repair was cleaned, and the incision was sutured. Culture identified bacteria as MRSA. The patient was also diagnosed with osteomyelitis.

3 Days post-op Necrotic tissue was not removed at the first surgery and is visible.

The second surgery to remove necrotic tissue and the hardware in the lower tibia and fibula was performed a few days after the initial surgery. Wound culture grew MRSA. A wound vac was placed after the dressing was removed.

2 Months post-op after the second surgery. Note: the tendon is visible.

Image taken 2 years after initial MRSA infection and surgeries. The patient has been treated with multiple types of therapies, such as wound vac, IV antibiotic, hyperbaric oxygen chamber treatments, several skin substitutes, amniotic cell treatments, and fish skin treatments.

2 years 6 months after initial MRSA infection and surgeries. The size is smaller, but still there is an open wound. The patient has not been able to wear normal shoes in over 2 years or shower without a cover on his foot. At the time of writing of this text, the patient still sees a wound care specialist weekly.

(Information and images in this case study courtesy John Wesley Griffin Jr.)

Advances in technology have resulted in better management of these types of infections. Teams of infectious disease doctors are able to isolate the DNA in bacteria and prescribe specific antibiotics orally, intravenously, or both. Occasionally toxic and resistant strains of MRSA have been termed *flesh-eating bacteria* because of the rapid spread of infection, resulting in the destruction of human skin. MRSA continues to be a leading cause of surgical wound infections in hospitals (see Enrichment box on MRSA Progression).

MRSA is easily transmitted from person to person and can survive for a long time, nearly anywhere in the environment. About 2 in 100 people in the United States have the organisms in their body without showing signs of infection; however, they may transmit MRSA bacteria to others. Because of the constant threat of infection, everyone must be considered at risk for MRSA, particularly hospitalized patients.

Excellent hygiene practices help prevent the spread of MRSA. Washing hands with alcohol-based hand sanitizer or soap and water before and after patient care is effective in reducing bacterial infections. Participating medical facilities have implemented active surveillance testing, such as nasal swab tests on patient admission. Individuals with a history of MRSA may be placed in isolation in some instances.

MRSA receives a lot of attention, but it is only one concern in today's health care environment. The CDC has identified many other pathogenic bacteria that are antibiotic resistant. The lists changes because of the bacteria's capability of changing with the use of antibiotics. Antibiotics should only be prescribed when necessary to treat bacterial

• **Fig. 1.2** Examples of karyotypes. (A) Normal female (46,XX). (B) Normal male (46,XY). (From Damjanov I: *Pathology for the health professions,* ed 4, St. Louis, 2011, Saunders.)

infections. Antibiotics are not effective in treating viral infections. Prescribing antibiotics is not recommended in treating viral infections in individuals or animals, as this contributes to the problem of resistance.

Genetic Diseases

Genetics, the study of genes and their heredity, will continue to occupy center stage in the practice of medicine. Genetic factors can guide treatment decisions and preventive strategies. The application of genetics may influence genetic counseling, newborn screening, and carrier screening. At this point, several thousand human genetic disorders have been described and cataloged.

Every cell in the body is coded with genetic information arranged on 23 pairs of chromosomes; one chromosome from each pair is inherited from the father and the other from the mother. The X and Y chromosomes are known as the *sex chromosomes*, whereas the remaining 22 pairs are called *autosomes*. Each cell in an individual's body contains the same chromosomes and genetic code (genotype). A karyotype is an ordered arrangement of photographs of a full chromosome set (Fig. 1.2). Genes, the basic units of heredity, are small stretches of a DNA molecule situated at a particular site on a chromosome.

Genetic diseases are (1) produced by an abnormality in, or a mutation of, the genetic code in a single gene; (2) caused by several abnormal genes (producing the so-called *polygenic diseases*); (3) caused by the abnormal presence or absence of an entire chromosome; or (4) caused by an alteration in the structure of chromosomes. Harmful genetic mutations, or changes in the genetic code, passed from one generation to the next may occur spontaneously or be caused by agents known to disrupt the normal sequence of DNA units.

Agents (called *mutagens*) that can damage DNA include certain chemicals, radiation, and viruses.

The main modes of inheritance for genetic diseases are as follows:
- Autosomal dominant: The gene in question is located on an autosome, and the mutant *phenotype* is seen even if a normal gene is present on the other chromosome in the pair. Examples include Marfan syndrome and Huntington disease.
- Autosomal recessive: The gene is located on an autosome but is insufficient to produce the mutant phenotype in the presence of a normal gene on the paired chromosome. Both genes must be mutated for the disease to occur. Examples include cystic fibrosis and phenylketonuria.
- X-linked (sex-linked) recessive: The gene is located only on the X chromosome. Males are much more commonly affected by these diseases than females. Examples include Duchenne muscular dystrophy and hemophilia A. Red-green color blindness is also more common in males than females.

Individuals with only one copy of a recessive gene and appear outwardly normal are known as *carriers* of the defective gene. The mutant gene may produce an abnormal protein that causes a disease or may fail to produce its normal cellular function. Hereditary diseases are often noted at birth, but they may not appear until later in life. Many genetic mutations are compatible with life, but some are not.

Genetic Counseling

For many genetic diseases, the responsible gene or chromosomal abnormality has been identified, and it is possible to test for the presence of the mutation in an individual. The discovery of a genetic disease in a family member

TABLE 1.2   Comparison of Benign and Malignant Tumors

Characteristics	Benign Tumors	Malignant Tumors
Mode of growth	Relatively slow growth by expansion; encapsulated; cells adhere to each other	Rapid growth; invade surrounding tissue by infiltration
Cells under microscopic examination	Resemble tissue of origin; well differentiated; appear normal	Do not resemble tissue of origin; vary in size and shape; abnormal appearance and function
Spread	Remain localized	Metastasis; cancer cells carried by blood and lymphatics to one or more other locations; secondary tumors occur
Other properties	No tissue destruction; not prone to hemorrhage; may be smooth and freely movable	Ulceration and/or necrosis; prone to hemorrhage; irregular and less movable
Recurrence	Rare after excision	A common characteristic
Pathogenesis	Symptoms related to location with obstruction and/or compression of surrounding tissue or organs; usually not life threatening unless inaccessible	Cachexia; pain; fatal if not controlled

Gross appearance of benign (A) and malignant (B) tumors.

often raises questions as to whether other family members are affected, whether others are carriers of the disease, and whether future offspring will be affected by the genetic disease. Genetic counseling is a communication process that is centered on the occurrence or risk of occurrence of a genetic disorder in a family. Such counseling should be offered to all families affected by the diagnosis of a genetic disease in one or more members.

If genetic testing is available for the disorder, the counselors first explain the test and the benefits of taking or not taking the test. They help prepare the family for any outcome of the genetic test. Common feelings experienced after receiving a diagnosis of a genetic disorder are a sense of being "labeled," guilt that other family members may be affected, and feeling hopeless if there is no cure. As a result of the Genetic Information Nondiscrimination Act (GINA) of 2008, insurance companies are prohibited from using any type of genetic information when deciding if they will cover an individual or how much the premium for coverage will be. Individuals should understand that the protection of the GINA law does not cover long-term care, disability, or life insurance coverage or premiums.

Cancer

Cancer, a leading cause of death in the United States, refers to a group of diseases characterized by uncontrolled cell proliferation. This abnormal growth leads to the development of tumors or *neoplasms*, a relentlessly growing mass of abnormal cells that proliferate at the expense of the healthy organism. Tumors are characterized as malignant or benign according to the cell type and tissue of origin (Tables 1.2

> ✦ **NOTE**
>
> What follows is a general introduction to the pathology and pathogenesis of cancer, including prognosis, as demonstrated by *staging* and *grading* of tumors. Broad measures of prevention, diagnosis, and treatment are also discussed.

TABLE 1.3   Classification of Neoplasms by Tissue of Origin

Tissue of Origin	Benign	Malignant
Connective tissue		Sarcoma
Embryonic fibrous tissue	Myxoma	Myxosarcoma
Fibrous tissue	Fibroma	Fibrosarcoma
Adipose tissue	Lipoma	Liposarcoma
Cartilage	Chondroma	Chondrosarcoma
Bone	Osteoma	Osteogenic sarcoma
Epithelium		Carcinoma
Skin and mucous membrane	Papilloma	Squamous cell carcinoma
Glands		Basal cell carcinoma Transitional cell carcinoma
	Adenoma	Adenocarcinoma
	Cystadenoma	Cystadenocarcinoma
Pigmented cells (melanocytes)	Nevus	Malignant melanoma
Endothelium		Endothelioma
Blood vessels	Hemangioma	Hemangioendothelioma Hemangiosarcoma Kaposi sarcoma
Lymph vessels	Lymphangioma	Lymphangiosarcoma Lymphangioendothelioma
Bone marrow		Multiple myeloma Ewing sarcoma Leukemia
Lymphoid tissue		Malignant lymphoma Lymphosarcoma Reticulum cell sarcoma
Muscle Tissue		
Smooth muscle	Leiomyoma	Leiomyosarcoma
Striated muscle	Rhabdomyoma	Rhabdomyosarcoma
Nerve Tissue		
Nerve fibers and sheaths	Neuroma Neurinoma Neurilemmoma	Neurogenic sarcoma
	Neurofibroma	Neurofibrosarcoma
Ganglion cells	Ganglioneuroma	Neuroblastoma
Glial cells	Glioma	Glioblastoma
Meninges	Meningioma	Malignant meningioma
Gonads	Dermoid cyst	Embryonal carcinoma Embryonal sarcoma Teratocarcinoma

From Black JM, Matassarin-Jacobs E: *Medical-Surgical Nursing*, ed 6, Philadelphia, 2001, Saunders.

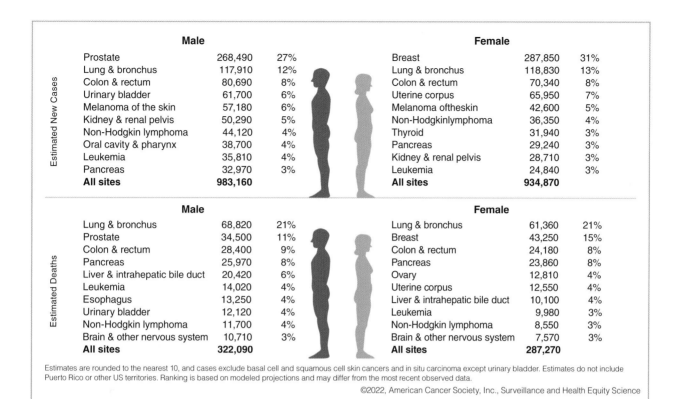

Male				Female		
Estimated New Cases						
Prostate	268,490	27%		Breast	287,850	31%
Lung & bronchus	117,910	12%		Lung & bronchus	118,830	13%
Colon & rectum	80,690	8%		Colon & rectum	70,340	8%
Urinary bladder	61,700	6%		Uterine corpus	65,950	7%
Melanoma of the skin	57,180	6%		Melanoma oftheskin	42,600	5%
Kidney & renal pelvis	50,290	5%		Non-Hodgkinlymphoma	36,350	4%
Non-Hodgkin lymphoma	44,120	4%		Thyroid	31,940	3%
Oral cavity & pharynx	38,700	4%		Pancreas	29,240	3%
Leukemia	35,810	4%		Kidney & renal pelvis	28,710	3%
Pancreas	32,970	3%		Leukemia	24,840	3%
All sites	**983,160**			**All sites**	**934,870**	
Estimated Deaths						
Lung & bronchus	68,820	21%		Lung & bronchus	61,360	21%
Prostate	34,500	11%		Breast	43,250	15%
Colon & rectum	28,400	9%		Colon & rectum	24,180	8%
Pancreas	25,970	8%		Pancreas	23,860	8%
Liver & intrahepatic bile duct	20,420	6%		Ovary	12,810	4%
Leukemia	14,020	4%		Uterine corpus	12,550	4%
Esophagus	13,250	4%		Liver & intrahepatic bile duct	10,100	4%
Urinary bladder	12,120	4%		Leukemia	9,980	3%
Non-Hodgkin lymphoma	11,700	4%		Non-Hodgkin lymphoma	8,550	3%
Brain & other nervous system	10,710	3%		Brain & other nervous system	7,570	3%
All sites	**322,090**			**All sites**	**287,270**	

Estimates are rounded to the nearest 10, and cases exclude basal cell and squamous cell skin cancers and in situ carcinoma except urinary bladder. Estimates do not include Puerto Rico or other US territories. Ranking is based on modeled projections and may differ from the most recent observed data.

©2022, American Cancer Society, Inc., Surveillance and Health Equity Science

• **Fig. 1.3** Leading sites of new cancer cases and deaths, 2022 estimates. (American Cancer Society: *Cancer facts and figures 2022*, Atlanta, 2022, American Cancer Society, Inc.)

and 1.3). Some of the main general types of cancer are carcinoma, cancer of the epithelial cells; sarcoma, cancer of the supportive tissues of the body, such as bone and muscle; lymphoma, cancer arising in the lymph nodes and tissues of the immune system; leukemia, cancer of blood cell precursors; and melanoma, cancer of the melanin-producing cells of the body.

Benign tumors usually develop slowly and can arise from any tissue. They tend to remain encapsulated and do not infiltrate surrounding tissue. When examined microscopically, benign tumor cells are well differentiated; they resemble the tissue of origin. Because these tumors take up space, complications can result from compression of tissue by the lesion or obstruction of organs. Benign tumors rarely recur after surgical removal.

Malignant tumors can represent a serious threat to the health, life, and well-being of a person. Cancer cells are variable in appearance and disorderly (anaplastic) with irreversible changes in structure. Malignant tumors have the ability to invade the surrounding tissue. Often malignant cells enter the bloodstream or the lymphatic vessels and lead to tumor growth in other areas of the body. These secondary tumors are known as *metastases*. Metastasis makes the neoplasm more difficult to eradicate from the body.

Cancer is actually one of the many different diseases with numerous causes. Cancer may be caused by both external exposure to *carcinogens* (chemicals, radiation, and viruses) and internal factors (hormones, immune conditions, and inherited mutations). Many years may pass between exposures or mutations and the onset of detectable cancer. Cancer can develop in anyone, but the frequency increases with age. Fig. 1.3 shows the leading sites of cancer incidence and death.

Recommendations for decreasing the risk of cancer encompass guidelines and appropriate screening tests for early detection and treatment. Primary prevention guidelines include the following:

- Consume a diet rich in fruits, vegetables, and whole grains. Limit consumption of processed and red meats
- Eliminate active and passive exposure to cigarette smoke
- Limit skin exposure to sunlight
- Limit the use of alcohol
- Avoid excessive exposure to radiation and radon
- Avoid chemical agents known to be carcinogenic
- Increase physical activity
- Maintain a healthy weight
- Protect against sexually transmitted infections, including getting the human papillomavirus (HPV) vaccine

Cancer is very prevalent in the United States. According to statistics from the American Cancer Society in 2022, 1,918,030 new cancer cases and 609,360 cancer deaths are projected to occur in the United States. This is the most current data projection at the time of authoring this book.

Early cancer detection employs physical examination, medical history taking, and laboratory screening tests.

Screening examinations can detect cancers of the breast, rectum, colon, prostate, cervix, testis, oral cavity, and skin early, which is when treatment is more likely to succeed.

Some tumor cells produce and secrete substances called *tumor markers*. Screening tests for elevation of blood serum levels of tumor markers, when considered with other diagnostic data, are shown to have clinical value in (1) helping determine the diagnosis of cancer, (2) evaluating response to therapy, and (3) screening for disease recurrence. For example, in primary and metastatic prostate cancer, elevated prostate-specific antigen (PSA) may be found.

If cancer is suspected, additional diagnostic investigation is achieved by using high-technology imaging techniques and, most decisively, by performing a *biopsy* of the lesion.

After a cancer diagnosis has been confirmed, the patient undergoes an evaluation to determine the stage of the neoplasm. The *stage* reflects tumor size and the extent of tumor spread. It has important implications for prognosis and in the determination of treatment choice. Staging is a terminology that institutions can use to communicate patient information. The TNM Classification of Malignant Tumors (TNM) is recognized globally as the standard for classifying the extent of the spread of cancer. It is published by the Union for International Cancer.

TNM staging assesses the neoplasm in three different areas: (1) the size or extent of the primary tumor (T); (2) the extent of regional lymph node involvement by the tumor (N); and (3) the number of distant metastases (M). Once all three parameters are defined, they are combined to assign a stage number: I, II, III, or IV to the cancer. Stage I is an early-stage tumor and carries the best prognosis, whereas stage IV is the most advanced stage. Within each stage, subcategories are defined (Ia, Ib, and so on) to further aid in treatment planning and facilitate communication among institutions and physicians. Some cancers also have stage 0, which is carcinoma in situ.

See Table 1.4 for an example of staging.

The stage usually offers the best indicator of prognosis. The prognosis reflects the estimation of the likelihood of cancer recurrence and death, independent of the treatment given. In general, the diagnosis of cancer in an early stage offers a greater chance for cure. The prognosis is usually reported statistically as the percentage of patients with that cancer who are still alive after a certain period. The patient may be cured of the disease, in remission, or still undergoing treatment. Survival periods may typically be reported in 5- or 10-year increments. Survival periods can be reported as "overall 5-year survival," which takes into account all the people, regardless of stage, with that cancer who are still alive, or it can be reported to reflect the 5-year survival rate for people in the various stages of cancer.

Depending on the type of neoplasm, other factors can impact prognosis. Examples include the age of the patient, serum concentration of any tumor markers, time between diagnosis and treatment, and grade of the tumor. Tumor grade is determined through microscopic evaluation of the tumor or a biopsy specimen by a pathologist. Grade is assigned on the basis of the degree of differentiation of the

TABLE 1.4 Melanoma Staging System of the American Joint Committee on Cancer

Primary Tumor (pT)

TX	Primary tumor cannot be assessed
TO	No evidence of primary tumor
Tis	Melanoma in situ (atypical melanotic hyperplasia, severe melanotic dysplasia)
T1	Tumor ≤1 mm in thickness, a = without ulceration and mitosis <1/mm^2; b = with ulceration and mitoses ≥1/mm2
T2	Tumor >1 mm but not >2 mm in thickness, a = without ulceration; b = with ulceration
T3	Tumor >2 mm but not >4 mm in thickness, a = without ulceration; b = with ulceration
p4	Tumor >4 mm in thickness, a = without ulceration; b = with ulceration

Lymph Node (N)

NX	Regional lymph nodes cannot be assessed
NO	No regional lymph node metastasis
N1	One positive lymph node, a = intralymphatic micrometastasis; b = macrometastases
N2	Two to three positive lymph nodes, a = micrometastasis; b = macrometastases; c = in transit metastasis without metastatic nodes
N3	≥4 metastatic nodes or matted nodes or in transit metastasis with metastatic nodes

Distant Metastasis (M)

MX	Presence of distant metastasis cannot be assessed
MO	No distant metastasis
M1a	Metastases to skin, subcutaneous tissue, or distant lymph nodes; normal LDH
M1b	Metastases to lung, normal LDH
M1c	All other visceral metastases with normal LDH, any distant metastasis with elevated LDH

Clinical Stage Grouping

Stage 0	Tis	NO	MO
Stage IA	T1a,	NO	MO
Stage IB	T1b, T2a	NO	MO
Stage IIA	T2b,T3a	NO	MO
Stage IIB	T3b, T4a	NO	MO
Stage IIC	T4b	NO	MO
Stage III	Any T	N1, N2, or N3	MO
Stage IV	Any T	Any N	M1

LDH, Lactate dehydrogenase.

tumor cells. The higher the grade, the more different the cells look when compared to normal cells. A tumor with a Grade 4 rating has more abnormal-looking cells than a Grade 1 tumor, which is composed of cells that resemble normal tissue.

One type of cancer in which grade is a very important indicator of prognosis is prostate cancer. The grading system is known as the *Gleason grade*, and this system was designed with the knowledge that prostate cancer has different patterns of growth and that multiple patterns coexist in the prostate. Analysis of prostate tumor histology is performed, and the two predominant patterns are recorded and scored from 1 to 5 (1 represents a well-differentiated histology; 5 is the most poorly differentiated). Both scores are summed to give a Gleason score from 2 to 10. The Gleason grade correlates with the extent of disease throughout the body and with prognosis.

The goal of cancer treatment is to eradicate every cancer cell in the body. Treatment options involve primary treatment, adjuvant treatment, or palliative treatment. Any treatment can be used for primary treatment; however, with many types of cancer, surgery is the recommended choice. The tumor is removed, along with the margins around the tumor, to see if the cells surrounding it are affected.

Adjuvant treatment involves destroying cancer cells that may remain after the primary treatment. Even when eradicated, there is always a chance cancer will come back. Adjuvant treatment will help reduce those instances when used with primary treatment options. Radiation, chemotherapy, and hormone therapy are types of adjuvant treatment options.

Neoadjuvant therapy is similar, but treatments are used before the primary treatment to make the primary treatment easier or more effective. There are also times when the recommendation is to treat the tumor with neoadjuvant therapy before primary treatment. One example is using radiation to shrink a tumor, which can result in the primary treatment being more effective or easier.

Palliative treatment involves measures to lessen the symptoms that result from cancer or other serious chronic diseases. A patient receiving palliative care may also be undergoing treatment for cancer, whereas a patient under hospice services would not. Palliative care is also helpful for the patient's family members and caregivers.

Each patient with cancer will have an individualized plan, including localized therapy (e.g., surgery and radiation) along with systemic modalities (e.g., chemotherapy, hormonal therapy, and immunotherapy) based on the type and location of the cancer and their specific situation. Surgery alone is curative only for some early-stage tumors. Usually, more than one treatment option is employed. *Neoadjuvant therapy* may be administered preoperatively to shrink the tumor before surgical removal.

Surgery is important for the treatment of solid cancers and is often used in the staging evaluation as well. As a treatment modality, the goal is either cure or palliative symptom control. When surgery is employed as a curative measure,

surgeons try to achieve negative margins around the tumor—that is, the surgeon will remove a certain amount of normal tissue along with the tumor to ensure that the entire tumor has been removed. If negative margins are not achieved, surgery must be performed again, or another type of treatment must be tried. At the time of surgery, the regional lymph nodes may be evaluated to determine whether the cancer cells have entered the lymphatic system and invaded the nodes. Affected nodes are generally removed. Palliative surgery is performed to relieve troublesome symptoms, such as an obstruction. Relief can be achieved by tumor resection, bypass, stenting, or laser *ablation*.

Chemotherapy involves the use of medicines to destroy cancer cells. Most of the drugs affect cell replication, so chemotherapy is most effective against rapidly dividing cells, such as cancer cells. Normal cells in other parts of the body that are known to divide rapidly are also destroyed, and this accounts for many of the classic side effects of chemotherapy. These cell populations (and the related side effects) include hair (alopecia), GI mucosal (anorexia, vomiting, and diarrhea), hematopoietic (anemia and bruising), and reproductive organs (infertility). Often drugs that affect different steps in cell replication are administered at the same time (combination chemotherapy). Chemotherapy usually is given in cycles that include a treatment period followed by a recovery period and is often performed in an outpatient setting. Although cancer cells may be initially responsive to the drugs, cells tend to develop resistance to the drugs over time, and new drugs or different treatment modalities must then be employed.

The use of hormone therapy and immunotherapy in the treatment of cancer has evolved over the past few years and continues to evolve. Hormone therapy can be effective in hormone-dependent cancers, such as breast cancer and prostate cancer. It may involve the administration of drugs that suppress hormone synthesis, such as luteinizing hormone–releasing hormone antagonists or aromatase inhibitors that are used to treat prostate cancer; drugs that block the action of hormones, such as the estrogen receptor modulator tamoxifen used to treat breast cancer; or surgical removal of hormone-producing glands, such as an *oophorectomy* and *orchiectomy*.

Immunotherapy stimulates the body's immune system to fight cancer. It can involve the use of cancer vaccines (see the Enrichment box on Cancer Vaccines), infusion of cellular products, such as T cells or natural killer cells, which may or may not be modified prior to administration, or *monoclonal antibodies* to target certain products of cancer cells that are not found in normal cells. These antibodies may generate an anticancer effect in one of three ways: (1) they can trigger an immune response against the tumor cell, (2) deliver a lethal dose of radiation to the cell, or (3) release a deadly chemical inside the cell. Several antibodies are currently approved by the US Food and Drug Administration (FDA). They include trastuzumab (Herceptin), approved for use in breast and gastric cancers that overexpress the human epidermal growth factor receptor 2 (HER2/neu) protein;

rituximab (Rituxan) for use in non-Hodgkin lymphoma; for use in chronic lymphocytic leukemia; and ipilimumab (Yervoy) for metastatic melanoma. Newer-generation medications to treat breast cancer include three newer drugs, which are CDK4 and CDK6 inhibitors (cyclin-dependent kinases). Abemaciclib (Verzenio), palbociclib (Ibrance), and ribociclib (Kisqali) all belong to this class of drugs.

For patients with metastatic disease, a cure may not be possible, but these same treatment modalities may be useful in prolonging life or improving the quality of life for the patient. Even after the patient has achieved remission, they must be followed up closely for several years. Micrometastases may exist at the time of diagnosis that can lead to eventual recurrence of the cancer if they are not eradicated by systemic therapy.

Advances in radiation and chemotherapy have diminished the need for radical surgery. However, these modalities have significant side effects that require constant surveillance and management. Pain management, both during and after treatment, is a major concern in patients and includes generous use of various analgesics and noninvasive techniques that promote relaxation and distraction. Terminally ill persons can be referred to hospice care for compassionate, holistic case management.

Research continually provides useful information about new, promising approaches to cancer treatment. Certain forms of cancer are inherited; thus much of the current research is focused on cancer at its genetic roots. Scientists are investigating genetic switches that cause healthy cells to become disorderly. It has been observed that broken genes can send cells into spirals of cancerous growth. Such oncogenes and tumor suppressor genes are proposed targets for therapy. One drug currently targeting an oncogene is imatinib (Gleevec) that inhibits the *BCR-ABL* tyrosine kinase (an abnormal enzyme) in chronic myelogenous leukemia.

Immune Disorders

The immune system is a complex network of specialized cells and organs that has evolved to defend the body against attacks by foreign organisms. Immune disorders are the result of a breakdown in the body's defense system that may generate (1) hypersensitivity (allergy), (2) autoimmune diseases, or (3) immunodeficiency disorders.

Allergic disease is a hypersensitivity of the body to a substance (allergen) ordinarily considered harmless. Common allergens include inhalants (dust, molds, and fungi), food, animal dander, drugs, insect venom, chemicals, and physical agents (heat, cold, and radiation). Initial exposure to an allergen, which acts as an antigen (a substance that causes the allergic response), stimulates the production of immunoglobulin E (IgE) antibodies, and the person thus is sensitized. Subsequent exposures trigger the allergic response,

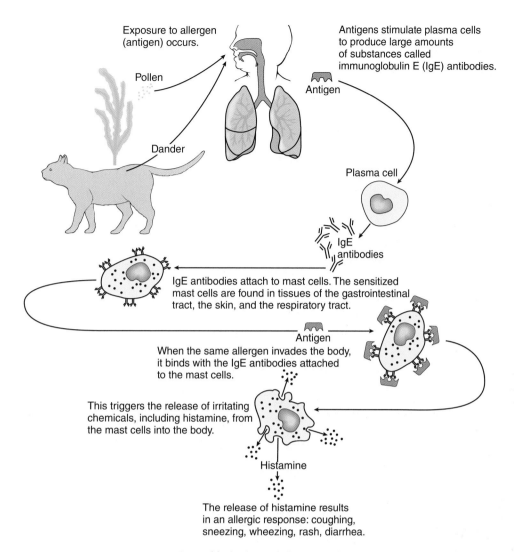

Exposure to allergen (antigen) occurs.

Pollen

Dander

Antigens stimulate plasma cells to produce large amounts of substances called immunoglobulin E (IgE) antibodies.

Antigen

Plasma cell

IgE antibodies

IgE antibodies attach to mast cells. The sensitized mast cells are found in tissues of the gastrointestinal tract, the skin, and the respiratory tract.

Antigen

When the same allergen invades the body, it binds with the IgE antibodies attached to the mast cells.

This triggers the release of irritating chemicals, including histamine, from the mast cells into the body.

Histamine

The release of histamine results in an allergic response: coughing, sneezing, wheezing, rash, diarrhea.

• **Fig. 1.4** Mechanisms of allergic reaction.

which is an antigen-antibody reaction causing the release of histamine and other chemicals (Fig. 1.4). The chemicals cause symptoms including nasal congestion, sneezing, coughing, wheezing, itching, burning, swelling, and diarrhea. Common allergic conditions include seasonal allergic rhinitis (hay fever), allergic sinusitis, bronchial asthma, urticaria (hives), and eczema.

Although allergies cannot be cured, they can usually be controlled with proper diagnosis and treatment. Diagnosis includes allergy blood testing and/or allergy skin testing. When the offending allergens can be identified, they are eliminated from the diet or the environment. Symptomatic treatment includes the use of antihistamines, bronchial dilators, and corticosteroids. Desensitization with a series of injections may be recommended to build immunity to some antigens.

Severe systemic manifestations of allergic responses include **anaphylaxis**, serum sickness, arthralgia, and status asthmaticus. For example, anaphylaxis (anaphylactic shock), the result of a severe systemic allergic reaction, calls for emergency life-saving intervention. Common causes of anaphylaxis include insect stings, food, latex, and medications.

Epinephrine kits can be used for self-administration until they can reach an emergency facility.

Autoimmune diseases represent a large group of disorders marked by an inappropriate or excessive response of the body's defense system that allows the immune system to become self-destructive. Normally the immune system is able to distinguish self-antigens, which are harmless, from foreign antigens, which present a threat to the body. In autoimmune diseases, antibodies are formed against self-antigens mistakenly identified as foreign.

Immunodeficiency disorders result from a depressed or absent immune response. Causative factors can be primary, manifested by a characteristic decrease in the number of T cells and B cells, leaving the body unable to adequately defend itself against infection and tumors. Immunodeficiency also may be secondary to disease, infection, and aging or may be the result of damage to the immune system caused by drugs, radiation, or surgery. Acquired immunodeficiency syndrome (AIDS), a prominent example of an immunodeficiency state, is caused by infection by the human immunodeficiency virus (HIV).

Chapter 3 discusses specific diseases of the immune system.

Physical Trauma and Chemical Agents

Physical trauma is the major cause of death in children and young adults. Common mechanisms of acute injury are falls; motor vehicle accidents, including those involving pedestrians; physical abuse; physical injury from incidents of domestic violence; penetrating injuries; multiple types of injuries sustained in military combat; drowning; and burns. Emergency management begins with triage to determine the priorities of care. Persons who sustain trauma require precise assessment and management to prevent infection, minimize the insult to the body's tissues, combat shock and hemorrhage, and restore homeostasis.

Chemical agents or irritants that are potentially injurious include pollutants, poisons, drugs, preservatives, cosmetics, and dyes. There are known bioterrorism infectious agents that can cause severe toxic trauma to humans in a bioterrorism attack. Extreme heat or cold, radiation, electrical shock, and insect and snake bites are other instruments of injury to the body.

Malnutrition

Disorders of nutrition, as discussed in Chapter 8, may be the result of a deficient diet or of disease conditions that do not allow the body to break down, absorb, or use food. An example of a severe deficiency disease is protein-calorie malnutrition (kwashiorkor), the starvation associated with famine. Other nutritional disorders include eating disorders, iron deficiency, anemia, obesity, and hypervitaminosis.

Aging

Because of the gradual diminishment of body functions, the aging process, although not considered a disease in itself, is a risk factor for the onset of many health problems. With aging comes *immunosenescence*, which is a gradual deterioration of the functions of the immune system. As a result, older adults are at higher risk for infections and less able to achieve full protection from vaccinations. This, along with other age-related risk factors, explains why bacterial community-acquired pneumonia is responsible for illness in older adults. A yearly physical examination with specific screening tests is recommended. Some tests are ordered after a patient turns a specific age. Screening examinations include determination of blood cholesterol levels for hyperlipidemia, electrocardiography for heart disease, rectal examination for bowel cancer and prostate enlargement, PSA serum blood test to determine prostate health, blood pressure check for hypertension, Papanicolaou (Pap) smear for cervical cancer, mammography for breast cancer, and urinalysis for possible diabetes and renal disease.

The nature of geriatrics is changing as the life span in the United States has reached an all-time high because of preventative health care and innovations in medical management. Knowing the special needs of older people is becoming a more critical component of health care. Common concerns are substance abuse, overmedication, loss of mental acuity, depression, and nutritional problems. Regular exercise three to five times a week, proper nutrition, and creating a hazard-free environment to prevent falls should all be emphasized. Each year, one in three adults age 65 years and older falls, causing moderate to severe injuries.

Adults can have many significant life stresses, such as financial hardship, relocation, loss of normal roles in life, and death of loved ones and friends. Skyrocketing health care costs and medical insurance premiums are troubling to seniors living on fixed incomes and younger people who do not have insurance. Such added stress in a person's life may be a contributing factor in disease development or progression. Drug therapy is another major issue because many older adults take several different prescribed medications, in addition to nonprescription drugs and supplements, that health care professionals providing care might not know about. When taking an antibiotic, some adults are often given daily doses of intestinal probiotics to ward off antibiotic-associated diarrhea and infection with *Clostridioides difficile,* which can cause life-threatening bowel inflammation.

Older adults also may not be able to tolerate the standard dose of medications because of metabolic and other changes in body composition (increased adipose tissue, decreased total body water, and so on) that occur with aging. Severe cognitive impairment from any one of several forms of dementia may present substantial hardship to the older person and to family members and caregivers. Other conditions frequently associated with aging include urinary incontinence and sensory isolation because of visual and/or hearing impairment. The state of frailty makes older people more vulnerable to infection, injury, and inability to tolerate invasive therapies.

Psychological Factors

The constant interaction between mind and body can potentially affect a person's wellness or illness. Psychological evaluation encompasses the observation of behavior, appearance, mood, communication, judgment, and thought processes. Because people react differently to disease or the threat of illness, treatment plans must also be tailored to meet their psychological needs. Preservation of self-esteem is of great importance.

Illness can disrupt daily activities, and it can significantly change a patient's life and the lives of involved family members. In the face of disease, the person experiences an altered body image and emotional and social changes that are best understood in terms of past personal experience and perception. For example, when the patient was a child, did illness elicit empathy and a "chicken soup" approach, or was illness met with aversion and a "tough it out" attitude?

Chronic disease is a stressor that can affect a person's self-esteem and behavior. Fear, helplessness, and lack of control are typical feelings. Patients pass through stages of anxiety, shock, denial, anger, withdrawal, and depression as they adjust to the presence of disease. If these stages are sustained

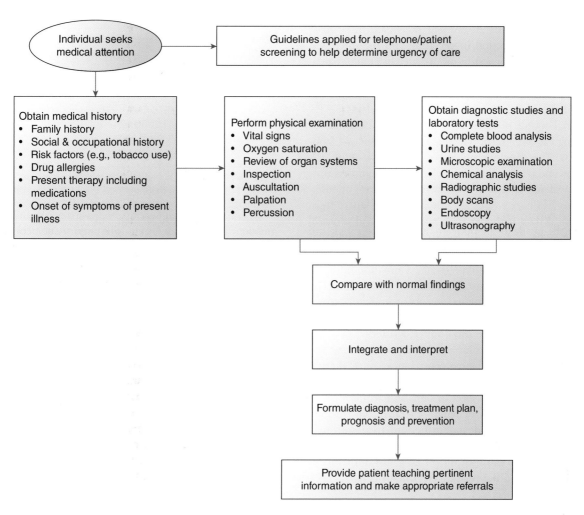

• **Fig. 1.5** Essential steps in diagnosis.

and the person fails to accept the reality of the disease, the patient may develop psychological disturbances in addition to physical alterations.

Mental Disorders

Generally, mental disorders are described as clinically significant behavioral or psychological syndromes that are associated with psychic pain, distress, or impairment of function. Although sometimes cloaked in mystery, the common occurrence of mental disorders and their potential to cause disability dictate the need for the same careful handling as any other sickness. Chapter 14 discusses mental disorders in more detail, including grief response, dementia, mood disorders, and somatoform disorders. Of importance, too, is the fact that some infections can alter the behavior of a patient. Urinary tract infections can cause a change in behavior, which may be mistaken for a cognitive decline or mental problem. Caregivers should also understand that dementia does not occur overnight, within days or weeks, but typically progresses over the course of years. In some cases though, dementia can progress faster over several months.

Diagnosis of Disease

When a person seeks medical attention and describes symptoms and/or exhibits signs of disease, the clinician begins an orderly series of steps to investigate the cause and make a diagnosis (Fig. 1.5). Establishing a diagnosis is a decision-making process in which data collected from the medical history, physical examination, and diagnostic tests are analyzed, integrated, and interpreted. A diagnosis provides a logical basis for determining treatment and prognosis.

The importance of the patient's medical history cannot be overstated. As the primary source of data, it provides vital clues and background information that help direct the remainder of the assessment. During the patient interview, medical information (e.g., family history, predisposing factors or preexisting conditions, drug allergies, and current therapies) is carefully noted. This can provide the foundation for an individualized treatment plan. And, finally, the clinician focuses questions on the onset and nature of the present illness.

Next, a methodical physical examination of the patient from head to toe (a systems review) is performed to detect the physical signs of disease. Assessment skills used to evaluate health status are inspection (observation and measurement, including vital signs), **auscultation** (trained listening), palpation (investigation by sense of touch), and percussion (tapping that produces vibration and sound). The information gathered is then measured against norms or standards.

The final source of assessment data can be obtained by conducting various appropriate diagnostic studies and laboratory tests. These include microscopic examination of cells and tissues and chemical analysis. Although diagnostic testing is considered an important scientific measure of function, these laboratory data are not interpreted apart from other clinical data gathered from the history and physical examination. In deciding or confirming the identification of a disease, the results of diagnostic studies are integrated with the medical history and physical examination findings. In fact, physicians now have computerized systems that can analyze large numbers of patient records to quantify probabilities and devise an orderly approach to diagnosis (a decision tree). As a result, the physician is reminded of a full range of possible diagnoses for a given set of symptoms and signs; in other words, the physician is aided in making a *differential diagnosis*, especially when two or more diseases resemble one another in respect to signs and symptoms.

Laboratory tests, particularly biochemical profiles obtained by testing blood and urine, are used routinely to screen for imbalances or to detect early signs of disease. They are also used to monitor the effectiveness of therapeutic medications and other medical treatments (Box 1.1).

Treatment of Disease

After the initial assessment is completed and a diagnosis is established, appropriate medical intervention is implemented. The plan of treatment is directly related to an identified expected outcome. The goal may be specifically to cure, control symptoms, or be supportive, or may be a combination of these. Therapeutic elements of a conventional medical care plan may be used conservatively or aggressively and include one or more of the following: preventive measures, therapeutic procedures, administration of medications, measures for the relief of pain, surgery, physical therapy, diet modification, psychotherapy, patient education, and follow-up care.

After a medical treatment plan is implemented, it is evaluated and modified as needed. The current trend is to involve patients directly in the choices of treatment and to emphasize their responsibility to make choices that promote their recovery. The physician is the expert advisor who must inform and empower the patient. A team approach to medical treatment, involving the patient, medical personnel, family, and community support systems, is optimal for complicated cases.

The concept of holistic medicine is comprehensive care that focuses on the needs of the whole person (Fig. 1.6). The physical and psychological well-being of the individual are dependent on each other. This established mind-body

• BOX 1.1   Key Physical Guidelines for Adults

All adults should be active and get some type of exercise. A sedentary lifestyle has been linked to an increased risk for health problems. Some physical activity is beneficial for better health compared to no physical activity.

For substantial health benefits, adults should do at least 150 minutes (2.5 hours) to 300 minutes (5 hours) of moderate-intensity aerobic activity each week. Exercise of vigorous-intensity aerobic physical activity of 75 minutes (1.25 hours) to 150 minutes (2.5 hours) a week provides benefits. An individual may also use a combination of both types of exercise. Spreading the activity throughout the week is recommended. Additional health benefits are gained by engaging in physical activity beyond this amount.

Muscle-strengthening activities that involve all the major muscles performed 2 or more days a week are also beneficial.

From U.S. Department of Health and Human Services: 2018 Physical activity guidelines for Americans, ed 2, *health.gov* (website): www.health.gov/paguidelines.

• **Fig. 1.6** Holistic health views the individual as an integrated system rather than one or more separate ones. (From Leonard P: *Quick & easy medical terminology*, ed 9, 2020, Elsevier Inc.)

interaction compels the holistic health care provider to consider the patient as a whole person. Rather than narrowly defining a disease *only* in terms of physical pathologic changes, the clinician also considers the patient's social, emotional, intellectual, and spiritual components. Individualizing care is important; the personality, environment, and lifestyle of the patient need to be factored into the care plan. The holistic practitioner acknowledges the uniqueness of the patient with regard to their needs, aspirations, perception, comprehension, and insight.

Holistic care encourages the patient to consciously pursue the highest possible expressions of being, including those of spirit, mind, emotion, environment, socialization, and physical being. Although integrating all the needs of a patient is compatible with the comprehensive treatment plans of traditional medicine, holistic medicine may also incorporate several nontraditional methods of treatment, which may be empirical or experimental.

One important aspect of holistic medicine is the recognition of the cultural diversity of patients. The United States continues to grow more culturally diverse. Health care providers must be aware of the challenges of caring for such a diverse population, which may include language, religious beliefs, views about health issues, and life experiences. Stereotyping and bias can be misleading while caring for a patient. Health care providers should embrace the differences of individuals and recognize the "one size fits all" approach is not realistic in today's society.

Overcoming the challenges that cultural diversity presents begins with a willingness on the part of the health care provider to learn about cultural issues, overcome language barriers, and take the time necessary to understand what the patient is trying to convey. Many hospitals and clinics have interpreters available to facilitate communication with more prominent minority groups in their communities. Cultural competence in caring for all individuals takes time, patience, and flexibility to acquire knowledge of different cultures and their ways of explaining, understanding, and treating health problems.

Gene Therapy

Gene therapy refers to changing or altering the genes inside cells in the body in hopes of treating or eradicating disease. Genes are made of an individual's DNA. Some diseases result from genes that do not function the way they are supposed to function. A therapeutic gene is delivered by using a vector (a chaperone molecule that accompanies and aids in the safe delivery of DNA). Most of the vectors used for DNA delivery involve viruses or plasmids. Researchers continue to study the best way to alter DNA in genes. Fixing or replacing mutated genes is the goal of gene therapy. Another measure is altering genes so the immune system can recognize which genes pose potential problems.

Stem Cell Research

Scientists study stem cells to investigate their potential to repair damaged tissue in a field called *regenerative medicine*. A stem cell is an unspecialized cell that has the potential to give rise to cells specialized for any tissue in the body. When the stem cell divides, the daughter cell has the potential to become another stem cell or to differentiate into liver, lung, heart, or other specific types of cells. In the human embryo, stem cells give rise to the specialized cells that comprise the lungs, heart, brain, and other tissues. Stem cells still exist in many adult tissues, such as bone marrow, skin, and liver, to replace cells lost through disease, injury, or normal use. As long as a person is alive, their stem cells can divide, differentiate, and replenish the various cells in the body. Specialized cells, in contrast, can only give rise to other specialized cells.

Patients are experiencing the results of this research. Osteonecrosis treatment is one example. Bone marrow is removed from one area of the body and transplanted into another area where bone death has occurred, typically due to loss of blood supply. This helps with the regeneration of cells, but more importantly, is effective in helping the patient's pain.

Another example involves treating single-tract fistulas in patients with Crohn's disease. This trial, conducted by the Mayo Clinic, involved using a dissolvable plug to deliver stem cell therapy to patients with single-tract perianal fistulas, with promising results. Another example is bone marrow transplantation. Stem cells from the bone marrow are used in this procedure to treat several types of cancer, aplastic anemia, sickle cell anemia, immunodeficiencies, and other diseases.

Stem cells are also beneficial to patients with problematic wounds and are being used to ensure better outcomes for burns, cancer surgeries, tissue loss, corneal transplants, and trauma patients.

The processes developed can allow the patient's own cells to be used to correct what is wrong.

These stem cell successes continue to spur on researchers who hope to use stem cells to treat humans suffering from Parkinson disease, cancer, organ failure, and other diseases. Important questions stem cell research hopes to answer include:

- What are the signals involved in getting a stem cell to differentiate?
- Can stem cell lines be used to test the efficacy and safety of new drugs?
- Can stem cells be used to generate new human tissue that can be used to treat disease?

If scientists can reliably direct the differentiation of stem cells into specific cell types, the resulting cells could be used to treat diabetes, spinal cord injury, muscular dystrophy, heart disease, and many other conditions. The use of stem cells and regenerative medicine holds exciting promise for novel therapies, but much research still needs to be done to understand the full potential this can provide for patients.

Pain

All of us experience pain at some time in our lives. What is pain? How do we describe pain? How do we interpret pain? What are the types of pain? Why are tolerance levels different for different people? Why do we have pain at all? Knowing the answers to these questions is a necessary component of understanding pain and how the health care provider can facilitate relief of pain for patients. In addition to established medical options for pain management, there are doctors who specialize in pain management and offer new approaches for those who suffer from chronic discomfort, such as back pain.

Describing Pain

Pain is subjective, individualized, and perceived only by the individual experiencing it. It can be physiologic or psychological. The vocabulary people use to express their sensations of pain varies widely; pain may be described as an

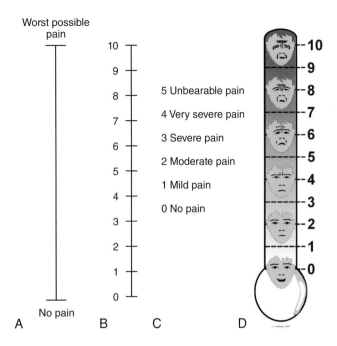

Worst possible pain

5 Unbearable pain

4 Very severe pain

3 Severe pain

2 Moderate pain

1 Mild pain

0 No pain

No pain

A   B   C   D

• **Fig. 1.7** Pain intensity scales (vertical format). (A) Visual analog scale. (B) Numeric rating scale. (C) Descriptive rating scale. (D) Faces pain thermometer. (From Urden L: *Priorities in critical care nursing*, ed 9, 2024, Elsevier Inc. Courtesy Céline Gélinas, Ingram School of Nursing, McGill University, Canada.)

uncomfortable sensation, an unpleasant experience, distress, strong discomfort, suffering, agony, or simply hurting. *Dull* and *aching* are words used often to describe pain resulting from overuse of the musculoskeletal system. Pain along a nerve route that is described as "burning" is often an indication of peripheral nerve insult. Patients use the term *cramping* to characterize an abdominal-visceral type of pain. Head pain or pain felt along a blood vessel commonly is described as *throbbing*. Other descriptive terms include *shooting, stabbing*, and *stinging*. In reference to thermal injury, pain may be described as a burning sensation. When expressing concern about how pain is affecting them, patients may use such terms as *frightening, sickening, tiring, discomforting, intense, unbearable, mild, excruciating*, and *vicious* to categorize the pain.

Because pain interpretation is subjective, the intensity with which it is felt depends on many factors. An individual's perception of pain and response to pain may be based on cultural values, past experiences, religious beliefs, emotional support or lack thereof, anxiety, level of education, and the specific situation in which pain is being felt. Various pain rating scales, using numbers and figures, are sometimes used to help measure an individual's perception of pain intensity and quality (Fig. 1.7). Often the patient may be asked to use a numerical scale from 0 to 10 to classify the intensity of pain: 1 to 3 as mild, 4 to 5 as moderate, or 6 to 10 as severe or "as bad as you can imagine." In the clinical setting, assessment of a patient's pain is noted when vital signs are taken. This information is helpful in tracking the patient's response to treatment.

Physiology of Pain

Pain is a necessary phenomenon in life. The physiology of pain involves the stimulation of specialized nerve endings called **nociceptors**. These pain receptors are found on free sensory nerve endings in the superficial portions of skin, in some tissues of internal or visceral organs, in joint capsules, in the periosteum of bones, surrounding the walls of blood vessels, and in certain deep tissues. Pain is often a signal of injury or tissue damage and, as such, is a protective mechanism that makes people aware of tissue insult.

Pain is the result of tissue insult from noxious (harmful) stimuli, including heat and cold, pressure, chemicals, electrical shock, and trauma. Pain receptors respond to three types of stimuli: (1) temperature extremes, (2) mechanical damage, and (3) dissolved chemicals, including potassium, acids, histamines, acetylcholine, bradykinin, and prostaglandins. A very strong stimulus may excite all three types, creating a burning-type sensation. Additional causes of painful stimuli include hypoxia and ischemia to the tissue and muscle spasms.

Pain impulses travel from the nerve ending through the spinal cord to the thalamus and then proceed to the sensory cortex in the parietal lobe of the brain. Adaptation to painful stimuli does not occur because the receptors continue to respond as long as the stimulus remains, stopping only when the tissue damage has ended.

Pain is a signal that helps locate and eliminate or reduce the source of tissue damage. Pain may also be a part of the normal healing process as a reaction to the inflammatory process. It is also possible for pain to occur in the absence of physical injury; this is referred to as *psychological pain*. Psychological or emotional pain is as real as pain with a physical cause to the person experiencing it. This type of pain can also be acute, chronic, transient, or *intractable*.

Pain is not always reported accurately. Stress can alter both perception and response to pain. The cerebral cortex is responsible for the interpretation of pain and therefore must be functioning at normal capacity for interpretation to occur. Many of the internal organs are poorly supplied with nociceptors, and therefore the tissue insults in these organs are not always reported as such. The free nerve endings have large receptive fields, consequently making it difficult to determine the true source of the pain stimuli. Additionally, neurons from certain organs may travel a parallel pathway along the spinal cord to the brain, resulting in *referred pain*. Generally referred pain follows a *dermatome* that is supplied by the same spinal nerve as the nerve that has been stimulated by the insult, causing the pain to be projected to the body surface. For example, the patient experiencing myocardial ischemia or angina describes the pain as chest pain radiating to the left arm. Likewise, the nervous tissue of the brain has no pain receptors; nevertheless, headaches are commonly reported. Often the pain is caused by pressure on the blood vessel walls or the meninges. Tissue insult or inflammation of the gallbladder often results in pain referred to the right scapular region (Fig. 1.8).

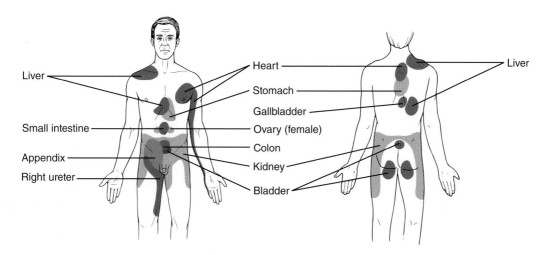

• **Fig. 1.8** Referred pain, anterior and posterior views. (From Miller-Keane BF: *Encyclopedia and dictionary of medicine, nursing, & allied health*, ed 7, Philadelphia, 2003, Saunders.)

Pain Classification

Pain may be classified as acute, chronic, transient, or intractable. Acute pain usually has a sudden onset and is severe in intensity. It also usually is of short duration. Individuals with acute pain have a tendency to guard the painful area; may exhibit distractive behavior, such as crying or moaning; are restless, anxious, or listless; and may have altered thought processes. Blood pressure and pulse often increase, whereas respiratory rates may increase or decrease. Occasionally the sudden onset of very severe pain may cause vascular collapse and a resulting state of shock. Facial movements may indicate a grimace, and the skin may become *diaphoretic*. Chronic pain is usually less severe, with a duration of greater than 6 months. Pain from inflammatory conditions, such as arthritis and bursitis, is considered chronic. Patients with chronic pain often exhibit weight loss or gain, insomnia or altered sleep patterns, anorexia, inability to continue normal activities, and guarded movements. Psychosocial relationships may be altered. Chronic intractable pain, usually generated by nerve damage or cancer, is debilitating and can cause depression. Transient pain comes and goes, usually has a brief duration, and often is not significant.

Pain can also be classified as superficial, deep, or visceral. Superficial pain is described as being located on the body's surface. Deep pain is usually correlated with muscles, joints, or tendons. Visceral pain is attributed to internal organs.

Pain Relief

Acute pain, such as the pain experienced as a result of myocardial infarction, postoperative pain after surgical intervention, pain resulting from severe trauma, and pain felt during a terminal illness, can be treated with narcotics or opioid-related drugs. A device called a *patient-controlled analgesia pump* allows a prescribed dose of an analgesic to be dispensed intravenously at safe intervals for effective control of acute pain. Cannabis and cannabidiol oils and preparations are also used to treat pain.

Chronic pain often is treated with acetaminophen, steroids, or antiinflammatory agents, such as nonsteroidal antiinflammatory drugs. More recently, evidence-based guidelines for the treatment of chronic pain have suggested that antidepressants and anticonvulsants can be used for chronic neuropathic pain. Transcutaneous electrical nerve stimulation sends types of electrical impulses to the nerve endings with the intention of blocking nerve transmission to the brain and may be of benefit to persons experiencing acute or chronic pain. In some cases, surgical intervention is necessary to remove the source of pain or block the transmission of pain.

Complementary and alternative methods of pain control include physical therapy and massage of the painful area to increase the blood flow to and from the area and to increase the flow of lymph from the area. Acupuncture, an ancient therapeutic treatment, is thought to elicit pain relief by way of the needles used to stimulate nerves deep in the tissue, thus arousing the pituitary gland and other parts of the brain to cause the release of *endorphins*, the brain's own natural opioids. Endorphins reduce the perception of pain while the stimulus remains.

Preventive Health Care

Preventive health care emphasizes strategies for preventing disease and injury. Included is the trend to be proactive in one's own health care. Current statistical evidence indicates that positive personal health behavior, in conjunction with prophylactic medical services, may reduce the mortality rate associated with certain diseases, such as cardiovascular disease. Identifying risk factors and employing specific screening tests to detect alterations give individuals information they can use to modify their lifestyles. Using available medical measures can help prevent the onset of disease or at least minimize complications.

One risk factor is smoking and exposure to secondhand smoke. Smoking tobacco and exposure to secondhand smoke is the *single greatest avoidable cause of death and disease*. Public education in this regard has led to laws that prohibit smoking in many restaurants and other public arenas.

Preventing patients from hospital-acquired infections (known as nosocomial infections) is another measure of preventive health care. Health care institutions are challenged daily to uphold infection control measures that protect patients against hospital-acquired infections (known as *nosocomial infections*). Approximately 5% of patients have MRSA in their nose or on their skin in the US hospitals. Continuing education requirements fulfilled by physicians and other health care providers give them the skills that help diminish occasions of *iatrogenic* infections or disorders, that is, those diseases or conditions that are a result of medical procedures or treatment.

Some US companies are embracing wellness program initiatives that motivate employees to improve their health and overcome problems, which may have an effect on their overall well-being and health. Losing weight, tobacco use cessation, and routine exercise lead to lower health risks and healthier individuals. These onsite programs provide the worker with tools and incentives to improve health, which results in lower rates of absenteeism and overall reduced health risks.

On-the-job injuries are prevented by implementing training all employees: (1) improved safety measures involving the operation of machinery and automobiles; (2) protective labeling and packaging of food, drugs, and toxic products; and (3) general public safety education.

Family violence, another possible threat to an individual's health, is a serious and growing epidemic in the United States, resulting in both psychological stress and physical trauma. In many cases, early intervention may prevent such abuse. Involving legal, social, and medical authorities early on can serve to identify and protect those caught up in the cycle of domestic violence before serious medical consequences result. Chronic stress can affect certain functions within the brain and adversely impact health. Interventions to help reduce and manage stress include meditation and ways to increase confidence in one's ability to self-regulate emotion and mood. Exercise that involves a structured program to improve physical fitness has proven to be health enhancing to the body and mind as well (Box 1.1).

Vaccines are important for adults, adolescents, and children for protection against many communicable diseases. Vaccine recommendations for adolescents and adults are based on various factors, including age, overall health status, and medical history. Contraindications and precautions associated with each specific vaccine are factored in for the individual before immunization is begun. In general, vaccines for adults include:

- Tetanus-diphtheria vaccine (all adults, every 10 years)
- Seasonal influenza (flu) vaccine (adults age 50 years and older)
- COVID-19 vaccine and boosters as recommended by age
- Pneumococcal vaccine (adults age 65 years and older)
- Hepatitis B vaccine (adults at risk), three doses
- Hepatitis A (two doses)

- Measles-mumps-rubella vaccine (susceptible adults) contraindicated in HIV infection and pregnancy
- Varicella (chickenpox) vaccine (susceptible adults but contraindicated in pregnancy)
- Meningococcal vaccine (college freshmen living in dormitories)
- HPV vaccine (all previously unvaccinated females and males through age 26 years)
- Gardasil (HPV) vaccine (can be given to young males)
- Shingrix vaccine to help prevent shingles (herpes zoster) in adults 60 years of age or older except when contraindicated (pregnancy and HIV infection)
- Tetanus toxoid, reduced diphtheria toxoid, and acellular pertussis (Tdap) vaccine are recommended for adults 19 to 64 years of age and for certain adults 65 years of age and older (specific recommendations for Tdap vaccine exist for persons 11–18 years of age)
- Respiratory syncytial virus vaccine using shared decision-making criteria
- Vaccines for travelers (specific recommendations are found on the CDC website)
- Special recommendations for the polio vaccine

No vaccine is completely risk free or completely effective. Side effects can occur. The national program that monitors the safety of vaccines after they are licensed is called the *Vaccine Adverse Event Reporting System (VAERS)*. Although unexpected reactions are rare, anyone can report a possible problem to VAERS, where the information is monitored by the FDA and the CDC.

Nontraditional Medicine

Many patients and practitioners now accept safe complementary and alternative medicine (CAM) as an adjunct to conventional medicine. Patient demand for integrative medicine (integrating mainstream medicine with CAM) is evident by the big gain in the percentage of hospitals offering one or more types of CAM services. The National Center for Complementary and Alternative Medicine, a component of the National Institutes of Health, is the government's lead agency for the classification and scientific research of CAM.

By definition, *complementary* medicine is used *together with* conventional medicine. An example of complementary therapy is using aromatherapy to help lessen a patient's discomfort following surgery. *Alternative* medicine is used *in place of* conventional medicine. An example of an alternative therapy is using a special diet to treat cancer instead of undergoing surgery, radiation, or chemotherapy that has been recommended by a conventional doctor.

Osteopathy is probably the most widely accepted form of alternative medicine. In the United States, osteopathic physicians (doctors of osteopathy) are trained medical doctors who emphasize the stimulation of the body's natural processes as a means to promote healing and well-being. In addition to traditional medical and surgical concepts, osteopathic physicians use manipulation techniques to realign body structure, thereby restoring balance and promoting healing.

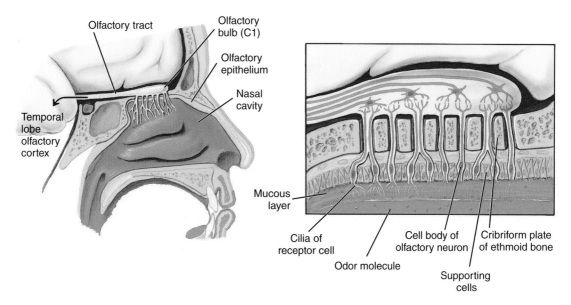

• **Fig. 1.9** Structure of the olfactory receptors. (From Applegate EJ: *The anatomy and physiology physical learning system*, ed 4, St. Louis, 2011, Saunders.)

Chiropractic medicine is based on the concept that the body's nervous system is the foundation of health and that undue pressure on or an insult to the nervous system may result in pain and disease. Correct alignment of the spinal vertebrae is emphasized; therefore many chiropractic adjustments involve manipulation of the spine.

Massage, although not a new concept, is just now being recognized by the US medical community as a valid alternative therapy or type of medicine. According to Eastern philosophy and also Swedish concepts, massage encourages drainage of the lymphatic system and increases circulation to the tissue.

Reflexology, a form of massage, primarily involves massage of the feet and sometimes the hands. The theory is that the body is divided into zones and these zones are reflected in specific areas of the feet or hands. Manipulation of these areas is expected to have a therapeutic effect on the organ or system represented in that zone.

Aromatherapy uses essential oils to promote wellness and healing and to relieve stress. Although this therapy mainly involves inhalation and the olfactory system (Fig. 1.9), the oils used are absorbed through the skin and transported to the various body tissues and systems by the circulatory system as well. The essential oils are diluted and then massaged into the skin or placed in a steam inhaler for inspiration. Some of the more common essential oils used in aromatherapy are chamomile, clary sage, clove, eucalyptus, geranium, ginger, lavender, orange, peppermint, rosemary, sage, tea tree, evening primrose, and ylang-ylang. Often aromatherapists mix the oils to meet the specific needs of their patients.

Herbs have been used as medicines for many centuries, with ancient Egyptians being the first known to record lists of herbs. Sometimes called *natural medicines*, herbs are now being substituted for pharmaceutical products by some. Common herbal products include ginkgo biloba, garlic, saw palmetto, ginseng, passion flower, angelica, chamomile, fennel, lavender, peppermint, rosemary, sage, St. Johns wort, valerian, and yarrow. Herbs may be purchased in a pharmacy, in a herbal drug store, or by mail. Herbal remedies are professed to treat allergies, arthritis, gastrointestinal (GI) problems, headaches, hypertension or hypotension, insomnia, urinary problems, menstrual or menopausal symptoms, and skin diseases. Many of these products do not have FDA approval and may damage health if taken unwarily or in conjunction with prescription drugs. For example, one of the most used herbal supplements, ginkgo biloba, was recently studied for evidence of positive effects on memory and other clinical uses. Results were mixed and inconclusive, resulting in narrowed indications for its use and a list of contraindications and cautions. Lack of FDA regulation also means that the ingredients stated on the outside of the bottle may not necessarily be inside the bottle or may not be present in the amounts indicated.

Diet and nutrition therapy certainly is not a new concept; however, many follow special diets and address nutritional needs, hoping to eliminate toxins from the body and allow it to function at the optimal level. Diet therapy may include fat-free, low-saturated-fat, low-sugar, high-protein, low-carbohydrate, vegetarian, no- or low-caffeine, and seafood diets. Vitamin and mineral supplements are often added to the daily routine, but this should be done with caution because megadoses may be toxic. Patients should check with a physician or pharmacist before starting any nutritional supplement regimen.

Cupping is used to increase blood circulation to an area of the body. Cupping may be performed with plastic or glass and other objects to help relieve pain in conjunction with other therapies (Fig. 1.10A).

Acupuncture, an Asian therapy that uses meridians, attempts to adjust the body's energy (*chi* [chee]) flow by

• **Fig. 1.10** (A) Cupping placement for tendonitis of the shoulder, (B) meridians for acupuncture, and (C) acupuncture. (A, Courtesy Kaitlynn S. Fuqua; B, From Phillps N, et al: *Berry & Kohn's operating room technique*, ed 14, 2021, Elsevier; C, From Penman ID, et al: *Davidson's principles and practice of medicine*, ed 23, 2018, Elsevier.)

inserting needles into acupuncture points (Fig. 1.10B and C). After insertion, the needles are manipulated by twirling or by a gentle pumping action. Recent advances in techniques use electrical or laser stimulation and only professionals trained in acupuncture should attempt this procedure. Patients with cardiac pacemakers and other electronic devices are advised to talk with their doctor before beginning acupuncture.

Acupressure, similar to acupuncture, involves the manipulation of acupoints by means of finger pressure. The intent is to balance the flow of energy along the meridians to promote healthy functioning of internal organs. Acupressure is often incorporated into massage as a method of muscle relaxation and stress reduction.

Therapeutic touch is derived from an ancient technique called *laying-on of hands*. It is based on the premise that it is the healing force of the therapist that affects the patient's recovery; healing is promoted when the body's energies are in balance; and, by passing their hands over the patient, healers can attempt to identify energy imbalances.

Shiatsu (she-AT-sue), a form of therapy from Japan that is similar to acupressure, is usually performed on a mat on the floor. The patient remains clothed, and the therapist applies pressure to the acupoints and along the meridians using the fingertips, knuckles, elbows, knees, or even the feet.

A magnetic therapy called transcranial magnetic stimulation has been approved by the FDA for use in some cases of certain types of migraine headaches and as a treatment for major depression. However, it is being used extensively in veterinary medicine, especially in equine veterinary medicine. It is believed that magnets increase circulation to the area being treated, thereby increasing the available amount of oxygen (O_2) and nutrients while at the same time transporting away the waste products of metabolism and the inflammatory process. It is also postulated that the magnetic field interferes with the conduction of the sensory nerves by preventing movement of the sodium (Na^+) and potassium (K^+) ions in and out of the nerve cell; this reduces the conduction capability of the sensory nerve. Advocates of this therapy state that magnets are useful in relieving muscle and nerve pain, reducing inflammation, and mitigating migraines.

Hypnosis and hypnotherapy have been accepted as means of psychological therapy. The therapist places the patient in a trance-like state, often resembling sleep. While in this trance, the subject follows acceptable suggestions. Often, relaxation and pain relief can be achieved by using this therapy. Only a qualified practitioner who is trained specifically in the performance of hypnosis should attempt this therapy.

Relaxation can be thought of as a form of self-hypnosis. Many techniques for achieving relaxation are available to the individual. Physical relaxation usually is the starting point for the subject, with psychological relaxation often being the next step. Relaxation is used to treat stress-related physical and emotional problems, pain, anxiety, asthma, arthritis, depression, panic attacks, and hypertension. Many forms of relaxation include the repetition of an action, images, or sounds that then passively erase everyday thoughts from the mind. Some meditation techniques can be used to establish a relaxation response and are used in stress reduction programs. However, meditation is contraindicated for patients with certain personality disorders or active psychosis.

Prayer is considered a mind-body therapy used by many as a source of healing and comfort. Some recent studies link positive patient outcomes to prayer; other studies report uncertain scientific evidence of a relationship between prayer and recovery. Nevertheless, some schools are including the value of spirituality in holistic models of care.

Reiki (ray-KEE) claims to transfer healing energy from the practitioner to the patient. Usually the practitioner starts the ritual at the patient's head and either touches the head or moves the hands close to the head within the patient's aura. The practitioner's hands then touch other parts of the patient's body, or the hands move into the aura space outlining the body. The healing energy is then transferred to the patient. The intention of this therapy is the promotion of physical, emotional, and spiritual well-being.

Music therapy recognizes the involvement of vibrations, rhythms, and sound in the well-being of individuals. Listening to music by composers of the Baroque period, such as Mozart,

can help achieve relaxation. Music, along with anesthesia or pain medication, is used to elevate mood, create a calming effect, lessen muscle tension, and alleviate feelings of fear and anxiety by manifesting a state of relaxation. Patients undergoing chemotherapy for cancer can benefit from music that induces relaxation. Trained and qualified music therapists design the therapy to fit the particular patient's needs.

Homeopathy, polarity therapy, Rolfing, *tai chi* (tie-CHEE), iridology, naturopathy, hydrotherapy, and Ayurveda are some additional forms of alternative medicine. Although any of these therapies may be considered a form of alternative medicine, the patient and practitioner should check with the physician before attempting to include these therapies in the course of treatment. When used, they should be considered adjunct treatments and not necessarily proven medical treatments. Health care providers should inquire routinely about a patient's use of alternative therapies because a large percentage of the population does use them, and many do not think to report this use to their physicians.

Patient Teaching

It is important, and in the patient's best interests, that all health care workers, as members of a team, understand the principles, goals, and specifics of patient teaching. ***Licensing regulations and state practice acts should be followed in regard to patient teaching***. Under these regulations, medical assistants often contribute significantly to patient education, according to the discretion of the supervising physician or licensed professional.

> **◆ NOTE**
>
> Please consult your state code regarding licensing regulations for an explanation of the rules and regulations governing medical assistant practice in your location. Practice laws address what tasks a properly prepared medical assistant can perform; these laws differ from state to state. It is important that medical assistants know who their legally responsible supervisor is in a medical office; it may be the physician. Medical assistants should ask to see the written office policy regarding any delegation of tasks by the health care provider.

General Principles of Patient Teaching

- The concept of patient teaching is based on patient-centered care, with the patient being a partner in the process of learning skills, solving problems, and preventing complications.
- Effective patient teaching requires skillful listening as patients express their understanding of their situations, worries, and hopes. The education process is ongoing, interactive, and directed toward achieving the patient's plan of care.
- Patient teaching is a course of action that involves assessment, critical thinking, and compromise directed toward successful compliance.

- Effective patient teaching policies indicate who has primary legal responsibility for patient teaching and documentation (outlined in nurse state practice acts).

Goals of Patient Teaching

- Encourage the patient to comply with the personalized medical treatment plan to ensure recovery.
- Offer guidance, support, and clear instructions to the patient who requires medical attention and the family or caregiver.
- Develop a trusting relationship with patients through empathy, effective communication, and knowledge about the subject matter being taught.
- Help patients learn how to effectively deal with their conditions by making healthy lifestyle choices.
- Give the individual the confidence needed to take responsibility for their health or recovery.

Reasons for Patient Teaching

- Ease anxiety
- Answer questions
- Instill confidence through individualized education
- Evaluate the patient's perception of the treatment plan, and make any necessary adjustments
- Reinforce the physician's instructions
- Highlight reasonable goals for recovery
- Encourage the individual to take responsibility for their health care
- Help build the esteem that creates a sense of self-sufficiency and control
- Educate the primary caregiver or family about specific aspects of the care plan
- Improve patient/family coping
- Provide an opportunity to practice skills associated with care
- Reduce clinic visits and hospitalization
- Supply the patient and caregiver with educational materials (booklets, websites, and community resources)
- Suggest participation in appropriate social support groups
- Supply a list of phone numbers to call for answers to questions or medical concerns during recovery
- Stress the importance of keeping future appointments for follow-up care

NOTE

Modern information technology is an essential component of all health care and a powerful tool for patient education. Electronically generated materials can be customized according to almost any patient's need for knowledge and practical application of the prescribed treatment plan. Electronic learning (e-learning) teaching methods include videos or educational websites that demonstrate activities for rehabilitation or using home equipment, such as an oxygen support system or a glucose monitoring system. It is wise to integrate e-learning with face-to-face or telephone contact for reinforcement of patient education to help ensure a safe and positive outcome.

The Specifics of Patient Teaching: Addressing the Patient's Concerns

"What's wrong with me?"

Answering this question provides an opportunity to reinforce or explain *only what has been expressed to the patient by the medical professional with primary responsibility for care*. It is not appropriate to "second guess" or give false or unsubstantiated information to a patient.

"What are these tests for?"

Again, your response will depend on guidelines given by the medical professional ordering the tests.

- Explain any special preparation and the purpose of the test
- In plain words, explain the procedure and what to expect during and after the procedure
- Make sure the patient understands the warning signs of complications that may occur, if any
- Tell the patient when to expect the test results, and advise when to call or wait to be called for those results
- Be prepared to discuss the cost with the patient or insurance company, if asked

"What is this disease?"

You should review and explain the physician's diagnosis. When possible, use illustrations and plain language to explain the pathophysiology of the disease. Try to point to the history of symptoms that may relate to the disease. This will help the patient monitor changes in symptoms during recovery.

"What causes this disease?"

Review the physician's explanation of the cause(s) and contributing factors. This could include the source of infection, genetic influences, lifestyle, age, diet, trauma, or epidemic factors. Understanding prevention measures is helpful in some cases.

"Why do I need this medication?"

Explain the purpose and expected results. Review the dosage schedule and route of administration. Discuss the common side effects and what side effects to report to the physician. Give special instructions, such as how to handle skipped doses, and explain why some medications must not be stopped abruptly without the advice of the doctor. Be sure to mention which over-the-counter drugs to avoid.

"When should I call the doctor?"

Review warning signs of possible complications from the disease or any medical intervention that require notification of the nurse or physician: sudden increase in pain, signs of infection or bleeding, neurologic changes, muscle pain or weakness, and so on. Advise the patient on how to obtain refills for medications.

"How long do I have to undergo this therapy?"

Explain the goal(s) of treatment or therapy: physical therapy, therapeutic topical applications of heat or ice, eye drops, wound care, extra rest, or avoidance of certain activities. Demonstrate and give the patient time to practice a prescribed treatment or evaluation, such as glucose monitoring or the use of an inhaler.

"Would you explain this diet?"

Instruct the patient on the relationship between diet and recovery and health. Warn the patient about the possible interactions between specific herbs and certain medications. List the signs of dehydration. Refer to a dietitian, as needed.

"The doctor says I need an operation."

Preoperative Care

- Offer reasonable assurance, because preoperative anxiety is universal.
- Review the preoperative instructions given by the physician.
- Ask the patient if they understands what to expect from the operation, and offer as much information as possible to the family or caregiver. Determine whether the patient needs further clarification about the benefits and risks of the operation.
- Arrange for any preoperative blood work, radiology, or scans. Answer related questions. Give laboratory phone numbers and hours of service.
- Give the patient complete directions and parking instructions.

Postoperative Care

- After surgery, make sure the patient understands the medical plan: wound care, how to take medications, and when to resume activity and return to work.
- The patient needs reassurance about pain control and what to expect during the recovery process.
- Explain warning signs of complications: fever, bleeding, infection, shock, dehydration, and emotional depression.
- The patient and caregiver should be given written instructions and the phone numbers of the nurse or physician to call for answers to questions.
- Make appropriate referrals to support groups.

  "When do I have to be seen again?"

  Make a follow-up appointment for the patient. Explain the importance of ongoing care during the recovery process. Encourage the patient to ask questions about any aspect of his or her medical care. Long-term treatment and medical concerns are addressed on an ongoing basis.

Special Considerations for the Patient With Cancer or a Life-Threatening Disease

When the clinician interrelates with patients and families faced with life-shortening illness, the provider has many opportunities to offer important responses and guidance. Seriously ill patients benefit from an interdisciplinary approach to the clinical management of their diseases. Clinicians can expect to address many special needs of the people diagnosed with the disease itself and also with the side effects of therapeutic interventions. The issues to be addressed are many and varied:

- Keep patients and families from feeling abandoned by providing support based on their personal needs and goals.
- Give verbal and written instructions.
- Welcome feedback on all aspects of the care plan.
- Encourage discussion about the side effects of medications, especially chemotherapy, radiation, or any therapeutic procedures.
- Review warning signs to report to the physician (i.e., weight loss, dehydration, or pain that is not controlled by prescription medication).
- Address the physical, psychological, social, and spiritual aspects of care.
- Bear in mind the two main fears of those with life-threatening illnesses: being in pain and becoming a burden to others.
- Make appropriate and timely referrals to support groups or comprehensive programs of end-of-life care, such as hospice.
- Reinforce the concept of palliative care being prescribed when curative treatment offers no hope; the goal is to prevent and ease suffering and can be delivered at any time in the course of an illness.
- If spiritual distress is identified, offer a referral to a hospital chaplain.
- Address the caregiver's concerns, including adjusting to role changes, providing physical care, and ethical issues and dilemmas.

Patient and Family Support

Throughout this text, the diseases and disorders discussed may be mild to debilitating or cause death. For this reason, many patients and families need resources to help them navigate their condition. For each condition or disease, support for the patient is imperative in the care of the patient. The caregiver also needs support, and the health care worker plays an integral part in the support system. From those who provide direct or indirect patient care to those who handle billing and insurance for medical claims, each person plays a role.

Patients may need three types of care in response to different diseases or even just age progression. At some point, most of us will need some type of help. Home health agency services and outpatient and inpatient hospice care are helpful.

Home Health

Home health agencies provide skilled nursing and health care providers and may also provide resources for other types of services that will help support patients in the comfort of their homes. Some of the services provided include at-home blood pressure and vital sign monitoring, laboratory testing, and testing for therapeutic drug levels for blood thinners such as sodium warfarin. Home health agencies may also provide physical and occupational therapists to visit the client in the home. Language and speech therapy may also be a service provided. These agencies send health care providers to care for those who are unable to leave the home for treatment. Clients who have had strokes, heart attacks, motor vehicle accidents, and other medical problems may benefit from home health services. Bathing care can also be provided. The home health agency is not an elder client-sitting service. They provide specialized care based on the patient's health care provider's orders and support the needs of the patient.

Hospice Care

There are two types of hospice care. Outpatient hospice care allows a client with a terminal illness to live their last days at home with palliative care, or care focused on pain relief and comfort surrounded by family and those individuals who are important to them.

Inpatient hospice is also centered around palliative care. It is another option if "at-home" care is not possible or if the patient's pain cannot be controlled at home. Nursing care,

personal care, and support for family members and caregivers are provided. Hospice care has been instrumental in making the process of transitioning from life to death easier on the client, and the client's family.

Conclusion

Human pathologic processes involve complex mechanisms that can be weighed separately as elements of the disease process but that ultimately converge into the total picture of how and why an individual is sick and what is required as a remedy.

It is worth the effort to strive to understand the nature and impact of human disease on people and humankind. One can expect to find great personal and professional satisfaction in knowing the nature, signs, symptoms, causes, and treatment of the pathologic conditions that alter or seriously threaten health. This knowledge also fosters insight into the scenario imposed by diseases and compassion for the people affected by them.

Review Challenge

Answer the following questions:

1. How may the following predisposing factors make a person more vulnerable to disease?
   a. Age
   b. Sex
   c. Lifestyle
   d. Environment
   e. Heredity
2. Describe three ways that genetic diseases are caused.
3. Name three of the body's natural defense mechanisms.
4. How does acute inflammation protect against infection?
5. Discuss the behavioral characteristics of malignant neoplasms.
6. What is the goal of cancer treatment, and what therapeutic measures may be used?
7. What is an allergic disease? What are the symptoms, and how may they be treated?
8. List the normal sequence of steps in formulating a diagnosis.
9. What is the difference between benign and malignant tumors?
10. What is the emphasis on preventive health care?
11. Explain the importance of knowing the types of pain, the possible causes, and how it may be described by the patient.
12. List some of the stresses and special needs of older people.
13. What are the components of the holistic concept of medical care?
14. Discuss osteopathy as a form of alternative medicine.
15. How does genetic counseling help families?
16. How does good patient teaching affect the positive outcome of disease?
17. What are some of the harmful health effects of exposure to tobacco smoke?
18. What does the acronym MRSA stand for? Why is MRSA considered a threat to public health?

Internet Assignments

1. Explore the plethora of information available for research from the National Cancer Institute (www.cancer.gov). Report on your personal points of interest on this subject.
2. Navigate the website for the Centers for Disease Control and Prevention (www.cdc.gov), available in English or Spanish, and explore the available materials, such as the Health Topics A-Z page.
3. Explore the Genetic Alliance website (www.geneticalliance.org) for available resources regarding any particular genetic disease.
4. Access the American Academy of Allergy and Immunology website (www.aaaai.org) and explore the pages, such as the National Allergy Bureau report on pollen and mold.

Critical Thinking

1. Explain this statement: "The absence of illness does not necessarily indicate optimal health."
2. It is said that *cancer* refers to a group of diseases with numerous causes. Explain.
3. Describe some challenges a health care worker might encounter caring for a person from a foreign culture.
4. Suggest ways in which chronic and/or severe stress can adversely affect health.
5. Generally speaking, why is good communication in patient teaching an essential component of all health care?
6. What is implied in the statement: "The physician is the expert advisor who must inform and empower the patient?"
7. Choose one of the goals of patient teaching as listed in the textbook. Explain how you or someone you know has benefited from such patient teaching.

Credentialing Examination Questions

1. Which option best describes the term homeostasis?
   A. Equal with bad and good
   B. A state of internal stability
   C. Individuals who have an infection
   D. Individuals with good mental health despite other health conditions
2. Which factors may predispose an individual to being susceptible to a disease or condition?
   A. Age
   B. Lifestyle
   C. Genetics
   D. All of the above
3. Which acronym stands for an infection that does not respond to antibiotic treatment and is to blame for aggressive skin and soft tissue infections?
   A. NSRM
   B. NOSO
   C. MRSA
   D. INFE
4. What is the purpose of the Genetic Information Nondiscrimination Act of 2008?
   A. Prohibits insurance companies from discriminating against individuals who have a hereditary disease.
   B. Ensures veterans will have good health care benefits.
   C. Allows people who were injured to obtain health insurance coverage for free.
   D. Expands Medicare coverage after the age of 75.
5. Which statement describes the concept of holistic medicine?
   A. Focuses on the mental health of a patient.
   B. Centers around the physical health of a patient.
   C. Used when caring for a patient who has cancer.
   D. Focuses on the needs of the whole person.
6. Which classification of pain has a sudden onset and is severe in intensity?
   A. Chronic
   B. Acute
   C. Transient
   D. Intractable
7. Which vaccine is administered to prevent chickenpox?
   A. Gardasil
   B. Shingrex
   C. Varicella
   D. Pneumococcal
8. Which test can measure overall kidney function?
   A. 24-Hour urine collection
   B. Urinalysis with microscopy
   C. Urine culture and sensitivity
   D. Urinalysis without microscopy
9. A patient is diagnosed with a terminal illness and is expected to live approximately 4 weeks. The patient wishes to die at home. Which type of service will be most beneficial for this patient?
   A. Home health
   B. Inpatient hospice
   C. Outpatient hospice
   D. Palliative care
10. Cancer is staged according to which criteria?
    A. Size and extent of primary tumor
    B. Extent of regional lymph node involvement
    C. Number of distant metastases
    D. All of the above

2

Developmental, Congenital, and Childhood Diseases and Disorders

CHAPTER OUTLINE

LEARNING OBJECTIVES

After studying this chapter, you should be able to:

1. List the possible causes of congenital anomalies.
2. Discuss genetic disorders and syndromes.
3. Discuss the purpose and procedure of amniocentesis.
4. Describe the condition of prematurity and associated disorders: the causes and treatments.
5. List possible risk factors of retinopathy of prematurity.
6. List symptoms and signs of Down syndrome.
7. List and discuss diseases of the pediatric nervous system.
8. Distinguish between muscular dystrophy and cerebral palsy.
9. Describe patent ductus arteriosus.
10. Name and describe the most common congenital cyanotic cardiac defect.
11. List and discuss the musculoskeletal conditions of newborns and young children.
12. List and discuss pediatric genitourinary conditions.
13. List and discuss pediatric diseases of the digestive system.
14. List and discuss pediatric metabolic disorders.
15. List the major clinical manifestations of cystic fibrosis.
16. Distinguish between Klinefelter syndrome and Turner syndrome.
17. List and discuss contagious diseases of children.
18. Describe the clinical condition of congenital rubella syndrome.
19. Discuss the possible causes and prevention of sudden infant death syndrome.
20. Distinguish between croup and epiglottitis.
21. Describe the symptoms, signs, and treatment for tonsillitis and adenoid hyperplasia.
22. Identify measures used in the treatment of asthma.
23. Discuss the causes and treatment of bronchiolitis.
24. List the types of worms that may infest the gastrointestinal tract.
25. List the symptoms and signs of anemia; describe the pathology of leukemia.
26. Explain the etiology of erythroblastosis fetalis.
27. Name some warning signs of lead poisoning.
28. Describe the infant born with fetal alcohol syndrome.

KEY TERMS

acetabulum (ass-eh-TAB-u-lum)
acyanotic (a-sigh-ah-NOT-ik)
adenosarcoma (ad-eh-no-sar-KO-mah)
amniocentesis (am-nee-o-sen-TEE-sis)
anencephalic (an-en-seh-FAL-ik)
ataxic (ah-TACH-sik)
azoospermia (azo-SPIR-me-a)
bicornuate (bye-KOR-nate)
contracture (kon-TRACK-chur)
dysplasia (dis-PLAY-zee-ah)
dystrophy (DIS-troe-fee)

electromyography (e-LECK-tro-my-og-ra-fee)
foramen ovale (for-A-men o-VAL-a)
meconium (meh-KOH-nee-um)
meninges (men-IN-jeez)
neonates (NEE-o-nates)
pylorus (pye-LOR-us)
stenosis (ste-NO-sis)
syncope (SIN-koh-pee)
tachypnea (tack-ip-NEE-ah)
trisomy (TRY-so-me)

Developmental and Congenital Disorders

Developmental Characteristics and Congenital Anomalies

The developmental process begins with conception (Fig. 2.1A) and progresses as a gradual modification of the structure and characteristics of the individual (see Fig. 2.1B). The first 2 months of the gestational period is considered the embryonic period, after which the developing human being is considered a fetus. At any point in this prenatal development, during the birth process (perinatal period) or during the neonatal and postnatal periods, development may diverge from normal, generating a developmental dilemma. The causes of these dilemmas can be many or even unknown. Pregnant females are encouraged to abstain from smoking, consuming alcohol, and taking any form of

medication or drugs without their physician's knowledge and consent and to prevent any situation that may expose the developing fetus to toxic substances. Pregnant females should also consult their physician regarding herbal medication and other foods to avoid eating during pregnancy, such as uncooked shellfish and fish, which contain high levels of mercury. Any type of uncooked meat and eggs has the potential to expose the pregnant female to bacterial food poisoning and should be avoided.

Congenital Anomalies

Congenital anomalies can be physical, mental, or both and can vary in severity. They are present at birth but might not be detected until later in infancy or childhood. The limbs or organs may be malformed, duplicated, or entirely absent. Organs sometimes fail to move to their proper location or

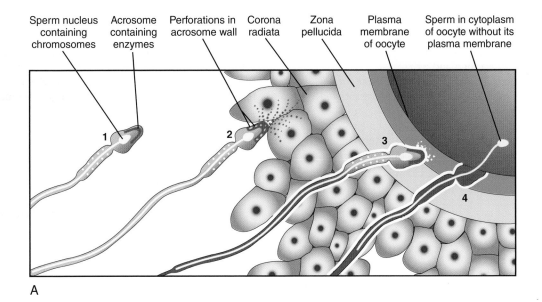

• **Fig. 2.1** (A) Acrosome reaction and sperm penetration of an oocyte. *1,* Sperm during capacitation. *2,* Sperm undergoing the acrosome reaction. *3,* Sperm forming a path through the zona pellucida. *4,* Sperm entering the cytoplasm of the oocyte.

• **Fig. 2.1, cont'd** (B) Normal prenatal development can be divided into several stages. (A, From Moore KL, et al: *Before we are born: essentials of embryology and birth defects*, ed 8, St. Louis, 2013, Saunders; B, From Damjanov I: *Pathology for the health professions*, ed 4, St. Louis, 2011, Saunders.)

fail to open or close at the right time. Anomalies are seldom isolated and are likely to occur in multiple forms and/or organs or organ tissues. One example is amniotic band syndrome which results when there is a sheet or band of amnion tissue loose in the uterus. This can become a wound around the fetus or extremities. The bands can constrict blood flow and growth, resulting in amputation or physical deformity depending on the developmental stage, and obstruction of blood flow.

The causes and risk factors of congenital defects may be genetic or unknown. Environmental, socioeconomic, and demographic factors can also contribute to anomalies. Nongenetic causes include infection in the mother, drugs taken by the mother, the age of the mother, radiographic examination made early in pregnancy, or injury to the pregnant female or the fetus. The cause often is unknown. However, prenatal care and advanced surgical techniques have greatly improved the management of anomalies that are compatible with life. Parents may face emotional and physical challenges and rely on support from the medical community. A team approach is ideal, including medical assessment by physicians and appropriate therapy for the child, as well as family involvement and participation in a support group for the parents. Support groups are also available online, which can be of benefit to caregivers who do not have a local in-person support group. Health care workers are important navigators in assisting those individuals caring for patients with congenital conditions.

Genetic Disorders and Syndromes

Genetic syndromes are a form of congenital anomaly. Genetic information is contained in microscopic threadlike structures in the nucleus of human body cells. The genetic material contained within the genes is responsible for inheritance traits. Each normal cell within the human body contains 46 chromosomes arranged in 23 pairs. Twenty-two pairs of the chromosomes are termed *homologous pairs*, and the remaining pair comprises the sex chromosomes.

Genetic disorders and syndromes are the result of an abnormal gene taking up residence on one of the 22 pairs of nonsex chromosomes. The 22 pairs of homologous pairs are also identified as autosomes. When the abnormal gene that causes the condition is on one of the 22 pairs of autosomes, the condition is termed an *autosomal inherited condition*.

Some of the autosomal inherited conditions have a dominant pattern of inheritance; other conditions may be the result of autosomal recessive traits. Dominant inheritance occurs when only one gene of the pair has the ability to produce symptoms, thus making it dominant over the normal gene. The parent who carries the abnormal gene has a 50% chance of transmitting the defective gene to each of their offspring. When the condition is considered autosomal recessive inheritance, the parent's abnormal genetic makeup must have genetic errors on both of the genes of the pair, resulting in the carrier usually having no symptoms of the disorder. The autosomal recessive disorder has a 25% chance of surfacing when two carrier parents conceive a child. The child could be affected by the autosomal inherited condition when the pair of affected genes is present.

Methods of Prenatal Diagnosis

Congenital anomalies in a fetus can be diagnosed by taking a fluid sample from the amniotic sac between the 14th and 20th weeks of pregnancy. This procedure, known as **amniocentesis**, allows amniotic fluid to be tested and cells to be microscopically examined for abnormal substances or chromosomal abnormalities. An example of an abnormal substance is an elevated alpha-fetoprotein (AFP) level. Amniocentesis is not without risk to the mother and the baby.

Abnormalities of the spine, skull, and many organs, such as the heart and kidneys, may be discovered during ultrasound studies of the fetus which is usually performed at 19 to 21 weeks of gestational age. An alternative procedure called *chorionic villus biopsy* or chorionic villus sampling (CVS) can be performed as early as 10 weeks of pregnancy but is usually performed during the 11th and 14th week. This procedure also has risks which will be discussed thoroughly with the mother. Two methods of specimen collection may be used. The transabdominal method involves the insertion of a needle into the uterus by going through the abdomen. The transcervical method involves catheter insertion through the cervix and removal of a tissue sample from the placenta. Potential complications include bleeding, cramping, leaking of amniotic fluid, infection, miscarriage, preterm labor, and limb defects. The risk for limb defects, although rare, is higher if the CVS is performed before 9 weeks of gestation.

Many, but not all, congenital disorders can be detected through prenatal diagnosis (Fig. 2.2). The diagnosis of potential genetic or neural tube deficit disorders may

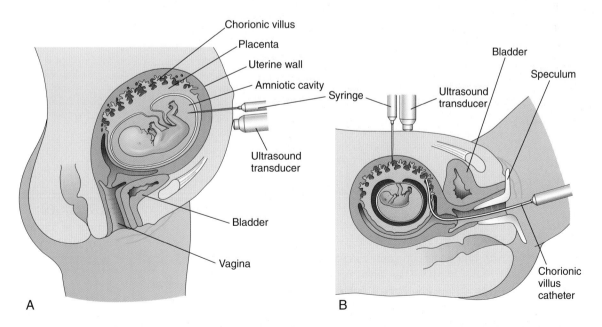

• **Fig. 2.2** (A) Illustration of amniocentesis. A needle is inserted through the lower abdominal and uterine walls into the amniotic cavity. A syringe is attached, and amniotic fluid is withdrawn for diagnostic purposes. (B) Drawing illustrating chorionic villus sampling. Two sampling approaches are illustrated: through the maternal anterior abdominal wall with a needle dend through the vagina and cervical canal using a malleable catheter. A speculum is an instrument for exposing the vagina. (From Moore KL, et al: *The developing human, 11e-South Asia edition: clinically oriented embryology*, ed 11, 2020, Elsevier.)

❖ **ENRICHMENT**

Conjoined Twins

During the conception process, the fertilized egg (the embryo) may divide, creating identical twins. Conjoined twins result when the separation process of identical twins fails to complete before the 13th day after fertilization resulting in fused twins in utero. As with identical twins, the embryo originates from a single fertilized ovum and occupies one placenta. For an unidentifiable reason, however, the normal separation of the embryo into twins stops before completion, resulting in a partially separated embryo that continues to mature into conjoined fetuses. Conjoined twins occur more often in female embryos than in male embryos and result in two fetuses that are joined at some point on their bodies. Conjoined twins can be diagnosed during prenatal ultrasound, and some conjoined twins are born alive as a result of specific prenatal diagnosis and surgical intervention to facilitate the delivery (Fig. 2.3A).

Conjoined twins may be joined at different locations of the body and may share various organs. The attachment to each other may involve a small portion of tissue or may be as extensive as fusion at the head or sharing of an organ or body part. Common types or variations are usually categorized by the location and involvement of the junction through the term pagus, meaning fastened, included in the classification terminology.

Twins with a cranial union are called *craniopagus twins*. Those with anterior junctions at the thorax or chest, often sharing the heart and vital portions of the chest wall and internal organs, are called *thoracopagus conjoined twins*. *Thoracopagus* is the most common form of conjoined twins. The term *thoraco-omphalopagus* refers to twins joined at the abdomen and thorax. The term *pygopagus twins* describes those joined at the sacrum and perineum. Twins attached at the pelvic region, either face to face or back to back, is termed *ischiopagus* (see Fig. 2.3B). When the connection proceeds from the breastbone to the waist, the term *omphalopagus* describes the junction. A very rare form, *dicephalus*, is the condition in which the individual has one body and two separate heads and necks. Conjoined twins that are joined along the spine, back to back are called *rachipagus*. Cephalopagus twins are joined from the umbilicus to the head. Parasitic twins are referred to as *heteropagus*.

Modern technology and medical advances have helped physicians and surgical teams to successfully separate some of these twins. In some separation procedures, one or both of the children have died during or shortly after the surgery. The children and their families require emotional support and education about the possible outcomes of the condition.

• **Fig. 2.3** (A) Conjoined twins at 12 weeks of development. (B) Photo of ischipagus conjoined twins at the age of 2 months (1983. Pécs, Hungary). (A, From Moore KL, Persaud TVN, Shiota K: *Color atlas of clinical embryology*, ed 2, Philadelphia, 2000, Saunders; Courtesy Dr. D.K. Kalousek, Department of Pathology, University of British Columbia, Children's Hospital, Vancouver, British Columbia, Canada; B, From Tarnoki A, et al: *Twin Research for Everyone*, ed 1, 2022, Elsevier.)

provide future parents with time to obtain counseling and to prepare for the many health needs of the infant before the child's birth. When the testing indicates a potential abnormality, the delivery and nursery staff are provided with the opportunity to prepare for the delivery. There are also times when births are planned to occur in a specific city where medical teams are better equipped to handle the infants' needs if the needed medical resources are not available locally.

Prematurity

Preterm Birth or Prematurity

Description

Preterm birth, or prematurity, is the result of birth before the 37th gestational week. The condition of prematurity describes the birth of a low-weight, underdeveloped, and short-gestation infant and is considered the leading cause of death during the neonatal period. These high-risk infants are born with incomplete development of organ systems. Compared with full-term infants, these infants are at a greater risk for developing serious health problems such as digestive problems, lung or breathing problems, and bleeding within the brain.

ICD-10-CM Code   P07.00 *(Extremely low birth weight newborn, unspecified weight)*
(P07.00–P07.03 = 4 codes of specificity)
P07.10 *(Other low birth weight newborn, unspecified weight)*
(P07.10–P07.18 = 6 codes of specificity)

ICD-10-CM Code   P07.00 *(Extremely low birth weight newborn, unspecified weight)*
(P07.00–P07.03 = 4 codes of specificity)
P07.10 *(Other low birth weight newborn, unspecified weight)*
(P07.10–P07.18 = 6 codes of specificity)

Weeks of Gestation

ICD-10-CM Code   P07.20 *(Extreme immaturity of newborn, unspecified weeks)*
(P07.20–P07.26 = 7 codes of specificity)
P07.3 *(Preterm newborn, other, unspecified weeks of gestation)*
(P07.31–P07.39 = 9 codes of specificity)
P07.21 *(Extreme immaturity of newborn, gestational age less than 23 completed weeks)*
P07.22 *(Extreme immaturity of newborn, gestational age 23 completed weeks)*
P07.23 *(Extreme immaturity of newborn, gestational age 24 completed weeks)*
P07.24 *(Extreme immaturity of newborn, gestational age 25 completed weeks)*
P07.25 *(Extreme immaturity of newborn, gestational age 26 completed weeks)*
P07.26 *(Extreme immaturity of newborn, gestational age 27 completed weeks)*
P07.31 *(Preterm newborn, gestational age 28 completed weeks)*
P07.32 *(Preterm newborn, gestational age 29 completed weeks)*
P07.33 *(Preterm newborn, gestational age 30 completed weeks)*
P07.34 *(Preterm newborn, gestational age 31 completed weeks)*
P07.35 *(Preterm newborn, gestational age 32 completed weeks)*
P07.36 *(Preterm newborn, gestational age 33 completed weeks)*
P07.37 *(Preterm newborn, gestational age 34 completed weeks)*
P07.38 *(Preterm newborn, gestational age 35 completed weeks)*
P07.39 *(Preterm newborn, gestational age 36 completed weeks)*
P07.30 *(Preterm newborn, unspecified weeks)*

Symptoms and Signs

Premature babies may weigh as low as 12 ounces or less at the time of birth. Their physical development is at various stages, depending on the length of gestational time. The smaller of these infants have little subcutaneous fat, palms and soles with few creases, possible undescended testes in males, and a prominent clitoris in females. Many of these very tiny and immature babies lack the ability to suck or swallow or have weakened sucking or swallowing reflexes. The lungs are often underdeveloped, leading to respiratory dangers. The immature neurologic system can lead to some difficulties in the maintenance of body temperature, problems in controlling cardiac function, and spontaneous episodes of apnea or may result in seizure activity. An immature immune system increases the risk of infection.

Patient Screening

Pregnant patients who contact the physician to say they may be in labor require prompt attention. When the pregnant patient thinks she is in labor more than 3 weeks before her due date, she must be assessed as quickly as possible. Many physicians prefer that these patients go directly to the hospital where the delivery is planned to take place. Others prefer to see the patient in the office as soon as possible.

Etiology

There are many reasons that premature infants enter the world before reaching the traditionally accepted gestational age of 40 weeks and thus have very low birth weights. Causes of premature labor resulting in a premature infant are an

Uterus having a single horn (unicornuate) and only one fallopian tube

Single uterus with a midline septum

Uterus having two horns (bicornuate) with an indentation at the top

Double uterus with one vagina

Double uterus and vagina

• **Fig. 2.4** Types of uterine malformations that can cause infertility or repeated pregnancy loss. (From McKinney E, et al: *Maternal-Child Nursing*, ed 6, 2022, Elsevier.)

• **Fig. 2.5** Infant in neonatal intensive care unit born at 28 weeks, weighing 2 lb 6 oz. (Courtesy Kim and LilliAnna Kervin.)

incompetent cervix; **bicornuate** uterus (Fig. 2.4); toxic conditions; maternal infection; trauma; premature rupture of the amniotic membranes; history of previous miscarriages; multiple gestations; intrauterine fetal delayed growth; and other physical conditions of the mother, such as pregnancy-induced or chronic hypertension. Diabetes, heart disease, kidney disease, poor nutrition, substance abuse, and lack of prenatal care also contribute to the incidence of the mother giving birth to a preterm infant. In some cases, the etiology is never identified. Attempts may be made to halt premature labor by having the mother on complete bed rest or using drug therapy to slow or halt contractions. The mother is often given a short course of steroids to aid fetal lung maturation.

Diagnosis

Diagnostic criteria include a gestational age of less than 37 weeks. **Neonates** diagnosed as small for gestational age are low-weight infants (<5 lb 8 oz) that may or may not be premature.

Treatment

Treatment varies, depending on the gestational age, weight, present or subsequent conditions, anomalies, and nutritional status. Intravenous (IV) fluids and hyperalimentation are necessary to encourage the growth and development of the premature infant. Airway management and pulmonary functioning are monitored very closely. Many of the smallest babies are intubated endotracheally, and respiration is maintained by mechanical ventilation. Recent advances in respiratory care for tiny premature infants permit extubation

of the infant and maintenance of the airway by continuous positive airway pressure (CPAP) through the nose. Pulse oximeters constantly monitor oxygen (O_2) saturation levels and heart rate. Body temperature is monitored closely and maintained at normal levels (Fig. 2.5). When infection is a risk caused by maternal prenatal infection or extended time of ruptured amniotic sac, close monitoring is required for the onset of any symptoms of infection, and antibiotics are often started presumptively. When early signs of infection occur, aggressive treatment is introduced. Monitoring of blood glucose, blood pressure, and body temperature is performed on a frequent and regular basis, and any treatment necessary is instituted to maintain optimal levels.

Comfort measures include placing an article with the mother's scent in the crib with the infant. These tiny babies are also swaddled to simulate the closeness and feeling of the womb. Lights are kept at a dim level, and harsh auditory stimuli are kept at a minimum.

Prognosis

Advances in technology have made the survival of low-weight and short-gestation infants possible. The prognosis for these children varies, depending on gestational age, weight, and the occurrence of anomalies and developmental deficits. There are documented cases of a 7.48-ounce and/or 21 to 22 gestational-week babies surviving. They fall into the 1% of premature babies born at that weight and gestational age. Because they are born before the normal prenatal development is complete, these children often have many problems to overcome (Fig. 2.6).

One of the primary risks is cerebral bleeding, which may occur during the labor and delivery process or may result from handling after delivery. The cerebral bleeding may cause the development of CP, mental functioning deficiencies, or other neurologic conditions.

Another major concern is the underdevelopment of the pulmonary system, including the lung tissue and the airway. Some pulmonary conditions these infants experience

• **Fig. 2.6** Four-day-old premature infant. Weight is 14.6 oz, and gestational age is 22 weeks.

• **Fig. 2.7** (A) Same premature infant from Fig. 2.5 at age 9 months; weight 11 lb 8 oz. (B) Same infant at age 10 months, weight 13 lb. (Courtesy David L. Frazier, 1999.)

are infant respiratory distress syndrome (IRDS), broncho-pulmonary dysplasia (BPD), laryngomalacia, tracheomalacia, and bronchomalacia. Lack of body fat can affect the maintenance of body temperature. Any stress or increased or high supplemental O_2 flow may be responsible for retinopathy of prematurity (ROP) and possible blindness. Necrotizing enterocolitis (NEC) is a danger to the digestive system because of the reduced tolerance of the alimentary tract. Atrial septal defect (ASD) and patent ductus arteriosus (PDA) often are present because the fetal circulatory system has failed to mature.

The generally accepted gestational age for 50% of infants to survive the birth process and perinatal period is 24 weeks, with a greater percentage of infants surviving as gestational age increases. Improvements in technology are making it possible for more and more of these tiniest infants to survive (Fig. 2.7).

Prevention

Preventing prematurity requires good prenatal care, adequate nutrition, and assessment of the pregnant patient's risk factors for premature labor. Abstaining from consuming any alcohol and smoking cigarettes helps reduce the risk of premature birth and/or low birth weight. Additionally, bed rest of the expectant mother may delay the onset of premature labor and create more time for the fetus to develop. Drug therapy may be used in an attempt to stop premature labor that results in premature birth (see Chapter 12).

Patient Teaching

Encouraging pregnant females to obtain prenatal care and follow guidelines is important. Pregnant females should be instructed to contact their physicians at the first sign of labor, especially labor before the 37th week of gestation.

Parents should be educated regarding potential problems or symptoms to watch for when the infant is released from the hospital.

Infant Respiratory Distress Syndrome

Description

IRDS, or hyaline membrane disease, is similar to adult respiratory distress syndrome in that the patient suffers acute hypoxemia caused by infiltrates within the alveoli. This is one of the most common problems in premature infants.

ICD-10-CM Code	P22.0 *(Respiratory distress syndrome of newborn)* *(P22.0-P22.9 = 4 codes of specificity)*

Symptoms and Signs

Shortly after birth, the neonate exhibits signs of respiratory distress, including nasal flaring, grunting respirations, and sternal retractions. Blood gas studies indicate reduced oxygen tension and ineffective gas exchange. The infant becomes cyanotic with mottled skin. The symptoms get worse over the first two to three days and then begin to improve with appropriate treatment.

Patient Screening

The infant is hospitalized, usually in a neonatal intensive care unit (NICU). The NICU staff observes the infant for signs of respiratory distress, and immediate intervention is instituted at the first signs of distress.

Etiology

The neonate's lungs lack the surfactant needed to allow the alveoli to expand. The surfactant is normally produced relatively late in fetal life; consequently, premature infants are at risk. The outcome of this inability of the lungs to expand is an inadequate surface area for proper gas exchange and a potentially fatal lack of oxygen in the blood.

Diagnosis

The first indications of IRDS are increased respiratory efforts of the newborn and a history of prematurity. Blood gas studies demonstrate the reduced potential for adequate gas exchange. Radiographic chest films indicate the presence of the infiltrate or hyaline membrane.

Treatment

Treatment consists of the administration of carefully titrated supplemental oxygen, usually administered by mechanical ventilation and positive end-expiratory pressure, and is of primary importance. Drug therapy, including the administration of an exogenous surfactant, such as beractant (Survanta) or poractant alfa (Curosurf), into the pulmonary tree via an endotracheal tube as soon as possible after birth helps provide an artificial surfactant, allowing the alveoli to expand. This treatment should begin within the first 8 hours of life and be repeated once or twice if needed, until the alveoli are expanded.

Prognosis

The infant survival rate has increased throughout the years due to advancements in drug and respiratory therapies.

Prevention

Prevention is the best treatment; therefore if time permits, the mother is injected with a corticosteroid (betamethasone [Celestone Soluspan]) 24 hours before delivery in an attempt to mature the surfactant-synthesizing system.

Patient Teaching

Online and written medical resources are helpful for parents and caregivers. The information should be provided and available in the parents' native language. Allow the parents to verbalize their anxieties and fears to a compassionate and understanding individual to validate their feelings regarding the situation. Some parents may benefit from support groups.

Unfortunately, the occurrence of IRDS, along with its treatment modalities, often predisposes premature infants to the development of BPD.

Bronchopulmonary Dysplasia

Description

BPD is a serious lung disease that develops or occurs after another breathing condition. It may be a sequela to IRDS, a lung infection, or extreme prematurity. The lungs are stiff, obstructed, and hard to ventilate.

ICD-10-CM Code	P27.0 *(Wilson-Mikity syndrome)*
	(P27.0-P27.9 = 4 codes of specificity)
	P27.1 *(Bronchopulmonary dysplasia originating in the perinatal period)*
	P27.8 *(Other chronic respiratory diseases originating in the perinatal period)*

Symptoms and Signs

The infant experiences periods of dyspnea, including tachypnea, wheezing, cyanosis, nasal flaring, and sternal retractions. O_2 saturation decreases, as does heart rate. The infant may experience coughing and difficulty feeding. These babies appear to be working very hard to breathe, and they exhibit poor posture of the neck, shoulders, and upper body. Wet or crackling sounds are heard on auscultation of the lungs with a stethoscope.

Patient Screening

The infant is hospitalized, usually in a NICU. The NICU staff observes the infant for signs of respiratory distress, and immediate intervention is instituted at the first signs of distress.

Etiology

BPD occurs in many premature infants after IRDS, mechanical ventilation with supplemental oxygen, and infection or pneumonia. The pressure and oxygen needed to maintain life-sustaining oxygen levels can damage soft and fragile lung tissue, causing overinflation or scarring.

Diagnosis

Observation of the infant reveals early respiratory distress. Radiographs of the chest are abnormal, indicating alveolar damage, either scarring or overinflation, sometimes described as a "ground-glass" appearance. Arterial blood gas (ABG) levels indicate a problem. Oxygen levels in the lungs may be low, and carbon dioxide (CO_2) levels may be high.

Treatment

A pediatric pulmonologist should be consulted to ensure the best individual treatment plan is developed based on the infant's needs. The goal of treatment is the replacement of the damaged alveoli. Children grow new alveoli until about 8 years of age. Infants who have BPD need to grow new alveoli to replace those damaged by scarring. As this replacement occurs, the severity of the condition lessens. Supportive treatment includes supplemental oxygen and adequate nutritional support. Medications such as diuretics, bronchodilators, corticosteroids, and theophylline can be used to treat BPD.

Supplemental O_2 therapy may be needed for several weeks, occasionally for more than 1 year. This therapy is usually given via a nasal cannula; however, if the infant has a tracheostomy, it may be delivered via the tracheostomy collar or via CPAP. O_2 saturation levels must be monitored with a pulse oximeter so that they can be maintained at 90% or greater. The pulse oximeter also monitors heart rate. As the infant grows and matures, blood oxygen saturation levels may be maintained on room air, usually by the age of 1 year.

Diuretics help reduce fluid accumulation in the lungs and reduce the incidence of pulmonary hypertension and right-sided heart failure. Bronchodilators are administered to reverse the narrowing of the bronchi resulting from inflammation or bronchospasm, thus allowing more oxygen to reach the lung tissue. These drugs may be administered orally as syrups or via aerosol inhalation. Antiinflammatory drugs help prevent the inflammatory process from becoming severe.

Adequate nutrition is needed for the infant's growth and to meet the increased caloric demand resulting from difficult breathing. High-calorie formulas are used. The infant must be held with the head raised slightly and frequently given the formula given in small amounts to prevent gastroesophageal reflux disease (GERD). Some infants are given medications to prevent GERD and other medications, such as antacids or histamine-2 blockers, to reduce gastric acid.

Prognosis

A prognosis is good with early and aggressive intervention, prudent monitoring, and maintenance of adequate O_2 saturation levels and heart rate. The resolution of the condition is slow, and improvement is gradual. Complications include pulmonary edema and hypertension, right-sided heart failure (cor pulmonale), respiratory infections, apnea, tracheomalacia, asthma, GI reflux, and aspiration. These children are particularly susceptible to respiratory infections, such as bronchiolitis caused by the respiratory syncytial virus (RSV). They may experience poor growth or delayed development. Some children outgrow the condition, but others may be susceptible to respiratory distress for life. Apneic periods and low oxygen saturation levels for an extended period may cause hypoxia of the brain, which may result in developmental deficits. Some infants may not survive.

Prevention

There is currently no way to prevent BPD, but since premature infants are at the highest risk, trying to prevent early labor in pregnant females is a step toward preventing the development of BPD. Early weaning from mechanical respiratory support may reduce its incidence in premature infants. Early and aggressive intervention and treatment may prevent complications and permanent conditions, even death.

Patient Teaching

Help parents find community support groups and agencies to help deal with emotional and financial stressors, and there are also online support groups. Parents should be encouraged to become as involved as possible in the care of their infant, helping them become familiar with the infant's health care needs and promoting bonding with the infant.

Retinopathy of Prematurity

Description

ROP, or retrolental fibroplasia, is an abnormal growth of blood vessels in the retinas of the infant's eyes. The condition occurs in the eyes of premature infants.

ICD-10-CM Code	H35.179 *(Retrolental fibroplasia, unspecified eye)* (H35.171-H35.179 = 4 codes of specificity)

Symptoms and Signs

ROP occurs most often in infants born before 28 weeks of gestation. There are no visible symptoms. Screening examinations are performed routinely on premature infants weighing less than 1500 g or at a gestational age of less than 30 weeks. The entire retina is visualized to determine the stages of development of the blood vessels supplying it. These examinations are first performed when the infant is 4 to 6 weeks old (Fig. 2.8).

• **Fig. 2.8** Advanced retinopathy of prematurity (retrolental fibroplasia). (From Yanoff M, et al: Ophthalmology, ed 5, 2019, Elsevier.)

Patient Screening

An ophthalmologist performs routine examinations of the retina.

Etiology

The vascularization of the retina begins at the back central part of the eye, as vessels grow out toward the edges. The blood vessels to the retina do not begin development until about the 28th week of gestation. In premature infants, this vascularization is incomplete. Regardless of gestational age at birth, most ROP originates 34 to 40 weeks after conception.

No specific risk factors for the development of ROP have been identified. Therefore there is a group of risk factors that contribute to it. The more premature and the lower the birth weight of the infant, the greater the risk of ROP. High supplemental oxygen concentrations are responsible for many incidents of ROP. Therefore close monitoring of oxygen saturation levels and appropriate adjustment and titration of oxygen concentration levels in the infant reduces the risk. Certain drugs, such as surfactant and indomethacin, administered to the neonate for the treatment of immature lungs, as well as PDA, may increase the risk for the premature infant.

Diagnosis

A diagnosis is made by an ophthalmologist using an indirect ophthalmoscope and scleral depression to visualize the retina. The lens and iris are also examined at this time.

Treatment

Most mild forms of ROP resolve without treatment. Laser treatment of the area anterior to the vascular shunt eliminates abnormal vessels before they deposit enough scar tissue to cause retinal detachment. Severe cases may require other procedures.

Prognosis

Blindness may result from serious damage. ROP that has been resolved can have later complications. These include crossed or wandering eyes (strabismus), "lazy eye" (amblyopia), nearsightedness (myopia), glaucoma, and late-onset retinal detachment. Corrective glasses may be needed. A partially or completely detached retina may occur in the most serious cases. Prompt intervention may result in the repair of the detachment and prevention of blindness.

Prevention

There is no way to prevent ROP in premature infants. Close monitoring and titration of oxygen concentrations have reduced the incidence of the condition. NICUs now protect premature infants' eyes from excessive exposure to artificial lighting. Attempts are made to avoid exposing premature infants to stress factors.

Patient Teaching

Parents should be informed of the risk of this condition in premature infants. Either printed or digital resources with accurate information should be shared with caregivers. Online support groups may also be available when communities do not have local groups that meet in person where the family lives. Encourage follow-up eye examinations for infants as prescribed by the ophthalmologist.

Necrotizing Enterocolitis

Description

NEC is an acute inflammatory process caused by ischemic necrosis or death of the mucosal lining of the small intestine, the large intestine, or both. It is a condition of premature infants or sick neonates that develops after birth when the fragile intestinal tract of the premature or compromised newborn becomes active.

ICD-10-CM Code	P77.9 (Necrotizing enterocolitis in newborn, unspecified) (P77.1, Stage 1; P77.2, Stage 2; P77.3, Stage 3 = 4 codes of specificity)

Symptoms and Signs

Feeding intolerance, abdominal distention, bile-colored emesis, diarrhea, blood in the stool, decreased or absent bowel sounds, lethargy, and body temperature instability a few days after birth are some of the initial symptoms exhibited by the preterm or low birth weight infant. The state of well-being declines as these infants experience respiratory problems related to brief apneic periods, reduced urine output, hyperbilirubinemia, and erythema. The abdomen is tender to palpation (Fig. 2.9).

Patient Screening

The infant is hospitalized, usually in the NICU. The NICU staff observes the infant for signs of NEC, and the

• **Fig. 2.9** A Preterm neonate with severe necrotizing enterocolitis and intestinal necrosis. (A) Abdominal discoloration consistent with dead bowel. (B) Necrotizing enterocolitis with a segment of dead bowel (top) and evidence of free stool in the abdomen (*arrow*). These infants often have bowel perforation and hemorrhage from the bowel or liver. They can have severe hypotension requiring vasopressor support and enormous volume requirements. Moreover, because of hemorrhage and disseminated intravascular coagulopathy, these infants will generally require transfusions of blood, platelets, and fresh frozen plasma. Some practitioners also advocate administration of vitamin K. (Courtesy Dr. Daniel P. Doody.)

neonatologist is notified of any signs of distress so that immediate intervention can be instituted.

Etiology

The etiology of NEC is not fully understood; however, it is thought to be a breakdown in the normal defense systems of the GI tract, allowing the *normal flora* of the GI tract to invade the intestinal mucosa. This can happen when there is poor circulation to the GI tract, resulting in convulsive vaso-constriction of the mesenteric vessels and diminished blood supply, interfering with the normal production of protective mucus. In simple terms, portions of the intestines do not get oxygen and will die. In addition to prematurity, factors that may predispose infants to NEC include an inability to digest food and a failure to keep dangerous bacteria out.

Diagnosis

Observation of changes in the infant's feeding patterns or activity level, impaired body temperature maintenance, and respiratory difficulties, along with abdominal distention and tenderness, call for further investigation. A complete blood count (CBC) indicates an elevated white blood cell (WBC) count, and guaiac test results of stool specimens for occult blood are positive. Blood and stool cultures are performed, and radiography of the intestine confirms the condition.

Treatment

Aggressive and immediate intervention is necessary if the infant has to survive. Feedings are stopped, making the infant's status NPO (nothing by mouth). A small tube is inserted into the stomach through the nose or mouth for decompression. Fluids are administered IV, as are antibiot-ics. Respiratory status and pH are monitored by measur-ing ABGs. The infant's weight and intake and output are monitored closely, and fluid and electrolyte balance are maintained. Abdominal distention is monitored through frequent measurements of the abdomen by a tape measure. Radiographic monitoring of the intestinal tract is also per-formed. Complications of intestinal perforation or perito-nitis require surgical intervention with the removal of the necrotic tissue. An ileostomy or colostomy may be necessary until the infant grows, and closure with anastomosis can be performed.

Prognosis

The survival rate for NEC is better than in years past due to immediate and aggressive intervention; however, it is still a serious complication of prematurity, and some babies die even with aggressive treatment. Resection of a portion of the bowel can lead to an obstruction of the bowel or malabsorp-tion syndrome. Perforation of the bowel can lead to sepsis and death due to the bacteria from the colon being released into the abdomen.

Prevention

Most of these babies are still in the hospital when NEC develops. Prudent nursing observations and reporting of any symptoms of NEC are essential. Infections that cause NEC may be transmitted from one infant to another, so strict infection control procedures will be necessary. Breast milk appears to offer some protection from this condition. Awareness of the high-risk infant is fundamental to the pre-vention and early intervention of this disease.

Patient Teaching

Parents require emotional support along with informa-tion about the condition. Meticulous hand washing should be emphasized, and the dangers of infection should be explained to the parents.

Cri-du-Chat Syndrome (Cat's Cry Syndrome, 5p-syndrome)

The deletion of genetic material from the small p arm of chromosome 5 results in the condition called *cri-du-chat*. The majority of infants born with this rare disorder will die during the first month of life. "Cat's cry" syndrome usually results in stillborn children or those who die shortly after birth. Those who survive the perinatal and neonatal periods may progress to maturity. These individuals may have various medical and mental problems.

Infants with cri-du-chat syndrome have an abnormally small head (microcephaly), with a deficiency of cerebral brain tissue, and usually experience some level of intellectual developmental disorder. Those who are born alive have a weak, mewing, catlike cry. The orbits of the eyes are spaced far apart. Surviving children usually experience slow growth patterns, a small head, and poor muscle tone. Development of motor and language skill may be delayed. Mental development may be slow, and behavioral problems may develop. Cri-du-chat syndrome is a hereditary condition and the result of a chromosomal aberration caused by the deletion of part of the short arm of chromosome 5 of the B group. A genetic study indicating the chromosomal defect confirms the diagnosis.

Parents' awareness of the condition usually occurs when the child is born. Generally, parents are anxious to discuss why the syndrome is present in the child and the possibility of subsequent children also having the same syndrome. Discussions should take place as soon as possible. Should the child survive and be in the home environment, the child should be seen immediately for any problems that arise.

Because there is no cure, treatment supports body functions as long as the infant survives. Many fetuses with this chromosomal aberration die in utero. Those infants who survive and progress into childhood need support from educational systems and other resources. These individuals can possibly experience a normal life span.

There is no cure for this hereditary condition. Parents are encouraged to contact support groups for rare genetic disorders (Fig. 2.10).

• **Fig. 2.10** Facial view of a 2-year-old boy with cri-du-chat syndrome. (From Turnpenny PD, et al: *Emery's elements of medical genetics and genomics*, ed 16, 2022, Elsevier.)

Genetic Syndromes and Conditions

Hypertrophic Cardiomyopathy

Description

Hypertrophic cardiomyopathy (HCM), a congenital disorder, occurs when a portion of the heart muscle thickens, changing the heart's ability to function appropriately. A change in the heart's electrical system may also take place, resulting in sudden cardiac death in young athletes or other active young adults who appear to be healthy.

ICD-10-CM Code	I42.2 *(Other hypertrophic cardiomyopathy)*
	(I42.0-I42.9 = 10 codes of specificity for cardiomyopathy)
	I42.5 *(Other restrictive cardiomyopathy)*
	I42.8 *(Other cardiomyopathies)*

Symptoms and Signs

Tragically, the first sign is the collapse of a seemingly healthy young athlete during a strenuous sporting event or other period of stressful exercise. This collapse can be followed by a cardiac arrest caused by cardiac arrhythmia. Many people with this condition have no symptoms until they collapse. It should also be noted that death can occur when the patient is resting or performing light exercise. It is possible that some individuals experience no symptoms. Signs may be discovered during a physical examination. Symptoms may include chest pain, syncope, hypertension, palpitations, or shortness of breath. Some report experiencing fatigue, shortness of breath when lying down, or reduced tolerance of activity.

Etiology

A portion of the myocardium becomes thickened without any obvious cause. The normal alignment of the myocardial cells is disturbed (myocardial disarray), resulting in disruption of cardiac electrical impulses. Children with a parent who has this condition have a 50% chance of a mutation of a gene, which results in hypertrophic cardiomyopathy.

Diagnosis

The diagnosis of young people who had a sudden cardiac arrest is made during an autopsy. Before a collapse, the condition may be diagnosed with an investigation of a report involving any of the following symptoms: a drop in blood pressure may be noted during exercise; the person has a family history of cardiac arrest or sudden death at a young age, along with a history of the individual experiencing palpitations or unexplained syncope; and the presence of life-threatening arrhythmias.

Electrocardiography may indicate the presence of hypertrophy. Echocardiography, radiography, or cardiac magnetic resonance imaging (MRI) may also indicate the thickness of areas of the myocardium (Fig. 2.11). A genetic test can be done to look for any of the known mutations leading to HCM.

Treatment

When arrhythmias are present, medications, including beta-blockers and calcium channel blockers, may be prescribed. Some patients may require the implantation of a pacemaker or implantable cardioverter-defibrillator. Should the thickening obstruct the flow of blood, a surgical myectomy may be performed. Patients should avoid strenuous exercise and stressful situations.

Prognosis

Young people with HCM are at a high risk for sudden cardiac death. The prognosis of the young person who has collapsed is very guarded because most do not respond to immediate cardiac resuscitation. Those who are diagnosed before a catastrophic event and who can follow medical guidelines, such as avoiding strenuous exercise, have a fair outlook. Some may not experience symptoms and may live a normal life span.

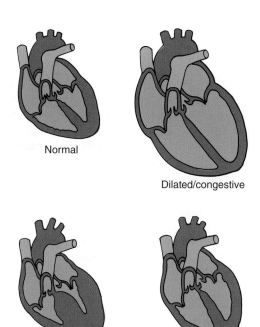

Normal

Dilated/congestive

Hypertrophic

Restrictive

• **Fig. 2.11** Drawing of heart with cardiomyopathy. (From Black JM, Hawks JH: *Medical-surgical nursing: clinical management for positive outcomes*, ed 8, St. Louis, 2009, Saunders.)

Prevention

There is no prevention for this genetic disorder. Genetic counseling is advised for the individual and their relatives. Electrocardiography performed during a sports physical can help identify those who are at risk for HCM.

Patient Teaching

Patients who have been diagnosed with HCM should be encouraged to follow their physician's advice about avoiding strenuous exercise. They should continue follow-up care with their physician and be compliant regarding medications that have been prescribed.

Down Syndrome

Description

Down syndrome is a genetic syndrome in which the individual has an extra or partial chromosome instead of the usual 46. This results in a congenital form of mild-to-severe intellectual developmental disorder that is accompanied by characteristic facial features and distinctive physical abnormalities.

ICD-10-CM Code	R00.0 *(Tachycardia, unspecified)*

Symptoms and Signs

Down syndrome, in addition to being a mild-to-severe intellectual developmental disorder, is associated with heart defects and other congenital abnormalities. Typically, the infant has a small head with a flat back skull, a characteristic slant to the eyes, a flat nasal bridge, small low-set ears, a small mouth with a protruding tongue, and small, weak muscles. The hands are short, with stubby fingers and a deep horizontal crease across the palm (simian line). There is an exaggerated space between the big and little toes.

Patient Screening

Down syndrome is usually diagnosed prenatally via ultrasonography, blood tests, and/or amniocentesis or during the neonatal period. Patients are monitored closely through normal infant and childhood office visits. When the parent of a child with Down syndrome calls requesting an appointment, an assessment should be made depending on the complaint. Consider the anxiety level of the parent, and schedule an appointment for the next available time.

Etiology

Infants with Down syndrome have an extra or partial chromosome number 21 (**trisomy** 21). It occurs in 1 in 700 live births, and more often in infants born to females of 35 years old (Fig. 2.12).

Diagnosis

Infants with severe Down syndrome usually are identified at or before birth; milder forms are diagnosed later. The physical characteristics may be blatantly obvious. Findings on examination of the eyes may include the presence of small

• **Fig. 2.12** Down syndrome. These clinical photographs show several minor anomalies associated with this disorder. (A) Characteristic facial features with up-slanting palpebral fissures, epicanthal folds, and flat nasal bridge. (B) Brushfield spots. (C) Bridged palmar crease, seen in some affected infants. Two transverse palmar creases are connected by a diagonal line. (D) Wide space between first and second toes. (E) Short fifth finger. (F) Small ears and flat occiput. (G) Head-to-toe common characteristics of down syndrome. (H) Karyotype of a Down syndrome female patient showing trisomy 21. There is an extra copy of chromosome 21, in addition to the usual pair, for a total of three (tri-). (A–F, From McIntire S, et al: *Zitelli and Davis' atlas of pediatric physical diagnosis*, ed 8, 2023, Elsevier.)

white dots on the iris. A karyotype showing the chromosomal abnormality can confirm the diagnosis.

Treatment

Care for a child with Down syndrome depends on the severity of the physical defects and the degree of mental impairment. There is no known cure. The treatment plan is individualized and includes a multidimensional approach to maximize the development of motor and mental skills. Life expectancy has been improved through surgical correction of cardiac defects and antibiotic therapy for susceptibility to pulmonary disease.

Prognosis

There is no known cure for Down syndrome. Down syndrome may have an effect on an individual's learning style. Research shows the increase in life span compared to the life span of previous years, increases the chance of developing Alzheimer disease. The correlation between the two has been linked to a gene that is present on chromosome 21. Amyloid is produced by the gene and causes a disruption in the normal communication between brain cells. Amyloid has been identified in almost all patients over 40 years old who have Down syndrome, but not all patients who have increased amyloid buildup get Alzheimer disease.

Severe heart problems can also affect the prognosis of the patient, as approximately 50% of patients with Down syndrome are at a higher risk of early-onset dementia. The individual also may experience problems usually seen in the older population because they age quicker than those without Down syndrome.

Prevention
There is no prevention for this condition.

Patient Teaching
Help parents find and contact local or online support groups. Be available to answer parents' questions and to provide up-to-date information and resources.

Diseases of the Nervous System

Cerebral Palsy

Description
Cerebral palsy (CP) is the most common motor disability diagnosed in children and the most common crippling condition in children. It is a collection of disorders involving cerebral and nervous system functions that deal with movement, learning, hearing, sight, and thinking. This disorder may be congenital or acquired and may be bilateral or unilateral in the form of a nonprogressive paralysis that results from damage to the central nervous system (CNS).

ICD-10-CM Code	G80.9 *(Cerebral palsy, unspecified)*
	(G80.0-G80.9 = 7 codes of specificity)

Infantile CP is coded by type. Refer to the physician's diagnosis and then to the current editions of the ICD-9-CM and ICD-10-CM coding manuals to ensure the greatest specificity of pathology.

Symptoms and Signs
This syndrome affects primarily motor performance and might be noticed shortly after birth when the infant has difficulty with sucking or swallowing. The muscles may be floppy (like a rag doll) or stiff, with reduced voluntary movement. When the infant is lifted from behind, the legs may be difficult to separate, and the infant may cross its legs. There are three major types of CP:
- **Spastic CP** is characterized by hyperactive reflexes or rapid muscle contractions. The older child manifests the scissor gait by walking on the toes and crossing one foot over the other. This is the most common type of CP.
- **Athetoid CP** is characterized by involuntary muscle movements, especially during times of stress, and reduced muscle tone. The child has difficulty with speech.
- **Ataxic CP** is characterized by a lack of control over voluntary movements, poor balance, and a wide gait.

A patient may exhibit signs of all three types in varying degrees, from mild to severe. The symptoms tend to be more exaggerated as the child grows; however, they may be static (i.e., they neither get worse nor improve). Some patients have other related complications, including visual and auditory deficits, seizure activity, and intellectual developmental disorders.

Patient Screening
Most times, CP is suspected during routine well-baby or well-child visits. However, when a parent calls the office about previously mentioned symptoms, the child should be scheduled for an evaluation as soon as possible.

Etiology
CP usually stems from inadequate blood or oxygen supply to the brain during fetal development, during the birth process, or after birth. In the majority of patients, the brain insult occurs before an infant is 28 days old, while in very few cases, the damage occurs after that age. Most insults to the brain result from an interruption in the circulation of blood to the brain during labor and delivery and can also result from the mother having an infection during pregnancy. Research shows that the following factors also put one at higher risk for this syndrome. Low birth weight, prematurity, being one of the set of multiples (triplets, twins, etc.), being conceived by assisted reproductive technology, and when an infant has an excessive level of bilirubin in the blood that goes untreated.

Diagnosis
Diagnosis is made from screening for developmental delay, monitoring, and neurological tests, which include brain imaging tests and referrals to pediatric neurologists. The diagnosis is made based on the results of tests performed and screenings that help determine the degree of physical and mental impairment.

Treatment
There is no cure for CP. Early treatment helps the child reach optimal accomplishments. In mild or severe cases, the goal of treatment is to minimize the handicap by providing every possible therapeutic measure to help the child reach their potential. This takes a team effort involving the family or the caregiver and various medical specialists. Physical therapy, speech therapy, and special education may be required. Orthopedic intervention with casts, braces, and traction or surgery may be indicated. If the child experiences seizure activity, anticonvulsant agents are prescribed. Muscle relaxants help reduce spastic muscle activity.

Prognosis
The brain damage cannot be reversed; therefore there is no cure for CP. Supportive treatment is important and intended to provide the child with the best attainable quality of life.

Prevention

Measures to prevent oxygen deprivation in the developing brain are essential during the prenatal, perinatal, and neonatal periods. Additional steps are important to prevent head injury or brain infection during these periods of cerebral development.

Patient Teaching

Encourage and help parents to contact community support or credible online support groups. Reinforce the fact that there is no cure for CP and that parents should take advantage of support services available in the community. When possible, assist parents by giving them the names of agencies that provide services to children with CP and their families, and assist with referrals to those agencies.

Muscular Dystrophy

Description

Muscular dystrophy (MD) is a progressive degeneration and weakening of the skeletal muscles where muscle fibers are abnormally vulnerable to injury. There are several types of the disease, but all are rare. The most common and best-known type is Duchenne MD, which is diagnosed soon after birth or during early childhood, usually before the age of 5 years.

ICD-10-CM Code   G71.0 *(Muscular dystrophy)*
MD is coded by type. Refer to the physician's diagnosis and then to the current editions of the ICD-9-CM and ICD-10-CM coding manuals to ensure the greatest specificity of pathology.

Symptoms and Signs

MD initially affects the muscles of the shoulders, hips, thighs, and calves of the legs, causing the characteristic waddling gait and toe walking. Affected muscles sometimes look larger than normal because fat replaces atrophied muscles. The child also may have lordosis or other spinal deformities. In addition, the child has difficulty climbing stairs and running, tends to fall easily, and has difficulty getting up. As the disease progresses, it involves all the muscles, causing crippling and immobility (Fig. 2.13). Contractures typically develop, and the child becomes increasingly susceptible to serious pulmonary infections, such as pneumonia. Children with Duchenne MD are often also impaired mentally.

Patient Screening

MD is usually first suspected during routine well-baby or well-child visits. However, when a parent calls the office about the previously mentioned symptoms, the child should be scheduled for an evaluation as soon as possible. The condition usually is not a life-threatening one; nevertheless, the parents' anxiety will be high, and the condition may appear as an emergency to them.

Etiology

Duchenne MD is the result of a genetic defect caused by the absence of dystrophin, a protein involved in maintaining the integrity of muscle. As is the case for hemophilia and color blindness, the disease affects only males and is generally inherited through female carriers. In one-third to one-half of cases, there is no family history of MD. This means that the disease may be caused by a newly acquired mutation.

Diagnosis

Characteristic symptoms, along with family history of MD, suggest the diagnosis. A muscle biopsy and electromyography (EMG) confirm the diagnosis. Also, an elevated serum creatine kinase (CK) level is evident in the blood. Another

• **Fig. 2.13** (A and B) Clinical photograph of two brothers with severe scoliosis secondary to muscular dystrophy. The boy on the right underwent a successful posterior spinal instrumentation and fusion, achieving good sitting balance. His older brother had already lost too much pulmonary function to tolerate surgery. He is unable to sit well, even with support. (From Herkowitz HN, et al: *Rothman-Simeone the spine*, ed 6, 2011, Elsevier.)

diagnostic test is the deoxyribonucleic acid (DNA) blood test, which can indicate the presence of an abnormality of the protein dystrophin.

Treatment

The US Food and Drug Administration approved the drug deflazacort (Emflaza) for the treatment of Duchenne MD. Experimental drugs based on genetic mutations are also being developed, so genetic research will play a role in future treatment options. Physical therapy, exercise, surgery, and in some cases, the use of orthopedic appliances minimize deformities and preserve mobility. Metal rods may be implanted into the spine to assist the patient with staying upright, which assists with breathing. When swallowing becomes difficult, some patients require a feeding tube to prevent asphyxiation. Corticosteroids may be prescribed to slow muscle degeneration. Seizures and some muscle activity may be controlled with anticonvulsants. Delaying some damage to dying muscle cells may occur with the use of immunosuppressants, and respiratory infections can be warded off with the use of antibiotics.

Prognosis

There is no cure for Duchenne MD, but the average life span has increased with advances in technology and treatment. Some patients with Duchenne MD live into adulthood, and historically, death usually results from cardiac or respiratory complications within 10 to 15 years of the onset of the disease. Mild cases have been known to progress slowly, allowing the child to attain early adulthood with only a mild disability.

Prevention

MD is genetic and, therefore, not preventable.

Patient Teaching

With no cure for MD available at present, parents and family members need emotional support. Help them contact support groups and services for patients with MD and their families. Offer families educational material on the supportive treatment and care of the child with MD. As the child gets older, he or she will need wheelchair-access vehicles for physician office visits. The patient may also need other assistive devices and walk-in shower access for rolling a bath wheelchair in for bathing.

Spina Bifida

Description

Spina bifida is a group of malformations of the spine in which the posterior portion of the bony canal containing the spinal cord (usually in the lumbar region) is completely or partially absent (Fig. 2.14A). Also called *neural tube defects*,

SPINA BIFIDA
Posterior vertebral arches have not fused; there is no herniation of the spinal cord or meninges

A

MENINGOCELE
External protruding sac contains meninges and CSF

MYELOMENINGOCELE
External sac contains meninges, CSF, and the spinal cord

C

B

• **Fig. 2.14** (A) Congenital spinal cord defects. (B) Myelomeningocele. (C) Radiograph of myelomeningocele. *CSF,* Cerebrospinal fluid. (B, From Shiland B: *Mastering healthcare terminology*, ed 6, St. Louis, 2019, Mosby; C, From Frank ED, Long BW, Smith BJ: *Merrill's atlas of radiographic positioning and procedures*, ed 12, St. Louis, 2012, Mosby.)

the three different levels of the condition originate during the early weeks of gestation as the spinal cord and bony canal develop. During this developmental stage, there is a failure of the posterior spinal processes to close, usually in the lumbar region. This failure of complete closure allows the meninges and, in severe cases, the spinal cord to herniate. Depending on the extent of the herniation and the amount of the neural tube that has herniated, various degrees of neural deficits or impairment occur. The three types of spina bifida are spinal bifida occulta, meningocele, and myelomeningocele.

Spina Bifida Occulta

Description. In the defect called spina bifida occulta, the posterior arches of the vertebrae, commonly in the lumbosacral area, fail to fuse, but there is no herniation of the meninges or spinal cord. Usually there is no spinal cord or spinal nerve involvement.

ICD-10-CM Code	Q76.0 *(Spina bifida occulta)*
	Q05.8 *(Sacral spina bifida without hydrocephalus)*
	(Q05.0–Q05.9 = 10 codes of specificity) (codes for Cervical, Thoracic, Lumbar, and Sacral)

Spina bifida is coded according to involvement of hydrocephalus and region affected. Refer to the physician's diagnosis and then to the current editions of the ICD-9-CM and ICD-10-CM coding manuals to ensure the greatest specificity of pathology.

Symptoms and Signs. When this malformation occurs without displacement of the cord or the meninges, spina bifida occulta is asymptomatic. At other times, the only evidence of the neural tube defect is a dimpling, a tuft of hair, or a hemangioma over the site where the vertebrae have not completely fused.

Patient Screening. Most cases are discovered during the newborn examination. Parents requesting an appointment to discuss the condition should be scheduled as soon as possible. It is important to remember the amount of anxiety the parents may experience.

Etiology. The etiology of this congenital anomaly is unknown, but risk factors have been identified. These risk factors include folate deficiency, a familial history of neural tube defects, antiseizure medications, diabetes, obesity, and hyperthermia.

Diagnosis. Maternal blood levels of AFP may be measured to detect possible neural tube defects. Diagnosis is made by using prenatal ultrasonography or with postnatal physical examination, detection of neurologic symptoms, visual inspection of the spine, and spinal ultrasonography. If the infant is asymptomatic, the condition may not be discovered unless medical attention is sought.

Treatment. Spina bifida occulta usually requires no intervention other than prudent observation throughout the child's growth and development. Treatment depends on the degree of neurologic involvement. If the child becomes symptomatic with neurologic problems, surgical intervention to repair the defect is necessary.

Prognosis. The prognosis is good for children with spina bifida occulta.

Prevention. Avoiding exposure to ionizing radiation during pregnancy is a wise precaution and significant in the prevention of this disorder. As a precaution for that risk factor, increased intake of folic acid is encouraged in females while planning to become pregnant and during the early stages of pregnancy. Because many pregnancies are unplanned, all females of childbearing age capable of becoming pregnant are encouraged to take the recommended amount of folic acid each day.

Patient Teaching. The value of regular observation during the growth and development period should be emphasized to both the child and the parents. In addition, the parents and the child should be urged to watch for and report any neurologic symptoms.

Meningocele

Description. The second level of failure of the spinal column to fuse during the developmental stage is called meningocele. The meninges protrude through an opening in the spinal column, thus forming a sac that becomes filled with cerebrospinal fluid (CSF) (see Fig. 2.14B).

ICD-10-CM Code	Q05.8 *(Sacral spina bifida without hydrocephalus)*

Meningocele is coded according to the region affected. Refer to the physician's diagnosis and then to the current editions of the ICD-9-CM and ICD-10-CM coding manuals to ensure the greatest specificity of pathology.

Symptoms and Signs. There is no nerve involvement; therefore the infant usually has no neurologic problems. The sac formed over the defect permits the passage of light during transillumination, indicating no spinal cord or neurologic involvement. The skin over the area may be fragile, and rupture of the sac is a potential problem.

Patient Screening. Most cases are discovered during the newborn examination. When parents request an appointment to discuss the condition, it should be scheduled as soon as possible. It is important to remember the anxiety parents may be experiencing. As the child grows and matures, the parents may detect the onset of neurologic symptoms. When this happens, the child requires an immediate assessment.

Etiology. As in spina bifida occulta, the posterior portion of the neural tube fails to close. The exact cause is not known. However, genetic and environmental factors may play a role. It is possible that a metabolic abnormality in which there are reduced levels of vitamin A and folic acid may contribute to the incidence of spina bifida.

Diagnosis. A diagnosis is made by visual examination of the spinal area and verification of the presence of a sac. Radiographic studies of the spine confirm the clinical findings. The infant is assessed for hydrocephalus, which often is associated with neural tube defects.

Treatment. Treatment usually consists of surgical intervention to correct the defect in the first 24 to 48 hours of life. Because the spinal cord is not involved, paralysis usually does not occur.

Prognosis. With early surgical intervention, the outlook for these children is good.

Prevention. Avoiding exposure to ionizing radiation during pregnancy is a wise precaution and significant in the prevention of this disorder. Increased intake of folic acid is encouraged for females planning to become pregnant and during the early stages of pregnancy. Because many pregnancies are unplanned, all females of childbearing age capable of becoming pregnant are encouraged to take the recommended amount of folic acid each day.

Patient Teaching. The value of regular observation during the growth and development period should be emphasized to both the child and the parents. In addition, the parents and child should be urged to watch for any neurologic symptoms and report them.

Myelomeningocele

Description. Myelomeningocele (also known as spina bifida cystica) is a protrusion of a portion of the spinal cord and the meninges through a defect in the spinal column, usually in the lumbar region (see Fig. 2.14A and B).

ICD-10-CM	Q05.8 *(Sacral spina bifida without*
Code	*hydrocephalus)*

Myelomeningocele is coded according to the region affected. Refer to the physician's diagnosis and then to the current editions of the ICD-9-CM and ICD-10-CM coding manuals to ensure the greatest specificity of pathology and any appropriate modifiers.

Symptoms and Signs. Myelomeningocele is the most severe form of spina bifida. Because spinal nerves or the spinal cord are present in this herniation, the infant exhibits neurologic symptoms. The infant may have musculoskeletal malformations, immobile joints, or paralysis of the lower extremities. Depending on the level of the anomaly, bowel or bladder control may be affected.

Patient Screening. This condition is apparent during the newborn examination. Parents requesting an appointment to discuss the condition should be scheduled as soon as possible. It is important to remember the amount of anxiety the parents may be experiencing. As the child grows and matures, the parents may detect the onset of increased neurologic symptoms. When this happens, the child requires immediate assessment.

Etiology. As in spina bifida occulta and meningocele, the neural tube fails to close during fetal development. This allows the meninges, spinal nerves, and spinal cord to herniate through the opening of the posterior aspect of the spinal column. The etiology may include genetic factors; spinal cord defects are more common when prior offspring of the mother have had a similar defect.

According to the Agent Orange Benefits Act, Public Law 104-204, which became law in 1996, the federal government and the US Department of Veterans Affairs recognized the possibility that exposure of a parent to Agent Orange before conception could result in the child being born with a form of spina bifida.

Diagnosis. Diagnosis is made on the basis of a physical examination and imaging findings. EMG is used to determine the extent of neurologic involvement. Surgical exploration verifies the severity of the disorder (see Fig. 2.14C).

Treatment. Treatment is surgical intervention, usually within the first 24 hours of life, to prevent further deterioration of the involved nerves, infection, and rupture of the herniation. As the child grows, additional procedures may be required to correct evolving problems. Children with myelomeningocele may have other anomalies, including hydrocephalus. Many of these children have no bowel or bladder control and may never be able to walk. A large number of these children die before the age of years.

Prognosis. Nerve damage is irreversible. Surgical intervention in early life may halt the progression of any paralysis. Physical therapy, including leg braces, crutches, and ambulation training, helps increase the child's mobility. Bladder and bowel problems will not improve, and the child and family must be educated to provide care.

Prevention. As with other spina bifida conditions, avoiding exposure to ionizing radiation during pregnancy is a wise precaution and significant in the possible prevention of this disorder. Increased intake of folic acid is encouraged for females planning to become pregnant and during the early stages of pregnancy. Because many pregnancies are unplanned, all females of childbearing age capable of becoming pregnant are encouraged to take the recommended amount of folic acid each day.

Patient Teaching. Parents are told that nerve damage is irreversible. Parents should be given information about spina bifida, along with help in locating and contacting support groups.

The value of regular observation during the growth and development period should be emphasized to both the child and the parents. In addition, the parents and child should be urged to watch for and report any neurologic symptoms.

Hydrocephalus

Description

In hydrocephalus, the amount of CSF is increased greatly or its circulation is blocked, resulting in an abnormal enlargement of the head and characteristic pressure changes in the brain. Hydrocephalus affects both pediatric and adult patients.

ICD-10-CM Code	Q05.4 *(Unspecified spina bifida with hydrocephalus)*
	Q07.01 *(Arnold-Chiari syndrome with spina bifida)*
	Q07.02 *(Arnold-Chiari syndrome with hydrocephalus)*
	Q07.03 *(Arnold-Chiari syndrome with spina bifida and hydrocephalus)*
	G91.0 *(Communicating hydrocephalus)*
	(G91.0-G91.9 = 7 codes of specificity)
	G91.1 *(Obstructive hydrocephalus)*

• **Fig. 2.15** Hydrocephalus. (From Kliegman R, Stanton BF, St. Geme JW, et al: *Nelson textbook of pediatrics*, ed 19, St. Louis, 2011, Saunders/Elsevier.)

Symptoms and Signs

The fontanels begin to bulge, the sutures of the skull separate, and the scalp veins become distended. Head circumference increases at a faster rate than expected for normal growth. The infant has a high-pitched cry, is irritable, and may have episodes of projectile vomiting. Eventually there is downward displacement of the eyes. Neurologic signs include abnormal muscle tone in the legs.

Patient Screening

Many cases of hydrocephalus are apparent during the newborn examination, and others may be detected during well-baby examinations. The head circumference should be measured and plotted on a growth chart at each office visit. Parents requesting an appointment to discuss the condition will have great anxiety, so the appointment should be scheduled as soon as possible. When a parent contacts the office with concern about the child's head appearing to be unusually large, the child requires prompt assessment. The same policy should apply to parents contacting the office with concerns about possible neurologic signs. When a parent or a patient with a shunt in place calls about possible problems with the shunt, an immediate appointment is required, or the patient should be sent to the nearest emergency facility for evaluation.

Etiology

In hydrocephalus, a large amount of CSF accumulates in the skull, causing increased intracranial pressure. An impairment of the circulation of the CSF in the ventricular circulation (obstructive hydrocephalus) may be caused by a lesion within the system or by a congenital structural defect. Impairment of the flow of CSF in the subarachnoid space (communicating hydrocephalus) prevents CSF from reaching the areas where it normally would be reabsorbed by the arachnoid villi. This may be the result of intracranial hemorrhage resulting from head trauma, a blood clot, prematurity, or infection (meningitis) (Figs. 2.15 and 2.16).

Diagnosis

Diagnosis is made on the basis of the clinical picture, physical examination, and radiographic skull studies. CT and MRI scans demonstrate the condition.

Treatment

Treatment consists of surgical intervention to place a shunt in the ventricular or subarachnoid spaces to drain off excessive CSF. Some catheters empty into the peritoneal cavity, and other shunt catheters empty into the right atrium of the heart (Fig. 2.17).

One-way valves help shunt the excessive CSF away from the cerebrospinal canal and maintain a normal pressure. If left untreated, the increasing intracranial pressure of hydrocephalus causes intellectual developmental disorder and eventually death.

Prognosis

The prognosis for these children varies, depending on the extent of the condition and the success of corrective interventions. Most children can function normally in society. Parents and the child must watch for the onset of neurologic symptoms and seek medical assessment and treatment.

Prevention

There is no known prevention for the congenital form of this disorder. Good prenatal care, along with prudent observation and assistance during labor and delivery, helps prevent damage to the brain. Preventing infections and injuries to the head during childhood, although challenging, may prevent some incidences.

Patient Teaching

Parents and child should be taught to recognize signs of malfunctioning shunts. In addition, they should be told the importance of promptly reporting any neurologic signs or symptoms to the physician.

Arachnoid villus

Superior sagittal sinus (venous blood)

Arachnoid mater

Cerebral cortex

Bone of skull

Dura mater

Pia mater

Arachnoid layer

Falx cerebri (dura mater)

Subarachnoid space

B

Arachnoid villus

Subarachnoid space

Superior sagittal sinus

Choroid plexus of third ventricle

Cerebral aqueduct

Lateral foramen

Choroid plexus of fourth ventricle

Median foramen

Choroid plexus of lateral ventricle

Interventricular foramen

Cisterna magna

Central canal of spinal cord

Dura mater

A

• **Fig. 2.16** Flow of cerebrospinal fluid. (From Patton KT, Thibodeau GA: *Anatomy and physiology*, ed 9, St. Louis, 2016, Mosby.)

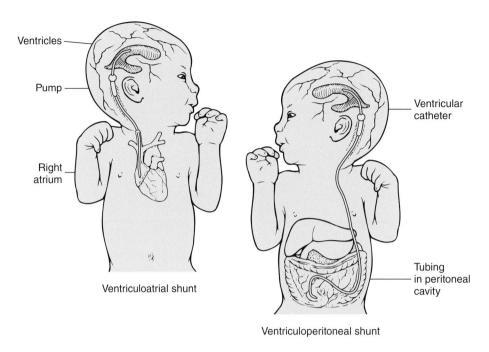

• **Fig. 2.17** Shunting procedures for hydrocephalus. Ventriculoperitoneal shunt is the preferred procedure.

• **Fig. 2.18** Anencephaly. (From Damjanov I: *Pathology for the health professions*, ed 4, St. Louis, 2011, Saunders.)

Anencephaly

Description

This most severe form of neural tube defect occurs early in gestation, when the cephalic aspect of the neural tube fails to close.

ICD-10-CM Code	Q00.0 *(Anencephaly)*

Symptoms and Signs

The anencephalic fetus or neonate has no cranial vault and little cerebral tissue. Bones of the base of the skull and the orbits are present (Fig. 2.18). The microcephalic fetus or neonate has very small amounts of cerebral tissue and may survive for a few hours or days. Most of these infants die before birth or during the birth process.

Patient Screening

This anomaly may be found during prenatal ultrasonography. The mother or both parents should be scheduled for an office visit, at which the physician should discuss the ultrasonographic findings. When the anomaly is not apparent until birth, the infant usually is stillborn or dies shortly after birth. This event produces great anxiety, and parents may request an appointment for additional information. An appointment should be scheduled promptly.

Etiology

The etiology is essentially unknown, but this anomaly is characterized by failure of the neural tube at the cephalic (cranial) end to close completely during the second or third week of gestation. The occurrence of this defect tends to be familial; females are affected more often compared with males. It is possible that the mother's diet and vitamin intake may be involved; therefore females of childbearing age are encouraged to take folic acid supplements regularly to prevent neural tube deficits in their offspring.

Diagnosis

Diagnosis is made by ultrasonographic examination of the fetal head when blood tests of the mother indicate an elevated AFP level. The ultrasonogram shows a symmetric absence of normal cranial bone structure and brain tissue.

Treatment

There is no effective treatment for this anomaly. Infants who survive the birth process die shortly afterward because many have several other neural tube anomalies incompatible with life.

Prognosis

These fetuses or neonates lack sufficient cerebral tissue to sustain life.

Prevention

As with other neural tube defects, the etiology is unclear. All females of childbearing age and capability are urged to avoid radiation exposure and take the recommended amount of folic acid daily.

Patient Teaching

Patient teaching includes answering the parents' questions. Encourage and help parents learn about appropriate community resources.

Congenital Cardiac Defects

Fetal Circulation

Oxygen and nutrients are supplied by the mother's blood to the developing fetus. The maternal blood supply also carries away waste products. The exchange takes place in the placental tissue. The umbilical vessels, two arteries and one vein, transport the blood between the placenta and the fetus (Fig. 2.19).

The umbilical vein transports oxygen-rich blood and nutrients to the fetus. The umbilical vein enters the fetal body by passing through the umbilical ring and then goes on to the liver. Fifty percent of this blood passes into the liver, and the other 50% bypasses the liver by way of the ductus venosus. The ductus venosus soon joins the inferior vena cava, allowing the oxygenated placental blood to mix with the deoxygenated blood coming from the lower fetal body. This blood then travels to the right atrium through the vena cava.

Because the fetal lungs are not functioning, this blood mostly bypasses the lungs. Most of the blood entering the right atrium by the inferior vena cava is shunted directly into the left atrium through the foramen ovale. On the left side of the atrial septum, there is a small valve called the *septum primum*. This valve keeps blood from going back into the right atrium. The remaining fetal blood that has entered the right atrium contains a large amount of oxygen-poor

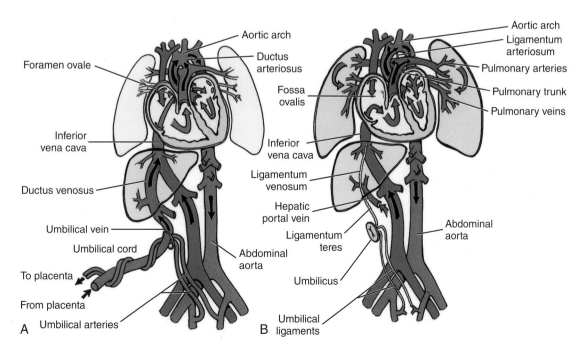

• **Fig. 2.19** Circulation patterns before and after birth. (A) Fetal circulation. (B) Circulation after birth. (From Applegate EJ: *The anatomy and physiology learning system*, ed 4, Philadelphia, 2011, Saunders.)

blood from the superior vena cava and travels to the right ventricle and into the pulmonary trunk. The pulmonary blood vessels have a high resistance to blood flow because of the collapsed state of the lungs; thus they only allow a small amount of blood to enter the pulmonary circulation. This small amount is enough to nourish the pulmonary tissue.

The blood that has been shunted away from the pulmonary circulation bypasses the lungs through the fetal vessel, the ductus arteriosus. This vessel connects the pulmonary trunk to the descending area of the aortic arch. The ductus arteriosus allows the blood with low oxygen concentration to bypass the lungs and also prevents it from entering the arteries leading to the brain.

The blood that has a high oxygen concentration and has been shunted to the left atrium by way of the foramen ovale mixes with the small amount of blood returning from the pulmonary circulation by way of the pulmonary veins. This blood flows into the left ventricle and then into the aorta. From the aorta, some blood travels to the coronary and the carotid arteries. A portion travels on through the descending aorta to other parts of the fetal tissue. The remaining blood travels into the umbilical arteries and back to the placenta for the exchange of gases, nutrients, and waste.

After the birth process, the infant's respiratory effort, and the initial inflation of the lungs, the circulatory system undergoes important changes. The resistance to blood flow through the lungs is reduced by the inflation of the tissue, allowing an increased blood flow from the pulmonary arteries. An increased volume of blood now flows from the right atrium into the right ventricle and the pulmonary arteries. In addition, the volume of blood flowing through the foramen ovale into the left atrium is reduced. The volume of blood returning by way of the pulmonary veins from the lungs to the left atrium is increased, causing an increase in the pressure in the left atrium. Blood is forced against the septum primum by decreased right atrial pressure and increased left atrial pressure, and the foramen ovale closes. If this does not occur, the infant has an ASD (discussed subsequently under congenital anomalies). In most cases, however, the heart now is a two-sided pump.

With the lungs expanded and taking over the function of gas exchange, the infant no longer needs the ductus arteriosus to shunt blood from the pulmonary trunk to the descending aorta. Normally the ductus arteriosus closes in the first few days after birth. If it does not close, it is termed patent. PDA is a congenital birth defect (discussed subsequently).

Symptoms and Signs

Congenital cardiac defects are developmental anomalies of the heart or the great vessels of the heart. They are present at birth, and the defects cause mild to fatal stress on the cardiac muscle. Signs and symptoms vary, depending on the nature of the anomaly, the severity of the defect, and its effect on the heart and the circulatory system. One defect can be present, or a combination of defects can complicate the case. The common defects generally are categorized as follows: **acyanotic**, in which deoxygenated and oxygenated

blood do not mix, and cyanotic, in which oxygenated and deoxygenated blood mix. The greatest medical concern for infants with acyanotic cardiac defects is congestive heart failure. The greatest concern for infants with cyanotic cardiac defects is hypoxia. Occasionally when the defects are minor, they may not be discovered until adulthood (Fig. 2.20).

Acyanotic Defects

Description

In this condition, oxygenated blood does not mix with deoxygenated blood, and the infant usually maintains a fairly normal pink skin color. Cyanosis is not prevalent.

Patient Screening

Most cases are discovered during the newborn examination. When parents request an appointment to discuss the condition, it should be scheduled as soon as possible. The parents may be experiencing great anxiety. Those cases not detected during the neonatal period of hospitalization may develop symptoms after discharge from the hospital. When parents contact the office to relay concerns and symptoms, the infant requires prompt assessment.

Ventricular Septal Defect

ICD-10-CM Code	Q21.0 *(Ventricular septal defect)*
	(Q21.0-Q21.9 = 7 codes of specificity)

The most common congenital cardiac disorder, VSD, is an abnormal opening between the right and the left ventricles (Fig. 2.21). When the defect is small, there is little functional disease; when it is large, the results are serious. In this condition, blood is shunted from the left to the right side of the heart as a result of higher pressure in the left ventricle. The characteristic murmur of VSD is described as harsh and holosystolic. The murmur is loudest when the defect is small because a relatively large amount of blood is passing through a tiny opening. Clinical features include failure to gain weight, restlessness, irritability, sweating when feeding, and increased heart rate and respiration. This condition may go undetected until later in childhood, adolescence, or adulthood.

Patent Ductus Arteriosus

ICD-10-CM Code	Q25.0 *(Patent ductus arteriosus)*
	(Q25.0-Q25.9 = 10 codes of specificity)

PDA results when the ductus fails to functionally close. During normal fetal circulation, the patent ductus short circuits, shunting the circulation from the lungs and instead directing blood from the pulmonary trunk to the aorta. If

MAJOR CYANOTIC DEFECTS

Tetralogy of Fallot

Transposition of the great arteries

Tricuspid atresia

MAJOR ACYANOTIC DEFECTS

Atrial septal defect

Coarctation of the aorta

Ventricular septal defect

Patent ductus arteriosus

• **Fig. 2.20** Chart comparing acyanotic and cyanotic heart defects in a newborn. (A) Tetralogy of Fallot. (B) Transposition of the great arteries. (C) Tricuspid atresia. (D) Atrial septal defect. (E) Coarctation of the aorta. (F) Ventricular septal defect. (G) Patent ductus arteriosus. (From Goodman CC, Fuller KS: *Pathology for the physical therapist assistant*, ed 1, St. Louis, 2012, Saunders.)

PDA continues after birth, circulation of oxygen is compromised because this abnormal opening is a shunt that allows oxygenated blood to recirculate through the lungs

(Fig. 2.22). PDA is detected during a physical examination when a classic "machinery" murmur is heard on auscultation and palpitation reveals a thrill. The infant's growth

• **Fig. 2.21** Ventricular septal defects: anatomic classification. (Modified from Hockenberry MJ, Wilson D, Rodgers CC: *Wong's nursing care of infants and children*, ed 11, St. Louis, 2019, Elsevier.)

Ventricular septal defect

• **Fig. 2.23** Coarctation of the aorta. (Used with permission of Ross Products Division, Abbott Laboratories, from Congenital heart abnormalities [Clinical Education Aid No. 7], 1992.)

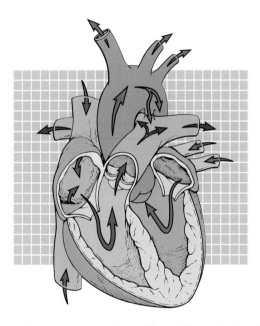

• **Fig. 2.22** Patent ductus arteriosus. (Used with permission of Ross Products Division, Abbott Laboratories, from Congenital heart abnormalities [Clinical Education Aid No. 7], 1992.)

and development may be slowed, and various signs of heart failure may be present. Closure may be attempted by drug therapy using an antiprostaglandin or ibuprofen. The other option is surgical closure of the ductus.

This condition is fairly common in premature infants and often is accompanied by ASD with failure of the foramen ovale to close.

The prognosis for these infants depends on the presence of other anomalies. Closure by using either drug therapy or surgical intervention establishes a normal postnatal circulation path and gives the infant the opportunity to grow and thrive. Currently no prevention is known.

Coarctation of the Aorta

ICD-10-CM Code   Q25.1 *(Coarctation of aorta)*

This defect is characterized by a narrowed aortic lumen, causing a partial obstruction of the flow of blood through the aorta (Fig. 2.23). The result is increased left ventricular pressure and workload, with decreased blood pressure distal to the narrowing. Signs and symptoms can be evident shortly after birth or may not surface until adolescence. They include signs of left ventricular failure with pulmonary edema. The patient is pale and cyanotic with weakness, dyspnea, and tachycardia. Systemic blood pressure is elevated when measured in the arms but decreased in the lower extremities. This defect is often associated with Turner syndrome.

Atrial Septal Defect

ICD-10-CM Code   Q21.1 *(Atrial septal defect)*

ASD is an abnormal opening between the right and left atria (Fig. 2.24). Although the defect can vary in size and location, blood generally shunts from left to right in all ASDs. Small defects may be undetected or cause symptoms such as fatigue, shortness of breath, and frequent respiratory tract infections. A large defect causes pronounced cyanosis, dyspnea, and syncope. A classic systolic cardiac murmur can be heard with a stethoscope. This condition often is associated with prematurity and PDA, and closure is achieved with surgical repair.

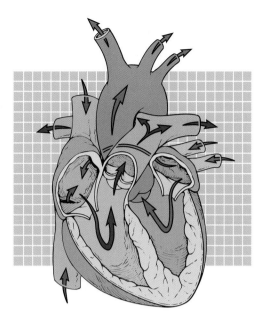

• **Fig. 2.24** Atrial septal defect. (Used with permission of Ross Products Division, Abbott Laboratories, from Congenital heart abnormalities [Clinical Education Aid No. 7], 1992.)

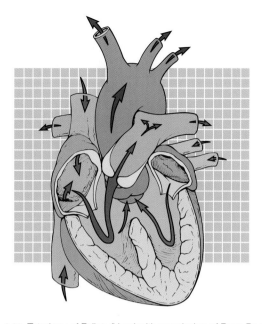

• **Fig. 2.25** Tetralogy of Fallot. (Used with permission of Ross Products Division, Abbott Laboratories, from Congenital heart abnormalities [Clinical Education Aid No. 7], 1992.)

Cyanotic Defects

Description

Central cyanosis is a sign that the atrial blood is not fully oxygenated. The infant appears cyanotic, with a blue tinge to the lips, tongue, and nail beds. The five main cardiac causes of central cyanosis are tetralogy of Fallot, transposition of the great arteries, truncus arteriosus, tricuspid atresia, and total anomalous pulmonary venous return. The two most common defects are discussed here.

Patient Screening

Some defects can be detected in prenatal ultrasonography. Most cases are discovered during the newborn examination. Appointments for parents seeking to discuss the condition should be scheduled as soon as possible. One must consider the great anxiety in the parents. Those cases not detected during the neonatal period of hospitalization may develop symptoms after discharge from the hospital. When parents contact the office to relay concerns and symptoms, the infant requires prompt assessment.

Tetralogy of Fallot

ICD-10-CM Code   Q21.3 *(Tetralogy of Fallot)*

The most common cyanotic cardiac defect is a combination of four congenital heart defects: (1) VSD, an abnormal opening in the ventricular septum; (2) pulmonary stenosis, a tightening of the pulmonary valve or vessel; (3) dextroposition (displacement to the right) of the aorta, which overrides (receiving circulation from both ventricles) the VSD; and (4) right ventricular hypertrophy, caused by increased pressure in the ventricle (Fig. 2.25).

Affected infants with severe obstruction are "blue babies" at birth. Deoxygenated blood enters the aorta, causing the symptoms of hypoxia: tachycardia, tachypnea, dyspnea, and seizures. Bone marrow hypoxia causes polycythemia, or increased total red blood cell (RBC) mass. Physical examination may reveal delayed physical growth and development along with clubbing of the fingers and toes. Cardiac murmurs can be heard. Older children assume a squatting position after exercise to relieve breathlessness caused by hypoxia.

Transposition of the Great Arteries

ICD-10-CM Code   Q20.3 *(Discordant ventriculoarterial connection)*

In this defect, the aorta and the pulmonary artery are reversed: the aorta originates from the right ventricle, and the pulmonary artery originates from the left ventricle. The result is two closed-loop circulatory systems: one between the heart and the lungs and the other between the heart and systemic circulation (Fig. 2.26). Within a few hours of birth, neonates with this defect exhibit cyanosis and tachypnea, followed by signs of heart failure.

Immediate surgical intervention is indicated. Prostaglandins are administered to the infant in an effort to keep the ductus arteriosus patent and the foramen ovale from closing. As soon as surgery is possible, the blood flow is redirected by the correction of the defect.

The prognosis for these infants is poor unless a pediatric surgical unit is readily available and transportation to it is swift. Another factor in the survival of the infant with this condition is the infant's response to the drug therapy

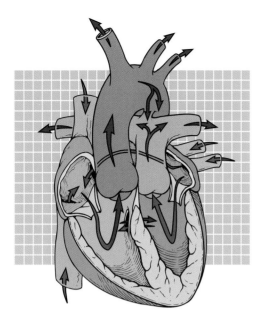

• **Fig. 2.26** Transposition of the great arteries. (Used with permission of Ross Products Division, Abbott Laboratories, from Congenital heart abnormalities [Clinical Education Aid No. 7], 1992.)

to maintain fetal circulation and prevent the change to the normal postbirth circulatory system.

Methods of preventing this condition are unknown.

Etiology. The cause of congenital cardiac defects remains unknown. They may result from several factors, including chromosomal abnormalities and environmental conditions, such as maternal infections and the mother's use of certain drugs during gestation. Several congenital disorders result from the failure of the circulatory system to shift from the fetal route of blood flow at the time of birth.

Diagnosis. Physical examination and patient history are essential. The physician palpates the neck vessels and auscultates for blood pressure and murmurs. Diagnostic procedures depend on the initial findings and may include chest radiography, blood tests, cardiac catheterization, echocardiography, and electrocardiography. Many defects can be detected in prenatal ultrasonography. The diagnostic investigation determines the presence and severity of any structural or functional abnormality or defect.

Treatment. The medical management of congenital cardiac defects is determined by the type of defect, the degree of symptoms and signs, and the presence of life-threatening complications. Advances in surgical techniques enable surgeons to close septal defects, reconstruct or replace a valve, and repair or join blood vessels. These procedures make it possible to save, improve, and extend the lives of individuals born with congenital cardiac defects. Medications are available to strengthen and regulate the heartbeat. Supportive measures include prophylactic antibiotic administration before dental procedures in some cases to ward off infection.

Prognosis. The prognosis varies and depends on the severity, the number of defects, and the gestational age of the infant or child. Most defects can be surgically repaired.

Prevention. There is no known prevention for these defects. Good prenatal care accompanied by good nutrition is always wise during any pregnancy.

Patient Teaching. Parents and caregivers need understanding, encouragement, and teaching to cope with changes in individual and family lifestyles imposed by these conditions. Help and encourage parents to find and contact support groups in the community or online. It is recommended that individuals who have had surgical repair of cardiac defects maintain regular follow-up care with a cardiologist.

Musculoskeletal Conditions

Clubfoot (Talipes Equinovarus)

Description

Clubfoot is an obvious, nontraumatic deformity of the foot of the newborn in which the anterior half of the foot is adducted and inverted.

ICD-10-CM Code	Q66.0 (Congenital talipes equinovarus)

Symptoms and Signs

Besides the previously mentioned description, the heel is drawn up, with the lateral side of the foot being convex and the medial aspect being concave (Fig. 2.27A). A true clubfoot cannot be manipulated to the proper position, whereas distortions caused by intrauterine position usually can.

Patient Screening

Most cases are discovered during the newborn examination. Appointments for parents seeking to discuss the condition should be scheduled as soon as possible. Remember the great anxiety the parents may be feeling. As treatment progresses, routine examinations are scheduled.

Etiology

Some sources suggest that fetal position is the cause, and other studies implicate genetic factors because of abnormal development of the germ plasma during the embryonic stage.

Diagnosis

The deformity is obvious at birth, with a resistance of the foot to return to a neutral position during manipulation. In addition, the Achilles tendon is shortened.

Treatment

Treatment consists of either cast application or the use of splints. Treatment must start early in the neonatal period. Casts are reapplied at frequent intervals as the correction increases and the infant grows (see Fig. 2.27B). Splints include a bar affixed to shoes; the infant is placed in the shoes, which hold the feet and legs in position. Many physicians employ a combination of manipulative methods, with cast application followed by the use of splints as the child matures. The child must be observed throughout childhood for reversal of the improvement. If casting and splinting are unsuccessful, surgery may be indicated to correct the condition. In many

Bilateral clubfoot
(talipes equinovarus)

Congenital hip dysplasia

C

• Fig. 2.27, cont'd

cases a procedure called Achilles tenotomy is performed to release the tightness of the Achilles tendon.

Prognosis
The prognosis is good when casting is performed or splints can be used early in life. When these modes of treatment do not completely resolve the condition, surgical intervention usually corrects the deformity.

Prevention
No prevention of this deformity is known.

Patient Teaching
Parents will be extremely anxious and need information about this condition. Instruction on cast care and skin care is important. The importance of observing continuously for any reversal of correction is stressed.

Developmental Dysplasia of the Hip

Description
Developmental dysplasia of the hip (DDH), previously known as *congenital hip dysplasia*, is an abnormal development of the hip joint, ranging from an unstable joint to the dislocation of the femoral head from the acetabulum.

ICD-10-CM Code	Q65.8 *(Other congenital deformities of hip)*
	(Q65.0-Q65.9 = 15 codes of specificity)
	Q65.2 *(Congenital dislocation of hip, unspecified)*

Refer to the physician's diagnosis and then to the current edition ICD-10-CM coding manual to ensure the greatest specificity of pathology.

Unilateral cleft lip

• **Fig. 2.27** (A–E) Congenital musculoskeletal diseases. (A, From Zitelli BJ, McIntire SC, Davis HW: *Zitelli and Davis' atlas of pediatric physical diagnosis*, ed 6, St. Louis, 2012, Saunders; B, From Perry S, Hockenberry M, Lowdermilk D, et al: *Maternal-child nursing care*, ed 3, St. Louis, 2007, Mosby; C and E, From Behrman RE, Kliegman RM, Arvin AM: *Slide set for Nelson textbook of pediatrics*, ed 15, Philadelphia, 1996, Saunders; D, Courtesy Texas Scottish Rite Hospital for Children, Dallas, Texas.)

Symptoms and Signs

Physical examination reveals asymmetric folds of the thigh of the newborn, with limited abduction of the affected hip. A shortening of the femur is noted when the knees and hips are flexed at right angles (see Fig. 2.27D).

Patient Screening

This dysplasia is apparent during the newborn examination. When parents request an appointment to discuss the condition, it should be scheduled as soon as possible. Remember the great anxiety the parents may be feeling. As treatment progresses, routine examinations are scheduled.

Etiology

The exact cause is unknown. Typical DDH occurs shortly before, during, or shortly after birth, possibly as a result of softening of the ligaments caused by the maternal hormone relaxin. DDH may result from a breech presentation and is more common in female infants.

Diagnosis

Abnormal signs, including positive Ortolani and Barlow maneuvers, may be detected at birth. Diagnosis is made during the physical examination and is confirmed with ultrasonography of the hip.

Treatment

Treatment includes the use of various devices to reduce the hip dislocation. After the femoral head is returned to its proper position in the acetabulum, the legs are held in place by a Pavlik harness, a splint, or a cast, allowing stable maintenance of the hip in a position of flexion and abduction. Early treatment offers the best results and may help avoid surgical intervention.

Prognosis

The prognosis for this deformity is good when therapy is instituted early in the neonatal period. If this therapy is unsuccessful, surgical intervention may be required.

Prevention

No prevention for this condition is known.

Patient Teaching

Parents should be taught to care for the skin and the correctional device. In addition, the need for compliance with the treatment should be stressed. After the condition appears to have been corrected, parents should be told of the importance of follow-up assessments of the child.

Cleft Lip and Palate

Description

Cleft lip is a congenital birth defect consisting of one or more clefts in the upper lip (see Fig. 2.27E). Cleft palate is a birth defect in which there is a hole in the middle of the roof of the mouth (palate).

ICD-10-CM Code	Q37.9 *(Unspecified cleft palate with unilateral cleft lip)*

(Q37.0–Q37.9 = 8 codes of
specificity)
*Cleft palate and lip are coded by type. Refer to the
physician's diagnosis and then to the current editions
of the ICD-9-CM and ICD-10-CM coding manuals to
ensure the greatest specificity of pathology and any
appropriate modifiers.*

Symptoms and Signs
The cleft may extend completely through the hard and soft palates into the nasal area. The defects appear singularly or may be linked and vary in severity. Some infants have difficulty with nasal regurgitation and feeding because of air leaks around the cleft. The infant's face has an abnormal appearance.

Patient Screening
These birth defects are apparent during newborn examination after birth. At times the condition may be diagnosed before birth during ultrasound beginning the 13th week of gestation. Parents may want an appointment to discuss the condition and treatment with the physician. Because of the great anxiety that the parents may be feeling, a prompt appointment should be scheduled. As the repair and correction of conditions progress, the parents may contact the office about problems the child is having, especially with feeding. Prompt response to their requests is required.

Etiology
The cause is a failure in the embryonic development of the fetus. It is considered a multifactorial genetic disorder and may result from environmental factors the mother comes into contact with during pregnancy, or what she drinks, foods, and medications she takes.

Diagnosis
Cleft abnormalities are obvious during clinical examination at birth.

Treatment
Cleft deformities are usually repaired surgically as soon as possible. Extensive deformities require a second repair and multiple surgeries may be needed. Special feeding devices can be tried. The child often requires speech therapy.

Prognosis
The prognosis for this disorder is good with surgical repair. Advances in plastic surgery have made the repair look as natural as possible. Individuals may have self-esteem issues due to looking different than others.

Prevention
No prevention of this disorder is known, but risk factors have been identified. Smoking, diabetes, and use of medications that treat epilepsy pose a higher risk with mothers than those who do not smoke, are not diabetic, and those who are not taking seizure medications.

Patient Teaching
Parents need instruction on care of the surgical repair and feeding of the infant. Help and encourage them to find and contact support groups in the community. There are devices that are specifically made to enable the infant to nurse and keep food and liquid from entering an open palate. Encourage parents to seek organizations with medical care specializing in care, treatment, and financial assistance in infants and children with cranial-facial defects, primarily cleft deformations.

Genitourinary Conditions

Cryptorchidism (Undescended Testes)
Description
Cryptorchidism is the failure of one or both of the testicles to descend from the abdominal cavity into the scrotum.

ICD-10-CM Code	Q53.9 *(Undescended testicle, unspecified)*
	(Q53.0–Q53.9 = 10 codes of specificity)

Symptoms and Signs
Cryptorchidism, or failure of the testicles to descend from the abdominal cavity into the scrotum, is detected at birth or shortly thereafter (Fig. 2.28A and B). The condition may be unilateral or bilateral. During infancy and early childhood, there are no symptoms besides the absence of the testes. The condition is more common in premature infants.

Patient Screening
This condition is palpable and observed during the newborn examination. Parents may request an appointment to discuss the condition and possible treatment. The anxiety of the parents calls for an appointment at the earliest convenience of the parents and the physician.

Etiology
The cause of failure of the testes to descend during the final fetal development is not clearly understood. Genes, the mother's health, and exposure to substances in the environment that can lead to an imbalance of hormones are believed to play a part. Prematurity, decreased birth weight, family history of developmental issues of genitals, drinking alcohol, exposure to secondhand smoke, smoking during pregnancy, and the parents' exposure to pesticides are risk factors for this condition.

Diagnosis
Diagnosis is by visual inspection and by palpation, starting above the inguinal ring and pushing downward on the inguinal canal toward the scrotum. The examination reveals

• **Fig. 2.28** (A) Cryptorchidism and (B) cryptorchidism in left testicle of a neonate. (A, From Niedzwiecki B, et al: *Kinn's the medical assistant: an applied learning approach*, ed 14, 2020, Elsevier; B, From Zitelli BJ, Davis HW: *Atlas of pediatric physical diagnosis*, ed 5, St. Louis, 2007, Mosby/Elsevier.)

no evidence of one or both testes in the scrotal sac. When the condition is bilateral, the scrotum appears underdeveloped.

Treatment
The testes often descend spontaneously during the first year of life. If this does not happen by age 4 years, the treatment is to place the undescended testes into the scrotum by either surgical manipulation (orchiopexy) or hormonal drug therapy (beta-human chorionic gonadotropin or testosterone). Treatment is important because untreated cryptorchidism may lead to sterility in the adult male. There is an increased risk of testicular cancer in untreated cryptorchidism.

Prognosis
The prognosis is good when surgical intervention can move the testicles down into the scrotum and secure them. This procedure is necessary in early childhood to prevent sterility and possible cancer later in life.

Prevention
There is no known method of prevention.

Patient Teaching
Parents need to be told about the dangers of not utilizing the suggested surgical intervention. After the procedure, they need instructions on caring for the incisions.

Wilms Tumor
Description
Wilms tumor, or nephroblastoma, is a highly malignant neoplasm of the kidney that affects children younger than

10 years of age. It is the most common kidney tumor in childhood and the fourth most common childhood cancer.

ICD-10-CM Code	C64.9 *(Malignant neoplasm of unspecified kidney, except renal pelvis)* (C64.1–C64.9 = 3 codes of specificity)

Symptoms and Signs
The most common presentation is a mass in the kidney region, which is often discovered by a parent or an examining physician. The mass is firm, non-tender, and usually confined to one side of the body. The patient may experience other symptoms resulting from compression caused by the tumor mass, metabolic alterations resulting from the tumor, or metastasis. These signs and symptoms may include hematuria, abdominal pain or swelling, hypertension, nausea, vomiting, loss of appetite, constipation, shortness of breath, and fever.

Patient Screening
A child who is experiencing hematuria, pain, and vomiting and has a noticeable mass in the kidney region requires prompt assessment.

Etiology
Wilms tumor is an **adenosarcoma** (Fig. 2.29). This type of tumor is associated with several congenital anomalies, such as aniridia (absence of the iris) and genitourinary anomalies (e.g., cryptorchidism and ambiguous genitalia), and is a part of some familial cancer syndromes.

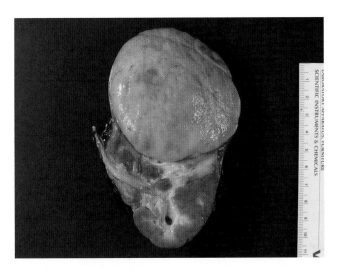

• **Fig. 2.29** Nephroblastoma (Wilms tumor). This well-circumscribed tumor has a bulging cut surface and a thin fibrous pseudocapsule. (From Fogo A, et al: *Diagnostic Atlas of Renal Pathology*, ed 4, 2023, Elsevier.)

• **Fig. 2.30** Photo showing phimosis. (From Lewis SL, et al: *Medical-surgical nursing: Assessment and management of clinical problems*, ed 8, St. Louis, 2011, Mosby.)

Diagnosis

A child suspected of having Wilms tumor often undergoes a physical examination to palpate the kidney mass, to seek associated congenital anomalies, and to look for signs of malignancy (e.g., increased size of liver and spleen and lymphadenopathy). Blood tests are done to assess for anemia and kidney and liver function. Specific tests that help determine the extent of the disease include abdominal ultrasonography, CT, and urinalysis. Surgery is necessary for the complete staging of the tumor. Staging is based on the degree the tumor extends beyond the kidney capsule, the presence of metastasis, and whether there is bilateral kidney involvement.

Treatment

Prompt recognition and treatment are imperative because the tumor is locally invasive and tends to metastasize. Surgical removal of the tumor and accessible metastatic sites is followed by chemotherapy with or without radiation therapy. Most children are treated according to research protocols at pediatric cancer centers. The specific treatment choice is guided by tumor stage and histology.

Prognosis

Wilms tumor has one of the highest survival rates of all childhood cancers. The prognosis is largely based on stage and tumor histology.

Prevention

No prevention is known.

Patient Teaching

Help and encourage parents to find and contact support groups in the community and resources that provide services to the child and the family.

Phimosis

Description

Phimosis is stenosis, or narrowing, of the opening of the foreskin in the male that leads to an inability to retract the foreskin. It is rare for the foreskin to be retractable in the neonatal period. This is normal and, in some cases, can persist into adolescence. Phimosis can be problematic if acquired after the neonatal period.

ICD-10-CM Code	N47.0 *(Adherent prepuce, newborn)*
	N47.1 *(Phimosis)*
	N47.2 *(Paraphimosis)*
	(N47.0–N47.8 = 9 codes of specificity)

Symptoms and Signs

The child may experience difficulty with urination, or the parents may have difficulty with cleaning the area under the prepuce of the glans penis, resulting in accumulation of secretions. These symptoms may develop later in uncircumcised males, even into adulthood.

Etiology

Many male infants are born with phimosis; the cause is unknown.

Diagnosis

Diagnosis is made by visual examination and the inability to slide the prepuce back over the glans penis (Fig. 2.30).

Treatment

Definitive treatment is circumcision, the surgical removal of the prepuce. This procedure, which used to be routine for male newborns, is usually performed in the first few days of life. An alternative treatment, when parents decide not to have the surgery performed on the male infant, is for the parents to gently wash the glans and prepuce with soap and water and gently slide the prepuce back over the glans. This procedure is done on a regular schedule, and the prepuce is never forced over the glans. Topical steroid cream may also be useful.

Prognosis

The prognosis is good.

Prevention

Newborn circumcision prevents this condition.

Patient Teaching

Parents require instruction in caring for the incised area. When the parents decide to attempt manual manipulation of the prepuce, instruction is provided, with emphasis on never forcing the prepuce over the glans. Parents must also be encouraged to cleanse and dry the area daily.

Diseases of the Digestive System

Congenital Pyloric Stenosis

Description

Pyloric stenosis (Fig. 2.31A and C), a congenital disorder, is a gastric obstruction associated with narrowing of the pyloric sphincter at the exit of the stomach. This condition may also be called *congenital hypertrophic pyloric stenosis*.

ICD-10-CM Code	Q40.0 *(Congenital hypertrophic pyloric stenosis)*

Symptoms and Signs

The infant has episodes of projectile vomiting after feedings (Fig. 2.31B) and fails to gain weight. Symptoms usually begin when the infant is 2 to 3 weeks of age. The infant appears hungry, continues to feed, and yet fails to gain weight. If left untreated, the infant becomes dehydrated and experiences electrolyte imbalances. A small olive-shaped hard mass may be palpated in the region of the pyloric sphincter, and left to right peristalsis may be noted, followed by reverse peristalsis. The emesis contains no bile.

Patient Screening

The infant with sudden onset of projectile vomiting requires prompt assessment.

Etiology

There is a slight hereditary tendency, but the exact cause is unknown. It occurs four times more often in male than in female infants.

Diagnosis

The condition is diagnosed from the history and the patient's physical condition. Diagnostic studies include upper GI radiographic studies and ultrasonography of the pylorus.

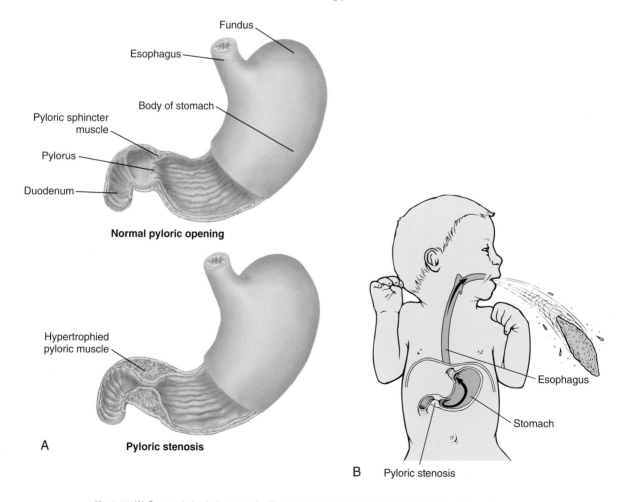

• **Fig. 2.31** (A) Congenital pyloric stenosis. (B) The abnormal narrowing of the opening of the pylorus causes episodes of projectile vomiting.

• **Fig. 2.31, cont'd** (C) Pyloric stenosis. (A, From Ashwill JW, Droske SC: Nursing care of children: principles and practice, ed 3, Philadelphia, 2007, Saunders; C, From Lakshmanaswamy A: *Textbook of pediatrics*, ed 1, 2022, Elsevier.)

Treatment
Treatment consists of surgical intervention, in which the constricted pylorus is incised (pyloromyotomy) and sutured to relieve the obstruction.

Prognosis
The prognosis is good with prompt surgical intervention.

Prevention
No prevention is known.

Patient Teaching
Parents need instruction in the care of the incision. Reinforce the importance of postoperative visits.

Hirschsprung Disease (Congenital Aganglionic Megacolon)
Description
Hirschsprung disease, a congenital condition, is an impairment of intestinal motility that causes obstruction of the distal colon (Fig. 2.32A and B).

ICD-10-CM Code   Q43.1 *(Hirschsprung disease)*

Symptoms and Signs
The symptoms and signs vary slightly, depending on the age of the child experiencing an exacerbation of the condition. In the neonatal period, the newborn fails to pass meconium within 48 hours after birth. The infant may have bile-stained or fecal vomitus and does not want to feed. The abdomen becomes distended and swollen.

After the neonatal period, the symptoms and signs include a failure to thrive, with obstinate constipation, vomiting, and abdominal distention. When the condition worsens, the infant may become feverish and may have explosive, watery diarrhea.

The older child exhibits more chronic symptoms, such as constipation, abdominal distention, ribbonlike stools that are foul smelling, easily palpable fecal masses, and visible peristalsis. The child appears malnourished and anemic.

Patient Screening
Infants or children with GI symptoms of bile-stained or fecal vomitus require prompt assessment, as do those children with obstinate constipation, especially when combined with vomiting and abdominal distention. Any child experiencing ribbonlike stools should also have a prompt assessment.

Etiology
The defect lies in the abnormal innervation of the intrinsic musculature of the bowel wall. In Hirschsprung disease, the parasympathetic nerve ganglion cells are absent in a segment of the colon, usually in the rectosigmoid area. This deficiency of innervation results in a lack of peristalsis in the affected portion of the colon and the succeeding backup of fecal material. The proximal portion of the colon becomes grossly distended, and intestinal obstruction results.

Statistics indicate that males are more likely than females to have a megacolon and that the risk is increased in children with Down syndrome. It is believed to be a familial congenital disease.

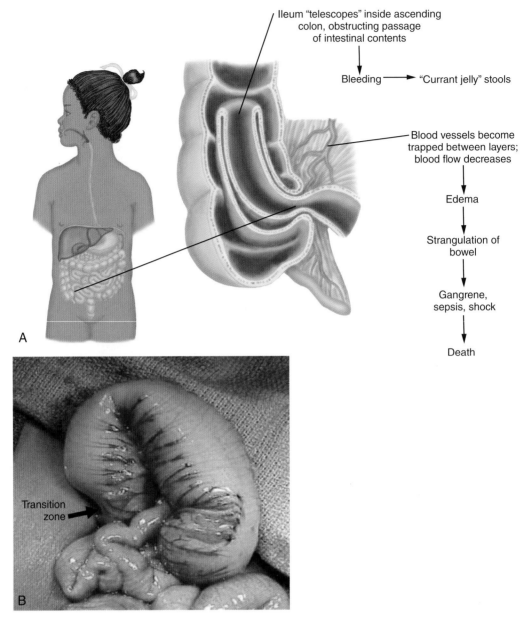

Ileum "telescopes" inside ascending colon, obstructing passage of intestinal contents

Bleeding ⟶ "Currant jelly" stools

Blood vessels become trapped between layers; blood flow decreases

Edema

Strangulation of bowel

Gangrene, sepsis, shock

Death

Transition zone

• **Fig. 2.32** (A) Hirschsprung disease. (B) The absence of intramural ganglion cells prevents intestinal peristalsis through segments affected by Hirschsprung disease, causing a functional bowel obstruction. The involved segment appears narrow when compared with the distended, obstructed proximal bowel, which possesses normal ganglion cells. (A, From James K, et al: *Nursing care of children*, ed 4, St. Louis, 2013, Saunders; B, From McIntire S et al: *Zitelli and Davis' atlas of pediatric physical diagnosis*, ed 8, 2023, Elsevier.)

Diagnosis

Diagnosis is based on family history, the clinical picture, radiographic studies of the bowel, and, finally, biopsy to confirm the absence of the ganglionic cells.

Treatment

Treatment consists of relief of the obstruction by surgical intervention; the affected bowel is excised, and the normal colon is joined to the anus. A temporary colostomy is performed proximal to the aganglionic section of the colon. Electrolyte and fluid balance must be maintained. After the colon recovers function (6 months to 1 year), the colostomy is closed.

Prognosis

The prognosis varies, depending on the extent of colon involvement and the success of surgical intervention. Ideally the colon will heal and the colostomy can be closed.

Prevention

No prevention is known for this apparently familial congenital disease.

Patient Teaching

The parents and the child require training on caring for the stoma, as well as dealing with the colostomy bags and drainage. Help and encourage families to find and contact support groups and other community resources. The parents, the family, and the child may require counseling. Provide nutritional and dietary information.

Metabolic Disorders

Cystic Fibrosis

Description

Cystic fibrosis (CF), an autosomal recessive inherited disorder, is a chronic dysfunction of a gene called *cystic fibrosis transmembrane conductance regulator (CFTR)* that affects multiple body systems. It is the most common fatal genetic disease.

ICD-10-CM Code	E84.9 *(Cystic, fibrosis, unspecified)*
	(E84.0–E84.9 = 5 codes of specificity)

Cystic fibrosis is coded according to the region involved. Refer to the physician's diagnosis and then to the current edition of the ICD-10-CM coding manual to ensure the greatest specificity of pathology.

Symptoms and Signs

Symptoms may become apparent soon after birth or may develop in childhood. The disease primarily attacks the lungs and the digestive system, producing copious thick and sticky mucus that accumulates and blocks glandular ducts. The clinical effects of CF can be immense and include dry paroxysmal cough, exercise intolerance, pneumonia, bulky diarrhea, vomiting, and bowel obstruction. Pancreatic changes occur, with fat and fiber replacing normal tissue. Involvement of sweat glands causes increased concentrations of salt in sweat. Normal growth and ability to thrive are reduced (Fig. 2.33). Sinus infections and diarrhea often accompany the other symptoms. Infertility is common.

Patient Screening

In many of these children, the disease is suspected during the neonatal period while they are still in the newborn nursery. The condition may become apparent during routine well-baby examinations. When parents report that the child has developed a cough producing thick, sticky mucus, or failure to thrive despite adequate intake, prompt assessment of the child is indicated.

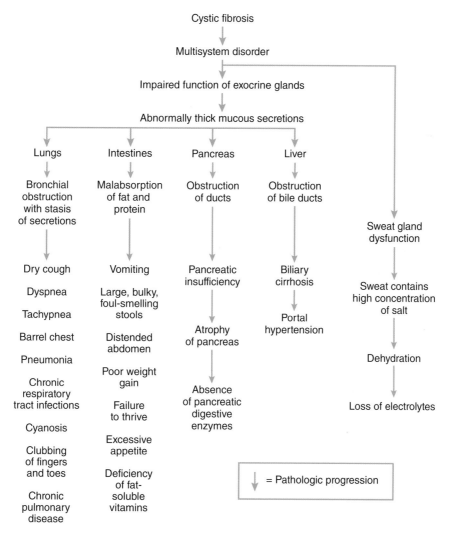

• **Fig. 2.33** Major clinical manifestations of cystic fibrosis in a child.

Etiology

CF is an inherited disorder and is transmitted as an autosomal recessive trait (see the Genetic Disorders and Syndromes section).

Diagnosis

Genetic testing can be done prenatally if parents are known to be carriers of a genetic mutation for this disorder. The diagnostic workup includes family history, pulmonary function test, chest radiography, and stool studies. The sweat test reveals elevated levels of sodium and chloride and confirms the diagnosis.

Treatment

CF is considered a fatal disease. However, early diagnosis and treatment have greatly increased life expectancy in the past few decades. Treatment includes supportive measures that help the child lead as normal a life as possible and that prevent pulmonary infections. These measures include the use of a high-calorie, high-sodium chloride diet; chest physiotherapy; supplementation of vitamins A, D, E, and K; increased fluid intake; and pancreatic enzyme supplementation to aid in digestion. Patients may require insulin to treat CF-associated diabetes. Broad-spectrum antibiotics are used aggressively to treat infection, and drugs that thin the mucus are given. Percussive therapy to dislodge mucus is helpful. Breathing treatments with aerosols using nebulizers is also helpful. Oxygen therapy may be required. Some patients with CF may be candidates for lung transplantation. Patients with CF are encouraged to avoid exposure to dust, dirt, household chemicals, smoke, fumes, fireplace smoke, mold, and mildew.

Prognosis

Because CF is considered a fatal disease, the long-term prognosis is not favorable. Early diagnosis and compliance with treatment have improved the chances for these children to have as near normal a life as possible and an increased life expectancy. Many have graduated from high school, and some have completed a college degree. At the present time, the projected life expectancy of a patient born between the years of 2015 and 2019 with CF in the United States has extended into the 40s, according to the Cystic Fibrosis Foundation registry data.

Prevention

CF is genetic, and no prevention is known.

Patient Teaching

The family needs emotional support and teaching about the disease; referral to genetic counseling is helpful. Help and encourage the family to find and contact support groups and other resources in the community and reputable online resources.

Phenylketonuria

Description

Phenylketonuria (PKU) is an inborn error in the metabolism of amino acids and, when not corrected, causes brain damage and intellectual developmental disorder.

ICD-10-CM Code	E70.0 *(Classical phenylketonuria)*

Symptoms and Signs

In this defect, an enzyme needed to change an amino acid (phenylalanine) in the body into another substance (tyrosine) is lacking. As a result, phenylalanine accumulates in blood and urine and is toxic to the brain. Symptoms may not begin until the infant is 4 months old when a characteristic musty odor of the child's perspiration and urine is noted. Other signs include rashes, irritability, hyperactivity, personality disorders, and evidence of arrested brain development.

Patient Screening

Screening of all newborns is mandatory in all states, and a positive result on screening indicates immediate dietary intervention. Prompt assessment is indicated when a parent or caregiver reports that the infant emanates a musty smell, especially in urine.

Etiology

PKU is inherited as an autosomal recessive trait and causes defective enzymatic conversion in protein metabolism, resulting in the accumulation of phenylalanine in blood (see the Genetic Disorders and Syndromes section).

Diagnosis

PKU is detected by mandatory screening of blood in the newborn. A positive Guthrie test result indicates the presence of phenylalanine in the blood. The urine is tested for phenylalanine derivatives.

Treatment

The treatment is to place the infant on a phenylalanine-free diet, which allows the infant to grow with normal brain development. Individuals with PKU must eat a diet low in phenylalanine for the rest of their lives. Because natural proteins contain phenylalanine, the patient must remain on a protein-restricted diet. Restrictions or elimination of the following foods is required: meat, chicken, fish, cheese, nuts, and dairy products. The newborn cannot have breast milk because of its high levels of phenylalanine. Intake of some starchy foods, including potatoes, corn, pasta, and bread, requires close monitoring. The sweetener aspartame used in diet soda and diet food is metabolized into substances including phenylalanine.

Prognosis

The prognosis is excellent when the infant is placed on a phenylalanine-free diet soon after birth. Late dietary intervention does not reverse the brain damage.

Prevention

No prevention is known.

Patient Teaching

Close follow-up with testing for phenylalanine levels in the blood may allow for some modification of the difficult dietary restrictions. Emotional support is important for the child and the parents. Genetic counseling is recommended. Help parents find the essential dietary information listing foods and substances high in phenylalanine.

Endocrine Syndromes

Klinefelter syndrome and Turner syndrome are examples of genetic, chromosomal diseases that are not inherited. They result from nondisjunction, or the failure of a chromosome pair to separate, during *gamete* production (Fig. 2.34).

Humans normally have 46 chromosomes: 22 pairs of autosomes and two sex chromosomes. The technical notation for a human female is 46,XX and for a male, 46,XY. In a fertilized ovum, one chromosome from each pair of autosomes originates from the mother's ovum and the other from the father's sperm. Each ovum normally contains a single X chromosome. Sperm cells may contain either an X or a Y chromosome. If a sperm bearing the X chromosome fertilizes the ovum, the fetus develops into a female. A sperm carrying the Y chromosome produces a male fetus. Sometimes, through what may be described as an accident of nature, extra chromosomes or the absence of chromosomes in the fertilized ovum cause congenital syndromes with a variety of physical and mental developmental effects (Fig. 2.35).

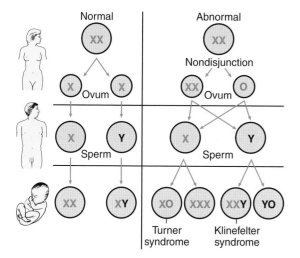

• **Fig. 2.34** Pathogenesis of sex chromosome abnormalities (Turner and Klinefelter). (From Damjanov I: *Pathology for the health professions*, ed 4, St. Louis, 2011, Saunders.)

Klinefelter Syndrome

Description

Klinefelter syndrome (KS; XXY condition) is male hypogonadism that appears in males after puberty with at least two X chromosomes and one or more Y chromosomes (typically the 47,XXY pattern).

ICD-10-CM Code	Q98.4 *(Klinefelter syndrome, unspecified)* (Q98.0–Q98.9 = 9 codes of specificity)

Symptoms and Signs

The presence of two X chromosomes in affected males causes abnormal development of the testes and reduced levels of the male hormone testosterone. Puberty begins at the usual time and usually results in a normal-sized penis, but the testes are small, and body hair is scant. In general, the person appears normal, except for exceptionally long legs, above-average height, and reduced muscle development. The most significant problem associated with KS is infertility resulting from azoospermia. Only rarely are these patients fertile; they have the mosaic form that carries the extra X chromosome in only one cell line. Other alterations include a mild delay in language acquisition and an increased risk of behavioral and learning disabilities. Some affected individuals have mild to more significant intellectual impairment. The mammary glands may be enlarged in about half the cases. Possible complications include osteoporosis and chronic pulmonary diseases. Other complications may include autoimmune disorders, venous disease, osteoporosis, breast cancer, or tooth decay.

Patient Screening

The male infant appears normal at birth, and symptoms are usually not noted until puberty. The condition may be discovered during a routine sports or precamp physical examination. In other situations, parents may call to discuss the delay in sexual maturation of the young male. Considering the anxiety that the family may be experiencing, an assessment should be performed promptly.

Etiology

KS results from the presence of at least two X chromosomes, typically the 47,XXY pattern. The extra X chromosome may be of either maternal or paternal origin. Other variants include XXYY, XXXY, and XXXXY. The disease is not inherited but results from a nondisjunction during gamete formation. This disorder affects an estimated 1 in 500 liveborn males.

Diagnosis

The diagnostic workup includes a physical examination, serum and urine gonadotropin level determination, and semen analysis. A chromosomal smear analysis confirms the

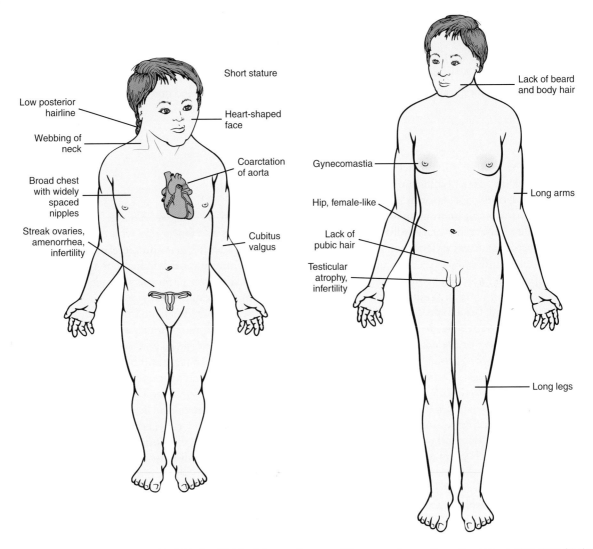

• **Fig. 2.35** Line art comparing features of individuals with Klinefelter syndrome and Turner syndrome. (From Damjanov I: *Pathology for the health professions*, ed 4, St. Louis, 2012, Saunders.)

diagnosis and differentiates between the mosaic and true forms of Klinefelter syndrome.

Treatment

At the time of normal puberty, long-term hormone replacement with testosterone is given by injection or a transdermal patch, usually under the supervision of an endocrinologist. Testosterone is necessary for the maintenance of normal sexual function and normal muscle and bone mass. However, fertility cannot be restored. Many patients report an improvement in energy and emotional stability with hormone therapy. Supplemental calcium intake is prescribed to help prevent osteoporosis.

Prognosis

There is no cure for the syndrome, and natural fatherhood probably will never be achieved. Alteration of intelligence correlates with the number of extra X chromosomes. Many of these males achieve their goals in their chosen professions and are productive members of society.

Prevention

Because KS is a chromosomal disorder, no prevention is known.

Patient Teaching

Inform the patient and the family of the importance of follow-up appointments to monitor hormone replacement and identify the target dosage. Explain the importance of adhering to the prescribed dosage schedule of medication to maintain proper blood levels. Describe the possible adverse effects of testosterone therapy, such as insomnia, anxiety, tremors, and dizziness; tell the patient to report these or other symptoms to the attending physician. Refer the patient and the family to Klinefelter Syndrome and Associates for support, meetings, and conventions.

Turner Syndrome

Description

Turner syndrome is a chromosomal disease that occurs in females with a single sex chromosome, 45,XO.

ICD-10-CM Code	Q55.4 *(Other congenital malformations of vas deferens, epididymis, seminal vesicles, and prostate)*
	Q96.9 *(Turner syndrome, unspecified)*
	(Q96.0–Q96.9 = 7 codes of specificity)

Symptoms and Signs

Turner syndrome is a disorder of gonadal dysgenesis in females. At birth, the ovaries are immature or absent, and the female infant appears short, with low-set ears, swollen hands and feet, and webbing of the neck. As these children grow, there is an absence of sexual maturation, along with amenorrhea, sterility, dwarfism, and cardiac and kidney defects. Cardiac defects may include coarctation of the aorta in the infant and, in adulthood, aortic dissection caused by cardiovascular disease. If ovaries were present at birth, they slowly begin to disappear, leaving only small amounts of tissue. If the ovaries do not disappear, they typically contain no eggs. Most of these female children may experience delayed speech and ambulation; however, they usually are of normal intelligence.

Patient Screening

Well-baby examinations may reveal signs of the disorder. The baby is referred for chromosome studies to confirm the diagnosis. As the child matures, appointments may be needed to assess possible cardiac or renal disorders.

Etiology

Turner syndrome results from a missing or partially missing X chromosome.

Diagnosis

Chromosomal smear studies show only one X chromosome instead of the normal 46,XX chromosomal pattern. The syndrome can be diagnosed by prenatal testing or after birth.

Treatment

Symptoms can be reduced by estrogen and growth hormone therapy. Surgical correction may be indicated for certain anomalies, such as webbing of the neck. Emotional support for the patient and the family helps them develop strategies for coping with low self-esteem and body image disturbance. Potential cardiac or renal disorders that may develop will need to be managed by specialists in those areas of medicine. Referrals to a geneticist and endocrinologist are also helpful for managing the symptoms.

Prognosis

There is no cure for this genetic disorder; however, the prognosis is good if the patient has no other complicating conditions, including cardiac or kidney disorders. The ovaries may fail to develop at birth or slowly throughout their growth and development. Sexual development may be slowed down or even stopped when they become a teenager. Menses may cease. Most females with Turner syndrome are unable to conceive without the aid of fertility treatment.

Prevention

Because Turner syndrome is a chromosomal disorder, there is no prevention.

Patient Teaching

Help the child and the parents find and contact support groups and community resources that are available online and in person. Networking with other individuals who are diagnosed with the syndrome can be beneficial and there are support groups that offer services and information that will support information given by the health care provider.

Childhood Diseases

Nothing causes more anxiety than a seriously ill child. Pathologic processes in children pose special threats because children are constantly changing physically and functionally. The journey through childhood normally results in the maturation and expansion of the body's natural immune defense mechanisms. In addition, rapid advances in treatment and preventive medicine have enabled us to control many infectious diseases that formerly caused serious illness, disabling complications, and even death. However, many infections and disease syndromes can interrupt the normal growth and development of any child. The following section describes common diseases that affect children.

Infectious Diseases

Although the infant acquires limited natural immunity from the mother, the growing child is vulnerable to many infectious diseases and the disabilities that they cause. Many of these communicable diseases can be prevented. Dramatic results have been achieved in pediatric medicine through routine prophylactic immunization with vaccines that build specific and prolonged protection. To prevent epidemics of contagious diseases, all states in the United States require that children receive vaccinations before entering school (Fig. 2.36) (see the discussion of immunity in Chapter 3).

Chickenpox (Varicella Zoster)
Description
Chickenpox is a highly contagious, acute viral infection that is common in children and young adults.

ICD-10-CM Code	B01.9 *(Varicella without complication)*
	(B01.0–B01.9 = 7 codes of specificity)

Table 1	COVID-19 vaccination recommendations have changed. Find the latest recommendations at www.cdc.gov/covidschedule																

Recommended Child and Adolescent Immunization Schedule for ages 18 years or younger, United States, 2023

These recommendations must be read with the notes that follow. For those who fall behind or start late, provide catch-up vaccination at the earliest opportunity as indicated by the green bars.
To determine minimum intervals between doses, see the catch-up schedule (Table 2).

Vaccine	Birth	1 mo	2 mos	4 mos	6 mos	9 mos	12 mos	15 mos	18 mos	19–23 mos	2–3 yrs	4–6 yrs	7–10 yrs	11–12 yrs	13–15 yrs	16 yrs	17–18 yrs
Hepatitis B (HepB)	1st dose	←---- 2nd dose ----→			←----------------------- 3rd dose -----------------------→												
Rotavirus (RV): RV1 (2-dose series), RV5 (3-dose series)			1st dose	2nd dose	See Notes												
Diphtheria, tetanus, acellular pertussis (DTaP <7 yrs)			1st dose	2nd dose	3rd dose			←---- 4th dose ----→				5th dose					
Haemophilus influenzae type b (Hib)			1st dose	2nd dose	See Notes		3rd or 4th dose, See Notes										
Pneumococcal conjugate (PCV13, PCV15)			1st dose	2nd dose	3rd dose		←---- 4th dose ----→										
Inactivated poliovirus (IPV <18yrs)			1st dose	2nd dose	←------------------------ 3rd dose ------------------------→							4th dose					See Notes
COVID-19 (1vCOV-mRNA, 2vCOV-mRNA, 1vCOV-aPS)					2- or 3- dose primary series and booster (See Notes)												
Influenza (IIV4)					Annual vaccination 1 or 2 doses									Annual vaccination 1 dose only			
or													**or**				
Influenza (LAIV4)											Annual vaccination 1 or 2 doses			Annual vaccination 1 dose only			
Measles, mumps, rubella (MMR)					See Notes		←---- 1st dose ----→					2nd dose					
Varicella (VAR)							←---- 1st dose ----→					2nd dose					
Hepatitis A (HepA)					See Notes		2-dose series, See Notes										
Tetanus, diphtheria, acellular pertussis (Tdap ≥7 yrs)														1 dose			
Human papillomavirus (HPV)														See Notes			
Meningococcal (MenACWY-D ≥9 mos, MenACWY-CRM ≥2 mos, MenACWY-TT ≥2years)							See Notes							1st dose		2nd dose	
Meningococcal B (MenB-4C, MenB-FHbp)																See Notes	
Pneumococcal polysaccharide (PPSV23)												See Notes					
Dengue (DEN4CYD; 9-16 yrs)														Seropositive in endemic dengue areas (See Notes)			

Range of recommended ages for all children	Recommended vaccination can begin in this age group	Recommended vaccination based on shared clinical decision-making
Range of recommended ages for catch-up vaccination		No recommendation/ not applicable
Range of recommended ages for certain high-risk groups		

• **Fig. 2.36** Centers for Disease Control and Prevention (CDC) schedule of recommended childhood and adolescent immunization.

Symptoms and Signs

Chickenpox is a systemic disease with superficial cutaneous lesions that begin as red macules that progress to *papules* and then finally become *vesicles* that form crusts. The lesions are first seen on the face or the trunk and then spread over the extremities; they can be distributed everywhere on the body and even have been found internally. A day or two before the rash appears, the patient may experience fever, malaise, and anorexia. The lesions can continue to erupt for 3 to 4 days and cause intense itching. Recovery is usually complete within 2 weeks, leaving the person with lifetime immunity. Some possible complications include secondary bacterial infection, viral pneumonia, conjunctival ulcers, and Reye syndrome (Fig. 2.37).

Patient Screening

Contagious diseases present a challenge in the patient screening process. Many physicians prefer not to have the contagious patient in the regular reception area. Many pediatricians have a sick child waiting room and a regular waiting room. At offices that have no sick child waiting area, the child is immediately placed in an examination room and the physician is notified. Some physicians prefer

• **Fig. 2.37** Chickenpox. The rash begins with macules, which turn into severe papules. Symptoms can last a few days to 2 weeks. (From Callen JP, et al: *Color atlas of dermatology*, ed 2, Philadelphia, 2000, Saunders.)

to have a staff person make a telephone call to the parents ahead of the clinic appointment to obtain information on symptoms, body temperature, and so on, as well as the telephone number where the parent can be reached. The physician reviews the information and calls the parent back to discuss the situation.

Etiology

The causative organism is varicella zoster virus (VZV), also known as *human herpes virus 3*, a member of the herpes virus group. The virus is transmitted via direct or indirect spread of droplet nuclei from the respiratory tract of the infected person or a carrier. Fluid from cutaneous lesions is also infectious, but dried crusty lesions are not contagious. The patient is considered contagious for 1 to 2 days before the eruptions until about 6 days after the eruptions. The incubation period is 2 to 3 weeks.

Diagnosis

Chickenpox usually is diagnosed on the basis of the history of exposure and the presence of characteristic cutaneous eruptions. Although laboratory testing is not usually necessary, VZV can be visualized when a culture of vesicular fluid is examined microscopically. After the infection, antibodies are found in the serum.

Treatment

Palliative treatment to alleviate pruritus includes cool bicarbonate of soda baths, followed by cornstarch dusting or the application of calamine lotion. This helps control scratching that can lead to secondary infection and scarring. Other comfort measures include the administration of acetaminophen for fever and pain. *Caution*: Aspirin is *not* given to children with chickenpox because of the risk of Reye syndrome. In some cases, treatment with antiviral drugs (e.g., acyclovir) may be prescribed. The patient must be isolated until all lesions have crusted.

Prognosis

The prognosis for recovery from chickenpox is good. The patient may have scarring resulting from the eruptions. Individuals who have had chickenpox are at risk of developing herpes zoster (shingles) later in life.

Prevention

A varicella virus vaccine (varicella virus vaccine [Varivax]) is available for protection against chickenpox. For children, an injection of the vaccine at age 12 to 15 months is recommended, with a second dose between 4 and 6 years of age. Another vaccine that can protect against varicella is ProQuad; a combination of measles, mumps, rubella, and varicella vaccine.

Patients who are immunocompromised or otherwise at high risk can be given the varicella zoster immune globulin within 10 days of exposure.

Patient Teaching

Reinforce the need for thorough hand washing, use of tissues during coughing or sneezing episodes, and proper handling and disposal of soiled tissues. Encourage parents to minimize contact between these children and others during

ENRICHMENT

Prevention of Disease Spread During Athletic Events

Precautions to be taken during athletic events or participation help prevent the spread of bacteria and viruses. Observe ball handlers to see if they have a tendency to put their saliva on their hands to have a better grip on the ball. This has been banned in some areas of the world due to the COVID-19 outbreaks. Encourage individuals to wash their hands with soap and water, use hand sanitizer, and shower after athletic activities. Wrestling or any contact sport where a mat is used creates an area that holds body perspiration and saliva. After each contact set, it is important that the mat be washed down with a 10% bleach solution. Any uniform or piece of equipment that has blood on it must be cleansed with the 10% bleach solution. Athletes should shower after contact sports, such as wrestling.

ENRICHMENT

Vaccines

A vaccine is a suspension of dead or attenuated organisms given to stimulate an active immune response that produces more or less permanent resistance to pathogenic organisms and viruses. Booster doses are smaller amounts of the original vaccine given at specified intervals to maintain serum antibody levels. Vaccines are controlled for potency and stability and are tested for safety and effectiveness. Some vaccines are grown in bird eggs or in animal organs or are weakened with chemicals. The patient is screened for certain allergies or previous reactions to vaccines. Local responses of soreness, redness, and swelling at the site of injection are common. Untoward responses include high fever, generalized swelling, difficulty breathing, severe headache, arthralgia, and seizures. Any of these symptoms should be reported immediately to the physician.

Toxoids contain altered forms of bacterial toxins to stimulate antibody production and thereby impart protection against toxins. Individuals who are severely immunocompromised must not be given vaccines containing live microorganisms. It is also recommended that pregnant females not receive live attenuated vaccines.

the contagious period, which is 1 to 2 days before the eruptions until about 6 days after the eruptions.

Diphtheria

Description

Diphtheria is an acute communicable disease that causes necrosis of the mucous membrane in the respiratory tract.

ICD-10-CM Code | A36.9 *(Diphtheria, unspecified)*

(A36.0–A36.9 = 12 codes of specificity)
Refer to the physician's diagnosis and then to the current edition ICD-10-CM coding manual to ensure the greatest specificity of pathology.

Symptoms and Signs

The patient, most often a child, has a sore throat, dysphagia, a cough, hoarseness, and chills. Fever, swollen regional lymph nodes, foul breath, and, in some cases, cyanosis can be noted. As the bacteria invade the nasopharynx, they multiply and produce a powerful exotoxin that travels in blood throughout the body. Locally, the infection and inflammation cause grayish patches of thick mucous membrane, known as *pseudomembrane* or *false membrane*, to appear along the respiratory tract. The membrane, which can be extensive, is composed of bacteria, inflammatory cells, dead tissue, and fibrin; it is surrounded by inflammation and swelling that can interfere with airway function, impairing swallowing and speech. As the toxin is absorbed, it affects other vital organ systems, with many possible complications, including otitis media, pneumonia, myocarditis, and paralysis.

Carriers, although infected, remain asymptomatic and do not experience active infection themselves.

Patient Screening

Children with fever, chills, and respiratory difficulties require prompt assessment. When a parent reports a child with respiratory difficulties, most protocols recommend that the child be seen in an emergency facility.

Etiology

The causative organism, *Corynebacterium diphtheriae*, is present in the nasopharynx of infected individuals or carriers and is transmitted via airborne respiratory droplets. The incubation period is 2 to 5 days, however the range may be from 1 to 10 days. The patient is contagious for 2 to 6 weeks if untreated. Carriers of the disease remain asymptomatic but can infect the inadequately immunized individual.

Diagnosis

The presence of the characteristic membrane adhering to the throat is diagnostic. A culture of the throat and staining would be positive for *C. diphtheriae*, and antibodies are found in the serum. Immunity or susceptibility can be determined by the Schick test.

Treatment

Diphtheria antitoxin is given as soon as possible. The administration of antibiotics, such as penicillin and erythromycin, is indicated to kill the organism. The patient is isolated, restricted to bed rest, and given a diet as tolerated. The patient is observed for possible complications related to systemic involvement. Carriers are given antibiotics to eliminate the organisms from the respiratory tract.

Prognosis

With prompt intervention and completion of antibiotic drug therapy, the prognosis is good.

Prevention

Diphtheria, once common in North America and Europe, can be prevented by the administration of diphtheria toxoid to produce active immunity. Vaccination begins at 2 to 3 months in the form of the diphtheria-tetanus-pertussis vaccine, with booster doses given at appropriate intervals during childhood. Adults should receive booster vaccinations to ensure that immunity is maintained. Therefore when an injection to prevent tetanus is administered to adults, the inoculation tetanus-diphtheria-pertussis (TDaP) should be administered. This is also helpful in preventing outbreaks of whooping cough.

Patient Teaching

Reinforce the need for good hand washing and the use of tissues during coughing or sneezing episodes. Instruct on the handling and disposal of soiled tissues. Encourage parents to minimize contact between these children and others during the contagious period, which continues for 1 to 2 days after starting antibiotic therapy. Emphasize the importance of routine immunizations for children.

Mumps (Epidemic Parotitis)

Description

Mumps is an acute communicable viral disease causing inflammation and swelling of one or both parotid glands.

ICD-10-CM Code	B26.9 *(Mumps without complication)*
	(B26.0–B26.9 = 11 codes of specificity)

Refer to the physician's diagnosis and then to the current edition of the ICD-10-CM coding manual to ensure the greatest specificity of pathology.

Symptoms and Signs

The patient, usually a child, has tenderness in the neck in front of and below the ears in the region of the parotid glands and pain on swallowing (Fig. 2.38). Patients also may experience a rash, headache, muscle aches, and a low-grade fever, with loss of appetite and an earache that is aggravated by chewing. A common complication of the disease in the adult male is mumps orchitis, which may lead to sterility. Often the infection is subclinical, without noticeable symptoms.

Patient Screening

Contagious diseases present a challenge in the patient screening process. Many physicians prefer not to have the contagious patient in the reception area. When the parents feel an office visit is warranted, the child is immediately placed in an examination room and the physician is notified. In some situations the provider may wish to perform a telehealth visit to decrease exposure among patients who are in the office.

• **Fig. 2.38** Mumps. This young boy with mumps has unilateral parotid swelling on the right side. (From Patton K, et al: *Anatomy & physiology*, ed 11, 2022, Elsevier.)

Etiology

The causative agent of mumps is an airborne virus that is spread by droplet nuclei from the respiratory tract. The average incubation period is long, usually 16 to 18 days with a range of 12 to 25 days. The patient is considered contagious for 2 days before onset of the swelling of the parotid glands and up to 5 days thereafter. Lifelong immunity develops after a clinical or subclinical infection; active immunization with the mumps vaccine also affords prolonged immunity. Quarantining is recommended to keep the illness from spreading.

Diagnosis

Diagnosis is made from a history of exposure and a clinical picture that includes swelling of the parotid glands. The male patient is assessed for tenderness of the testes. Serum amylase is often elevated. Reverse transcription polymerase chain reaction tests are performed to diagnose the condition. CSF and urine may also be used for diagnosing this condition.

Treatment

Acetaminophen is given, and warm or cold compresses are applied for pain. A soft or liquid diet can help minimize discomfort when eating. A male patient experiencing testicular tenderness and swelling may need scrotal support. Isolation of the patient is helpful in preventing the spread of the disease.

Prognosis

Most children recover from mumps; however, orchitis, meningitis, and encephalitis are possible complications of mumps.

Prevention

Childhood immunization is the best prevention. Children should receive the first MMR (measles, mumps, rubella) immunization at age 12 to 15 months of age. The second dose should be given at age 4 to 6 years and before the child enters school. An unimmunized person should be referred to a physician for active immunization within 48 hours of contact to prevent or alter the severity of the disease. Good hand washing and proper handling of soiled tissues help prevent the spread of the disease among family members and other contacts.

Patient Teaching

Reinforce the need for good hand washing and proper handling and disposal of soiled tissues. Discuss the airborne viruses responsible for mumps and the means of preventing the spread of the disease. Emphasize the importance of routine immunizations for children.

Pertussis (Whooping Cough)

Description

Whooping cough is a highly contagious bacterial infection of the respiratory tract.

ICD-10-CM Code	A37.90 (*Whooping cough, unspecified species without pneumonia*) (A37.0–A37.91 = 8 codes of specificity)

Symptoms and Signs

The disease has three stages: (1) the highly contagious catarrhal stage, when the child seems to have a common cold; (2) the paroxysmal stage, when the cough becomes violent, ending in a high-pitched inspiratory whoop, often followed by vomiting of thick mucus; and (3) the convalescent stage, when the cough gradually diminishes.

Patient Screening

A child exhibiting symptoms of violent coughing with a high-pitched inspiratory whoop and vomiting of thick mucus requires prompt attention.

Etiology

The pertussis bacillus *Bordetella pertussis* reproduces in the respiratory tract, where it releases a toxin that leads to necrosis of the mucosa, producing a thick exudate. It is transmitted by droplet nuclei spread via direct or indirect contact with the nasopharyngeal secretions of the contagious patient.

Diagnosis

Bacterial studies of nasopharyngeal mucus are positive for the pertussis bacillus. A PCR test can also be performed. The patient's WBC count usually is elevated.

Treatment

Macrolide antibiotics such as erythromycin, azithromycin, and clarithromycin are the preferred treatment. Fluid intake is encouraged to prevent dehydration, and a nutritious diet is important to prevent weight loss. Quiet and rest are required because episodes of prolonged coughing cause exhaustion and weakness. The patient should be observed closely for respiratory distress. Bronchopneumonia, convulsions, or hemorrhages are possible complications of severe disease.

Prognosis

With prompt intervention, hydration monitoring and maintenance, and antibiotic therapy, the prognosis is good. However, if untreated, pertussis can be fatal.

Prevention

Pertussis can be prevented by immunization with the pertussis vaccine. Childhood immunization is the best prevention, and a booster is recommended in early adolescence. Good hand washing and proper handling of soiled tissues help prevent the spread of the disease among family members and other contacts. Emphasize the importance of routine immunizations for children. The newly developed acellular vaccine has been shown to be safer with fewer side effects. An increase in the incidence of whooping cough in adults has been noted. It is recommended that all adults receive TDaP or Td immunization every 10 years to reduce the incidence of whooping cough.

Patient Teaching

Reinforce the need for good hand washing and proper handling and disposal of soiled tissues. Discuss the airborne microbe responsible for pertussis and the methods of preventing airborne spread of the disease. Emphasize the importance of routine immunizations.

Measles (Rubeola)

Description

Measles is an acute, highly contagious viral disease.

ICD-10-CM Code	B05.9 *(Measles without complication)* (B05.0–B05.9 = 7 codes of specificity)

Symptoms and Signs

Early symptoms include cough, coryza, conjunctivitis, and photophobia. The child has a fever, followed, in 3 to 7 days, by a red, blotchy rash. The rash starts behind the ears, hairline, and forehead and then progresses down the body (Fig. 2.39). Before the eruption of the rash, Koplik spots can be detected on the oral mucosa as tiny white spots on a red background (Fig. 2.40).

Patient Screening

Contagious diseases present a challenge in the patient screening process. Many physicians prefer not to have the contagious patient in the reception area. When the parents feel an office visit is warranted, the child is immediately placed in an examination room and the physician is notified. Some physicians prefer to have a staff person telephone the parents to obtain information on symptoms, body temperature, and so on, as well as a contact telephone number. The physician reviews the information and either calls the

• **Fig. 2.39** Rubeola (measles). (From Hockenberry M, Wilson D, Rodgers C: *Wong's nursing care of infants and children,* ed 11, St. Louis, 2019, Elsevier.)

• **Fig. 2.40** Koplik spots. Gray-white papules of the buccal mucosa in a patient with measles. (From Paller A, Mancini A: *Paller and Mancini - Hurwitz clinical pediatric dermatology: a textbook of skin disorders of childhood and adolescence,* ed 6, 2023, Elsevier.)

parent back or has the staff person call the parent back with instructions for care.

Etiology

The causative agent of measles is the measles virus, specifically a *paramyxovirus* of the genus *Morbillivirus*. The infection is airborne, spread by direct contact with secretions from the nose or throat of the infected person. The rash appears about 14 days after the patient is exposed. The patient is contagious from about 4 days before the onset of the rash until about 4 days after the onset.

Diagnosis

Diagnosis is based on a history of exposure and the clinical picture, which includes a rash and the presence of Koplik spots on the oral mucosa.

Treatment

Acetaminophen, ibuprofen, or other nonaspirin medications may be given to treat the fever. If the fever is persistently high, tepid sponge baths may be given. Treatment is aimed at making the patient more comfortable during the outbreak. Increasing fluids will help prevent dehydration and rest is recommended. Lowering lights may help the patient feel more comfortable. If a secondary infection occurs, antibiotics are prescribed to treat the infection.

Prognosis

The prognosis for uncomplicated measles is good. Complications of measles include pneumonia, otitis media, conjunctivitis, and encephalitis. Refer to the Alert box about Subacute Sclerosing Panencephalitis regarding the delayed complications of the disease.

Prevention

Inoculation with the live measles vaccine is given during childhood to protect the individual and prevent epidemics of the disease. The first combination MMR vaccine is given at age 12 to 15 months, with a booster vaccine given between 4 and 6 years. Measles immune globulin given 5 days after exposure to the disease creates passive immunity in unimmunized individuals at high risk. An attack of the disease usually creates immunity for life.

Patient Teaching

Reinforce the necessity of good hand washing and proper handling and disposal of soiled tissues. Discuss the airborne microbe responsible for measles, and discuss methods of preventing airborne spread of the disease. Emphasize the importance of routine immunizations for children.

❶ ALERT!

Recent outbreaks of measles, as well as mumps, have occurred in communities where parents have refused immunizations for their children.

Rubella (German Measles, 3-Day Measles)

Description

Rubella, a highly contagious viral disease, resembles measles clinically but it has a shorter course and fewer complications.

ICD-10-CM Code	B06.9 *(Rubella without complication)* (B06.0–B06.9 = 8 codes of specificity)

Symptoms and Signs

In this viral disease, the child has a rose-colored, slightly elevated rash that appears first on the face and head and then progresses downward on the body (Fig. 2.41). In addition, the child has a low-grade fever and can have tenderness and enlargement of the lymph nodes. Complications include transient arthritis, myocarditis, and hemorrhagic manifestations.

❶ ALERT!

Subacute Sclerosing Panencephalitis

Parents are encouraged to have their children immunized against measles.

Subacute sclerosing panencephalitis (SSPE), an infectious condition of the CNS, is considered a rare disorder and is listed as such in the National Organization for Rare Disorders. SSPE, one of three forms of encephalitis occurring secondary to the measles virus, evolves after reactivation of the dormant measles virus. The reactivation of the latent measles virus causes a cerebral infection. This infectious process causes atrophy of the cortical areas of the brain, demyelination of the nerves, or ventricular dilation. The brain tissue is diffusely inflamed. Symptoms of this progressive neurologic disorder emerge with an insidious onset and are identified by progressive motor and mental or intellectual deterioration, including personality changes and neurologic deterioration, subsequently resulting in severe dementia. Seizures, blindness, and fever are additional symptoms. Motor involvement leads to periodic involuntary movements and eventual decerebrate rigidity. This can occur approximately 6 to 8 years after a child under the age of 2 has measles. Very rarely, the onset of this inappropriate immune response follows measles immunization.

SSPE is diagnosed on the basis of symptoms and a history of previous occurrences of measles or a recent measles immunization. CSF shows elevated gamma globulin levels. The antibody titer is elevated, indicating the presence of measles virus antibodies.

There is no effective therapy or cure for SSPE. Measles vaccination is the best way to prevent this from occurring. The treatment includes supportive measures, including drug therapy for seizure control. The duration of this disorder is several years, with progressive deterioration of the CNS. The patient usually is nonresponsive and unable to care for himself or herself for some time before ultimate death.

The mother of a young English singer who was afflicted by this rare disorder at the age of 18 years urges all parents to have their children immunized against measles in the hope of preventing the condition that left her daughter blind and unable to speak. The daughter died 14 years after the onset of SSPE.

• **Fig. 2.41** Rubella (German measles). (A) Note the pinkish-red, maculopapular eruption. (B) Red palatal lesions (Forchheimer spots) are seen in some patients on day 1 of the rash. (From James WD, et al: *Andrews' diseases of the skin clinical atlas*, ed 2, 2018, Elsevier.)

Rubella causes great danger to the fetuses of pregnant females who contract the disease.

Patient Screening

Contagious diseases present a challenge in the patient screening process. Many physicians prefer not to have the contagious patient in the reception area. When the parents feel an office visit is warranted, the child is immediately placed in an examination room and the physician is notified.

Etiology

The causative agent is the rubella virus, which is spread by direct contact with nasal or oral secretions. The incubation period after exposure is 14 to 21 days. The patient is contagious from 1 week before the eruption of the rash until 1 week after the onset of the rash. Although rubella is preventable through immunization, sporadic epidemics still arise, often on college campuses.

Diagnosis

Diagnosis is made on the basis of a history of exposure and the clinical picture, including the rash. Because rubella resembles other diseases, a definitive diagnosis includes a throat culture for the rubella virus and serologic studies to detect antibodies.

Treatment

Treatment consists of supportive measures, including the administration of a mild analgesic for fever and joint pain. The patient is isolated until the rash disappears.

Prognosis

The prognosis is good. (Refer to the Enrichment box about Congenital Rubella Syndrome.)

◆ ENRICHMENT

Congenital Rubella Syndrome

Females of childbearing age who have not been immunized against rubella or who have not had the disease can transmit rubella to their fetus if they become infected during pregnancy. When the virus is transferred to the fetus during the first few weeks of pregnancy 85% of infants will have a variety of congenital deformities, known as *congenital rubella syndrome*. The risk is lower if infection occurs later in pregnancy. Anomalies caused by congenital rubella syndrome include congenital cardiac disease, blindness, deafness, and intellectual developmental disorder.

Pregnant females should be isolated from individuals infected with rubella to prevent perinatal infection; in addition, pregnant females must not be given the rubella vaccine. The best protection against congenital rubella syndrome is universal routine immunization with live rubella vaccine during infancy or as soon as possible in adulthood. Rubella causes great danger to the fetuses of pregnant females who contract the disease.

Prevention

Active immunity conferred by the rubella vaccine in a patient older than 12 months of age prevents the disease. (Refer to Fig. 2.36 for CDC guidelines for childhood immunizations.)

Patient Teaching

Reinforce the need for good hand hygiene, and proper handling and disposal of soiled tissues. Discuss the microbe responsible for rubella and the methods of preventing the spread of the disease via the nasal and mucous routes. Emphasize the importance of routine immunizations for children.

Tetanus

Description

Tetanus is an acute, potentially deadly, systemic infection characterized by painful involuntary contraction of skeletal muscles.

ICD-10-CM Code	A35 (Other tetanus)

Symptoms and Signs

The patient is extremely febrile (temperature >101 °F), is irritable, and sweats profusely. He or she has a stiff neck, a tight jaw ("lockjaw"), spasms of the facial muscles, and difficulty swallowing. As the infection progresses, the muscles of the back and abdomen become rigid with generalized convulsive muscle spasms (opisthotonos). These tonic spasms may cause death caused by asphyxiation.

Patient Screening

Patients who have experienced a soft tissue wound, including animal bites and punctures from nails, burns, and abrasions, should be assessed for tetanus prophylaxis and instructed about the importance of receiving the tetanus shot. Patients experiencing high fever, irritability, and profuse perspiration accompanied by stiff neck, tight jaw (lockjaw), spasms of the facial muscles, and difficulty swallowing require immediate assessment and intervention.

Etiology

The bacillus Clostridium tetani is found in contaminated soil and animal excreta and enters the skin through a puncture wound, laceration, abrasion, burn, or other injury. Puncture wounds are excellent breeding grounds for the bacillus because they lack a good oxygen supply and the bacillus thrives in dead tissue, producing a powerful exotoxin that attacks the nervous system. The incubation period is 3 to 21 days, with the onset commonly occurring at about 8 days. Tetanus antitoxin immunizations followed by booster doses every 10 years create immunity.

Diagnosis

The patient's history may indicate inadequate immunization. The patient is acutely ill, as described previously. Laboratory test results do not always produce conclusive data for diagnosis.

Treatment

The medical management is chiefly supportive, with the administration of sedatives and muscle relaxants to relieve spasms and seizures; a quiet, dark environment promotes rest. If the patient suffers convulsions, respiratory integrity must be preserved.

The unimmunized patient at risk is given human tetanus immune globulin within 72 hours of injury for temporary immunity. A booster injection of tetanus toxoid is needed if the injured person has not had tetanus immunization within 5 years.

Prognosis

There is no cure for tetanus. Adults 60 years of age and older are at the highest risk for death from tetanus.

Prevention

The best course is childhood immunizations, timely booster doses, and prompt cleaning of wounds with hydrogen peroxide.

Patient Teaching

Encourage and stress the importance of tetanus booster immunizations. Cleansing of soft tissue injuries also should be stressed.

Influenza

Influenza is an acute, highly contagious viral infection of the respiratory tract. Its highest incidence is in school children, and it is more severe in young children. Influenza occurs sporadically or as an epidemic and is transmitted by droplet nuclei or direct contact with moist secretions. Children tend to have high fevers with influenza and are susceptible to pulmonary complications and Reye syndrome. Because of the latter, acetaminophen, and *not* aspirin, is given to children and adolescents for fever and pain.

Common Cold

Young children have several colds each year, and most colds are self-limiting and run their course in 4 to 5 days. In infants, nasal congestion can cause difficulty with eating and breathing. Supportive treatment consists of rest, increased fluid intake, and diet as tolerated. The possibility of secondary bacterial infection or extension of the infection into the lower respiratory tract or into the middle ear is potentially dangerous for the child. These complications warrant antibiotic therapy.

Respiratory Diseases/Disorders

Sudden Unexpected Infant Death

Description

Sudden unexpected Infant deaths are responsible for infants less than 1 year of age. These deaths are classified three ways: (1) SIDS, (2) unexpected deaths, and (3) accidental suffocation and strangulation in bed.

ICD-10-CM Code	R99 (Ill-defined and unknown cause of mortality)

Sudden Infant Death Syndrome

Symptoms and Signs

SIDS, formerly called *crib death*, is defined officially as the sudden death of an infant younger than 1 year of age, for which a cause cannot be established. It is the number one cause of death among infants 1 to 12 months of age; 1 in 2000 infants dies mysteriously during the first year of life. Death occurs within seconds during sleep without sound or struggle, and the baby does not suffer. Most infants with SIDS appear healthy before death. When found, the dead infant may have a mottled complexion and cyanotic lips and fingertips.

Known causes and contributing factors for the sudden death of an infant are ruled out. These may include an immature respiratory control system, a susceptibility to deadly arrhythmias, congenital heart disease, and myocarditis.

Patient Screening

Any call regarding an infant not breathing is an emergency, and 911 emergency services should be called to the scene. When an infant dies, the situation usually becomes a coroner's case, and an autopsy is ordered. The parent desiring an appointment for an infant with near-miss SIDS should be seen as soon as possible. Adequate information should be obtained to determine whether the situation is an emergency and whether the child needs to be entered into the emergency care system or can be seen in the office. If the parent of a child who has died of diagnosed SIDS calls for an appointment, remember the magnitude of the situation, and schedule an appointment as soon as possible. During the entire process, remaining nonjudgmental is important.

Etiology

Although there are many theories and much misinformation about SIDS, the exact cause remains uncertain. Research studies and autopsies point to certain pathologic findings and have suggested more than one cause. There may be an abnormality in the area of the brain that controls breathing and the ability to wake up from sleep. Many maternal and infant risk factors are known: mother's age being less than 20 years, poor prenatal care, smoking and drug abuse during pregnancy, exposure of the infant to secondhand smoke, prematurity, recent upper respiratory tract infection in the infant, sleeping in the prone position, and a sibling who had SIDS or failure to thrive. Overheating or bundling of the infant during sleep are also risk factors.

Diagnosis

When a complete postmortem investigation, including autopsy, a review of the child's medical history, and examination of the scene of death, has failed to identify the cause of death, it is diagnosed as SIDS.

Treatment

Resuscitation attempts fail. Currently, SIDS is not predictable or preventable The American Academy of Pediatrics (AAP) has added sleeping in the prone position or on the side to the list of risk factors. To reduce that risk, the AAP recommends placing babies in bed on their backs instead of on their stomachs or sides.

Prognosis

Infants with near-miss SIDS are at risk for additional episodes and should be placed on their backs to sleep. Parents who have had an infant die as a result of SIDS are at risk of having another infant with SIDS.

Prevention

Recent studies have isolated the risk factors for SIDS. Although these risk factors may play a role in SIDS, parents must understand that of themselves, these factors do not cause SIDS.

As previously mentioned, the supine sleeping position carries the lowest risk for SIDS. Infants should not be placed in the prone position unless they are actively monitored by an adult. Exposure to cigarette smoke should be prevented. The use of firm bedding materials in a safety-approved crib is prudent. All blankets and pillows should be removed from the crib. Research shows that overheating an infant by dressing in excessive clothing, especially during illness, is to be avoided. Other important factors include good prenatal care and breastfeeding. Breastfeeding is a source of immunity to the newborn infant. An additional prevention is to avoid any contact of the infant with anyone with an upper respiratory illness or a GI upset, even if it is considered a minor episode. All individuals touching or handling the infant should wash their hands before any encounter with the infant. Infants who are high risk may be placed on apnea monitors during the first year of life.

Pregnant females should be advised not to smoke during their pregnancy.

Patient Teaching

Survivors of SIDS should be offered sensitive interventions to help them deal with the grief and possible feelings of guilt and anger. The Sudden Infant Death Syndrome Alliance is a national voluntary organization in the United States dedicated to eliminating SIDS through medical research. Help families find and contact SIDS support groups.

Unknown cause: Infants less than 1 year old die with no explanation of death, or cause which can be determined.

Accidental suffocation and strangulation in bed: These infant deaths are determined to be caused by something in the crib or bed with the infant, which gets caught around the infant's neck, or gets in front of their nose and mouth and blocks air. For this reason, it is recommended not to place toys, stuffed animals, bumper pads, or anything in the crib with an infant. Bed-sharing, where an infant and adult share the same surface for sleeping such as in a bed, is not recommended as the infant may accidentally be smothered.

Croup

Description

Croup is an acute, severe inflammation and obstruction of the respiratory tract.

ICD-10-CM Code	J05.0 *(Acute obstructive laryngitis [croup])*

Symptoms and Signs

It usually is preceded by an upper respiratory tract infection. The symptoms include hoarseness, fever, a harsh, high-pitched cough, and stridor during inspiration caused by narrowing of the upper airways. The child may experience dyspnea (fast and difficult respirations) that may be accompanied by a grunting noise or wheezing. When the child is not receiving enough oxygen, the skin becomes pale with circumoral cyanosis (a slight blue tinge around the mouth). It is possible for the bronchi and lungs to become involved. The child may be anxious and frightened by the respiratory distress.

Patient Screening

Children experiencing signs and symptoms of respiratory distress, including hoarseness, fever, a harsh, high-pitched cough, and stridor during inspiration, require prompt, if not immediate, assessment and intervention.

Etiology

Croup is usually a viral disease that involves the larynx, trachea, and bronchi. Clinical manifestations are caused by edema and spasm of the vocal cords, creating varying degrees of obstruction (Fig. 2.42A).

Diagnosis

Croup must be distinguished from epiglottitis. If necessary, blood or throat cultures may be performed to identify certain bacterial causes. A laryngoscopy may be performed. Radiographs of the airway may show a characteristic "steeple sign" or be necessary to rule out an obstruction by a foreign body.

Treatment

The patient is treated symptomatically, with the administration of antipyretic agents, rest, increased fluid intake, cool humidification of air, and, if the cause is bacterial, antibiotic therapy. The steam from a warm shower may be beneficial. A dose of steroids may decrease airway edema. In severe cases, the patient is hospitalized for endotracheal intubation and oxygen therapy until the respiratory crisis passes. In most instances, the illness subsides in 3 to 4 days.

Prognosis

The prognosis is good with prompt intervention. The child is likely to experience recurrences of the condition.

Prevention

Because croup is a viral disease, the only prevention is through avoidance of contact with respiratory viruses. Replace toothbrushes regularly and after any infectious process.

Patient Teaching

Instruct the parents *not* to place anything in the child's mouth until the child is assessed by a health care professional and epiglottitis is ruled out. Additional teaching includes instruction on handling and disposal of soiled tissues and the importance of good hand washing.

Epiglottitis

Description

Epiglottitis is inflammation of the epiglottis, the thin, leaf-shaped structure that covers the entrance of the larynx during swallowing.

ICD-10-CM Code	J05.10 *(Acute epiglottitis without obstruction)*
	J05.11 *(Acute epiglottitis with obstruction)*
	J37.0 *(Chronic laryngitis)*

Symptoms and Signs

Epiglottitis typically strikes children between ages 3 and 7 years. The symptoms include a sore throat, croupy cough, fever, and respiratory distress caused by laryngeal obstruction. Visual inspection reveals a red and swollen epiglottis. Rapidly increasing dyspnea and drooling are the most significant signs of this critical respiratory emergency (see Fig. 2.42B).

• **Fig. 2.42** Acute inflammation of the larynx. (A) Inflammation of the entire larynx, causing diffuse laryngeal swelling and laryngospasm (croup). (B) Inflammation localized to the epiglottis (so-called *acute epiglottitis*). (From Damjanov I: *Pathology for the health professions*, ed 4, St. Louis, 2011, Saunders.)

Patient Screening

Children experiencing any form of respiratory distress require immediate assessment and intervention. Instruct the parents *not* to place anything in the child's mouth until the child is assessed by a health care professional because airway spasms may result.

Etiology

Epiglottitis may follow an upper respiratory tract infection. The most common cause is *Haemophilus influenzae* type B (Hib). Other organisms that may be responsible for epiglottitis include *Streptococcus pneumoniae*, VZV, *Haemophilus parainfluenzae*, *Staphylococcus aureus*, and herpes simplex virus type 1. Another form of epiglottitis, thermal epiglottitis, may be caused by heat damage to the epiglottis from ingestion of very hot liquids or food.

Diagnosis

Radiography of the neck may reveal an enlarged epiglottis. If the obstruction is not significant, the throat is examined to inspect the epiglottis. Nothing is placed in the child's mouth without the presence of a health care professional with the capability, equipment, and supplies needed to perform endotracheal intubation and tracheostomy.

Treatment

If the airway is obstructed, the child is hospitalized and given intensive care. The airway is established with tracheostomy or endotracheal intubation. Broad-spectrum antibiotics may be given parenterally, and the patient is closely monitored.

Prognosis

Although this condition can be fatal if not treated, prompt treatment affords a good prognosis.

Prevention

The incidence of this potentially life-threatening condition has dramatically decreased following the introduction of the Hib conjugate vaccine. The AAP recommends that all children receive the Hib vaccine. Replace toothbrushes regularly and after any infectious process.

Patient Teaching

Instruct the parents *not* to place anything in the child's mouth until the child is assessed by a health care professional. Additional teaching includes instruction in the handling and disposal of soiled tissues and the importance of good hand washing. Reinforce the recommendation for immunization with the Hib conjugate vaccine.

Acute Tonsillitis

Description

Acute tonsillitis is a painful inflammatory and infectious process affecting the tonsils.

ICD-10-CM Code	J03.90 (*Acute tonsillitis, unspecified*) (J03.0–J03.91 = 9 codes for specificity)

Symptoms and Signs

Tonsillitis, or inflammation of the tonsils, usually has a sudden onset. The patient has a mild-to-severe sore throat, chills, fever, headache, malaise, anorexia, and muscle and joint pain. The tonsils appear inflamed and swollen, with yellowish exudate projecting from crypts. Lymph glands in the submandibular area are tender and enlarged (Fig. 2.43).

Patient Screening

An individual with pain, fever, and a sudden onset sore throat requires prompt assessment, with a culture and sensitivity test of the exudate obtained to determine the causative agent.

Etiology

Tonsillitis is caused by many organisms, with group A beta-hemolytic streptococci being the most common cause.

Diagnosis

The throat is examined, and a throat culture is performed to identify the causative organism. The WBC count may be elevated in response to the infection.

Treatment

When the throat culture result is positive for group A streptococci ("strep throat"), a full course of a penicillin antibiotic regimen is typically given. This strict regimen is

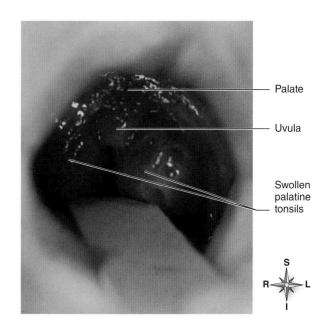

— Palate

— Uvula

Swollen palatine tonsils

• **Fig. 2.43** Tonsillitis. Enlarged palatine tonsils can be seen nearly meeting at the midline of the pharynx. (From Patton K, et al: *The human body in health & disease*, ed 8, 2024, Elsevier.)

necessary to prevent rheumatic fever, rheumatic heart disease, and renal complications. If the pain is debilitating, the child may need a liquid diet or saline throat irrigations. Tonsillectomy may be recommended for chronic tonsillitis.

Prognosis
The prognosis is good with drug therapy. Surgery may be the option for chronic tonsillitis. Recovery from the surgical procedure usually is uneventful, although significant postoperative bleeding may occur. The patient should be evaluated in the emergency department should this occur.

Prevention
As with any infectious process, good hand washing and proper handling and disposal of soiled tissues help prevent exposure to microbes.

Patient Teaching
Teach the patient and family about the importance of hydration during illness. In addition, emphasize the importance of completing the entire recommended regimen of antibiotic therapy. Sharing of drinking glasses and eating utensils should be discouraged, and old toothbrushes should be replaced.

Adenoid Hyperplasia

Description
Adenoid hyperplasia is an abnormal enlargement of the lymphoid tissue located in the space above the soft palate of the mouth, causing a partial breathing blockage, especially in children.

ICD-10-CM Code	J35.2 *(Hypertrophy of adenoids)*
	(J32.0–J35.9 = 8 codes of specificity)

Refer to the physician's diagnosis and then to the current edition of the ICD-10-CM coding manual to ensure the greatest specificity of pathology.

Symptoms and Signs
Adenoids (and tonsils) are present at birth and play a role in the formation of immunoglobulins. After puberty, they normally atrophy.

Adenoid hyperplasia can contribute to recurrent otitis media and conductive hearing loss, resulting from obstruction of the eustachian tube. The child is usually a mouth breather and snores during sleep. In extreme cases, the obstruction may cause the child to experience episodes of sleep apnea. The child's speech has a nasal quality.

Patient Screening
Mouth-breathing children who snore should be evaluated for adenoid enlargement. Schedule the child for an assessment of adenoids, tonsils, nasopharynx, and oropharynx.

Etiology
The cause of adenoid hyperplasia is unknown. Contributing factors include repeated infections, chronic allergies, and heredity.

Diagnosis
The abnormal enlargement may be visualized on lateral pharyngeal radiographs or with a nasopharyngoscopic examination.

Treatment
Adenoidectomy is indicated for obstructive adenoids with recurrent otitis media or chronic serous otitis media with conductive hearing loss. It may also be indicated if the child is experiencing obstructive sleep apnea.

Prognosis
Surgical removal of the adenoids usually corrects the condition.

Prevention
No prevention is known.

Patient Teaching
Instruct the patient and the family about the importance of hydration during illness. Teach comfort measures and routine postoperative care when the adenoids have been removed.

Asthma

Description
Asthma is a chronic reversible obstructive disease caused by increased reactivity of the tracheobronchial tree to various stimuli. Two major processes are at work: constriction of the bronchioles and inflammation of the airway. It is a leading cause of chronic illness and school absenteeism in children.

ICD-10-CM Code	J45.909 *(Unspecified asthma, uncomplicated)*
	(J45–J45.998 = 18 codes of specificity)
	J45.998 *(Other asthma)*

Refer to the physician's diagnosis and then to the current edition of the ICD-10-CM coding manual to ensure the greatest specificity of pathology. Coding is done by extent of inflammation and type.

Symptoms and Signs
The child has an incessant productive or nonproductive cough, a pronounced expiratory wheeze, and rapid shallow respirations. The labored breathing results in a rapid pulse, pallor, profuse perspiration, and an inability to speak more than a few words without halting to breathe. The child often has nasal flaring and intercostal or sternal retractions.

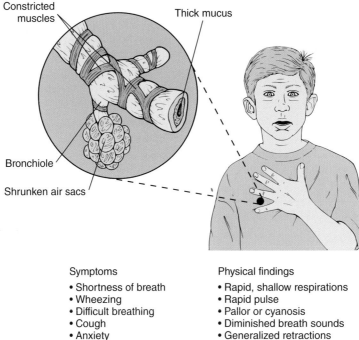

Symptoms
- Shortness of breath
- Wheezing
- Difficult breathing
- Cough
- Anxiety

Physical findings
- Rapid, shallow respirations
- Rapid pulse
- Pallor or cyanosis
- Diminished breath sounds
- Generalized retractions
- Frequent pausing to catch the breath when talking
- Hyperexpansion of the chest

• **Fig. 2.44** An asthma attack with respiratory distress.

The patient often is anxious, exhausted, and reports a "tight chest." The examining physician hears diminished breath sounds, with wheezes and rhonchi in the lungs. The bronchial spasms trap air and thick mucus in the lungs. An asthma exacerbation (Fig. 2.44) can be mild to severe, can last minutes or days, and may become a medical emergency. The attack may or may not have been preceded by a respiratory infection (Fig. 2.45) or exposure to a known trigger.

Patient Screening
Patients with asthma present an alarming clinical situation. A possible respiratory compromise requires prompt assessment and intervention.

Etiology
A hereditary factor is strongly associated with the disease. Asthma is the result of hyperactive and hypersensitive bronchial tubes. The bronchial spasms of asthma can be triggered by many extrinsic (allergic) or intrinsic (nonallergic) factors, including stress, heavy exercise, infection, and inhalation of allergens or other substances. Allergens may include pollen, cockroaches and their excrement, molds, household dust mites, and pet dander. Additional "triggers" include air pollutants and irritants (perfumes, colognes, and aftershaves), smoke and secondhand smoke, cold air, emotional upset, and exercise.

Diagnosis
The best tool available to reveal the degree of airway obstruction is the pulmonary function test. However, this

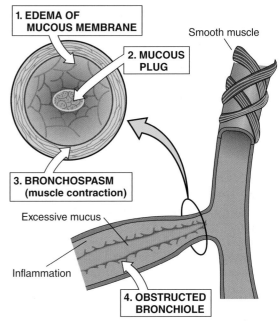

• **Fig. 2.45** Asthma—acute episode. (From Gould BE: Pathophysiology for the health professions, ed 4, St. Louis, 2011, Saunders.)

test may show normal results between attacks. Chest radiography may show hyperinflation and changes in the lungs associated with mucous plugging. Specialists may order intradermal skin testing to identify inhalant and food allergies. Blood tests include a CBC with a differential leukocyte count, which may show an increased eosinophil count and elevated serum immunoglobulin E (IgE) levels (Fig. 2.46).

• **Fig. 2.46** Radiograph of lungs of child with asthma attack. (From Des Jardins T, Burton GC: Clinical manifestations and assessment of respiratory disease, ed 6, St. Louis, 2011, Mosby.)

Treatment

Many individuals with chronic asthma require medical management under the care of an expert. Strict compliance with a regimen of medications to relax and widen the bronchi and release excessive mucus is important. Some of the drugs used are cromolyn sodium, albuterol, theophylline, and aerosol corticosteroids. Allergy evaluation and skin testing may indicate immunotherapy by desensitization injections, commonly called *allergy shots*. Avoiding infection, known allergens, and other triggers is strongly advised. Individuals with asthma are encouraged to avoid smoking and exposure to secondhand smoke.

Severe acute asthma attacks are treated with injections of steroids and inhalation therapy. Steroids can reduce airway inflammation, whereas inhaled albuterol decreases bronchoconstriction. The patient may require supplemental oxygen. In a severe attack that is refractory to drug therapy, a condition called *status asthmaticus* may lead to fatal respiratory failure and thus the need for endotracheal intubation. The patient requires hospitalization for aggressive medical treatment and follow-up. Occasionally some children may develop pneumonia concurrent with the asthma attack.

Prognosis

The prognosis varies depending on the extent of the asthmatic attack and the causative factor. The use of prophylactic medications helps. Medication inhalers should be kept readily available at all times. Allergy testing may reveal the irritant, and allergy serum injections may help alleviate or reduce the severity of the attack. As previously mentioned, unresponsive asthma (status asthmaticus) may result in death.

Prompt medical intervention is necessary when an attack cannot be resolved by usual and available methods.

Prevention

The patient should take all controller medications as prescribed. Use of a daily controller medication helps to reduce the incidence and severity of the attacks. Avoiding any stimulating allergens and environments containing cigarette smoke is suggested. Vaping should be avoided.

Patient Teaching

Encourage patients to use prophylactic medications and to avoid known triggering allergens. Teach caregivers the importance of seeking medical help when an attack does not resolve quickly with normal intervention.

Bronchiolitis

Description

Bronchiolitis is inflammation of the bronchioles, the smallest air passages of the lungs, and is usually caused by viruses. It is a common disease in infancy.

ICD-10-CM Code	J21.8 (*Acute bronchiolitis due to other specified organisms*) (J21.0–J21.9 = 4 codes of specificity)

Symptoms and Signs

The infant or small child has a cough and nasal congestion that evolve into a wheeze, tachypnea, and respiratory distress. Fever and posttussive emesis may be present. The patient may be breathing too fast to feed properly and can become dehydrated. In very young infants, especially in those who were premature, apnea may occur.

Patient Screening

Any infant with a wheeze or respiratory distress must be evaluated immediately.

Etiology

Bronchiolitis is most commonly caused by infection with RSV. Many other viruses can cause this disease, including parainfluenza virus and adenovirus. Bronchiolitis is most common during the winter months (October through April). Infants in daycare or who have school-age siblings are at highest risk. The natural progression of the infection is that symptoms worsen over the first few days of infection, peaking in severity around day 4 or 5, and then slowly improve.

Diagnosis

The diagnosis is made on the basis of patient history and physical examination. A chest radiograph may be obtained to rule out pneumonia. Rapid RSV testing is available in most emergency room settings to help with grouping of patients, but it does not affect management of the disease. Viral culture from the nasopharynx may also be obtained to determine etiology. Chest x-rays may be obtained.

Treatment

Treatment is supportive care. Albuterol, racemic epinephrine, or hypertonic saline given via a nebulizer may improve respiratory symptoms. Supplemental oxygen may be required. If the patient is unable to feed, administration of IV fluids is necessary. In extreme cases, the patient experiences respiratory failure and must be intubated and mechanically ventilated until the infection runs its course. Even after the acute infection, the airways may be sensitive for several weeks, leading to recurrent wheeze and cough.

Prognosis

The prognosis depends on the severity of the infection and early evaluation and initiation of supportive measures when needed. Premature infants and those with cardiac disorders or lung disease are at the greatest risk for complications. Children who receive prompt and appropriate care usually do quite well. There is a possible link between bronchiolitis and the later development of asthma.

Prevention

Measures that reduce the spread of viruses, such as hand washing and avoidance of individuals symptomatic with respiratory infections, are the best ways of prevention. Infants who meet certain qualifications, such as prematurity, lung disease, and exposure to school-age siblings, may be able to receive vaccination with palivizumab, a monoclonal antibody against RSV. This immunization must be given monthly during the winter months when RSV infection is most prevalent. The qualification criteria are quite stringent because of the high cost of the vaccine.

Patient Teaching

Provide printed or online resources in the parents' native language. Parents need emotional support and understanding, especially when the child is hospitalized for treatment. Allow the parents to verbalize their anxieties and fears to a compassionate and understanding individual, thus validating their feelings in the situation.

Gastrointestinal Disorders

Infantile Colic

Description

Colic is intermittent distress in the newborn or during early infancy and has an unclear etiology.

ICD-10-CM Code	R10.9 *(Unspecified abdominal pain)*
	(R10.0–R10.9 = 29 codes of specificity)

Refer to the physician's diagnosis and then to the current edition of the ICD-10-CM coding manual to ensure the greatest specificity of pathology.

Symptoms and Signs

The infant intermittently draws up the legs, clenches the fists, and cries as if in pain. During the episode, the infant may pass gas via the mouth and the rectum. The episodes of colic are likely to occur in the late afternoon and evening. These babies usually thrive, gain weight, and appear to tolerate formula or mother's milk.

Patient Screening

Although not life threatening, infantile colic is a very disruptive state in the life of the family with an infant with the condition. This child requires prompt assessment, and an appointment should be scheduled as soon as convenient for all.

Etiology

The etiology of colic is unknown, although several theories have been advanced. One hypothesis suggests that improper feeding techniques may be responsible, and another theory blames overfeeding or swallowing of excessive air. Sensitivity to cow's milk may be the causative factor, even for the nursing infant. In this case, the nursing mother is urged to eliminate cow's milk from her own diet. Regardless of the cause, the infant is extremely uncomfortable and cries a great deal, with sleep pattern disturbance.

Diagnosis

Diagnosis is made by the symptoms and a physical examination to rule out other causes of the infant's fussiness.

Treatment

Investigation into possible causes is the first step in treatment. Eliminating any of the possible causative factors may help lessen the symptoms. The infant usually outgrows the condition at about age 3 months. Probiotics or simethicone can provide relief in some cases.

Prognosis

The prognosis for the child outgrowing colic type of symptoms is good. Parents can become exhausted both physically and emotionally with the colicky, constantly crying baby. Intervention by another family member or support person may be advised to prevent abuse of the baby.

Prevention

Because the etiology is unknown, prevention is also undetermined.

Patient Teaching

Encourage the use of support persons so that parents can get the needed rest. Many theories of treatment have been proposed; encourage parents to discuss these with their physician.

Helminth (Worm) Infestation

Description

Roundworms, pinworms, hookworms, and tapeworms all can take up residence in the GI tract. All of these worms are classified as helminths, and the term *helminth infestation* describes the presence of these parasites in the intestinal tract.

ICD-10-CM Code	B83.9 *(Helminthiasis, unspecified)*
	(B83.0–B83.9 = 7 codes for specificity)

Symptoms and Signs

Worm infestations in children occur as the eggs of parasites are introduced into their mouths from contaminated hands. After the pinworm *(Enterobius vermicularis)* eggs are swallowed, they hatch in the intestine. The female worms migrate to the perianal area at night, where they lay their eggs. This process causes mild to intense itching and irritation in the area. The itching and scratching contaminate the fingers with the eggs and allow reingestion by the host (Figs. 2.47 and 2.48).

Patient Screening

Children exhibiting behaviors that suggest the presence of intestinal worms require prompt assessment and intervention.

Etiology

E. vermicularis (pinworm) is one of many possible parasitic worms. It is the most common cause of helminth infestation in the United States, and most patients are preschool or school-age children and the mothers of infected children. Pinworms are transmitted directly or indirectly from human to human.

CNS
Taenia solium (pork tapeworm),
Echinococcus granulosus
(hydatid cyst), *Trichinella spiralis*

EYE
Onchocerca volvulus, Loa-loa,
Toxocara

LUNG
Paragonimus westermani (liver fluke),
Strongyloides stercoralis,
Wuchereria bancrofti (filariasis),
Ascaris lumbricoides (roundworm),
Echinococcus granulosus (hydatid cyst)

LYMPHOID TISSUE
Wuchereria bancrofti (filariasis)

HEART
Trichinella spiralis

LIVER
Clonorchis sinensis, Fasciola hepatica
(liver fluke), *Schistosoma,*
Echinococcus granulosus (hydatid cyst)

LARGE INTESTINE
Enterobius vermicularis (pinworm),
Trichuris trichiura (whipworm)

SMALL INTESTINE
Ascaris lumbricoides (roundworm),
Necator americanis (hookworm),
Ancylostoma duodenale (hookworm),
Taenia solium (pork tapeworm),
Taenia saginata (beef tapeworm)

BLADDER
Schistosoma

SKELETAL MUSCLE
Trichinella spiralis, Taenia solium
(pork tapeworm)

SKIN
Onchocerca volvulus, Loa-loa,
Toxocara

• **Fig. 2.47** Helminthic infestations. *CNS*, Central nervous system. (From Stevens A, et al: Core pathology, ed 3, London, 2010, Mosby.)

• **Fig. 2.48** Intestinal worms. (A) Tapeworm. Two main features of the tapeworm are the scolex, which has muscular suckers surrounded by hooks for attachment, and the individual body segments called proglottids. (B) Pinworms (*Enterobius vermicularis*). (C) Ascariasis, gross. Most *Ascaris lumbricoides* infections are asymptomatic, but a large worm burden may produce obstruction from a large mass of worms as shown here. An adult female worm is 20 to 35 cm in size, and an adult male 15 to 30 cm long; these worms can survive for up to 2 years in the human intestine. (A, From VanMeter K, Hubert R: *Microbiology for the healthcare professional,* St. Louis, 2010, Mosby; B, From Anofel: *Parasitoses et mycoses: des régions tempérées et tropicales,* ed 5, 2016, Elsevier Masson; Courtesy Ashutosh Mohapatra, MD, Bhubaneswar, India; C, From Klatt, E: *Robbins & Cotran Atlas of Pathology,* ed 4, 2021, Elsevier.)

Diagnosis

The diagnosis is made by detection of eggs or worms in the anal opening on transparent adhesive tape placed in the perianal area. A stool specimen examined microscopically may be positive.

Treatment

A complete course of anthelmintic agents is given; some physicians treat the entire family. Frequent showering and hand washing are advised. The worms and eggs also can be destroyed by laundering clothing and linens in hot water with bleach.

Prognosis

The prognosis is good when the entire family is treated.

Prevention

Good hand washing and frequent showering help prevent infestation. Children should be encouraged not to touch or scratch the anus and not to put their hands in their mouths.

Patient Teaching

Stress the importance of good hand washing, using hand sanitizer when appropriate, and other cleanliness measures.

Point out to parents the importance of teaching children good hygiene habits, especially in the toileting process.

Diarrhea

Description

Diarrhea is the rapid passage of stool through the intestinal tract, with a noticeable change in frequency, fluid content, appearance, and consistency.

ICD-10-CM Code	K52.2 *(Allergic and dietetic gastroenteritis and colitis)* (K52.0–K52.9 = 7 codes of specificity) K52.89 *(Other specified noninfective gastroenteritis and colitis)* R19.7 *(Diarrhea, unspecified)*

Refer to the physician's diagnosis and then to the current edition of the ICD-10-CM coding manual to ensure the greatest specificity of pathology.

Symptoms and Signs

Diarrhea may be mild or severe, acute or chronic. In the infant or child, diarrhea can rapidly cause dehydration and electrolyte imbalance when fluid loss is profuse. Severe or prolonged diarrhea can produce metabolic acidosis; the patient may be lethargic and may hyperventilate. Depending on the cause, the symptoms could include intestinal cramping, weakness, nausea, irritability, and fever. Stool passage may become painful as a result of excoriation of the anus or skin in the diaper area.

Patient Screening

Children with diarrhea can become dehydrated rapidly. Prompt assessment is indicated.

Etiology

Diarrhea has multiple causes: infection (viral, bacterial, or parasitic), medications, allergic reactions, emotions, anatomic abnormalities, malabsorption syndromes, mechanical or chemical irritation resulting from the diet, and toxicity. The cause may be unknown.

Diagnosis

The clinician attempts to determine the degree of diarrheal disease, the underlying cause, and the fluid and electrolyte status of the patient. This requires a specific history of the onset and severity of symptoms, laboratory blood testing, stool cultures, and analysis of the stools.

Treatment

The treatment of diarrhea is directed at the cause, if known. Blood components are monitored for fluid and electrolyte balances. The frequency, color, consistency, and general composition of the stools are observed. Oral intake may be restricted to rest the intestinal tract and to reduce intestinal irritability. When infection is the cause, appropriate antibiotics may be given. Ignoring prolonged diarrhea in the infant or small child is dangerous. The patient may require hospitalization for IV fluid and electrolyte therapy.

Prognosis

The prognosis is good with prompt intervention. Dehydration and electrolyte imbalance are factors in the outcome of the condition. Hospitalization may be necessary to maintain hydration, stable electrolytes, and nutrition.

Prevention

Prevention is multifaceted because of the cause. Good hand washing is important in preventing microbial infections. Avoiding known allergens, certain medications, and dietary factors helps. Mechanical and chemical irritations in the diet may be eliminated. When the cause is anatomic abnormalities or malabsorption syndromes, preventive steps are probably few.

ⓘ ALERT!

Childhood Obesity

Childhood obesity has become a major health concern in the United States. Children with weights significantly beyond the average weight for age or height are often identified as having this serious health condition. As children become more and more obese, they are beginning a pattern that may plague them for the rest of their lives. Additionally, this condition may lead to health problems, such as diabetes, hypertension, hypercholesterolemia, respiratory ailments, and orthopedic problems. Another concern is that poor self-esteem and depression may occur in these children. They also may become targets for teasing and bullying by their peers.

The most common cause of childhood obesity is the combination of eating too much food and not getting enough exercise. Types of food also play an important role in weight gain. Fast-food restaurant type of food often has a content that is high in sugar and fat. Snacks, such as cookies, crackers, candy, and sodas, are high in calories and low in nutritional value. Many families consume prepared meals that are high in sodium and calories. Children today spend several hours a day sitting in front of a television screen or computer, communicating with peers or others on a cell phone or tablet, limiting quality exercise and the burning of calories.

Because parents usually make decisions regarding food and activity, they are encouraged to provide nutritious food for their children, as well as limiting the time the child spends watching TV, playing computer games, and sitting at a computer. Schools are being encouraged to provide nutritious meals containing fruits and vegetables and less fat and sugar. The schools also are urged to increase student physical activity with quality exercise. In addition to burning calories, exercise is essential for building strong bones and muscles.

During a well-child examination, the health care provider compares the child's weight and height with the Centers for Disease Control and Prevention (CDC) standard growth charts, and the child's body mass index (BMI) is measured as well. A child who has a BMI-for-age between the 85th and 94th percentiles is considered overweight. When a child has a BMI-for-age that is in the 95th percentile or above, he or she is considered obese. The health care provider takes into consideration the child's growth and development, family weight-for-height history, and skeletal and muscular structure of the body before making a diagnosis of obesity.

Five or more daily servings of fruit and vegetables are recommended. Many children consume fried potatoes as their five daily servings. Drinking sodas high in sugar content has increased steadily, whereas intake of milk has declined. Missed breakfasts, eating dinners outside the home, and increased snacking also contribute to the increasing incidence of obesity. Another factor in the increased incidence of obesity is a change in lifestyle. Many children ride buses or are driven to school rather than walking. Numerous children have no safe place to be physically active because of a lack of outdoor lighting or a protected place to play or because of high rates of crime or unrestrained dogs in the neighborhood. Some neighborhoods do not have sidewalks where children can walk safely.

There is no simple answer to dealing with childhood obesity. It is a complex situation that involves lifestyle, intake of too much food, consumption of high-calorie foods and beverages, economic status, environmental circumstances, home location, transportation versus walking, decreased or restricted exercise activities, and increased TV, computer, or electronic game time. Family history, body structure, ethnic background, social factors, and genetics all play a role, along with diet and exercise, in the incidence of childhood obesity.

Patient Teaching

Emphasize the importance of hydration to the parents. Care of the anal area may be required as a result of the irritation caused by the loose and irritating stools. Good hand washing is necessary after handling soiled diapers or any other clothing that may contain stool. Teach the parents to observe urinary output for volume and color. When the child is in diapers, have the parents count the number of soiled or wet diapers within a set time and report this to the physician's office.

Vomiting

Description

Vomiting, or ejection of stomach contents through the mouth, is a common symptom in infants and children.

ICD-10-CM Code	R11.10 *(Vomiting, unspecified)*
	(R11.0–R11.2 = 6 codes of specificity)
	R11.11 *(Vomiting without nausea)*
	R11.12 *(Projectile vomiting)*

Symptoms and Signs

Vomiting can range from a mild regurgitation to projectile expulsion. The infant has a distended abdomen, is irritable, and often has a fever. Aspiration of vomitus into the lungs can result in pneumonia.

Patient Screening

Chronic or severe vomiting deserves special attention as a warning sign of disease or possible dehydration. Assessment is essential. Projectile vomiting requires prompt assessment.

Etiology

Vomiting, which is more common in infants than in children, usually results from trivial or temporary factors. However, it has a host of possible causes, including overfeeding, food allergy, gastric irritation, infection, drug poisoning, elevated intracranial pressure, defects (e.g., pyloric stenosis), and habitual voluntary vomiting.

Diagnosis

Vomiting in the infant or child must always be evaluated in the context of the child's total state of health. One assesses causative factors by performing a physical examination, taking the history, and monitoring the patient's vital signs, weight, nutritional status, and fluid and electrolyte balance. Radiographic studies of the intestinal tract may be indicated.

Treatment

Most vomiting can be expected to abate spontaneously. Food may be withheld for a time to rest the upper GI tract and to reduce gastric irritation. When treatment is indicated, it depends on the cause, severity, and nature of the vomiting. Infant feeding problems require changes in technique or intake. Other more serious causes, such as infection, poisoning, and congenital anomalies of the GI tract, may require direct medical or surgical intervention.

Prognosis

The prognosis varies depending on the cause. Most vomiting subsides in a few hours. Longer periods of vomiting requiring medical or surgical intervention may or may not be corrected. Hydration, nutrition, and electrolyte balance are important factors in resolving the condition.

Prevention

Prevention varies depending on causative factors. Avoiding overfeeding, known food allergens, and substances that cause gastric irritation is often all that is necessary to prevent recurrence. Infection, drug poisoning, elevated intracranial pressure, defects (e.g., pyloric stenosis), and habitual voluntary vomiting may not be preventable.

Patient Teaching

Emphasize the importance of hydration and nutrition along with thorough hand washing after handling emesis.

Blood Disorders

Anemia

Description

Anemia is an abnormal reduction in the concentration of RBCs or in the hemoglobin content of circulating blood. It is not a disease, but a symptom of various diseases. Anemia can lead to tissue hypoxia. See Chapter 10 for additional information on anemias.

ICD-10-CM Code	D64.9 *(Anemia, unspecified)*
	(D64.0–D64.9 = 9 codes of specificity)

Refer to the physician's diagnosis and then to the current edition of the ICD-10-CM coding manual to ensure the greatest specificity of pathology.

Symptoms and Signs

Pallor, weakness, fatigability, and listlessness are noted initially in the child or infant with anemia. Palpitations, tachycardia, cardiac enlargement, jaundice, and mental sluggishness are symptoms of severe anemia.

Laboratory studies show reduced hematocrit and hemoglobin concentration. Other laboratory results vary, depending on the underlying cause or type of anemia.

Patient Screening

When parents report that their child appears pale, weak, easily fatigued, and listless, prompt assessment is required.

Etiology

Iron deficiency is the most common cause of anemia in children. Other causes include acute or chronic blood loss, decreased blood formation, nutritional deficiency disorders, hemolytic diseases, inhibition or loss of bone marrow, and sickle cell disease.

Diagnosis

Diagnosis is based on findings from physical examination and laboratory testing for signs and symptoms of anemia. Diagnostic tests include the determination of hemoglobin concentration, hematocrit levels, serum iron levels, RBC count, mean corpuscular hemoglobin levels, and bone marrow studies. It is often helpful to view a blood smear under a microscope.

Treatment

The first priority of treatment is to determine the cause of anemia. For iron deficiency anemia, iron-rich foods and oral preparations of ferrous sulfate are administered. When blood loss is the cause, blood volume is restored by transfusion. Replacement therapy is indicated in deficiency states (e.g., vitamin B_{12}, folic acid, and ascorbic acid deficiency). Specific hemolytic blood disorders are treated when the anemia is caused by excessive blood cell destruction. A planned program of activity balanced with rest is recommended during treatment.

Prognosis

The prognosis varies, depending on the cause. When diet modification can be recommended and followed, the prognosis is good. When the problem is bleeding and the source of the bleed can be determined and corrected, the prognosis is good with blood replacement and dietary supplements. Hemolytic disorders have a fair prognosis with aggressive treatment once the hemolytic disorder is identified.

Prevention

Diets meeting the daily requirement of iron and other vitamins and minerals help prevent iron deficiency anemia. Prompt exploration of any unexplained type of bleeding helps reveal underlying conditions and allows for prompt treatment.

Patient Teaching

Encourage parents to provide children with nutritious diets and the recommended nutritional supplements and pediatric vitamins and minerals. Emphasize the importance of follow-up appointments for these children.

Leukemia

Description

Leukemia, a cancer of blood-forming tissues, is the most common childhood malignancy. It is characterized by an abnormal increase in the number of immature WBCs or undifferentiated blastocytes.

ICD-10-CM Code	C95.9 (Leukemia, unspecified)

(C90.1–C95.92 = 105 codes of specificity)

Refer to the physician's diagnosis and then to the current edition of the ICD-10-CM coding manual to ensure the greatest specificity of pathology.

Symptoms and Signs

Bone marrow infiltration by leukemic cells leads to anemia, susceptibility to infection resulting from neutropenia, and prolonged bleeding time resulting from the reduction in the amount of platelets. Common signs and symptoms include fever, easy bruising, pallor, weakness, weight loss, and bone and joint pain. The abnormal cells can invade various organs of the body, causing pressure symptoms in those areas. Lymph nodes and the spleen may become enlarged.

Patient Screening

When the parents report that their child has a fever, frequent infections, easy bruising, pallor, and weakness, prompt assessment is required.

Etiology

Two general types of leukemia are found in children, acute lymphoid leukemia (ALL) and acute myelogenous leukemia (AML). These main types are further divided into subtypes based on the specific aberrations of the WBCs. About 75% of childhood leukemias are ALLs. The etiology is unknown. Predisposing factors include congenital disorders, such as Down syndrome and radiation exposure. The peak age of incidence is between 2 years and 6 years. See Chapter 10 for additional discussion of leukemia.

Diagnosis

A peripheral blood smear shows immature forms of WBCs. Leukocytosis, neutropenia, anemia, and thrombocytopenia are often present. Laboratory studies also include measurement of uric acid levels, electrolytes, kidney and liver function, and coagulation studies. A specimen from bone marrow aspiration is examined. Chromosome analysis of the leukemic cells is performed for diagnosis and because the presence of different characteristic abnormalities has prognostic value. A lumbar puncture is performed to determine whether the CNS is involved because this determination can guide therapy.

Treatment

The disease is treated through systemic chemotherapy to eradicate leukemic cells and to induce remission. Chemotherapy may also be administered as a prophylaxis against CNS invasion. The patient must be followed up closely for signs of tumor lysis syndrome, a group of metabolic complications that develop because of the destruction of leukemic cells when chemotherapy is initiated. Bone marrow transplantation is a possible treatment for children with a poor prognosis or relapsed ALL or for children with AML (because AML carries a poorer prognosis than ALL when treated solely with chemotherapy). Psychological support for the child and the family must be provided.

Prognosis

The best prognostic indicators in determining long-term survival are the patient's age at diagnosis, WBC count at diagnosis, cytogenetics, and immunophenotype (T cell or B cell) play a role in the outcome for the patient.

Prevention

There is no known prevention. Smoking is one risk factor that has been identified in adult patients and should be avoided.

Patient Teaching

Provide reputable online resources and written information. Allow the patient to ask questions and provide appropriate responses.

Erythroblastosis Fetalis (Hemolytic Disease of the Newborn)

Description

Erythroblastosis fetalis stems from the incompatibility of fetal and maternal blood, resulting in excessive rates of RBC destruction.

ICD-10-CM Code	P55.8 *(Other hemolytic diseases of newborn)* (P55.0–P55.9 = 4 codes of specificity) P55.9 *(Hemolytic disease of newborn, unspecified)*

Symptoms and Signs

Erythroblastosis fetalis is characterized by anemia, jaundice, kernicterus, and enlargement of the liver and the spleen. In the most severe form, called *hydrops fetalis*, the fetus or infant is in great jeopardy because of extreme hemolysis. If the infant survives, the condition is marked by heart failure, edema, pulmonary congestion, lethargy, seizures, and intellectual developmental disorder.

Patient Screening

Physicians caring for expectant mothers who have had prenatal care should understand the possibility of Rh incompatibility. New patients aware of possible Rh incompatibility because they know their Rh factor is negative should be scheduled to discuss the matter with the physician as soon as convenient for all parties. Newborn infants with hemolytic disease of the newborn are identified during the newborn examination if not before birth, and treatment will be instituted as soon as possible.

Etiology

The cause is Rh factor incompatibility. Rh factor is the antigen found on the RBCs of the Rh-positive individual. The mother, through a prior pregnancy, has become sensitized to the Rh factor (Rh isoimmunization) of the fetal RBCs. When sensitized maternal blood finds its way into fetal circulation, particularly during delivery, the antibodies in the mother's blood destroy the RBCs of the fetus (Figs. 2.49 and 2.50).

With an Rh-negative female and an Rh-positive male, some or all of the infants will be Rh positive. During pregnancy, blood from the Rh-positive fetus may move from fetal circulation into the mother's bloodstream, where it stimulates the mother's body to form antibodies against the Rh factor. When sufficient quantities of the antibodies pass back into the infant's circulation, the antibodies can clump and destroy Rh-positive cells, causing the symptoms of erythroblastosis fetalis.

Diagnosis

Blood typing of the mother and the father is essential. The maternal history includes pregnancy, elective and spontaneous abortions, and blood transfusions. The direct Coombs test of the umbilical cord blood measures Rh-positive antibodies in the newborn; the bilirubin test for bilirubinemia and hematocrit determination are also performed on the infant's blood. The amniotic fluid may be analyzed for hemolysis.

Treatment

The treatment is dictated by the degree of erythroblastosis fetalis and its effect on the fetus or the newborn. Intrauterine transfusions may be indicated when the fetus shows signs of distress. When necessary, the delivery of the infant is planned 2 to 4 weeks before term. Through exchange transfusion, the infant is given fresh group-O, Rh-negative blood. Phototherapy and albumin infusion are used to reduce the amount of circulating bilirubin in the newborn.

Prognosis

The prognosis is good when the disease is discovered early in pregnancy and closely monitored. Early delivery with immediate transfusion usually treats this condition successfully. Mothers with Rh-negative blood factor need to continue Rho-GAM injections for protection in subsequent pregnancies, including any spontaneous or induced abortions.

Prevention

Protection is now available for Rh-negative mothers who have never been sensitized, preventing the possibility of harm to an Rh-positive baby. Rho(D) immune globulin is given at 28 weeks in the Rh-positive identified pregnancy and as soon as possible to the female at risk after each exposure to Rh-positive blood (most often by giving birth to an Rh-positive infant) to prevent maternal Rh isoimmunization and complications in subsequent pregnancies.

Maternal
circulation

Maternal
Rh-negative
erythrocyte

Fetal
Rh-positive
erythrocyte
enters
maternal
circulation

Fetal
Rh-positive
erythrocyte

A

Maternal
circulation

Maternal
Rh-negative
erythrocyte

Rh
antibodies

B

Maternal
circulation

Agglutination of
fetal Rh-positive
erythrocytes
leads to hemolytic
disease of
the newborn

Maternal
Rh antibodies
cross the
placenta

C

D antigen

Hemolysis

D

• **Fig. 2.49** Hemolytic disease of the newborn. (A) Before or during delivery, Rh-positive erythrocytes from the fetus enter the blood of an Rh-negative female through a tear in the placenta. (B) The mother is sensitized to the Rh antigen and produces Rh antibodies. Because this usually happens after delivery, there is no effect on the fetus in the first pregnancy. (C) During a subsequent pregnancy with an Rh-positive fetus, Rh-positive erythrocytes cross the placenta, enter the maternal circulation, and (D) stimulate the mother to produce antibodies against the Rh antigen. (From McCance K, et al: Pathophysiology: the biological basis for disease in adults and children, ed 6, St. Louis, 2010, Mosby.)

• **Fig. 2.50** The Rh antibodies from the mother cross the placenta, causing agglutination and hemolysis of fetal erythrocytes, and hemolytic disease of the newborn develops. (From McCance K, Huether S: Pathophysiology: the biological basis for disease in adults and children, ed 6, St. Louis, 2010, Mosby.)

Patient Teaching

Emphasize the importance of Rh screening to all pregnant females. Those who are Rh-negative require information about Rh-negative mothers with Rh-positive babies. Provide help with finding and contacting community support groups.

Lead Poisoning

Description

Lead poisoning is an environmentally caused blood toxicity resulting from ingestion or inspiration of lead dust or particles.

ICD-10-CM Code	M1A.10X1 (*Lead-induced chronic gout, unspecified site, with tophus [tophi]*) (M1A.10–M1A.19X1 = 24 codes of specificity)

T56.0X1A *(Toxic effect of lead and its compounds, accidental [unintentional], initial encounter)*

T56.0X2A *(Toxic effect of lead and its compounds, intentional self-harm, initial encounter)*

T56.0X3A *(Toxic effect of lead and its compounds, assault, initial encounter)*

T56.0X4A *(Toxic effect of lead and its compounds, undetermined, initial encounter)*

Refer to the physician's diagnosis and then to the current edition of the ICD-10-CM coding manual to ensure the greatest specificity of pathology.

Symptoms and Signs

Children exposed to toxic levels of lead, a poisonous metallic element, exhibit signs of lead poisoning. Some warning signs are loss of appetite, vomiting, irritability, and ataxic gait. Chronic symptoms include anemia, weakness, colic, and peripheral neuritis. Evidence of intellectual developmental disorder resulting from brain damage is possible. A child with acute lead intoxication presents as a medical emergency. The child has symptoms of encephalopathy with vomiting, headache, stupor, convulsions, and coma resulting from cerebral edema (Fig. 2.51).

Patient Screening

Children exhibiting fatigue, headaches, irritability, stomachaches, cramps, muscle and joint pain, and changes in behavior require prompt assessment.

Etiology

Any level of lead in the blood is abnormal. Exposure results from breathing or swallowing substances containing lead. The condition has been reported to develop in children who eat flakes of peeling lead paint, drink water from lead pipes, or ingest lead salts in certain foods. Some imported toys have been found to contain lead or are painted with lead-based paint. Lead dust may remain in soil contaminated by exhaust from previous use of leaded gasoline. Lead taken into the body is stored in many tissues; it is released into the blood and excreted in the urine.

Diagnosis

The history of lead exposure and the presence of previously listed symptoms suggest the diagnosis. Blood tests reveal anemia and a blood lead level greater than 5 µg/dL. Lead excretion through urine is increased. Radiographs note characteristic changes in the ends of growing bones.

Treatment

The source of poisoning must first be eliminated. Subsequent treatment is based on lead level and symptoms. For patients with levels greater than 45 mcg/dL, an attempt

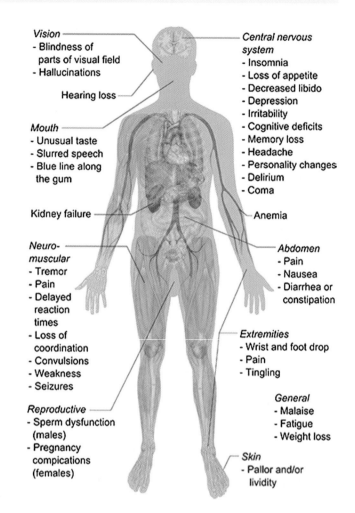

• **Fig. 2.51** Manifestations of lead poisoning. (From Kathiah R: Textbook of pathology, ed 1, 2022, Elsevier (India).)

may be made to remove the lead from the body by giving substances, known as *chelating agents*, that tie up the lead in a chemically inactive form in the bloodstream while it is transported to the kidneys for elimination. Antiemetics help control nausea and vomiting, and sedation is given for convulsions.

Prognosis

The prognosis varies, depending on the extent of damage and the promptness in discovering the toxicity. Aggressive intervention and removal of the child from the contaminated environment help prevent additional damage.

Prevention

An awareness of the environmental sources of lead, such as lead paint, lead plumbing, and other sources of lead dust is prudent. An act, Title X, or the Lead-Based Paint Hazard Act of 1992, has helped prevent exposure to lead in homes built before 1978 by requiring disclosure of lead-based paint hazards in the home. Dust on vinyl mini-blinds may contain lead deposits. Caution must be used with imported toys that may contain lead or be painted with lead-based paint.

Patient Teaching

Teaching the parents about the hazards of lead poisoning and how to recognize toxic sources is essential.

Miscellaneous Diseases, Syndromes, and Disorders

Reye Syndrome

Description

Reye syndrome is a combination of brain disease and fatty invasion of the inner organs, especially the liver.

> ICD-10-CM Code G93.7 *(Reye syndrome)*
> *Refer to the physician's diagnosis and then to the current edition of the ICD-10-CM coding manual to ensure the greatest specificity of pathology.*

Symptoms and Signs

This rare syndrome is an acute, often fatal illness that may affect children through age 15 years. The pathogenesis includes a disruption in the urea cycle that causes swelling of the brain, resulting in increased intracranial pressure. The symptoms of Reye syndrome progress through five stages: (1) lethargy, listlessness, irritability, combativeness, vomiting, and hepatic dysfunction; (2) hyperventilation, hyperactive reflexes, hepatic dysfunction, disorientation, convulsions, and delirium; (3) organ changes and coma; (4) deeper coma and loss of cerebral functions; and (5) seizures, loss of deep tendon reflexes, and respiratory arrest.

Patient Screening

Children who begin vomiting 3 to 6 days after a viral illness, such as chickenpox, are possible candidates for Reye syndrome and require immediate assessment and intervention.

Etiology

The cause of Reye syndrome is unknown. However, it typically follows infection with influenza A or B viruses or chickenpox. It has been linked to the use of aspirin during these infections.

Diagnosis

The medical history and the patient's clinical features suggest the disease. Laboratory blood studies show elevated serum ammonia levels. Liver function tests show elevated enzyme levels. Other tests include liver biopsy and CSF analysis.

Treatment

The early recognition and treatment of Reye syndrome has reduced the mortality rate. Successful management with early diagnosis involves hospitalization to stabilize the patient, control cerebral edema, monitor blood chemistries, manage seizures, and provide mechanical ventilation if needed. Complete recovery is possible.

Prognosis

The prognosis is good with prompt intervention and aggressive treatment.

Prevention

For prevention, the use of nonsalicylate analgesics and antipyretics, such as acetaminophen, is recommended, instead of aspirin.

Patient Teaching

Caution all parents or caregivers that children should not be given aspirin during possible viral infections.

Fetal Alcohol Syndrome

Description

According to the Fetal Alcohol Spectrum Disorders (FASD) United website, "Fetal alcohol spectrum disorders (FASD) is an umbrella term describing the range of effects that can occur in an individual prenatally exposed to alcohol. These effects may include physical, mental, behavioral, and/or learning disabilities with lifelong implications. The term FASD is not intended for use as a clinical diagnosis."

> ICD-10-CM Code P04.3 *(Newborn [suspected to be] affected by maternal use of alcohol)*
> Q86.0 *(Fetal alcohol syndrome [dysmorphic])*

Symptoms and Signs

Intrauterine exposure to sufficient levels of alcohol has been associated with delayed fetal growth, in which the infants are short and below average in weight. Facial characteristics of FAS include smaller eye openings, with eyes spaced widely apart, and a thin upper lip. The infant may experience growth deficiencies and CNS problems. Heart defects, including ASD and VSD, may be present. FAS also is associated with intellectual developmental disorder. The infant may exhibit signs of alcohol withdrawal shortly after birth.

These children may experience learning difficulties, including decreased attention span and memory, visual and auditory problems, and communication difficulties. Poor development of social skills may be present.

Patient Screening

Maternal history and newborn examination usually reveal the condition. Parents seeking medical attention for their child at any stage of development should be scheduled for the earliest possible appointment.

Etiology

FASD is caused when alcohol enters the fetal blood while in the womb.

Diagnosis

Typical clinical features present in the newborn and a maternal history of chronic alcoholism determine the diagnosis (Fig. 2.52).

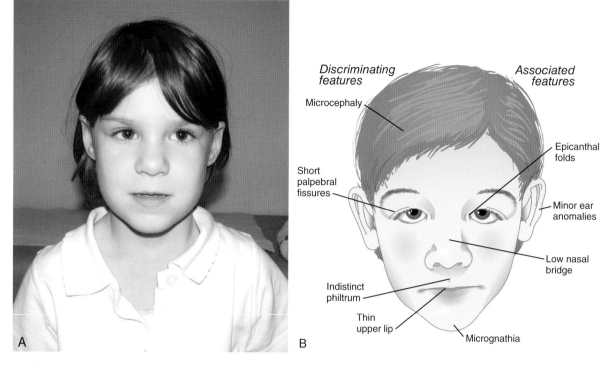

• **Fig. 2.52** (A) Face of a young girl with fetal alcohol syndrome showing a long, thin upper lip; shortened, upwardly slanting palpebral fissures; and epicanthic folds. (B) Commonly expressed facial characteristics of fetal alcohol syndrome in a young child. (A, From Turnpenny P, et al: Emery's Elements of Medical Genetics. Philadelphia, 2012, Elsevier; B, Adapted from Streissguth AP: Alcohol Health Res World, 1994.)

Treatment

The treatment depends on the defects present in the newborn. Much of the treatment is supportive because neurologic damage cannot be reversed. Proper nutrition is vital. Because the baby may have a poor sucking reflex, special adaptation may be necessary to ensure proper intake. The psychosocial needs of the infant and the mother must be addressed.

Prognosis

As previously mentioned, neurologic damage cannot be reversed; therefore the prognosis varies, depending on the amount of neurologic damage sustained.

Prevention

Preventive measures include prenatal care and education. Females are advised not to consume any amount of alcohol during pregnancy.

Patient Teaching

Drinking is not advised at any point during pregnancy. Females who are trying to become pregnant should also avoid drinking. In addition, good prenatal care should be emphasized.

Diaper Rash

Description

Diaper rash, considered a contact dermatitis, is evident in the diaper area as an irritation or rash.

ICD-10-CM Code   L22 *(Diaper dermatitis)*

Symptoms and Signs

Diaper rash can vary from mild to severe and can be self-limiting or a chronic source of discomfort to the infant and dismay to the parent or caregiver. Diaper rash takes multiple forms: from a mild excoriation, or maculopapular rash, to blisters and ulceration.

Patient Screening

Infants and toddlers with diaper rash that does not clear require prompt assessment.

Etiology

Infants with sensitive skin seem to have a hereditary predisposition to diaper rash, or irritant dermatitis. Diaper rash may be triggered by friction or prolonged exposure to moisture, feces, or the ammonia produced by bacterial action in urine. Poorly washed or rinsed diapers and the use of occlusive plastic pants over the diapers may be contributing factors. Poor hygiene or overzealous cleaning could irritate the diaper area.

Diagnosis

One may need to differentiate diaper rash from seborrheic dermatitis, eczema, and secondary skin infection.

Treatment

In addition to frequent diaper changes and proper cleaning and drying of the diaper area, a bland protective agent, such as zinc oxide or hydrated petrolatum, may promote healing.

If possible, allowing the infant to remain without a diaper for some time will promote healing. Topical antimicrobial agents are used for secondary skin infections. Cloth diapers should be rinsed of irritating residue.

Prognosis
The prognosis is good.

Prevention
Frequent changing of diapers accompanied by thorough cleansing of the diaper area helps prevent the rash. Leaving the area exposed to air for short periods often allows the area to dry and helps prevent the rash from returning.

Patient Teaching
Stress the importance of changing the infant's or toddler's diaper on a regular schedule and not leaving the child in a soiled diaper for extended periods. If necessary, demonstrate the method of cleansing the diaper area.

Neuroblastoma

Description
Neuroblastoma, a cancer of the sympathetic nervous system, is the third most common childhood malignancy. It arises from primitive sympathetic ganglion cells.

ICD-10-CM Code	C74.90 *(Malignant neoplasm of unspecified part of unspecified adrenal gland)* (C74.0–C74.92 = 9 codes of specificity)

Refer to the physician's diagnosis and then to the current edition of the ICD-10-CM coding manual to ensure the greatest specificity of pathology.

Symptoms and Signs
Neuroblastoma can arise from any site in the sympathetic nervous system, with the adrenal gland and the abdomen being the most common areas. Symptoms include abdominal mass, abdominal pain or fullness, anemia, bone pain, fever, hypertension, and weight loss. Periorbital ecchymosis ("raccoon eyes") is not uncommon (Fig. 2.53).

Patient Screening
When the parents report that their child has an abdominal mass or unexplained fever and weight loss, the child should be evaluated promptly.

Etiology
Most cases of neuroblastoma are diagnosed in the first few years of life. The etiology is unknown, but because of the early age at onset, maternal factors or exposures during pregnancy could play a role.

• **Fig. 2.53** Neuroblastoma: neuroblastoma metastatic to the orbit may present with an abrupt onset of unilateral or bilateral proptosis and ecchymosis of the eyelids. Neuroblastoma is the most common lesion to metastasize to the orbit in childhood. (From McIntire S, et al: *Zitelli and Davis' Atlas of Pediatric Physical Diagnosis*, ed 8, 2023, Elsevier.)

Diagnosis
Laboratory studies include measurement of urine and serum catecholamine levels, as well as electrolytes and kidney and liver functions. Biopsy of the mass gives a definitive diagnosis. For staging evaluation, bone marrow aspirate and biopsy, radionuclide bone scan, abdominal CT, and chest radiography are all performed. Chest and head CT may be indicated, depending on the patient's symptoms.

Treatment
For patients with low-risk tumors, surgical removal is the only treatment required. For higher-stage tumors, chemotherapy with or without radiation therapy is employed. For children with high-risk disease, high-dose chemotherapy followed by autologous hematopoietic stem cell rescue may be beneficial. Even after therapy is completed, the patient needs to be followed up closely to monitor for the development of any late effects of treatment, including second malignancies.

Prognosis
The best prognostic indicators include younger age at diagnosis, localized disease, and certain cytogenetic abnormalities. It should be noted that there is a stage 4S that includes children younger than 1 year of age with disseminated disease. This actually confers a better prognosis because these tumors may regress spontaneously without any therapy.

Prevention
There is no known prevention.

Patient Teaching
Work with parents to contact support groups.

Review Challenge

Answer the following questions:

1. List the possible causes of congenital anomalies.
2. What is the purpose of amniocentesis? Describe the procedure.
3. Describe the condition of prematurity, and list its causes. List the associated disorders, identify their causes, and discuss the treatment options.
4. List some genetic syndromes.
5. What often is a cause of sudden death in a teenage athlete?
6. What is the cause of Down syndrome?
7. Describe neural tube defects, and list the conditions resulting from them.
8. How is hydrocephalus treated?
9. Trace fetal circulation.
10. Explain the difference between cyanotic and acyanotic defects.
11. Name and describe the most common congenital cyanotic cardiac defect.
12. Describe patent ductus arteriosus and its treatment.
13. Explain the differences between muscular dystrophy and cerebral palsy.
14. List the major clinical manifestations of cystic fibrosis.
15. Explain cryptorchidism, how it is treated, and what may happen if left untreated.
16. Explain the symptoms of Wilms tumor.
17. What is congenital pyloric stenosis, and how is it treated?
18. Explain the differences between Klinefelter syndrome and Turner syndrome.
19. Describe the symptoms of chickenpox.
20. Why is it important for parents to follow the recommended schedule of childhood immunizations?
21. Discuss the importance of childhood immunizations, and list the schedule for the first year of life.
22. Describe the symptoms of mumps, and discuss the progression of the disease.
23. What vaccine is important for parents and grandparents to be up to date with?
24. Compare rubeola and rubella.
25. Describe the clinical condition of congenital rubella syndrome.
26. What are the symptoms of sudden infant death syndrome?
27. Compare croup and epiglottitis.
28. Why is throat culture important for a child with tonsillitis?
29. What does adenoid hyperplasia cause?
30. Discuss the incidence, etiology, treatment, and risks of asthma.
31. Discuss the types of worm infestations that may occur and how they are treated.
32. Childhood obesity is a major health concern. List some recommended guidelines to assist parents in providing proper nutrition for their children.
33. List the signs of childhood anemia.
34. List the symptoms and signs of anemia; describe the pathology of leukemia.
35. Explain the etiology of erythroblastosis fetalis.
36. Name some warning signs of lead poisoning.
37. Describe the infant born with fetal alcohol syndrome.
38. List the possible causes of diaper rash.

Real-Life Challenge: Asthma

A 6-year-old male has coughing with audible expiratory wheezes and dyspnea. The child is pale, the skin is moist and cool, and the child has difficulty speaking more than a few words before stopping to catch his breath. His parents state that the difficulty breathing had a rapid onset approximately 1 hour earlier when he was playing with the neighbor's dog. The child has a history of previous asthma attacks, primarily after visiting his aunt's home where there are cats.

Assessment of the child shows temperature (T), 98.6°F; pulse (P), 120 beats per minute; and respiratory rate, 40 breaths per minute and labored. Bilateral rales are heard on auscultation, louder on expiration but also present on inspiration. Cromolyn sodium had been prescribed to be taken prophylactically before visits to the aunt's home. The child also has an albuterol sulfate inhaler to be used PRN (as needed). The use of the inhaler has brought no relief.

Questions

1. Which diagnostic procedures would be ordered to reveal the degree of airway obstruction?
2. Which immediate intervention may be ordered to relieve the symptoms and provide comfort to the child?
3. What future testing may be ordered?
4. What is the cause of the dyspnea?
5. List the allergens commonly responsible for asthma attacks.
6. Explain why asthma attacks are considered medical emergencies and what steps should be taken on arrival of a patient experiencing an asthma attack.

Real-Life Challenge: Patent Ductus Arteriosus

A 1-week-old premature infant weighing 1 lb 10 oz begins exhibiting reduced oxygen saturation levels, bradycardia, and cyanosis. The infant's respirations are being maintained with mechanical ventilation. Increased oxygen concentration is required to maintain oxygen saturation levels at 90%. The chest radiograph reveals infant respiratory distress syndrome (IRDS) as resolving. The echocardiogram indicates patent ductus arteriosus (PDA).

Questions

1. Explain the two treatment options, drug therapy and a surgical procedure, used to close the PDA.
2. Explain the complication that could occur as a result of high concentration levels of oxygen.
3. What is the prognosis for the cardiac status of this child once closure has been achieved?
4. Which other congenital cardiac defect may be present?
5. Trace fetal circulation, and explain the role of the ductus arteriosus before birth.

Internet Assignments

1. Go to the Asthma and Allergy Foundation of America website to ascertain and report on recent treatment options for asthma.
2. Go to the Cystic Fibrosis Foundation website to research new treatment options and support systems for patients and their families.
   Prepare to discuss the Critical Thinking case study exercises for this chapter that are posted on Evolve.

Credentialing Examination Questions

1. Which food should be avoided by pregnant patients?
   A. Fruits
   B. Raw shellfish
   C. Cooked shrimp
   D. Beef
2. How many pairs of chromosomes are present in a normal human cell?
   A. 20
   B. 21
   C. 22
   D. 23
3. During which gestational age, in weeks, does amniocentesis usually take place?
   A. 19th to 21st
   B. 15th to 17th
   C. 10th to 12th
   D. 6th to 8th
4. Which term refers to conjoined twins that are attached at the pelvic region?
   A. Craniopagus
   B. Thoracopagus
   C. Rachipagus
   D. Ischiopagus
5. Which organ system is affected by hyaline membrane disease?
   A. Cardiac
   B. Urinary
   C. Respiratory
   D. Endocrine
6. Which condition involves ischemic necrosis or death of the lining of the small or large intestine?
   A. Malnutrition
   B. Necrotizing enterocolitis
   C. Cri-du-chat syndrome
   D. Retrolental fibroplasia
7. Which amount of alcohol can be consumed without a potential risk to an unborn child?
   A. None
   B. 4 oz per week
   C. 1 oz per day
   D. 3 oz per week
8. Down syndrome results from which genetic anomaly?
   A. Deletion of two chromosomes resulting in 44
   B. Two X chromosomes and one Y chromosome
   C. An extra or partial chromosome number 21 (trisomy 21)
   D. An extra or partial chromosome on number 11
9. A child with a diaper rash is considered to have which diagnosis?
   A. Pediculosis
   B. Contact dermatitis
   C. Folliculitis
   D. Erythroblastosis
10. In which organ system does a neuroblastoma occur?
    A. Endocrine
    B. Pulmonary
    C. Nervous
    D. Integumentary

3

Immunologic Diseases and Conditions

CHAPTER OUTLINE

LEARNING OBJECTIVES

After studying this chapter, you should be able to:

1. Name the functional components of the immune system.
2. List the examples of inappropriate responses of the immune system.
3. Characterize the three major functions of the immune system.
4. List the five immunoglobulins and explain complement fixation.
5. Trace the formation of T cells and B cells from stem cells.
6. Explain how T cells and B cells specifically protect the body against disease.
7. Identify the difference between active immunity and passive immunity.
8. Explain the ways that human immunodeficiency virus is transmitted.
9. List the guidelines for universal precautions and infection control.
10. Describe the primary absent or inadequate response of the immune system in the following diseases:

- Common variable immunodeficiency
- Selective immunoglobulin A deficiency
- Severe combined immunodeficiency disease

11. Explain the destructive mechanisms in autoimmune diseases.
12. Describe the symptoms and signs of pernicious anemia. Name the primary treatment.
13. Recall the systemic features of systemic lupus erythematosus. Recall the diagnostic criteria.
14. Detail the pathology of rheumatoid arthritis (RA).
15. Specify the primary objectives of the treatment for RA.
16. List the distinguishing diagnostic features of ankylosing spondylitis.
17. Compare the pathology of multiple sclerosis with that of myasthenia gravis.
18. Describe the pathology of vasculitis in general terms.

KEY TERMS

anticholinesterase (an-tee-koh-lyn-ES-ter-ase)
autoimmune (aw-tow-im-YOON)
candidiasis (kan-dih-DIE-ah-sis)

collagen (KOLL-ah-jen)
hematopoietic (hem-ah-toh-poy-ET-ik)

hypogammaglobulinemia (hye-poh-gam-a-glob-you-lyn-
    EE-me-ah)
immunocompetent (im-you-no-KOM-peh-tent)
immunodeficiency (im-you-no-deh-FISH-en-see)
immunoelectrophoresis (im-you-no-ee-lek-troh-foh-REE-
    sis)
immunogen (IM-you-no-jen)
immunoglobulin (im-you-no-GLAHB-you-lyn)

immunosuppressive (im-you-no-sup-PRESS-iv)
keratoconjunctivitis (ker-ah-toh-kon-junk-tih-VIE-tis)
lymph (limf)
lymphadenopathy (lim-fad-eh-NOP-ah-thee)
lymphocyte (LIM-foh-sight)
macrophage (MACK-roh-fayj)
phagocytes (FAG-oh-sights)
phagocytosis (fag-oh-sigh-TOH-sis)

Orderly Function of the Immune System

The immune system, a major defense mechanism, is responsible for a complex response of the body to invasion by foreign substances. The concept of the immune system arose from the observation that a person who recovers from a specific infection may not get sick from that infection again. The person is thereafter considered "immune" to that particular infectious agent. Immunity is very specific in that a person has developed immunity to a certain virus. Historically, the United States had many cases of the rubella virus, but this was eradicated in 2004 after the vaccine became available in 1969. Prior to the vaccination program, rubella was widespread, and 12.5 million people were reported as having the disease between 1964 and 1965, which caused illness and death. Hence, those vaccinated became immune, and the disease was not transmitted, which led to a huge decline each year in cases. The very rare cases in the United States today have been linked to visiting a foreign country or traveling.

If a person was vaccinated against the rubella virus, they are still susceptible to infection by other viruses, such as the measles virus. The immune response assists the body in maintaining its functional integrity, and it battles infection caused by bacteria, viruses, fungi, and parasites. The immune system involves lymphoid tissues classified as primary (thymus and bone marrow) or secondary (tonsils, adenoids, spleen, Peyer patches, appendix, etc.) (Fig. 3.1).

When the immune system reacts appropriately to an antigen and homeostasis is maintained, a person is immunocompetent. If the immune system's response is inappropriate, either too weak or too strong, it results in the disruption of homeostasis. This malfunction in the system is referred to as *immunoincompetence*. Disruption of homeostasis is the cause of many diseases. When the immune system does not work in the intended way, an autoimmune system disorder occurs.

Inappropriate responses or malfunctioning of the immune system are classified as follows:

- Hyperactive responses (e.g., allergies), in which the immune response is excessive and triggered by specific allergens.
- Immunodeficiency disorders (e.g., acquired immunodeficiency syndrome [AIDS]), in which the immune response is inadequate.
- Autoimmune disorders (e.g., systemic lupus erythematosus [SLE]), in which the immune response is overactive and misdirected against one's own tissues.
- Attacks on beneficial foreign tissue (e.g., reaction to blood transfusions or transplanted organ rejection) (see Enrichment box about Transplant Rejection and Fig. 3.2).

The immune response is normally activated whenever foreign substances, or antigens, enter the body by evading its first line of defense—the skin and mucous membranes. The body recognizes the antigen or immunogen, usually a protein, as foreign, or nonself, and produces antibodies in response to that specific antigen. Antibody molecules have combining sites on its surface and can combine with threatening cells, such as microorganisms or cancer cells. This forms an antigen-antibody complex that renders the antigen harmless. It is crucial that the immune system be able to differentiate between self and nonself or foreign molecules. When this differentiation does not occur as it should, an autoimmune disease is the result. In autoimmune disease, the body mistakenly recognizes molecules of its own tissues as foreign and then attacks them.

The mechanisms of nonspecific defense involve preformed and fully activated components that launch a nonspecific attack on a foreign organism as soon as it is detected. The main cells involved in nonspecific defense include the following:

- Natural killer (NK) cells kill virus-infected cells and tumor cells by secreting certain toxins
- Macrophages that phagocytose bacteria, viruses, and other foreign substances
- Polymorphonuclear neutrophils (or simply *neutrophils*) also phagocytose bacteria

The development of the components required for immunity begins early in fetal life when the fetal liver produces stem cells, which, in turn, produce all cells of the hematopoietic system. Bone marrow assumes this role after birth (Fig. 3.3). Some of the stem cells migrate to the thymus gland, where they become T cells (T^c), which multiply and develop the capacity to combine with specific foreign antigens derived from viruses, fungi, tumors, or transplanted tissue (Fig. 3.4). Those T cells, coded to recognize self-antigens, are destroyed. The remaining T cells are coded to seek

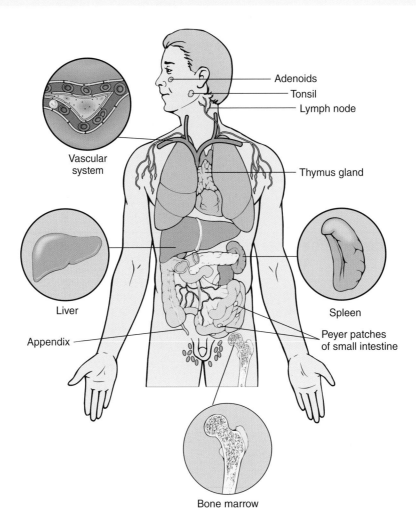

Vascular system

Adenoids

Tonsil

Lymph node

Thymus gland

Liver

Spleen

Appendix

Peyer patches of small intestine

Bone marrow

• **Fig. 3.1** Immune system.

out foreign invaders. The body produces several types of T cells; each has a different function:

- Cytotoxic T cells (killer T cells) directly destroy virus-infected cells, tumor cells, and allograft cells by releasing certain toxins or by inducing apoptosis. These cells also may be referred to as *CD8 cells* because they carry the CD8 glycoprotein on their surface.
- Helper T cells stimulate the B cells to differentiate into plasma cells and to produce more antibodies. They also activate cytotoxic T cells and macrophages. Helper T cells carry the CD4 glycoprotein on their surface.
- Suppressor T cells inhibit both B- and T-cell activities and moderate the immune response.
- Memory T cells remain dormant until they are reactivated by the original antigen, allowing a rapid and more potent response years after the original exposure.

T cells are the major component of the type of acquired immunity known as *cell-mediated immunity*. The mononuclear phagocytic system, formerly termed the *reticuloendothelial system*, initiates this immune response. Macrophages, which develop from monocytes, a type of white blood cell (WBC), are found in the tissue of the liver, lungs, and lymph nodes. These large cells intercept and engulf the

foreign invader antigens and then process and present them to the T cells. Cell-mediated immunity defends the body against viral and fungal attacks, mediates graft rejection and tumor cell destruction, and helps or suppresses an antibody-mediated response to infection.

The remaining stem cells develop into B cells (B lymphocytes) to produce antibody-mediated (humoral) immunity, which protects the body against bacterial and viral infections and reinfections (see Fig. 3.4). Once activated by exposure to an antigen, B cells are stimulated to proliferate and form a clone of cells that respond to that specific antigen. Some B cells become antibody-secreting plasma cells, whereas others become memory B cells, ready for a quick response if the target antigen presents itself again. The plasma cells are responsible for producing antibodies that attach to invading foreign antigens, thus marking the antigens for destruction by other cells of the immune system.

B cells are coated with **immunoglobulins**, giving them the ability to recognize foreign proteins and stimulate an antigen-antibody reaction. The five classes of immunoglobulins or antibodies are immunoglobulin M (IgM), IgG, IgA, IgD, and IgE (Table 3.1). These immunoglobulins are usually all present during an antigenic response, although

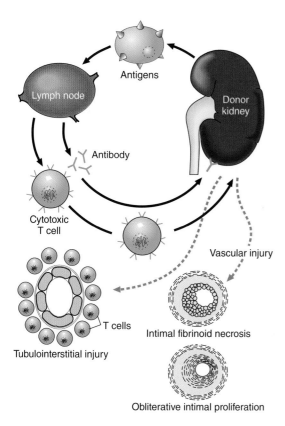

• **Fig. 3.2** Transplant rejection. (Modified from Damjanov I: *Pathology for the health-related professions*, ed 5, St. Louis, 2017, Elsevier, Inc.)

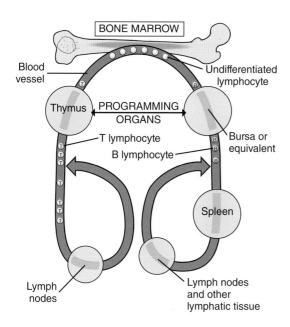

• **Fig. 3.3** Bone marrow formation of lymphocytes.

in varying amounts, depending on the stimulant and the health of the patient. Actions of the antigen-antibody complex include the following:
• Inactivation of the pathogen or its toxin through direct binding.

• Stimulation of phagocytosis through complement fixation, the process by which an antibody targets an infected cell for destruction by binding to the cell surface. (Phagocytic cells recognize the antibody marker and engulf the infected cell.)

Activation of the complement system (complement fixation) involves several proteins found in plasma or body fluids. The antigen-antibody reaction initiates a series or cascade of reactions that activate the complement system, fixing the complement system and consequently permitting the destruction of pathogens by the process of phagocytosis or lysis of the pathogen's cell membrane (Fig. 3.5). This activation occurs during an immune reaction mediated by IgG or IgM.

The human body is protected by two types of acquired specific immunity: active immunity and passive immunity. *Active immunity* results when a person has had previous exposure to a disease or pathogen or when a person receives immunizations against a disease to stimulate the production of a specific antibody. Active immunity affords the person permanent protection. *Passive immunity* bypasses the body's immune response to afford the benefit of immediate antibody availability. A person gains passive immunity by being given immune substances created outside that person's body for temporary immunity, such as antibodies received through the placenta, breast milk, or when immune

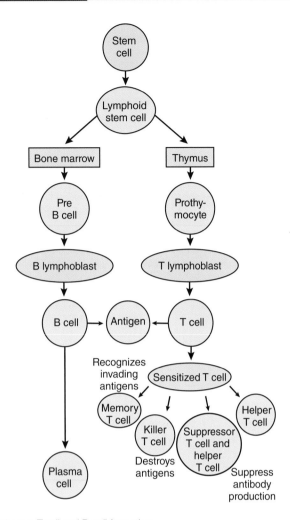

• **Fig. 3.4** T-cell and B-cell formation.

globulin, an antibody-containing preparation made from the plasma of healthy donors, is given to help a person combat disease (Fig. 3.6).

Immunodeficiency Diseases

An absent or inadequate response of the immune system results in immunodeficiency conditions and increased susceptibility to other diseases and opportunistic infections. **Immunodeficiency** can occur in any of the following major components of the immune system: B cells, T cells, complement, or **phagocytes**. Although the deficiency may be in either the humoral (antibody-related) or the cell-mediated responses, the consequences are similar: The individual does not have the capability to eliminate foreign and harmful substances. In general, an increased susceptibility to bacterial infections results from a B-cell deficiency, whereas recurrent viral, fungal, and protozoan infections are usually caused by decreased T-cell function. Some of the conditions are genetic and present at birth, whereas other defects are not manifested until later in life or are acquired. Acquired immunoincompetence may result from a bacterial or viral insult to the body, malnutrition, or exposure to radiation or certain drugs. The severity of the immunodeficiency disease depends on the type of cell or cells that are affected. It can range from annoying chronic infections to severe life-threatening or fatal conditions.

Acquired Immunodeficiency Syndrome

Description

AIDS is a progressive impairment of the immune system caused by the human immunodeficiency virus (HIV). This gradual destruction of the immune system affects many organ systems and is potentially life threatening for the person infected.

TABLE 3.1 Classes of Antibodies

Class	Percent of Total	Location	Function
IgG	75–85	Blood plasma	Major antibody in primary and secondary immune responses; inactivates antigen; neutralizes toxins; crosses the placenta to provide immunity for newborn; responsible for Rh reactions
IgA	5–15	Saliva, mucus, tears, breast milk	Protects mucous membranes on body surfaces; provides immunity for newborn
IgM	5–10	Attached to B cells; released into plasma during immune response	Causes antigens to clump together; responsible for transfusion reactions in the ABO blood typing system
IgD	0.2	Attached to B cells	Receptor sites for antigens on B cells; binding with antigen results in B-cell activation
IgE	0.5	Produced by plasma cells in mucous membranes and tonsils	Binds to mast cells and basophils, causing release of histamine; responsible for allergic reactions

Ig, Immunoglobulin.
From Applegate EJ: *The anatomy and physiology learning system*, ed 4, St. Louis, 2011, Saunders.

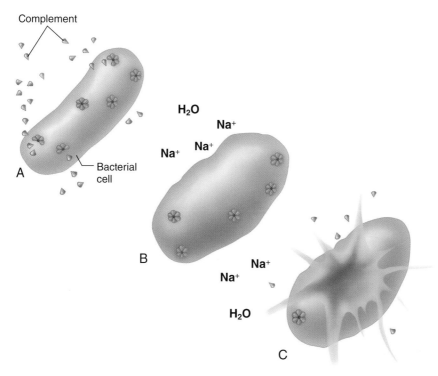

• **Fig. 3.5** Complement cascade. (A) Complement molecules activated by antibodies form doughnut-shaped complexes in a bacterium's plasma membrane. (B) Holes in the complement complex allow sodium (Na^+) and then water (H_2O) to diffuse into the bacterium. (C) After enough water has entered, the swollen bacterium bursts. This is just one of many functions of the complement proteins. (From Patton KT, Thibodeau GA: *The human body in health and disease*, ed 6, St. Louis, 2014, Mosby.)

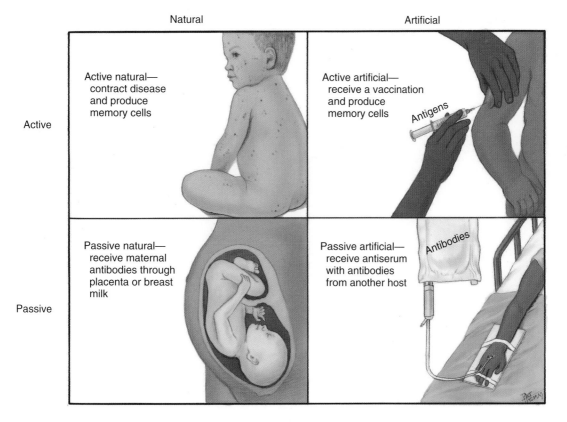

• **Fig. 3.6** Acquired immunity. (From Applegate EJ: *The anatomy and physiology learning system*, ed 4, St. Louis, 2011, Saunders.)

ICD-10-CM Code   B20 *(Human immunodeficiency virus [HIV] disease)*

Symptoms and Signs

A person infected with HIV may remain healthy for years during the latent period and may unknowingly transmit the virus to other people. Within 1 to 4 weeks after exposure, the patient may experience a flu-like illness with sore throat, fever, and body aches that often lasts about 2 weeks. Lymphadenopathy, weight loss, fatigue, diarrhea, and night sweats are common as the clinical course progresses. The body's number of T cells becomes lower and allows for frequent infections, especially opportunistic infections, pneumonia, fever, and malignancies (see the Enrichment box about Malignancies and Common Opportunistic Infections and Conditions in Patients with AIDS; Fig. 3.7).

Often, in the later stages, encephalopathy and malignancy lead to dementia and death (Fig. 3.8).

Patient Screening

An individual who complains of weight loss, fatigue, swollen glands, night sweats, and/or a persistent flulike syndrome needs an appointment with a physician for a medical evaluation as soon as possible. When an individual reports known HIV exposure through unprotected sexual contact or puncture with a contaminated needle, immediate medical care should be arranged.

Etiology

AIDS is caused by HIV, type 1 or 2 (HIV-1 is found worldwide, and HIV-2 is mainly found in West Africa) retroviruses that contain RNA; they cannot survive apart from human

• **Fig. 3.7** Clinical symptoms of acquired immunodeficiency syndrome. (A) Severe weight loss and anorexia. (B) Kaposi sarcoma lesions. (C) Perianal lesions of herpes simplex infection. (D) Deterioration of vision from cytomegalovirus retinitis leading to areas of infection, which can lead to blindness. (From Rogers J: *McCance & Huether's pathophysiology: the biologic basis for disease in adults and children*, ed 9, 2024, Elsevier; A and D, From Taylor PK: *Diagnostic picture tests in sexually transmitted diseases*. London, 1995, Mosby; B and C, From Morse SA, et al., editors: *Atlas of sexually transmitted diseases and AIDS*, ed 4, London, 2011, Saunders.)

Malignancies and Common Opportunistic Infections and Conditions in Patients With AIDS

- Kaposi sarcoma is an aggressive malignancy of the blood vessels that appears as purple or blue patches on the skin, in the mouth, or anywhere else on the body.
- Lymphomas are cancerous lesions of lymphoid tissues.
- *Pneumocystis carinii* pneumonia (PCP) is a lung infection that can progress to be life threatening. It is the most common lung disease in persons with AIDS.
- Tuberculosis is a bacterial infection of the lungs or other organs.
- Herpes simplex infection consists of painful blisterlike lesions of the mouth, genitalia, or anus caused by the herpes virus.
- Herpes zoster (shingles) is characterized by clusters of red, blisterlike skin lesions that are distributed along the distribution of an inflamed nerve.
- *Candida albicans* causes a fungal infection of the mucous membranes of the mouth, genitalia, or skin.
- Toxoplasmosis is an infection caused by a protozoan intracellular parasite. A rash and lymphadenopathy can be present, and the central nervous system (CNS), heart, or lungs can become involved.
- Neurologic complications include inflammation of nerves, neuropathy, neoplasms, and AIDS dementia complex.
- Diarrhea is a symptom of a host of bacterial and viral infections of the gastrointestinal (GI) tract, liver, or gallbladder.
- Epstein-Barr virus causes hairy leukoplakia that is characterized by white plaque visible on the tongue.

cells. HIV attacks helper T lymphocytes (CD4 cells), the body's safeguard against tumors, viruses, and parasites. The destruction of T cells and the proliferation of HIV leave the body defenseless against infection and malignancy by reducing cell-mediated immunity. The virus also directly damages the nervous system. AIDS was first recognized in the United States in 1981. Since then, it has become a top killer of young males and a worldwide threat to humankind. It is estimated that more than 38 million people worldwide are currently infected by HIV. To date, neither a cure nor an effective vaccine has been found for this disease. The virus mutates rapidly. The use of highly active antiretroviral therapy (HAART) has significantly prolonged the life span of those infected.

HIV is spread most readily by direct contact with the blood or semen of an infected person. Individuals may contract HIV through vaginal or anal intercourse, sharing syringes, needles, and other items used for administering drugs. It is not transmitted by casual contact, such as touching, shaking hands, and hugging. It should also be noted that AIDS also can be transmitted through blood and blood products, but the risk is extremely low since blood and blood products are currently tested for HIV prior to infusion. In years past, this was not the case, and blood was not

checked for HIV. Infants of infected mothers are at minimal risk for contracting HIV if the mother is being treated for HIV and has an undetectable viral load. Sharing of needles by HIV-positive intravenous drug users also leads to infection. The risk of transmission of HIV to and from health care workers and patients is minimized by strict adherence to the universal precautions for infection control.

Diagnosis

A common laboratory screening test used to detect the presence of HIV antibodies in blood is enzyme-linked immunosorbent assay (ELISA). If the findings are positive, the test is repeated, and the result is then confirmed by using the western blot test. A positive result on the p24 antigen test indicates circulating HIV antigen. ELISA results are often negative during the first month of infection, although results of the p24 antigen test or the polymerase chain reaction assay may be positive. Rapid HIV antibody testing has become the preferred method of testing because the results are often available within 5 minutes. Although a negative test is regarded as a true negative, a positive result requires confirmatory testing with a western blot. A viral titer and CD4 T-cell count are usually obtained after a positive test result to determine the patient's disease burden and risk for opportunistic infections. Transmission of HIV is possible during all stages of infection, even before it can be detected by laboratory tests, which is called the *window period*.

Home testing kits for HIV have evolved in recent years. A few years ago, the US Food and Drug Administration approved an over-the-counter saliva test. Individuals can perform these self-tests using saliva samples and obtain results in less than an hour without the need for the specimen to be sent to a laboratory. When an at-home test indicates a positive result, the patient should follow up with their health care provider. As with any test, there may be false-positive and false-negative results.

With advances in technology, there is a nucleic acid test (NAT) that identifies the virus in the blood. This test involves the collection of a blood sample, which is sent to a laboratory for testing. The test provides results of HIV status and also determines the amount of the virus in the blood or HIV viral load. The NAT is used to detect HIV in people who have been recently exposed or in those individuals who have symptoms of HIV but have negative test results from other types of screening methods. If someone was recently exposed to HIV and contracted the virus, the NAT provides positive results sooner after exposure to HIV than other tests.

Treatment

Currently, no cure exists for AIDS. After a patient has been diagnosed with it, he or she will undergo periodic measurements of the number of CD4 T cells and the amount of HIV RNA (viral load) present in the bloodstream. These are both markers of disease progression from the initial infection with HIV to the development of AIDS. These numbers can also be used to determine when to begin HAART,

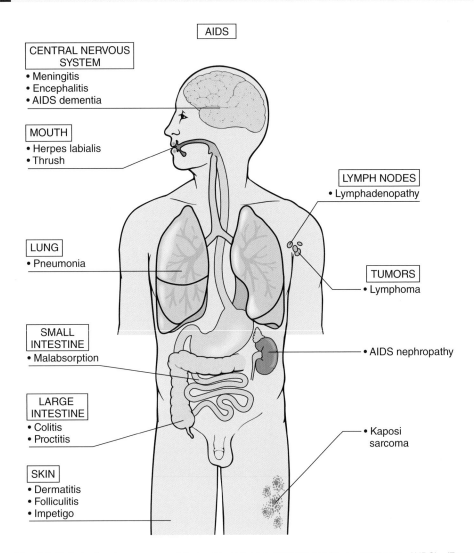

AIDS

CENTRAL NERVOUS SYSTEM
• Meningitis
• Encephalitis
• AIDS dementia

MOUTH
• Herpes labialis
• Thrush

LYMPH NODES
• Lymphadenopathy

LUNG
• Pneumonia

TUMORS
• Lymphoma

SMALL INTESTINE
• Malabsorption

• AIDS nephropathy

LARGE INTESTINE
• Colitis
• Proctitis

• Kaposi sarcoma

SKIN
• Dermatitis
• Folliculitis
• Impetigo

• **Fig. 3.8** Pathologic changes associated with acquired immunodeficiency syndrome (AIDS). (From Damjanov I: *Pathology for the health-related professions*, ed 4, St. Louis, 2011, Saunders.)

although currently, in the United States, it is recommended that HAART be started in all patients with HIV infection irrespective of the CD4 count or the viral load.

HAART consists of a three-drug combination, which is typically a combination of nucleoside reverse transcriptase inhibitors (NRTIs), and either a non–nucleoside reverse transcriptase inhibitor (NNRTI) or a protease inhibitor. HAART therapy may also consist of integrase strand transfer inhibitors, fusion inhibitors, and chemokine receptor antagonists (CCR5 antagonists). There are currently more than 20 antiretroviral drugs approved for use in HAART; therefore many different drug combinations are possible. Although these drugs have been effective in prolonging life and maintaining the quality of life for patients, they are associated with a number of toxicities and serious side effects, so patients on HAART must be followed closely. In the later stages of the disease, patients require prophylactic antibiotics. Addressing the psychological needs of the patient with AIDS is essential.

Health care practitioners who are involved in various forms of patient care with exposure to body fluids and blood should follow the principles of infection control and universal precautions (see the Alert box about Infection Control and Universal Precautions). All body fluids and blood from any patient should be handled with extreme care as if the patient were known to be infected by HIV or other potential viral infections contracted via blood or blood products.

The results of an 8-year, London-based research study involving almost 1000 gay male couples were released in May 2019. During the 8 years, no partner became infected with HIV even though the couples were not using barrier protection. "A European study of nearly 1000 gay male couples who had sex without condoms—where one partner had HIV and was taking antiretroviral drugs to suppress it—has found the treatment can prevent sexual transmission of the virus."

Prognosis

Although AIDS is ultimately a fatal disease, the number of Americans dying of AIDS each year has dropped. A person who has been diagnosed with AIDS is more prone to opportunist infections and has difficulty fighting those infections.

ⓘ *ALERT!*

Infection Control and Universal Precautions

Guidelines: Treat blood and all body fluids as if infected, and remember to use the following precautions:

1. Practice frequent and thorough handwashing
2. Report any accidental needlesticks
3. Wear personal protective equipment, including a mask or face shield, gown, gloves, and goggles. Change equipment between patients
4. Use caution with laboratory specimens
5. Dispose of contaminated sharps in designated biohazard containers. *Caution:* Do not recap or break needles
6. Use proper linen disposal containers.
7. Use clean mouthpieces and resuscitation bags
8. Obtain hepatitis B vaccination to protect against occupational exposure to blood
9. Use proper decontamination techniques
10. Absorb blood spills with paper towels, clean the area with soap and water, and disinfect it with a 1:10 solution of household bleach

Note: Pathogens can be bloodborne or airborne. Standard precautions, which correlate with universal precautions, are recommended and posted for hospitals and patient care institutions.

Treatment strategies that result in better prognosis include the use of HAART, the use of prophylactic antibiotics, and care by a physician experienced in HIV care.

Prevention

Because HIV is transmitted directly from human to human, prevention measures relate to avoiding risk factors for sexually transmitted diseases and practicing infection control through the use of universal precautions. The use of HAART significantly decreases the risk of HIV transmission to an HIV-seronegative sexual partner. Use of condoms and not sharing needles are highly recommended. The drugs used in HAART can be administered as postexposure prophylaxis after a needlestick injury. Patients who test positive for HIV infection should be encouraged to inform their sexual partners because they may be at high risk for contracting the disease.

There are many people who are considered to be at high risk for contracting HIV infection. In addition to avoiding risk factors, preexposure prophylaxis, or PrEP, may be recommended. PrEP has been effective in reducing the risk of HIV infection from sexual intercourse by 99% when used consistently every day. PrEP is effective in reducing the risk of HIV by intravenous drug use by 74%. There are two approved pills for PrEP and one injection. Truvada is recommended for people at high risk due to injectable drug use and exposure during sexual intercourse. Descovy is effective in individuals who are at high risk due to sexual intercourse. An injectable PrEP drug called Apretude has been approved for individuals weighing over 77 pounds and is also effective for individuals at high risk due to sexual intercourse. Apretude is not recommended for individuals who use injectable drugs.

Patient Teaching

Describe the diagnostic tests, and inform the patient about when to expect test results. Assure the patient of medical confidentiality. Make sure that the HIV-positive individual knows how the disease is transmitted. Stress the important aspects of the medication regimen and the dangers of noncompliance. Explain the side effects of the therapeutic drugs, and encourage the patient to contact the health care worker with questions or concerns. Other teaching points include how to minimize infections, the need for lifelong therapy, and the responsibility to inform health care providers about the HIV diagnosis. The psychological, social, and financial ramifications of having HIV require referrals for community support. Results may be typically given to the patient in person to provide in-person support and answer all questions regarding both positive and negative results.

Common Variable Immunodeficiency (Acquired Hypogammaglobulinemia)

Description

Common variable immunodeficiency (CVID) is an acquired B-cell deficiency that results in decreased antibody production and/or function. Deoxyribonucleic acid (DNA) analysis can determine if a person inherited the gene responsible for causing this deficiency.

ICD-10-CM Code	D83.8 *(Other common variable immunodeficiencies)* D83.9 *(Common variable immunodeficiency, unspecified)* (D83.0-D83.9 = 5 codes of specificity)

Symptoms and Signs

The person with CVID has a history of chronic or recurrent infections, such as pneumonia, bronchitis, sinusitis, and otitis media. GI disease is often seen with such symptoms as diarrhea, abdominal pain, and weight loss. Lymphadenopathy, splenomegaly, and hepatomegaly often are observed. Chronic lung disease and granulomatous disease are common. CVID is associated with an increased frequency of autoimmune disorders, such as autoimmune hemolytic anemia or immune thrombocytopenia. As the disease progresses, susceptibility to opportunistic and viral infections and malignancies escalates.

Patient Screening

When a child or young teenager is susceptible to frequent infections, it is recommended that an appointment to discuss potential reasons for infections be made with the health care provider. When the individual experiences frequent bacterial infections, an appointment for an in-depth medical investigation is indicated.

Etiology

CVID has two peaks of incidence: one between ages 18 and 25 years, and a smaller peak between ages 1 and 5 years. Although the exact cause of **hypogammaglobulinemia** is not known, it is thought to be a result of genetic defects leading to immune system dysregulation and a failure of B-cell differentiation. The number of circulating B cells is often normal, but the ability of the B cells to produce all types of immunoglobulins is reduced. Some patients have impaired T-cell signaling as well. Cell-mediated immunity usually remains intact.

Diagnosis

A history of repeated and chronic infections should lead to further investigation of immunoglobulin levels and T-cell quantities. When tested, antibody responses to vaccines are poor. Hypogammaglobulinemia and IgA and/or IgM deficiency in this clinical setting are indicative of the disease; however, other causes of these findings must be ruled out.

Treatment

Treatment aims to prevent infections and implement early treatment with appropriate antibiotic administration when infections occur. Regular immunoglobulin replacement decreases the number of infections, antibiotic usage, and hospitalizations. Patients should be monitored closely because they are at an increased risk for the development of autoimmune disease and lymphoma. Live virus vaccines are often not given to people known to have CVID. Otherwise, appropriate vaccination is recommended, although vaccine response may be poor.

Prognosis

Although the use of immunoglobulin has improved the prognosis, patients often succumb to chronic lung disease or malignancies. Lower levels of immunoglobulin and a lower percentage of B cells are associated with a poorer prognosis.

Prevention

No methods of prevention are known.

Patient Teaching

Teaching points include steps to prevent infection and ensure good nutrition, adequate rest, and regular follow-up care.

Selective Immunoglobulin A Deficiency

Description

Patients with selective IgA deficiency fail to produce the normal levels of IgA. Selective deficiencies of IgM or IgG have been reported but are rare. Immunoglobin A is present in respiratory, digestive, and other mucous membranes. It is also present in tears, breast milk, and saliva.

ICD-10-CM Code	D80.2 (Selective deficiency of immunoglobulin A [IgA]) (D80.0–D80.9 = 10 codes of specificity)

Symptoms and Signs

The majority of patients with IgA deficiency are asymptomatic and healthy. A smaller number of patients experience symptoms of recurrent sinopulmonary infections, GI infections, and/or autoimmune disease. Food allergies are also common. Anaphylactic reactions to blood transfusions may occur. Children with IgA deficiency typically exhibit recurrent otitis media, eye, skin, and bronchial infections including pneumonia, and the child may have asthma.

Patient Screening

Frequent recurrent infections in a child or adult necessitate an appointment for a medical investigation to determine a possible underlying cause. The patient may also report allergies and digestive problems. Patients with a family history of IgA deficiency or CVID should be screened or may schedule an appointment with a genetic counsellor about the risks of potentially transmitting it to children.

Etiology

Failure of B cells to produce adequate levels of IgA is the most common immunologic defect in the general population. The most common risk factor for the disease is a family history of either IgA deficiency or CVID.

Diagnosis

In patients with recurrent infections, levels of immunoglobulins should be measured. Children younger than 4 years old will have lower levels of IgA than normal. A newborn will have very little IgA, and it takes time for the immune system to produce IgA in normal amounts. For this reason, children younger than 4 years old are not diagnosed with IgA deficiency. Complete blood count (CBC), complement assay, and vaccine response testing are used to rule out other immunodeficiencies.

Treatment

No cure for this condition is known. Treatment is geared toward the prevention and management of infections. Prophylactic antibiotics may be given. If these do not reduce the number of infections, intravenous immune globulin (IVIG) with low concentrations of IgA (to reduce the risk of anaphylaxis) may be tried. Patients should be monitored for the development of autoimmune disease and progression to CVID. Patients must be monitored closely when given blood products because of the increased risk of an anaphylactic reaction. Screening for anti-IgA antibodies can help identify those who may have an adverse reaction.

Prognosis

In most cases, no significant medical problems are expected and the prognosis is good. In some children, slow, spontaneous resolution of the condition may occur.

Prevention

No method of prevention is known. Limiting exposure to harmful pathogens by practicing frequent hand sanitization and avoiding large crowds may decrease the number of infections.

Patient Teaching

Teaching points include steps to prevent infection and ensure good nutrition, adequate rest, and regular follow-up care. Explain the purpose of prophylactic antibiotic therapy, as prescribed. Encourage patients with severe IgA deficiency to obtain a medical alert bracelet because of the risk of allergic reactions to blood products. This should be specifically noted on the medical alert bracelet.

X-Linked Agammaglobulinemia
Description

X-linked agammaglobulinemia (XLA) (Bruton agammaglobulinemia) is a condition characterized by near absence of serum immunoglobulins and increased susceptibility to infection.

ICD-10-CM Code   D80.0 *(Hereditary hypogammaglobulinemia)*

Symptoms and Signs

Infant with XLA are usually healthy after birth due to the antibodies from their mother. Small tonsils and the absence of lymph nodes are indicators of this condition. If lymph nodes are present, they are small. The infant is susceptible to recurrent infections, including bacterial otitis media, bronchitis, pneumonia, osteomyelitis, and meningitis. The inability to fight infection can lead to serious consequences when the infant has an infection. These are usually first noted between 3 and 18 months of age, when the natural transplacental immunity from the mother has been depleted.

Patient Screening

Recurrent severe bacterial infections in an infant signal the need for in-depth medical investigation to determine the possible underlying cause(s). The health care provider can order tests to reveal the cause of these recurrent infections.

Etiology

This congenital X-linked disorder almost always affects males. Females can be carriers. It is caused by a defect in the Bruton tyrosine kinase *(BTK)* gene, which is normally expressed in B cells during all stages of development. All five immunoglobulin classes are usually absent, along with the absence of circulating B cells and the presence of normal numbers of circulating T cells. This leads to increased infection with encapsulated bacteria and certain viruses. Most affected individuals present with symptoms by 5 years of age, and almost all have symptoms by age 5 years. Around 40% of patients have an affected family member.

Diagnosis

The clinical findings, along with a thorough history, including a family history of relatives who died of severe infections, suggest XLA. Immunoelectrophoresis indicates decreased levels of serum IgM, IgA, and IgG; however, relying on this method of diagnosis is not valid before the infant

is 6 to 8 months of age. Serum antibody titers in response to immunizations are low. Other findings suggestive of this disease are normal T-cell numbers along with low or absent B-cell numbers. It may be useful to assess for the *BTK* gene mutation if there is no significant family history to aid diagnosis. B-cell defects can be detected on newborn screening, but such testing is not routine in most states in the United States at this time.

Treatment

Treatment is directed at improving the child's immune defenses and controlling infections. Intravenous infusions or subcutaneous administrations of immune globulin every 2 to 4 weeks and appropriate antibiotics are administered. Antibiotics may be administered continuously as a preventative to keep bacterial infection from occurring. In other individuals, the antibiotics may only be administered when the patient has an infection, but the course of treatment may be longer than usually deemed necessary. *These patients must never be immunized with live virus vaccines, nor should corticosteroids or immunosuppressive drugs be administered.* Killed vaccines should be administered, however, because they may provide T-cell–mediated protection for the patient.

Prognosis

Although this condition cannot be cured, regular infusions of immune globulin may provide the patient with a near-normal lifestyle. Affected individuals tend to miss more days of school or work and are hospitalized more frequently than males in the general population, however.

Prevention

No methods of prevention are known, although parents of affected children are encouraged to seek genetic counseling regarding future pregnancies.

Patient Teaching

Discuss the importance of preventing infections. Explain the procedure for administering immune globulin. Discuss the need for administering antibiotics. Caution the parents about the contraindications for live virus vaccines and immunosuppressive drugs.

Severe Combined Immunodeficiency
Description

Severe combined immunodeficiency (SCID) is a group of disorders that result from a disturbance in the development and function of T cells with or without B cells. Because T-cell signaling is needed for B cells to produce antibodies, this leads to an absence of both cell-mediated (T-cell) immunity and antibody-mediated (B-cell) immunity. NK cells may or may not be present. This disease has been referred to as *Bubble Boy disease.*

ICD-10-CM Code   D81.0 *(Severe combined immunodeficiency [SCID] with reticular dysgenesis)*

D81.1 *(Severe combined immunodeficiency [SCID] with low T- and B-cell numbers)*
D81.2 *(Severe combined immunodeficiency [SCID] with low or normal B-cell numbers)*
D81.89 *(Other combined immunodeficiencies)*
D81.9 *(Combined immunodeficiency, unspecified)*
(D81.0–D81.9 = 13 codes of specificity)

Symptoms and Signs

SCID manifests as severe, recurrent infections with bacteria, viruses, fungi, and protozoa; chronic diarrhea; and failure to thrive. This occurs by age 3 to 6 months, when the natural maternal placental immunity begins to be depleted. Common infections are PCP and persistent mucocutaneous candidiasis. Discernible lymphoid tissue (enlarged tonsils, palpable lymph nodes, and so on) may be absent. Abnormal laboratory findings often include hypogammaglobulinemia and very low or absent T cells.

Patient Screening

Abnormal newborn screening tests are reported to the patient's pediatrician. A history of pneumonia in the first weeks of life, followed by frequent, severe infections, is indicative of underlying conditions that need a complete medical evaluation. These infections are potentially life threatening in the infant, and immediate medical care is required.

Etiology

There are several variations of genetic defects that result in SCID. The type of SCID is determined by the defective gene.

Diagnosis

Testing for SCID is now part of the recommended uniform newborn screening panel in the United States. Screening tests are also performed in many countries throughout the world. It is one of many tests performed after birth by collecting a few drops of blood on a screening form.

If the clinical picture indicates suspicion of SCID, many laboratory tests are performed. These include measurement of immunoglobulin levels, antibody titers, and numbers of T cells and B cells. Lymphopenia is a common finding. T-cell response is also tested. Usually, there is an absence of the thymic shadow on a chest radiograph.

Treatment

BMT from a sibling donor has resulted in positive results, but there are many children who do not have an appropriate match.

St. Jude Children's Research Hospital has had success with their gene therapy treatment protocol. The treatment includes removing bone marrow, which contains the mutated gene, then putting in a normal or corrected version of the gene into a viral vector. The vector, with the corrected version of the gene, is then put into the bone marrow cells that were taken from the child. Those cells are then frozen by means of cryonics or at an extremely low negative Celsius temperature. The child will then receive small doses of chemotherapy drugs to make room for the new cells. The new corrected version of the bone marrow cells is then administered to the child so their own bone marrow will begin to make normal immune cells that will be able to fight infection.

Prognosis

The clinical trial has had positive effects on the children treated with this protocol. Unless the underlying gene defect is corrected, the outlook is not favorable for children with SCID. Death will occur before 2 years of age.

Prevention

No methods of prevention are known, although routine newborn screening aids in a timely diagnosis which leads to earlier treatment.

Patient Teaching

Explain the medical interventions used to protect against infection and restore immune response. Refer the parents to available community support organizations that can help with the psychological, physical, and financial burdens precipitated by the infant's prognosis of severe illness and early death. Refer the parents to a genetic counselor.

DiGeorge Anomaly (Thymic Hypoplasia or Aplasia)

Description

DiGeorge anomaly is a congenital condition of immunodeficiency that results from defective development of the pharyngeal pouch system and presents with cardiac anomalies, hypoplastic thymus, and hypocalcemia. In some coding manuals, this disease may be listed as *DiGeorge syndrome*.

ICD-10-CM Code   D82.1 *(DiGeorge syndrome)*
(D82.0–D82.9 = 7 codes of specificity)

Symptoms and Signs

Children with DiGeorge anomaly often have a set of structural abnormalities. These include abnormally wide-set, downward-slanting eyes; low-set ears with notched pinnae; a small mouth (Fig. 3.9); abnormalities of the palate; and cardiovascular defects, such as tetralogy of Fallot. The thymus and parathyroid glands are absent or underdeveloped. The infant exhibits signs of *tetany* resulting from hypocalcemia caused by hypoparathyroidism. Some degree of cognitive impairment often is present. Some patients are susceptible

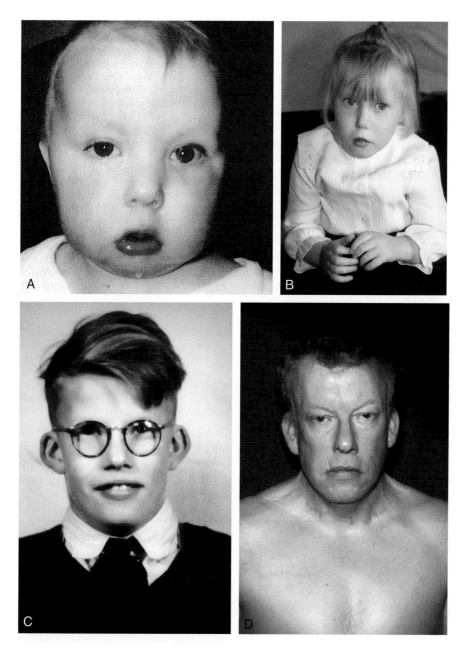

• **Fig. 3.9** Deletion 22q11.2 (DiGeorge/Sedlác̆ková/velocardiofacial) syndrome. (A) A young infant. (B) A young child. (C) An older child. (C) The same individual shown in (C) as an adult aged 49 years. (From Turnpenny P et al: *Emery's elements of medical genetics and genomics*, ed 16, 2022, Elsevier.)

to infections, such as sinopulmonary infections and thrush. Some of the symptoms may be present at birth; however, problems may be identified at well-baby visits and then an investigation of the cause of symptoms may be confirmed with further testing.

Patient Screening

Infants or children with DiGeorge syndrome anomalies need prompt medical treatment when signs of infection occur.

Etiology

DiGeorge anomaly results when an infant has a microdeletion on a part of chromosome 22. This may be referred to as

22q11.2 deletion syndrome. This may be considered a complete DiGeorge anomaly or partial. This causes the thymus gland to be underdeveloped or absent, cardiac defects, and parathyroid hypoplasia. This leads to defects in T-cell number function and, in some cases, decreased B-cell function as well. Although some of these children will not be clinically immunodeficient, others will have increased sinopulmonary infections, and a small percentage will have life-threatening SCID as a result of the absent thymus.

Diagnosis

A definitive diagnosis requires a laboratory test to determine if there is a deletion in chromosome 22.

Treatment

Hypocalcemia should be treated to stabilize the myocardium and reduce the risk of seizures. Vitamin D and parathyroid hormone replacement therapy are also necessary. Repair of cardiac anomalies may be attempted. Thymic transplantation or BMT may reconstitute immune function in patients with the most severe form of DiGeorge anomaly. Appropriate developmental interventions should be instituted. Before administering live vaccines, the health care provider will determine safety on a case-by-case basis.

Prognosis

Complete DiGeorge anomaly is usually fatal within the first year of life. For some patients with partial DiGeorge anomaly, the prognosis depends on the severity of the cardiac and parathyroid defects. Immune function, however, may improve with age and should be monitored regularly.

Prevention

No methods of prevention are known. Genetic counseling is recommended if there is a family history of DiGeorge Syndrome because there is a possibility of transmission from parent to child.

Patient Teaching

Congenital structural anomalies, their complications, and the child's susceptibility to infections determine what information is most helpful to parents and caregivers. Procedures, such as those given to treat hypocalcemia, are explained.

Chronic Mucocutaneous Candidiasis

Description

Chronic mucocutaneous candidiasis (CMC) refers to a group of disorders characterized by persistent and recurrent candidal (fungal) infections of the skin, nails, and mucous membranes. These disorders are unified by the inclusion of deficient cell-mediated immunity to *Candida* organisms.

> ICD-10-CM Code   B37.9 *(Candidiasis, unspecified)*
> (B37.0–B37.9 = 16 codes of specificity)
> *Refer to the physician's diagnosis and then to the current edition of the ICD-10-CM coding manuals to ensure the greatest specificity of pathology.*

Symptoms and Signs

Symptoms usually develop during the first 2 or 3 years of life or, if late-onset CMC, in young adulthood. Large circular lesions appear on the skin, mucous membranes, nails, or vagina. Sores in the mouth make eating difficult (Fig. 3.10). Recurrent thrush or diaper rash is often the first symptom of the disease in infants. Patients in the late stages of the disease experience recurring respiratory tract infections. Associated endocrine disorders or autoimmune conditions can be found depending on the type of CMC. Later onset

• **Fig. 3.10** Oral candidiasis, or thrush, manifests with a whitish, curd-like substance on the tongue or inside the mouth. (From Cooper K, Gosnell K: *Adult health nursing*, ed 9, 2023, Elsevier; Courtesy Deborah Greenspan, DSC, BDS, University of California, San Francisco, and US Department of Veterans Affairs.)

CMC can be associated with myasthenia gravis, thymoma, or bone marrow abnormalities. Interestingly, systemic *Candida* infections are not seen in these patients.

Syndromes of CMC are as follows:
- Chronic oral candidiasis (disease affecting the mucosa of the lips, tongue, and buccal cavity)
- CMC with endocrinopathy (hypoadrenalism, hypothyroidism, hypoparathyroidism, and ovarian failure in females)
- Chronic localized candidiasis (cutaneous lesions with hyperkeratosis)
- Chronic diffuse candidiasis (widespread infection of the skin, nails, and mucous membranes) (Fig. 3.11)
- Candidiasis with thymoma (candidiasis accompanied by hypogammaglobulinemia, neutropenia, aplastic anemia, or myasthenia gravis)

Patient Screening

Frequent, persistent fungal infections of the mouth, skin, or nails in the young child necessitate a prompt appointment with the physician for medical evaluation and to begin treatment.

Etiology

In the immunocompetent individual, *Candida albicans* is a nonpathogenic normal flora. Patients with CMC have a T-cell deficit specific to *Candida* that makes them susceptible to infection. Other T-cell and B-cell functions are usually normal. Mutations in the autoimmune regulator gene *(AIRE)* or the *STAT1* gene have been implicated in CMC pathogenesis. These mutations also lead to susceptibility to various autoimmune diseases.

• **Fig. 3.11** Chronic mucocutaneous candidiasis. (From James WD et al: *Andrews' diseases of the skin clinical atlas*, ed 2, 2018, Elsevier.)

Diagnosis

Evaluation for CMC is prompted by a history of recurrent *Candida* infections. Potassium hydroxide preparations of scrapings from a lesion show yeast pseudohyphae (a string of atypical fungal cells) when examined under the microscope. Fungal culture grows *Candida*. Blood studies indicate normal T-cell circulation and normal antibody response to all organisms except *Candida*. Patients have normal immunoglobulin levels, normal lymphocyte numbers, and normal responses to non-*Candida* antigens. Genetic testing for *AIRE* mutations can be done. Other immunodeficiency diseases need to be ruled out, and all endocrine functions should be evaluated. Any other abnormalities are evaluated according to the organs involved.

Treatment

Treatment is directed at eliminating the infections along with correcting the immunologic defects. Systemic therapy with antifungal agents is the mainstay of treatment. Chronic use of antifungals may prevent recurrences. Transfer factor, a protein of T lymphocytes isolated from donors sensitized to *Candida*, has been shown to increase the immune response to *Candida* in patients with CMC. Topical treatment with antifungal agents appears to improve skin and nail lesions.

Associated endocrine or autoimmune diseases should be treated appropriately.

Prognosis

Death caused by CMC is unusual because infections are usually localized. Treatment with antifungals has good results, but most patients relapse after cessation of these agents. The associated endocrinopathy or autoimmune disease is usually the major factor affecting prognosis.

Prevention

No method of prevention is known.

Patient Teaching

Give written instructions to the patient or the parents on the medication regimen. Teach comfort measures for mouth lesions, such as a soft diet and the use of a mild mouthwash and a soft toothbrush. Instruct the patient or parents not to delay medical attention for any infections or signs of relapse. Address questions regarding any endocrine involvement, as appropriate to the diagnosis.

Wiskott-Aldrich Syndrome

Description

Wiskott-Aldrich syndrome is a very rare genetic disorder characterized by inadequate B- and T-cell function. The B and T cells do not work the way they should in a normal immune response and are unable to fight infections. The bone marrow does not produce platelets as it should resulting in thrombocytopenia.

ICD-10-CM Code   D82.0 *(Wiskott-Aldrich syndrome)*

Symptoms and Signs

The child with Wiskott-Aldrich syndrome experiences eczema, thrombocytopenia with severe bleeding, and an increased susceptibility to bacterial and viral infections. Bleeding manifestations include petechiae, purpura, hematemesis, epistaxis, hematuria, and more serious GI and intracranial bleeding. These children are predisposed to the development of autoimmune disorders (hemolytic anemia, vasculitis, etc.), and lymphoma.

Patient Screening

Severe bleeding manifestations call for immediate assessment and medical care. If the child is being treated for Wiskott-Aldrich syndrome and signs of infection are reported, prompt medical attention is indicated.

Etiology

This rare immunodeficiency disorder is inherited as an X-linked trait affecting males, however females may be carriers of the gene. It arises from mutations in the gene encoding the Wiskott-Aldrich syndrome protein, which is expressed in hematopoietic cells. The thymus gland is normal at birth but decreases in size as the child grows up, resulting in decreased B- and T-cell functions. Additionally, metabolic defects in platelet synthesis that cause platelets to be short lived, and phagocytes to be incompetent are both present.

Diagnosis

A diagnosis is suspected in a boy with thrombocytopenia and small platelet size, especially when accompanied by eczema and frequent infections. The diagnosis is supported by finding a mutation in the *WAS* gene. The numbers of T cells and B cells may be low. Vaccine response may be defective. Regulatory T-cell function is impaired.

Treatment

Bone marrow stem cell transplant is the only curative therapy. Stem cells from bone marrow, umbilical cord, and peripheral blood are an option. The success of stem cell transplant depends on the overall health of the child at the time of transplant, performing the transplant before the age of 5, and the matched donor. Siblings are the best potential matches for stem cell transplants.

Gene therapy or gene transfer is another treatment method. The patient receives their own bone marrow, which has been removed, and infused with a healthy copy of the gene that is responsible for the disease.

Prognosis

Long-term survival is good for patients who receive a bone marrow stem cell transplant before 5 years of age. Successful gene therapy provides the same result as a stem cell or bone marrow transplant.

Prevention

No methods of prevention are known.

Patient Teaching

Encourage the parent or caregiver to express concerns about episodes of bleeding. Discuss the signs of bleeding that require emergency care, such as signs of shock. Explain the importance of timely and aggressive treatment for infections. If BMT is scheduled, discuss the procedure and reinforce the physician's explanation of the expected results. If the child is experiencing symptoms of eczema, demonstrate the topical application of medication as prescribed. All family members and caregivers, as well as other individuals who are in close contact with the child, should practice good handwashing. Follow the health care provider's instructions regarding preventative medications and which vaccinations the child may or may not receive. Eliminating the potential chance of injury from playing contact sports should be discussed.

Autoimmune Diseases

Autoimmune diseases occur when the body's normal immune system mistakenly is misdirected against its own tissues. Autoimmunity is characterized by the presence of abnormal autoantibodies that bind to various portions of

the body's own tissues. Tolerance to self-antigens is believed to commence during fetal life. As the body ages and experiences various disease processes or environmental exposures, persons with a variety of genetic risks can have changes in their immune system, because of which the system misidentifies body tissues and develops autoantibodies that result in self-destruction. Certain gene markers identify patients at increased risk for many autoimmune diseases.

Autoimmune diseases can occur in many body systems when lymphocytes and antibodies are sensitized to develop against the self, that is, against the constituents of the body's own tissues. For example, if a patient has an organ transplant, it is understood the body will try to reject the new organ because it recognizes this new organ is not a part of "self" or its own body. When one has an autoimmune disease, the body reacts this same way, even though the tissue is a part of the individual, as stated above. The production of autoantibodies may occur by means of several mechanisms, including disease, injury, metabolic change, and a mutation of immunologically competent cells. Additionally, viral infection, trauma, and certain drugs or chemicals may alter specific body proteins, thereby thwarting recognition and resulting in their rejection as if they were foreign proteins.

Hematopoietic Disorders

Autoimmune Hemolytic Anemia

Description

Autoimmune hemolytic anemia is an autoimmune condition in which red blood cells (RBCs) are destroyed by antibodies.

ICD-10-CM Code	D59.0 *(Drug-induced autoimmune hemolytic anemia)* D59.1 *(Other autoimmune hemolytic anemias)* (D59.0–D59.9 = 9 codes of specificity)

Symptoms and Signs

Autoimmune hemolytic anemia causes fatigue, weakness, chills, fever, dyspnea, and itching. The skin is pale and jaundiced and bruises easily. Additionally, the patient may be hypotensive.

Patient Screening

Scheduling a same-day appointment for the patient experiencing the symptoms listed above leads to a quicker diagnosis and treatment. Patients with mild or fewer symptoms may be scheduled with less urgency.

Etiology

Because of a misguided immune response, B cell–produced antibodies do not identify RBCs as self, resulting in agglutination of RBCs and an attack on and destruction of the red corpuscles. The two types of hemolytic anemia are warm antibody hemolytic anemia (wAIHA) and cold antibody hemolytic anemia. wAIHA may be idiopathic or caused by an autoimmune disease, medications, infection, lymphoma, or pregnancy. It is associated with an excess of IgG antibodies that react with protein antigens on the RBC surface at 37°C or higher body temperature. Pinpointing an exact cause of wAIHA is helpful in determinng treatment. Cold antibody hemolytic anemia results from fixation of complement proteins on IgM that occurs at colder temperatures less than 37°C. This condition can result from an unknown cause, or be due to another autoimmune disease, infections, or some type of cancer.

Diagnosis

A direct Coombs test indicates antibody-coated RBCs that agglutinate when antiglobulin is added to the medium. Some RBCs appear spherical (spherocytes) as visualized under a microscope; serum bilirubin levels are elevated; and RBC count, platelet count, hemoglobin (Hgb) concentration, and hematocrit usually are all decreased. The reticulocyte (immature RBC) count is usually elevated. Examination of a peripheral blood smear for agglutination of RBCs and flow cytometry may be performed. In mild or sporadic disease, these previously mentioned findings might be less evident.

Treatment

Treatment should first address any underlying disease or medication use that could be causing the hemolytic anemia. Warm and cold antibody anemias are treated differently. In warm antibody anemia, corticosteroids and immunosuppressant drugs are administered to reduce antibody production. Splenectomy or IVIG administration may be done to reduce antibody effectiveness. RBC transfusions may be attempted. Cold antibody hemolytic anemia is treated with rituximab (Rituxan). While rituximab may be used as monotherapy for patients with comorbidities, it is most effective when combined with cytotoxic medications such as fludarbine (Fludara) and bendmustine (Bendeka).

Prognosis

Anemia resulting from infection or drug use usually abates after the infection resolves or the drug is discontinued. Anemia resulting from other causes is often chronic and poorly responsive to therapy. Warm antibody anemia is generally self-limited in children, disappearing within 1 to 3 months.

Prevention

No methods of prevention are known.

Patient Teaching

Explain the diagnostic tests, and tell the patient when to expect results. If the cause has been determined, explain how the RBCs are being destroyed and how the treatment regimen is expected to help. Discuss expected results from IVIG administration or, if indicated, the removal of the spleen. Instructions on monitoring blood tests can be helpful.

Pernicious Anemia

Description

Pernicious anemia is caused by chronic atrophic gastritis, resulting in decreased gastric production of hydrochloric acid and a shortage of intrinsic factor. Additionally, the antibodies produced block the intrinsic factor and parietal cells. These two factors lead to impaired vitamin B_{12} absorption, resulting in vitamin B_{12} deficiency.

ICD-10-CM Code	D51.0 (Vitamin B_{12} deficiency anemia due to intrinsic factor deficiency) (D51.0–D51.9 = 6 codes of specificity)

Symptoms and Signs

Patients with pernicious anemia can develop a sore tongue, weakness, and tingling and numbness in the extremities. The lips, tongue, and gums appear pale, whereas the sclera and skin appear slightly jaundiced (Fig. 3.12). Because of the decreased hydrochloric acid production and atrophy of the gastric mucosa, the patient experiences disturbances in digestion, such as anorexia, nausea, vomiting, diarrhea, constipation, flatulence, and weight loss. In this condition, the individual is more vulnerable to infections. Vitamin B_{12} deficiency causes neurological symptoms such as demyelination of the peripheral nerves and, eventually, the spinal cord. This leads to neuritis, peripheral weakness, numbness, and paresthesia. Ataxia (muscular incoordination), light-headedness, altered vision, tinnitus, and optic muscle atrophy are additional symptoms that may occur as the anemia progresses. CNS changes may cause headaches, irritability, confusion, and depression. Reduced Hgb levels cause decreased oxygen-carrying capacity, leading to fatigue, weakness, and light-headedness. The patient may experience palpitations, dyspnea, tachycardia, premature ventricular contractions, and even congestive heart failure.

Patient Screening

Initially, the patient may have insidious and vague symptoms; unless the symptoms are severe, the patient is scheduled for a medical evaluation as soon as it is convenient. Patients complaining of weakness or cardiovascular symptoms (e.g., a rapid heart rate) require prompt medical care. A same-day appointment is scheduled for the patient being treated for pernicious anemia if physical or psychological complications develop.

Etiology

Greater than 90% of patients with pernicious anemia have gastric parietal cell antibodies. In the majority of patients, anti-intrinsic factor antibodies are also present. Intrinsic factors must be present in the gastric mucosa for vitamin B_{12} absorption to occur. Vitamin B_{12} is necessary for RBC

Light-headedness
Headaches
Optic muscle atrophy
Ringing in ears
Sclera slightly jaundiced
Lips, gums, tongue pale
Sore tongue
Dyspnea
Skin slightly jaundiced
Palpitations and cardiac arrhythmias
Stomach—decreased production of hydrochloric acid
Generalized weakness
Disturbances in digestion (i.e., nausea, anorexia, vomiting, diarrhea, constipation)
Tingling and numbness in extremities

• **Fig. 3.12** Symptoms and signs of pernicious anemia.

formation, and a deficiency causes RBCs to be deformed and reduced in number. Pernicious anemia is often associated with other autoimmune diseases, such as Graves disease or Hashimoto thyroiditis. It is particularly common in people of Northern European descent ages 40 to 70 years, but it can be seen in any ethnic group.

Diagnosis

Diagnosis is confirmed by the clinical findings and laboratory tests. Vitamin B_{12} level, CBC, reticulocyte count, and other laboratory tests may be performed.

An upper endoscopy may also be performed in order for the provider to visualize the lining of the stomach. Health care providers use a thin, tube-like instrument with a light and lens for viewing called an endoscope to look for signs of degeneration or atrophy (wasting away) of the lining of your stomach. Blood tests reveal a decrease in Hgb level, decreased RBC count, and increased mean cell volume (MCV). The

RBCs and the platelets are large and malformed. Bone marrow studies indicate abnormal RBC production and other changes typical of vitamin B_{12} deficiency. Reduced amounts or absence of gastric acid are found in gastric analysis. Hypersegmented neutrophils (megaloblasts) on a peripheral blood smear are characteristic. Vitamin B_{12} also is necessary for proper myelin formation; a myelin deficiency can cause damage to the nerves (neuropathy).

Treatment

Initially weekly and then monthly intramuscular injections of vitamin B_{12} are the primary treatment for pernicious anemia, and they are often continued for life. B_{12} is also available in a sublingual form and a nasal spray. Blood replacement may be indicated in severe cases. Supportive measures include adequate rest, gentle nonirritating mouth care, a well-balanced diet high in vitamin B_{12}, and the use of tranquilizers for behavioral problems.

Prognosis

No cure for pernicious anemia is known, but early detection and treatment with vitamin B_{12} help with most symptoms in the majority of patients.

Prevention

No method of prevention for the primary condition is known. Patients who have had extensive gastric surgery may also benefit from vitamin B_{12} replacement because they often cannot produce the intrinsic factor necessary for B_{12} absorption.

Patient Teaching

If bone marrow studies are ordered, explain the procedure. Once diagnosed, inform the patient that improvement is likely within weeks of treatment and good compliance with the treatment regimen. To promote compliance, explain the importance of lifelong vitamin B_{12} replacement therapy; demonstrate the injection technique to the patient or caregiver, if required. Review the signs of any complications that should be reported to the physician.

Idiopathic Thrombocytopenic Purpura

Description

Idiopathic thrombocytopenic purpura (ITP) is an acquired disorder that results from an isolated deficiency of platelets (i.e., other blood counts are normal). It is believed that platelet destruction and/or inhibition of platelet production is the result of autoantibodies against platelets.

ICD-10-CM Code	D69.3 *(Immune thrombocytopenic purpura)* (D69.0–D69.9 = 11 codes of specificity)

Symptoms and Signs

Symptoms are related to an inability of the blood to clot and include spontaneous hemorrhages in the skin, mucous membranes, or internal organs. Petechiae, small spiderlike hemorrhages under the surface of the skin (Fig. 3.13), and ecchymoses, larger hemorrhagic areas, are apparent. The patient may experience epistaxis (nosebleeds), GI bleeding, menorrhagia, hematuria, and easy bruising. The clinical symptoms vary with patient age, with older patients exhibiting more severe bleeding symptoms.

Patient Screening

Multiple bruising of unknown cause in a child or an adult requires prompt medical attention. (Note: An event of spontaneous bruising in a child can cause a parent to become extremely alarmed and also precipitates in medical personnel a natural concern about the child's welfare. Care must be taken by medical personnel to avoid judgmental attitudes toward parents unless a sound reason to suspect child abuse has been established.)

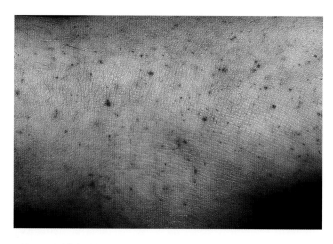

• **Fig. 3.13** Idiopathic thrombocytopenic purpura. This school-age child was seen with a chief complaint of a rash after a viral upper respiratory tract infection. Examination revealed diffuse petechiae, shown here over her ankle, and scattered purpuric lesions. Her hemoglobin and white blood cell count and differential were normal, but her platelet count was markedly reduced. (From McIntire SC, et al: *Zitelli and Davis' atlas of pediatric physical diagnosis*, ed 8, 2023, Elsevier.)

Etiology

Thrombocytopenic purpura is often considered idiopathic (of unknown cause), although antibodies that reduce the life of platelets have been found in most cases. Some cases may occur after a viral infection, especially rubella or mumps. Additionally the spleen may be destroying the damaged platelets.

Diagnosis

The diagnosis of ITP is often one of exclusion; therefore other causes of thrombocytopenia must be ruled out first. CBC and peripheral blood smear analysis are performed. The clinical symptoms, along with prolonged bleeding time and reduced platelet count, suggest the diagnosis. The size and shape of the platelets may be abnormal. Circulating platelet time is reduced to hours instead of normal days. Testing for other diseases, such as HIV infection and SLE, is often performed to rule out other causes of thrombocytopenia.

Treatment

Steroids and IVIG are used. In children who are Rh positive and still have their spleen, intravenous Rho (D) immune globulin may be administered. In older children or adults, surgery to remove the spleen (splenectomy) may be considered. Chronic ITP may be treated with an immune-suppressing drug that reduces platelet destruction. In some cases, hormone therapy may be used, and if a patient has an infection that causes ITP, antibiotics are prescribed.

Prognosis

In general, the prognosis for ITP is good for both adults and children. There is a risk of serious bleeding with ITP as a result of such low platelet counts. This can have an effect on the prognosis due to hemorrhage.

Prevention

No methods of prevention are known.

Patient Teaching

Explain the purpose and procedure of prescribed infusion therapy. The parents of a young child will benefit from reassurance that complete remission is likely. Adults with chronic ITP who fail to respond to initial treatment with corticosteroids may require preoperative instructions for splenectomy.

Immune Neutropenia

Description

The term *immune neutropenia* is used to describe neutropenia, which is a decrease in the number of circulating neutrophils usually caused by the production of antineutrophil antibodies.

ICD-10-CM Code	D70.9 *(Neutropenia, unspecified)*
	(D70.0–D70.9 = 7 codes of specificity)

Symptoms and Signs

The patient with immune neutropenia experiences malaise, fatigue, weakness, fever, and stomatitis. Recurrent infections are common, especially upper respiratory infections and otitis media in infants.

Patient Screening

Schedule an infant with a respiratory infection for a prompt medical evaluation. Follow office policy regarding referral to a pediatrician. The adult patient complaining of the above symptoms needs a medical evaluation at the first available opportunity.

Etiology

Immune-mediated neutropenia is often associated with an accelerated turnover of neutrophils (increased neutrophil production), but there is an even greater increase in destruction mediated by the antineutrophil antibodies. There is almost complete absence of neutrophils in blood. The neutropenia may be associated with infection, drug exposure, ITP, autoimmune hemolytic anemia, or connective tissue diseases, including SLE and rheumatoid arthritis (RA). A type of immune neutropenia, isoimmune neutropenia, is a rare disorder caused by the transplacental transfer of maternal IgG that reacts with fetal neutrophils. This type of neutropenia usually resolves in 12 to 15 weeks.

Diagnosis

Neutropenia is confirmed by the significantly reduced number of neutrophils displayed in a WBC count. Detection of antineutrophil antibodies is possible using in many patients using assays, such as immunofluorescence, agglutination tests, and antiglobulin analysis.

Treatment

Infants with idiopathic neutropenia usually require no specific treatment because their disease typically resolves spontaneously. Children, adults, and infants with severe disease may be treated with corticosteroids, immune globulin, or granulocyte colony–stimulating factor (a hematopoietic growth factor). Appropriate antibiotics are administered to treat bacterial infections. Transfusions of WBC concentrates may be indicated. Care must be taken to prevent exposure to any type of infection.

Prognosis

In infants, the disease usually resolves spontaneously. Neutropenia in children and adults often follows a benign course, especially with appropriate treatment.

Prevention

No methods of prevention are known.

Patient Teaching

The parents of infants with immune neutropenia can benefit from understanding the relationship between frequent infections and the condition. When treatment is required, explain the effect of immune therapy, transfusion, or the need for antibiotics as prescribed.

Renal Disorders

Goodpasture Syndrome

Description

Goodpasture syndrome, also known as *antiglomerular basement membrane [GBM] antibody disease,* is an autoimmune kidney disease characterized by the presence of antibodies directed against an antigen in the GBM.

ICD-10-CM Code	M31.0 *(Hypersensitivity angiitis)*
	(M31.0–M31.9 = 11 codes of specificity)

Symptoms and Signs

The patient with Goodpasture syndrome may experience extreme tiredness, nausea, problems breathing and may exhibit a pale appearance to the skin. With the progression of the syndrome, the patient's symptoms will become more severe, and the patient may cough up blood and experience dysuria, hematuria, and proteinuria.

Patient Screening

Symptoms of acute renal failure, such as oliguria, hematuria, and systemic complaints, signal a critical illness that requires immediate medical care.

Etiology

The cause of this rare disease is obscure, but it does sometimes occur in families, so genetics may play a role as well as environmental factors leading to the disease. Antibodies cause complement-mediated tissue damage in the glomerular and alveolar basement membranes, resulting in glomerulonephritis and pulmonary hemorrhage. The toxic weed killer paraquat, which is only available in the United States to licensed applicators, and other chemicals may play a role in this syndrome. Certain medications may also be involved in the development of this disease.

Diagnosis
The diagnosis is suspected in any patient with acute glomerulonephritis, especially if accompanied by pulmonary hemorrhage and acute renal failure. Blood and urine testing is performed. Detection of anti-GBM antibodies in the serum or the kidney is necessary for a definitive diagnosis. This can be done by performing ELISA, immunofluorescence, or renal biopsy. Chest radiographs are performed to determine if there is lung involvement.

Treatment
The treatment may include plasmapheresis (to remove anti-GBM antibodies), corticosteroids to reduce pulmonary hemorrhages, and immunosuppressants.

Prognosis
The prognosis for Goodpasture syndrome is better now than in previous years with early diagnosis. Bleeding in the lungs and kidney failure are both life threatening. Early treatment is effective in increasing life expectancy and physician monitoring is also necessary. There are some patients who will need dialysis and kidney transplants.

Prevention
No methods of prevention are known. Regular dosing of medication according to prescribed intervals can help minimize chances of reflaring.

Patient Teaching
Explain the purpose and procedure for the diagnostic studies. After the diagnosis has been made, discuss the effects of renal impairment on body systems, as appropriate to the patient's symptoms. Explain the purpose of plasmapheresis and the expected results from the medical regimen. Refer the patient to a dietitian for instruction on how best to maintain optimal nutritional status. Teach the patient how to monitor weight, intake, and output of fluids, and warning signs of complications. Encourage questions regarding treatment options as presented by the physician and emphasize communicating with the physician if symptoms worsen or if there are changes in health that take place.

Connective Tissue Diseases

The main component of connective tissue, an essential part of all structures in the body, is a fibrous, insoluble protein called collagen. Collagen constitutes 30% of the total body protein.

Connective tissue diseases are autoimmune disorders. In autoimmune disorders, the immune system malfunctions and works against itself. In these connective tissue diseases, the immune system attacks and destroys the collagen, resulting in damage to some of the body's connective tissues. The precise reason for this malfunction of the immune system is unknown, but genetic factors do play some role. The immune system incorrectly identifies the body's own tissues as foreign and attacks them.

No cures for connective tissue diseases are known; treatment is directed at quieting the overactive immune system and reducing inflammation through medications. In some patients, serious damage to the heart, lungs, or kidneys occurs.

Two well-known examples of the many connective tissue diseases are SLE and RA.

Systemic Lupus Erythematosus
Description
SLE, also known as *lupus*, is a chronic, inflammatory autoimmune disease characterized by unusual autoantibodies in the blood that target tissues of the body.

ICD-10-CM Code	M32.10 *(Systemic lupus erythematosus, organ or system involvement unspecified)* (M32.0–M32.9 = 10 codes of specificity)

Symptoms and Signs
SLE can inflame and damage connective tissue anywhere in the body. SLE most commonly produces inflammation of the skin, joints, nervous system, kidneys, lungs, and other organs. The degree to which any of these tissues are involved varies from patient to patient. A characteristic butterfly rash, or erythema, may be present on the face, spreading from one cheek across the nose to the other cheek (Fig. 3.14A). Similar rashes may appear on other exposed areas of the body. Exposure to the sun can aggravate the rash, a feature known as *photosensitivity*. SLE may begin acutely with fever, fatigue, joint pain, and malaise or may develop slowly over a period of years, with intermittent fever, malaise, joint deformities, and weight loss. Raynaud phenomenon and hair loss are common in SLE.

Patient Screening
The manifestation of an unexplained cluster of symptoms, as described earlier, requires a complete medical evaluation. After the initial diagnostic evaluation, follow the office policy for referral to a rheumatologist.

Etiology
SLE is an autoimmune disorder. Genetic, environmental, and hormonal factors may predispose a person to this disease.

Diagnosis
Patients with symptoms of SLE are diagnosed through the results of physical examination, radiographs, laboratory

• **Fig. 3.14** (A) The characteristic butterfly-like rash of systemic lupus erythematosus (SLE). (B) SLE in black skin. (A, From Everest: *Medical assistant: skeletal and muscular system, infection control, minor office surgery and pharmacology—module* B, ed 2, 2016, Elsevier; B, From Hill MJ: *Skin disorders—Mosby's clinical nursing series*, St. Louis, 1994, Mosby.)

tests, bloodwork, and their symptoms. Some of the symptoms are similar to other symptoms The formal diagnosis of SLE can be made if four or more of the following symptoms or positive laboratory tests are present either at the same time or sequentially: a butterfly rash on the face, a discoid skin lesion, photosensitivity. The visual appearance of SLE may be impacted by natural skin color (see Fig. 3.14B).

People with SLE may experience a variety of symptoms, including fatigue, skin rashes, fevers, and pain or swelling in the joints. Among some adults, having a period of SLE symptoms—called flares—may happen every so often, sometimes even years apart, and go away at other times—called remission.

Other symptoms or positive laboratory tests include nasopharyngeal ulceration, polyarthritis without deformity seizures or psychosis, chronic pleuritis or pericarditis, a false-positive serologic test result for syphilis or DNA or Sm (Smith, an uncharacterized nuclear antigen) antibodies in blood or cardiolipin antibody, greater than 0.5 g of protein in urine in a 24-hour period, the presence of cellular casts in urine, hemolytic anemia, thrombocytopenia, the presence of abnormal antibodies in the bloodstream, and the characteristic leukocytes (WBCs) called *LE cells*, which are not found in the circulation but are created in the laboratory as part of the testing. Diagnostic tests include CBC with differential leukocyte count, platelet count, erythrocyte sedimentation rate (ESR), antinuclear antibody determination, anti-DNA antibody, anti-Sm antibody, and anti-chromatin antibody. The anti-DNA test is the most specific test for SLE, but it is reliably positive more often with active disease.

Treatment

In mild cases, antiinflammatory drugs, including aspirin, nonsteroidal antiinflammatory drugs (NSAIDs), or prednisone, are effective in relieving constitutional symptoms, such as fever and joint pain. Antimalarial agents are commonly added to control skin involvement and arthralgia. For more substantial symptoms, corticosteroids are indicated. Immunosuppressive medications are useful when organ-threatening disease is present. Immunosuppressive agents are also helpful when the patient fails to respond to conventional therapy or when intolerable side effects develop. Monoclonal antibodies (mAbs) such as belimumab (Benlysta) and anifrolumab-fnia (Saphnelo) may also be utilized.

Prognosis

The outlook for patients with systemic lupus continues to improve with the development of more accurate monitoring tests and treatments. Some individuals have mild cases and other people have more severe cases. With treatment, the majority of patients diagnosed with SLE live a normal life span. The prognosis also depends on internal organ involvement. Patients with lupus are at a somewhat increased risk of developing cancer as well as heart disease. The cancer risk is most dramatic for blood cancers, such as leukemia and lymphoma, but is also increased for breast cancer.

Prevention

It is essential that patients diligently adhere to their medication regimens. Flare-ups of disease can be prevented by not missing doses of prescribed medications and avoiding unnecessary exposure to sunlight.

• **Fig. 3.15** Skin involvement in scleroderma is subdivided into "limited" and "diffuse" cutaneous forms. (A) Sclerodactyly in limited cutaneous disease. (B) Truncal changes in diffuse cutaneous disease. (C) Inflammatory signs in early active skin disease. (D) Finger contracture in the chronic fibrotic phase of skin involvement in scleroderma. (From Firestein GS et al: *Kelly's textbook of rheumatology*, ed 9, Philadelphia, 2013, Saunders.)

Patient Teaching

Teaching the patient and the family about the elements of the disease and laboratory testing can beneficially impact the health of patients with lupus. When appropriate, reinforce the physician's advice to avoid stress, decrease exposure to sunlight, cease smoking, and perform moderate exercise.

Scleroderma (Systemic Sclerosis)

Description

Scleroderma is a chronic, progressive disease characterized mostly by sclerosis (hardening) of the skin; scarring of certain internal organs can occur as well. Scleroderma is classified as either diffuse or limited, depending on the extent and location of skin involvement. The diffuse form involves symmetric thickening of the skin of the extremities, face, and trunk, whereas the limited form tends to be confined to the skin of the fingers and face.

ICD-10-CM Code   M34.0 *(Progressive systemic sclerosis)*
M34.1 *(CR[E]ST syndrome)*
M34.9 *(Systemic sclerosis, unspecified)*
(M34.0–M34.9 = 8 codes of specificity)

Symptoms and Signs

Hardening and shrinking of the skin and certain internal organs, including the GI tract, heart, lungs, and kidneys are seen with scleroderma. Involved skin becomes taut, firm, and edematous and is firmly attached to the subcutaneous tissue (Fig. 3.15). The skin feels tough and leathery; it may itch; and pigmented patches may occur. Raynaud phenomenon is often the first symptom of scleroderma. This is followed by swelling, stiffness, and pain in the joints.

Patient Screening

Arrange an appointment for a consultation and medical evaluation to determine options for a person describing unexplained skin changes.

Etiology

The cause of scleroderma is unknown, but it appears to be an autoimmune disease. It features abnormal activation of scar-forming cells (fibroblasts), vascular endothelial abnormalities, and immune dysregulation. There is excessive production of collagen in the body tissues which accumulates. Those diagnosed with scleroderma may have another type of immune disorder.

Diagnosis

A complete history and physical examination are all that are necessary for a diagnosis to be made. Laboratory testing, including Scl-70 and centromere antibodies, can be supportive of the diagnosis. A skin biopsy is only rarely necessary. Blood tests and urinalysis are performed to rule out complications or accompanying conditions. Patients are also evaluated for signs of SLE, polymyositis, Sjögren disease, and hypothyroidism. Lung function testing is helpful in detecting pulmonary disease, and echocardiography can be helpful in screening for pulmonary hypertension. Further testing may include high-resolution computed tomography (high-res CT) of the chest and right heart catheterization.

Treatment

No specific treatment for scleroderma is known. A large number of drugs have been tried, including corticosteroids, vasodilators, and immunosuppressive agents, but their effects are merely palliative. Treatment is directed to the area(s) of the body affected. A rheumatology referral is recommended. Physical therapy helps patients maintain muscle strength but does not change the course of joint disease.

Prognosis

The prognosis for patients with scleroderma depends on which organs are affected and the severity of organ involvement. Patients with pulmonary hypertension, interstitial lung disease, and uncontrolled blood pressure have a higher risk of mortality.

Prevention

How to prevent scleroderma is not known. Preventing its complications, such as those from Raynaud phenomenon and esophageal reflux, may require medications and lifestyle changes.

Patient Teaching

Teaching the patient and the family about the elements of the disease and laboratory testing can be beneficial to the health of patients with scleroderma.

Sjögren Syndrome

Description

Sjögren (pronounced sho′-gren) syndrome is an autoimmune disease that manifests inflammation in the

• **Fig. 3.16** Bilateral parotid gland enlargement. Marked enlargement of both parotid glands is evident in this young female with Sjögren syndrome. (From Hochberg MC et al: *Rheumatology*, ed 8, 2023, Elsevier.)

moisture-secreting glands of the body (Fig. 3.16). This glandular problem results in dryness in the affected areas.

ICD-10-CM Code   M35.00 *(Sicca syndrome, unspecified)*
M35.01 *(Sicca syndrome with keratoconjunctivitis)*
(M35.0–M35.9 = 15 codes of specificity)

Symptoms and Signs

Sjögren syndrome symptoms include xerostomia and **keratoconjunctivitis** sicca. This dryness of the nasal, oral, and laryngeal pharynx causes difficulty talking, chewing, and swallowing. The patient may experience sores on or in the mouth and nose, and dental decay may occur. Sjögren syndrome can follow or precede the onset of RA.

Patient Screening

The onset of symptoms may be insidious or present with much discomfort caused by dryness in the eyes or the oral cavity. When discomfort is present, offer the patient the first available appointment for a medical evaluation.

Etiology

The exact cause of Sjögren syndrome is not known. Genetic (inherited) factors seem to play a role in predisposing a person to Sjögren syndrome. It is found more commonly in families that have members with other autoimmune illnesses. Most patients with Sjögren syndrome are females. It is also believed that a bacterial or viral illness precedes the syndrome.

Diagnosis

Patients with symptoms of Sjögren syndrome are screened for medication side effects, autoimmune thyroid disease, RA,

• **Fig. 3.17** Schirmer's test to detect tear deficiency. A filter paper strip is permitted to remain in contact with the eye for 5 minutes. The wetting effect is measured. (From Stein HA, et al: *The ophthalmic assistant: a text for allied and associated ophthalmic personnel*, ed 11, 2023, Elsevier.)

• **Fig. 3.18** Advanced rheumatoid arthritis. Small muscle wasting, subluxation, and ulnar deviation at the metacarpophalangeal joints, boutonnière deformities at the ring and little fingers, and swelling and deformity of the wrist. (From Dover A et al: *Macleod's clinical examination*, ed 15, 2024, Elsevier.)

SLE, sarcoidosis, and scleroderma associated with Sjögren syndrome. Dry eyes can be defined as abnormal results on the Schirmer test for dryness (Fig. 3.17). Enlarged salivary glands may prompt further investigation, including a lower lip biopsy, which may indicate a characteristic infiltration of lymphocytes. Blood studies often demonstrate anemia, decreased WBC count, and elevated ESR. Additional blood testing shows autoantibodies, called *Sjögren syndrome antibodies* (SSA and SSB antibodies), and high rheumatoid factor titers.

Treatment

There is no cure for Sjögren syndrome. Treatment will vary according to the severity of symptoms; however, many patients are able to control symptoms by using drops or gel to help with dry eyes. Increasing fluid intake, chewing sugarless gum, and using oral sprays help relieve oral dryness. Artificial tears are used in the eyes, and wearing sunglasses is recommended. Sometimes ophthalmologists block the tear ducts with silicone or by cautery to maintain adequate eye moisture. Occasionally prednisone and/or antimalarial medications, such as hydroxychloroquine, are used to lessen the immune inflammation.

Prognosis

The prognosis depends on what complications develop, such as infections in the respiratory tract. The most frequent complications include problems with vision, cavities in teeth, and yeast infections. More serious but rare complications of Sjögren syndrome include lymphoma, lung, liver, peripheral neuropathy, and kidney problems for which patients are monitored.

Prevention

Prevention focuses on avoiding irritation of tissues caused by dryness, monitoring for the development of cancer, and the early management of infections.

Patient Teaching

Patients with Sjögren syndrome can benefit by learning about the immune system and precisely how their bodies are affected by the condition. Awareness of the early warning signs of infection can prevent many serious complications. Moisturizing products for the mouth, eyes, and vagina are available over the counter.

Rheumatoid Arthritis

Description

RA is a chronic, inflammatory, systemic disease that affects the joints (Fig. 3.18). It is one of the most severe forms of arthritis, commonly causing deformity and disability. RA affects 1.5 million Americans; females are affected three times more often than males. RA may begin at any age, but it most commonly strikes individuals in their 30s and 40s.

ICD-10-CM Code	M06.9 *(Rheumatoid arthritis, unspecified)* (M06.00–M06.9 = 97 codes of specificity)

Symptoms and Signs

RA causes inflammation and edema of the synovial membranes surrounding a joint. Eventually this inflammation spreads to other parts of the affected joint and, if left untreated, has the capacity to destroy cartilage, deform joints, and destroy adjacent bone (Fig. 3.19). Most commonly, many joints (polyarthritis) or one or two on both sides of the body are affected by RA. When the neck is involved, the spinal cord can be at risk for damage, potentially leading to

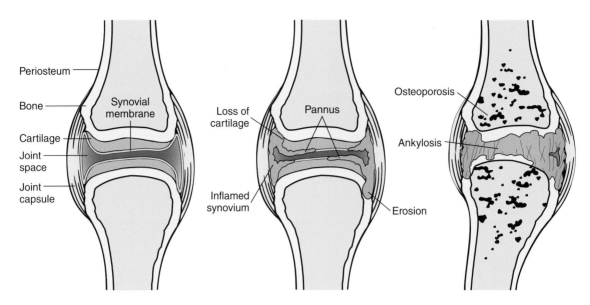

• **Fig. 3.19** Schematic presentation of the pathologic changes in rheumatoid arthritis. The inflammation (synovitis) leads to pannus formation, to the obliteration of the articular space, and finally ankylosis. The periarticular bone shows diffuse atrophy in the form of osteoporosis.

paralysis or death. RA is called a *systemic disease* because it can affect the entire body. It can cause generalized inflammation around or in the lungs, in the cardiac muscle, in blood vessels, and within the skin layers.

RA may begin without any obvious symptoms in the joints. The person may have unexplained weight loss, fatigue, a persistent low-grade fever, and general malaise. This may accompany or precede joint stiffness, which is noticed especially on wakening and during periods of inactivity. Edema, pain, tenderness, erythema, and warmth in one or more joints occurring in a symmetric pattern gradually emerge as the principal symptoms. Joints typically affected are those of the fingers, wrists, knees, ankles, and toes. RA occurs less often in the spine or the hips, which are more susceptible to osteoarthritis (see the Osteoarthritis section in Chapter 7).

In some patients, the joint symptoms appear suddenly without any precursor symptoms. In other cases, joint symptoms are accompanied by bursitis or anemia.

Patient Screening

RA may have an insidious onset with vague systemic symptoms and joint pain, but occasionally the onset is abrupt. Initially, the patient should be seen for diagnostic evaluation. Follow office policy regarding referral to a rheumatologist as soon as possible.

Etiology

RA is an autoimmune disorder. Genes may predispose some people to the disease, and a viral infection may trigger the disease process in some patients.

Diagnosis

Patients with symptoms of RA are evaluated for SLE, Sjögren syndrome, scleroderma, polymyositis, hormone disorders, cancer, and other possible causes of polyarthritis.

Diagnosis is based on a review of the symptoms, patient and family histories, physical examination, radiographic studies, and blood tests that show elevated levels of rheumatoid factor in most patients. Other useful laboratory tests include CBC, synovial fluid analysis, serum protein electrophoresis, ESR, citrulline antibody, and antinuclear antibody titer. Occasionally the diagnosis of RA is achieved only after observation of disease progression for several weeks or months.

Treatment

The primary objectives of treatment are the reduction of inflammation and pain, the preservation of joint function, and the prevention of joint deformity. These require a combination of medication, rest, special exercises, and joint protection. Antiinflammatory medications, including high doses of aspirin, are among the first choices to ease pain and stiffness, reduce edema, and control inflammation. NSAIDs are prescribed as an alternative to aspirin. Corticosteroids, by mouth or by local injection, often are given to control acute flare-ups. Even more potent disease-modifying antirheumatic drugs (DMARDs), such as hydroxychloroquine (Plaquenil), sulfasalazine (Azulfidine), immunosuppressive agents, and newer biologic response modifiers, may slow the disease process or even stop its progression. These treatments, which can prevent damage, work most effectively when started earlier in the disease. Give the patient information about the Arthritis Foundation website and other online resources that are available.

Juvenile Idiopathic Arthritis

Description

Juvenile idiopathic arthritis, formerly referred to as *juvenile rheumatoid arthritis*, is the most common childhood arthritis and affects children less than 16 years of age.

ICD-10-CM   M08.00 *(Unspecified juvenile rheumatoid*
    Code   *arthritis of unspecified site)*
            (M08.0–M08.99 = 121 codes of
                specificity)

Symptoms and Signs

There are subtype classifications for juvenile idiopathic arthritis. The main subtypes are oligarticular, polyarticular, and systemic, which is also known as Still disease.

One or more joints can be affected, but it is more typical in large joints, and symptoms can vary from one patient to another. Patients will have periods of time without as severe symptoms and other times with more painful symptoms (Fig. 3.20). Symptoms include:

- Swollen, stiff, and painful joints, most commonly involving the neck, elbows, knees, and ankles. Limping may be noticed by the parent
- Temperature that fluctuates from mild to high
- Poor appetite, with resulting weight loss
- A blotchy, salmon-colored rash over the limbs and trunk of the body
- Swollen, stiff, and painful joints, most commonly involving the neck, elbows, knees, and ankles. Limping may be noticed by the parent or caregiver

Other possible symptoms include red, painful eyes; swollen cervical or axillary lymph glands; irritability; and acute pericarditis. Skeletal development may be impaired if the epiphyseal, or growth, plates of the long bones are damaged because of the inflammation around the joints.

Sites of arthritis vary considerably from child to child, and girls are affected more often compared with boys. The inflammation usually develops gradually but can be abrupt. In a few cases, the inflammation in the joints leads to partial or crippling deformity as a result of the recurring attacks. Unlike adult RA, remission does occur in some individuals with JRA.

Patient Screening

A young child with fever, rash, and/or swelling and stiffness in the joints should be seen for medical evaluation as soon as possible.

Etiology

Juvenile idiopathic arthritis is an autoimmune disease with an unknown cause; however, genes and environment seem to be factors that play a role in the process.

Diagnosis

There is not a specific test to determine if JIA is present. The diagnosis is based on history, physical examination, and ruling out other diagnoses. While adult patients will test positive for rheumatoid factors, pediatric patients do not always have a positive result, so bloodwork alone cannot be a sole indicator of the condition.

Treatment

Treatment of children with JIA is achieved through resources, and pediatric rheumatologists are the best providers to manage the disease process. Physical and other therapists may be

• **Fig. 3.20** Juvenile rheumatoid arthritis. (A) Child with juvenile rheumatoid arthritis. (B) Frontal view of the child's knees. (From Zitelli BJ, Davis HW: *Atlas of pediatric physical diagnosis,* ed 5, Philadelphia, 2007, Mosby/Elsevier.)

able to help. Managing symptoms and preventing "flare-ups" is a goal that the care providers work together to achieve. Medication dosages are based on the child's weight. Parents should encourage the child's independence. Participation in school and social activities that do not increase joint pain or cause undue fatigue is also important for the child.

Prognosis

With proper therapy, children with all forms of arthritis usually improve over time. Indeed, the vast majority of children with arthritis grow up to lead normal lives without significant physical limitations.

Prevention

Aggressive early medical intervention is mandatory to prevent joint damage, loss of function, and disability. This

• **Fig. 3.21** Ankylosing spondylitis. (A) Frontal view. (B) Lateral view. (From Seidel HM, Ball JW, Dains JE et al: *Mosby's guide to physical examination*, ed 7, St. Louis, 2011, Mosby/Elsevier.)

generally means the early use of DMARDs under the guidance of a qualified physician. A physical therapist can play a central role in helping the child maintain optimal function.

Patient Teaching

Patients and families must have as good an understanding of the disease and its management as possible. Stress the importance of follow-up care and regular eye examinations. The child should be encouraged to be as independent as possible. Give the family information about the Arthritis Foundation and its support programs.

Ankylosing Spondylitis

Description

AS is a systemic, progressive, inflammatory disease affecting primarily the spinal column.

ICD-10-CM Code	M45.9 (Ankylosing spondylitis of unspecified sites in spine) (M45.0–M45.9 = 10 codes of specificity)

Symptoms and Signs

AS commonly affects young males. It is several times more common in males than in females. Typically, it first affects the sacroiliac area of the spine and adjacent soft tissue structures. The patient may have recurring morning low back pain and stiffness that improves with activity. Constitutional symptoms, such as fatigue, weight loss, fever, and/or diarrhea, also may be present at the onset, along with eye pain and photophobia caused by uveitis. Pain and tenderness may be noted over the site of inflammation. The history may include heel pain, inflammatory bowel disease, or family incidence of arthritic conditions. Less often, patients have cervical or thoracic axial pain and stiffness with paraspinal muscular spasms. Peripheral large joints can be involved, particularly in females. Females often have more mild forms of the disease; however, each patient is different.

As the disease progresses, perhaps over many years, the physical examination can reveal a limited range of motion in affected joints resulting from fusion (ankylosis). The inflammation and ossification can progress up the spine, greatly inhibiting the activities of daily life. Chronic pain is experienced in some patients. Eventually, the spinal vertebrae become fused, inflexible, and rigid; the patient's posture exhibits the typical forward flexion of the spine (Fig. 3.21).

Patient Screening

Schedule the patient having back pain and morning stiffness for a medical evaluation. AS is an underdiagnosed cause of low back pain in teens and young adults. Follow office policy regarding referral to a rheumatologist. Patients with known family members who have been diagnosed with AS should be evaluated as soon as possible.

Etiology

The exact cause of AS is not known. Studies support a genetic basis and an association with several genes, including human leukocyte antigen (HLA)-B27. These immunogenic factors may predispose a person to the development of an immune response directed at joint tissue after exposure to particular infectious agents, which have yet to be clearly defined. According to the Spondylitis Association of America: "Identified risk factors that predispose a person to AS include testing positive for the HLA-B27 genetic marker, a family history of AS, and frequent gastrointestinal infections." While not every patient who is positive for HLA-B27 will develop ankylosing spondyliatis, over 90% of patients diagnosed with AS are positive for this gene.

Diagnosis

AS shares a number of diagnostic features with other arthritic diseases; thus early clinical diagnosis is often missed, especially in females. The clinical evaluation includes back pain and stiffness, joint pain with limitation of motion, and positive family history. Laboratory results reveal a negative rheumatoid factor and confirm the inflammatory nature of the disease with a mildly elevated ESR or cross-reactive protein. The HLA-B27 antigen marker is present in the blood of 95% of White individuals with AS; however, not all patients who are HLA-B27 positive will develop the disorder. According to the Spondylitis Association of America, "Scientists suspect that other genes—along with a triggering environmental factor, such as a bacterial infection, for example—are needed to activate AS in susceptible people. HLA-B27 likely accounts for about 30% of the overall risk, but there are numerous other genes working in concert with HLA-B27. Researchers have identified more than 60 genes that are associated with AS and related diseases. Among the newer key genes identified are *ERAP 1, IL-12, IL-17*, and *IL-23*."

Radiographic evaluation of all areas of symptoms is useful initially and later for monitoring. Characteristic radiographic findings are noted years after the onset and include bilateral sacroiliitis, "squaring" of the vertebrae, fusion of joints, and generalized osteoporosis. These changes produce the classic appearance of a "bamboo spine."

Treatment

No cure for AS is known. The goal of drug treatment is to relieve pain, swelling, and inflammation. NSAIDs are the preferred first-line therapy for the treatment of AS. Medications such as corticosteroids, sulfasalazine, or methotrexate may be utilized if NSAIDs are ineffective. Newer generations of medications such as tumor necrosis factor inhibitors, etanercept (Enbrel), adalimumab (Humira), and IL-17 inhibitors, secukinumab (Cesentyx) and ixekizumab (Taltz) have also proven effective in treating the symptoms associated with AS. Patients benefit from physical therapy and moderate exercise to maintain good posture and maximize mobility. Surgical procedures are rarely indicated.

Prognosis

The course of AS is variable with periods of remission and episodes of exacerbation. A poorer prognosis is associated with the early onset of the disease and the male gender. Occasionally the disease takes a severe and rapid course, resulting in systemic complications and severe deformity.

Prevention

No preventive measures for AS are known, but its complications can be prevented or at least lessened with adequate exercise and medications. Because AS is occasionally associated with lung scarring and decreased chest expansion, patients with AS must not smoke.

Patient Teaching

Discuss the importance of maintaining prescribed medication and keeping follow-up appointments. Counsel the patient on individual comfort measures and positional modification in the work environment, as indicated. Stress the importance of moderate, low-impact exercise, such as swimming, to maintain range of motion and good posture. Maintaining a healthy weight will prevent the patient from placing additional stress on the joints, and a regular exercise regimen will prevent fusion of the spine. Discuss the progressive nature of the disease, and encourage the patient to contact credible online support groups.

Polymyositis

Description

Polymyositis is a disease of the muscles that features inflammation of the muscle fibers. The muscles affected are mostly those closest to the trunk or torso. This results in weakness that can be severe. It is a chronic illness with periods of increased symptoms, called *flare-ups* or *relapses*, and decreased symptoms, known as *remissions*.

ICD-10-CM Code	M33.20 *(Polymyositis, organ involvement unspecified)* (M33.00–M33.99 = 16 codes of specificity)

Symptoms and Signs

Muscle weakness is the most common symptom of polymyositis, usually involving the muscles closest to the trunk of the body. The onset can be gradual or rapid. This results in varying degrees of loss of muscle power and atrophy. The loss of strength can be noted as difficulty getting up from chairs, climbing stairs, or lifting above the shoulders. Trouble with swallowing and weakness in lifting the head from the pillow can occur. Occasionally the muscles ache and are tender to the touch. This disease may be accompanied by skin inflammation, in which case it is referred to as *dermatomyositis*. In such cases, a rash may appear and spread over the face, shoulders, arms, and bony prominences (e.g., knuckles, elbows, and knees).

Patient Screening

The patient will have diffuse muscle weakness. Schedule the first available appointment for medical evaluation.

Etiology

The cause of polymyositis is unknown; however, it is thought to be an autoimmune disorder. Polymyositis occurs when WBCs, the immune cells of inflammation, spontaneously invade and injure muscles.

Diagnosis

The history and physical examination should include a thorough search for muscle conditions, such as muscular dystrophy, drug toxicity (e.g., toxicity caused by statin cholesterol drugs), thyroid disorder, sarcoidosis, and infections (e.g., HIV infection and parasites). Moreover, because polymyositis can sometimes accompany cancers, an intense screening for underlying cancer is crucial. A medical history and physical examination document weakness. Blood analysis is used to detect elevated levels of muscle enzymes (creatinine phosphokinase, aldolase, serum glutamate oxaloacetate transaminase, serum glutamate pyruvate transaminase, and lactate dehydrogenase). Electromyography (EMG) demonstrates a typical abnormal pattern of electrical activity in the inflamed muscle, and muscle biopsy confirms the diagnosis.

Treatment

Treatment of polymyositis is directed toward stopping the inflammation and inhibiting the overactive immune system. High doses of steroids usually are prescribed to suppress the inflammation. Immunosuppressive agents, such as cyclophosphamide and methotrexate, as well as IVIG, are also used. Gradually exercise therapy is added to rebuild strength and prevent muscle atrophy.

Prognosis

Patients can ultimately recover with early medical treatment of the disease and its flare-ups. The disease often becomes inactive. Rehabilitation of atrophied muscle can be accomplished with long-term physical therapy. Complications of this disease process can cause problems with swallowing, which may cause one to choke and aspirate food or liquids into the lungs, which will result in pneumonia. Breathing problems due to muscle weakness are also a complication.

Prevention

It is essential that patients be diligent in taking their medications and closely monitor their muscle symptoms. Optimal outcomes are achieved with intervention at the earliest sign of activation of muscle inflammation.

Patient Teaching

Patients should be instructed clearly about the purpose and importance of regular medications. Physical therapy and occupational therapy instructions play major roles in the recovery process.

Common sites of MS lesions in brain and brainstem

Myelin and nerve cell damage

• **Fig. 3.22** Myelin degeneration in multiple sclerosis (MS).

Neurologic Disorders

Multiple Sclerosis

Description

Multiple sclerosis (MS) is an inflammatory disease of the CNS. It attacks the myelin sheath, a fatty substance covering most of the nerves in the brain and spinal cord, and ultimately causes scarring (sclerosis) that debilitates the nerves (Fig. 3.22).

ICD-10-CM Code   G35 *(Multiple sclerosis)*

Symptoms and Signs

The sclerosis of nervous tissue prevents the transmission of stimuli to the brain and spinal cord and causes the following sensory and motor abnormalities (Fig. 3.23): weakness or numbness in one or more limbs, optic neuritis, visual disturbances, unsteady gait, vertigo, difficulty with urination, facial numbness or pain, speech problems, dysphagia, hearing loss, impotence, fatigue, emotional disturbances including depression, irritability, and short temperedness.

The most common characteristic of MS is relapse, the onset of clinical dysfunction, followed by a remission during which the symptoms resolve for a period. MS can be defined as one of several types:

1. Relapsing remitting: relapses followed by recovery with no progression of neurologic dysfunction between relapses
2. Primary progressive: disease progression with no remissions
3. Secondary progressive: disease begins as relapsing remitting but later becomes progressive with few remissions
4. Progressive relapsing: progressive disease from the onset, with relapses and disease progression during the period between relapses

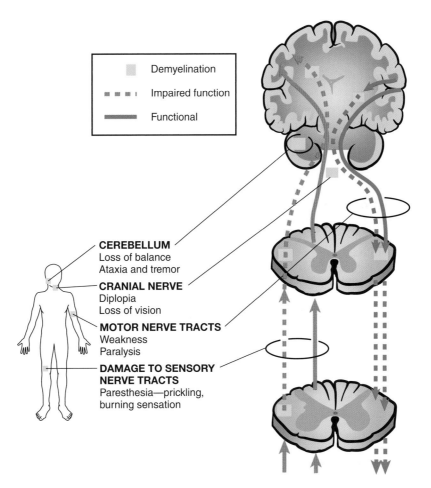

• **Fig. 3.23** Multiple sclerosis (MS)—distribution of lesions. (From Gould BE: *Pathophysiology for the health professions*, ed 4, St. Louis, 2011, Saunders.)

Patient Screening

Initially, a patient with undiagnosed or possible MS may report variable and sporadic symptoms, such as those listed earlier. Schedule an appointment for a clinical evaluation.

Etiology

The cause of MS is unknown. It is thought that the immune system is involved; an inherited trait that increases one's susceptibility to the disease may be a factor as well. A common theory holds that an unknown virus triggers the immune system to turn against the body and attack the myelin, which eventually results in MS. No virus has been conclusively implicated, however. The incidence of MS varies geographically. The risk is also greater in white populations. MS is rare in children and usually develops in people between ages 20 and 40 years but it can occur at any age. MS occurs more often in females than in males.

Diagnosis

MS can be challenging to diagnose because the symptoms are so variable and sporadic. A physical examination done in the early stages may elicit completely normal findings. Often

the diagnosis is determined by eliminating other possible causes of the symptoms. Usually the patient has had two or more distinct episodes of CNS dysfunction with resolution of symptoms between episodes. The diagnosis is made clinically and supported by other test findings. Magnetic resonance imaging is the modality of choice for supporting the diagnosis. A characteristic cerebral or spinal plaque is often found. Examination of cerebrospinal fluid often results in normal findings, although it may reveal elevated immunoglobulin levels and oligoclonal bands on an MS panel.

Treatment

Acute attacks are treated with corticosteroids. Those with diagnosed relapsing-remitting disease may be started on medications approved for treatment of this form of MS, including (interferon beta-1a [Avonex, Rebif], interferon beta-1b [Betaseron], glatiramer [Copaxone], and mitoxantrone [Novantrone]). Immunosuppressive therapies (radiation, steroids, immune globulin, and cytotoxic drugs) may be useful in the treatment of progressive disease. mAbs such as natalizumab (Tysabri) can decrease reflare rates and progressive brain injury. Disease-modifying drugs such as siponimod (Mayzent) and cladribine Mavenclad) were approved in 2019 for treating both secondary-progressive MS and relapsing-remitting MS. They are orally administered medications, unlike some of the other more effective injectable treatments, such as Avonex and Betaseron.

Otherwise, the disease is treated symptomatically. This may include taking muscle relaxants; taking vitamin supplements to prevent a vitamin B deficiency, which might contribute to nerve damage; undergoing physical therapy to help preserve as much muscle function as possible; wearing braces; and using a cane, walker, or wheelchair. Adequate rest and a well-balanced diet are also important.

Prognosis

No cure for MS is known, and the duration of the disease is variable. Some patients die within a few months after the onset of the disease; the average duration is 30 years or longer. Several prognostic indicators are known. A more favorable prognosis is seen in females, with young age at onset, relapsing (rather than progressive) disease, and impairment of sensory pathways as an initial symptom.

Prevention

No method of prevention is known.

Patient Teaching

Describe diagnostic procedures and treatments prescribed. Explanations of the possibility of remission and exacerbations are helpful. Discuss the medications that are prescribed and how they will be monitored for side effects. Make referrals to community support groups, such as the National Multiple Sclerosis Society.

Myasthenia Gravis

Description

Myasthenia gravis is a chronic, progressive neuromuscular disease that is caused by autoantibodies to the acetylcholine receptor at nerve synapses. There is an interruption in communication between the nerves and muscle tissue.

ICD-10-CM Code	G70.00 *(Myasthenia gravis without (acute) exacerbation)* (G70.00–G70.01 = 2 codes of specificity)

Symptoms and Signs

Myasthenia gravis is characterized by extreme muscular weakness (without atrophy) and progressive fatigue. Drooping eyelids, diplopia, and difficulty with talking, chewing, and swallowing may be the first signs that something is wrong. The degree of weakness varies considerably from hour to hour, day to day, and year to year. Muscle weakness typically occurs late in the day or after strenuous exercise. Short periods of rest characteristically restore muscle function. Muscle weakness is progressive in myasthenia gravis, and eventually paralysis occurs. A myasthenic crisis (sudden inability to swallow and respiratory distress) may be so severe that mechanical ventilation becomes necessary. Prolonged exposure to sunlight, cold, infections, and emotional stress exacerbates the symptoms.

Patient Screening

Abrupt onset of the symptoms listed earlier can be disconcerting to the patient and might be confused with symptoms of stroke, indicating prompt medical attention.

Etiology

The disease mainly affects females between ages 20 and 40 and males older than 60 years of age. Myasthenia gravis is thought to be caused by an autoimmune mechanism in which a faulty transmission of nerve impulses to and from the CNS occurs, especially at the neuromuscular junction. Autoantibodies against the acetylcholine receptor are found in 80% to 90% of patients. A majority of patients have either thymus hyperplasia or thymoma, and this may play a role in the development of the disease.

Diagnosis

When myasthenia gravis is suspected, a physical examination is done to test for the fatigability of different muscle groups. The Tensilon test, intravenous administration of a short-acting acetylcholinesterase inhibitor, is performed to see whether the administration improves muscle strength. Tests are done to check for the presence of antibodies against the acetylcholine receptor. EMG may also be performed.

Treatment

The treatment of myasthenia gravis is symptomatic and supportive. Restricted activity, complete bed rest for severe cases, and a soft or liquid diet may be necessary. Anticholinesterase drugs are effective initial treatment for fatigue and muscle weakness, but they become less effective as the condition worsens. Pyridostigmine bromide (Mestinon) is the drug of choice for treatment. If a thymus gland tumor (thymoma) is present, a thymectomy is needed. Corticosteroids are effective in patients who have not improved with thymectomy. A useful adjunct to alternate-day therapy with corticosteroids is immunosuppression. Myasthenic crisis is treated with intubation and withdrawal of anticholinesterase medications, followed by reintroduction of the drugs and plasmapheresis.

Prognosis

Unexplained, spontaneous remissions can occur; however, the disease is usually a lifelong condition, characterized by remissions and exacerbations. The prognosis for patients who experience myasthenic crisis has improved over the years, but such an event can still leave many patients who had been independent before the crisis functionally dependent afterward.

Prevention

No methods of prevention are known.

Patient Teaching

Give the patient information about the diagnostic tests prescribed. Explain the medical management of symptoms and what side effects to report. Encourage the patient to take the initiative in deciding on his or her own supportive care. List the warning signs of an impending myasthenic or cholinergic crisis.

Vasculitis

Vasculitis is inflammation in the walls of blood vessels. The affected vessel becomes necrotic when it is obstructed by a thrombus, and an infarct of adjacent tissue results. Biopsies of an involved vessel can demonstrate the presence of inflammation in the blood vessel wall. Any blood vessel can be involved, and the many forms of vasculitis are each characterized by the particular vessels affected. Vasculitis can be classified into two main types: small-vessel vasculitis and systemic necrotizing vasculitis. Each of these types has many subtypes.

Small-Vessel Vasculitis

Description

Small-vessel vasculitis is the category of vasculitis that primarily affects the capillaries, arterioles, and venules.

ICD-10-CM Code	I77.9 *(Disorder of arteries and arterioles, unspecified)*
	(I77.0–I77.9 = 14 codes of specificity)

Symptoms and Signs

Inflammation of the small vessels causes petechiae (nonblanching), purpura, erythema, ulcerations, and edema, which are most often found on the skin of the lower extremities. Pain and a burning sensation can accompany these lesions. Additionally, depending on the type of small vessel syndrome that the patient experiences, symptoms can include ocular lesions, genital or oral ulcerations, abdominal pain, arthralgia, and weakness.

Patient Screening

The patient with a rash, joint pain, fatigue, and weakness needs prompt medical evaluation. Follow office policy regarding referral to a rheumatologist.

Etiology

Although the exact cause is unknown, vasculitis often accompanies other immune disorders. A reaction to medication or drugs may also be a factor, as well as having an infection such as hepatitis B, hepatitis C, or a cancer of the blood.

Diagnosis

The diagnosis is confirmed by biopsied tissue. Blood tests such as C-reactive protein, CBC, angiography of the vessels, and imaging tests are helpful. The presence of immunoglobulins and complement in the blood vessels, as well as the pattern of vascular involvement and the cell types present, can help define the subtype of small vessel vasculitis. Bleeding disorders, anticoagulant medication, and even aspirin can cause skin findings that mimic small vessel vasculitis.

Treatment

Treatment consists of identifying and preventing exposure to the causative agent or managing the underlying disease. Corticosteroid therapy may afford relief; analgesics are prescribed, and rest is encouraged.

Prognosis

The outlook for patients with small vessel vasculitis is generally very good. The condition tends to readily respond to treatment.

Prevention

For those patients who have developed small vessel vasculitis as a result of reaction to certain medications, avoidance of those medications in the future is the key to prevention.

Patient Teaching

The importance of regular medical follow-up and adherence to the medication regimen cannot be overemphasized.

Systemic Necrotizing Vasculitis

Description

Systemic necrotizing vasculitis tends to primarily affect medium and large arteries.

ICD-10-CM Code	I77.3 *(Arterial fibromuscular dysplasia)*
	I77.8 *(Other specified disorders of arteries and arterioles)*

Symptoms and Signs

Systemic necrotizing vasculitis occurs in a number of cutaneous and systemic conditions. Symptoms vary, depending on the body system involved; they can include headaches, fever, weakness, fatigue, malaise, anorexia, and weight loss. Patients also may experience muscle and joint pain, angina, dyspnea, hypertension, and visual disturbances. Impaired tissue perfusion causes ischemic pain in the system or tissues involved. Ulceration of the skin can result. Paralysis of an affected nerve can lead to weakness or numbness.

Patient Screening

Rapid evaluation by a qualified physician experienced in the evaluation and management of vasculitis is crucial.

Etiology

It is not clear how the inflammation and necrosis of blood vessels develop. Each subtype of systemic necrotizing vasculitis has specific clinical features with several probable mechanisms involved. Autoimmune responses play a role and are mediated by cellular and humoral (antibody-related) immunity. Illicit drug use, including cocaine and amphetamines, and hepatitis B and C have been associated with the development of some forms of systemic vasculitis.

Diagnosis

A complete history and a thorough physical examination are important. Comprehensive blood studies, including CBC, ESR, RA factor determination, and serum tests for immunoglobulins, are done. The CBC indicates anemia and usually elevated WBC and platelet counts. The ESR is elevated during the acute stage. The CRP test shows an earlier and more intense increase compared with ESR. When the pulmonary system is involved, chest radiographs show pulmonary infiltrates. Hematuria and proteinuria are present with renal involvement. Aneurysms and myocardial ischemia are indicators of cardiac involvement. Biopsy specimens of involved vessels ultimately confirm the diagnosis by demonstrating the invasion of leukocytes in the blood vessel wall. An alternative to biopsy, in some cases, can be angiography, a radiographic examination of blood vessels.

Treatment

Treatment focuses on decreasing the inflammation of the arteries and improving the function of the affected organs. Treatment addresses the underlying causative factors and systemic involvement. Corticosteroids and analgesics afford relief from the effects of inflammation. Immune-suppressing medications, such as azathioprine and cyclophosphamide, and plasmapheresis are also used to lessen the immune activation. Hypertension is treated with antihypertensive drugs, for example, angiotensin-converting enzyme (ACE) inhibitors. Ocular problems should be closely monitored.

Prognosis

The outlook for patients with systemic necrotizing vasculitis is guarded until the condition is controlled with medications to suppress inflammation and immune activity. This category of vasculitis can permanently damage organs.

Prevention

No method of prevention for systemic necrotizing vasculitis is known, other than avoiding known causes, including cocaine, amphetamines, and hepatitis B and C.

Patient Teaching

The importance of regular medical follow-up, monitoring for signs of activation of disease, and adherence to the medication regimen cannot be overemphasized. Patients with skin damage should be taught good skincare, and those who smoke should be encouraged to stop.

Review Challenge

Answer the following questions:
1. Name the functional components of the immune system.
2. Describe the three major functions of the immune system.
3. List examples of inappropriate responses of the immune system.
4. Explain the difference between active immunity and passive immunity, and give examples for each.
5. Trace the formation of T cells and B cells from stem cells.
6. Explain how T cells and B cells specifically protect the body against disease.
7. List the five immunoglobulins.
8. Explain complement fixation and its importance in the immune system.
9. Describe the invasion of T-helper cells by HIV.
10. Explain the ways that HIV infection is transmitted.
11. Discuss the treatment of HIV infection.
12. List the guidelines for universal precautions and infection control.
13. Describe the primary absence or inadequate response of the immune system in the following diseases:
    - Common variable immunodeficiency
    - Selective immunoglobulin A deficiency
    - Severe combined immunodeficiency disease
14. Explain the destructive mechanisms in autoimmune diseases.
15. Describe the symptoms and signs of pernicious anemia. Name the primary treatment.
16. Describe the systemic features of SLE. Recall the diagnostic criteria.
17. Detail the pathology of RA.
18. Specify the primary objectives of the treatment for RA.
19. Compare the pathology of MS to that of myasthenia gravis.
20. Explain the cause of the typical forward flexion of the spine in the patient with advanced ankylosing spondylitis.
21. Discuss the treatment and prognosis for patients with polymyositis.

Real-Life Challenge: Pernicious Anemia

A 46-year-old female patient reports fatigue, loss of appetite with occasional nausea and vomiting, a sore tongue, and weight loss. She also mentions weakness, numbness, and loss of feeling in her hands, lower arms, feet, and lower legs.

She has recently experienced lightheadedness, visual disturbances, ringing in the ears, shortness of breath, rapid pulse, and palpitations. In addition, she mentions experiencing headaches, irritability, and depression. Examination shows pale-appearing lips, tongue, and gums. Her skin and sclera appear jaundiced.

Hematology tests reveal reduced Hgb, RBCs, WBCs, platelets, and increased MCV. The RBCs and platelets appear large and malformed. Studies of bone marrow are indicative of abnormal RBC production. Gastric acid is either reduced or absent.

Questions

1. What is meant by pernicious anemia?
2. What is the importance of the intrinsic factor?
3. Why would the patient experience GI type of symptoms?
4. What is the cause of the neurologic symptoms?
5. Why would the patient experience lightheadedness, fatigue, and weakness?
6. How long must the patient continue treatment after the symptoms abate?
7. Why is the patient unable to take vitamin B_{12} orally?
8. At the present time, what is the cure for pernicious anemia?

Real-Life Challenge: Rheumatoid Arthritis

A 33-year-old female reports a recent onset of pain in the joints of her fingers and hands. She has also experienced weight loss, fatigue, and a persistent low-grade fever. On examination, the joints of the hands and fingers display tenderness, redness, warmth, and swelling. Blood tests indicate an elevated level of rheumatoid factor. Further observation over a period of a few months shows a continuation of the symptoms with the involvement of additional joints. The patient has been diagnosed with RA.

Questions

1. Compare the incidence of RA in males and females.
2. Compare the symptoms and signs of RA and osteoarthritis (see the Osteoarthritis section in Chapter 7).
3. Describe the projected course of RA that is left untreated.
4. What is the cause of RA?
5. Which diagnostic tests are usually ordered when RA is suspected?
6. Because the primary treatment is to reduce inflammation and pain, preserve joint function, and prevent deformities, what is the usual prescribed treatment?
7. Explain the side effects the patient may experience with NSAID therapy.
8. Explain why early referral to a rheumatologist is recommended.

Real-Life Challenge: Ankylosing Spondylitis

A 28-year-old patient has complained of lower back pain for several months. She sees her health care provider and is prescribed antiinflammatory medications and physical therapy for muscle strain. The pain continues, and there is no relief after completion of physical therapy. The patient is then referred to an orthopedist. The physician orders a bone scan and also a series of laboratory tests, including the HLA-B27 marker test. The test results are positive for this genetic marker. Which health care provider will need to see the patient with this result? Which disease or disorder may be the source of the patient's pain?

Internet Assignments

1. Explore the Lupus Foundation of America website for breaking news. Learn how to use the website to locate the chapter of the Lupus Foundation nearest to you.
2. Explore the National AIDS Hotline and report on a top story in the What's New section.
3. Go to the National Multiple Sclerosis Society to identify promising areas of disease research, and list some current clinical trials.

Critical Thinking

1. Why does patient teaching need to be very specific for a patient diagnosed with an immunodeficiency disease?
2. What is the understanding of the "window period" stage of infection with HIV?

3. Explain how autoantibodies cause diseases.

4. What is the relationship between pernicious anemia, shortage of intrinsic factors, and the impairment of vitamin B_{12} adsorption?

5. How does the immune system malfunction in connective tissue diseases?

6. Why is scleroderma difficult to diagnose?

7. Which gene is known to be associated with autoimmune disorders, such as AS?

8. A patient who has undergone heart transplantation shows immediate signs of organ rejection despite an accurate tissue match prior to the transplantation. What are some of the reasons for this type of rejection?

Prepare to discuss Critical Thinking case study exercises for this chapter that are posted on the Evolve website.

Credentialing Examination Questions

1. Which class of drugs must patients who have received an organ transplant take to help ensure they do not have a rejection of their new organ?
 A. Antibiotic
 B. Antihypertensive
 C. Immunosuppressive
 D. ACE Inhibitor

2. Which method is not included in ways that HIV can be transmitted?
 A. Sexual intercourse
 B. Blood products
 C. Shared needles
 D. Casual contact

3. Which disease has been referred to as Bubble Boy disease?
 A. Severe combined immunodeficiency disease
 B. X-linked agammaglobulinemia
 C. DiGeorge anomaly
 D. Wiskott-Aldrich syndrome

4. Which condition refers to persistent and recurrent candidal (fungal) infections of the skin, nails, and mucous membranes?
 A. Selective immunoglobulin A deficiency
 B. Chronic mucocutaneous candidiasis
 C. Systemic *Candida* infection
 D. Autoimmune hemolytic anemia

5. Which condition is included in hematopoietic disorders?
 A. Autoimmune hemolytic anemia
 B. Selective immunoglobulin A deficiency
 C. Human immunodeficiency virus
 D. X-linked agammaglobulinemia

6. Which deficiency causes recurrent otitis media, eye, skin, and bronchial infections, including pneumonia?
 A. IgA
 B. IgM
 C. IgG
 D. CVID

7. Which type of counseling is beneficial when a child has a diagnosis of DiGeorge syndrome?
 A. Psychological
 B. Genetic
 C. Pediatric
 D. Behavioral

8. Which person is typically the best match for a patient who needs a bone marrow transplant?
 A. Mother
 B. Father
 C. Child
 D. Sibling

9. Which option most accurately describes connective tissue diseases?
 A. Acute conditions that resolve with treatment.
 B. Caused as a result of an untreated bacterial infection.
 C. The immune system malfunctions and works against itself.
 D. Results from a viral infection.

10. Which condition has symptoms of inflammation of the joints, nervous system, kidneys, lungs, and organs in addition to a characteristic butterfly rash on the face?
 A. Goodpasture syndrome
 B. Scleroderma
 C. Sjögren syndrome
 D. Systemic lupus erythematosus

4

Diseases and Conditions of the Endocrine System

CHAPTER OUTLINE

LEARNING OBJECTIVES

After studying this chapter, you should be able to:

1. Describe the importance of hormones and explain some of the critical body functions that they control.
2. List the major glands of the endocrine system.
3. Explain the importance of normal pituitary function.
4. Compare gigantism with acromegaly.
5. Describe the condition of dwarfism and its etiology.
6. Explain the cause of diabetes insipidus.
7. Explain the treatment for a simple goiter.
8. Compare the signs and symptoms of thyroid hypofunction with those of thyroid hyperfunction.
9. List the signs and symptoms of Graves disease.
10. Distinguish between cretinism and myxedema.
11. Describe the signs and symptoms of thyroid malignancy, and discuss the most important prognostic factor.
12. Compare and contrast hyperparathyroidism and hypothyroidism.
13. Describe Cushing syndrome and Addison disease.
14. Explain the pathogenesis of diabetes mellitus.
15. Identify the two major types of diabetes mellitus.
16. Distinguish between diabetic coma and insulin shock.
17. Explain the medical management of all three types of diabetes mellitus.
18. Discuss why early recognition of metabolic syndrome offers the patient an advantage in focusing on intervention.
19. Explain why hypoglycemia can be a serious medical condition.
20. Define precocious puberty.

KEY TERMS

acidosis (ass-ih-DOE-sis)
corticotropin (kor-tih-ko-TRO-pin)
epiphyseal (eh-pih-FEEZ-e-al)
gonadotropin (go-nad-oh-TRO-pin)
hyperglycemia (hye-per-gli-SEE-me-ah)
hyperkalemia (hye-per-ka-LEE-me-ah)
hypocalcemia (hye-poh-kal-SEE-me-ah)
hypothalamus (hye-poh-THAL-ah-mus)
panhypopituitarism (pan-high-poh-pih-TOO-ih-tair-ism)
polydipsia (pahl-ee-DIP-see-ah)

polyphagia (pahl-ee-FAY-jee-ah)
polyuria (pahl-ee-U-ree-ah)
pruritus (pruh-RI-tus)
radioimmunoassay (ray-dee-oh-IM-u-no-ass-a)
somatotropin (soh-mat-oh-TROH-pin)
thyrotoxicosis (thye-roh-tox-ih-KOH-sis)
thyrotropin (thye-ro-TRO-pin)
thyroxine (thye-ROKS-in)
triiodothyronine (try-eye-oh-doh-THYE-row-neen)
vasopressin (vaz-oh-PRES-in)

Orderly Function of the Endocrine System

Body activities, homeostasis, and the stress response are communicated and controlled by two distinct but interacting systems: the nervous system and the endocrine system. The systems interact as one system starts, ends, or extends the activity of the other. The nervous system (discussed in Chapter 13) creates an immediate but short-lived response, operating on the principles of electricity through impulse conduction. The endocrine system has a slightly slower onset and a longer duration of action and uses highly specific and powerful hormones to control its response chemically. Hormones are chemical messengers classified as either amino acids (proteins) or steroids.

The endocrine system is composed of many glands scattered throughout the body; these glands secrete unique and potent chemicals called *hormones* directly into the bloodstream (Fig. 4.1). Most hormones direct their action to target glands or tissues at distant receptor sites, thereby regulating critical body functions, such as urinary output, cellular metabolic rate, and growth and development. Hormonal secretions are typically regulated by negative feedback; information about the hormone level or its effect is fed back to the gland, which then responds accordingly (Fig. 4.2).

Certain endocrine glands are stimulated to secrete hormones in response to other hormones. Hormones that stimulate the secretion of other hormones are called *tropic hormones*. For example, in females, **gonadotropins** stimulate the synthesis of ovarian hormones. In diagnostic analysis, when excessive hormones are produced by an ectopic source (e.g., a malignant tumor), the tropic hormones are low. Other secreting cells that perform endocrine functions may be scattered in the tissue, such as in the digestive tract, where local hormones regulate the motility and secretions of other hormones. The influence of hormones is of vital importance because they regulate body function to promote health.

Endocrine diseases result from an abnormal increase or decrease in the secretion of hormones. Symptoms of disease vary with the degree of increase or decrease in hormonal secretion and the age of the patient. This divergence from normal hormone quantities may be the result of hyperplasia, hypertrophy, or atrophy of an endocrine gland. Changes in gland size that affect the gland's production and secretion of a hormone often result from an insult to the gland, such as infection, radiation, trauma, surgical intervention, and inflammation. Dysfunction of an endocrine gland is associated with many physical and mental symptoms that can affect a person's quality of life.

Some common symptoms are as follows:
- Growth abnormalities
- Emotional disturbances or psychiatric problems
- Skin, hair, and nail changes
- Edema
- Hypertension or hypotension
- Arrhythmia
- Changes in urine output
- Muscle weakness and atrophy
- Menstrual irregularity or amenorrhea
- Impotence or changes in libido
- Sterility
- Changes in energy level

To appreciate the effect of endocrine gland function on health and disease, review the main glands and their primary hormones (Table 4.1). The pituitary gland, which is intricately connected to the **hypothalamus**, plays a central role in regulating most of the endocrine glands; it has a cascading effect on the glands that it stimulates. The pituitary gland is divided into anterior and posterior lobes; the anterior lobe accounts for about 80% of the gland. The hypothalamus, a part of the brain that also has endocrine functions, controls

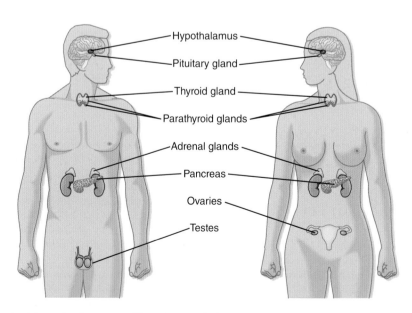

• **Fig. 4.1** Glands of the endocrine system. (From Koeppen B, Stanton B: *Berne & Levy Physiology*, ed 8, 2024, Elsevier.)

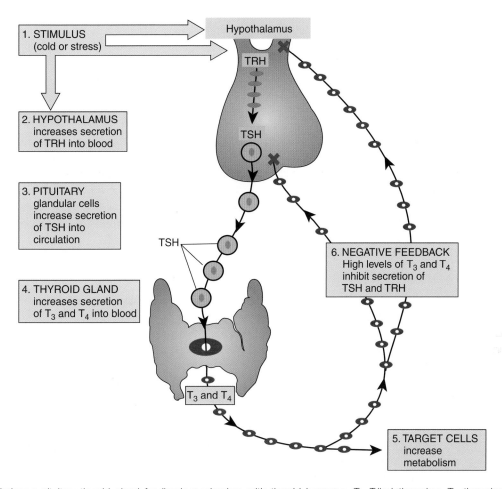

1. STIMULUS
(cold or stress)

Hypothalamus

TRH

TSH

2. HYPOTHALAMUS
increases secretion
of TRH into blood

3. PITUITARY
glandular cells
increase secretion
of TSH into
circulation

TSH

6. NEGATIVE FEEDBACK
High levels of T_3 and T_4
inhibit secretion of
TSH and TRH

4. THYROID GLAND
increases secretion
of T_3 and T_4 into blood

T_3 and T_4

5. TARGET CELLS
increase
metabolism

• **Fig. 4.2** Hypothalamus-pituitary-thyroid gland feedback mechanism with thyroid hormone. T_3, Triiodothyronine; T_4, thyroxine; *TRH*, thyrotropin-releasing hormone; *TSH*, thyroid-stimulating hormone. (From Gould B: *Pathophysiology for the health professions*, ed 3, Philadelphia, 2006, Saunders.)

many activities of the pituitary gland by neural and chemical stimuli. Pituitary dysfunction can affect some or all of the glands that are targets of pituitary hormones, thereby indirectly affecting body structure and function (Fig. 4.3).

Diagnosing endocrine disorders requires correctly matching the patient's symptoms with a specific hormone dysfunction and obtaining laboratory confirmation of overproduction or underproduction of a particular hormone or hormones.

Hormone levels can be detected by using blood serum or plasma, which is collected by phlebotomy . Whole blood can also be used when performing blood spot testing, which requires capillary blood. Urine and saliva testing are also methods for evaluating hormone levels.

Newer research indicates that blood and plasma levels only reflect a small amount of hormones actually being used by the body because these tests measure the levels of circulating hormones rather than the hormones that are available for use by organs. Historically, hormone levels have been measured by serum blood tests using **radioimmunoassay** or immunometric assay and occasionally by using a 24-hour urine test. Blood spot testing requires only a drop of blood.

Hormone testing can also be accomplished with saliva testing, and patients themselves may even order hormone tests online to check levels with kits that require saliva for testing.

Computed tomography (CT), ultrasonography, and magnetic resonance imaging (MRI) can help determine the type and location of a lesion. In some cases, a positron emission tomography (PET) scan may also be used as a diagnostic tool. A biopsy is performed to determine whether a lesion is malignant.

After an endocrine problem is identified, treatment is initiated to replace the hormone deficit or reduce a lesion by surgical removal or radiation therapy. Newer medical therapies also inhibit the synthesis of hormones. However, therapeutic drugs may have substantial side effects. Neuroendocrine cells relay messages by using hormones to different areas of the body. At times, these cells multiply and become neuroendocrine tumors.

Bioidentical Hormone Replacement

Currently, hormones called *bioidentical hormones* are available. Bioidentical hormones are made from plants. They

TABLE 4.1 **Major Endocrine Gland Secretions and Functions**

Endocrine Gland	Hormone	Target Action
Anterior pituitary	Growth hormone	Promotes bone and tissue growth
	Thyrotropin (thyroid-stimulating hormone)	Stimulates thyroid gland and production of thyroxine (T_4)
	Corticotropin (adrenocorticotropic hormone)	Stimulates adrenal cortex to produce glucocorticoids
	Gonadotropins	
	Follicle-stimulating hormone	Initiates growth of eggs in ovaries; stimulates spermatogenesis in testes
	Luteinizing hormone	Causes ovulation; stimulates ovaries to produce estrogen and progesterone; stimulates testosterone production
	Prolactin	Stimulates breast development and formation of milk during pregnancy and after delivery
	Melanocyte-stimulating hormone	Regulates skin pigmentation
Posterior pituitary	Vasopressin (antidiuretic hormone)	Stimulates water resorption by renal tubules and has antidiuretic effect
	Oxytocin	Stimulates uterine contractions; stimulates ejection of milk in mammary glands; causes ejection of secretions in male prostate gland
Thyroid	Thyroid hormone (TH): T_4 and triiodothyronine (T_3)	Regulates rate of cellular metabolism (catabolic phase)
	Calcitonin	Promotes retention of calcium and phosphorus in bone; opposes effect of parathyroid hormone
Parathyroid	Parathyroid hormone	Regulates metabolism of calcium; elevates serum calcium levels by drawing calcium from bones
Adrenal cortex	Mineralocorticoids, primarily aldosterone	Promote retention of sodium by kidneys; regulate electrolyte and fluid homeostasis
	Glucocorticoids: cortisol, corticosterone, cortisone	Regulate the metabolism of carbohydrates, proteins, and fats in cells
	Gonadocorticoids: androgens, estrogens, progestins	Govern secondary sex characteristics and masculinization
Adrenal medulla	Catecholamines: epinephrine and norepinephrine	Produce quick-acting "fight or flight" response during stress; increase blood pressure, heart rate, and blood glucose level; dilate bronchioles
Pancreas	Insulin	Regulates metabolism of glucose in body cells; maintains proper blood glucose level
	Glucagon	Increases concentration of glucose in blood by causing conversion of glycogen to glucose
Ovaries	Estrogens	Cause development of female secondary sex characteristics
	Progesterone	Prepares and maintains endometrium for implantation and pregnancy
Testes	Testosterone	Stimulates and promotes growth of male secondary sex characteristics and is essential for erections
Thymus	Thymosin	Promotes development of immune cells (gland atrophies during adulthood)
Pineal gland	Melatonin	Regulates daily patterns of sleep and wakefulness; inhibits hormones that affect ovaries; other functions unknown

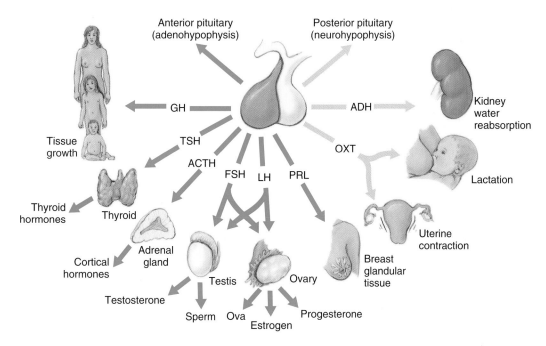

• **Fig. 4.3** The effect of pituitary hormones on target tissues. *ACTH,* Adrenocorticotropic hormone; *ADH,* antidiuretic hormone; *FSH,* follicle-stimulating hormone; *GH,* growth hormone; *LH,* luteinizing hormone; *OXT,* oxytocin; *PRL,* prolactin; *TSH,* thyroid-stimulating hormone. (From Applegate EJ: The anatomy and physiology learning system, ed 4, St. Louis, 2011, Saunders.)

are processed and imitate natural hormones. The US Food and Drug Administration (FDA) has approved some bioidentical hormones; however, there are other bioidentical hormones which are compounded by a compounding pharmacy. These are currently not FDA approved, and there are risks with using them. Some bioidentical hormones that are compounded may have the exact formula as those approved by the FDA, but there are other hormones added that have not been approved. The companies that make these hormones claim that they are better and that their use has certain advantages over traditional hormone replacement therapy. While there may be advantages in some cases and for some patients to use bioidentical hormones, research has not indicated, at this point, that they are safer or more effective.

Pituitary Gland Diseases

Excess Pituitary Hormone Secretion

Inflammation or tumor of the pituitary gland can lead to a chronic and progressive disease resulting from the excessive production and secretion of pituitary hormones, for example, human growth hormone (hGH). Excessive hGH produces one of two distinct conditions, gigantism or acromegaly, depending on the time of life at which the dysfunction begins.

Gigantism

Description

Gigantism describes an abnormal pattern of growth and stature. This is a rare condition.

ICD-10-CM Code	E22.0 *(Acromegaly and pituitary gigantism)*

Symptoms and Signs

When the hypersecretion of growth hormone (GH, **somatotropin**) occurs before puberty, the result is gigantism, a proportional overgrowth of all body tissues (Fig. 4.4A). The affected child experiences abnormal and accelerated growth, especially of the long bones, because **epiphyseal** closure has not begun. Typically an accelerated linear growth prompts an initial investigation in children. Sexual development and mental development are often delayed.

Patient Screening

Symptoms usually appear over time; signs of the condition may be discovered during a routine examination. Follow office policy for referral to an endocrinologist.

Etiology

An anterior pituitary adenoma is most often the cause of oversecretion of GH, which results in gigantism. Although a genetic link has not been identified, gigantism sometimes affects multiple members of a family. In children, a genetic change in AIP gene deletions or mutations has been discovered, which causes a pituitary tumor to form. Carney complex, McCune-Albright syndrome, multiple endocrine neoplasias (MEN) type 1 or type 4, neurofibromatosis, and familial isolated pituitary adenomas are genetic conditions that can lead to this condition. Hypogonadism may lead to tall stature, but not gigantism, by delaying puberty and the closure of the epiphyses.

Diagnosis

The clinical picture of abnormal growth in a prepubescent child leads the physician to order diagnostic investigations. Levels of GH are elevated on the laboratory test result. Age-reference norms for insulin-like growth factor 1 (IGF-1) are the best indicators of endogenous secretion of GH. The best imaging study is pituitary MRI; CT can also detect the presence of a pituitary lesion. Bone radiographs show thickening of the cranium, enlargement of the jaws, and elongation of the long bones.

Treatment

The objective of treatment is to reduce the amount of GH secreted. This is performed ideally through surgery (transsphenoidal approach) (Fig. 4.4B), with or without the addition of medication or radiation to the pituitary gland to reduce its size. Appropriate gonadal hormones may be needed in children or adolescents exhibiting hypogonadism. Yearly follow-up examinations are recommended.

Prognosis

Correction of the disorder prevents further physical changes.

Prevention

No prevention is known.

Patient Teaching

Explain the diagnostic tests and surgical interventions as appropriate. Give the child and parents visual aids depicting the pituitary gland and its functions. Emphasize the importance of getting follow-up care and adhering to the dosage schedule for medications.

Acromegaly

Description

Acromegaly is a chronic metabolic condition in adults caused by hypersecretion of GH by the pituitary gland.

ICD-10-CM Code	E22.0 *(Acromegaly and pituitary gigantism)*

Symptoms and Signs

When hypersecretion of GH occurs after puberty, acromegaly (overgrowth of the bones of the face, hands, and feet) occurs, with an excessive overgrowth of soft tissue because epiphyseal closure has already occurred (Fig. 4.5). It is often seen in those 30 to 40 years of age after they experience years of excess GH. The patient notices that they must wear larger gloves, shoes, or both. Excessive jaw growth causes larger spaces between teeth. The individual may experience

• **Fig. 4.4** (A) Growth hormone abnormalities. The 22-year-old male on the left with gigantism is much taller than his identical twin on the right. (B) Hypophysectomy. Surgical removal of the pituitary gland may be performed to excise a pituitary tumor or to slow the growth and spread of endocrine-dependent malignant tumors. It is done only if other treatments fail to destroy all pituitary tissues. (A, Courtesy Robert F. Gagel, MD, and Ian McCutcheon, MD, University of Texas, MD Anderson Cancer Center, Houston, Texas; From Black JM, Hawks JH: *Medical-surgical nursing: clinical management for positive outcomes*, ed 8, St. Louis, 2009, Saunders; B, From Leonard P: *Building a medical vocabulary:with Spanish translations*, ed 11, 2022, Elsevier.)

• **Fig. 4.5** Acromegaly. (From Forbes CD, Jackson WF: *Color atlas and text of clinical medicine*, ed 3, London, 2003, Mosby, Elsevier Science Ltd.)

joint pain resulting from osteoarthritis and other clinical problems in the body systems.

Patient Screening
Symptoms usually appear over time; signs of the condition may be discovered during a routine examination. Follow office policy for referral to an endocrinologist.

Etiology
As with gigantism, a pituitary tumor or adenoma is often the cause of acromegaly. It affects females and males with equal frequency.

Diagnosis
The clinical picture of abnormal thickening of the bones of the face, hands, and feet leads the physician to order diagnostic tests. Levels of GH and IGF-1 are elevated. In conjunction, another reliable test is the glucose tolerance test because increased glucose levels cause failure to supress GH levels. As with gigantism, MRI of the pituitary and CT can detect the presence of a pituitary lesion.

Treatment
The objective of treatment is to reverse or prevent tumor mass effects and reduce the amount of GH secreted. Correcting the disorder prevents further disfigurement and reduces the mortality that results from excess GH. This is performed ideally through surgery (transsphenoidal approach), with or without the addition of medication or radiation to the pituitary gland to reduce its size. The success of medical therapies depends on the response of the tumor cells to the intervention.

Prognosis
Acromegaly can cause an increase in mortality due to cardiovascular and cerebrovascular diseases. Reduction in the

levels of GH is associated with improvement in symptoms and signs.

Prevention
No prevention is known.

Patient Teaching
Offer the patient teaching website links and visual aids that explain the anatomy and function of the pituitary gland and its hormones. Reinforce the physician's explanation of the cause, treatment of acromegaly, and purpose of the required diagnostic tests. Describe the surgical procedures, if appropriate. Explain the medication dosage schedule and the possible adverse effects to report. Encourage the patient to express concerns and questions about changes in body image.

Hypopituitarism

Description
Hypopituitarism is a condition caused by a deficiency or absence of any of the pituitary hormones, produced by the anterior pituitary lobe.

ICD-10-CM Code	E23.0 *(Hypopituitarism)*
	(E23.0–E23.7 = 6 codes of specificity)

Symptoms and Signs
Because the anterior pituitary secretes several major hormones, the syndrome can be complex and marked by metabolic dysfunction, sexual immaturity, or delayed growth. Physical findings vary, depending on the specific hormone deficiency. A deficiency of pituitary hormones that stimulate other endocrine glands can result in the atrophy of those glands. When **thyrotropin** (thyroid-stimulating hormone [TSH]) secretion is reduced, the functioning of the thyroid gland is affected and the patient experiences symptoms of hypothyroidism. When the secretion of **corticotropin** (adrenocorticotropic hormone [ACTH]) dwindles, salt balance and nutrient metabolism are affected. Gonadotropin deficiency impairs sexual functions, including sexual development, menstruation, and libido.

Hypopituitarism causes delayed growth in children. Headache and blindness are signs of tumor infringement on the optic nerve.

Patient Screening
The symptoms of the complex syndromes associated with this disorder usually have an insidious onset. Schedule a complete medical evaluation, and follow office policy for referral to an endocrinologist.

Etiology
The cause of hypopituitarism may be a pituitary tumor. Some causes are genetic and congenital deficiencies, and some are acquired. A physical injury to the pituitary gland can also

cause this condition. Traumatic brain injury is an example that can damage the pituitary gland. Radiation; surgical removal; and ischemia resulting from an infarct, tumor, or basilar skull fracture can also cause this condition. If the ischemia is severe and not reversed, permanent destruction of glandular tissue begins. Destruction of the entire anterior lobe results in panhypopituitarism, a decline in multiple anterior pituitary hormone secretion. The condition is most common in females, and sometimes the cause is unknown.

Diagnosis

When the patient has clinical symptoms of hyposecretion of any of the anterior pituitary hormones, a complete medical evaluation is necessary to detect partial or selective hormone deficiencies and to pinpoint the diagnosis. A history of head trauma, previous radiation, or a surgical procedure to the gland or nearby tissue contributes to the diagnosis. Plasma levels of all or some of the pituitary hormones are low. Radiographic films of the skull, cranial CT, and MRI are used to identify the tumor. The clinical investigation must rule out diseases of the target glands themselves.

Treatment

The course of treatment is determined by the patient's age, the severity and type of deficiency, and the underlying cause of hypopituitarism. When neoplasia is the cause, removal of the tumor alleviates the symptoms. Replacement therapy with hormonal supplements, including thyroxine (T_4), cortisone, sex hormones, or somatropin (hGH), is usually effective. Hormone levels must be continually monitored during hormone replacement therapy.

Prognosis

The prognosis varies because of the many possible causes of hypopituitarism and the complex functions of the pituitary gland itself.

Prevention

No prevention is known.

Patient Teaching

Emphasize the importance of following any instructions given by the endocrinologist regarding hormone replacement therapy, warning signs of overreplacement, and necessity of follow-up visits to monitor the results of therapy and drug doses.

Dwarfism

Description

The deficiency of pituitary GH in children results in short stature. Dwarfism is generally defined as an abnormal underdevelopment of the body in children, with adult height reaching only 4 feet 10 inches or less (Fig. 4.6).

ICD-10-CM Code	E34.3 *(Short stature due to endocrine disorder)*

• **Fig. 4.6** Dwarfism (hypopituitarism). The child on the left has dwarfism and is 25 inches tall compared with the child on the right, who is 39 inches tall. Both children are 4 years of age. (Brashear H, Raney R: *Shand's handbook on orthopaedic surgery*, ed 10, St. Louis, 1986, Mosby.)

Symptoms and Signs

Hyposecretion of the pituitary gland hormones, especially GH, results in delayed growth. As a result, the child is extremely short, with a body that is small in proportion. The prepubescent child does not develop secondary sex characteristics. The condition may be linked to other defects and a varying degree of intellectual developmental disorder.

Patient Screening

Children deficient in GH require regular follow-up appointments during therapy. Follow office policy for referral to an endocrinologist.

Etiology

Dwarfism can be caused by a genetic abnormality, and there are many different types, with achondroplasia being the most common. Occasionally there is no identifiable cause. A deficiency of the growth hormone–releasing hormone produced by the hypothalamus is termed *secondary hypopituitarism* and results from head trauma, tumor, or infection.

Diagnosis

Physical examination shows that the child fails to grow at a normal rate and is short in stature. The child's general health appears to be good. Secondary tooth eruption is delayed, and fat deposits may be noted in the lower trunk area. Persistently low serum GH levels are found. CT may confirm the presence of a cranial tumor.

Treatment

Somatotropin (hGH) is administered until the child reaches a height of 5 feet. When multiple hormone deficiencies are found, these children may also need replacement thyroid and adrenal hormones. If necessary, sex hormones are administered as they approach puberty.

Prognosis

Clinical manifestations of GH deficiencies depend on the time of onset and the degree of hormone deficiency. GH replacement is effective in children with well-documented GH deficiency. Treatment is essential to help reach final adult height. Safety for long-term GH administration indicates negligible adverse effects.

Prevention

Known causes are not preventable, but common precautions may be taken to prevent head trauma and infection.

Patient Teaching

Digital resources and support groups for the patient may be helpful. It is also important to educate the patient and family members on safety and learn how to do things differently due to short stature.

Diabetes Insipidus

Description

Diabetes insipidus is a disturbance of water metabolism, resulting in extreme thirst and excessive secretion of dilute urine.

ICD-10-CM Code   E23.2 *(Diabetes insipidus)*

Symptoms and Signs

Diabetes insipidus is a deficiency in the release of **vasopressin** (antidiuretic hormone [ADH]) by the posterior pituitary gland, resulting in the excretion of copious amounts of dilute urine (**polyuria**). The patient experiences excessive thirst (**polydipsia**), fatigue, and symptoms of dehydration, including dry mucous membranes, hypotension, dizziness, and poor skin turgor. The onset of symptoms may be abrupt.

Patient Screening

An abrupt onset of excessive thirst and excessive urination, together with the symptoms of dehydration, merits prompt medical attention.

Etiology

In diabetes insipidus, the posterior pituitary gland releases reduced amounts of vasopressin. The condition may be hereditary, or it may be the result of an insult to the hypothalamus or the pituitary gland resulting from head trauma, cerebral edema, or an intracranial lesion. Nephrogenic diabetes insipidus results from renal tubular resistance to the action of vasopressin. More common in males than females, this disease may occur in childhood or early adulthood. In many cases, the cause is unknown.

When the amount of vasopressin is insufficient, the distal tubules of the nephron do not reabsorb water from the filtrate back into the bloodstream; consequently, the volume of urine is excessive.

Diagnosis

The presence of polyuria and polydipsia leads the clinician to investigate the composition of the urine through laboratory tests. Urinalysis that reveals almost colorless urine with a low specific gravity (<1.005) suggests diabetes insipidus. The patient may be given the water-restriction test, during which the kidneys exhibit an inability to concentrate urine despite the patient being deprived of fluid intake for several hours. When the urine concentration (osmolality) is stable on consecutive measurements or the blood osmolality is above normal, vasopressin (ADH) is administered. Urine volume is compared with specific gravity. Reduced output and increased specific gravity of urine after the administration of vasopressin indicate diabetes insipidus.

Treatment

Treatment consists of vasopressin injections, nasal spray, or oral desmopressin acetate (trade name DDAVP). In nephrogenic diabetes insipidus, thiazide diuretics act by inducing mild volume depletion. In the kidneys, hypovolemia induces an increase in proximal sodium and water resorption, diminishing water delivery to the vasopressin-sensitive collecting tubules, thus reducing urine output. Any underlying cause should be identified and treated. When excessive diuresis is the result of trauma to the pituitary gland, the symptoms begin to subside as the insult resolves.

Prognosis

Patients who are bedridden or unable to drink enough water to compensate for urinary loss of water can become dangerously dehydrated. Individuals with uncomplicated diabetes insipidus respond to treatment and return to a normal life.

Prevention

The causes and contributing factors cannot be prevented.

Patient Teaching

Give the patient guidelines for monitoring fluid intake and output to ensure adequate water replacement. Instruct the patient to notify the physician of any increase in symptoms, including weight loss or gain. Encourage the patient to wear a medical alert bracelet (Fig. 4.7).

Thyroid Gland Diseases

Thyroid diseases present as functional disturbances that produce excessive or reduced secretions of thyroid hormones—thyroxine (T_4) and **triiodothyronine** (T_3)—and mass lesions of the thyroid. Table 4.2 lists types of thyroid diseases and their signs and symptoms. Fortunately, diseases of the thyroid gland may be resolved through medical and surgical interventions.

The thyroid gland is the endocrine organ that most often produces pathology. Under the control of TSH from the pituitary gland, the thyroid gland produces two types of hormones: T_4 and T_3. Iodine in the diet is necessary for the synthesis of thyroid hormone. Released into the systemic circulation, thyroid hormones affect the metabolism of all body tissues, the function of the pituitary gland's essential GH, and many body systems. The size and superficial location of the thyroid gland in the neck make it uniquely available for inspection and palpation. A goiter is often the first sign of thyroid disease.

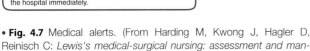

• **Fig. 4.7** Medical alerts. (From Harding M, Kwong J, Hagler D, Reinisch C: *Lewis's medical-surgical nursing: assessment and management of clinical problems*, ed 12, 2023.)

Simple Goiter

Description
The term *goiter* refers to any enlargement of the thyroid gland, usually evidenced by a swelling in the neck.

ICD-10-CM Code	E04.0 *(Nontoxic diffuse goiter)*
	OR
	E01.2 *(Iodine-deficiency related (endemic) goiter, unspecified)*
	(E01.0–E01.8 = 4 codes of specificity)
	E04.9 *(Nontoxic goiter, unspecified)*

Disorders of the thyroid gland are coded according to the underlying pathology. Refer to the physician's diagnosis and then to the current edition of the ICD-10-CM coding manual to ensure the greatest specificity of pathology.

Symptoms and Signs
Simple goiter, or hyperplasia of the thyroid gland, may be asymptomatic in the early stages. The patient, who is usually female, may be unaware of the condition until the anterior aspect of the neck enlarges with conspicuous swelling of the

TABLE 4.2	Comparison of Hypothyroid and Hyperthyroid Disorders	
	Hypofunction of Thyroid	**Hyperfunction of Thyroid**
Names or types	Congenital, untreated can become cretinism or thyroid dwarfism	Hyperthyroidism
	Myxedema coma	Thyrotoxicosis
	Hashimoto thyroiditis	Graves disease: autoimmune with or without exophthalmos
	Iodine deficiency: simple goiter	Toxic nodular hyperplasia
	Idiopathic hypothyroidism	Toxic adenoma, thyroid tumors
Symptoms and signs	Decreased activity, sleepiness, lethargy	Restlessness, irritability, easy fatigability, nervousness
	Reduced mental alertness, easy fatigability	Tremors
	Dry skin and hair, decreased sweating	Moist skin, increased sweating
	Cold intolerance	Heat intolerance
	Bradycardia	Tachycardia and palpitations
	Constipation	Diarrhea
	Weight gain	Weight loss, increased appetite
	Edema, bloated face, puffy eyelids	Polydipsia
	Poor circulation, extremity edema	Loss or thinning of hair
	TSH levels increased	TSH levels decreased
	T_3, T_4 levels decreased	T_3, T_4 levels increased
	I^{131} uptake decreased	I^{131} uptake increased

I^{131}, Radioactive iodine; T_3, triiodothyronine; T_4, thyroxine; *TSH*, thyroid-stimulating hormone.

• **Fig. 4.8** Goiter. (From Swartz MH: *Textbook of physical diagnosis*, ed 4, Philadelphia, 2002, Saunders.)

thyroid gland, called a *goiter* (Fig. 4.8). As the hyperplasia increases, it presses on the esophagus, producing difficulty swallowing, and occasionally it can enlarge further, pressing onto the trachea and producing dyspnea. Weight loss despite a hearty appetite, heat intolerance, tachycardia, anxiety, and increased sweating may be reported by the patient when there is excessive production of thyroid hormones.

Patient Screening
The patient who complains of enlargement in the area of the thyroid gland, with or without accompanying discomfort in the area, should be scheduled for a thorough patient history and physical examination.

Etiology
A simple, or nontoxic, goiter results from a deficiency of iodine in the diet. Iodine is necessary for the synthesis of both T_3 and T_4. Together, they are known as *thyroid hormones*, which are produced by the thyroid gland. The inadequate blood level of thyroid hormone causes the anterior pituitary gland to increase its secretion of thyrotropin (TSH). Thyrotropin keeps attempting to stimulate the thyroid gland to produce thyroid hormone. This continued stimulation, in turn, causes the thyroid gland to increase in size.

In the past, there were high rates of simple goiter among people living in geographic regions where the soil had low levels of iodine and where seafood was not readily available. The regular addition of iodine to salt and the advent of rapid refrigerated transport of seafood and fresh vegetables from areas where soil and water iodine levels are high have reduced the endemic aspects of this condition. Simple goiter can be exacerbated as a result of the ingestion of large amounts of goitrogenic foods, such as cassava and cabbage, or drugs, such as lithium.

Diagnosis
Diagnosis is made by examination of the neck, noting the enlargement of the thyroid gland (goiter). A goiter may also be found when a patient has an x-ray or imaging study for another reason not related to the goiter itself. Blood studies indicate elevated thyrotropin levels and occasionally reduced levels of T_3 and T_4. Measurement of radioactive iodine uptake by the thyroid gland is often helpful in determining the cause of the abnormality. Thyroid ultrasonography can confirm the presence of thyroid nodules.

Treatment
Treatment will depend on how large the goiter is and what type of symptoms the patient has. If the goiter is very large, surgical intervention may be needed to keep the airway open from the goiter pressing on soft tissues in the neck. Prevention calls for the addition of iodine to the diet; there are no longer any iodine-deficient areas in the United States because of the introduction of iodized salts. There has been an increase in the use of sea salt for seasoning foods. Sea salt has some iodine but not as much as table salt, which has added iodine. Sporadic goiter requires avoidance of goitrogenic drugs or foods. Thyroid hormones, such as T_4, sometimes help.

Prognosis
The prognosis is good when treatment to reduce the goiter is successful.

Prevention
Adequate dietary intake of iodized salt prevents this deficiency. Some individuals should be advised to avoid goitrogenic drugs or foods. Examples of goitrogenic foods include broccoli, cauliflower, turnips, Brussels sprouts, cabbage, and radishes.

Patient Teaching
Instruct the patient to take the prescribed thyroid hormone medication at the same time each day to maintain a constant level of the medication in the blood. Make sure the patient and the family know the symptoms of the adverse effects of a thyroid preparation that should be reported to the physician: palpitations, increased pulse rate, anxiety, insomnia, sweating, and tremors.

Hashimoto Thyroiditis
Description
Hashimoto thyroiditis (chronic lymphocytic thyroiditis) is a chronic disease of the immune system that attacks the thyroid gland.

ICD-10-CM Code1	E06.3 *(Autoimmune thyroiditis)* (E06.0–E06.9 = 7 codes of specificity)

Symptoms and Signs
The condition occurs more in females than in males. It is the leading cause of goiter and hypothyroidism. The outstanding

clinical feature is the gradual and painless lumpy enlargement of the thyroid gland, which causes a feeling of pressure in the neck and may result in difficulty with swallowing. Symptoms of hypothyroidism, such as sensitivity to cold, weight gain, fatigue, depression, puffiness in the face, brittle nails, hair loss, and problems with concentration or memory, may occur.

Patient Screening

Schedule a physical examination for a patient with a "lump in the throat" or a swelling in the neck. Follow office policy for referral to an endocrinologist.

Etiology

Heredity plays a prominent role in Hashimoto thyroiditis. Antibodies appear to destroy thyroid tissue instead of stimulating it. The gland enlarges as a result of an inflammatory process, with infiltration by lymphocytes and plasma cells. As a result, gland tissue is replaced by fibrous tissue, and a significant number of patients with Hashimoto thyroiditis become hypothyroid.

Diagnosis

Serum TSH levels are elevated in patients with hypothyroidism. Autoantibodies against thyroid tissue, such as thyroid peroxidase antibodies, are found in the blood. In Hashimoto thyroiditis, characteristic changes can be seen in the thyroid gland through needle biopsy and examination of the gland tissue, but these procedures are not necessary.

Similarly, a radioactive iodine uptake scan will show a low uptake, but it usually is not needed to make the diagnosis.

Treatment

The treatment is the lifelong replacement of thyroid hormones in patients with hypothyroidism, which also prevents the goiter from growing further.

Prognosis

Mild hypothyroidism is common and usually responds well to thyroid replacement therapy.

Prevention

No prevention is known.

Patient Teaching

Explain each diagnostic test and procedure, medications, and follow-up guidelines. Written and digital information according to the patients' preferences should be provided.

Hyperthyroidism

Graves Disease

Description

Graves disease, a condition of primary hyperthyroidism, occurs when the entire thyroid gland hypertrophies, resulting in a diffuse goiter and an overproduction of thyroid hormones.

• **Fig. 4.9** Thyroid eye disease (Graves disease) with characteristic exophthalmos and eyelid retraction. (From Goldman L, Cooney K: *Goldman-Cecil medicine*, ed 27, 2024, Elsevier.)

ICD-10-CM Code	E05.00 *(Thyrotoxicosis with diffuse goiter without thyrotoxic crisis or storm)*
	OR
	E05.0 *(Thyrotoxicosis with diffuse goiter)*
	(E05.0–E05.91 = 14 codes of specificity)

Refer to the physician's diagnosis and then to the current edition of the ICD-10-CM coding manual to ensure the greatest specificity of pathology.

Symptoms and Signs

Overproduction of thyroid hormone causes increased metabolism and multisystem changes. The patient has rapid heartbeats and palpitations, nervousness, excitability, and insomnia. Despite excessive appetite and food consumption, the patient loses weight. Profuse perspiration and warm, moist skin cause the person to be intolerant of hot weather. Other symptoms include muscular weakness and nail changes (onycholysis). General hyperactive behavior, tremors, and loss of hair are noted. Sometimes, the eyes develop exophthalmos, an outward protrusion, which gives the patient a staring expression (Fig. 4.9), and sometimes skin changes called *dermopathy* are noted. Changes in menstrual cycle may also occur. A sudden exacerbation of symptoms may signal **thyrotoxicosis**, or thyroid storm, resulting from exaggerated thyroid hormone levels, can be life threatening.

Patient Screening

A patient with mild or vague symptoms should be scheduled for a complete physical examination. An acute manifestation of severe symptoms (e.g., notable tachycardia, manic behavior, vomiting, confusion, or coma) can indicate a life-threatening condition. Prompt consultation with the physician is necessary.

Etiology

Graves disease is caused by a disorder of the immune system. Antibodies to thyroid antigens stimulate the hyperactivity of the thyroid gland. A familial predisposition strongly suggests genetic causation.

Diagnosis

Taking the clinical picture and a thorough history are the first steps in the diagnosis. Laboratory tests are performed. Serum T_3 and T_4 levels are typically elevated, and TSH levels are low. Radioiodine uptake tests, ultrasound, and in some cases, MRI or CT scan are necessary. A thyroid scan is diagnostic and shows an increased uptake of radioiodine. Blood tests may reveal elevated levels of certain antithyroid immunoglobulins, such as thyroid-stimulating immunoglobulin.

Treatment

Treatment begins with the administration of antithyroid drugs, such as propylthiouracil and methimazole (Tapazole), to block the synthesis of thyroid hormones. β-Blockers, such as propranolol hydrochloride (Inderal) and atenolol (Tenormin), are given to treat tachycardia. Alternative treatments include radioactive iodine therapy or surgery (thyroidectomy), which is used to reduce the activity of the thyroid gland. Patients require ongoing medical supervision to monitor thyroid hormone levels. Some patients need help coping with the anxiety, stress, and physical discomfort associated with Graves disease.

Prognosis

Therapeutic intervention almost always restores the balance of thyroid hormone in the body and relieves symptoms. Some patients are more difficult to treat, especially older patients with concomitant underlying heart disease, and complications may arise. Some patients experience spontaneous remission. Relapses do occur; thus lifelong follow-up is recommended.

Prevention

There is no known prevention.

Patient Teaching

Explain the effects of hyperthyroidism on the body and on emotional stability. Discuss the diagnostic procedures and their purposes. Explain the dosage schedule of medications and the adverse effects to report. Give preoperative and postoperative instructions as appropriate. Emphasize the importance of follow-up appointments to monitor treatment.

Hypothyroidism

Hypothyroidism refers to any state in which thyroid hormone production is below normal. There are several possible causes that must be considered, including familial tendencies. At first, the symptoms may be subclinical or subtle and take time, even years, to be noticed. Fatigue, cold intolerance, constipation, and dry, flaky skin may be experienced initially (see Table 4.2). A simple blood test measures the level of TSH secreted by the pituitary gland and the levels of the thyroid hormones (T_3 and T_4). An increase in TSH and below-normal levels of T_3 and T_4 or free T_4 are indicative of the condition. With a proper diagnosis of hypothyroidism, the patient can be treated with hormone replacement and expect excellent results. In most cases, lifelong treatment with a form of T_4 (levothyroxine) is indicated, along with careful monitoring for therapeutic blood levels. Failure to treat the condition can lead to an increase in symptoms and/or severity of the disease.

Although more common in females, hypothyroidism can strike either sex and at any age. Much of the world's population lives at high risk in iodine-deficient areas, resulting in congenital hypothyroidism, a cause of mental deficiency.

Cretinism

Description

Cretinism is a congenital hypothyroidism developing in infancy or early childhood.

ICD-10-CM Code	E00.9 (Congenital iodine-deficiency syndrome, unspecified) (E00.0–E00.9 = 4 codes of specificity)

Symptoms and Signs

Cretinism is a congenital hypothyroid condition in which the thyroid gland is absent or thyroid hormone is not synthesized by the thyroid gland; this causes intellectual developmental disorder and delayed growth in the infant or young child. The child is stocky in stature and has a protruding abdomen. Other physical characteristics include a short forehead, a broad nose, and small wide-set eyes with puffy eyelids; a wide-open mouth with a thick, protruding tongue; an expressionless face; and dry skin. The sex organs fail to develop. A lack of muscle tone contributes to an inability to stand or walk.

Patient Screening

Follow office policy for referral of newborns or children with endocrine conditions or with suspected developmental disorders.

Etiology

An error in fetal development may cause the thyroid gland to fail to develop or to function. The patient may have a congenital absence of one of the enzymes necessary for T_3 and T_4 synthesis. Maternal thyroid deficiency or antithyroid drugs taken during pregnancy may be an etiologic factor. Cretinism occurs in areas where the diet is deficient in iodine.

Diagnosis

Blood test results showing the absence or abnormally low amount of T_4 in the presence of an elevated TSH level indicate cretinism. A thyroid scan confirms the absence of thyroid tissue. If cretinism is not detected during the neonatal period, the infant will be slow to smile, and intellectual developmental disorder will occur.

Treatment

Early treatment with thyroid hormone promotes normal physical growth but may not prevent intellectual developmental disorders. This replacement therapy must continue throughout the life of the patient.

Prognosis

The prognosis is good when cretinism is discovered early in life and T_4 replacement is begun. Even skeletal abnormalities are reversible with treatment. The condition may be associated with other endocrine abnormalities.

Prevention

The use of iodized salt greatly reduces the incidence of cretinism in a population. Public education about the importance of good prenatal care that manages any maternal endocrine disease is important.

Patient Teaching

The response to hormone replacement takes time; give the parent reasonable expectations for the child taking the medication. Giving the parents and/or caregivers educational materials in print and digital resources provides a blended experience.

Myxedema and Myxedema Coma

Description

Myxedema (hypothyroidism) is a disease characterized by clinical manifestations associated with a low metabolic rate caused by thyroid hormone deficiency.

Myxedema coma is the result of severe untreated hypothyroidism exacerbated by an acute event, such as myocardial infarction, infection, or the use of sedatives.

ICD-10-CM Code	E03.9 *(Hypothyroidism, unspecified)* (E03.0–E03.9 = 8 codes of specificity)

Symptoms and Signs

Severe hypothyroidism with significantly reduced levels of T_4 and T_3, especially in older adults, leads to a slowing of function in multiple organs. Excessive fatigue, muscular weakness, loss of hair, weight gain, constipation, and intolerance to cold are common symptoms. The skin is dry and scaly, and there is puffiness of the hands and face, in addition to an enlarged tongue (Fig. 4.10). Sometimes the term *myxedema* is also used synonymously with severe

• **Fig. 4.10** Myxedema facies. (From Patton KT, Thibodeau G: *Human body in health & disease*, ed 7, St. Louis, 2018, Mosby.)

hypothyroidism. Rarely does it progress to a myxedema coma when severe hypothyroidism is accompanied by signs of hypothermia and altered mental status: slurred speech and drowsiness, followed by profound lethargy or even unconsciousness. Myxedema coma has a high mortality rate.

Patient Screening

Complaints vary, depending on age at onset. When a parent reports slowing of physical and mental activities in a child or an adult reports the same, an appointment for a complete physical examination is needed. Keep in mind that the symptoms may mimic depression.

Etiology

The thyroid gland's ability to synthesize T_4 is impaired. This can be the result of reduced amounts of thyrotropin, radiation destruction of the thyroid gland, surgical removal of the gland without T_4 replacement therapy, tumors, or failure of the thyroid gland to function. The disorder may also be secondary to the failure of the pituitary to produce thyrotropin. A common cause of hypothyroidism in females is Hashimoto thyroiditis.

Diagnosis

The clinical features of myxedema in adults or the delayed physical and mental development in children may lead the physician to order diagnostic tests. Blood studies indicate abnormally low levels of thyroid hormones (total T_4, total T_3, and free T_4) and, in most cases, significantly elevated TSH levels. Rarely is the TSH level low as a result of a pituitary condition.

Treatment

The goal of medical management is to achieve normal thyroid function with the lowest possible dose. The patient should be told that replacement therapy is required for life.

Myxedema coma is treated as an emergency. Levothyroxine sodium (T_4), a therapeutic agent, is administered orally or intravenously. Additionally, it is important to treat any coexisting medical condition, including adrenal insufficiency, with corticosteroids.

Prognosis

The response to hormone replacement therapy is usually good, and the symptoms improve. If myxedema coma develops, the mortality is high.

Prevention

Endocrinologists and other health care providers recommend screening (testing for TSH levels) in identified high-risk groups, at age 35, and every 5 years thereafter as part of a periodic health examination.

Patient Teaching

Patients on medications should be taught the importance of taking the medication at the same time each day on an empty stomach and recognizing the signs of overmedication. Inform the patient that a clinical response to the medication may take several weeks to appear and that blood tests will be required to monitor for therapeutic blood levels of the medication. Demonstrate and encourage periodic self-examination of the thyroid gland. Use customized electronically generated educational materials, when available, to reinforce the treatment plan.

Thyroid Cancer

Description

Thyroid cancer is a neoplasm of the thyroid gland. The term includes primary thyroid tumors, thyroid lymphoma, and metastases from breast, colon, kidney, or skin cancers to the thyroid gland.

ICD-10-CM Code	C73 (Malignant neoplasm of the thyroid gland)

Refer to the physician's diagnosis and then to the current edition of the ICD-10-CM coding manuals to ensure the greatest specificity of pathology.

Symptoms and Signs

Thyroid malignancies often do not cause symptoms until the disease is advanced. Signs of cancer include palpation of a hard, painless lump or nodule on the thyroid gland, vocal cord paralysis, obstructive symptoms, and cervical lymphadenopathy. Some patients exhibit dysphagia or hoarseness resulting from compression of the upper aerodigestive tract. A rapidly enlarging neck mass may be a sign of anaplastic thyroid cancer.

Patient Screening

When patients complain of persistent hoarseness, difficulty swallowing, or a painless lump in the neck, schedule an appointment with the physician as soon as possible.

Etiology

Thyroid cancer accounts for a small percentage of all thyroid nodules. Other causes include multinodular goiter, Hashimoto thyroiditis, cysts, and follicular adenomas. The four main types of thyroid cancer are papillary (small nipple-like projections), follicular (saclike ball of cells), medullary (affecting the interior portion of the gland), and anaplastic (loss of differentiation of cells). Papillary and follicular carcinomas are the most common types of thyroid cancer. Anaplastic tumors are rare, invasive, and occur mainly in patients older than 60 years of age. Females are nearly three times more likely to have thyroid cancer compared with males. Relatives of patients with thyroid cancer have a 10-fold higher incidence of thyroid cancer, which indicates a genetic basis for tumor susceptibility. Previous head and neck radiation exposure, especially in early childhood, is the only other established risk factor. A diet deficient in iodine may contribute to follicular cancer. Although 80% of cases of medullary carcinoma are sporadic, some are caused by inherited genetic mutations, resulting in MEN type 2, a rare, heritable disorder characterized by various types of endocrine tumors. Inherited medullary cancer usually presents in the third decade of life.

Diagnosis

Thyroid nodules are usually discovered by the patient, found incidentally on a physical examination, or detected by a radiologic procedure performed for another reason. TSH is measured in all patients with thyroid nodules. Fine-needle aspiration and histologic examination of the nodule tissue are needed to confirm the diagnosis and type of cancer. Medullary thyroid carcinomas often secrete calcitonin and occasionally secrete carcinoembryonic antigen (CEA), both of which can serve as tumor markers. Patients with this type of thyroid cancer should undergo testing for mutations in the *RET* gene to evaluate for MEN type 2. Tests used for staging include CT or ultrasonography of the neck and chest radiography. All anaplastic tumors are considered stage IV tumors and require a PET to better determine the extent of tumor spread (see Chapter 1 for a discussion of the staging of cancer).

Treatment

The primary therapy mode for papillary, follicular, and medullary thyroid cancers is surgery. Most patients undergo total thyroidectomy with the removal of any involved lymph nodes, followed by the administration of radioiodine to destroy any remaining thyroid tissue and tumor and to image any recurrent disease. Aggressive initial therapy yields lower rates of local and regional recurrence and lower overall mortality. Thyroid surgery is associated with the risk of vocal cord paralysis resulting from damage to the recurrent laryngeal nerve and the risk of hypoparathyroidism. After surgery, patients are started on T_4 therapy to prevent TSH stimulation of tumor growth and to prevent hypothyroidism. However, excessive T_4 therapy carries risks of accelerated bone loss, atrial fibrillation, and cardiac dysfunction, so the amount of T_4 administered is carefully regulated. Because thyroid cancers are largely resistant to conventional chemotherapy, new agents are being investigated to treat this disease. Tyrosine kinase inhibitors can be used to delay progression in patients with metastatic disease.

Anaplastic tumors are the most aggressive form of thyroid cancer. They are resistant to most therapies. Nonsurgical treatment (e.g., radiotherapy and/or chemotherapy) may prolong survival. Total thyroidectomy is indicated to reduce symptoms caused by the tumor mass if the disease is confined to the local area.

Most recurrences of any type of thyroid neoplasm appear within 5 years of initial treatment, although they can occur decades afterward. All patients should periodically undergo a physical examination and measure serum thyroglobulin, TSH, and T_4 levels after treatment. Patients with medullary thyroid cancer with preoperatively elevated levels of calcitonin and/or CEA should have the levels of these tumor markers measured periodically as well.

Prognosis

Most patients with differentiated thyroid carcinomas have a very good prognosis. The most important prognostic factors are age at diagnosis, size of the primary tumor, and the presence of tissue invasion or metastases.

If the cancer has spread to other organs or tissues close to the thyroid gland, it is referred to as *regional thyroid cancer*. The 5-year survival rate for regional follicular cancer is 98%, and the 5-year survival rate for regional papillary thyroid cancer is 99%. The 5-year survival rate for individuals with regional medullary cancer is 92%, and those with regional anaplastic cancer have a poor 5-year survival rate of 11%.

If thyroid cancer metastasizes and spreads to other distant organs, the percentage for 5-year survival drops. Anaplastic and medullary cancers spread more frequently compared with follicular or papillary tumors.

Prevention

Patients who have been exposed to radiation should receive follow-up screening for thyroid cancer, depending on their estimated risk level. Those at low risk should undergo thyroid palpation every year or every other year. Those at high risk should undergo annual palpation and thyroid ultrasonography on a regular basis. Those at high risk usually have been exposed to high-dose radiation of the thyroid at a young age.

Patient Teaching

Give the patient preoperative instructions, and encourage the patient to ask questions about the risks the surgeon identifies. Tell the patient what to expect after surgery, including symptoms of low calcium or a temporary loss of voice. Explain postoperative instructions, including hormone therapy, chemotherapy, and/or radiotherapy, as prescribed by the physician. Refer the patient to the attending physician for questions about the prognosis after treatment.

Emphasize the need for follow-up appointments, and review the schedule for these appointments.

Parathyroid Gland Diseases

The parathyroid glands are found on the back of the thyroid gland (Fig. 4.11). They secrete parathyroid hormone (PTH), the main hormone the body uses to maintain calcium homeostasis. A feedback loop regulates blood calcium levels to maintain a normal level. Disorders of parathyroid secretion result in serious disturbances throughout the body.

Hyperparathyroidism

Description

Hyperparathyroidism is a condition caused by the overactivity of one or more of the four parathyroid glands, which results in the overproduction of PTH.

ICD-10-CM Code	E21.3 *(Hyperparathyroidism, unspecified)*
	(E21.0–E21.5 = 6 codes of specificity)

Symptoms and Signs

Hyperparathyroidism increases the breakdown of bone from the skeletal system (demineralization), which results in excessive calcium in the blood (hypercalcemia). Hypercalcemia produces the symptoms of hyperparathyroidism. Hypercalcemia reduces the irritability of nerve and muscle tissues, and this causes the patient to experience muscle weakness and atrophy, gastrointestinal pain, and nausea. High serum calcium levels can produce conduction defects in the heart. An increased calcium deposit in soft tissue causes low back pain and renal calculi. Bone tenderness, arthritis-type of pain, and easy fracturing of the bones are the results of demineralization of the bone (Fig. 4.12).

Patient Screening

Some patients may have vague symptoms, such as fatigue, weakness, or mental disturbance. Schedule a complete physical examination. The patient experiencing symptoms of hypercalcemia is very ill and requires prompt medical intervention.

Etiology

The cause of primary hyperparathyroidism is increased activity of the parathyroid gland, usually as a result of an excessive growth of one of the parathyroid glands (adenoma) or an idiopathic hyperplasia of the gland. Females are more likely than males to have hyperparathyroidism. Secondary hyperparathyroidism may be caused by an increased secretion of PTH induced by a low level of serum calcium or serum vitamin D as a result of renal disease or other disorders.

Diagnosis

The serum's intact PTH level is elevated with an increased calcium and reduced phosphorus levels in serum. The alkaline

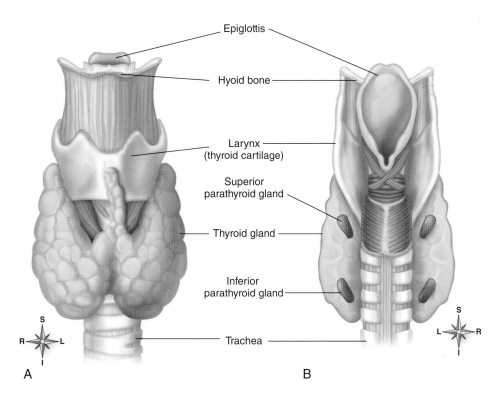

• **Fig. 4.11** Thyroid and parathyroid glands. Note their relationship to each other and to the larynx (voice box) and trachea. (A) Anterior view and (B) posterior view. (From Patton K, Bell F, Thompson T, Williamson P: *The human body in health & disease*, ed 8, 2024.)

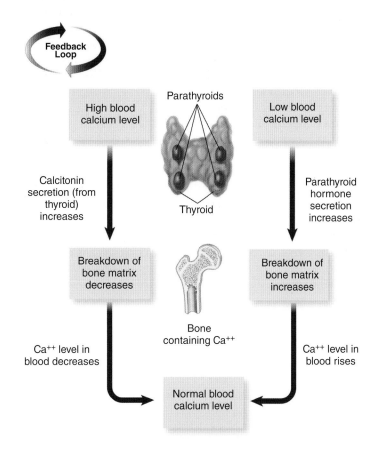

• **Fig. 4.12** Regulation of blood calcium levels. Calcitonin and parathyroid hormones have antagonistic (opposite) effects on calcium concentration in blood. (From Patton KT, Thibodeau GA: *Anthony's textbook of anatomy & physiology*, ed 20, St. Louis, 2013, Mosby.)

phosphatase levels tend to be increased, and urine calcium is high. Low bone mineral density, especially at sites richer in cortical bone (i.e., femoral neck and forearm), is noted through the appearance of bone on radiographic films.

Bone demineralization leads to osteoporosis, which can be detected by dual-energy x-ray absorptiometry (a bone density test).

Treatment
The treatment plan for hyperparathyroidism varies with the cause and is highly individualized. If the hypersecretion of PTH is caused by an adenoma, the tumor can be removed by minimally invasive parathyroid surgery. If hyperplasia is the cause of the hypersecretion, usually three and a half of the four glands are removed. When the condition is secondary, the underlying cause must be treated, and blood serum calcium levels must be reduced. Drugs that increase the excretion of calcium by the kidneys or inhibit the reabsorption of calcium from bone may be used.

Prognosis
After successful surgery, calcium replacement prevents hypocalcemia and allows skeletal remineralization in patients with bone disease.

Prevention
No prevention is known.

Patient Teaching
Use visual aids to explain the location and function of the parathyroid glands. Explain hyperparathyroid disease and the treatment plan. Fractures can occur easily, and the patient is advised to take care to avoid trauma. Give preoperative and postoperative instructions as indicated. Explain the dosage schedule for prescription medication and the adverse side effects to report. Caution against using over-the-counter medications containing excessive calcium. Refer the patient to a dietitian, as required.

Hypoparathyroidism

Description
Hypoparathyroidism is a condition in which the secretion of PTH by the parathyroid glands is greatly reduced.

ICD-10-CM Code	E20.9 *(Hypoparathyroidism, unspecified)* (E20.0–E20.9 = 4 codes of specificity)

Symptoms and Signs
PTH increases the blood calcium level by stimulating bone demineralization and increasing the absorption of calcium in the digestive tract and the kidneys. When the level of this hormone is insufficient, circulating levels of calcium are reduced, resulting in hypocalcemia, with the occasional possibility of excessive deposits of calcium into tissue. A consequence of hypocalcemia is a hyperexcitable nervous system, resulting in

• **Fig. 4.13** Signs of hypocalcemia. (A) Chvostek sign (facial twitch). (B) Trousseau sign (carpopedal spasm). (From Ignatavicius DD, Workman ML: *Medical-surgical nursing: patient-centered collaborative care*, ed 8, St. Louis, 2016, Saunders.)

an overstimulation of the skeletal muscles (Fig. 4.13). Initial symptoms include numbness and tingling of fingertips, toes, ears, or nose, followed by muscular spasms or twitching of the hands and feet. Tetany, or severe, sustained muscular contractions, may develop. The patient may experience emotional changes, confusion, and irritability. Sustained hypocalcemia leads to laryngospasm, arrhythmias, respiratory paralysis, and death.

Patient Screening
Acute, symptomatic hypocalcemia requires emergency treatment.

Etiology
The most common cause of hypoparathyroidism is the surgical destruction of the parathyroid glands. Accidental surgical removal of the parathyroid gland during a thyroidectomy can induce hypocalcemia. Acquired hypoparathyroidism can result from injury to one or more of the

parathyroid glands, ischemia from an infarct, accidental radiation, neoplasia, or various disease processes. The condition may result from an autoimmune genetic disorder or from a congenital absence of the parathyroid glands.

Diagnosis

The clinical picture of neuromuscular hyperexcitability, along with a history of possible insults to the parathyroid glands, leads the physician to further investigation. The presence of the Trousseau phenomenon is a sure indication of hypocalcemia. Blood studies indicate reduced serum calcium levels and increased serum phosphate levels. Electrocardiography shows increased QT and ST intervals. PTH levels are reduced.

Treatment

Calcium replacement therapy with vitamin D reduces hypocalcemia. This replacement therapy usually is given for life unless the condition is reversible. In the case of a life-threatening deficiency (tetany), calcium gluconate is administered intravenously. The patient is encouraged to follow a high-calcium diet.

Prognosis

Reversible forms of the condition respond to appropriate treatment. Some cases are transient.

Prevention

No prevention is known.

Patient Teaching

Answer questions about the location and function of the parathyroid gland. Explain hypocalcemia and the way it affects the nervous system. Refer the patient to a dietitian, as indicated. Emphasize the importance of follow-up care to monitor renal function and serum calcium levels.

Adrenal Gland Diseases

Cushing Syndrome

Description

Cushing syndrome is a condition of chronic hypersecretion of the adrenal cortex, which results in excessive circulating cortisol levels.

ICD-10-CM Code	E24.0 (Pituitary-dependent Cushing disease)
	E24.2 (Drug-induced Cushing syndrome)
	E24.3 (Ectopic ACTH syndrome)
	E24.8 (Other Cushing syndrome)
	E24.9 (Cushing syndrome, unspecified)

Symptoms and Signs

The patient with Cushing syndrome experiences fatigue, muscular weakness, weight gain, and changes in body appearance.

• **Fig. 4.14** Clinical manifestations in a patient with Cushing syndrome. (From Forbes CH, Jackson WF: *Color atlas and text of clinical medicine*, ed 3, St. Louis, 2003, Elsevier Science Limited/Mosby.)

Fat deposits form in the scapular area (buffalo humps) and the trunk, causing a protruding abdomen (Fig. 4.14). Salt and water retention result not only in hypertension and edema but also in the characteristic moon face noted in patients with Cushing syndrome. The patient may show clinical evidence of hyperlipidemia, hyperglycemia, osteoporosis, and atherosclerosis. Changes in mood and cognition and decreased short-term memory are common. The skin becomes thin, tends to bruise easily, and develops red or purple striae (stretch marks). The individual is predisposed to infection as a result of suppression of the immune response. Other symptoms include excessive hair growth, amenorrhea, and impotence.

Patient Screening

Early manifestations include weight gain, hypertension, and emotional instability. These symptoms warrant a medical evaluation. Follow office policy for referral to an endocrinologist.

Etiology

Excessive levels of circulating cortisol can be caused by hyperplasia of the adrenal gland, excessive secretion of corticotropin (ACTH) from the pituitary gland, a tumor of the adrenal cortex, or production of corticotropin in another organ (e.g., cancer cells in the lungs). Iatrogenic factors, such as prolonged administration or large doses of glucocorticoids used to treat other diseases, can induce Cushing syndrome.

Diagnosis

The typical picture of the moon face, buffalo hump, and gross obesity of the trunk, particularly the abdomen, leads the physician to further investigation. A continuous elevation of serum cortisol levels is found in Cushing syndrome.

Free cortisol levels are elevated in a 24-hour urine collection. CT or MRI may detect adrenal tumors. Saliva testing and inferior petrosal sinus sampling may be performed.

Treatment

Treatment of Cushing syndrome depends on the cause of the oversecretion of cortisol. When a tumor is the cause, surgical removal or radiation of the tumor in the pituitary gland or adrenal gland is indicated. Drug therapy to suppress ACTH secretion can be used separately or as an adjunct to radiation.

Prognosis

The prognosis depends on the underlying cause. Without treatment, or when the condition is caused by ectopic carcinoma, the prognosis is poor.

Prevention

Generally, there is no prevention; however, the patient on large doses of glucocorticoids is monitored closely.

Patient Teaching

Appropriate computer-based health education about Cushing syndrome can be helpful, when available, for patient teaching. If surgery is indicated, give the patient information about the procedures and what to expect after surgery. If medication and hormone replacement therapy are planned, give careful instructions; the medication must be taken exactly as directed and never discontinued abruptly. Refer the patient to a dietitian, as indicated. Teach the patient about recognizing symptoms of adrenal hypofunction: apathy, fatigue, weakness, and syncope.

Addison Disease

Description

Addison disease is a partial or complete failure of adrenocortical function.

ICD-10-CM Code	E27.1 *(Primary adrenocortical insufficiency)*
	E27.2 *(Addisonian crisis)*
	E27.40 *(Unspecified adrenocortical insufficiency)*
	(E27.0–E27.9 = 8 codes of specificity)

Symptoms and Signs

Addison disease, primary adrenal insufficiency or hypoadrenalism, gradually manifests as symptoms of fatigue, weakness, anorexia, agitation, confusion, weight loss, and gastrointestinal disturbances. The patient can experience cardiovascular difficulties, including irregular pulse, reduced cardiac output, and orthostatic (postural) hypotension. Depression, anxiety, and emotional distress are often experienced. Reduced levels of aldosterone cause an inability to retain salt and water. When dehydration, **hyperkalemia** (high blood potassium level), and electrolyte imbalance

occur, the condition is life threatening. The patient needs to seek treatment immediately.

Patient Screening

The onset is usually gradual over weeks or months. However, in acute cases when complications, such as fever, profound weakness, or confused behavior, prompt the call for medical attention, life-threatening conditions may follow, requiring emergency care.

Etiology

The onset of Addison disease is usually gradual, with progressive destruction of the adrenal gland and reduction in its important hormones. The destruction can result from an autoimmune process, tuberculosis, hemorrhage, fungal infections, neoplasms, or surgical resection of the gland. An autoimmune response is the most common cause. There are familial tendencies. The disease also can be secondary to hypopituitarism, in which there is reduced output of corticotropin.

Diagnosis

Blood tests include cortisol, potassium, sodium, and ACTH. The ACTH stimulation test involves the administration of artificial ACTH to see how the patient's adrenal glands respond to the injection. If the cortisol level is low after the injection, there can be a problem. Another test is an insulin-induced hypoglycemia test. The patient receives an injection of insulin. The blood glucose level should decrease, and the cortisol level should increase. This test provides information regarding whether the issue results from the pituitary gland or the adrenal gland. CT scan also provides information regarding damage to the adrenal or pituitary glands.

Treatment

Treatment includes the replacement of the natural hormones. Aldosterone is replaced with the drug fludrocortisone, and cortisol may be replaced by the drugs hydrocortisone, prednisone, or methylprednisolone. Hormone replacement therapy with close medical supervision must continue for life. The patient must be educated about the symptoms of overdosing and underdosing and the role of stress and infection in Addison disease. Insufficiency or a sudden decrease in adrenocortical hormone levels, such as from the sudden withdrawal of replacement therapy, can result in a life-threatening emergency called an *addisonian crisis*.

Prognosis

Early diagnosis and strict adherence to the treatment regimen can result in a good prognosis, and the patient's resistance to infection and general well-being can be maintained. Some individuals diagnosed with Addison disease will develop other autoimmune diseases.

Prevention

There is no known prevention. After diagnosis, the individual will need lifelong hormone replacement therapy, which needs to be monitored closely.

Patient Teaching

Instructions regarding the medication regimen are important. Patients will be advised not to discontinue medications abruptly. Emphasize the importance of getting follow-up care from the health care provider and medical alert jewelry.

Endocrine Dysfunction of Pancreas

Diabetes Mellitus

Description

Diabetes mellitus is a chronic disorder of carbohydrate, fat, and protein metabolism caused by inadequate production of insulin by the pancreas or faulty use of insulin by the cells.

ICD-10-CM Code	E11.9 *(Type 2 diabetes mellitus without complications)* (E08.0–E13.9 = 205 codes of specificity)

Diabetes mellitus is coded in the fourth digit according to clinical manifestations and with a fifth-digit modifier for non-insulin-dependent or insulin-dependent state. Refer to the physician's diagnosis and then to the current edition of the ICD-10-CM coding manual to ensure the greatest specificity of pathology.

Symptoms and Signs

A reduction in insulin results in **hyperglycemia** and deprives cells of fuel. Cells begin to metabolize fats and proteins; this process allows wastes called *ketone bodies* to accumulate in the blood (ketosis). Ketonuria develops as excess ketone bodies are excreted in urine. This leads to **acidosis**. Hyperglycemia is at the root of the principal symptoms: polyuria, **polyphagia**, polydipsia, weight loss, and fatigue. The patient may have **pruritus**, especially in the genital area, and a fruity odor to the breath may be noted when ketosis occurs in type 1 diabetes. Diagnostic tests of blood and urine point to the common signs of diabetes mellitus. Some patients with diabetes are referred to as "brittle diabetics."

There are two primary forms of diabetes mellitus:

1. Type 1 (formerly known as *juvenile-onset diabetes* or *insulin-dependent diabetes mellitus*) has an early, abrupt onset and occurs during childhood or teenage years, but it can occur at any age with little or no insulin being secreted by the patient and can be difficult to control.
2. Type 2 (formerly known as *adult-onset diabetes* or *non-insulin-dependent diabetes mellitus*), the most common form, has a gradual onset in adults older than 40 years of age; however, it is becoming more common in children and younger adults. In this form, some pancreatic function remains, permitting control of symptoms by dietary management; in addition, an oral hypoglycemic medication is often prescribed.

• **Fig. 4.15** Diabetic ulcer, dorsal aspect of the foot. (From Hill MJ: *Skin disorders—Mosby's clinical nursing series*, St. Louis, 1994, Mosby.)

Untreated or poorly managed diabetes has many systemic complications: retinopathy, which leads to blindness; neuropathy; renal failure; atherosclerosis, leading to myocardial infarction; and cerebrovascular accidents. Hyperglycemia delays healing and impairs resistance to infection. Patients with diabetes require careful attention to foot care to prevent damage from circulatory disorders and infections Fig. 4.15. Improved glycemic control and adequate blood pressure and lipids control prevent diabetic complications such as diabetic pressure sores and ulcers.

Patient Screening

Individuals known to be at high risk require screening for the signs of diabetes as part of regular medical checkups. Known patients with diabetes having warning signs of diabetic coma or insulin reaction need instructions for immediate medical intervention (Table 4.3). Anyone complaining of weight loss, excessive thirst, excessive hunger, and frequent urination needs a prompt appointment for diagnostic evaluation. In addition, patients diagnosed with diabetes should remove both shoes and socks at each appointment for foot assessment since the patient with neuropathy does not feel a change when they start developing a pressure sore or ulcer. This can result in gangrene and loss of limbs.

Etiology

The disease is often familial but may be acquired. Metabolic abnormalities can induce the diabetic disease process, causing insulin resistance, abnormal insulin secretion by the pancreas, or inappropriate glucose production by the liver. Both forms of diabetes are linked genetically. In type 1 diabetes, an infection early in life may trigger an autoimmune process that produces antibodies that destroy the β-cells of the pancreas. Type 2 tends to occur in older, overweight adults. Destruction of the pancreas by tumor, trauma to the pituitary gland, or other endocrine disorders can induce diabetes mellitus. Some drugs also may suppress insulin

TABLE 4.3	Warning Signs and Interventions for Diabetic Coma and Insulin Reaction	
Diabetic Coma	**Insulin Reaction**	
Causes		
Undiagnosed diabetes	Excessive insulin	
Skipped insulin dose	Delayed meal	
Excessive food	Insufficient food	
Infection or stress	Excessive exercise	
Symptoms and Signs		
Slow onset	Rapid onset	
Thirst	Hunger	
Increased urination	Trembling and paleness	
Nausea and vomiting	Feeling of faintness	
Abdominal pain	Cold sweat	
Drowsiness	Headache	
Lethargy	Anxiety	
Flushed appearance	Rapid heartbeat	
Dry skin	Irritability	
Fruity breath odor	Impaired vision	
Dehydration	Hypoglycemia	
Heavy respirations	Confusion	
Dilated, fixed pupils	Seizures	
Hyperglycemia	Loss of consciousness	
Ketoacidosis		
Loss of consciousness		
Coma		
Intervention		
Give insulin, fluids, and salt	If awake, give simple sugar, candy, orange juice, or soda	
If severe, give intravenous fluids, insulin, and sodium bicarbonate	If unconscious, give intravenous dextrose or glucagon	

production. Some genetic disorders render the body's insulin receptors insensitive to insulin.

Diagnosis

The diagnosis of diabetes mellitus is straightforward and the patient is carefully assessed for cardinal symptoms. At least two positive tests of fasting blood plasma glucose and the presence of glucose and acetone in the urine confirm the diagnosis. Other tests include blood insulin level determination and an ophthalmic examination for diabetic retinopathy. Glycated hemoglobin testing is also used to determine the range of the patient's glucose level over the preceding 2 to 3 months before the test is collected.

Treatment

Management of diabetes is multifactorial, including a well-balanced diet closely integrated with insulin administration or oral medication, exercise, blood and urine testing, and hygienic measures. Patient compliance and education are vital to the control of symptoms and complications.

Patients with type 1 diabetes require insulin replacement therapy that correlates closely with calculated carbohydrate intake on a regular schedule. Methods of insulin delivery include injection, insulin pump therapy (see the Enrichment box about Insulin Pump Therapy), and insulin pens. Insulin preparations can be short-acting, intermediate-acting, long-acting, or premixed insulins. Researchers are investigating other insulin delivery methods. Patients with type 2 diabetes usually do not necessarily require insulin injections to control blood glucose levels. Their therapeutic regimen includes restricted caloric intake and exercise, along with oral hypoglycemic medications.

Various forms of oral drug therapy currently are used to treat type 2 diabetes. Sulfonylureas such as glipizide (Glucotrol) and glyburide (DiaBeta or Micronase) and meglitinide drugs such as nateglinide (Starlix) are oral hypoglycemic drugs that stimulate the pancreas to produce insulin. These medications are usually taken once or twice a day, and blood glucose levels must be monitored on a strict schedule. Because sulfonylureas stimulate the pancreas to increase insulin production, the increased insulin levels tend to lower blood glucose levels, often resulting in symptoms and complications of hypoglycemia.

Metformin (Glucophage) works in several ways. It primarily prevents the liver from producing hepatic glucose but also helps enhance the benefits of the available insulin. Under normal circumstances, metformin hydrochloride does not elevate blood insulin levels and, therefore, does not produce hypoglycemia. See the Alert box for special information and warnings about antidiabetic agents.

Acarbose, an α-glucosidase inhibitor, works in the gastrointestinal tract to delay the digestion of carbohydrates and lengthen the time needed to convert carbohydrates to glucose. It mainly affects blood sugar levels after eating. An annoying side effect is the formation of intestinal gas and resulting flatus.

Rosiglitazone (Avandia) and Pioglitazone (Actos) belong to the thiazolidinedione class of drugs. They work as insulin sensitizers by binding to the peroxisome proliferator–activated receptors (PPARs) of cells, making them more responsive to insulin.

Pramlintide (Symlin) is an injectable drug that resembles human amylin produced by the pancreas. It has four mechanisms of action. Symlin inhibits glucagon production

Insulin Pump Therapy

More recent technology offers an alternative to multiple insulin injection regimens for patients with type 1 diabetes as well as some patients with type 2 diabetes on insulin. The insulin pump is a small computerized device that delivers small doses of insulin at regular intervals 24 hours a day. The pump is programmed to deliver fast-acting insulin at a rate calculated for that individual. Some devices function to monitor the blood sugar level as well. It is necessary to test the blood sugar level throughout the day and then enter the data into the pump. Then adjustments can be made to accommodate food intake and balance the delivery of insulin to maintain proper blood sugar.

An insulin pump unit is about the size of a deck of cards or smaller. These devices are clipped to a belt or directly applied to the skin. Insulin is delivered from small cartridges within the pump, either directly through the skin via a microscopic cannula or through a plastic cannula inserted and secured into the tissue just under the skin. The pump is monitored by the patient or, in the case of a child or a very sick patient, by a trained caregiver. This trained observer can monitor the functioning of the unit and can help distinguish between symptoms of hyperglycemia or hypoglycemia. An insulin pump requires a prescription from a physician.

There are lifestyle benefits and more freedom for many patients with diabetes who can manage their own care in this way with fewer side effects. Management of diabetes in children and teenagers who respond well to training in the use of an insulin pump can achieve tighter blood sugar control and reduce the risk for long-term complications in patients with diabetes.

⚠ ALERT!

Antidiabetic Agents: Information and Warnings

Metformin (Glucophage), an antidiabetic agent used for type 2 diabetes, should not be taken by patients with a history of kidney disease, congestive heart failure, liver disease, or alcohol use disorder. Patients should be instructed to stop taking metformin before undergoing any imaging procedures with injectable contrast agents. Patients needing a procedure to place stents will have to wait 3 days until it is safe for an iodine dye to be in the blood.

A rare but serious side effect of metformin is lactic acidosis. It is a rare side effect and is seen in patients with renal failure, liver failure, and congestive heart failure.

The symptoms and signs of lactic acidosis are weakness, fatigue, unusual muscle pain, dyspnea, unusual stomach discomfort, dizziness or lightheadedness, and bradycardia or cardiac arrhythmias. With any of these symptoms, the patient should stop metformin immediately and contact the physician.

Rosiglitazone maleate (Avandia) was transiently removed from the US market because of heart disease risks but has been reinstituted. Pioglitazone (Actos) is in the same therapeutic drug class as Avandia. Both medications require an FDA Black Box warning regarding the potential for increased risk of congestive heart failure. Patients should talk to their health care professionals if they have concerns regarding these medications.

(therefore reduces hepatic glucose production), delays gastric emptying, increases pancreatic insulin production, and reduces appetite.

The mechanism of action of incretin hormones is similar to that of pramlintide (Symlin). It increases the production of insulin right after eating, inhibits postprandial hepatic glucose production, delays gastric emptying, and induces satiety. Exenatide (Byetta, Bydureon) and liraglutide (Victoza) are injectable medicines in the class of drugs called *incretin mimetics*.

Incretin hormones regulate glucose levels through the mechanism of action mentioned above. They are broken down within minutes in the bloodstream by enzymes called *DPP IV*. A new class of oral drugs called *DPP IV inhibitors* inhibit this enzyme and therefore regulate blood glucose. Sitagliptin (Januvia), saxagliptin (Onglyza), linagliptin (Tradjenta), and alogliptin (Nesina) are the approved medications in this class of drugs.

Bromocriptine (Cycloset) works by increasing dopamine receptor activity in the morning, and this lowers blood sugar without increasing insulin levels. The drug is taken once each morning when dopamine levels are low.

Sodium-glucose–linked transporter 2 inhibitors prevent the function of sodium-dependent glucose transport proteins in the kidney to reabsorb filtered glucose. This leads to a reduction in blood glucose levels and a concomitant loss of calories and, therefore, weight. Canagliflozin (Invokana) and dapagliflozin (Farxiga) are the first approved drugs in this class.

Early implementation and use of combination medications seem to be the most effective way to treat patients with diabetes. The goal is to normalize glucose control by optimizing hemoglobin A1c (HbgA1c) while avoiding hypoglycemia.

Prognosis

People with diabetes mellitus are now living longer than in the past. When people with diabetes mellitus practice appropriate self-care, the symptoms are eased, blood glucose levels are controlled, and there are fewer complications and fewer hospitalizations. Without treatment and when blood sugar levels remain high over a long period, the eyes, blood vessels, kidneys, and nerves sustain serious damage.

Prevention

The precise causal mechanism of diabetes mellitus remains unknown; however, screening for diabetes mellitus is recommended for those with risk factors, such as genetic susceptibility, obesity, a history of gestational diabetes, and age 45 years or greater. Prediabetes has been identified as a risk factor for the progression of type 2 diabetes. Education about lifestyle changes known to delay the onset of diabetes is an appropriate prevention strategy when the blood glucose level is higher than normal (see the Alert box about prediabetes).

Patient Teaching

Diabetes control is monitored daily mainly by measuring blood glucose levels through the use of a device for that purpose, a glucose meter.

A continual glucose monitoring system may be a supplement to traditional glucose monitoring. The system consists of a sensor inserted via needle and a transmitter device. Each sensor is single use and is designed to remain in place for 14 consecutive days; however, the length of time the sensor can stay in place may vary from one manufacturer to another.

Sensors can be read from a cell phone app or the manufacturer's monitor. The sensor records can also be downloaded and reviewed at the physician's office for a detailed log of results. Insurance approval for payment is usually obtained prior to ordering sensors. There are criteria that must be met in order for insurance approval. A sensor may need to be removed during patient diagnostic imaging tests and in those cases, the patient will monitor their glucose levels using the fingerprick method until another sensor can be ordered, if the sensors cannot be worn for the intended length of time due to early removal.

All patients with diabetes are encouraged to reach and maintain the appropriate body weight. In addition, patients must be taught that the balance between insulin and glucose requirements is upset easily by trauma and infection. Regular medical supervision is encouraged, especially for insulin-dependent patients. Patients and caregivers are taught the proper techniques of insulin administration; special training in the use of an insulin pump is offered when appropriate. Premeasured insulin pens are also available, and patients should be taught how to accurately use these for insulin administration. The patient and caregivers must be educated to recognize the

symptoms of diabetic coma (high blood glucose with the release of ketone levels) and insulin shock (excessive insulin) and to take immediate action to correct these serious complications (see Table 4.3).

The patient must understand the importance of preventing infection and injury. Give the patient written material that explains the importance of skin care, foot care, and dental care. Instruct the patient to carry some form of fast-acting sugar, such as glucose tablets, to combat the onset of hypoglycemia. Advise the patient to obtain a medical alert jewelry (see Fig. 4.7).

Gestational Diabetes

Description

Gestational diabetes mellitus (GDM) is a condition of damaged ability to process carbohydrates that has its onset during pregnancy.

ICD-10-CM Code	O99.810 *(Abnormal glucose complicating pregnancy)* (O99.810–O99.815 = 3 codes of specificity)

Symptoms and Signs

GDM is detected between 24 and 28 weeks of pregnancy. The pregnant patient may be asymptomatic or may exhibit the usual signs of diabetes mellitus: polyuria, polydipsia, and polyphagia. Routine blood or urine screening indicates the presence of excessive glucose.

Patient Screening

The patient exhibiting the onset of the above symptoms is scheduled for a same-day appointment. With a prior diagnosis of GDM, prompt medical attention is necessary for any increase in symptoms or onset of new complaints. Strict adherence to scheduled follow-up appointments is important for careful monitoring.

Etiology

Increased destruction of insulin by the placenta plays a role in causing GDM. There is a reduced effectiveness of maternal insulin during pregnancy. The fetus takes its glucose from the mother, stressing the balance of glucose production and glucose use. Elevated levels of estrogen and progesterone block the action of insulin. Risk factors include a family history of diabetes, obesity, and age above 25 years.

Diagnosis

The first indication of GDM is the presence of glucose in urine, as demonstrated by a routine prenatal urine glucose test. Fasting blood glucose determination indicates elevated levels of glucose. Other serum tests are the glucose tolerance test, 2-hour postprandial (oral glucose tolerance) test, and glycated hemoglobin test. Elevations above normal levels yield a positive diagnosis.

❗ *ALERT!*

Prediabetes

Prediabetes is defined as a blood glucose level that is moderately elevated but not high enough to meet the diagnostic values indicating diabetes. When this condition is identified, it is considered a risk factor for the later development of type 2 diabetes. Prediabetes is considered a significant health problem itself. Many health risks are associated with prediabetes, such as hypertension, abnormal cholesterol, obesity, and increased risk for cardiovascular disease. It is important to help those showing signs of prediabetes understand their risk of progressing to type 2. There are known steps that can be taken to reduce or prevent this progression.

Lifestyle interventions such as weight management, nutritional interventions, and exercise can be challenging but effective first steps in the prevention of diabetes. These lifestyle changes must be maintained by the patient taking responsibility for their self-care decisions; however, positive social support from an individual or a group increases the success of compliance and health. The Centers for Disease Control and Prevention authorized the establishment of a National Diabetes Prevention Program.

Treatment

Treatment is started as soon as possible to preserve a healthy pregnancy. The medical management of GDM is similar to the treatment of any type of diabetes, with close surveillance of the mother and fetus because of the increased risk of complications, control of the diet, and limits on the intake of simple sugars. Consistent moderate exercise, such as walking, is encouraged. Oral hypoglycemic agents may be prescribed, or insulin may be indicated. The patient is instructed to monitor blood glucose levels frequently.

Prognosis

The risk of cesarean delivery and neonatal complications, including large body size and hypoglycemia, is increased. The condition usually disappears right after delivery; however, half develop diabetes later in life.

Prevention

GDM is a common enough complication of pregnancy to warrant regular monitoring of glucose levels in urine and blood during the pregnancy.

Patient Teaching

Emphasize the importance of regular prenatal checkups to monitor weight, proper nutrition, and blood glucose levels. Teach self-monitoring of blood glucose and insulin administration, as required. Dietary management depends on the severity of the disease and the amount of insulin therapy required. Go over the prescribed diet, or assist with referral to a dietitian if indicated.

Hypoglycemia

Description

Hypoglycemia is an abnormally low glucose level in the blood.

ICD-10-CM Code	E16.2 *(Hypoglycemia, unspecified)* (E16.0–E16.2 = 3 codes of specificity)

Symptoms and Signs

Hypoglycemia, a deficiency of glucose (sugar) in the blood, can be a serious condition. It occurs when excessive insulin enters the bloodstream or when the glucose release rate falls below tissue demands. This condition may occur despite adequate food intake. Symptoms include sweating, nervousness, weakness, hunger, dizziness, trembling, headache, and palpitations. Because glucose is the primary fuel of the brain, the consequences of hypoglycemia can be severe. Extremely low blood glucose levels can cause central nervous system manifestations, including confusion, visual disturbances, behavior that may be mistaken for drunkenness, stupor, coma, and seizures. Hypoglycemic syndromes are classified as drug induced (the most common) or non–drug induced.

Patient Screening

An individual with severe symptoms of acute reactive hypoglycemia requires emergency medical attention. For the individual experiencing milder episodes of hypoglycemia, an appointment should be scheduled as early as possible for a diagnostic evaluation of the cause. Follow office policy for referral of an infant or child to a pediatrician.

Etiology

The major cause of drug-induced hypoglycemia is insulin overdose. Failure to eat a meal or excessive exercise also can trigger hypoglycemia in an insulin-dependent patient with diabetes. A person with a significantly elevated blood alcohol level can experience alcoholic hypoglycemia. Sulfonylureas can induce hypoglycemia. Nondrug–induced hypoglycemia can result from fasting, delayed or excessive secretion of insulin by the pancreas, adenoma or carcinoma of the pancreas, gastrointestinal disorders, or various hereditary or endocrine disorders.

Diagnosis

Diagnosis requires evidence that the symptoms correlate with a low blood glucose level and can be remedied by raising the blood glucose level. The glucometer can be used as a quick screening test to detect abnormally low blood glucose levels in patients with symptoms of hypoglycemia. The blood glucose level is further evaluated through the glucose tolerance test. Fasting blood plasma glucose levels below 70 mg/dL indicate hypoglycemia, and further testing is indicated for a final diagnosis. Hypoglycemia is uncomplicated when the initial assessment suggests a probable cause, such as a history of insulin use, excessive ingestion of alcohol, or the use of sulfonylureas in treatment.

Treatment

In acute hypoglycemia, the priority is to restore the normal blood glucose level through intravenous infusion of glucose. The hormone glucagon may also be given to counteract the effects of insulin. As the patient's condition is stabilized, a complex carbohydrate and protein snack is given to keep the blood glucose level within normal limits. When hypoglycemia is associated with a tumor, surgery may be required. The diet is modified to correct hereditary fructose intolerance or gastrointestinal conditions that provoke the symptoms.

Prognosis

The underlying cause of hypoglycemia dictates the long-term management of the disorder. In most cases, the signs and symptoms of hypoglycemia resolve with the ingestion of food or glucose. Severe, prolonged hypoglycemia can cause irreversible brain damage.

Prevention

Proper adjustment of diet, insulin, and exercise in the individual with diabetes. Insulin-dependent patients benefit from a conscientious application of self-management skills.

Metabolic Syndrome

Metabolic syndrome (previously known as *syndrome X*) is a collection of signs and/or conditions that together may increase an individual's risk for type 2 diabetes and cardiovascular disease. Early recognition of this syndrome can help determine suitable interventions to correct the individual mechanisms of metabolic syndrome.

Metabolic syndrome has five main components:
1. Central obesity is defined as a collection of excess fat around the abdomen (a waist circumference of greater than 35 inches for females and greater than 40 inches for males.)
2. Increased blood pressure, that is, greater than 130/80 mm Hg.
3. Abnormal triglyceride levels above 150 mg/dL.
4. Abnormal high-density lipoprotein cholesterol levels below 40 mg/dL.
5. Fasting glucose levels above 100 mg/dL.

These components, especially obesity, have metabolic consequences. Although the exact cause is not known, poor nutrition and inadequate physical exercise contribute to the risk factors of metabolic syndrome. Recognition of metabolic syndrome offers a patient the opportunity to focus on interventions that may prevent the premature onset of cardiovascular disease and/or type 2 diabetes.

Patient Teaching

Teach the patient to watch for signs of hypoglycemia. Instruct the insulin-dependent patient with diabetes to be prepared to counter an attack of hypoglycemia by carrying glucose tablets to take at the first sign of hypoglycemia. Address the effects of alcohol intoxication and adverse reactions to medications. Assist with referral to a dietitian as indicated.

Precocious Puberty

Precocious Puberty in Boys

Description

Precocious puberty in boys is defined as the onset of puberty before age 9 years.

ICD-10-CM Code	E30.1 *(Precocious puberty)*
	E30.8 *(Other disorders of puberty)*
	(E30.0–E30.9 = 4 codes of specificity)

Symptoms and Signs

Precocious, or earlier-than-expected, sexual maturity in the male manifests as early development of secondary sex characteristics, gonadal development, and spermatogenesis. The patient's history may include altered growth patterns or emotional disturbances. Pubic hair and facial hair begin to grow, the gonads and the penis increase in size, and sebaceous gland activity increases. Male puberty normally begins between ages 13 and 15 years; onset before 9 years of age is considered precocious.

Patient Screening

Schedule a physical examination with the health care provider. Then follow office policy regarding referral to an endocrinologist.

Etiology

Idiopathic precocity may be transmitted genetically. The hypothalamus normally initiates puberty by stimulating the pituitary gland. Because the pituitary gland secretes vital gonadotropic hormones that stimulate the testes to produce sex hormones, many problems involving sexual development can be traced to pituitary dysfunction. Intracranial pituitary or hypothalamic neoplasia can cause excessive or premature secretion of gonadotropin. Testicular tumors and other endocrine disorders can induce precocious development. The history may reveal inadvertent ingestion of sex steroids through therapeutic medications or deliberate ingestion of sex steroids.

Diagnosis

Obvious physical and emotional signs of precocity are noted. Diagnostic tests include MRI, blood tests for elevated hormone levels, brain scans, skull and bone radiographic studies, chromosomal karyotype studies, and testing of blood for male hormone levels.

Treatment

The therapy depends on the cause of precocious puberty. When the condition is idiopathic, no specific treatment may be needed. One treatment is to take hormones to suppress sexual maturation until the appropriate time for the onset of puberty. Gonadotropin-releasing hormone agonists, medications that inhibit androgen action (spironolactone), inhibit androgen synthesis (ketoconazole), or block the conversion of androgens, have been used. When the cause is a testicular tumor or brain tumor, the treatment is more invasive, and the prognosis is guarded. Other endocrine disorders may require lifelong hormone therapy.

Prognosis

Early diagnosis and treatment of true precocious puberty offers a positive outcome. More complicated cases have a guarded prognosis.

Prevention

In almost all cases, no prevention is known.

Patient Teaching

Emphasize the importance of following the exact medication regimen and keeping follow-up appointments. Refer the patient to genetic counseling and psychological support, as indicated by the treatment plan.

Precocious Puberty In Girls

Description

Precocious puberty in girls is defined as the onset of puberty before age 8 years.

ICD-10-CM Code	E30.1 *(Precocious puberty)*
	E30.8 *(Other disorders of*
	puberty)

Symptoms and Signs

Precocious, or earlier-than-expected, sexual maturity in the female is marked by increased growth rate, breast enlargement, and the appearance of pubic hair and underarm hair before age 8 years; the onset of menstruation (menarche) may occur before age 10 years. The ovarian function makes pregnancy a possibility. Emotional problems may occur.

Patient Screening

Schedule a physical examination with the health care provider. Then follow office policy regarding referral to an endocrinologist.

Etiology

In most cases, precocious puberty in girls is idiopathic, without associated abnormalities. Uncommon causes include intracranial tumors, encephalopathy, meningitis, and endocrine disorders. The ingestion of oral contraceptives and other estrogen-containing drugs is a rare cause. Hormone-secreting ovarian or adrenal neoplasms are infrequent causes.

Diagnosis

Blood serum levels of follicle-stimulating hormone, luteinizing hormone, and sex steroids are in the normal adult range. Urinalysis of hormone levels and excretion of 17-ketosteroids show elevated levels. Other diagnostic studies to determine the cause include ultrasonography, CT, and MRI.

Treatment

The treatment depends on the cause. Tumors may require surgery or radiation. Hormone therapy may be used to suppress the secretion of gonadotropins and to prevent menstruation in true precocious puberty. The patient may need assistance to develop coping skills for handling emotional problems. Caregivers must understand that physical maturity may occur with psychological immaturity. Precocious puberty does not necessarily trigger sexual behavior.

Prognosis

The outcome depends on the early diagnosis and treatment of true precocious puberty; certain causes prompt a more guarded prognosis.

Prevention

In almost all cases, no prevention is known.

Patient Teaching

Emphasize the importance of following the exact medication regimen and keeping follow-up appointments. Provide a referral for psychological support as indicated by the treatment plan.

Review Challenge

Answer the following questions:

1. Name the major glands of the endocrine system.
2. What are some ways in which the endocrine system affects health and disease?
3. Describe two conditions that are the result of increased production and secretion of pituitary hGH.
4. What pathologic changes may result from hypopituitarism? Why is the age of the individual significant?
5. What causes diabetes insipidus?
6. What causes the thyroid gland to enlarge in a patient with a simple goiter?
7. Which hypothyroid condition (or chronic thyroiditis) is thought to be caused by autoimmune factors?
8. Describe the signs and symptoms of Graves disease.
9. What disease may be induced by prolonged administration or large doses of corticosteroids?
10. What are the possible causes of Addison disease?
11. Compare the cause and treatment of type 1 and type 2 diabetes mellitus.
12. Distinguish between diabetic coma and insulin shock.
13. How are hypoglycemic syndromes classified?
14. Name the important prognostic factors for thyroid malignancy.
15. What are the possible causes of precocious puberty in boys and girls?
16. Which benefits do bioidentical hormones provide versus traditional hormone replacement therapy?

Real-Life Challenge: Hypothyroidism

A 40-year-old female reports tiredness, loss of hair, and weight gain. She has not had a menstrual period for 3 months. Her skin appears dry and scaly. On questioning, the patient reports episodes of constipation and being unable to tolerate the cold. Her speech is somewhat slow and slurred. A blood test for thyroid functioning shows low thyrotropin levels. A thyroid scan shows no uptake of iodine. The diagnosis for this patient is hypothyroidism.

Questions

1. Severe untreated hypothyroidism with onset at maturity can lead to *myxedema coma*. What is the term describing hypothyroidism with onset in infancy or early childhood?
2. What causes the insidious onset of the various complaints and conditions of the patient with hypothyroidism?
3. What can be the cause of the reduced production of thyroxine (T_4) by the thyroid gland?
4. Hormone replacement is the usual drug therapy of choice. Research levothyroxine sodium (Synthroid) and explain its side effects.
5. For patient teaching, how long will the patient be instructed to take the medication?

Real-Life Challenge: Diabetes Mellitus

A 50-year-old male became lethargic and drowsy with flushed dry skin after eating a large meal. His family became concerned when he was difficult to rouse and had a fruity odor to his breath. He was transported to an emergency facility, where he gave a history of extreme thirst, hunger, and frequent urination. He recently had an upper respiratory infection that was slow to clear. Adult-onset diabetes mellitus is suspected.

Questions

1. Which blood test would be ordered?
2. Identify the normal results of blood glucose and glycated hemoglobin levels.
3. What are some of the possible causes of adult-onset type 2 diabetes mellitus?
4. In addition to the symptoms previously described, what else might be observed?
5. What determines the course of the treatment prescribed?
6. Why is glucose level monitoring important?
7. What patient teaching should be considered?
8. Why is a diet important?
9. Explain how insulin works.
10. What is the therapeutic action of the sulfonylureas?
11. How does metformin (Glucophage) reduce blood glucose levels?

Internet Assignments

1. Choose a related topic (an endocrine disorder) from the National Institute of Diabetes and research the latest health information on that topic. Review the easy-to-read and/or Spanish-language options.
2. Visit the American Thyroid Association website and report on a recent public health statement related to the treatment of thyroid disease.

Critical Thinking

1. What factors are considered essential in the diet plan for the insulin-dependent patient with diabetes?
2. Discuss the circumstances that can cause diabetic coma in a patient with diabetes. What circumstances can cause insulin shock?
3. What are the clinical manifestations in the patient with Cushing syndrome caused by excessive levels of circulating cortisol? Which gland(s) may be responsible for the disease? Why must the patient on large doses of glucocorticoids for another disease be monitored for Cushing syndrome?
4. Why is it wise for patients with endocrine diseases (e.g., diabetes, thyroid gland disease, or hypoglycemia) to wear a medical alert bracelet?
5. What known medical history information indicates a high risk for thyroid cancer?
6. Prepare to discuss the Critical Thinking case study exercises posted on Evolve for this chapter.

Credentialing Examination Questions

1. Which role best describes the endocrine system?
   A. Secretes hormones directly into tissues.
   B. Acts alone in maintaining homeostasis.
   C. Interacts with the nervous system to control homeostasis by secreting hormones.
   D. Produces only short-lived hormone responses.

2. From which source are bioidential hormones created?
   A. Plants
   B. Humans
   C. Animals
   D. All of the above

3. Which condition, characterized by excessive overgrowth of the bones of the face, hands, and feet, is a chronic metabolic condition in adults caused by hypersecretion of GH by the pituitary gland?
   A. Cretinism
   B. Acromegaly
   C. Graves disease
   D. Cushing syndrome

4. Patients with an iodine deficiency can increase their iodine intake by eating which food?
   A. Fish
   B. Beef
   C. Chicken
   D. Tofu

5. A patient presents with fat deposits in the scapular area and the trunk, which causes a protruding abdomen. Which disorder caused by excessive circulating cortisol levels results in which condition?
   A. Cretinism
   B. Acromegaly
   C. Graves disease
   D. Cushing syndrome

6. In addition to glucose, which other substance may be measured on the urine dipstick when the patient is metabolizing fats and proteins?
   A. Ketones
   B. Leukocytes
   C. Erythrocytes
   D. Bilirubin

7. A patient with diabetes administers their prescribed dose of insulin but does not eat any breakfast. Which condition may occur due to not eating?
   A. Hyperglycemia
   B. Hypoglycemia
   C. Hypercholesterolemia
   D. Hypocholesterolemia

8. At which age is puberty onset considered precocious in male patients?
   A. Before age 9
   B. Age 11
   C. Age 13
   D. After age 14

9. Which condition may cause exophthalmos or a protrusion of the eyes?
   A. Cretinism
   B. Acromegaly
   C. Graves disease
   D. Cushing syndrome

10. Which hormone plays a role in blood calcium level regulation?
    A. Thyroid
    B. Parathyroid
    C. Estrogen
    D. Progesterone

5

Diseases and Disorders of the Eye and Ear

CHAPTER OUTLINE

LEARNING OBJECTIVES

After studying the chapter, you should be able to:

1. Recall and define the four main refractive errors of vision.
2. Compare the pathology and etiology of nystagmus with those of strabismus.
3. Name the possible causes of conjunctivitis.
4. List the possible causes of "dry eye syndrome."
5. List the causes of cataracts.
6. Explain the importance of early treatment of glaucoma.
7. Characterize the visual disturbance caused by macular degeneration.
8. Explain the susceptibility of patients with diabetes to diabetic retinopathy.
9. Explain why early diagnosis and treatment are important in retinal detachment.
10. Using a diagram or an anatomic model, describe the process of hearing.
11. Compare conductive hearing loss with sensorineural hearing loss.
12. List the symptoms of otitis externa.
13. Describe the treatment of otitis media.
14. Explain the signs and symptoms of Ménière disease.
15. Describe the symptoms of benign paroxysmal positional vertigo.
16. Discuss the importance of preventing sensorineural hearing loss.

KEY TERMS

amblyopia (am-blee-OH-pee-ah)
blepharitis (blef-ar-RIE-tis)
cryotherapy (kry-o-THER-ah-pee)
diplopia (dih-PLO-pee-ah)
iridotomy (ir-ih-DOT-oh-me)
labyrinth (LAB-ih-rinth)
macula (MACK-you-la)
meibomian (my-BO-mee-an)
myringotomy (mir-in-GOT-oh-me)

otoscopy (oh-TOSS-ko-pee)
retinopathy (ret-ih-NOP-ah-thee)
seborrhea (seb-oh-RHEE-ah)
sensorineural (sen-so-ree-NEU-rol)
tinnitus (tih-NIE-tus)
tonometry (tohn-AHM-eh-tree)
tympanoplasty (tim-pan-oh-PLAS-tee)
vertigo (VER-tih-go)

Disorders of the Eye

Functioning Organs of Vision

Focusing a clear image on the retina is vital for good vision. The functional process of vision takes place in the presence of light in the following manner: (1) an image is formed on the retina; (2) the rods and cones are stimulated; and (3) nerve impulses are conducted to the brain. The area of the brain that involves the sense of sight is much larger than the areas involved in the other senses. Before discussing the pathophysiology of ocular disease, a review of the complex structure of the eye is in order (Fig. 5.1).

The eyeball, similar in shape to a sphere, is composed of a wall of primary structures in three concentric layers—the sclera, the choroid, and the retina—and is connected to the brain by way of the optic nerve.

The sclera, the outermost layer, consists of tough fibrous connective tissue visible as the white of the eye. Attached to the sclera are the six extrinsic muscles that move the eye (Table 5.1). The cornea, the colorless transparent structure on the front of the eye, is continuous with the sclera on the anterior aspect of the globe. This transparent structure uses its curvature to help focus light rays as they enter the eye.

Next to the sclera is the middle layer of tissue called the *choroid*. This layer is continuous with the ciliary body and the iris. These vascular structures supply the tissues of the eye with oxygen and nutrients. Anteriorly, the choroid joins the ciliary body, which contains ciliary muscles used to focus the lens of the eye. The ciliary processes in the ciliary body secrete aqueous humor, the fluid found in the anterior portion of the eye. The ciliary body is connected by suspensory ligaments to the biconvex, transparent lens of the eye. Contraction of the ciliary muscles causes the suspensory ligaments to relax. The lens then bulges, allowing the focusing that is necessary for close vision.

Also attached to the ciliary body is the iris, or colored portion of the eye, which helps regulate the amount of light entering the eye. In a brightly lit environment, the iris contracts, causing the opening in the center of the iris, the pupil, to become smaller. In limited light conditions, the iris relaxes and the pupil enlarges, permitting more light to enter the eye.

The innermost layer, covering the posterior three-quarters of the eye, is called the *retina*. The retina is a light-sensitive layer made up of photo-receptive cells called *rods* and *cones*. The rods function best in dim light, thereby enabling night vision, whereas the cones function in bright light and also detect color and fine detail. Within the rods and cones, the image initiates a chemical reaction and sends messages through the nerve fiber layer of the retina to the optic nerve. The optic nerve penetrates the fibrous layers at the optic disc and continues on to the brain. The optic disc contains no receptor cells and often is called the *blind spot* of the eye. The optic nerve transmits the image to the portion of the brain that is used for vision. The brain interprets the impulses from each eye and produces a single three-dimensional image. The macula lutea, a yellow spot, lies lateral to the optic disc. In the center of the macula lutea is the fovea centralis, the area that produces the sharpest image.

Covering the anterior externally visible portion of the sclera is a thin, transparent membrane called the *conjunctiva*. It begins at the edge of the cornea, extends over the exposed sclera, and folds anteriorly to line the inside portion of the lids. This creates both a superior cul-de-sac and an inferior cul-de-sac, where the conjunctiva reflects images from the sclerae to the lids. The space between the iris, the colored portion of the eye, and the anterior clear cornea is called the *anterior chamber*. The fluid occupying the anterior chamber is a watery substance called the *aqueous humor*, which is produced by the ciliary body. The fluid exits the anterior chamber through the trabecular network, a drainage system located at the junction of the base of the iris and the cornea. Appropriate pressure within the eye is maintained by the aqueous humor, which ultimately enters the general circulation of the body. The large cavity behind the lens is the vitreous body; it contains a jellylike fluid called the *vitreous humor*, which helps maintain the globular shape of the eyeball.

The internal lens of the eye is elastic and therefore can focus images whether viewed close by or at a distance. The focusing is accomplished by contraction and relaxation of the muscles of the ciliary body. This action makes it possible for the lens to assume either a more rounded spherical shape or a flatter elongated shape, depending on the focus length

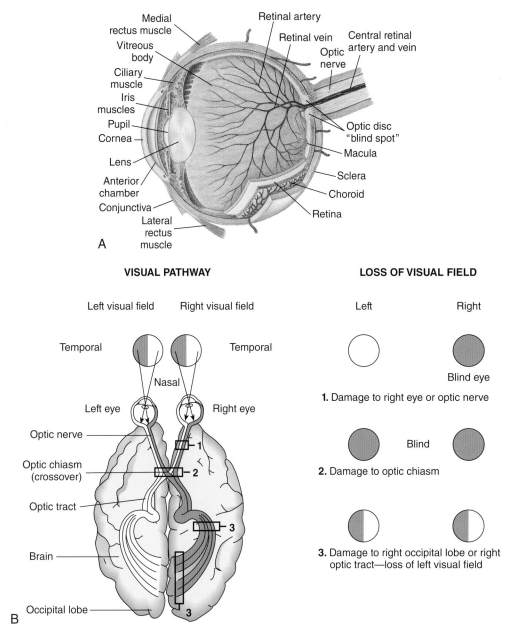

• **Fig. 5.1** (A) Anatomy of the human eye. (B) The visual pathway. (A, From Seidel HM, et al.: *Mosby's guide to physical examination*, ed 8, St Louis, 2014, Mosby. B, From Gould B: *Pathophysiology for the health professions*, ed 3, St Louis, 2006, Mosby.)

required. The lens is attached to the ciliary body by small strands of tissue called *zonules*. These are attached at points all the way around the lens. When the ciliary body relaxes, the zonules are pulled, causing flattening of the lens, the configuration needed for focusing on a distant image.

Light rays are the key to sight. The light rays enter the eye and pass through the cornea, aqueous humor, lens, and finally the vitreous humor. These rays can travel in a straight line or be bent at an angle. The process of bending light rays is known as *refraction*. The cornea and the lens are capable of bending or refracting the light rays so that they can be focused on the retina. The image that forms on the retina is reversed both in the up/down and right/left directions.

The image is turned right side up and forward in the brain as the brain interprets the visual concept. Another step in the process of vision involves accommodation. Adjustments must be made in the eye to facilitate the image in relation to the viewer's distance from the object. The process of accommodation involves changing the shape of the lens, making it either flatter or thicker. The ciliary muscle and the suspensory ligaments contract and relax in opposition to accomplish this task.

The intrinsic muscles of each eye respond to light levels and change the size of the pupil to regulate the amount of light that enters the eye and reaches the retina. Each eye has six extrinsic muscles that control the movements of the eye;

TABLE 5.1 Muscles of the Eye

Muscle	Function	Cranial Innervation
Extrinsic Muscles of the Eye		
Inferior rectus	Rotates eyeball downward and medially; adducts	Oculomotor nerve (CN III)
Lateral rectus	Rotates eye laterally; abducts eyeball	Abducens nerve (CN VI)
Medial rectus	Rotates eye medially; adducts eyeball	Oculomotor nerve (CN III)
Superior rectus	Causes eye to look up	Oculomotor nerve (CN III)
Inferior oblique	Rotates eyeball upward and outward; abducts	Oculomotor nerve (CN III)
Superior oblique	Rotates eyeball downward and outward; abducts	Trochlear nerve (CN IV)
Intrinsic Smooth Muscles of the Eye		
Ciliary muscle	Regulation of lens shape for close vision	Oculomotor (CN III)
Iris (radial muscles)	Sympathetic stimulation; dilation of pupil	Oculomotor (CN III)
Iris (circular muscles)	Parasympathetic stimulation; contraction of pupil	Oculomotor (CN III)

CN, Cranial nerve.

TABLE 5.2 Functions of the Major Parts of the Eye

Structure	Function
Sclera	External protection
Cornea	Light refraction
Choroid	Blood supply
Iris	Light absorption and regulation of pupillary width
Ciliary body	Secretion of vitreous fluid; in addition, its smooth muscles change the shape of the lens
Lens	Light refraction
Retinal layer	Light receptor that transforms optic signals into nerve impulses
Rods	Means of distinguishing light from dark and perceiving shape and movement
Cones	Color vision
Central fovea	Area of sharpest vision
Macula lutea	Blind spot
External ocular muscles	Movement of the globe
Optic nerve (cranial nerve II)	Transmission of visual information to the brain
Lacrimal glands	Secretion of tears
Eyelid	Eye protection

these muscles pull on the eyeballs, making the two move together to converge on one visual field (see Table 5.1). Normally, the eyes work together in unison, so an assessment of the functioning of these muscles often is included in a neurologic assessment. Table 5.2 summarizes the functions of the major parts of the eye.

Some eye disorders are signs of systemic diseases, such as hypertension, diabetes mellitus, or certain autoimmune arthritic diseases. Common symptoms of eye diseases and conditions that should be called to the attention of the physician include the following:

- Redness of the eye
- Pain, itching, or burning in or around the eye
- Swollen red eyelids
- Drainage from the eyes
- Lesions/sores in or around the eyes
- Visual disturbances
- Unequal pupils, sudden loss of vision, persistent pain, or other symptoms associated with eye injury
- Repetitive, involuntary movements of the eye

Diagnostic tests for eye diseases and conditions include the following:

- Eye charts, such as the Snellen chart, to measure visual acuity.
- Visual field tests to check central and peripheral vision.
- Tonometry to measure intraocular pressure (IOP).
- Eye cultures to identify viral or bacterial infectious agents.
- Dilation to directly view the posterior structures of the eye, including the retina and the optic nerve.
- Lectronystagmography (ENG) to measure the direction and degree of nystagmus.
- Electroretinography to measure the electric activity of the retina in response to the flashing of light.
- Fluorescein angiography to assess the vasculature of the eye.
- Optical coherence tomography (OCT) scans to capture three-dimensional images and to measure the dimensions of structures in the posterior chamber, such as epiretinal membranes and optic disks.
- Ocular and orbit ultrasonography is another excellent method to detect and evaluate many diseases and conditions of orbital and posterior orbital structures.

Many systemic medications taken for a variety of diseases can have ocular side effects. It is important for patients

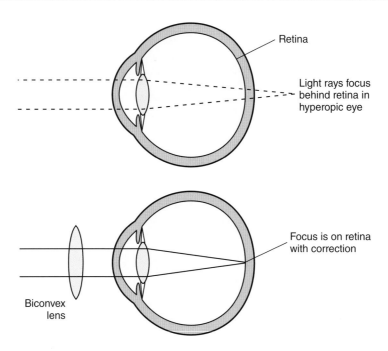

• **Fig. 5.2** Hyperopia and correction.

taking certain systemic medications to be monitored periodically for ocular toxicity. These include hydroxychloroquine (Plaquenil), used in the treatment of lupus and rheumatoid arthritis, ethambutol used in the treatment of tuberculosis, and steroids used in the treatment of various conditions.

Refractive Errors

Refractive errors are the most common cause of diminished visual acuity. Refractive errors that result in the eye being unable to focus light effectively on the retina are identified as hyperopia, myopia, astigmatism, and presbyopia as discussed next.

Hyperopia (Farsightedness)

Description

Hyperopia (farsightedness) occurs when light that enters the eye is focused behind the retina rather than on the retina, requiring refocusing by the internal lens or the use of an external corrective lens to reposition the viewed object on the retina to sharpen the image. With this condition, near vision is particularly impaired. Hyperopia occurs when the eyeball is abnormally short, as measured from front to back (Fig. 5.2).

ICD-10-CM Code H52.03 *(Hypermetropia, bilateral)*
(H52.00–H52.03 = 4 codes of specificity)

Myopia (Nearsightedness)

Description

Myopia (nearsightedness) occurs when light rays entering the eye are focused in front of the retina, causing blurred vision. Near objects can be seen clearly, but distant objects are blurry, and the image being viewed cannot be sharpened by the internal lens of the eye. Myopia occurs when the eyeball is abnormally long, as measured from front to back (Fig. 5.3).

ICD-10-CM Code H52.13 *(Myopia, bilateral)*
(H52.10–H52.13 = 4 codes of specificity)

Astigmatism

Description

Astigmatism is an irregular focusing of light rays entering the eye. It usually is caused by the cornea not being spherical. The front of the cornea may be more egg-shaped than spherical, thereby causing light rays to be unevenly or diffusely focused across the retina. This causes some images to appear clearly defined, whereas others appear blurred.

ICD-10-CM Code H52.209 *(Unspecified astigmatism, unspecified eye)*
(H52.20–H52.229 = 12 codes of specificity)

Refer to the physician's diagnosis and then to the current edition of the ICD-10-CM coding manual to ensure the greatest specificity of pathology.

Presbyopia

Description

Presbyopia is the inability of the internal lens of the eye to focus on near objects due to the loss of elasticity of the lens.

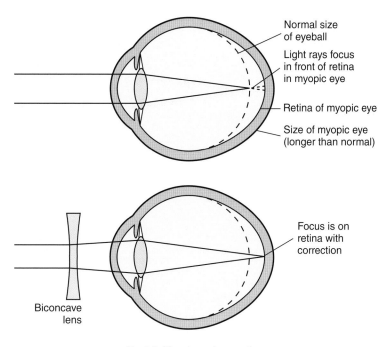

Normal size
of eyeball

Light rays focus
in front of retina
in myopic eye

Retina of myopic eye

Size of myopic eye
(longer than normal)

Focus is on
retina with
correction

Biconcave
lens

• **Fig. 5.3** Myopia and correction.

This condition is related to aging and usually starts in people in their mid-40s.

ICD-10-CM Code   H52.4 *(Presbyopia)*

Symptoms and Signs
The primary symptoms of a refractive error are blurred vision and eye fatigue, which can lead to squinting, frequent rubbing of the eyes, and headaches. Some patients may experience discomfort and have problems with night vision.

Patient Screening
Schedule a comprehensive eye examination for a patient who complains of changes in visual acuity, clarity, or sharpness of visual perception.

Etiology
Some refractive errors are influenced by genes. If the parents have these errors, they predispose the child to have a refractive error. When the lens ages, the shape of the cornea changes, and if the shape of the eyeball gets too long or short, refractive errors can occur.

Diagnosis
Eye health history and tests for visual acuity and refraction are used to diagnose refractive errors. Usually for children, the pupils are dilated with eye drops, and the eyes are then evaluated for refractive error with a retinoscope. The optimal lens adjustment needed to correct the deficit is determined by having the patient look through a series of corrective lenses of different powers.

Treatment
Correcting refractive errors involves fitting the patient with artificial lenses in the form of eyeglasses or contact lenses or performing corrective surgery. Radial keratotomy, a surgical procedure used to reshape the eye, has been replaced by laser surgery, which results in more precise visual correction and has fewer complications. The following refractive surgical procedures can be done to correct myopia, hyperopia, and astigmatism: laser-assisted in situ keratomileusis, astigmatic keratotomy (AK), photorefractive keratotomy, laser thermal keratoplasty, radial keratotomy (RK), automated lamellar keratoplasty, intracorneal ring (Intacs) conductive keratoplasty (CK), and intraocular contact lenses (lens permanently placed in the eye).

Prognosis
Correctly prescribed eyeglasses or contact lenses can produce excellent results. Elective refractive surgical procedures can benefit medically eligible individuals, and the risks for complications are generally low.

Prevention
Refractive errors, in general, cannot be prevented.

Patient Teaching
When a patient is to have refractive surgery, describe the procedure and advise the patient as to when to expect visual recovery, how to use preoperative and postoperative medications, and when to return to a regular work schedule is likely. Explain the importance of follow-up visits to monitor progress.

Nystagmus

Description

Nystagmus is involuntary, repetitive, rhythmic movements of one or both eyes.

| ICD-10-CM Code | H55.00 *(Unspecified nystagmus)* (H55.00–H55.09 = 6 codes of specificity) |

Refer to the physician's diagnosis and then to the current edition of the ICD-10-CM coding manual to ensure the greatest specificity of pathology.

Symptoms and Signs

Any repetitive or involuntary movement of one or both eyes is a sign of nystagmus. The eye movements can be horizontal, vertical, circular, or a combination of these. Blurred or decreased vision can also be associated with nystagmus. These movements may also cause a problem with depth perceptions and affect a person's balance.

Patient Screening

Schedule a comprehensive ophthalmic examination for a patient complaining of changes in visual acuity or of any involuntary or "jerky" movements of the eye. *Acquired nystagmus always necessitates a complete neurologic evaluation.*

Etiology

Spontaneous nystagmus can be congenital or acquired. Congenital nystagmus is manifested before age 6 months to 1 year and is the most common type. Acquired nystagmus results when a disease process produces lesions in the brain or inner ear. Alcohol use and abuse of certain drugs also may cause this condition. Brain tumors and cerebrovascular lesions can cause nystagmus, or it may instead be the result of abnormal development of the nervous system.

Diagnosis

Nystagmus can usually be diagnosed clinically by external examination of the eyes and observation of any involuntary movements. When needed for a definitive diagnosis, other, more specific, complex tests are available as well.

Treatment

Acquired nystagmus is managed by treating the underlying cause of the condition. Congenital nystagmus often can be lessened by using the Kestenbaum procedure, in which the eyes are surgically rotated toward the null point of the eye.

Prognosis

The outcome of acquired nystagmus depends on the treatment of the underlying cause. Surgical intervention for congenital nystagmus attempts to minimize nystagmus when the eyes are looking straight ahead.

• **Fig. 5.4** Strabismus. (From Zitelli BJ, Davis HW: *Atlas of pediatric physical diagnosis*, ed 6, Philadelphia, 2012, Mosby.)

Prevention

No specific method of prevention is known.

Patient Teaching

In acquired nystagmus, the patient benefits from understanding the underlying cause and treatment of nystagmus. Parents of a child with congenital nystagmus are given support and clear explanations about the condition and the surgical treatment, if indicated.

Strabismus

Description

Strabismus, a visual defect of misalignment, is a failure of the eyes to look in the same direction at the same time, which primarily occurs because of weakness in the nerves stimulating the muscles that control the position of the eyes (Fig. 5.4).

| ICD-10-CM Code | H51.9 *(Unspecified disorder of binocular movement)* (H51.0–H51.9 = 9 codes of specificity) |

Refer to the physician's diagnosis and then to the current edition of the ICD-10-CM coding manual to ensure the greatest specificity of pathology.

Symptoms and Signs

In esotropia (convergent strabismus, or cross-eye), both eyes turn inward; in exotropia (divergent strabismus, or wall-eye), both eyes turn outward. With either form, the main symptom is diplopia if strabismus is acquired in adulthood. Diplopia is usually not present when the strabismus is congenital.

Patient Screening

Schedule a comprehensive ophthalmic examination for a patient complaining of changes in visual acuity, clearness or sharpness of visual perception, or double vision. Parents may report the noted appearance of "crossed eyes" in an infant or young child.

Etiology

Esotropia usually develops in infancy or early childhood and may be associated with **amblyopia**. Amblyopia is reversible until the visual pathways fully develop at about age 7 to 8 years. In almost all cases, esotropia that develops in adults is caused by a condition or disease elsewhere in the body. The brain, the cranial nerves (CNs), or the muscles themselves are affected. These diseases and conditions include diabetes mellitus, temporal arteritis, muscular dystrophy, high blood pressure, trauma, aneurysm, or an intracranial lesion.

Diagnosis

To discover the underlying cause, the physician performs a complete ophthalmic examination and orders various appropriate radiographic studies and blood tests.

Treatment

Strabismus should be treated as soon as possible. Early intervention is the key. Corrective glasses, treatment to minimize or prevent amblyopia, or surgery to restore the eye muscle balance may be used in the course of the treatment. In some cases, preventing amblyopia involves covering the fixing eye to force the child to use the deviating eye.

Prognosis

In most cases, children respond well to early treatment. The prognosis of adults with acquired strabismus depends on the underlying cause.

Prevention

No specific method of prevention is known. Normal development of visual pathways begins in early childhood with appropriate retinal stimulation. Amblyopia may be prevented or at least minimized by early diagnosis and intervention.

Patient Teaching

Give parents of children with strabismus an explanation of the condition and the cause, if known. Parents are taught how to apply an eye patch. Reinforce the importance of early treatment to help prevent visual loss. The adult with acquired strabismus can benefit from an explanation of the relationship of the eye condition to the identified underlying cause.

Disorders of the Eyelid

Hordeolum (Stye)

Description

Hordeola (styes) are acute, painful abscesses of an eyelash follicle or in a sebaceous gland of the eyelids (Fig. 5.5).

ICD-10-CM Code   H00.019 (Hordeolum externum unspecified eye, unspecified eyelid) (H00.011–H00.029 = 14 codes of specificity)

• **Fig. 5.5** Hordeolum of upper eyelid. (From Roberts JR, Hedges JR: *Clinical procedures in emergency medicine*, Philadelphia, 2010, Saunders.)

H00.029 (Hordeolum internum unspecified eye, unspecified eyelid)
H00.039 (Abscess of eyelid unspecified eye, unspecified eyelid)
(H00.031–H00.039 = 7 codes of specificity)

Symptoms and Signs

Styes occur most often at the outside edge of the lid. Pain, swelling, redness, and formation of pus at the site are the main symptoms of a stye. Patients may report a feeling of having "something in the eye."

Patient Screening

Patients complaining of a lesion of the eyelid, with or without purulent drainage, require an appointment with their health care provider for an examination of the affected area. Follow office policy for referral to an ophthalmologist.

Etiology

Often styes are the result of a staphylococcal infection and can be associated with and secondary to blepharitis (see the Blepharitis section).

Diagnosis

Visual examination alone is usually sufficient for making the diagnosis.

Treatment

To hasten drainage, warm compresses over a period of days may be applied to the eye as soon as the inflammation is evident. Topical antibiotics are also effective at shortening the duration of symptoms. If surrounding soft tissue becomes infected (cellulitis), oral antibiotics may be needed. If persistent, these lesions need to be surgically drained.

Prognosis

Hordeola are usually self-limiting infections; thus the prognosis is good, but recurrence can be common.

Prevention

Face and eyelid hygiene and warm compresses can prevent recurrence. Practicing hand hygiene and avoiding touching the eyes and face can also help prevent infection.

Patient Teaching

Instruct the patient regarding the correct technique of applying an eye compress as prescribed. Inform the patient about the correct application and usage of topical or systemic antibiotic therapies.

Chalazion

Description

A chalazion is a small, firm, nonmobile, painless, subcutaneous nodule on the margin or body of the eyelid; it occurs with occlusion of the meibomian glands and may be referred to as a meibomian cyst.

ICD-10-CM Code	H00.19 *(Chalazion unspecified eye, unspecified eyelid)*
	(H00.11–H00.19 = 7 codes of specificity)

Symptoms and Signs

A chalazion can vary in size, from being barely visible to being the size of a pea. Chalazia can become infected, producing redness, swelling, and pain (Fig. 5.6).

Patient Screening

A brief visual examination by an ophthalmologist is sufficient for the diagnosis of a chalazion.

Etiology

Chalazia are caused by a blockage of fluid originating from one of the meibomian glands, which lubricate the eyelid margin.

Diagnosis

Visual examination and patient history are all that is necessary to make the diagnosis.

Treatment

Small chalazia usually disappear spontaneously over a month or two with regular application of warm compresses. Resolution may be facilitated by topical antibiotic treatment. Antibiotic therapy may vary from gentamicin or tobramycin to azithromycin or quinolone drops.

Isolated recurrent chalazia may respond to corticosteroid injection. Larger chalazia may not spontaneously disappear and may need to be removed surgically in the office setting.

• **Fig. 5.6** Chalazion. (From Zitelli BJ, Davis HW: *Atlas of pediatric physical diagnosis*, ed 6, Philadelphia, 2012, Mosby.)

Prognosis

Complete resolution is expected, but chalazia can be recurrent.

Prevention

Lid hygiene and warm compresses can help prevent recurrence.

Patient Teaching

The patient may be told a chalazion is not infectious. If surgical removal is recommended, reassure the patient that the procedure is minor.

Keratitis

Description

Keratitis is any inflammation or infection of the cornea.

ICD-10-CM Code	H16.9 *(Unspecified keratitis)*

Keratitis has many forms and therefore many ICD-10-CM codes. Refer to the physician's diagnosis and then to the current edition of the ICD-10-CM coding manual to ensure the greatest specificity of pathology.

Symptoms and Signs

Symptoms are decreased visual acuity, irritation, tearing, photophobia, and mild redness of the conjunctiva. Pain or numbness of the cornea may soon follow and is a significant sign.

Patient Screening

Scheduled for a prompt ophthalmic examination. Follow office policy for referral to an ophthalmologist.

Etiology

Keratitis often is caused by an infection resulting from herpes simplex virus. This is especially likely when the keratitis is preceded by an upper respiratory infection (URI) with facial cold sores (see the Herpes Simplex [Cold Sores] section in Chapter 8). Certain bacteria (i.e., *Pseudomonas, Streptococcus, and Staphylococcus*) and fungi also can be responsible for keratitis. Contact lens wear substantially increases the risk of bacterial keratitis, especially for those who sleep with lenses in place. Other forms of keratitis can be caused by corneal trauma or by exposure of the cornea to dry air or intense light, as occurs during welding. Cultures may be taken to identify the causative organism.

Diagnosis
Examination of the cornea with use of a slit lamp confirms the diagnosis. Medical history may indicate a recent URI, and visual acuity may be decreased.

Treatment
To avoid internal spread of the infection, urgent treatment is necessary. The administration of a broad-spectrum antibiotic or an antiviral agent can effectively eradicate the infection, depending on which type of organism is the causative agent. Ophthalmic moisturizing ointments and eye drops may be prescribed for symptomatic relief. An eye patch may be needed to relieve discomfort caused by photophobia. However, this is contraindicated in cases of fungal infection or contact lens wear.

Prognosis
Prompt treatment of the condition decreases the risk of ulceration that can erode the cornea and cause the formation of scar tissue that may interfere with vision.

Prevention
Following the recommended instructions for contact lens wear and care, such as proper handling and cleaning of the lenses, can reduce the risk of infection. Avoiding hand-to-eye contact can lessen the transfer of infection to the eye from contaminated medication, makeup, or contact lenses.

Patient Teaching
Explain how infections can be transferred to the eyes by the fingers. Encourage contact lens wearers to adhere to strict hand hygiene. Teach the patient the proper technique for the instillation of ophthalmic ointment and eye drops as prescribed; emphasize the importance of proper hand washing. Inform the patient of the increased risk of keratitis from wearing contact lenses while sleeping.

Blepharitis
Description
Blepharitis is inflammation of the margins of the eyelids involving hair follicles and glands.

ICD-10-CM Code	H01.009 *(Unspecified blepharitis unspecified eye, unspecified eyelid)* (H01.001–H01.029 = 21 codes of specificity) H01.019 *(Ulcerative blepharitis unspecified eye, unspecified eyelid)*

• **Fig. 5.7** Blepharitis. (From Zitelli BJ, Davis HW: *Atlas of pediatric physical diagnosis*, ed 6, Philadelphia, 2012, Mosby.)

H01.029 *(Squamous blepharitis unspecified eye, unspecified eyelid)*
Refer to the physician's diagnosis and then to the current edition of the ICD-10-CM coding manual to ensure the greatest specificity of pathology.

Symptoms and Signs
Blepharitis causes persistent redness and crusting on and around the eyelids (Fig. 5.7). Symptoms may include itching, burning, or foreign body sensation. The conditions are usually bilateral and symmetric. In severe cases, eyelashes can fall out, and the patient may experience persistent irritation of the eyes.

Patient Screening
The patient experiencing these symptoms needs a prompt clinical evaluation.

Etiology
The ulcerative form of blepharitis is usually the result of a staphylococcal infection but it can also be caused by a viral infection. Nonulcerative blepharitis can be caused by allergies or exposure to smoke, dust, or chemicals. This condition can also be secondary to seborrhea of the eyelid's sebaceous glands, and often the patient has a history of repeated hordeola and chalazia.

Diagnosis
Visual examination of the eyelids and culture.

Treatment
Use of warm wet compresses and cleansing of the lids is recommended. Antibiotic ophthalmic ointment (bacitracin or erythromycin) is indicated when the cause is from a bacterial infection.

Prognosis
The condition can sometimes be resistant to treatment and may become chronic if not properly treated. Untreated

• **Fig. 5.8** Entropion.

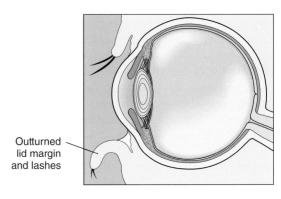

• **Fig. 5.9** Ectropion.

chronic cases may lead to corneal and conjunctival inflammation.

Prevention

It is prudent to protect the eyes from infection by adhering to proper hygiene. Avoid touching your eyes with unclean hands.

Patient Teaching

Describe eyelid hygiene, which includes rigorous cleaning of the eyelids and lashes with a clean warm washcloth daily. Teach the patient the proper technique for instilling ophthalmic ointment and eye drops as prescribed; emphasize the importance of hand washing before the procedure.

Entropion

Description

In the case of entropion, the eyelid margins (more often the margin of just the lower lid) turn inward, causing the lashes to rub the conjunctiva (Fig. 5.8).

ICD-10-CM Code	H02.009 *(Unspecified entropion of unspecified eye, unspecified eyelid)* (H02.001–H02.059 = 42 codes of specificity)

Refer to the physician's diagnosis and then to the current edition of the ICD-10-CM coding manual to ensure the greatest specificity of pathology.

Symptoms and Signs

The patient has the sensation of a foreign body in the eye, tearing, itching, and redness. Chronic irritation of the conjunctiva may cause conjunctivitis (see the Conjunctivitis section). Entropion can also damage the cornea, causing epithelial defects and vision problems, if not corrected.

Patient Screening

Schedule an appointment for the patient reporting the discomforting symptoms mentioned earlier.

Etiology

Entropion most often affects older people. With aging, the soft tissue on the lower eyelids loses elasticity, causing the eyelids to turn inward. This allows the lashes to irritate the conjunctiva and the cornea.

Diagnosis

Visual examination reveals an inversion of the eyelid. The lashes are visible on the conjunctiva, as is the redness that results from the irritation.

Treatment

For persistent irritation, the patient should be seen by a physician. A minor surgical procedure on the eyelid usually corrects the problem.

Prognosis

Surgical treatment usually corrects the problem.

Prevention

No specific method of prevention is known.

Patient Teaching

To avoid infection, advise the patient not to rub the eyes. If surgery is required to correct the condition, explain the minor procedure.

Ectropion

Description

Ectropion is a condition in which the lower eyelid everts from the eyeball and the exposed surface of the eyeball and the lining of the eyelid become dry and irritated (Fig. 5.9).

ICD-10-CM Code	H02.109 *(Unspecified ectropion of unspecified eye, unspecified eyelid)*

Refer to the physician's diagnosis and then to the current edition of the ICD-10-CM coding manual to ensure the greatest specificity of pathology.

Symptoms and Signs

Eversion of the eyelid exposes the conjunctival membrane lining the eyelid. Tears are diverted away from the tear duct and run down the cheeks instead. The patient reports dryness in the eye and tearing.

Patient Screening
Schedule a medical evaluation for a patient experiencing the symptoms listed earlier.

Etiology
This condition usually occurs in older adults as a result of decreased elasticity of the lower eyelid. A scar on the eyelid or cheek that contracts and pulls the eyelid downward can cause a cicatricial ectropion.

Diagnosis
The problem can be detected easily by visual examination, and a history of symptoms confirms the diagnosis.

Treatment
Ectropion rarely disappears without treatment; therefore a physician should be consulted. A minor surgical procedure is all that is needed to correct the condition.

Prognosis
If it is not treated, ectropion can cause the development of corneal ulcers and permanent damage to the cornea.

Prevention
No method of prevention is known.

Patient Teaching
Assure the patient that a minor surgical procedure can correct the problem. Teach the patient the proper technique for instilling ophthalmic ointment and eye drops as prescribed; emphasize the importance of hand washing before performing the procedure.

Blepharoptosis
Description
Blepharoptosis, also called *ptosis*, is a permanent drooping of the upper eyelid, such that it partially or completely covers the eye (Fig. 5.10).

ICD-10-CM Code	H02.409 *(Unspecified ptosis of unspecified eyelid)*

• **Fig. 5.10** Blepharoptosis.

Drooping eyelid

Refer to the physician's diagnosis and then to the current edition of the ICD-10-CM coding manuals to ensure the greatest specificity of pathology.

Symptoms and Signs
Blepharoptosis usually affects one eye, but both can be involved. The condition can vary in severity throughout the day. Blepharoptosis can occur at any age, is often familial, and, if severe, obstructs the vision of the affected eye.

Patient Screening
When vision is affected, or a previously normal upper eyelid has begun to droop, a physician should be consulted. Schedule the first available appointment.

Etiology
This condition is caused either by weakness of CN III or weakness of the muscle that raises the eyelid. Blepharoptosis also can occur when the muscle of the eyelid or the nerve that controls the muscle is damaged. Several diseases, such as muscular dystrophy and myasthenia gravis, can cause ptosis.

Diagnosis
In addition to an ophthalmic examination, blood tests and imaging may be ordered to rule out underlying disease.

Treatment
An operation can be performed to elevate the eyelid position, or in the case of myasthenia gravis, systemic medication may be prescribed.

Prognosis
Successful treatment of any underlying disease should help correct the blepharoptosis.

Prevention
No specific method of prevention is known.

Patient Teaching
Explain the relationship between the ptosis and the underlying disease, if known. If surgery is scheduled, describe the procedure to the patient, and provide written postoperative instructions, if appropriate.

Conjunctivitis
Description
Inflammation of the conjunctiva, the mucous membrane that covers the anterior portion of the eyeball and also lines the eyelids, is called *conjunctivitis*.

ICD-10-CM Code	H10.9 *(Unspecified conjunctivitis)* (H10.01–H10.9 = 68 codes of specificity)

Refer to the physician's diagnosis and then to the current edition of the ICD-10-CM coding manual to ensure the greatest specificity of pathology.

Symptoms and Signs

Conjunctivitis is common and can be either unilateral or bilateral. Symptoms include redness, swelling, foreign body sensation, and itching of the conjunctiva. The eyes may tear excessively and be extra sensitive to light. In the case of infectious conjunctivitis, a discharge ranging from watery to hyperpurulent can be present. This condition ("pink eye") is highly contagious (Fig. 5.11).

Vernal conjunctivitis can be caused by extreme allergies or sensitivity or by irritation by contact lenses. This type of conjunctivitis appears as bumps or cobblestones when the eyelid is turned up.

Patient Screening

Schedule a prompt ophthalmic examination for the patient presenting with swollen, red, itchy eyes.

Etiology

Conjunctivitis can be caused by infection, most commonly viral or bacterial, and also by irritation resulting from allergies or chemicals. Infections are often transmitted when contaminated fingers, washcloths, or towels touch the eyes. Conjunctivitis can also be produced through sexual contact with someone who has a sexually transmitted disease.

Diagnosis

Ophthalmic examination reveals inflammation of the conjunctiva. To identify bacterial or viral organisms, samples of the discharge can be taken for culture and sensitivity tests,

Treatment

The treatment varies, depending on the causative agents. The eyes should be kept free from discharge using cool compresses applied to the eyes. For bacterial infections, topical or systemic antibiotics are prescribed.

• **Fig. 5.11** Purulent conjunctivitis. (From Stein HA, Stein RM, Freeman MI: *The ophthalmic assistant: a text for allied and associated ophthalmic personnel*, ed 10, St. Louis, 2018, Elsevier.)

Prognosis

Except in severe instances, conjunctivitis is usually not a serious condition, although recurrences are common. Usually, 1 to 2 weeks of treatment clears up this type of infection. Viral infections usually are self-limiting.

Prevention

If the determined cause is irritants or allergens, avoiding the offending agents can result in resolution of the symptoms. Infectious conjunctivitis can be controlled by having the patient avoid contaminated washcloths and refrain from touching the eyes with contaminated fingers.

Patient Teaching

Give the patient written instructions on how to apply cool compresses and on the dosage schedule to be followed for medications. Teach the patient the proper technique for instilling ophthalmic ointment and eye drops as prescribed; emphasize the importance of hand washing before performing the procedure. When an oral antibiotic is ordered, advise the patient to be sure to take the entire course of medication.

Keratoconjunctivitis Sicca (Dry Eye Syndrome)

Description

Keratoconjunctivitis sicca (dry eye syndrome) is a condition in which tears do not adequately lubricate the eyes. Dry eye syndrome is uncomfortable and may cause irritation of the eye.

ICD-10-CM Code	H04.12 (*Dry eye syndrome*)
	H04.123 (*Dry eye syndrome of bilateral lacrimal glands*)
	H04.129 (*Dry eye syndrome of unspecified lacrimal gland*)

Symptoms and Signs

Symptoms include a feeling of having a foreign object in the eyes; scratchy, burning, or stinging sensation in the eyes; sensitivity to light; blurred vision; and/or redness of the eyes. Additionally, the individual may experience difficulty with nighttime driving or with the wearing of contact lenses.

Patient Screening

Individuals reporting scratchiness accompanied by visual difficulty require prompt assessment. Schedule an appointment that same day, or consult with a health care provider to add the patient to the schedule as a "work in" so that they can be seen promptly. In some cases, referral to their ophthalmologist or a facility where prompt assessment can occur may be necessary after the health care provider has made a recommendation for a referral.

Etiology

Lack of adequate tear production is often the cause. Aging, many medical conditions, medications, damage to the tear glands as the result of radiation or inflammation, or temporary damage related to laser eye surgery. Increased tear evaporation may be caused by blinking less often than usual, dry air, wind, smoke, or structural eyelid problems.

Risk factors include being female, being older than 50 years, wearing contact lenses, and consuming a diet low in vitamin A.

Diagnosis

The diagnosis is made from patient history and symptoms along with an examination of the eyes.

Treatment

Treatments include application of over-the-counter eye drops. Medications, including cyclosporin ophthalmic emulsion (Restasis) and lifitegrast ophthalmic solution (Xiidra), may be prescribed. Recommendations for relief include some changes in lifestyle, such as avoiding environments with smoke, wind, and dry air. Contact lens wearers should follow instructions regarding the length of time for wearing.

Prognosis

Instillation of eye drops will possibly be lifelong. Smokers may need to smoke less or avoid secondhand smoke. If lifestyle changes are made, symptoms may be reduced.

Prevention

The patient should follow instructions for wearing of contact lenses and avoid environments of dry air, wind, and smoke.

Patient Teaching

Instruct patients in the correct way to apply eye drops to prevent the possibility of eye injury or contamination of the solution. Patients should be instructed not to touch the tip of the applicator to the surface of the eye. Emphasize the importance of hand washing before performing the procedure.

Recommend situations where air is not blowing directly into the eyes. Have the patient establish a routine of using artificial tears on a regular basis; attempt to create a more humid environment by adding moisture to the air; and take breaks when performing long tasks with eyes (reading, computer use).

Disorders of the Globe of the Eye

Corneal Abrasion or Ulcer

Description

A corneal abrasion is the painful loss of surface epithelium or outer layer of the cornea. Corneal ulceration is an infection of the cornea.

ICD-10-CM Code	S05.00XA (*Injury of conjunctiva and corneal abrasion without foreign body, unspecified eye, initial encounter*)

H18.829 (*Corneal disorder due to contact lens, unspecified eye*) (H18.821–H18.829 = 4 codes of specificity)

Symptoms and Signs

The transparent outer covering of the eye is called the *cornea*. Because of its location, it is susceptible to injury and infection. Symptoms of abrasion and ulcer include pain, redness, and tearing. The patient may describe a sensation of having something foreign in the eye constantly and may report vision impairment as well. The patient may have a history of having a foreign body in the eye or of recent ocular trauma.

Patient Screening

The patient with corneal abrasion may experience significant persistent pain in the eye. Prompt medical care is indicated. The physician should be consulted for instructions immediately after documenting a thorough history of any chemicals the eye has been exposed to. Follow office policy for referral to an ophthalmologist.

Etiology

Abrasions may be caused by foreign bodies trapped between the cornea and the eyelid; by direct trauma to the cornea, such as being poked by a fingernail; or by the wearing of contact lenses that are scratched or poorly cleaned. Poorly fitting contact lenses can also cause corneal abrasions. If abrasions are not treated promptly, an ulcer can develop. A corneal ulcer is always a serious problem, and the patient should be referred to an ophthalmologist immediately in such cases.

Diagnosis

The diagnosis is confirmed by the presence of characteristic symptoms as well as by a visual examination of the patient. Corneal abrasions and ulcerations stain with fluorescein, which makes them readily detectable. In addition, corneal ulcers also demonstrate an opaque area on the cornea that represents the infiltration of immune cells.

Treatment

If a foreign body is present, it must be removed promptly to prevent further ulceration and infection. In cases of corneal abrasion, an ophthalmic antibiotic ointment or drops are often prescribed to prevent a secondary infection. Application of an eye dressing may be needed to promote healing if an abrasion is present. The dressing reduces the movement of the cornea against the eyelid. Corneal ulcers need to be treated with intensive broad-spectrum antibiotic therapy immediately.

Prognosis

Most corneal abrasions heal spontaneously. Early treatment of corneal ulcers results in healing and regeneration of tissue.

Complications can include secondary infection and scarring of tissue that may necessitate corneal transplantation.

Prevention

Abrasions can be prevented by wearing protective eyewear while working in hazardous situations. Occupations that involve working with metal, wood, or even yard work can lead to small particles getting into the eyes which is prevented by protective eyewear. Avoiding engaging in sports that might put a person at risk for ocular injuries and overnight wear of contact lenses can help prevent the development of corneal ulcers.

Patient Teaching

Teach the patient the proper care of an eye dressing and the technique for instilling ophthalmic ointment and eye drops, as prescribed; emphasize the importance of hand washing before performing the procedure. Stress the importance of keeping follow-up appointments to monitor the treatment of corneal ulcers. Contact lenses should be avoided during healing until the provider has given approval for contact lens use.

◆ ENRICHMENT

Spontaneous Subconjunctival Hemorrhage

A spontaneous subconjunctival hemorrhage is the result of a small blood vessel rupturing underneath the surface of the conjunctiva. All or a portion of the white part of the eye (sclera) appears bright red (Fig. 5.12). This event is usually painless and observed when looking in the mirror. It can be the result of an episode of violent sneezing or severe coughing, vomiting, straining. It also may be the result of trauma to the eye. Often the cause cannot be determined. The condition usually resolves spontaneously within 10 days to 2 weeks.

• **Fig. 5.12** Subconjunctival hemorrhage. (From Stein HA, Stein RM, Freeman MI: *The ophthalmic assistant: a text for allied and associated ophthalmic personnel*, ed 10, St Louis, 2018, Elsevier.)

Episcleritis/Scleritis

Description

Inflammation of the episclera (the external surface of the sclera) is called *episcleritis*; inflammation of the deeper sclera, the white outermost covering of the eyeball, is called *scleritis*. Episcleritis occurs far more commonly than scleritis.

ICD-10-CM Code	H15.009 *(Unspecified scleritis, unspecified eye)* (H15.001–H15.099 = 28 codes of specificity) H15.109 *(Unspecified episcleritis, unspecified eye)* (H15.101–H15.129 = 12 codes of specificity)

Refer to the physician's diagnosis and then to the current edition of the ICD-10-CM coding manual to ensure the greatest specificity of pathology.

Symptoms and Signs

Episcleritis usually affects only one eye and presents as swelling, redness, and irritation in an isolated portion of the eye. Scleritis can affect either one or both eyes; symptoms include intense redness in one or more areas of the sclera and are more commonly associated with pain and blurred vision. Inflammation can occur in the posterior portion of the eye, which may cause some loss of vision. If scleritis is left untreated, perforation of the globe and loss of the eye are possible outcomes.

Patient Screening

Eye pain and redness indicate the need for an ophthalmic examination as soon as possible.

Etiology

The cause of episcleritis is unknown. Scleritis, however, is often associated with autoimmune disorders, such as rheumatoid arthritis, and certain digestive disorders, including Crohn disease or ulcerative colitis.

Diagnosis

The patient should see an ophthalmologist as soon as possible if symptoms develop. Blood tests may be necessary to determine any underlying causes. Diagnostic evaluation may include ultrasonography, magnetic resonance imaging (MRI), or both to identify infectious or autoimmune connective tissue disease.

Treatment

Episcleritis and mild cases of scleritis usually respond well to the instillation of topical corticosteroid eye drops. Artificial tears and lubricating ophthalmic ointments may be used for palliative relief. Oral nonsteroidal antiinflammatory drug (NSAID) medications may also be used to reduce inflammation. For severe cases, immunosuppressive drugs may be prescribed. Perforation of the sclera, which is rare, necessitates surgical repair called *scleroplasty*.

Prognosis
The prognosis is good for mild cases.

Prevention
No method of prevention is known.

Patient Teaching
Teach the patient the proper technique for instilling ophthalmic ointment and eye drops as prescribed; emphasize the importance of hand washing before performing the procedure. If surgery is required, use visual aids to describe the anatomy of the eye to the patient, and explain the surgical repair procedure. Describe the postoperative regimen and stress the importance of follow-up care.

Cataract

Description
Cataract is the opacification of the natural lens of the eye.

ICD-10-CM Code	H26.9 *(Unspecified cataract)*
	(H25.011–H26.9 = 92 codes of specificity)

Additional digits are required. Refer to the physician's diagnosis and then to the current edition of the ICD-10-CM coding manual to ensure the greatest specificity of pathology.

Symptoms and Signs

Cataracts usually develop slowly and gradually reduce visual acuity. The primary symptom is the deterioration of vision in the affected eye. The patient may report poor night vision, yellowing or fading of colors, loss of brightness of color, and the need for bright light for reading. In advanced cases, the cataract may become readily visible, giving the pupil a white, opaque appearance and blocking light, thereby impairing vision (Fig. 5.13).

• **Fig. 5.13** Cataract. (From Black JM, Hawks JH, Keene AM: *Medical-surgical nursing: clinical management for positive outcomes*, ed 8, Philadelphia, 2009, Saunders. Courtesy Ophthalmic Photography, University of Michigan WK Kellogg Eye Center, Ann Arbor, MI.)

Patient Screening
Cataracts are often noted during a routine ophthalmic examination. Patients reporting changes in visual acuity and/or glare should be given the first available appointment for an ophthalmic examination. Follow office policy for referral to an ophthalmologist. Many patients are of the aging population, but cataracts can also develop in some younger patients.

Etiology
The most common cause of cataracts is opacification of the lens caused by the aging process, and in the United States, the condition is present in about 50% of persons aged greater than 75 years. According to the National Eye Institute, "the risk of cataract increases with each decade of life starting around age 40. By age 75, half of white Americans have cataracts." The numbers vary from one ethnic group to another.

Cataracts may be congenital, result from ocular trauma, drug toxicity (prolonged high-dose corticosteroid administration), or systemic diseases, such as diabetes mellitus, or as a complication of other ocular diseases. Long-term, unprotected exposure to sunlight is considered causative as well.

Diagnosis
Examination by an ophthalmologist should be considered if vision becomes distorted or seems to be deteriorating. Ophthalmoscopy, with dilation of the eye and a slit-lamp examination, confirms the presence of a cataract.

Treatment
Treatment depends on the amount of visual impairment and the age, health, and occupation of the patient. Surgery is advised when the cataracts begin to interfere with the lifestyle of the patient. The most common method of removing a cataract is phacoemulsification. In extracapsular surgery, the nucleus, or center, of the cataract is removed in one piece. This necessitates a larger incision and more sutures. With phacoemulsification, an ultrasonic probe vibrates to break up the cataract, which subsequently is aspirated through the small incision. With this method, often no sutures are required for wound closure.

In both extracapsular cataract extraction and phacoemulsification, the posterior capsule of the lens is left in place. This membrane helps support an artificial lens, which is placed into the eye after removal of the cataract. Often the posterior membrane becomes cloudy after surgery, and this again reduces visual acuity. If this does occur, a laser can be used to make an opening in the center of the cloudy membrane, thus immediately restoring good vision. This outpatient procedure is called *YAG capsulotomy* and entails local anesthesia.

Prognosis
After cataract surgery, the patient will need a change in eyeglass prescription. Cataract surgery currently is quite successful; however, as with all surgery, significant complications are possible, especially when other ocular diseases exist.

Prevention

Cataracts are primarily associated with the aging process, and no method of prevention is known. It is prudent for patients and physicians to consider the risk of cataracts associated with drug toxicity from certain medications.

Patient Teaching

Explain the preoperative tests and medications that are prescribed. Emphasize the importance of hand washing before performing the procedure. Give the patient written instructions regarding the technique for instilling eye drops and all other medications, how to apply the eye shield carefully, and any limitation of activities during recovery. Stress the importance of regular follow-up visits.

Glaucoma

Description

Glaucoma is damage to the optic nerve in the presence of elevated IOP. Glaucoma is one of the major causes of blindness.

ICD-10-CM Code	H40.9 *(Unspecified glaucoma)* (H40.0–H42 = 67 codes of specificity)

Additional digits are required. Refer to the physician's diagnosis and then to the current edition of the ICD-10-CM coding manual to ensure the greatest specificity of pathology.

Glaucoma is one of the major causes of blindness. It is more common in patients older than 60 years of age; however, it can occur at any age. The ciliary body in the eye continually produces a fluid called *aqueous humor*. This fluid circulates freely between the posterior and anterior chambers of the eye and passes through the trabecular meshwork and drains into the general circulation. Several different pathologic causes and abnormalities in fluid drainage lead to glaucoma. Risk factors include age greater than 60 years, nearsightedness, blood relatives with glaucoma, and African American descent.

The many types of glaucoma include chronic open-angle, acute angle-closure, secondary, and congenital (Fig. 5.14). Secondary glaucoma results from a specific disease in the eye and can occur after trauma or neovascularization in the anterior chamber and may occur after diabetes. Infantile glaucoma or congenital glaucoma causes the eye to distend. (Fig. 5.15).

Patient Screening

Encourage patients, especially those with the risk factors listed earlier, to have regular ophthalmic examinations and appropriate testing. Patients reporting the onset of headaches, changes in visual acuity, photophobia, nausea and vomiting, and/or eye pain need to see their ophthalmologist immediately; their condition should be treated as an emergency.

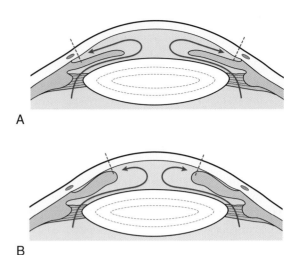

A

B

• **Fig. 5.14** Glaucoma. (A) In open-angle glaucoma the obstruction occurs in the trabecular meshwork. (B) In closed-angle glaucoma the trabecular meshwork is covered by the root of the iris or adhesions between the iris and the cornea. (From Damjanov I: *Pathology for the health-related professions*, ed 4, St Louis, 2011, Saunders.)

• **Fig. 5.15** Congenital glaucoma. Note enlargement of the eyes. (From Krachmer JH, Palay D. *Cornea atlas*, ed 3, Philadelphia, 2014, Elsevier.)

Chronic Open-Angle Glaucoma

ICD-10-CM Code	H40.10 *(Unspecified open-angle glaucoma)*

Refer to the physician's diagnosis and then to the current edition of the ICD-10-CM coding manual to ensure the greatest specificity of pathology.

Symptoms and Signs. Chronic open-angle glaucoma, a silent disease, is the most common form of glaucoma and is the most treatable cause of blindness. Patients can have open-angle glaucoma for a significant period before symptoms appear. By the time symptoms do appear, considerable damage usually has occurred. The best way to detect glaucoma is by having periodic routine ophthalmic examinations, which include IOP readings and optic nerve evaluations. If the IOP is somewhat elevated or the optic nerve shows signs of enlarging, glaucoma needs to be considered as a possibility. If chronic open-angle glaucoma goes untreated, the patient experiences characteristic loss of vision. The central vision may remain clear for a considerable period. However, if the condition progresses, the central vision is also lost, causing complete blindness.

Etiology. In chronic open-angle glaucoma, a block at the level of the trabecular meshwork impairs aqueous humor reabsorption. Chronic open-angle glaucoma can occur secondary to trauma, even years later. Overuse of topical steroids also can cause the condition. Risk factors include family history, the aging process, diabetes mellitus, ocular trauma, and obesity. Among blacks, glaucoma is the leading cause of blindness.

Diagnosis. The diagnosis of open-angle glaucoma is determined by patient history, ophthalmic examination with tonometry, examination of the optic nerves, and visual field analysis.

Treatment. Early treatment of glaucoma is essential; if not treated promptly, the disease can lead to blindness, because any vision lost as a result of the disease generally cannot be regained. This condition usually is treated with medication to decrease the production of aqueous humor (carbonic anhydrase inhibitors, beta-blockers, and alpha-adrenergic agents) or increased uveoscleral outflow (prostaglandin analogues). Different types of laser treatment, including argon laser trabeculoplasty and selective laser trabeculoplasty, also can be beneficial in opening the drainage system; occasionally, trabeculectomy or drainage implantation is necessary to bypass the drainage system. Fortunately, most of the time, chronic open-angle glaucoma can be controlled with eye drops.

> **NOTE**
> Beta-blockers used in glaucoma treatment can cause a rise in blood levels as the beta-blockers are absorbed through the tear duct. Eye drops in this class have been shown to affect heart rate and blood pressure and worsen symptoms of asthma. Beta-blockers are contraindicated in patients who suffer from heart failure.

Acute Angle-Closure Glaucoma

ICD-10-CM Code	H40.20 (Unspecified primary angle-closure glaucoma)

Refer to the physician's diagnosis and then to the current edition of the ICD-10-CM coding manual to ensure the greatest specificity of pathology.

Symptoms and Signs. Acute angle-closure glaucoma usually is associated with blurred vision, severe eye pain, headaches, and redness of the eye. The patient becomes photophobic and sees "halos" around light. With the full attack of acute glaucoma, the symptoms persist and become worse. Often severe pain develops and is associated with nausea and vomiting. The cornea of the eye becomes hazy because of the elevated pressure. The elevation of pressure in

acute angle-closure glaucoma is usually significantly higher than that associated with chronic open-angle (simple) glaucoma. If acute angle-closure glaucoma is left untreated, the patient can lose his or her vision.

Etiology. In acute angle-closure glaucoma, the mouth or opening of the drainage system is narrow and can close completely, causing a substantial increase in the IOP during a short time.

Diagnosis. The diagnosis is made on the basis of the patient's history and a notable increase in the IOP. With a special lens called a goniolens, the ophthalmologist can directly view the opening of the drainage system to determine whether it is open or closed. The eye is usually red, and the cornea can be hazy.

Treatment. The treatment of acute angle-closure glaucoma is primarily laser peripheral iridotomy, which creates a small opening in the iris, allowing the filtering angle to open. Often, the IOP is lowered with medication before the laser treatment. However, the definitive treatment of angle-closure glaucoma is virtually always a laser iridotomy.

Prognosis. The prognosis depends on the type of glaucoma, how early the condition is recognized and treatment is begun, and patient compliance with therapeutic regimens. Untreated glaucoma is a major cause of blindness.

Prevention. Regular ophthalmic examinations with testing appropriate to age and avoiding eye injury by wearing protective eyewear are recommended. Understanding family eye history and using eye drops accurately when prescribed are also important.

Patient Teaching. Explain the type of glaucoma and the treatment regimen. Teach the patient the proper technique for instilling ophthalmic ointment and eye drops as prescribed; emphasize the importance of hand washing before performing the procedure. Review the symptoms and signs that should be reported to the physician: severe eye pain, headache, blurred vision, halos, nausea, and vomiting. Stress the importance of good compliance with the medication regimen and follow-up care. Provide referrals for support services.

Macular Degeneration

Description
Macular degeneration is progressive deterioration or breakdown of the macula of the retina.

ICD-10-CM Code	H35.30 (Unspecified macular degeneration [age related]) (H35.30–H35.389 = 24 codes of specificity)

Refer to the physician's diagnosis and then to the current edition of the ICD-10-CM coding manual to ensure the greatest specificity of pathology.

Symptoms and Signs
The area of the retina near the optic nerve in the center of the field of vision that defines fine details is known as the

macula lutea. An early symptom of macular degeneration may be a mild distortion of central vision. As the condition progresses, the patient may describe seeing wavy lines when looking at lines that are straight and/or seeing semiopaque spots in the visual field. The condition is usually painless, develops slowly, and does not affect the peripheral vision. In most cases, both eyes are affected, either at the same time or one right after the other. As the condition worsens, reading and activities that require sharp vision become impossible. Age-related macular degeneration (AMD) is responsible for loss of central vision, which can impact a patient in many different ways, including their independence.

Patient Screening

Macular degeneration is often considered to be age related; therefore the mature adult is encouraged to have regular ophthalmic examinations. Patients reporting changes in visual acuity or loss of sharpness in central vision are scheduled for a prompt ophthalmic examination. Follow office policy for referral to an ophthalmologist.

Etiology

Age, genetic factors, and prolonged exposure to bright light are all causative factors. Macular degeneration usually is caused by degenerative changes in the pigment epithelium of the retina. Atrophic changes in the macula constitute dry macular degeneration; this is the more common type. The presence of abnormal fragile and hemorrhage-prone blood vessels can develop behind the macula and convert the disease to its wet form. Hemorrhage may occur when these abnormal vessels break and damage the retina. The result is loss of central vision. Smoking, hypertension, eating a diet high in saturated fats, and people over 50 years old are at higher risk for macular degeneration. There are patients who also are described as having geographic atrophy (GA). Geographic atrophy is used to describe the dry form of macular degeneration when it has progressed to the latest stage.

Diagnosis

The diagnosis of macular degeneration is made by an opthalmologist after a thorough examination with dilation. In nonexudative or dry macular degeneration, pigmentary changes are seen in the macular area, and drusen deposits are evident (Fig. 5.16A). In cases suspicious for wet macular degeneration, fluorescein angiography detects the presence and leakage of abnormal blood vessels.

Treatment

No definitive medical cure is known; however, a recent study has shown that vitamin supplements, especially vitamins C and E, beta-carotene, and zinc, can help slow the deterioration of moderate dry macular degeneration. Geographic atrophy can now be treated with the drug Pegcetacoplan (Syofovre). This is an injection that slows the progression of the disease. It is administered either every 2 months or each month. This is the first FDA-approved

• **Fig. 5.16** (A) The black arrows point to the drusen bodies in the image. Drusen bodies. (B) Handheld magnifier. (C) Amsler grid showing visual changes. (A, From Seidel HM, et al.: *Mosby's guide to physical examination*, ed 7, St Louis, 2011, Mosby. Courtesy Dr. Robert P. Murphy. B, Courtesy Eschenbach Optik, http://www.eschenbach.com. C, From Harding M, et al.: *Lewis's medical-surgical nursing*, ed 11, St. Louis, 2020, Elsevier.)

medication treatment. The wet form of this disease may be treated with traditional laser photocoagulation, photodynamic laser therapy, or the injection of antiangiogenic factors. Intraocular injection with an anti–vascular endothelial growth factor has become standard for the treatment of wet AMD. Clinical trials and new technology are providing new information that is being used to direct changes in the way the disease is being managed. Visual aids, such as handheld magnifiers (see Fig. 5.16B) and closed-circuit television, also may be beneficial. The patient is given an Amsler grid for home monitoring of visual changes that need to be reported (see Fig. 5.16C).

Prognosis

No cure is known, and the success of treatment has been limited; however, new treatment methods will hopefully provide a more positive prognosis in the future.

Prevention

The signs of early macular degeneration (tiny drusen) can be seen by the ophthalmologist during an eye examination before the patient is symptomatic. Taking a vitamin therapy called *AREDS 2* and protecting the eyes from ultraviolet rays and bright light are considered prudent measures. Smoking has been suggested to be a risk factor.

Patient Teaching

Patients benefit from an explanation of why their vision and depth perception have changed and how they can use visual aids to improve vision. Explain and demonstrate the use of the Amsler grid for home monitoring and when to call the physician. The patient's family should also be included in patient teaching, and simulation glasses may be helpful in educating the patient's family members on exactly what their family member sees. Driving will become difficult resulting in loss of some independence.

Diabetic Retinopathy

Description

Diabetic **retinopathy** is pathologic alterations of the retinal blood vessels and the pathologic proliferation of retinal vessels.

ICD-10-CM Code	E13.319 *(Other specified diabetes mellitus with unspecified diabetic retinopathy without macular edema)*
	E11.311 *(Type 2 diabetes mellitus with unspecified diabetic retinopathy with macular edema)*
	E11.36 *(Type 2 diabetes mellitus with diabetic cataract)*
	E11.39 *(Type 2 diabetes mellitus with other diabetic ophthalmic complications)*
	(E11.31–E11.39 = 12 codes of specificity)

Refer to the physician's diagnosis and then to the current edition of the ICD-10-CM coding manual to ensure the greatest specificity of pathology.

Symptoms and Signs

Diabetic retinopathy is characterized by microaneurysm, hemorrhages, dilation of retinal veins, macular edema, and the formation of abnormal new vessels (neovascularization). This condition usually occurs in both eyes, affecting the sharpness and clarity of vision. Diabetic retinopathy is a major cause of acquired blindness in the United States.

Patient Screening

The patient with diabetes is encouraged to have frequent ophthalmic examinations, at least annually. Any sudden change in visual acuity is to be reported to the primary care physician and the ophthalmologist immediately. The

• **Fig. 5.17** Diabetic retinopathy. (A) Nonproliferative retinopathy shows edema, microaneurysm, and exudates. (B) Proliferative retinopathy shows new blood vessel formation. (From Damjanov I: *Pathology for the health-related professions*, ed 4, St Louis, 2011, Saunders.)

RetinaVue is a handheld device that makes images of the retina. Many providers are now screening patients in the medical office and referring them to the ophthalmologist when this test identifies irregular images. This has been particularly helpful in populations of patients with diabetes who are not seeing their eye doctors for regular examinations as needed. Referrals are made from the health care provider's office, and patients follow up with the specialists.

Etiology

Diabetic retinopathy usually occurs a few years after the onset of diabetes mellitus. It occurs most often in those with diabetes who do not control their blood glucose levels, but all persons with diabetes are susceptible. Diabetes causes poor circulation in the retinal blood vessels and may cause leakage of exudate into the retina. Sometimes fragile new blood vessels (neovascularization) can grow and lead to leakage of blood into the vitreous humor. This may greatly reduce vision. In some cases, the blood is reabsorbed by the choroid; however, persistent vitreous hemorrhage necessitates surgical intervention (Fig. 5.17). There are four stages of this type of eye disorder, each one being progressively worse than the other. Mild nonproliferative, moderate nonproliferative, severe nonproliferative, and proliferative. Proliferative diabetic retinopathy can result in retinal detachment and permanent blindness.

Diagnosis

Complete ophthalmoscopic examination detects the retinal effects of diabetes.

Treatment

In mild cases, the patient may be monitored closely before treatment begins. Treatment with laser photocoagulation may be effective in controlling retinopathy. Panretinal photocoagulation may also be used. Shrinking and scarring of the abnormal vessels occur with this scatter laser treatment. The condition has a tendency to recur, but with treatment and tight control of blood sugar, vision often may be maintained. Medications such as Vabysmo (faricimab-svoa), Lucentis (ranibizumab), and Eylea (aflibercept) may also be used to inhibit the growth of blood vessels and reduce fluid buildup in the eye. These medications are administered using topical anesthesia and are injected into the vitreous of the eye. In cases of vitreous hemorrhage or proliferative disease, a vitrectomy may be necessary. Intravitreal steroid injection is also beneficial.

Prognosis

Diabetic retinopathy can be controlled with treatment; however, the prognosis is guarded.

Prevention

Maintaining blood glucose control can prevent the onset of diabetic retinopathy and can prevent any existing retinopathy from becoming worse.

Patient Teaching

Stress the importance of good diabetic care, especially good blood glucose control, to help prevent the complications of diabetic retinopathy and possible loss of vision.

Retinal Detachment

Description

Retinal detachment is the elevation (separation) of the retina from the choroid (Fig. 5.18).

ICD-10-CM Code	H33.20 (Serous retinal detachment, unspecified eye) (H33.20–H33.23 = 4 codes of specificity)

Refer to the physician's diagnosis and then to the current edition of the ICD-10-CM coding manual to ensure the greatest specificity of pathology.

Symptoms and Signs

Retinal detachment may be partial or complete and usually is associated with a retinal tear or a hole in the retina (Fig. 5.19). Early symptoms of detachment consist of the patient seeing many new floaters and light flashes. This persists and worsens and is followed by seeing a dark shadow that extends from the periphery inward. This may begin in any

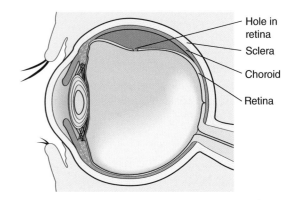

• **Fig. 5.18** Retinal detachment.

• **Fig. 5.19** Large retinal tear with associated retinal detachment. (From Kanski J, Bowling B: *Clinical ophthalmology—a systematic approach*, ed 7, Edinburgh, 2011, Saunders.)

of the visual fields. If the detachment extends to the central retina, the central vision also is blocked. The detachment often happens suddenly and without pain (Fig. 5.20).

Patient Screening

The patient reporting symptoms should be seen immediately for a dilated examination. They may describe a "wavelike pattern" in their visual field. This is a serious condition and the patient needs an evaluation as soon as possible.

Etiology

Certain retinal detachments are commonly associated with severe diabetic retinopathy. People who are extremely nearsighted are more susceptible to retinal detachments compared with the general population. Ocular trauma or retinal atrophy also can predispose a person to retinal detachment. A retinal detachment usually begins with a tear in the retina. Fluid then leaks under the retina and separates it from the choroid. After the retina is separated from the choroid, that portion of the retina no longer functions visually. As the retina continues to detach, more and more vision is lost.

• **Fig. 5.20** Retinal detachment. Folding of the retina, which is in focus anteriorly. (From Stein HA, Stein RM, Freeman MI: *The ophthalmic assistant: a text for allied and associated ophthalmic personnel*, ed 10, St Louis, 2018, Elsevier.)

Diagnosis

An ophthalmoscopic examination readily reveals the retinal detachment.

Treatment

Early treatment is advised; intervention is imperative. Treatment of a retinal detachment consists of either photocoagulation or surgery. This should be done without delay to prevent additional portions of the retina from detaching. If the detachment has extended to the macula, the central retina, permanent reduction in central acuity often occurs. Photocoagulation or cryotherapy can be used to treat retinal tears if no significant detachment occurs. Photocoagulation is a relatively simple procedure, which can be used to seal retinal tears before the development of retinal detachment. Early diagnosis is important in such cases. The treatment may include a period of bed rest.

Prognosis

Irreversible blindness can result from untreated retinal detachment.

Prevention

No specific method of prevention is known; however, preventing eye injury can be accomplished by wearing safety glasses or goggles to prevent cases resulting from eye trauma.

Patient Teaching

Use visual aids to explain the condition and the treatment to the patient. Prepare the patient for postsurgical procedures and treatments, including instruction on wearing a protective patch over the eye, taking pain medications, and executing measures to prevent raising IOP. Explain the importance of bed rest, if ordered. Teach the patient the proper technique for instilling ophthalmic ointment and eye drops as prescribed.

Uveitis

Description

Uveitis denotes inflammation of the uveal tract, including the iris, ciliary body, and choroid.

ICD-10-CM Code	H20.9 (*Unspecified iridocyclitis*)

Refer to the physician's diagnosis and then to the current edition of the ICD-10-CM coding manual to ensure the greatest specificity of pathology.

Symptoms and Signs

Uveitis may be either unilateral or bilateral. Pain, photophobia, blurred vision, and redness can occur. The photophobia is often pronounced.

Patient Screening

Having a complete ophthalmic examination performed as soon as possible is necessary for a patient experiencing the symptoms mentioned earlier. Follow office policy for referral to an ophthalmologist.

Etiology

Uveitis can be associated with autoimmune disorders such as juvenile rheumatoid arthritis and ankylosing spondylitis. Infections and injury can also cause uveitis. Often an exact cause for uveitis cannot be determined.

Diagnosis

A complete examination with the slit lamp is necessary for the diagnosis to be made. To detect some forms of disease, skin tests for tuberculosis, toxoplasmosis, and histoplasmosis may be needed. Certain blood tests also may aid in confirming the diagnosis.

Treatment

Treatment is specific to the type of uveitis and largely consists of topical or, in severe cases, systemic steroid use. Any underlying cause should be treated. Cycloplegic agents that cause paralysis of the ciliary muscle are often beneficial in reducing the pain associated with ciliary inflammation.

Prognosis

The prognosis is variable, depending on the clinical type and the underlying cause.

Prevention

No method of prevention is known.

Patient Teaching

Use visual aids to demonstrate what structure(s) of the eyes are involved in the inflammation. Explain the medical treatment. Teach the patient the proper technique for instilling ophthalmic ointment and eye drops as prescribed;

emphasize the importance of hand washing before performing the procedure.

Exophthalmos

Description
Exophthalmos is an abnormal protrusion or projection of the eyeballs.

ICD-10-CM Code	H05.20 *(Unspecified exophthalmos)* (H05.20, H05.241–H05.269 = 13 codes of specificity) Q15.8 *(Other specified congenital malformations of eye)* (Q15.0–Q15.9 = 3 codes of specificity)

Refer to the physician's diagnosis and then to the current edition of the ICD-10-CM coding manual to ensure the greatest specificity of pathology.

Symptoms and Signs
Exophthalmos exposes an abnormally large amount of the anterior eye. Patients report dryness and a gritty feeling in the affected eye or eyes. They also may note double vision and eye movement restriction. In severe cases, vision becomes seriously blurred.

Patient Screening
Schedule a prompt appointment for a complete medical evaluation and ophthalmic examination. Laboratory tests may be performed at these visits. Follow office policy for referral to an ophthalmologist.

Etiology
Exophthalmos is caused by multiple factors, including enlarged extraocular muscles, retrobulbar mass, or edema of the soft tissue that lines the bony orbit of the eye. This condition may be associated with hyperthyroid, hypothyroid, or euthyroid (normal thyroid) status (see the Hyperthyroidism section in Chapter 4). Sudden unilateral onset is usually a sign of retrobulbar hemorrhage or inflammation.

Diagnosis
To determine the underlying cause, a complete ophthalmic examination, blood tests, radiographic studies, computed tomography (CT), and echography are performed.

Treatment
The diagnosis determines the therapy. If the condition is caused by hyperthyroidism, the underlying disorder needs to be corrected. Severe cases may require surgical decompression of the orbit, and systemic steroids are beneficial in controlling edema.

Prognosis
The prognosis depends on the successful treatment of the underlying cause.

Prevention
No method of prevention is known.

Patient Teaching
Explain how exophthalmos relates to the underlying cause as diagnosed. Explain the purpose and dosage schedule of prescribed medication. Give emotional support, because the patient is likely to be distressed by the cosmetic effect of "bulging eyeballs."

Cancer of the Eye

Description
Cancer of the eye may involve the globe (ocular tumors), the orbit (the bone surrounding the orbital cavity and the soft tissues and muscles that lie between the globe and the bone), the optic nerve, or the eyelids. Neoplasms may be benign, malignant, or metastatic from another location (secondary tumors).

ICD-10-CM Code	C69 *(Malignant neoplasm of eye and adnexa)* (C69.00–C69.92 = 27 codes of specificity)

Neoplasms of the eye must be specified for location and type. Therefore it is not possible to list all applicable ICD-10-CM codes for neoplasms of the eye. Refer to the physician's diagnosis and then to the current edition of the ICD-10-CM coding manual to ensure the greatest specificity of pathology.

Symptoms and Signs
Tumors of the eyelid generally present as visible lesions (see Chapter 6 for a discussion of basal cell carcinoma [BCC], squamous cell carcinoma [SCC], and malignant melanoma lesions). Seborrheic keratosis presents as a skin tag (skin projection) on the eyelid. Ocular melanoma may present as a growing pigmented spot on the iris. Secondary eye tumors are usually associated with pain, which distinguishes them from most primary eye cancers.

Patient Screening
Patients reporting visible lesions around or "in" the eye, or those experiencing any unusual appearance or movement of the eye(s), with or without pain, need a timely appointment for a medical evaluation and an ophthalmic examination. In addition, infants and young children should be evaluated for leukokoria (white pupil) and strabismus at well-child examinations and referred urgently to an ophthalmologist, if noted.

Etiology
Ocular tumors include retinoblastoma, the most common primary malignancy of the eye in children, representing 2% of all childhood cancers (Fig. 5.21), and ocular (or

• **Fig. 5.21** Retinoblastoma. (From Michelson JB, Friedlaender MH: *The eye in clinical medicine*, London, 1996, Times Mirror International.)

uveal tract) melanoma and intraocular lymphoma, the most common ocular tumors in adults. Retinoblastoma is a neoplasm of the retina. Approximately 200 to 300 children are diagnosed each year. In approximately 40% of cases, it is due to an inheritable mutation on chromosome 13. Most cases of ocular melanoma are found in Caucasians. Orbital tumors are rarer and include rhabdomyosarcoma (malignant) and capillary hemangioma (benign) in children and cavernous hemangioma (benign) in adults.

Eyelid tumors include skin cancers (usually caused by sun exposure of the eyelid) and benign squamous papillomas (caused by human papillomavirus infection). BCC is the most common malignant eyelid tumor. Eyelid melanoma, on the other hand, accounts for only 1% of eyelid tumors. Optic pathway glioma is a low-grade tumor of the optic nerve that usually occurs in children under the age of 20 years. Approximately 3490 new cases of primary eye cancer occur each year, and 430 deaths result from this type of cancer. The most common tumor of the eye is cancer that has metastasized to the eye. The most common sites of origin are the lung in males and the breast in females, but many other types of cancer also are known to metastasize to the eye.

Diagnosis
The lesions of ocular melanoma may be first identified on routine eye examination, but ultrasound helps make the diagnosis. Eyelid tumors are diagnosed after a biopsy of the lesion. Other types of eye tumors may be seen on funduscopic examination and MRI. With or without a biopsy (depending on the tumor type and location), these are used for diagnosis and evaluation of the extent of disease. Additionally, CT and chest radiographs may be done for staging. Patients with retinoblastoma should have molecular genetic testing done in case they have a heritable form of the disease.

Treatment
Treatment may involve excision of the tumor, eyeball removal, radiation therapy, chemotherapy, proton therapy, or laser therapy. Proton therapy which uses protons rather than radiation, has fewer side effects than traditional radiation therapy. It is considered to be less toxic. Proton therapy is not available in all cities with only 43 regional facilities throughout the United States offering this method of treatment at the time of the authoring of this text due to the expense of equipment involved. Treatment of secondary eye cancer rarely improves patient survival, but chemotherapy or radiation therapy may be given for palliation of symptoms. Immunotherapy is another treatment.

Prognosis
Overall the 5-year survival rate for patients with primary eye neoplasms is generally good but largely depends on tumor type, size, and stage at diagnosis. There may be vision loss, depending on the treatment used.

Prevention
No methods of prevention are known for orbital and ocular eye tumors. Siblings and children of patients with retinoblastoma should have frequent evaluations by an ophthalmologist, because the disease can be hereditary. The skin neoplasms of the eyelid may be prevented by wearing sunglasses and wide-brimmed hats to reduce sun exposure to that area.

Patient Teaching
Information given to the patient is determined by the type of neoplasm, the treatment, and the prognosis. Patients, or the parents of children, benefit from clear explanations of all ongoing diagnostic and therapeutic procedures. In all cases, emotional support is imperative. Referral for genetic counseling is helpful for families of patients with the heritable form of retinoblastoma. Appropriate links to websites with accurate information for patient teaching are helpful to the patient and caregiver.

Disorders of the Ear

Functioning Organs of Hearing

The ear is the organ of balance and the organ of hearing. The ear is composed of three sections: the outer ear, the middle ear, and the inner ear (Fig. 5.22).

The outer section is made up of the external ear, also called the *pinna* or *auricle*, and the external auditory canal. The latter's function is to collect sound waves, or vibrations, from the air or environment and channel them to the tympanic membrane (eardrum), which then begins to vibrate.

The middle section contains the tympanic membrane and three ossicles (tiny bones) called the *malleus* (hammer), the *incus* (anvil), and the *stapes* (stirrup). Also in the middle ear is a canal, called the *eustachian tube*, which leads to a cavity (the pharynx) at the back of the nose. At the innermost

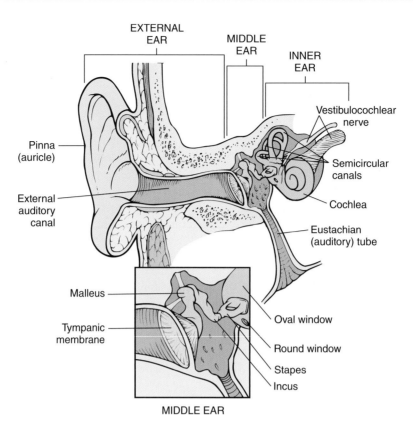

• **Fig. 5.22** Normal ear.

region of the middle ear is the oval window, the opening to the inner ear. The middle ear receives the sound waves from the vibrating eardrum and relays them along the three bones to the oval window (see Fig. 5.22).

The inner ear contains two membrane-lined chambers, each filled with fluid, called the *cochlea* and the labyrinth. The cochlea contains tiny hairs that change the sound waves in the fluid into nerve impulses, which then are transmitted to the brain via the auditory nerve. The labyrinth is responsible for maintaining balance. It consists of three connected tubes bent into half circles, called the *semicircular canals.* Their function is to detect movement of the head and relay this information to the brain.

Common symptoms of ear diseases and conditions that should receive attention from health care professionals include the following:

- Hearing loss
- Ear pain or pressure
- Tinnitus (ringing or buzzing noise)
- Vertigo (dizziness)
- Nausea and vomiting

Hearing loss or deafness is denoted by two basic types: conductive loss and sensorineural loss. Conductive deafness is caused by an impairment of the eardrum or bones in the middle ear, which conducts sound waves to the cochlea in the inner ear. Sensorineural deafness, or nerve deafness, results from impairment of the cochlea or the auditory nerve (see the Enrichment box about Cochlear Implants).

Central deafness results when the central nervous system (CNS) cannot interpret impulses because of a cerebrovascular accident or brain tumor.

Disorders of Conduction

Impacted Cerumen

Description

Impacted cerumen is an atypical accumulation of cerumen in the canal of the outer ear. The "earwax" that has accumulated hardens and has a tendency to prevent sound waves from reaching the tympanic membrane (eardrum), resulting in decreased hearing. Fig. 5.24A and B depicts a normal tympanic membrane and an ear canal occluded with cerumen.

ICD-10-CM Code	H61.23 *(Impacted cerumen, bilateral)* (H61.20–H61.23 = 4 codes of specificity)

Symptoms and Signs

The normal, soft, yellowish-brown, waxlike secretion produced by the glands of the external ear canal is called *cerumen,* or earwax. If this secretion accumulates excessively, gradual loss of hearing may occur, and the patient may feel that the ear is plugged and may experience tinnitus or

ENRICHMENT

Cochlear Implants

Individuals who experience severe sensorineural hearing loss that is not helped by hearing aids may have partial hearing restored by means of cochlear implants. Cochlear implants are electronic devices that use minute electrical currents to stimulate the auditory nerve and help the currents travel to the auditory cortex to be perceived as sound.

Cochlear implant systems are complex and include an electrode array, a receiver, a speech processor, a transmitting coil, and a microphone. The electrode array is placed surgically in the cochlea, and the receiver is implanted and fixed to the skull behind the mastoid bone. The surgical incision is allowed to heal for 4 to 6 weeks, after which the external components (the microphone, transmitting coil, and speech processor) are fitted to the patient. Fitting includes calibration of the transmitting coil and programming of the speech processor. Auditory and speech training are provided to the implant recipient.

Cochlear implants do not restore normal hearing; however, they can improve a deaf person's functioning in a hearing world. Candidates for the implants are selected carefully and should have severe to profound bilateral sensorineural hearing loss and be older than 2 years of age. Many still employ lip reading and American Sign Language as adjunct therapies to communicate.

An alternative implant device uses the principle of bone conduction to conduct sound waves to the inner ear. The bone conduction system is for individuals who experience conductive hearing loss, mixed, or single-sided hearing loss. Sound waves are transmitted to the inner ear by bone conduction bypassing outer or middle ear problems. A bone conduction system has an internal bone conduction implant (BCI) that is placed entirely subcutaneously. It contains a magnet to hold the externally placed audio processor above the BCI. The audio processor consists of a battery, microphones, and a digital processor. Fig. 5.23 shows cochlear implans.

• **Fig. 5.23** Cochlear implant. (From Patton KT, Thibodeau GA: *The human body in health & disease*, ed 6, St Louis, 2014, Elsevier.)

ALERT!

Ototoxicity

Ototoxicity occurs when a drug or chemical causes damage to CN VIII (acoustic nerve) or to the inner ear, resulting in temporary or permanent hearing loss or disturbances in balance. Symptoms and signs of ototoxicity usually have an insidious onset and include tinnitus, a feeling of fullness or pressure in the ears, hearing loss, vertigo, and occasionally nausea.

Drugs that can cause ototoxicity include salicylates (aspirin and aspirin-containing products); NSAIDs; certain antibiotics (aminoglycosides, erythromycin, and vancomycin); loop diuretics (furosemide [Lasix], bumetanide [Bumex], and ethacrynic acid [Edecrin]); chemotherapeutic agents (cisplatin, vincristine, and vinblastine); quinines (quinidine and quinine); and heavy metals, including mercury and lead.

The physician should be notified of any of the aforementioned symptoms when the individual is taking or going to receive any of the previously mentioned medications.

Discontinuing aspirin, aspirin-containing products, and NSAIDs often reverses the ototoxic effects of these drugs. None of the other drugs should be discontinued unless so ordered by the physician. Quinine ototoxicity, like aspirin-induced ototoxicity, can usually be reversed when the medication is stopped. Large dosages of antibiotics that may be ototoxic usually are administered in life-threatening situations.

Chemotherapeutic agents are monitored for any ototoxic side effects. In normal dosages, loop diuretics usually have very few ototoxic side effects; it is when they are given in massive doses for treatment of acute kidney failure or acute hypertension that ototoxicity may occur.

Environmental chemicals include butyl nitrite, carbon disulfide, hexane, styrene, toluene, trichloroethylene, and xylene, but they are not limited to these.

Once damage has occurred, it cannot be reversed. Hearing loss may be helped somewhat by hearing aids or cochlear implants. When the patient experiences loss of balance, physical therapy may be needed to help the patient regain the ability to balance.

• **Fig. 5.24** (A) Normal ear canal and tympanic membrane. (B) Cerumen impacted ear canal. (A, from Wareing MJ. Ear, nose, and throat. In: Glynn M, Drake WM, eds. *Hutchison's Clinical Methods*, ed 24, 2018, Elsevier; B, From Swartz MH. The ear and nose. In: Swartz MH. *Textbook of Physical Diagnosis: History and Examination*, ed 8, 2021, Elsevier.)

sometimes an earache (otalgia). Impacted cerumen is a common cause of conductive hearing loss.

Patient Screening

Individuals complaining of ear pain should be seen as soon as possible. Many times, the only complaint is one of reduced hearing levels. Schedule an appointment as soon as possible. Referral to an audiologist may be indicated. Awareness of the incidence of impacted cerumen may come about during a routine examination or during the course of an office visit for some other reason.

Etiology

Abnormal accumulation of cerumen can be caused by dryness and scaling of the skin or by excessive hair in the ear

canal. Some people have abnormally narrow ear canals, which may predispose them to this condition.

Diagnosis

The physician or specialist does an otologic examination, and the patient history of symptoms confirms the diagnosis.

Treatment

If impacted cerumen is found, it must be removed. If the cerumen adheres to the wall of the ear canal, it may have to be softened first with oily drops or hydrogen peroxide and then irrigated with water to accomplish the removal. Any hearing loss caused by the impaction is alleviated after removal of cerumen.

Prognosis

The prognosis for removal is positive. Hearing usually improves once the ear canal is clear of the impacted earwax. Recurrence is likely, so periodic examinations may be necessary.

Prevention

Prevention includes routine cleansing of the ear canal by the primary care physician or an ear care specialist. Other preventions include avoiding placing any object in the ear canal that may push the earwax down into the ear canal. The use of cotton-tipped applicators in the ear is often the cause of cerumen being packed into the ear canal.

Patient Teaching

Patient teaching involves reinforcement of not putting anything into the ear that would have the ability to push or pack the earwax down into the outer ear canal. Providing written information concerning proper ear care to the patient and family is helpful.

Infective Otitis Externa

Description

Inflammation of the external ear canal is called *otitis externa*. This condition is usually accompanied by an infectious process.

ICD-10-CM Code	H60.399 *(Other infective otitis externa, unspecified ear)*
	(H60.391–H60.399 = 4 codes of specificity)
	H60.00 *(Abscess of external ear, unspecified ear)*
	(H60.00–H60.03 = 4 codes of specificity)
	H60.10 *(Cellulitis of external ear, unspecified ear)*
	(H60.10–H60.13 = 4 codes of specificity)
	H60.319 *(Diffuse otitis externa, unspecified ear)*

(H60.311–H60.319 = 4 codes of
specificity)

H60.329 *(Hemorrhagic otitis externa,
unspecified ear)*

(H60.321–H60.329 = 4 codes of
specificity)

H60.399 *(Other infective otitis externa,
unspecified ear)*

(H60.391–H60.399 = 4 codes of
specificity)

*Designation by the physician of any special circumstances
determines the applicable code. Refer to the physician's
diagnosis and then to the current edition of the ICD-10-
CM coding manual to ensure the greatest specificity of
pathology.*

Symptoms and Signs

Severe pain; a red, swollen ear canal; hearing loss; fever; and
pruritus are common symptoms of otitis externa. Drainage
from the ear may be either watery or purulent.

Patient Screening

Individuals reporting pain in the ear accompanied by drainage require prompt attention.

Etiology

Accumulation of cerumen in the ear canal, when mixed with
water, acts as a culture medium for bacteria or fungi. Otitis
externa may also be caused by dermatologic conditions, such
as seborrhea and psoriasis. Trauma to the ear canal, caused by
attempts to clean or scratch inside the ear with a foreign object,
or frequent use of earphones and earplugs or hearing aids, can
predispose a person to the development of otitis externa.

Diagnosis

An otologic examination and a history of symptoms confirm the diagnosis. If a bacterial infection is suspected, a
culture of the material found in the canal may be needed to
determine how to properly treat the infection.

Treatment

The ear canal must be kept clean and free from water.
Antibiotic or steroid eardrops and systemic antibiotics may
be prescribed, depending on the severity. Otitis externa
tends to recur and can become chronic.

Prognosis

The prognosis is positive with treatment. Chronic otitis
externa may develop with repeated irritation by earphones,
earplugs, or hearing aids.

Prevention

Preventive measures include keeping the ear clean and dry.
It is important to also keep earphones, earbuds, and hearing

aids clean. Additionally, using another person's earphones
or earbuds is discouraged. Hearing aids or devices should be
cleaned according to the manufacturer's instructions.

Patient Teaching

Provide the patient or family with pictures of the anatomy
of the ear. Demonstrate how moisture trapped in the ear
by earphones, earplugs, or hearing aids can contribute to
infective otitis externa. Explain why sharing objects that are
placed in the ear may cause infective otitis externa.

Swimmer's Ear

Description

Inflammation and resulting infection of the outer ear canal
after water has been entrapped during swimming is termed
swimmer's ear.

ICD-10-CM   H60.339 *(Swimmer's ear,*
Code   *unspecified ear)*
            (H60.331–H60.339 = 4 codes of
            specificity)

Symptoms and Signs

Similar to infectious otitis externa, severe pain; a red, swollen ear canal; hearing loss; fever; and pruritus are common
symptoms of swimmer's ear. Any drainage from the ear may
be either watery or purulent. Typically, the onset of the condition occurs after the patient has been swimming.

Patient Screening

Individuals reporting pain in the ear accompanied by drainage require prompt attention.

Etiology

The accumulation of cerumen in the ear canal when mixed
with water, as during swimming, acts as a culture medium
for bacteria or fungi.

Diagnosis

An otologic examination and a history of symptoms confirm the diagnosis. If a bacterial infection is suspected, a
culture of the material found in the canal may be needed to
determine how to properly treat the infection.

Treatment

It is important that the ear canal be kept clean and dried after
swimming. Depending on the severity of the condition, antibiotic or steroid eardrops and systemic antibiotics may be prescribed. Swimmer's ear tends to recur and can become chronic
for those with repeated exposure to water, such as swimming.

Prognosis

The prognosis is positive with treatment. Swimmer's ear has
a tendency to recur with subsequent exposure to water during swimming or other water-related activities.

Prevention

Preventive measures include keeping the ear clean and dry. Earplugs may be used during water activities and swimming. Thorough drying of the ear canal after exposure to water is important.

Patient Teaching

Provide the patient or family with pictures of the anatomy of the ear. Demonstrate how moisture in the ear can contribute to swimmer's ear. Encourage compliance with any drug therapy prescribed and also report any symptoms of swimmer's ear as early as possible for treatment.

Otitis Media

Description

Otitis media is inflammation of the normally air-filled middle ear with the accumulation of fluid behind the tympanic membrane (eardrum), occurring either unilaterally or bilaterally.

ICD-10-CM Code	H65.90 *(Unspecified nonsuppurative otitis media, unspecified ear)* (H65.90–H65.93 = 4 codes of specificity) H66.009 *(Acute suppurative otitis media without spontaneous rupture of eardrum, unspecified ear)* (H66.001–H66.009 = 8 codes of specificity)

Refer to the physician's diagnosis and then to the current edition of the ICD-10-CM coding manual to ensure the greatest specificity of pathology.

Symptoms and Signs

Otitis media is the most common reason for visits to physicians by children and also can be experienced by adults.

Otitis media is classified as either serous or suppurative, according to the composition of the accumulating fluid. In serous (nonsuppurative) otitis media, the fluid is relatively clear and sterile. With suppurative otitis, the fluid is purulent. Symptoms vary according to the type. With serous otitis media, the only symptoms may be a feeling of fullness or pressure and some degree of impaired hearing. Suppurative otitis media, also referred to as *acute otitis media*, however, is painful and usually has sudden onset. General symptoms, such as infection, fever, chills, nausea, and vomiting, usually accompany this type. Children often rub or pull at the affected ear and lean the head sideways toward the affected side. Dizziness can be a symptom in either type. Muffled hearing may be present, or a significant loss of hearing may occur.

Patient Screening

The febrile individual or child experiencing ear pain and possible diminished hearing requires prompt assessment and pain relief. If it is not possible to see the patient the same day as the initial phone contact, refer the patient to another medical care facility where prompt assessment can be provided.

Etiology

Serous otitis media may be either acute or chronic. With acute serous otitis media (Fig. 5.25C), the cause is usually a virus from a URI that has spread through the eustachian tube into the middle ear. It can occur spontaneously or may result from an allergic reaction. Chronic otitis media can develop from an acute attack, hypertrophy of the adenoids, or chronic sinus infections. Suppurative otitis media is caused by bacteria, which also can enter the middle ear through the eustachian tube from the nose or throat or from a ruptured tympanic membrane. Variations in the normal structure of the eustachian tube can predispose a person to this disease. Often an allergic response is responsible for swelling of the eustachian tube and the resulting otitis media.

Diagnosis

Otoscopy reveals the presence of a fluid-filled middle ear. The normally pearl-gray eardrum is inflamed and may be bulging. Fluid bubbles may be visible through the membrane. If a culture of the fluid taken from the ear shows bacteria and the white blood cell count is elevated, suppurative otitis media is present. Audiometry may reveal mild to severe hearing loss. Measurement of the pressure in the middle ear with a tympanogram provides the physician with an estimation of how well the eustachian tube is functioning.

Treatment

Analgesics and decongestants may be ordered to provide pain relief and to promote drainage in both types of otitis media. Oral or topical antibiotics are ordered for cases of suppurative otitis media. In severe cases or in patients who fail to respond to medical treatment, surgical evacuation of the fluid (myringotomy) is necessary to prevent permanent hearing loss and the possible development of mastoiditis (see the Mastoiditis section) or a cholesteatoma (see the Cholesteatoma section). To keep the middle ear filled with air and to prevent fluid from accumulating, myringotomy tubes (Fig. 5.25D) may need to be inserted after the myringotomy (Fig. 5.26). Diagnosis and treatment of any allergic response involved is necessary. Removal of hypertrophic adenoids is a therapeutic measure.

Prognosis

Prognosis is positive with drug therapy. Otitis media often recurs; thus any indication of returning symptoms requires prompt attention. Surgical intervention, including placement of myringotomy tubes, usually helps promote a positive outcome. Identification of allergic-mediated responses and removal of enlarged adenoids is also helpful for a positive outcome.

• **Fig. 5.25** (A) Healthy tympanic membrane. (B) Tympanic membrane with cholesteatoma. (C) Tympanic membrane with acute otitis media. (D) Myringotomy with tympanostomy tube. (From Chabner D, *The language of medicine*, ed 13, 2025, Elsevier; A–C, Courtesy Richard A. Buckingham, Clinical Professor, Otolaryngology, Abraham Lincoln School of Medicine, University of Illinois, Chicago. From Barkauskas VH et al.: *Health and Physical assessment*, ed 3, St. Louis, 2002, Mosby; D, From Fireman P, Slavin RG: *Atlas of allergies*, ed 2, London, 1996, Glower Medical Publishing.)

Prevention

Prompt treatment of URI helps prevent the occurrence of otitis media. When the otitis is a result of an upper respiratory allergic reaction, diagnosis and control of the allergic response is helpful, as is the surgical removal of hypertrophied adenoids. A healthy diet can support the immune system. Avoiding secondhand smoke can help prevent ear infections.

Patient Teaching

If surgery is scheduled, provide patients and families with information regarding the care of the ear with myringotomy tubes in place. Stress the importance of drug therapy compliance and completion of the prescribed antibiotic regimen.

Otosclerosis

Description

Otosclerosis, an abnormal bone growth in the middle ear, primarily affects the stapes, the third bone or ossicle of the middle ear, as the individual ages. Movement of the ossicles is impaired, which causes diminished conduction of sound waves and resulting in hearing loss (Fig. 5.27).

ICD-10-CM Code   H80.93 *(Unspecified otosclerosis, bilateral)*
(H80.00-H80.93 = 20 codes of specificity)

Incision into
tympanic membrane

Placement
of tube with
forceps

Tube in place

• **Fig. 5.26** Myringotomy and insertion of a tympanoplast tube as a treatment for otitis media.

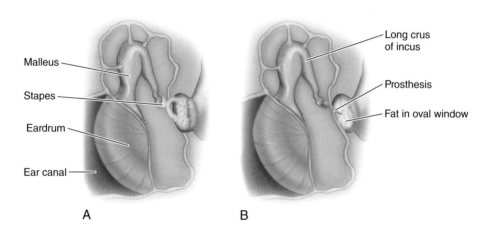

Malleus

Stapes

Eardrum

Ear canal

Long crus
of incus

Prosthesis

Fat in oval window

A

B

• **Fig. 5.27** Illustration of otosclerosis showing bones fusing. (A) Preintervention of otosclerosis. (B) Postintervention treatment for otosclerosis with prosthesis insertion. (From Black JM, Hawks JH: *Medical-surgical nursing: clinical management for positive outcomes*, ed 8, St Louis, 2009, Saunders.)

Designation by the physician of any special circumstances determines the applicable code. Refer to the physician's diagnosis and then to the current edition of the ICD-10-CM coding manual to ensure the greatest specificity of pathology.

Symptoms and Signs

With this condition, an abnormal growth of spongy bone forms around the oval window, causing ankylosis of the stapes, the third ossicle (small bone) in the middle ear.

Ankylosis produces conductive deafness because the ossicles cannot conduct the sound vibrations as they enter the ear. Symptoms of otosclerosis are tinnitus and a gradual hearing loss of low or soft sounds, which may be unilateral at first but usually affects both ears at some point. Patients usually report not being able to hear as well with the affected ear when talking on the telephone. Relatives may notice that patients turn their heads to hear well. Otosclerosis is a young person's disease, with onset usually beginning after puberty and before age 35 years.

Patient Screening

Individuals requesting an appointment for evaluation of decreased hearing are scheduled for the next available appointment that is convenient for them. It is important to realize that patients experiencing hearing loss may be anxious and worried.

Etiology

Otosclerosis is idiopathic, but genetic predisposition has been found to be a factor. The condition is more prevalent in femalesand can be aggravated by pregnancy.

Diagnosis

A diagnosis of otosclerosis is made by the physician using an audiogram, the patient's history, and an otoscopy. The audiogram shows moderate to severe hearing loss, especially in the low range.

Treatment

The only treatment that cures otosclerosis is a surgical procedure called *stapedectomy*. A stapedectomy involves the removal of the diseased stapes and replacement with a prosthesis. The composition of the prosthesis may be metal, ceramic, or plastic material. The use of ceramic or plastic is likely because these materials facilitate visualization with MRI for the purpose of diagnosing and because of the inability to perform an accurate test of the patient's hearing if the prosthesis is made of metal. If the condition is bilateral, only one ear is operated on at a time. Generally, hearing improves soon after the surgery. Stapedotomy can also be performed with a laser, which creates a hole in the stapes permitting placement of a prosthetic device. If surgery is not an option for the patient, a hearing aid may provide some improvement in hearing.

Prognosis

Surgical intervention usually has a positive outcome.

Prevention

Because this is an idiopathic condition, no method of prevention is known.

Patient Teaching

Provide patients and families with information concerning postsurgical care for surgical intervention. Assist patients and families in locating and contacting community support groups for those with diminished hearing.

Ménière Disease

Description

Ménière disease is a chronic disease of the inner ear that affects the labyrinth.

ICD-10-CM   H81.09 *(Ménière disease,*
Code   *unspecified ear)*

(H81.01–H81.09 = 4 codes of specificity)

There are specific codes for various states and sites of Ménière disease. Once the physician has established the pathologic evolvement of Ménière disease, refer to the physician's diagnosis and then to the current edition of the ICD-10-CM coding manual to ensure the greatest specificity of pathology.

Symptoms and Signs

Ménière disease is marked by a recurring syndrome of vertigo, tinnitus, progressive hearing loss, and a sensation of fullness or pressure in the affected ear. Symptoms have a sudden onset. Nausea, vomiting, tinnitus, sweating, and loss of balance can follow an acute attack of vertigo. Some individuals may be subjected to nystagmus, whereas others may experience an unusual sensitivity to noises (hyperacusis). These attacks can last from a few hours to several days and may become increasingly serious with each recurrence. Ménière disease usually affects just one ear, but both ears may become involved eventually. The disease usually manifests in individuals 40 to 60 years of age.

Patient Screening

Individuals reporting symptoms of vertigo, tinnitus, progressive hearing loss, and the sensation of fullness and pressure in the ear require prompt assessment and intervention. If an appointment time is not immediately available, refer the patient to an emergency facility for evaluation. Suggest that the patient not drive.

Etiology

The cause of this disease is unknown; however, the disease process seems to involve the destruction of the tiny hair cells inside the cochlea. Predisposing factors for Ménière disease are middle ear infections, head trauma, dysfunction in the autonomic nervous system, noise pollution, and premenstrual edema.

Diagnosis

The presence of four core symptoms (recurring vertigo, tinnitus, progressive hearing loss, and a sensation of fullness [aural fullness] in the ear) suggests the diagnosis of Ménière disease. Additional testing with audiometry; balance studies; radiographic studies, including MRI; and ENG may be necessary. Some of the tests which may be performed include Electrocochleograph, which is also used to measure inner ear fluid pressure. Rotary chair testing involves seeing how the inner ear works based on eye movement. Vestibular-evoked myogenic potentials testing involves using sound to cause parts of the inner ear to react or respond. Computerized dynamic posturography involves understanding which part of the balance system is used most. Electronystagmogram or videonystagmography (ENG or VNG) helps the provider to evaluate if there is an inner ear problem causing the dizziness. Video head impulse test determines if the inner ear and eyes work together the way they are supposed to, in addition to recording what the eyes do when sudden movement occurs.

Treatment

For acute attacks of Ménière disease, the physician usually prescribes medication to control the nausea, vomiting, and dizziness. Long-term treatment could include following a salt-free diet; restricting fluid intake; and using diuretics, meclizine, and mild sedatives. Limiting the amount of caffeine and alcohol in the diet and stopping smoking may be recommended. Patients are encouraged to avoid stressful situations if possible. If the disease does not respond to dietary restrictions and medications, surgical intervention may be needed. Surgical destruction of the affected labyrinth, using ultrasound, relieves the symptoms but also causes permanent hearing loss unless the cochlea is preserved.

Prognosis

No cure for Ménière disease is known. The goal of treatment is to improve or control symptoms. This condition has a tendency to recur.

Prevention

Presently, no etiology has been established, and therefore no preventive measures have been identified. Prompt treatment of otitis media is a prudent action and hopefully can ameliorate the condition. Genetic and environmental factors are believed to be factors.

Patient Teaching

Provide patients and families with information regarding the condition and its possible outcomes. Assist patients and families with locating and contacting appropriate community resource agencies for those with decreased hearing. Encourage patients to make changes in their lifestyles, such as avoiding caffeine and alcohol, stopping smoking, and avoiding possible stressful situations. Caution the patients not to drive or operate machinery while symptoms persist.

Benign Paroxysmal Positional Vertigo

Description

Benign paroxysmal positional vertigo (BPPV) is usually a vestibular system disorder. Patients complain of a spinning sensation, which becomes worse with movement of the head. They also may complain of a feeling that their surroundings are moving.

ICD-10-CM Code	H53.139 (Sudden visual loss, unspecified eye) (H53.131–H53.139 = 4 codes of specificity)

Symptoms and Signs

Patients with BPPV experience a spinning sensation with movement of the head. The dizziness experienced is that the room is spinning while the body is still; this is a false sensation. With closed eyes, the individual feels that the body is moving, and with the eyes open, the surroundings appear to be spinning. Nausea, vomiting, involuntary eye movement, and difficulty standing or walking may be present. The patient may report a feeling of dizziness, light-headedness, unsteadiness, and feeling faint. Although most of the episodes of vertigo are transient, lasting from 3 to 10 seconds (or slightly longer), the patient may experience an episode that feels much longer. Most report onset with change of position, turning over in bed, moving the head side to side, bending over, getting out of bed or a chair, and when looking up. An increased risk of falls is possible.

Patient Screening

An individual experiencing vertigo is usually in distress and will request prompt medical attention. Schedule the first available appointment. Advise the patient not to drive and to find assistance with transportation.

Etiology

The spinning sensation usually is the result of balance or equilibrium disorders. Normal functioning of the vestibular system occurs with movement of the head, causing transmission of impulses to the labyrinth in the inner ear. The labyrinth contains the three semicircular canals that are surrounded by fluid. This transmission of impulses causes a subsequent transmission to the vestibular nerve, which then transmits the impulse to the brainstem and the cerebellum. The brainstem and the cerebellum are responsible for the coordination of balance, movement, consciousness, and blood pressure. When the system is not functioning properly, problems with equilibrium, dizziness, light-headedness, and balance disorders occur. Head trauma may be a causative factor. Occasionally otitis media may be a precursor. Free-floating carbonate crystals that find their way into the semicircular canals may be the cause of the vertigo. Additional causes may be a viral infection, vascular in origin, or as an isolated symptom of unknown cause.

Diagnosis

Diagnosis is made from the history and examination. In addition to the false sensation of the room spinning or the patient spinning, nystagmus (involuntary eye movements) may be present. An audiogram or other means of hearing testing are used to determine the patient's level of hearing, which may be decreased. Lack of coordination may be detected, along with weakness and unsteadiness in the legs. Additional testing to rule out CNS involvement may include head CT, MRI of the head, or magnetic resonance angiogram of the brain's blood vessels. Another test is caloric stimulation, where, using a syringe, cool water followed by warm water is gently flushed against the eardrum to test eye reflexes. In a normal test, no abnormal eye movements are observed. During the test, BPPV can be detected if the eyes show involuntary movement from side to side. Blood tests may be ordered to rule out other disease conditions.

Treatment
Antihistamines (meclizine [Antivert], dimenhydrinate [Dramamine]), anticholinergics (scopolamine [Scopace]), and phenothiazines (prochlorperazine [Compazine]) may be prescribed to reduce the symptoms of positional vertigo. Exercises, such as the individual repeatedly turning the head from side to side, may also be helpful. Physical therapy may be ordered by the provider.

Prognosis
When the condition is benign, medication will often control the symptoms, as will the prescribed exercises. Often the vertigo resolves with time.

Prevention
There is no prevention for this condition.

Patient Teaching
Encourage the patient to take the medications as prescribed and instruct on how to perform the prescribed exercises. Caution the patient not to drive or operate machinery while symptoms persist.

Labyrinthitis

Description
Labyrinthitis is inflammation or infection of the labyrinth of the inner ear.

ICD-10-CM Code	H83.09 (Labyrinthitis, unspecified ear) (H83.01–H83.2X9 = 12 codes of specificity)

Additional digits are required. Once the physician has designated the pathology and type of labyrinthitis, refer to the physician's diagnosis and then to the current edition of the ICD-10-CM coding manual to ensure the greatest specificity of pathology.

Symptoms and Signs
The labyrinth is a group of three fluid-filled chambers (the semicircular canals) in the inner ear that control balance (Fig. 5.28). Inflammation or infection of these chambers is called *labyrinthitis*. The onset of infection is often acute and is associated with fever, with temperatures of 100°F to 101°F. The main symptom of this disease is extreme vertigo. Balance is affected, and nausea and vomiting may occur in some cases. The individual with labyrinthitis may experience tinnitus, loss of hearing in one ear, and difficulty focusing the eyes.

Patient Screening
Individuals reporting sudden onset of fever, vertigo, balance problems, and nausea and vomiting require prompt assessment. Refer the patient to an emergency facility for assessment to rule out a severe neurologic infection.

Etiology
Labyrinthitis is usually the result of a virus but can be caused by a bacterial infection that has spread from the middle ear. It also may be a result of meningitis.

Diagnosis
The diagnosis of labyrinthitis is based on the results of several tests, including audiometry and blood, neurologic, caloric, and possibly imaging studies.

Treatment
Bed rest for several days may be necessary. If a bacterial infection is present, prescriptions for a tranquilizer, an antiemetic

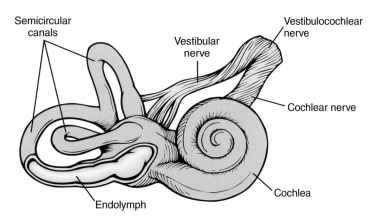
• **Fig. 5.28** The labyrinth or inner ear. Labyrinthitis is caused by a disturbance in the fluid in the semicircular canals.

agent, and an antibiotic may be necessary. Antihistamines and/or corticosteroids may also be prescribed. When properly treated, labyrinthitis is not a dangerous condition; however, it can be debilitating, and the labyrinth is delicate and easily damaged.

Prognosis
In most cases, labyrinthitis completely clears up within 1 to 3 weeks; however, a result of bacterial labyrinthitis may be permanent hearing deficiency or loss and/or balance problems.

Prevention
Prevention involves prompt medical treatment for otitis media or any other ear infection.

Patient Teaching
Stress the importance of seeking medical attention for ear infections. Provide written information about the condition. Encourage the patient to rest and be still when symptoms occur, to avoid sudden change of position, to avoid bright lights, and to try not to read while symptomatic.

Ruptured Tympanic Membrane (Ruptured Eardrum)

Description
Any type of tear or injury to the eardrum causes a breach in the integrity of the membrane. This may be the result of pressure, force, or insult from the exterior aspect, or it may be caused by increased pressure within the middle ear.

ICD-10-CM Code	H72.90 *(Unspecified perforation of tympanic membrane, unspecified ear)* (H72.00–H72.93, H73.811–H73.93 = 48 codes of specificity)

Refer to the physician's diagnosis and then to the current edition of the ICD-10-CM coding manual to ensure the greatest specificity of pathology.

Symptoms and Signs
Symptoms of a ruptured tympanic membrane (eardrum) are usually slight pain and partial loss of hearing and may include a slight discharge or bleeding from the ear. Buzzing in the ear and/or facial weakness or dizziness may be experienced. When an infectious process is involved, the drainage is usually purulent in nature. These symptoms may last only a few hours. The major risk is that an infection may develop in the middle ear.

Patient Screening
Individuals calling with complaints of diminished hearing, pain in the ear, ear infections, history of abrupt force or

• **Fig. 5.29** Tympanic membrane perforation. (Courtesy Michael Hawke, MD.)

pressure being incurred, and drainage from the ear require prompt assessment.

Etiology
The four most common causes of a ruptured eardrum are the insertion of sharp objects into the ear canal, a nearby explosion (including lightning strikes), a severe middle ear infection, and a blow to the ear. A ruptured eardrum also can occur as a result of a fractured skull. The eardrum occasionally ruptures spontaneously.

Diagnosis
A visual examination of the ear with an otoscope confirms the diagnosis of a ruptured eardrum (Fig. 5.29). Purulent drainage is usually present during an episode of suppurative otitis media complicated by rupture of the tympanic membrane. Audiometry also may be used.

Treatment
An antibiotic may be prescribed to prevent infection, and a patch may be applied to the eardrum to aid healing and to improve hearing. This procedure is similar to a **tympanoplasty** (tympanoplasty involves actual grafting of tissue for eardrum repair). Analgesics may be prescribed for pain.

Prognosis
The prognosis is good after treatment of the underlying cause. The eardrum heals naturally in about 1 to 2 weeks. After the eardrum has healed, hearing loss is minimal.

Prevention
Prompt intervention in otitis media may help prevent buildup of pressure in the middle ear. It is not possible to prevent many environmental causes of otitis media.

Patient Teaching

Provide an explanation and demonstration of the mechanism of ruptured tympanic membrane. Encourage patients and families to seek early treatment for otitis media.

Cholesteatoma

Description

A cholesteatoma is a pocket of skin cells located in the middle ear, normally shed by the eardrum, that collect into a cystlike mass or ball and become infected. As the infected material accumulates, the bone lining the middle ear cavity erodes, and the ossicles become damaged. Fig. 5.25A and B depicts normal tympanic membrane and cholesteatoma.

ICD-10-CM Code	H71.20 *(Cholesteatoma of mastoid, unspecified ear)*
	H71.21 *(Cholesteatoma of mastoid, right ear)*
	H71.22 *(Cholesteatoma of mastoid, left ear)*
	H71.23 *(Cholesteatoma of mastoid, bilateral)*
	H71 *(Cholesteatoma of middle ear)*
	(H71.00–H71.93 = 20 codes of specificity)

Cholesteatomas are located at various sites in the ear and therefore have specific codes for various sites. Refer to the physician's diagnosis and then to the current edition of the ICD-10-CM coding manual to ensure the greatest specificity of pathology.

Symptoms and Signs

The most common symptom of cholesteatoma is mild to moderate hearing loss. A purulent substance may drain from the affected ear, and earache, headache, vertigo, and some weakness of the facial muscles also may be present.

Patient Screening

Individuals with cholesteatomas usually have a history of otitis infections and are scheduled for routine reassessments. Often the condition is recognized during a routine follow-up examination. As with other ear conditions, drainage from the ear and diminished hearing require prompt assessment with the next available same-day appointment if possible.

Etiology

This condition often begins to develop in infancy, or it may be the result of chronic ear infection. The eustachian tube from the middle ear to the pharynx either fails to open properly or becomes blocked with material from recurring middle ear infections (see the Otitis Media section). As a result, this normally air-filled chamber develops a weak vacuum, causing the eardrum to become retracted. This forms the pocket in the eardrum that allows the cholesteatoma to develop.

Diagnosis

Patient history, otoscopy, and audiometry enable the physician to make the diagnosis. Radiographic studies, including CT, also may be useful, and a culture of the purulent drainage may be necessary to determine the most effective antibiotic for treatment.

Treatment

If the cholesteatoma is discovered early, before eroding begins, it can be removed fairly simply by a thorough cleaning of the middle ear cavity. Inflation of the eustachian tube may produce some improvement, and treatment with steroids and antibiotics helps prevent recurrence. If the cholesteatoma is discovered in an advanced stage, its removal becomes much more complicated. Damage to the middle ear structures may be extensive, necessitating surgical reconstruction of these structures. Complications may include deafness in one ear, persistent ear drainage, and vertigo. Badly damaged hearing may be improved with the use of a hearing aid. Additional complications may include erosion into the facial nerve with resulting facial paralysis and/or labyrinthitis. Untreated, a cholesteatoma erodes the roof of the middle ear cavity, making the development of an epidural abscess or meningitis possible.

Prognosis

Surgical intervention usually leads to a positive outcome.

Prevention

Prompt attention to otitis infections and problems of eustachian tube drainage helps delay the onset of this condition. Total prevention is not considered possible.

Patient Teaching

Encourage parents of children with chronic otitis media to schedule routine examinations that include audiology testing. Explain the origin and progression of the condition so that families understand how early intervention can help relieve it.

Mastoiditis

Description

Mastoiditis, whether acute or chronic, is inflammation of the mastoid bone, or mastoid process.

ICD-10-CM Code	H70.90 *(Unspecified mastoiditis, unspecified ear)*
	(H70.001–H70.13, H70.811–H70.93 = 28 codes of specificity)
	H70.009 *(Acute mastoiditis without complications, unspecified ear)*
	H70.10 *(Chronic mastoiditis, unspecified ear)*

Refer to the physician's diagnosis and then to the current edition of the ICD-10-CM coding manual to ensure the greatest specificity of pathology.

Symptoms and Signs

The mastoid is a round process of the temporal bone that can be felt immediately behind each ear and is porous or honey-combed in appearance. Pain and occasionally edema are present over and around the mastoid. Fever and chills, as well as head-ache and hearing loss, may be present. Some may experience drainage from the affected ear. A profuse discharge from the external canal is likely because of the middle ear involvement.

Patient Screening

Individuals reporting these symptoms accompanied by fever, chills, and pain in the mastoid region require prompt assessment. Schedule an appointment that same day, or if none is available, refer the patient to a facility where prompt assessment is possible.

Etiology

Acute mastoiditis is the result of neglected acute otitis media. Common causative organisms are *Streptococcus pneumoniae*, *Haemophilus influenzae*, and *Moraxella catarrhalis*. Less common causes are group A streptococci and *Staphylococcus aureus*. Chronic mastoiditis, necessitating radical or modified radical mastoidectomy, is associated with cholesteatoma.

Diagnosis

The diagnosis is made from patient history; otoscopy; audiometry; radiographic studies, including radiographs and CT of the mastoid; and the results of blood and culture studies.

Treatment

The treatment is based on the results of the sensitivity studies. Antibiotic or sulfonamide therapy is prescribed. Mastoiditis not responding to this treatment necessitates a surgical procedure called *simple mastoidectomy*, to prevent further complications and to preserve hearing. Radical mastoidectomy may be needed for chronic mastoiditis.

Prognosis

Prognosis is variable and depends on the degree of infection, extent of tissue involvement, and response to antibiotic and drug therapy. Surgical intervention usually corrects chronic involvement. Recurrence may occur when the infection is nonresponsive to antibiotic treatment. Complications may include partial or complete hearing loss of the affected ear. Additionally, there may be destruction of the mastoid bone, facial paralysis, and even meningitis. In severe nonresponsive cases, an epidural abscess may result, along with a spread of the infection to the brain.

Prevention

Because acute mastoiditis is the result of neglected acute otitis media, prompt medical intervention for otitis media is essential in preventing complications.

Patient Teaching

Stress the importance of prompt medical treatment of otitis media and completion of the prescribed antibiotic regimen.

Sensorineural Hearing Loss

Description

In sensorineural hearing loss (deafness), also often referred to as *occupational hearing loss*, sound waves reach the inner ear but are not perceived because the nerve impulses are not transmitted to the brain.

ICD-10-CM Code	H90.5 *(Unspecified sensorineural hearing loss)* (H90.3–H90.8 = 8 codes of specificity)

Refer to the physician's diagnosis and then to the current edition of the ICD-10-CM coding manual to ensure the greatest specificity of pathology.

Symptoms and Signs

Symptoms include tinnitus and partial to severe hearing loss.

Patient Screening

Sensorineural hearing loss usually has an insidious onset. Many times, the hearing loss is detected during a routine medical examination or preemployment screening. An abrupt onset of hearing loss is possible after exposure to a sudden loud explosive-type of noise or nearby lightning strike. Consider the anxiety level of these individuals when making an appointment for prompt assessment.

Etiology

The cause of sensorineural hearing loss is nerve failure or damage to the cochlea or the auditory nerve (CN VIII, or vestibulocochlear cranial nerve). This can be the result of the aging process (Table 5.3); however, loud music, machinery noise, or sometimes the side effects of medications—including aminoglycosides (tobramycin), loop diuretics, aspirin, or antimetabolites (methotrexate)—can cause such damage at any age. Other causes include mumps, measles, syphilis, meningitis, suppurative labyrinthitis, or viral infections. In addition, physical trauma from a fracture of the temporal bone may be a causative factor.

Diagnosis

The patient history and audiometry findings are usually all that is needed to make the diagnosis. Physicians are concerned that sensorineural hearing loss, tinnitus, and vertigo may be symptoms of a space-occupying mass, such as a tumor or an aneurysm; therefore these symptoms are investigated further to rule out such masses.

Treatment

Regardless of the amount of damage to the cochlea, steps must be taken to prevent further damage. Reducing noise levels by implementing measures, such as turning down the volume of loud music and wearing ear protectors at rock

TABLE 5.3 Changes In Hearing Caused By Aging[a]

Changes in Structure	Changes in Function
Cochlear hair cell degeneration	Inability to hear high-frequency sounds (presbycusis, sensorineural loss); interferes with understanding speech; hearing may be lost in both ears at different times
Loss of auditory neurons in spiral ganglia of organ of Corti	Inability to hear high-frequency sounds (presbycusis, sensorineural loss); interferes with understanding speech; hearing may be lost in both ears at different times
Degeneration of basilar (cochlear) conductive membrane of cochlea	Inability to hear at all frequencies but more pronounced at higher frequencies (cochlear conductive loss)
Decreased vascularity of cochlea	Equal loss of hearing at all frequencies (strial loss); inability to disseminate localization of sound
Loss of cortical auditory neurons	Equal loss of hearing at all frequencies (strial loss); inability to disseminate localization of sound

[a]Hearing loss affects about one-third of older people.
From McCance KL, Huether SE: *Pathophysiology: the biological basis for disease in adults and children*, ed 6, St Louis, 2010, Mosby.

concerts or in work areas with high noise levels, can prevent further or future damage to the ears.

Prognosis
Sensorineural hearing loss that is caused by damage to the cochlea is irreversible. Prevention is essential.

Prevention
No method of preventing hearing loss that results from the aging process is known. Preventing exposure to constant and extensive loud noise is essential in the prevention of sensorineural hearing loss. Use of ear protection at rock concerts and in work areas with high noise levels is helpful. It is prudent to limit the use of medications that affect the auditory nerve when possible.

Recommended noise exposure limit is 85 dB for an 8-hour time average, and any level above this is considered a risk factor for sensorineural hearing loss.

Patient Teaching
Provide patients with information about noise pollution and preventive measures that can be taken, including wearing ear protection when exposure to loud noise is possible.

Stress the importance of avoiding high volume on the radio or other audio equipment. Discuss sources of everyday noise pollution.

Cancer of the Ear

Description
Tumors of the ear can occur in any part of the ear and may be benign or malignant. They include skin cancers of the external ear, ceruminal gland neoplasms, acoustic and facial neuromas, and glomus tumors. Many cancers from other locations in the body may metastasize to the ear, resulting in secondary ear cancer.

ICD-10-CM Code	D49.2 *(Neoplasm of unspecified behavior of bone, soft tissue, and skin)*
	C41.0 *(Malignant neoplasm of bones of skull and face)*
	C79.89 *(Secondary malignant neoplasm of other specified sites)*

Neoplasms of the ear must be specified for location and type. Therefore it is not possible to list all applicable codes for neoplasms of the ear. Refer to the physician's diagnosis and then to the current edition of the ICD-10-CM coding manual to ensure the greatest specificity of pathology.

Symptoms and Signs
Symptoms of these neoplasms commonly include progressive hearing loss, chronic otic discharge, a visible mass or lesion on ear examination, loss of equilibrium, and tinnitus. Some cancers, such as SCC of the middle ear, are quite painful. Glomus tumors cause pulsatile tinnitus, that is, hearing a pulsing sound in the ear that has the tumor as a result of the tumor pressing on the bones of hearing.

Patient Screening
Symptoms may have an insidious onset with recognition of diminished hearing being thought of as troublesome rather than an acute symptom. Drainage from the ear, loss of equilibrium, and tinnitus require prompt assessment. Schedule patients with these symptoms for the next available appointment on the day of call. It is also important to consider the anxiety experienced by these patients and their families with the onset of these symptoms.

Etiology
Benign tumors of the ear include acoustic neuromas, facial neuromas, and glomus tumors. Acoustic neuroma arises from CN VIII, whereas facial neuroma is a tumor of the facial nerve. These tumors put pressure on the nerve fibers as they expand, causing hearing loss or facial paralysis, respectively, among other symptoms. Glomus tumors are the most

• **Fig. 5.30** Acoustic neuroma magnetic resonance T1-weighted axial. (A) and coronal (B) and T2-weighted axial (C) images show considerable contrast enhancement of the right-sided lesion (arrows and arrowheads). Note the normal neural structures on the left. (From Eisenberg RL, Johnson NM: *Comprehensive radiographic pathology*, ed 7, St Louis, 2021, Elsevier.)

common tumors of the middle ear and arise from the glomus bodies (tiny structures that serve as baroreceptors).

The most common malignant tumors of the external ear are the skin cancers: BCC, SCC, and melanoma. Another type of tumor found in the external auditory canal is the ceruminal gland neoplasm, a tumor arising from the glands producing cerumen, which can be either malignant or benign. Malignant tumors of the middle ear are very uncommon. SCC may arise in this location because of chronic inflammation of the middle ear, or mastoid.

Diagnosis
Tumors of the ear are often first identified because of the symptoms they cause. Examination of the ear may reveal a

BCC or SCC lesion, a mass in the external ear canal, or evidence of one of the other neoplasms. A biopsy is often performed to confirm the nature of the lesion, and CT and MRI are used to evaluate the extent of the disease (see Fig. 5.30).

Treatment
Treatment for all of these tumors is surgical excision. Radiation therapy is used if the tumor is known to be aggressive. A nerve graft may be performed after surgical excision of a neuroma.

Prognosis
The prognosis for many of these tumors is good after the patient receives appropriate treatment. However, SCC of

the middle ear has a very poor prognosis because it is often at an advanced stage at the time of diagnosis.

Prevention

No methods for prevention of most ear neoplasms are known. Skin cancers of the external ear may be prevented by reducing sun exposure to that area.

Patient Teaching

Encourage patients to be compliant with prescribed therapy. Provide information for postoperative care of any surgical excision site.

Review Challenge

Answer the following questions:
1. How does the process of normal vision take place?
2. List the three structures of the wall of the eye.
3. What is the function of the iris?
4. Discuss the function of the ciliary body.
5. What are the four main errors of refraction?
6. What is the difference between nystagmus and strabismus?
7. Name a common etiologic factor in hordeolum and blepharitis.
8. What are the pressing symptoms and signs of conjunctivitis? Is the condition contagious?
9. How is dry eye syndrome treated?
10. Name some possible causes of corneal abrasions.
11. How do cataracts interfere with vision?
12. Differentiate between the two primary types of glaucoma.
13. How is diabetic retinopathy detected and treated?
14. Explain the pathology involved in retinal detachment. How is this condition treated?
15. What are the possible causes of exophthalmos?
16. What is the primary symptom of refractive errors?
17. Name the etiologic factors of macular degeneration.
18. What is the best way to help control diabetic retinopathy?
19. Describe some ways cancer can affect the eye and adjacent structures.
20. Describe the three separate parts of the ear.
21. How does impacted cerumen cause deafness?
22. Precisely define *otitis media*. How is it classified? How is it diagnosed?
23. What is myringotomy?
24. What symptoms may an individual with Ménière disease experience?
25. Name the major symptom of labyrinthitis.
26. List common causes of a ruptured eardrum.
27. What causes occupational deafness?
28. List major symptoms of otitis media.
29. Define *otosclerosis*.
30. Which cranial nerve is damaged causing ototoxicity?
31. Which device can be used in the medical office to screen patients for diabetic retinopathy?

Real-Life Challenge: Acute Angle-Closure Glaucoma

A 61-year-old male has a sudden onset of blurred vision, head and eye pain, and nausea and vomiting. Upon questioning, he admits to seeing "halos" around lights and being especially sensitive to light. The examination confirms blurred vision and photosensitivity. Intraocular pressure (IOP) measures greater than 20 mm Hg on the tonometer. The patient is diagnosed with acute angle-closure glaucoma and referred to an ophthalmologist for immediate treatment.

Questions

1. Compare the symptoms of chronic open-angle glaucoma and acute angle-closure glaucoma.
2. Compare the reason for a buildup of IOP in chronic open-angle glaucoma and acute angle-closure glaucoma.
3. What history would suggest this patient is at risk for glaucoma?
4. Which type of treatment would you expect the ophthalmologist to institute?
5. If this were chronic open-angle glaucoma, which types of medications would you expect to be prescribed?
6. How would these medications help treat the disorder?
7. What is the danger of untreated glaucoma?

Real-Life Challenge: Otitis Media

An 18-month-old male child has been brought to the physician's office by his parents who say that he has been fussy and crying for the past 10 hours. The mother says she is having difficulty getting him to eat, and she has noticed that he sits with his head held to the right side. He has a history of a cold in the past few days with a runny nose and watering eyes.

Examination reveals a temperature of 103°F, pulse of 116 beats per minute, and respirations of 32 breaths per minute. The otoscopic examination is used to evaluate the condition of the tympanic membranes. The physician examines the left ear first, a method employed to see what the asymptomatic ear looks like. It reveals a normal translucent pearl-gray tympanic membrane. Examination of the right or symptomatic ear discloses a red, bulging eardrum. The mucous membrane of the nasal passages appears inflamed, as does the back of the throat.

An antibiotic (amoxicillin trihydrate [Amoxil] 125 mg four times daily [qid] × 10 days) is prescribed. The parents are instructed to give acetaminophen or ibuprofen (Motrin) for a temperature greater than 101°F and to call if the fever and pain persists beyond 24 hours. The child is scheduled for a follow-up visit in 1 week.

Questions

1. Why is it important to note that the child sits with his head held to the side?
2. What effect does the elevated temperature have on the other vital signs?
3. Why did the physician examine the left eardrum first?
4. What patient teaching would you offer the parents about the medication suggested for the elevated temperature?
5. What patient teaching would you offer the parents about the antibiotics?
6. Why are treatment and follow-up important?
7. Which surgical procedure may be indicated?
8. What long-term effects may the child experience if the otitis does not respond to treatment?

Real-Life Challenge: Sensorineural Hearing Loss

A 54-year-old retired male police officer presents with complaints that his hearing has diminished over the past few years. He is accompanied by his wife, who says he does not hear what she says anymore. She states that this has been getting progressively worse, but she has noted that he is turning up the sound on the television so loud that she cannot stand it. She also says that he cannot hear the phone ring, or what she is saying and confuses that information.

On examination, audiometry indicates a loss of hearing. The patient has difficulty hearing the examiner's commands or questions. He also complains of ringing in his ears (tinnitus). The patient has had a few experiences of dizziness or vertigo.

The physician attempts to discover a possible source of the condition and also to rule out other conditions, including tumors or aneurysms. The patient confirms previous exposure to extensive gun firing on a range without adequate ear protection. He also has worked in a machine shop where presses punch out metal objects on dies. Treatment includes reducing the source of damage, including reduction of noise levels. The reduction can be obtained by turning down the television volume and wearing earplugs.

Questions

1. What is the significance of the wife's complaints?
2. Why would an audiometric examination have been necessary?
3. What might have been some of the sources of the hearing loss?
4. What is the significance of shooting without adequate ear protection?
5. What will be the outcome if noise levels are reduced?
6. Why is it important for the physician to rule out a tumor or aneurysm?

Internet Assignments

1. Research facts about aging and vision by exploring the website of the American Foundation for the Blind (AFB). Choose a subject that considers older individuals and vision loss.
2. Visit the National Institute on Deafness and Other Communication Disorders website, choose the *News* and *Events* option, and research a current subject, such as new state guidelines for screening infant hearing.
3. Research a current topic, such as the danger of using illegal contact lenses, by visiting the American Academy of Ophthalmology website.

Critical Thinking

1. You read an online article written by a clinician suggesting that females replace their mascara product with a fresh unit at least once a month and to never share the mascara with anyone else. What is the concern behind these suggestions?
2. Why must close attention be paid to any changes in vision reported by a patient with age-related macular degeneration (AMD) before you schedule an appointment or contact the physician?
3. During an examination for employment, a small lesion is noted on the eyelid. The patient dismisses it as unimportant because it is not painful. What would be your necessary response, and why?

4. Discuss the effects of otitis media on school attendance of children.
5. Encourage a discussion about the psychological effect of otitis media.
6. Encourage a discussion as to how benign paroxysmal positional vertigo (BPPV) affects an individual's life.
7. Encourage a discussion about the causes of tympanic membrane rupture. Also promote discussion of teaching children not to place anything in their ears.

8. Encourage discussion of complications resulting from mastoiditis.
9. Encourage students to write a teaching plan for the prevention of sensorineural hearing loss.
10. Prepare to discuss Critical Thinking case study exercises for this chapter posted on Evolve.

Credentialing Examination Review Questions

1. Which eye structure is responsible for maintaining the shape of the eye?
   A. Retina
   B. Vitreous humor
   C. Iris
   D. Cornea
2. Which refractive error is also referred to as nearsightedness?
   A. Myopia
   B. Astigmatism
   C. Hyperopia
   D. Presbyopia
3. A patient experiences an involuntary, repetitive rhythmic movement of one or both eyes. Which term describes this condition?
   A. Nystagmus
   B. Esotropia
   C. Strabismus
   D. Hordeola
4. Which diagnosis is an infection of the eyelids?
   A. Conjunctivitis
   B. Blepharoptosis
   C. Ectropion
   D. Blepharitis
5. Clouding of the lens is one symptom of which disorder?
   A. Scleritis
   B. Presbyopia
   C. Cataracts
   D. Macular degeneration
6. Which section of the ear contains the malleus, incus, and stapes?
   A. Outer
   B. Middle
   C. Inner
   D. All of the above

7. Upon examination, a patient presents with pocket of skin cells located in the middle ear, which have collected into a cystlike mass. Which condition is most likely present?
   A. Mastoiditis
   B. Ménière disease
   C. Foreign object
   D. Cholesteotoma
8. Which type of cancer may be present on the outer ear?
   A. Squamous cell
   B. Melanoma
   C. Basal cell
   D. All of the above
9. Which ear problem is most likely to occur after a child visits a water park?
   A. Otitis Media
   B. Otitis Externa
   C. Swimmer's ear
   D. Cholesteotoma
10. Which test or procedure is performed to measure the amount of pressure in the middle ear?
    A. Tympanogram
    B. Audiometry
    C. Otoscopy
    D. Myringotomy

6

Diseases and Conditions of the Integumentary System

CHAPTER OUTLINE

LEARNING OBJECTIVES

After studying this chapter, you should be able to:

1. Explain the functions of the skin.
2. Recognize common skin lesions.
3. Describe how seborrheic dermatitis affects the skin.
4. Discuss the possible causes of contact dermatitis, atopic dermatitis, and psoriasis.
5. Describe the treatment of acne vulgaris.
6. Explain the pathologic course of herpes zoster.
7. Name the etiology of impetigo.
8. Explain why the treatment of cellulitis is important.
9. Cite examples of the classifications of fungal infections of the skin.
10. List preventive measures for decubitus ulcers.
11. Name the two most common parasitic insects to infest humans. Describe how infestation can occur.
12. Name two common premalignant tumors.
13. Differentiate the three types of skin cancer.
14. Describe the guidelines for avoiding excessive sun exposure.
15. List some conditions that are caused by the abnormal development or distribution of melanocytes.
16. Name some possible causes of alopecia.
17. State the cause of warts.
18. List some of the likely causes of deformed or discolored nails.

KEY TERMS

bulla (BUL-la)
cellulitis (sell-you-LIE-tis)
comedo (KOM-ee-doe)
dermatome (DER-mah-tome)
electrodesiccation (ee-leck-tro-des-ih-KAY-shun)
erythema (eh-rih-THEE-ma)
exudate (EKS-you-date)
exudative (EKS-you-day-tive)
fissure (FIS-ur)

keratolytic (ker-ah-toe-LIT-ik)
keratosis (ker-ah-TOE-sis)
nevus (NEE-vus)
papule (PAP-youl)
plaques (plaks)
sebaceous (seh-BAY-shus)
vesicle (VES-ih-kl)
vesicular (veh-SIK-you-lar)
wheal (WHEEL)

Orderly Functioning of the Integumentary System

The system comprising the skin and its accessory organs (hair, nails, and glands) is called the *integumentary system*. The skin, one of the largest organs, protects the body from trauma, infections, and toxic chemicals. When exposed to sunlight, the skin synthesizes vitamin D. Within the skin are millions of tiny nerve endings called *receptors*. These receptors sense touch, pressure, pain, and temperature. In addition to the skin's roles in the protection, sensation, and synthesis of vitamin D, it assists in the regulation of body temperature and in excretion.

The skin has three main structural layers (Fig. 6.1). The epidermis (outer layer) is a thin, cellular, multilayered membrane that is responsible for the production of keratin and melanin. The dermis, or corium (middle layer), is a dense, fibrous layer of connective tissue that gives skin its strength and elasticity. Within the dermis are blood and lymph vessels, nerve fibers, hair follicles, and sweat and sebaceous glands. The third layer is the subcutaneous layer, a thick, fat-containing section that insulates the body against heat loss.

Skin diseases frequently manifest as cutaneous lesions or alterations of the skin surface (Table 6.1). The diagnosis of a cutaneous disease is often based on the appearance of a specific type of lesion or group of lesions (Fig. 6.2).

Common presenting symptoms that need attention from health care professionals include:
- Cutaneous lesions or eruptions
- Pruritus (itching)
- Pain
- Edema (swelling)
- Erythema (redness)
- Inflammation

Many skin conditions are known to be aggravated by stress and anxiety. There are also some skin conditions that are affected by genes and lifestyle. Cosmetically, the skin is important to appearance. Much time and money are spent pursuing "beauty" and disguising the aging of the skin. Cosmetic surgeries are performed to alter the appearance of aging and to appear more youthful. Patients with skin conditions may feel anxious about their appearance. The treatment of many skin diseases is tedious, requiring strict compliance. Patient education and psychological support reduce the patient's anxiety and encourage good adherence to the treatment plan.

Dermatitis

Inflammation of the skin, or dermatitis, occurs in many types or forms. They all manifest as pruritus, erythema, and the appearance of various cutaneous lesions. The more common forms are seborrheic dermatitis, contact dermatitis, and atopic dermatitis (eczema). All forms of dermatitis can be acute, subacute, or chronic.

Seborrheic Dermatitis

Description

Seborrheic dermatitis, one of the most common skin disorders, is an inflammatory condition of the sebaceous, or oil, glands.

ICD-10-CM Code	L21.9 *(Seborrheic dermatitis, unspecified)*
	(L21.0–L21.9 = 4 codes of specificity)
	L21.0 *(Seborrhea capitis)*
	L20.83 *(Infantile [acute][chronic] eczema)*
	(L20.81–L20.9 = 6 codes of specificity)
	L21.8 *(Other seborrheic dermatitis)*

Symptoms and Signs

Seborrheic dermatitis is marked by a gradual increase in the amount of and a change in the quality of sebum, which is produced by the sebaceous glands. The inflammation occurs in areas with the greatest number of sebaceous glands. These include the scalp, eyebrows, eyelids, sides of the nose, the

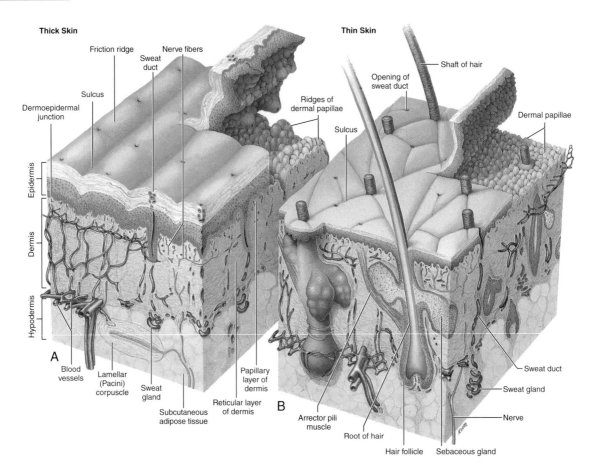

• **Fig. 6.1** Normal skin. (From Patton KT, Thibodeau GA: *Anatomy and physiology*, ed 9, St. Louis, 2016, Mosby.)

area behind the ears, and the middle of the chest. Affected skin is reddened and covered by yellowish, greasy-appearing scales. Itching may occur but is usually mild.

Seborrheic dermatitis can occur at any age but is most common during infancy, when it is called *cradle cap*. Cradle cap (Fig. 6.3) usually clears without treatment by age 8 to 12 months. Seborrheic dermatitis occurs at a higher rate in adults with disorders of the central nervous system, such as Parkinson disease. Patients who are recovering from stressful medical conditions, such as a myocardial infarction (heart attack); patients who have been confined to hospitals or nursing homes for long stays; and those who have immune system disorders, such as acquired immunodeficiency syndrome, appear to be more prone to this disorder. More intense forms of seborrheic dermatitis can be seen in patients with psoriasis (see the Psoriasis section).

Patient Screening
This condition has a gradual onset. The irritation becomes troublesome, and the patient or a caregiver calls to request an appointment. Schedule the patient to be seen at the earliest convenient time.

Etiology
This condition is idiopathic; however, heredity may predispose an individual to the condition, and emotional stress may be a precipitating factor. Evidence suggests that this skin disorder may be perpetuated or intensified by the yeast-like organism *Malassezia*, also called pityrosporum, which is normally found on the skin in small numbers. Whether diet or food allergies play a role in the development of seborrheic dermatitis in infants is still unknown.

Diagnosis
In most patients, blood, urine, and allergy tests are not necessary. In the rare case of chronic seborrheic dermatitis that does not respond to treatment, a skin biopsy, or more extensive testing may be performed to rule out the possibility of another disease.

Treatment
One of the more effective methods of treatment is the use of a low-strength cortisone or hydrocortisone cream applied topically to the affected area. *Caution:* Prolonged use of these medications should be avoided because of the possible side effects of steroids. When the scalp is involved, causing dandruff, frequent use of nonprescription shampoos containing tar, zinc pyrithione, selenium sulfide, sulfur, and salicylic acid is also recommended. Patients not responding to these treatments should consult a dermatologist, who can prescribe stronger medications.

TABLE 6.1 Description of Some Skin Lesions

Skin Lesion	Description
Macule	Small, flat circumscribed lesion of a color different from that of normal skin
Papule	Small, firm, elevated lesion
Nodule	Palpable elevated lesion; varies in size
Pustule	Elevated erythematous lesion, usually containing purulent exudate
Vesicle	Elevated, thin-walled lesion containing clear fluid (blister)
Plaque	Large, slightly elevated lesion with flat surface, often topped by scale
Crust	Dry, rough surface or dried exudate or blood
Lichenification	Thick, dry, rough surface (leather like)
Keloid	Raised, irregular, and increasing mass of collagen resulting from excessive scar tissue formation
Fissure	Small, deep, linear crack or tear in skin
Ulcer	Cavity with loss of tissue from the epidermis and dermis, often weeping or bleeding
Erosion	Shallow, moist cavity in epidermis
Comedo	Mass of sebum, keratin, and debris blocking the opening of a hair follicle

From Gould B: *Pathophysiology for the health professions*, ed 3, Philadelphia, 2006, Saunders.

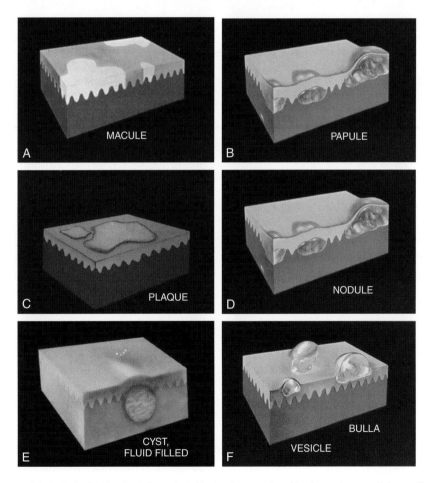

• **Fig. 6.2** Skin lesions. (A) Macule. A flat, colored lesion that may be white (hypopigmented), brown (hyperpigmented), or red (erythematous and purpuric). (B) Papule. A small elevated lesion less than 0.5 cm in diameter. (C) Plaque. A plateau-like elevated lesion greater than 0.5 cm in diameter. (D) Nodule. A marble-like lesion greater than 0.5 cm in depth and diameter. (E) Cyst. A nodule filled with either liquid or semisolid material. (F) Vesicle and **bulla**. Blisters containing clear fluid. Vesicles are less than 0.5 cm in diameter, and bullae are greater than 0.5 cm in diameter.

• **Fig. 6.2, (cont'd)** (G) Pustule. A vesicle containing purulent or cloudy fluid. (H) Crust. Liquid debris dried on the skin's surface, resulting from ruptured vesicles, pustules, or bullae. (I) Scale. A thickened outer layer of skin that is dry and whitish colored. (J) Fissure, erosion, and ulcer. A fissure is a thin tear. An erosion is a wide but shallow fissure. An ulcer involves the epidermis and dermis. (K) Burrow. A tunnel or streak caused by a burrowing organism. (L) Comedo. A lesion of acne. (From Marks JG, et al: *Lookingbill & Marks' principles of dermatology*, ed 4, Philadelphia, 2006, Saunders.)

• **Fig. 6.3** "Cradle cap," the most frequent form of seborrheic dermatitis in infants. The condition often begins in the first 2–3 weeks of life and usually disappears by age 12 months. (From Paller SA: *Hurwitz clinical pediatric dermatology: a textbook of skin disorders of childhood and adolescence*, ed 4 Philadelphia, 2012, Saunders.)

Treatment of cradle cap involves gentle massage of the scalp to loosen scales and improve circulation. When scales are present, shampooing daily with a mild soap is recommended. After the scales disappear, shampooing may be done twice a week. Care should be taken to rinse off all soap. The child's hair should be brushed with a soft brush after shampooing and several times during the day. When the scales do not loosen easily, mineral oil can be applied to the scalp, and a warm cloth used to cover the child's scalp for approximately 1 hour. The temperature of the cloth must be monitored so that it does not cool down too much and reduce the child's body temperature and the cloth should not be too hot to prevent potential burns. The scalp should be shampooed and dried. If this treatment is not successful in removing the scales, the physician may prescribe a lotion or cream to be applied to the child's scalp.

Prognosis

Most episodes resolve with treatment. Those who do not respond positively should be referred to a dermatologist for additional drug therapy. Whether treated or not, this condition tends to recur.

Prevention

No prevention is known, however good skin care may limit occurrence.

Patient Teaching

Teach the patient to properly apply the prescribed medication. For infants with cradle cap, instruct the parents to shampoo the scalp daily and perhaps gently massage the area with a soft brush designed for infants or a warm, wet cloth.

Contact Dermatitis

Description

Contact dermatitis is an acute inflammation response of the skin triggered by an exogenous chemical or substance.

ICD-10-CM Code	*L25.9 (Unspecified contact dermatitis, unspecified cause) (L25.0–L25.9 = 8 codes of specificity)*

Contact dermatitis has more than one form and therefore more than one ICD-10-CM code. The general code is L25.9 for the ICD-10-CM. Refer to the physician's diagnosis and then to the current edition of the ICD-10-CM coding manual to ensure the greatest specificity of pathology and any appropriate modifiers. A list of some of the specific codes follows:

Contact Dermatitis:

ICD-10-CM Code	*L24.0 (Irritant contact dermatitis due to detergents)*
	L24.1 (Irritant contact dermatitis due to oils and greases)
	L24.2 (Irritant contact dermatitis due to solvents)
	L25.1 (Unspecified contact dermatitis due to drugs in contact with skin)
	L25.3 (Unspecified contact dermatitis due to other chemical products)
	L25.4 (Unspecified contact dermatitis due to food in contact with skin)
	L25.5 (Unspecified contact dermatitis due to plants, except food)
	L56.0 (Drug phototoxic response)
	L56.1 (Drug photoallergic response)
	L56.2 (Photocontact dermatitis [berloque dermatitis])
	L25.8 (Unspecified contact dermatitis due to other agents)
	L25.9 (Unspecified contact dermatitis, unspecified cause)

• **Fig. 6.4** (A) Contact dermatitis. (B) Periorbital allergic contact dermatitis. Patient was patch-test positive to gold. Patient wears gold earrings and likely was touching eyelid skin after touching the earrings. (A, From Marks JG, et al: *Lookingbill & Marks' principles of dermatology*, ed 4, Philadelphia, 2006, Saunders; B, From Epstein E: *Common skin disorders*, ed 5, Philadelphia, 2001, Saunders/Elsevier.)

Symptoms and Signs

Contact dermatitis is caused either by the action of irritants on the skin's surface or by contact with a substance that causes an allergic response. Symptoms include erythema, edema, and small **vesicles** that ooze, itch, burn, or sting (Fig. 6.4A).

Patient Screening

The patient reporting symptoms of contact dermatitis feels the characteristic itching, burning, and stinging. If possible, these patients should be scheduled on the same day.

Etiology

Many substances can induce contact dermatitis, including plants, such as poison ivy, oak, or sumac. Poison ivy may be spread as an airborne irritant by burning plants. Other irritants are dyes used in soaps and facial and toilet tissues, other dyes, latex, furs, preservatives, drugs, detergents, cleaning compounds, cosmetics, chemicals, acids, and certain metals (e.g., nickel and other metals) used to make jewelry (Fig. 6.4B). Solar dermatitis from sun exposure, and other forms of radiation, including exposure through a tanning bed, may cause the dermatitis. If an irritant remains in constant contact with the skin, the dermatitis spreads.

Contact dermatitis develops in three ways:

1. It can develop through irritation, either chemical or mechanical, such as by latex gloves and wool fibers. If the irritant is strong, a single exposure may cause a severe inflammatory reaction.
2. Contact dermatitis may develop through sensitization. This means that the first contact with a substance causes no immediate inflammation. However, after the skin becomes sensitized, future contact or exposure results in inflammation.
3. Another interesting but uncommon mechanism for the development of this form of dermatitis is photoallergy. Some chemicals found in perfumes, soaps, suntan lotions containing para-aminobenzoic acid, or medications (e.g., tetracycline) can sensitize the skin to sunlight. The next time the individual uses the products and is exposed to sunlight, a rash develops.

Diagnosis
Diagnosis of a contact dermatitis is based on the appearance of the affected area; medical history, including prior outbreaks and their locations; and identification of the specific irritant or allergen with a patch test.

Treatment
If a patient has come in contact with a known irritant, thoroughly cleaning the skin surface should be the first step. This should be followed by the topical application of a corticosteroid cream. An oral steroid, such as methylprednisolone (Medrol) or prednisone, may be prescribed for 6 to 12 days, with a decreasing dosage. Some physicians believe that 6 days is typically not a long enough treatment for many contact dermatitis conditions. Poison plant dermatitis nearly always needs at least 12 days of medication. Oatmeal baths may provide some symptomatic relief. Sometimes dermatitis rebounds after short-course steroids.

Prognosis
The prognosis varies, depending on the amount of skin area involved and the likelihood of the causative agent being removed. The response to drug therapy is usually positive when combined with the removal of the offending substance.

Prevention
Identification of the offending or causative substance is primary in preventing recurrences.

Patient Teaching
Encourage patients to avoid substances or situations that trigger contact dermatitis. Give information about proper methods of cleansing the skin, affected clothing, and bed linens after contact with offending substances. Instruct patients to refrain from scratching affected skin to prevent additional damage or infection from developing in the skin tissue.

Atopic Dermatitis (Eczema)

Description
Atopic dermatitis (eczema) is a chronic inflammation of the skin that tends to occur in patients with a family history of allergic conditions.

ICD-10-CM Code	L20.0 *(Besnier prurigo)*
	L20.81 *(Atopic neurodermatitis)*
	L20.82 *(Flexural eczema)*
	L20.84 *(Intrinsic [allergic] eczema)*
	L20.89 *(Other atopic dermatitis)*

Symptoms and Signs
A rash develops, with **vesicular** and **exudative** eruptions in children and dry, leathery vesicles in adults (Figs. 6.5 and 6.6). The rash occurs in a characteristic pattern on the face, neck, elbows, knees, and upper trunk of the body and is accompanied by pruritus.

Patient Screening
When the individual calls for an appointment, consider the discomfort that he or she is experiencing, and schedule the patient to be seen at the earliest possible time.

Etiology
Eczema is an idiopathic disease. The tendency for it to develop is inherited, and an allergic connection is assumed. Eczema in some infants is believed to be traceable to sensitivity to milk, orange juice, or some other foods.

A flare-up of eczema can be triggered by stress, anxiety, or conflict. Stress can make the condition worse. Climate, especially sudden or extreme changes in temperature, can affect or aggravate the condition. Eczema may improve in summer and flare-up in winter. Wool clothing or blankets in contact with the skin may also cause a flare-up of the condition. Skin barrier disruption associated with transepidermal water loss from frequent bathing and/or hand washing without moisturizing is also an important trigger factor. Eczema in babies usually subsides by age 2 years. The rash may resolve during adolescence or persist into adulthood. Eczema generally tends to improve over time.

Diagnosis
A medical history, including a family history, along with an examination of the skin, confirms the diagnosis. Occasional skin testing for specific allergies is indicated to identify underlying causes.

Treatment
The main objective in treating atopic dermatitis is reducing the frequency and severity of eruptions and relieving the pruritus. Simple atopic dermatitis may be treated with skin

• **Fig. 6.5** (A) A common appearance of atopic dermatitis in children, with erythema and scaling confined to the cheeks, sparing the perioral and paranasal areas. (B) Extensive erythema and crusting in a baby with secondarily infected atopic dermatitis of the face. Of note, eczematous patches may look dark brown, purple, or gray on black or brown skin. (From Dinnulos JGH: Habif's *clinical dermatology: a color guide to diagnosis and therapy*, ed 7, Philadelphia, 2021, Elsevier.)

moisturizers, sunlight therapy, vitamin D, or calcipotriene. Unfortunately, no medications can eliminate eczema. Topical ointments and creams containing a cortisone derivative are the primary treatment for eczema. In addition, three unique nonsteroidal antiinflammatory drugs (NSAIDs), tacrolimus (Protopic) and pimecrolimus (Elidel), and Eucrisa, a phosphodiesterase type 4 inhibitor, are prescribed specifically to treat eczema. A newer class of injectables to block interleukin 4 (IL-4) and IL-13 (brand name Dupixent) is considered a biologic agent. Local and systemic medications, such as antihistamines, tranquilizers, and other sedatives, may be prescribed to prevent or control pruritus. Secondary bacterial or viral infections can result from scratching of the rash or lesions. A secondary bacterial infection is the most common complication. The physician usually prescribes an antibiotic to control the infection. A more serious complication of eczema can be caused by infection by certain viruses, especially herpes simplex virus. This is referred to as eczema herpeticum.

Prognosis
Reduction in the frequency and severity of eruptions and relief from pruritus are positive outcomes. There is no cure, and eczema cannot be eliminated with medications; however, they are prescribed to control the itch-scratch cycle that aggravates the condition.

Prevention
Eczema has no known prevention. An attempt should be made to prevent the secondary bacterial or viral infections that result from scratching of the rash or lesions.

• **Fig. 6.6** Atopic dermatitis in a dark-skinned patient. Note the typical papular variant commonly seen in dark-skinned individuals. (From Goldman L, et al: *Goldman-Cecil medicine, 2-volume set*, ed 26, 2020, Elsevier.)

Patient Teaching
Explain how scratching aggravates the condition. Emphasize following instructions for soaps and skin care products that are fragrance free and recommended by the physician for use.

Urticaria

Description
Urticaria, or hives, is associated with severe itching, followed by the appearance of redness and an area of swelling (**wheal**), in a localized area of skin (Fig. 6.7A and B).

• **Fig. 6.7** (A) Urticaria. (B) Hives as experienced by a 19 year-old female. (A, From Murphy GF, Herzberg AJ: *Atlas of dermatopathology*, Philadelphia, 1996, Saunders. B, Courtesy Margaret Frazier, 2019.)

ICD-10-CM Code   L50.9 *(Urticaria, unspecified)*

Urticaria has more than one form and therefore more than one ICD-10-CM code. The general code for urticaria is L50.9 for the ICD-10-CM. Refer to the physician's diagnosis and then to the current edition of the ICD-10-CM coding manual to ensure the greatest specificity of pathology and any appropriate modifiers. Some of the specific codes follow:

ICD-10-CM Code
- L50.0 *(Allergic urticaria)*
- L50.1 *(Idiopathic urticaria)*
- L50.2 *(Urticaria due to cold and heat)*
- L50.3 *(Dermatographic urticaria)*
- L50.4 *(Vibratory urticaria)*
- L50.5 *(Cholinergic urticaria)*
- L50.6 *(Contact urticaria)*
- L50.8 *(Other urticaria)*
- L50.9 *(Urticaria, unspecified)*

Symptoms and Signs

Hives of various sizes can erupt as a few lesions anywhere on the skin and often are scattered over the body or mucous membrane. In gastrointestinal involvement, the patient complains of abdominal colic. When hives develop in the pharyngeal mucosa, the airway can become obstructed, causing asphyxiation. When the swelling involves deeper tissues, the condition is called *angioedema* and is more serious. Urticaria is common, often acute, and self-limiting, lasting a few hours. In other cases, hives continue over months or years, becoming a chronic condition. A patient's complaint of itching is a significant symptom.

Patient Screening

Hives can develop into a life-threatening condition if they involve the respiratory system. Anyone experiencing respiratory difficulties should be brought into the emergency medical system for immediate assessment and intervention. Cutaneous symptoms make the individual very uncomfortable, and the patient should be seen immediately or referred to another facility, such as an emergency room, for prompt assessment.

Etiology

Urticaria affects the dermis and results from acute hypersensitivity and the release of histamine. This causes local inflammation and vasodilation of capillaries with substantial edema. Allergic reactions to food (e.g., shellfish, strawberries, or tree or ground nuts such as peanuts); drugs (e.g., antibiotics); or insect stings (frequently by bees) are some common causes. Infection can cause an attack of hives, as can some inhalants, sunlight, and temperature extremes. Sometimes the cause is not identified.

Diagnosis

Visual inspection of the urticaria is diagnostic. A prior episode in conjunction with a particular exposure to a known allergen is significant in the patient's history. If the medical history offers no clues to the cause, sensitivity testing, and blood tests for antibodies may help identify the causative agent.

Treatment

If known, the antigenic factor is removed and then avoided, if possible. Antihistamines quickly relieve symptoms. An injection of epinephrine is used in more severe cases.

In persistent cases, a course of prednisone or methylprednisolone is therapeutic. A variety of corticosteroid creams or ointments may also be used.

Prognosis

Immediate drug therapy usually resolves the allergic response, and the hives disappear.

Prevention

Prevention depends on identifying the offending allergen and avoiding it.

Patient Teaching

Teach patients the importance of avoiding the causative allergen and seeking proper and prompt medical intervention when the condition recurs.

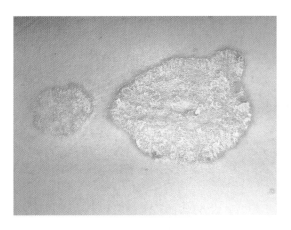

• **Fig. 6.8** Psoriasis. (From Marks JG, et al: *Lookingbill & Marks' principles of dermatology*, ed 4, Philadelphia, 2006, Saunders.)

Psoriasis

Description

Psoriasis is a chronic skin condition marked by thick, flaky, red patches of various sizes, covered with characteristic white, silvery scales (Fig. 6.8).

ICD-10-CM Code	L40.0 (Psoriasis vulgaris)
	L40.1 (Generalized pustular psoriasis)
	L40.2 (Acrodermatitis continua)
	L40.3 (Pustulosis palmaris et plantaris)
	L40.4 (Guttate psoriasis)
	L40.8 (Other psoriasis)

Psoriasis has more than one form and therefore more than one code. Refer to the physician's diagnosis and then to the current edition of the ICD-10-CM coding manual to ensure the greatest specificity of pathology.

Symptoms and Signs

Psoriasis is an inflammatory chronic and recurrent skin condition with silvery scales. The body makes new skin cells more quickly than it should resulting in extra layers of skin cells. These scales develop into dry **plaques** (see Fig. 6.2C), sometimes progressing to pustules (see Fig. 6.2G). They usually do not cause discomfort but might cause a slight itch or soreness. Affected skin typically appears dry, cracked, and encrusted. The most common areas where psoriasis develops are the scalp; the outer sides of arms and legs, especially elbows and knees; and the trunk of the body. In addition, the palms of hands and the soles of feet may be affected. In some patients, psoriasis spreads to the nail beds, causing the nails to thicken and crumble. Psoriasis plaques can also develop in areas of physical trauma (Koebner phenomenon). Psoriasis can occur at any age. It is noninfectious and does not affect general health.

Patient Screening

The patient calling for an appointment for these symptoms should be scheduled for the next available appointment.

Etiology

The cause of psoriasis is unknown, but it seems to be genetically determined. Psoriasis is now identified as an autoimmune disorder. Precipitating factors for the development of psoriasis include hormonal changes, such as those occurring with pregnancy, climate changes, emotional stress, and a period of generally poor health. Some drugs, including lithium, beta-blockers, and NSAIDs, are suspected of exacerbating psoriasis.

Diagnosis

The white, silvery scales of psoriasis are recognizable, making the condition easy to diagnose. Careful history taking, observation of the skin, or skin biopsy may help when the scales are not evident, as with patients who bathe and scrub frequently. Scratching of the lesions reveals the telltale scales.

Treatment

The goal of treatment is to reduce inflammation and to slow the rapid growth of skin cells that cause the condition. Keeping the involved skin moist and lubricated is beneficial. Treatment options include exposure to ultraviolet (UV) light to help delay cell reproduction; use of a psoralens medication (methoxsalen) in combination with UV light; application of topical steroid creams/ointments; application of coal tar preparations; application of cream containing retinoids (vitamin A derivative); administration of low-dosage antihistamines; and oatmeal baths. Additional treatments may involve the application of creams containing synthetic vitamin D analogs (calcipotriene 0.005%). Severe cases of psoriasis may require chemotherapy with methotrexate (Trexall) or acitretin, cyclosporine (Neoral), or the use of etretinate (Tegison), which is related to vitamin A. *Caution:* Pregnant females and nursing mothers should never take methotrexate, acitretin, or etretinate. Cyclosporine is in the US Food and Drug Administration (FDA) pregnancy category C. Antibiotics also may be prescribed. A new group of medications known as *monoclonal antibodies* and *fusion proteins (biologics)* have been approved for the treatment of psoriasis.

Recently a new drug, ustekinumab (Stelara), has been marketed as more effective than etanercept (Enbrel) for the treatment of psoriasis. Both drugs are biologic medications, and must be used with caution due to the potential for immune system suppression and severe infections. Biologic medications may not be considered for treatment unless the psoriasis is quite severe and the patient is not responsive to other therapies.

Prognosis

No cure for psoriasis is known, but it is controllable. Remissions and exacerbations occur often, and the condition may require lifelong treatment. Advise patients to

• **Fig. 6.9** Rosacea.

consider counseling for stress reduction, because stress may cause recurrence of the disorder.

Prevention

The condition has an autoimmune etiology; thus no prevention is known. Keeping the skin moist and lubricated; avoiding cold, dry climates; preventing stress and anxiety; limiting alcohol intake; and not scratching and picking at the skin help prevent recurrence of the condition.

Patient Teaching

Explain the concept of exposure to UV light and methods of timing the exposure. Demonstrate application of steroid creams, coal tar preparations, and other skin creams.

Rosacea

Description

Rosacea, a chronic inflammatory disorder of the facial skin, causes redness primarily in the areas that manifest blushing or flushing.

ICD-10-CM Code	L71.0 *(Perioral dermatitis)*
	L71.1 *(Rhinophyma)*
	L71.8 *(Other rosacea)*
	L71.9 *(Rosacea, unspecified)*

Symptoms and Signs

The onset of rosacea is insidious and often mistaken for a change in complexion, sunburn, or even acne. The redness becomes more noticeable and does not go away. The skin then may begin exhibiting dryness and pimples that may become inflamed or filled with pus. In addition, small blood vessels of the cheeks and face enlarge and show through the skin as red lines even after the redness diminishes (Figs. 6.9 and 6.10). Small knobby bumps occasionally appear on the nose, causing it to look swollen, mostly in the male with rosacea.

There are four major types of rosacea. The signs and symptoms vary from one form to the other. Ocular rosacea,

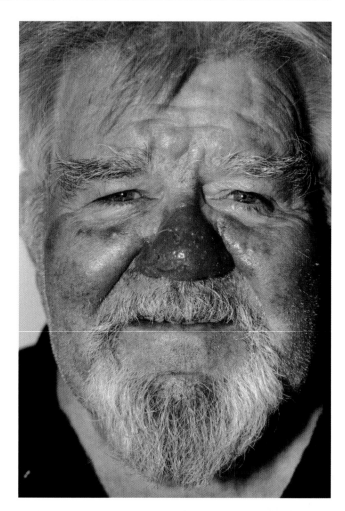

• **Fig. 6.10** Rosacea papules and pustules superimposed on the background of erythema. (From Marks JG, et al: *Lookingbill & Marks' principles of dermatology*, ed 4, Philadelphia, 2006, Saunders.)

• **Fig. 6.11** Patient with ocular rosacea. (From Habif TP, et al: *Skin disease diagnosis and treatment*, ed 3, St. Louis, 2011, Saunders.)

an inflammatory eye condition, is a less common form of rosacea. The blood vessels in the sclera become inflamed, and the eyelids appear to be reddened and swollen, often with small bumps that are inflamed and eyelashes that fall out. The individual may experience a burning or gritty feeling in the eyes. The eyes have a bloodshot appearance (Fig. 6.11).

Etiology

The etiology of rosacea, a chronic and often cyclic condition, is unknown. A possible correlation with the frequency of the individual's blushing or facial flushing has been suggested. Those with lighter complexions appear to have a greater incidence of the disorder, which possibly may be inherited. Rosacea is not considered infectious or contagious and is not spread through skin contact. The etiology of ocular rosacea is also unknown. It should be noted that some medications, such as those that treat hypertension by causing blood vessels to dilate, may trigger an occurrence.

Diagnosis

Rosacea is diagnosed on the basis of a history of facial blushing and flushing. Although rosacea often has many of the same symptoms as acne, the individual experiencing episodes of rosacea does not have the blackheads or whiteheads (comedones) typical of acne. A dermatologist should be consulted for a definitive diagnosis.

Ocular rosacea is diagnosed on the basis of a history of chronically bloodshot eyes, and examination of the eyes usually reveals inflammation and debris on the margins of the eyelids.

Treatment

Rosacea has no cure, but symptoms can be controlled through medical treatment with azelaic acid 15% (Finacea); metronidazole cream 1%; sodium sulfacetamide; topical antibiotics (erythromycin and clindamycin); and lifestyle changes. The patient is urged to identify situations that cause him or her to blush or experience facial flushing and attempt to avoid these triggers. These events may be different for various rosacea sufferers, so the patient would be wise to avoid sunlight, hard exercise, extreme heat or cold, stress, spicy foods, hot drinks, and alcohol. Sun exposure, hot weather, cold weather, and wind all have been identified as triggers, as have abrupt changes of season and weather extremes. The physician may prescribe medications to control the redness. Antibiotics (minocycline, doxycycline, or tetracycline) are prescribed in some cases. For stubborn cases, the redness can also be treated with laser surgery. Mild cleansers should be used, and moisturizers that do not contain alcohol or drying agents should be applied routinely. Use of sunscreen helps. Consistent treatment is necessary to prevent flare-ups. A topical gel, Mirvaso (brimonidine), works by constricting the blood vessels, thereby decreasing the appearance of redness.

The treatment of ocular rosacea is similar to that of facial rosacea and includes daily cleansing of eyelids with a form of diluted nontearing shampoo. If the individual is not allergic, antibiotics (minocycline, doxycycline, or tetracycline) are sometimes prescribed.

Prognosis

As previously mentioned, rosacea has no cure, but the patient may be able to control the symptoms with medical treatment and lifestyle modifications. Similar to facial rosacea, ocular rosacea has no cure.

Prevention

The etiology is unknown, so prevention is not possible. Identifying situations with the potential to cause blushing or facial flushing and avoiding these triggers is helpful. Avoiding sunlight, hard exercise, extreme heat or cold, stress, spicy foods, hot drinks, and alcohol also helps. The patient is urged to avoid triggers such as exposure to the sun, hot weather, cold weather, wind, abrupt changes of seasons, and weather extremes.

Patient Teaching

Work with patients to identify the causative factors and discuss ways to avoid them. Assist the patient in locating and contacting online or in person support groups.

Acne Vulgaris

Description

Acne vulgaris is an inflammatory disease of the sebaceous glands and hair follicles. Papules, pustules, and comedones are usually present (Fig. 6.12).

ICD-10-CM Code	L70.1 *(Acne conglobata)*
	L70.8 *(Other acne)*
	L70.9 *(Acne, unspecified)*

Symptoms and Signs

Acne vulgaris is marked by the appearance of papules, pustules, and comedones (see Fig. 6.2B, G, and L). Deeper, boil-like lesions, called *nodules*, sometimes can occur. Scars may develop if the chronic irritation and inflammation continue for a long period. Acne is found most often on the face but can also occur on the neck, shoulders, chest, and back (Fig. 6.13). Acne can appear at any age but is more common in adolescents during puberty.

Patient Screening

Many calls requesting appointments for the treatment of acne-type conditions will be for teenagers. Acne is not

• **Fig. 6.12** Acne. Inflammatory acne is characterized by erythematous papules and pustules with the possibility of eventual scarring. (From Cotran R, et al: *Robbins pathological basis of disease*, ed 6, Philadelphia, 1999, Saunders.)

• **Fig. 6.13** Acne vulgaris: comedonal. Closed comedones present as whiteheads. (From Paller AS, et al: *Hurwitz clinical pediatric dermatology, a textbook of skin disorders of childhood and adolescence*, ed 5, Philadelphia, 2016, Elsevier.)

a medical emergency, but an individual experiencing its symptoms may be feeling emotional stress. Schedule the next available appointment for these patients.

Etiology

The cause of acne vulgaris is not fully known. Research on the cause, however, links it to hormonal changes of adolescence that affect the activity of the sebaceous glands. Hereditary tendencies are also known to be predisposing factors. Precipitating factors may include food allergies, endocrine disorders, psychological factors, fatigue, and the use of steroid drugs. Pressure against the skin can also be a risk factor.

Sebum, an oily substance produced by the sebaceous glands, reaches the skin surface through the hair follicle. Overproduction of the oil seems to stimulate the follicle walls, causing a faster shedding of skin cells. This causes the cells and sebum to stick together and form a plug, which promotes the growth of bacteria in the follicles. This is the process by which pimples and nodules form.

Diagnosis

Examination of the characteristic lesions and patient history confirm the diagnosis.

Treatment

Therapy may include the use of topical or systemic antibiotics or both. Topically applied keratolytic agents may prove appropriate for many cases of acne. Topical application of medications chemically related to vitamin A (e.g., tretinoin [Retin-A] and adapalene) reduces the skin's natural oils and promotes drying and peeling of the acne lesions. Benzoyl peroxide gels are also effective. Antibiotics are prescribed to kill bacteria residing on the skin or in the lesions. Long-term antibiotic use for acne treatment, however, may have

side effects. Often combination therapy, including benzoyl peroxide, topical antibiotics, and retinoids, is the most effective.

For severe acne, isotretinoin (Accutane) may be indicated. Isotretinoin helps reduce the amount of sebum the body produces. Low-dose estrogen is prescribed to balance hormone levels. Optimal results usually are obtained by incorporating medications. Caution must be taken in the use of isotretinoin because it may produce serious psychological side effects, including depression, psychosis, and even suicide. Pregnant or nursing mothers should never take isotretinoin. Isotretinoin is a vitamin A derivative that is administered under an FDA program called IPLEDGE. Providers (physicians, nurse practitioners), patients, and pharmacists must participate in the modified IPLEDGE program for use of this agent. A newer treatment of intralesional dilute steroid injection can be done. This usually results in significantly decreased size and erythema in a matter of hours but can cause a depression.

Prognosis

The prognosis varies, depending on the extent of the acne and the individual's compliance with the medication regimen, including all topical and ingested medications prescribed.

Prevention

No prevention is known.

Patient Teaching

Give patients information about acne and its care. Teach patients the methods of applying dermal medications. Encourage patients to report any side effects resulting from oral medications. Emphasize the importance of not squeezing any pimples or pustules. In addition, emphasize the importance of good hand washing after touching involved skin areas. Scrubbing and washing the skin multiple times a day should be avoided as this may worsen the condition.

Herpes Zoster (Shingles)

Description

Herpes zoster, or shingles, is an acute inflammatory dermatomal eruption of extremely painful vesicles.

ICD-10-CM Code	B02.9 *(Zoster without complications)* (B02.0–B02.9 = 16 codes of specificity)

Herpes zoster has more than one form and location and therefore more than one code. Refer to the physician's diagnosis and then to the current edition of the ICD-10-CM coding manual to ensure the greatest specificity of pathology.

Symptoms and Signs

Shingles occurs in a bandlike unilateral pattern along the course of the peripheral nerves or dermatomes that are affected, and it does not cross the midline of the body (Fig. 6.14). Pain, often in the form of burning or tingling, begins a few days before the appearance of the lesions and sometimes is accompanied by a fever. The eruptions begin as a rash that rapidly develops into vesicles. The skin that overlies the affected dermatome or dermatomes becomes reddened and blistered. These vesicles often are grouped on a reddened area of the skin. After several days, the vesicles appear pustular, develop a crust, and then develop a scab.

The incubation period is usually a few days before the rash appears. The blisters typically become scabbed over in 7 to 10 days, and usually the condition is better or resolved approximately 2 to 4 weeks later. Although the commonly affected site is the skin-overlying thoracic dermatomes (see Fig. 6.14A), any area of the body may be affected. Shingles occasionally occur on the face, neck, and scalp (Fig. 6.14B). When nerves supplying the eye are involved, the disease may cause serious damage to the eye structure.

Patient Screening

Patients experiencing the onset of herpes zoster often experience excruciating pain in the affected area. Prompt assessment and intervention are required. An appointment should be scheduled as soon as possible for the day of the call. Drug therapy beginning immediately helps reduce the severity of symptoms.

Etiology

The cause is varicella-zoster virus (VZV), which is the same virus that causes chickenpox. After lying dormant in the dorsal root ganglia, it becomes reactivated in later years for unknown reasons. Stress appears to be a precipitating factor.

Diagnosis

Shingles (Fig. 6.15) is diagnosed by its characteristic pattern and painful vesicles. One can confirm the diagnosis by culturing the virus from vesicle scrapings. A blood sample containing VZV antibodies also aids in the diagnosis. Although shingles can affect any age group, those older than 50 years of age are more frequently affected. People who have compromised immune systems are also at greater risk of getting shingles.

Treatment

Treatment of shingles is directed toward making the patient comfortable. Analgesics, mild sedatives, antipruritics, steroids (e.g., methylprednisolone, prednisone, and betamethasone [Celestone Soluspan]), and a drying agent to be applied directly to the vesicles may be prescribed. Acyclovir (Zovirax), used orally, parenterally, or topically is also prescribed and is quite effective. Other antiviral agents that may be prescribed include famciclovir (Famvir), valacyclovir (Valtrex), or foscarnet sodium (Foscavir). Antibiotic therapy may be necessary to prevent secondary infections. If the eye is affected, early treatment with idoxuridine is necessary. An ophthalmologist should supervise the latter therapy. Topical treatment with capsaicin cream may provide relief in some cases. Caution is advised because capsaicin may burn when applied. There is also anecdotal evidence that certain essential oils applied to the vesicles can provide pain relief.

When the pain is intolerable, injections of lidocaine and nerve block agents may be attempted. If these steps do not provide relief, permanent nerve blocks via alcohol or nerve resection may be used as a last resort. Shingles occasionally recurs at later dates.

Prognosis

Most cases are resolved within a month. A common complication for some patients is postherpetic neuralgia (PHN). This chronic pain may persist from a month to years after the skin lesions have healed. Patients with chronic PHN may be treated with gabapentin (Neurontin) and are often referred to pain clinics for treatment.

Prevention

Two doses of the recombinant zoster vaccine Shingrix, is the recommended vaccine to prevent shingles. Shingrix is administered in two doses and is indicated for use in people who are 50 years or older and also in people who are 19 years of age and older who are immune compromised due to medications or illness. It is important to note that in the United States the vaccination Zostavax is no longer available for use to prevent shingles. A patient's immunization record may show that they received that immunization prior to discontinued use. Shingles is not contagious, but exposure to fluid in the blisters by an individual who has never had chickenpox may cause chickenpox in that individual. Immunocompromised patients and pregnant females should avoid contact with individuals diagnosed with shingles.

Patient Teaching

Give patients information about the disorder. Encourage patients to take their medications, including pain medications, as prescribed.

Impetigo

Description

Impetigo is a common, contagious, superficial skin infection. It manifests with early vesicular or pustular lesions that rupture and form thick yellow crusts (Fig. 6.16).

ICD-10-CM Code	L01.00 (Impetigo, unspecified) (L01.00–L01.09 = 5 codes of specificity) L01.03 (Bullous impetigo)

Impetigo has more than one form or location and therefore more than one code. Refer to the physician's diagnosis and then to the current edition of the ICD-10-CM coding manual to ensure the greatest specificity of pathology.

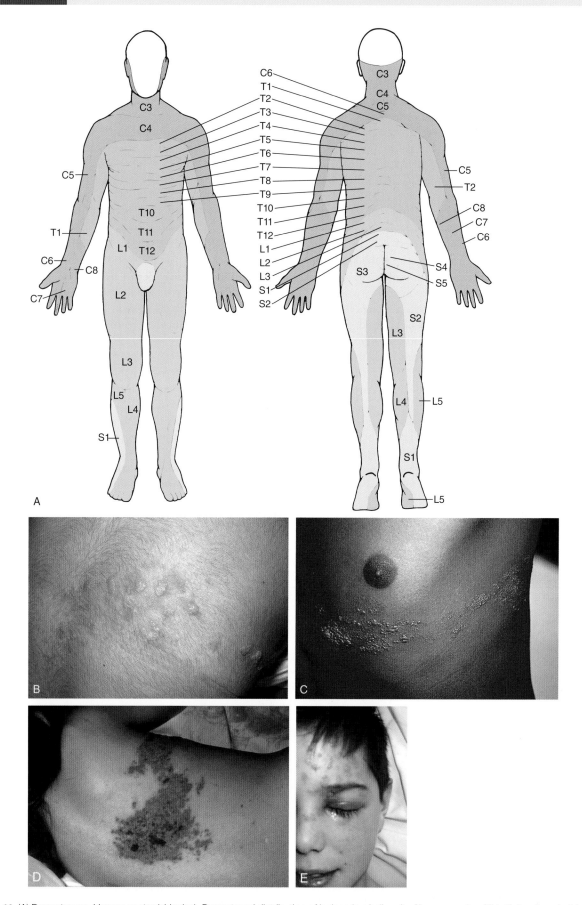

• **Fig. 6.14** (A) Dermatomes. Herpes zoster (shingles). Dermatomal distribution of lesions is a hallmark of herpes zoster. (B) Initially, discrete thin-walled vesicles on an erythematous base are seen. Vesicles coalesce over a few days (C), and lesions then evolve to a crusted stage (D). (E) Involvement of the ophthalmic branch of the trigeminal nerve produces lesions involving the forehead, eyelids, and nose. (From McIntire S, et al: *Zitelli and Davis' atlas of pediatric physical diagnosis*, ed 8, 2023, Elsevier; C, Courtesy Michael Sherlock, MD, Lutherville, Maryland.)

• **Fig. 6.15** Illustration of blisters of shingles. (From Brooks ML, et al: *Exploring medical language: a student-directed approach*, ed 8, St. Louis, 2012, Mosby.)

• **Fig. 6.16** Impetigo. (From Marks JG, et al: *Lookingbill & Marks' principles of dermatology*, ed 5, Philadelphia, 2014, Saunders.)

Symptoms and Signs

Impetigo lesions, a honey-colored crust, usually develop on the legs and are found less often on the face, trunk, and arms. Small vesicles are surrounded by a circle of reddened skin and usually are accompanied by pruritus. Adjacent lesions may develop as a result of autoinoculation resulting from scratching, but systemic symptoms are uncommon. Ulcerations with erythema and scarring also may result from scratching or abrading of the skin.

Patient Screening

Discovering the impetigo infection can be distressing to the individual or to the parent of an affected child. Urgent attention is also needed because impetigo can spread among children or other contacts. Because of the contagious nature of impetigo, the child's school may require immediate attention to the situation. Schedule the next available appointment for the patient following office or clinic policy.

Etiology

Impetigo is caused by either *Streptococcus* or *Staphylococcus aureus*. The infection is thought to originate from insect bites, scabies infestation, poor hygiene, anemia, malnutrition, and impairment in skin integrity related to eczema.

It is also highly contagious and so may be spread among children in schools or in the childcare environment. Cases of impetigo are common in temperate climates and occur more often in warm weather.

Diagnosis

The diagnosis is based on the appearance of the characteristic lesions.

Treatment

Systemic use of antibiotics and proper cleaning of lesions two or three times a day are effective treatments for impetigo. Mupirocin ointment (Bactroban) or cream, along with oral antibiotics such as penicillins, cephalosporins, and erythromycin, may be used in the treatment. If the infection does not respond to these treatments, a culture and sensitivity test may be necessary to determine which antibiotic will work better, since some strains of the bacteria can be antibiotic resistant.

Prognosis

With treatment, the prognosis is good. Most children recover without difficulty.

Prevention

Good hygiene is essential in preventing impetigo. Frequent and thorough hand washing with antibacterial soap is the first line of defense, as in many contagious conditions. Instruct children not to share towels, bedding, clothing, or other personal items.

Patient Teaching

Give parents or caregivers information about impetigo and the ways it spreads. Encourage them to teach children about the importance of good hygiene. All personal items should not be shared during an infection. Towels, bath cloths, sheets, and clothing should be laundered in hot water and detergent. Open lesions should be treated per the physicians' instructions and covered with bandages to prevent the spread.

Furuncles and Carbuncles

Description

A furuncle, or boil, is a pus-containing abscess that involves the entire hair follicle and adjacent subcutaneous tissue. A carbuncle is either an unusually large furuncle or multiple furuncles that develop in adjoining follicles, connected by many drainage canals under the skin.

ICD-10-CM Code   L02.92 *(Furuncle, unspecified)*
L02.93 *(Carbuncle, unspecified)*
(L02.01–L02.93 = 56 codes of specificity)

Furuncles and carbuncles are coded by the site or location. The code above is for unspecified site. Refer to the physician's diagnosis and then to the current edition of the and ICD-10-CM coding manual to ensure the greatest specificity of pathology.

ICD-10-CM Code   L02.02 *(Furuncle of face)*
L02.03 *(Carbuncle of face)*
L02.12 *(Furuncle of neck)*
L02.13 *(Carbuncle of neck)*
L02.221 *(Furuncle of abdominal wall)*
L02.222 *(Furuncle of back [any part, except buttock])*
L02.223 *(Furuncle of chest wall)*
L02.224 *(Furuncle of groin)*
L02.225 *(Furuncle of perineum)*
L02.226 *(Furuncle of umbilicus)*
L02.229 *(Furuncle of trunk, unspecified)*
L02.231 *(Carbuncle of abdominal wall)*
L02.232 *(Carbuncle of back [any part, except buttock])*
L02.233 *(Carbuncle of chest wall)*
L02.234 *(Carbuncle of groin)*
L02.235 *(Carbuncle of perineum)*
L02.236 *(Carbuncle of umbilicus)*
L02.239 *(Carbuncle of trunk, unspecified)*
L02.429 *(Furuncle of limb, unspecified)*
L02.439 *(Carbuncle of limb, unspecified)*
L02.529 *(Furuncle of unspecified hand)*
L02.539 *(Carbuncle of unspecified hand)*
L02.33 *(Carbuncle of buttock)*
L02.429 *(Furuncle of limb, unspecified)*
L02.439 *(Carbuncle of limb, unspecified)*
L02.629 *(Furuncle of unspecified foot)*
L02.639 *(Carbuncle of unspecified foot)*
L02.821 *(Furuncle of head [any part, except face])*
L02.828 *(Furuncle of other sites)*
L02.831 *(Carbuncle of head [any part, except face])*
L02.838 *(Carbuncle of other sites)*

Symptoms and Signs

Furuncles begin as the inflamed hair follicle becomes infected and the infection extends beyond the follicle. The affected area is red, swollen, and painful (Fig. 6.17A). Eventually, over several days, the pus-filled abscess either bursts through the skin or, less often, discharges internally. In either case, the pain is relieved and the boil heals. Erythema and edema may persist at the site for several more days or weeks. They typically form on the face, buttock, thigh, armpit, and the back of the neck. Boils are extremely common. They can affect almost everyone at some time. Carbuncles are much rarer (Fig. 6.17B). Both boils and carbuncles tend to recur.

Patient Screening

The individual reporting the symptoms of a furuncle or carbuncle will convey the degree of urgency to be seen. Give the patient some possible appointment times and allow them to choose the time that fits their schedule. When the patient reports pain and swelling, offer the next available appointment.

Etiology

The most common cause of furuncles and carbuncles is a bacterial infection with *Staphylococcus*, usually *S. aureus*. Both are localized infections and usually heal uneventfully. Predisposing factors include diabetes mellitus, nephritis, immunodeficiency, intravenous (IV) drug abuse, and other underlying diseases (e.g., digestive or gastrointestinal conditions). However, many have no underlying medical disease. In some cases, furuncles and carbuncles result from poor resistance to infection or from poor hygiene.

Diagnosis

The diagnosis is made by observing the characteristic lesion. An abscess may be cultured to isolate the causative organism. If recurring boils are a problem, the physician may order blood and urine analyses to rule out any underlying disease.

Treatment

Applying hot compresses every few hours helps relieve the discomfort and hasten the draining. Surgical incision and drainage (I&D) may be necessary. Antibiotic (cephalexin [Keflex] or dicloxacillin) treatment also may be needed for several weeks. There has been an increase in

• **Fig. 6.17** (A) Furuncle. (B) Carbuncle. (A, From LaFleur B: *Exploring medical language: a student-directed approach*, ed 9, St. Louis, 2014, Mosby; B, From Lawrence CM, Cox NH: *Physical signs in dermatology: color atlas and text*, London, 1993, Mosby Europe.)

methicillin-resistant *S. aureus* (MRSA) as a causative agent in recurring carbuncles. If MRSA is suspected, culture and alternative antibiotic therapy are recommended; either a sulfa-based antibiotic or doxycycline can be effective against most MRSA infections.

Prognosis

Most furuncles and carbuncles resolve with I&D and antibiotic therapy.

Prevention

Prevention requires thorough cleansing of the skin and application of good hand-washing techniques. Patients should be urged not to squeeze the lesions.

Patient Teaching

Give patients information on skin infections and how they spread. Emphasize the need for hand hygiene with antibacterial soap or hand sanitizer. Avoid sharing personal items such as towels and razors.

Cellulitis

Description

Cellulitis is an acute, diffuse, bacterial infection of the skin and subcutaneous tissue.

ICD-10-CM Code	L03.90 *(Cellulitis, unspecified)*
	L03.91 *(Acute lymphangitis, unspecified)*
	(L03.011–L03.91 = 86 codes of specificity)

Cellulitis appears in many forms and locations and thus has more than one code. Refer to the physician's diagnosis and then to the current edition of the ICD-10-CM coding manual to ensure the greatest specificity of pathology.

Symptoms and Signs

Cellulitis occurs most often in the lower extremities, but any part of the body can be affected. Clinically erythema and pitting edema develop, and the skin becomes tender and hot to the touch (Fig. 6.18). The infection develops and spreads gradually over a couple of days. Red lines or streaks may appear proximal to the infection and run along lymph vessels to nearby lymph glands. If the lymph glands become edematous, systemic symptoms of fever and malaise may be present.

Patient Screening

An individual reporting symptoms of edematous skin, reddened, hot, with streaks of red radiating from the site, requires prompt assessment. If the individual cannot be seen in the office within a few hours, a referral to another facility is appropriate according to office protocol.

Etiology

The cause of cellulitis is either *Streptococcus* or *Staphylococcus*, which enters the skin's surface via a small cut or lesion. The bacteria produce enzymes that break down the skin cells. As a result of the release of enzymes, the infection spreads locally. These enzymes prevent body responses that normally would reduce the local spread of infection by closing off the site.

Diagnosis

An examination of the affected body part, pitting edema, and other symptoms aid the physician in making the diagnosis. A blood culture may be indicated.

Treatment

The affected limb should be immobilized and elevated. Cool magnesium sulfate (Epsom salt) solution compresses may be used for discomfort. Warm compresses should be applied to increase circulation to the affected part. Systemic antibiotics, with penicillin being the drug of choice, are prescribed for the infection. Aspirin, NSAIDs, or acetaminophen alone or in combination with codeine is given for pain. Acetaminophen combinations with narcotics are also an option. Hospitalization is indicated when cellulitis is severe.

Prognosis

The prognosis is good with prompt intervention and drug therapy.

Prevention

Good hand washing is essential for prevention. Attention to small nicks and cuts helps prevent this infection.

Patient Teaching

Give patients information about skin infections and the importance of seeking medical attention promptly for an infected cut or scrape.

• **Fig. 6.18** Cellulitis of the left foot. (From Haskell A, et al: *Coughlin and Mann's Surgery of the Foot and Ankle*, ed 10, 2024, Elsevier.)

Dermatophytoses

Description

Dermatophytosis (tinea) is a chronic superficial fungal infection of the skin.

ICD-10-CM Code	B35.9 *(Dermatophytosis, unspecified)*
	(B35.0–B35.9 = 9 codes of specificity)

There are many codes for dermatophytosis, depending on site. Refer to the physician's diagnosis and then to the current edition of the ICD-10-CM coding manual to ensure the greatest specificity of pathology.

Symptoms and Signs

Dermatophyte infections are classified by the body region they inhabit. All dermatophytosis lesions are characterized by an active border and are marked by scaling with central clearing. Dermatophytosis occurring on the scalp is called *tinea capitis;* the body, *tinea corporis;* the nails, *tinea unguium;* the feet, *tinea pedis* (athletes foot); and the groin region, *tinea cruris.*

Patient Screening

Dermatophytosis is troublesome, worrisome, and annoying. The individual calling for an appointment for these symptoms should be seen at the next convenient appointment.

Tinea Capitis

ICD-10-CM Code	B35.0 *(Tinea barbae and tinea capitis)*

Tinea capitis is characterized by round, gray, scaly lesions on the scalp (Fig. 6.19). It is contagious and often epidemic among children. The infected child may have a slight pruritus of the scalp or may be asymptomatic. It is rarely seen in adults.

Tinea Corporis (Ringworm)

ICD-10-CM Code	B35.9 *(Dermatophytosis, unspecified)*

Tinea corporis is characterized by lesions that are round, ringed, and scaled with vesicles (Fig. 6.20A). This infection can occur in anyone who has skin contact with infected domestic animals, especially cats. It is more common in rural settings and in hot and humid climates. It can also be the result of autoinoculation from infections in other parts of the body, such as tinea pedis or tinea capitis, or of contact with contaminated soil.

Tinea Unguium

ICD-10-CM Code	B35.1 *(Tinea unguium)*

• **Fig. 6.19** Tinea capitis. (From Micheletti R, et al: *Andrews' diseases of the skin clinical atlas*, ed 2, 2023, Elsevier.)

Tinea unguium frequently begins at the tip of toenails, affecting one or more nails at a time. It also can affect fingernails, but this is less common. The affected nail or nails appear hypertrophic or thickened, brittle, and lusterless (Fig. 6.20B).

Tinea Pedis (Athletes Foot)

ICD-10-CM Code	B35.3 *(Tinea pedis)*

Tinea pedis is characterized by intense burning, and stinging pruritus between the toes and on the soles of feet (Fig. 6.21). The skin can become inflamed, dry, and peeling; and **fissures** (see Fig. 6.2J) may develop. This condition is rare in children.

Tinea Cruris (Jock Itch)

ICD-10-CM Code	B35.6 *(Tinea cruris)*

Tinea cruris is characterized by raised, red, pruritic vesicular patches with well-defined borders located in the groin area (Fig. 6.22). It is common in males, athletes, those with weakened immune systems, and those who have an increase in sweat. It can also be transmitted from the foot to the groin by towel use or other cross-contamination. Flare-ups are frequent in summer months and are aggravated by physical activity, perspiration, and tight-fitting clothes.

Etiology

Dermatophytosis is caused by several species of fungi that can invade the skin or nails, especially if the integrity of the skin is compromised. The infection is transmitted by direct contact with the fungus or its spores.

Diagnosis

The diagnosis is based on the appearance and location of the lesions. To isolate the causative fungus, a culture of the lesions is necessary. Trichoscopy may be used to diagnose tinea capitis by looking directly at the scalp and hair follicle under magnification.

• **Fig. 6.20** (A) Tinea corporis. (B) Tinea unguium. (A, From Hurwitz S: *Clinical pediatric dermatology: a textbook of skin disorders of childhood and adolescence*, ed 5, 2016, Elsevier; B, Courtesy Jean L. Bologna, MD.)

• **Fig. 6.21** Tinea pedis (athletes foot). (From Gawkrodger D: *Dermatology*, ed 5, New York, 2012, Churchill Livingstone.)

• **Fig. 6.22** Tinea cruris. (From Callen JP, Greer KE, Paller AS, Swinyer LJ: *Color atlas of dermatology*, ed 2, Philadelphia, 2000, W.B. Saunders.)

Treatment

Antifungal medications are prescribed either for topical application (ointment) or for oral use, depending on the severity of the infection. Selenium sulfide 2.5% (Selsun shampoo) is usually prescribed for treatment of tinea capitis, whereas terbinafine hydrochloride (Lamisil), butenafine (Lotrimin Ultra), and fluconazole (Diflucan) are normally prescribed for treatment of tinea pedis, tinea corporis, and tinea cruris, respectively. The affected skin must be kept as clean and dry as possible, clothing should be loose fitting and clean, and exercise should be limited to prevent excessive perspiration. Because all forms of dermatophytosis tend to be persistent and chronic, meticulous management is needed to correct this condition.

Prognosis

The prognosis is good with treatment that includes drug therapy and good skin care; however, because the condition tends to be chronic, recurrence is likely.

Prevention

Wearing loose-fitting cotton clothing helps prevent the condition. The patient must dry the skin after bathing or swimming, with special attention to drying the skin between the toes and in all folds of the skin. The use of a blow dryer on a low setting can aid in drying the area thoroughly.

Patient Teaching

Give the patient online resource information about the disorder. Encourage the patient to dry the skin after exposure to moisture, especially in the areas between the toes and in the folds of the skin. Explain the importance of wearing cotton clothing that absorbs moisture from the body. Advise patients with diabetes and those with compromised peripheral circulation to seek medical attention for athletes foot. Also, stress the importance of not sharing personal items with others.

Decubitus Ulcers

Description

A decubitus ulcer, commonly called a *pressure ulcer* or *bed sore*, is a localized area of dead skin that can affect the epidermis, dermis, and subcutaneous layers (Fig. 6.23).

• **Fig. 6.23** Decubitus ulcers. (A) Stage 1. (B) Stage 2. (C) Stage 3. (D) Stage 4. (From Elkin MK, Perry AG, Potter PA: *Nursing intervention and clinical skills*, ed 4, St. Louis, 2008, Mosby/Elsevier.)

ICD-10-CM Code L89.90 *(Pressure ulcer of unspecified site, unspecified stage)*
(L89.000–L89.95 = 151 codes of specificity)

Skin ulcers can occur in many locations. Refer to the physician's diagnosis and then to the current edition of the ICD-10-CM coding manual to ensure the greatest specificity of pathology.

Symptoms and Signs

An early sign of a decubitus ulcer is shiny, reddened skin appearing over a bony prominence in individuals with prolonged immobilization. Other signs that eventually occur include blisters, erosions, necrosis, and ulceration. If the decubitus ulcer becomes infected, a foul-smelling, purulent discharge is present. Pain may or may not accompany a decubitus ulcer. The ulcers are identified as Stage 1, 2, 3, 4, and 5 according to the tissue affected, deepness, and severitiy.

Patient Screening

Most patients experiencing decubitus ulcers are confined to a bed or are generally immobile. Some patients may not be capable of going to the office for a visit and are therefore seen in the hospital, nursing care facility, or home. Others are seen at a wound care facility by a physician who specializes in wound care. Schedule an appointment for the mobile patient to be seen at the earliest available time.

Etiology

Decubitus ulcers are caused by impairment or lack of blood supply to the affected area of skin. This is the result of constant pressure against the surface of the skin, as seen in people who are debilitated, paralyzed, unconscious, or those who have poor circulation.

Diagnosis

Visual examination of the ulcer is sufficient for a diagnosis. If infection is suspected, culture and sensitivity testing may be needed to isolate the causative organism.

Treatment

If not treated vigorously, the ulcer progresses from a simple erosion of the skin to complete involvement of all layers of skin. Eventually, the ulcer extends to the underlying muscle and bone tissue, and osteomyelitis, an infection of the bone, and/or gangrene may result.

Topical agents that have proved effective in the treatment of decubitus ulcers include absorbable gelatin sponges, granulated sugar, karaya gum patches, antiseptic irrigations, débriding agents, and antibiotics (when infection is present).

Prognosis

The prognosis is fair. Resolution and healing of the lesion depend on the patient's general health and potential for mobility and removal of pressure on the lesion site.

Prevention

Preventive measures include frequent inspection of the skin for signs of breakdown; alleviation of pressure points over bony prominences; good skin care; early ambulation, when possible; position changes every 2 hours; passive range-of-motion exercises; and the use of special pads and mattresses.

• **Fig. 6.24** (A) Scabies mite. Note the eggs within the body of the mite. (Live scabies mite, ×40 magnification.) (B) Scabies rash. (A, From Paller A, et al: *Hurwitz clinical pediatric dermatology: a textbook of skin disorders of childhood and adolescence*, ed 5, Philadelphia, 2016, Elsevier; B, From James WD, et al: *Andrews' diseases of the skin*, ed 11, Philadelphia, 2011, Saunders.)

Patient Teaching

Most teaching is directed to the caregivers. Encourage preventive measures and prompt reporting of any signs of impending skin breakdown.

Scabies and Pediculosis

Description

Itch mites (scabies) and lice (pediculosis) are the two most common parasitic insects to infest humans. Human scabies infestations are caused by the human itch mite, *Sarcoptes scabiei* (Fig. 6.24A). The three species of human lice are the head louse, *Pediculus humanus capitis* (Fig. 6.25A); the body louse, *P. humanus corporis;* and the pubic, or crab, louse, *Phthirus pubis* (Fig. 6.26A). Lice resemble insects, but they are wingless parasites with sucking mouths to feed on human blood. Body lice live in clothes and bedding and feed on the body and prefer to lay their eggs in folds or seams of clothing.

ICD-10-CM Code	B85.2 *(Pediculosis, unspecified)*
	(B85.0–B85.4 = 5 codes of
	specificity)
	B86.0 *(Scabies)*
	B85.0 *(Pediculosis due to*
	Pediculus humanus capitis)
	B85.1 *(Pediculosis due to*
	Pediculus humanus corporis)
	B85.3 *(Phthiriasis)*

Scabies and lice codes should be confirmed for accuracy with a coding manual. Refer to the physician's diagnosis and then to the current edition of the ICD-10-CM coding manual to ensure the greatest specificity of pathology.

Symptoms and Signs

Both scabies and pediculosis are *highly* contagious. They produce intense pruritus and a sensation of something crawling on the skin. With scabies, the most common symptom is a rash (see Fig. 6.24B) accompanied by intense itching that worsens at night. Scabies can occur anywhere on the body but usually are found on the hands, breasts, armpits, waistline, and genital area. Lice also can produce a rash or wheals, but the most common sign or symptom is the presence of nits (eggs) on hair shafts, skin, or clothing (see Figs. 6.25B and 6.26B).

Patient Screening

Patients reporting symptoms of scabies or lice should be seen according to office policy. Scabies mites cannot be seen with the naked eye, while lice can be observed. If a patient or caregiver has seen lice, then the physician will determine whether to have the child come into the office if the patient or caregiver knows what they are seeing is lice. The infestation in children may have been detected at a childcare facility or school. These children must be assessed, and treatment must be prescribed and started as soon as possible. Although not a life-threatening condition, scabies or lice can be spread to others through close contact, and the offending mites and lice should be brought under control quickly. In addition, the patient and or caregiver is typically upset when they call for an appointment.

Etiology

Itch mites and lice can infest anyone at any age. Both are spread easily from person to person via close physical contact. Transmission occurs most often among children playing together, family members, and sexual partners. In addition to physical contact, transmission may occur indirectly via infected clothing, bed sheets, towels, hats, scarves, and hair combs or brushes. Although the scabies mite can infest other mammals, it is not transmitted from pets to humans. Pubic lice, however, have been known to infest dogs and then migrate to humans. Both scabies and pediculosis are common in overcrowded areas that have inadequate facilities and where personal hygiene is poor.

Diagnosis

Visual examination can identify lice and nits on the hair, body, and clothing. When scabies is suspected, other skin disorders must be ruled out. A similar rash occurring about

• **Fig. 6.25** (A) Head louse (*Pediculus humanus capitis*) and an empty egg casing (the operculum is at the top) attached to a hair shaft. (B) Lice in hair. (A, From Ko C: *Dermatology: visual recognition and case reviews*, ed 2, 2022, Elsevier; B, From Lissauer T, et al: *Illustrated textbook of paediatrics*, ed 4, London, 2012, Mosby.)

• **Fig. 6.26** (A) *Phthirus pubis* (pubic or crab louse) has a short, oval body and prominent claws resembling those of sea crabs. (B) Pubic lice. (A, From Dinulos J, et al: *Dermatology DDX deck*, ed 3, 2020, Elsevier; B, From Long SS, et al: *Principles and practice of pediatric infectious diseases*, ed 4, Philadelphia, 2012, Saunders.)

the same time in several family members should suggest scabies, which can be confirmed by the physician's assessment.

Treatment

The goals of the treatment of scabies and pediculosis are to remove the mites, lice, and nits; to eliminate the pruritus; to provide emotional support to the patient, family, and contacts; and to treat the environment to prevent reinfestation.

To kill head lice, a permethrin creme rinse must be used to eliminate the lice and their nits. The patient must follow this with meticulous combing with a special fine-toothed comb to remove the nits. Body lice are removed with soap and water or the same shampoo used for head lice. Pubic lice may be treated with shampoo, creams, or lotions. Directions must be followed when using these special shampoos, because they may have residual toxic effects. Nonprescription treatments for head lice include permethrin, pyrethrins, or piperonyl butoxide. Prescription treatments include permethrin, malathion, as well as ivermectin and spinosad for resistant cases.

Scabies treatment includes the use of special shampoos, creams (permethrin cream [Elimite]), sulfur preparations, and topical steroids. Because of the intense pruritus and the

scratching associated with scabies and lice infestations, secondary infections may occur, necessitating treatment with oral antibiotics.

With both scabies and pediculosis, family members and others who have had direct contact with the infected person must be treated as well. All clothing and bedding belonging to the infected person must be washed in hot water or dry-cleaned. Any furniture that the person has been using also should be cleaned either with a surface cleaner or by vacuuming. Stuffed toys may be placed in plastic garbage bags and sealed tightly for a minimum of 2 weeks, allowing no air into the bag. This smothers the lice.

Prognosis

The prognosis is good with treatment and appropriate disinfection or decontamination of clothing, bedding, and furniture. To prevent reinfestation, those who have had contact with the patient must be made aware of the infestation and treated in a similar fasion.

Prevention

Prevention is difficult with the close social contact among people. Recommend that family members, including children, not share hats and hair-grooming equipment and that personal items are not shared at school or daycare. Infestation by pubic lice is considered a sexually transmitted disease, and suggested precautions are discussed in Chapter 12.

Patient Teaching

Give patients information about recognizing scabies and lice. Pictures of the offending organisms help in their recognition. Explain the importance of laundering clothing and bedding appropriately. Emphasize the importance of notifying all persons in contact with the patient about the infestation so that they can seek treatment. Teach the correct methods of using shampoos or scabicides. It is very important that all instructions are followed to treat the eggs as well as the adult parasites.

Benign and Premalignant Tumors

Description

Noncancerous growths or tumors of the skin fall into two categories: benign and premalignant. Benign tumors are usually a cosmetic problem only. Premalignant tumors must be identified and treated as early as possible to prevent them from developing into malignancies. Common benign and premalignant tumors include seborrheic keratoses, dermatofibromas, keratoacanthomas, keloids, and hypertrophic scars, epidermal (sebaceous) cysts, acrochordons (skin tags), actinic keratoses, and nevi.

Symptoms and Signs

Symptoms and signs vary according to the conditions experienced. Moles are the most common premalignant tumors. The following is a discussion of the conditions.

Patient Screening

Although benign tumors are usually only a cosmetic problem, they still present a source of anxiety to the patient. Premalignant tumors require early identification and treatment to prevent their development into malignancies. Recognize the patient's anxiety level, and schedule an appointment at the earliest convenient time.

Seborrheic Keratosis

ICD-10-CM Code	L82.0 (Inflamed seborrheic keratosis) (L82.0–L82.1 = 2 codes of specificity) L82.1 (Other seborrheic keratosis)

Seborrheic **keratoses** are benign growths originating in the epidermis, clinically appearing as tan-brown, greasy papules or plaques (see Fig. 6.2B and C) and having the appearance of being pasted onto the skin (Fig. 6.27). They are, for the most part, asymptomatic but may cause pruritus, especially in older people. These usually painless lesions may be black, brown, yellow, or other colors and may be

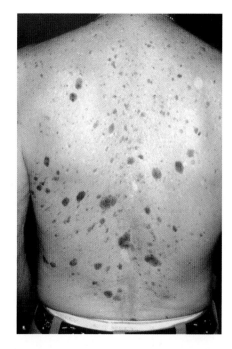

• **Fig. 6.27** Seborrheic keratosis. (From Micheletti R, James W, Elston D: *Andrews' diseases of the skin clinical atlas*, ed 2, 2023, Elsevier.)

located on the face, chest, back, shoulders, or other areas. Additionally, the lesions may have a rough, wartlike texture and may have a slightly elevated flat type of surface. The cause of seborrheic keratoses is unknown, and although they have no potential for developing into malignancy, they should be differentiated from other potentially malignant tumors. The appearance of a sudden increase in the number or size of these growths on uninflamed skin could indicate the presence of an internal malignancy, most commonly of the stomach.

Dermatofibroma

ICD-10-CM Code	D23.9 (Other benign neoplasm of skin, unspecified) (D23.0–D23.9 = 18 codes of specificity)

Dermatofibromas can have more than one site and therefore more than one code. Refer to the physician's diagnosis and then to the current edition of the ICD-10-CM coding manual to ensure the greatest specificity of pathology.

Dermatofibromas are benign and asymptomatic and can be found on any part of the body, particularly on the front of the lower leg. They are most often seen in young adults and are more common in females. These lesions are thought to be caused by fibrous reactions to viral infections. These growths also can be caused by a reaction to insect bites and trauma. Dermatofibromas are scaly, hard growths that are slightly raised and pinkish brown (Fig. 6.28).

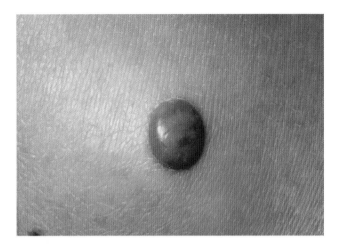

• **Fig. 6.28** Dermatofibroma. (Courtesy Steven Binnick, MD.)

• **Fig. 6.29** Keratoacanthoma. A nontender, well-demarcated nodule of the skin of the nose in an older female. The nodule demonstrates a central keratin plug. (From Neville B, et al: *Oral and maxillofacial pathology*, ed 5, 2024, Elsevier.)

Keratoacanthoma

ICD-10-CM Code	D48.5 *(Neoplasm of uncertain behavior of skin)*

Keratoacanthoma is a benign epithelial growth that may be caused by a virus and is generally seen in people in their 60s. The growth is a smooth, red, dome-shaped papule with a central crust that usually appears singly but may occur in multiple numbers (Fig. 6.29). Keratoacanthoma can disappear spontaneously, but scarring is common. It must be differentiated from squamous cell carcinoma (SCC).

Keloids and Hypertrophic Scars

ICD-10-CM Code	L91.0 *(Hypertrophic scar)* (L91.0–L91.9 = 3 codes of specificity)

Keloids and hypertrophic scars occur secondary to trauma or surgery. A keloid first appears normal, but after

• **Fig. 6.30** Keloid formation. Note the raised, thickened scar over the dorsum of the hand. Unlike a hypertrophic scar, keloids grow beyond the borders of the original wound. (From Lookingbill D, et al: *Principles of dermatology*, ed 3, Philadelphia, 2000, Saunders.)

several months, it becomes noticeably larger and thicker (Fig. 6.30). Keloids are harmless, but they can cause pruritus and sometimes deformities. They are more common in dark-skinned people. Keloids extend beyond the wound site and do not regress spontaneously. Hypertrophic scars, however, do not extend but stay confined to the site, and they generally regress over time. Keloids can be treated in a variety of ways. Compression dressings may be used for newer keloids. Corticosteroid creams or steroid injections may be used in some cases, or application of cryotherapy. Laser or low-dose radiation treatments may be successful in reducing the size of the keloid. Surgical removal may also be used in combination with other therapies, but if used independently, recurrence is common.

Epidermal (Sebaceous) Cyst

ICD-10-CM Code	L72.12 *(Trichodermal cyst)*

Sebaceous cysts develop when a sebaceous gland slowly fills with a thick fluid. This process can take many years but is usually painless and harmless. Some cysts, usually small ones, have a blackhead in the pore connecting the cyst to the skin's surface. Larger cysts most often are closed on the surface. The cysts are palpable and moveable and range in size from millimeters to several centimeters (Fig. 6.31). Sebaceous cysts commonly are found on the scalp, on the face, at the base of the ears, and on the chest. They also can develop in any area of the body that contains sebaceous glands. If bacteria enter the pore, the cyst becomes infected and enlarges, and inflammation and tenderness occur. The cyst eventually may burst, releasing a foul-smelling pus. Inflammation recedes, but the cyst remains and can become reinfected at another time. The cyst and sac that hold the cyst can be removed to prevent recurrence.

• **Fig. 6.31** Palpation of a sebaceous cyst. (From Bhuiyan N: *Surgery secrets: a manual of clinical surgery*, ed 4, 2018, Elsevier.)

• **Fig. 6.32** Acrochordons can be large and numerous, including in younger children. (From Paller A, et al: *Paller and Mancini - Hurwitz clinical pediatric dermatology: a textbook of skin disorders of childhood and adolescence*, ed 6, 2022, Elsevier.)

Acrochordon (Skin Tag)

ICD-10-CM Code	L90.9 *(Atrophic disorder of skin, unspecified)* (L90.0–L90.9 = 9 codes of specificity) L91.9 *(Hypertrophic disorder of the skin, unspecified)*

Acrochordons are common benign skin growths or tags. Painless and usually caused by friction, they are found mainly in the axilla, on the neck, and on the inguinal areas of the body. They can be brown or skin colored, flat or slightly elevated, and are attached to the body by a short stalk (Fig. 6.32).

Actinic Keratosis

ICD-10-CM Code	L57.0 *(Actinic keratosis)*

Actinic keratoses are common premalignant lesions and are seen on sun-exposed areas of the body. They are caused by long-term exposure to the UV portion of sunlight, and their numbers increase with age. Light-skinned people have a higher risk, as do those who do not use sunscreens or skin protection. Actinic keratosis initially appears as an area of rough, vascular skin, which later forms a yellowish-brown, adherent crust (Fig. 6.33).

Etiology
The causes vary, depending on the type of lesion.

Diagnosis
The diagnosis of these lesions is made through visual examination; a biopsy may be necessary to confirm the findings.

• **Fig. 6.33** Actinic keratosis. (From Dinulos J: *Habif's clinical dermatology: a color guide to diagnosis and therapy*, ed 7, 2021, Elsevier.)

Treatment
Treatment of these lesions varies, depending on the specific type of lesion. Seborrheic keratoses are treated with cryosurgery and curettage. Dermatofibromas can be surgically excised if symptomatic. Keratoacanthoma is treated with surgical excision, adrenocorticosteroids applied topically, and, for multiple lesions, oral isotretinoin and etretinate. Keloids and hypertrophic scars are treated with corticosteroids injected into the lesion once every 4 weeks or with surgery and scar compression. Epidermal, or sebaceous, cysts are excised surgically with sac inclusion and treated with antibiotics, if infected. Acrochordons (skin tags) also are treated with

excisional surgery. Actinic keratosis is frequently treated using cryotherapy. The frozen area blisters up, then the skin comes off and new skin replaces the old skin. Topical agents may also be used, such as tretinoin (Retin-A) alone or in combination with fluorouracil, and with curettage and desiccation.

Prognosis

The prognosis varies depending on the condition, the duration of the condition, the amount of skin involved, and the physical condition of the patient. Biopsy reports will indicate the possible outcome.

Prevention

Most of these lesions cannot be prevented. Avoiding direct exposure of the skin to sunlight helps prevent keratoacanthoma and actinic keratosis. Avoiding tanning beds is also beneficial in the prevention of skin lesions resulting from exposure to sun. The use of sunscreen is encouraged.

Patient Teaching

Give patients information about various benign and premalignant tumors. Encourage consistent use of sunscreen and regular evaluation of suspicious skin lesions by a physician. Patients should be taught to avoid tanning beds and to wear protective clothing such as hats when in the sun. Explain that many patients are referred to a dermatologist for follow-up care.

Skin Carcinomas

Collectively, skin cancers, basal cell carcinoma (BCC), SCC, and malignant melanoma, represent the most common types of malignancy. In fact, BCC is the most prevalent form of cancer worldwide. Because BCC and SCC usually do not metastasize, they often are not included in most cancer registries. Left untreated, however, these nonmelanoma skin cancers can be extremely locally destructive and can invade nerves, lymphatics, blood vessels, cartilage, and bone.

Nonmelanoma Skin Cancers

Description

Basal cell carcinoma, BCC, and squamous cell carcinoma SCC affect more than 3 million Americans each year. BCC arises in the basal (deepest) layer of the epidermis, and SCC arises in the epithelial (outer) layer. Merkel cell skin cancer (neuroendocrine carcinoma) is more rare and aggressive skin cancer.

ICD-10-CM Code	*(Refer to the Neoplasm Table in the current edition of the ICD-10-CM coding manual)*

Skin cancers are coded by body site and type. Refer to the physician's diagnosis and then to the current edition of the ICD-10-CM coding manual to ensure the greatest specificity of pathology. A morphology code is also required and is listed in the current edition of the coding manual.

Symptoms and Signs

BCC and SCC lesions can appear anywhere on the body. The most common sites are the sun-exposed areas: face, scalp, ears, back, chest, arms, and back of the hands (Fig. 6.34A and B). The BCC skin lesion can appear in several ways:

- A shiny bump or nodule that is pearly white, pink, red, or translucent. Blood vessels may appear on the surface.
- A sore that bleeds, heals, and recurs. It may be associated with ulceration and crusting.
- A reddish, irritated area, usually on the back, shoulders, extremities, or chest that may or may not be painful or cause pruritus.

• **Fig. 6.34** (A and B) Examples of basal cell carcinomas. (From James WD, et al: *Andrews' Diseases of the Skin: Clinical Dermatology*, ed 13, Philadelphia, 2020, Elsevier.)

• **Fig. 6.35** (A and B) Squamous cell carcinoma. (C) Merkel cell carcinoma on the cheek of a 90-year-old male. (A and B, Courtesy Kenneaster DG: Introduction to skin cancer, *Oral Maxillofac Surg Clin North Am* 17:133, 2005; C, From Saiag P, Blom A, Combined nivolumab and ipilimumab in nonresectable Merkel cell carcinoma, *Lancet* 400(10357), 2022. Credit: Dr P. Marazzi/Science Photo Library.)

- A smooth growth with an indented center and elevated, rolled edge, or border.
- A scarlike area, often with poorly defined edges, that is white, yellow, or waxy in appearance.

SCC lesions often present as a crusted or scaly area with a red, inflamed base; as a growing tumor; as a nonhealing ulcer; or as a raised, firm papule (Fig. 6.35A and B). Hyperkeratosis is an important feature that distinguishes SCC from BCC. The ulcerated lesions may be painful.

Merkel cell carcinoma (MCC) lesions usually appear on the neck, head, or face, but they can occur in other locations. They appear as painless nodules, or raised lesions that may have a purple, blue, or red color, or they may be the color of normal skin. They grow rapidly (Fig. 6.35C), and treatment depends on whether or not the cancer has spread to other tissues and organs.

Patient Screening

Patients reporting any of the following should be scheduled to be seen at the next available appointment: skin lesions, such as a sore that bleeds, heals, and recurs; a reddish, irritated area, usually on the back, shoulders, extremities, or chest, that may or may not be painful or cause pruritus; or a smooth growth with an indented center and elevated, rolled edge or border or a scarlike area, often with poorly defined edges, that is white, yellow, or waxy in appearance. If the patient has a bump or growth that is growing quickly in size they do need to be prioritized as this can indicate MCC. Although most of these skin conditions at an early stage are not life threatening, the patient's anxiety probably is quite high. Giving the patient the earliest possible appointment for assessment and treatment of the condition is a prudent approach to total patient care.

Etiology

These forms of skin cancer can develop in anyone, especially those with a history of sun exposure. People at the highest risk for both carcinomas have fair skin and light-colored hair and eyes. Chronic exposure to the UV radiation in sunlight has two main effects that can lead to tumor formation: (1) It causes mutations in deoxyribonucleic acid (DNA) and (2) it suppresses the skin's immune system, weakening its ability to fight any tumors that do form. Additional risk factors include therapeutic radiation treatment, immunosuppression, and chronic exposure to arsenic. Rare genetic syndromes, such as basal cell nevus syndrome, also increase the risk of nonmelanoma skin cancer. SCC often arises from actinic keratosis or chronically inflamed skin resulting from scar tissue or burns. Smoking increases the risk of development of these carcinomas. Although nonmelanoma skin cancers are not likely to metastasize, some forms of SCC are more aggressive and will spread to distant locations in the body. Both types will cause local destruction if left untreated.

Diagnosis

Unusual skin lesions are often identified by the patient or by the physician on examination of the skin. A biopsy (usually a punch biopsy) of the lesion is required for definitive diagnosis. Patients with SCC should have a lymph node examination to assess for nodal metastases. Those with high-risk SCC may also require computed tomography (CT), magnetic resonance imaging (MRI), or positron emission tomography (PET) examinations to evaluate for disease spread. SCC is staged according to the TNM (tumor-node-metastasis) staging system.

Treatment

Treatment consists of conventional or Mohs (surgery with intraoperative histologic evaluation) surgical excision (90% of cases), cryosurgery (tissue destruction by freezing), electrodesiccation (tissue destruction by heat), and curettage (ED&C), or radiation therapy. Topical therapy may include 5-fluorouracil or imiquimod. Systemic chemotherapy is reserved for those with distant metastases or locally advanced disease.

Patients should be monitored closely for 5 years after treatment to check for recurrence, metastasis, or a new skin cancer.

Prognosis

The overall 5-year survival rate for nonmelanoma skin cancer is 95%. SCC carries a worse prognosis if it occurs on the lip, ear, or scalp or is larger than 2 cm in diameter. About 50% of patients develop another skin cancer within 5 years. Although BCC carries an excellent prognosis because it rarely metastasizes, around 40% of patients with one BCC develop another lesion within 5 years. Having nonmelanoma skin cancer increases the risk of getting another BCC or SCC and developing malignant melanoma.

Prevention

Minimizing sun exposure, especially during childhood, is the key to prevention because people generally receive most of their lifetime UV exposure before adulthood. Any suspicious skin lesions should be evaluated by a physician.

Patient Teaching

Give patients written information about skin cancer. Help them find additional resources for more information. After excision of any lesion, give the patient information about care of the site. Encourage consistent use of sunscreen on exposed skin, and recommend that the patient limit the duration of exposure. Emphasize the importance of regular follow-up examinations.

Malignant Melanoma

Description

Malignant melanoma is the most serious of the three most common types of skin cancer, but it is not as common as squamous and basal cell carcinomas. It arises in epidermal melanocytes, cells that make the brown pigment melanin.

ICD-10-CM Code	C43.9 (Malignant melanoma of skin, unspecified)

Symptoms and Signs

Most melanomas occur as solitary lesions. They can be found anywhere on the skin but are most common on the backs in males and the legs in females. The most common symptom is change, either a newly pigmented area of the skin or a change in a mole that may have been present since birth or childhood (Fig. 6.36). Changes that may indicate the presence of malignant melanoma are as follows:

- Change in size, especially sudden or continuous enlargement
- Change in color, especially multiple shades of tan, brown, and black; mixing of red, white, and blue; or spreading of color from the border into adjacent skin
- Change in shape, especially the development of an irregular, notched border of an area with a previously regular border
- Change in the elevation of a previously flat pigmented area
- Change in the surface: scaliness, erosion, oozing, crusting, or bleeding
- Change in the surrounding skin: redness, swelling, or the development of colored areas adjacent to, but not part of, the pigmented area
- Change in sensation: tenderness, pain, or pruritus
- Change in consistency: softening or hardening

These changes are incorporated into a list known as the ABCDEs of melanoma (see the Enrichment box).

Patient Screening

Patients who report the previous warning signs or symptoms should be seen at the next available appointment. Consider that the patient's anxiety level is probably quite high. Giving the patient the earliest possible appointment for assessment and treatment of the condition is a prudent approach to total patient care.

• **Fig. 6.36** (A) A fully developed malignant melanoma of the left cheek in an older male. (B) Close-up of the lesion. (From Rigel DS, et al: *Cancer of the skin*, ed 2, London, 2012, Saunders.)

❖ ENRICHMENT

ABCDEs of Malignant Melanoma

- A = Asymmetry (lack of equality in the diameter)
- B = Border (notched, scalloped, or indistinct)
- C = Color (uneven, variegated ranging from tan, brown, or black to red and white)
- D = Diameter (usually greater than 6 mm)
- E = Evolving (any change in size, shape, color, elevation, or another trait; or any new symptom, such as bleeding, itching, or crusting)

Etiology

Risk factors for melanoma include a sun-sensitive skin type (fair skin, light-colored hair and eyes, and skin that burns easily), a history of severe sunburn (especially during childhood), geographic location closer to the equator, and use of tanning beds. Intermittent, intense exposures to UV light increase the risk more compared with continuous exposure. Apart from sun/UV radiation exposure, other factors that make certain people more prone to malignant melanoma are as follows:

- A family history of malignant melanoma
- A previous case of malignant melanoma or nonmelanoma skin cancer
- Having many atypical (irregular shape or color) moles
- Xeroderma pigmentosum, a genetic disorder associated with defects in DNA repair, leading to multiple skin cancers at a young age

Diagnosis

If a patient observes any of the ABCDE warning signs or notices an unusual growth, he or she should see a physician immediately. Greater than 50% of melanomas are first identified by the patient. Biopsy, usually excisional biopsy, is needed for histologic diagnosis and for staging. Staging is performed on the basis of the results of a full physical examination, chest radiography, liver function tests, and serum lactate dehydrogenase measurement. If distant metastases are expected, CT, MRI, and PET may be ordered. For patients with advanced melanoma, biopsy specimens may be tested for certain genetic mutations, such as mutation of the *BRAF* gene, which may help guide therapy choices.

Treatment

The treatment of choice is complete excision of the cancerous lesion with wide margins. Sentinel lymph node biopsy is often performed, with complete lymph node dissection if the sentinel node tests positive. Immunotherapy and targeted chemotherapy are becoming the mainstays of treatment for advanced melanoma. The goal of immunotherapy is to boost the body's own immune system to destroy cancer cells. Immunotherapeutic agents currently being used include ipilimumab, interferon-α, and interleukin-2. Recently drugs that specifically target the BRAF protein have been approved for the treatment of melanoma in individuals whose tumor harbors *BRAF* mutation. Many other targeted drugs are currently in clinical trials. Conventional chemotherapy and radiation therapy are still used in many cases.

Prognosis

The overall 5-year survival rate for all stages of melanoma is dependent upon the stage and if metastasis has occurred. According to the National Cancer Institute "The Surveillance, Epidemiology, and End Results (SEER) Program provides information on cancer statistics in an effort to reduce the cancer burden among the U.S. population. SEER is supported by the Surveillance Research Program (SRP) in NCI's Division of Cancer Control and Population Sciences (DCCPS)." Statistics can be accessed regarding different types of cancer. A poorer prognosis is associated with the presence of an ulcerated lesion, axial location of the melanoma, higher number of positive lymph nodes, age greater than 60 years, and male sex. The level of the S-100 protein, a tumor marker, can be used to determine the prognosis,

ENRICHMENT

Guidelines for Protecting the Skin Against Excessive Sun Exposure

- Avoid sunlight between 10:00 a.m. and 3:00 p.m., when UV rays are the strongest.
- Plan outdoor activities for early morning or late afternoon.
- Wear protective clothing, especially a hat with a brim to provide protection from the face and neck. Some clothing has an ultraviolet protection factor label which indicates how much UV radiation can penetrate the skin. Clothing that is darker or brighter in color absorbs more of the sun's UV rays.
- Use sunscreen with a sun protection factor of at least 15, applied 15 to 30 minutes before exposure and again after getting wet, especially after swimming.

with high levels after melanoma resection indicating a worse prognosis. In addition, the prognosis can be accurately correlated with tumor thickness (called *Breslow thickness*).

Prevention

Increased awareness of skin cancer and education about the dangers of excessive sun exposure greatly can improve the prevention and early detection of skin carcinomas and save lives. Adults should perform regular skin self-examinations. People at very high risk (those with familial melanoma syndromes, multiple atypical or common moles, or excessive sun exposure) should see their physicians for periodic whole-body examinations to look for early melanoma lesions. Patients who have had melanoma require close, regular follow-up to screen for recurrence.

Patient Teaching

As with BCC and SCC, give the patient written information about skin cancer. Help the patient find additional sources of information. After excision of any lesion, give the patient information about care of the site. Encourage consistent use of sunscreen on exposed skin, and recommend limiting the time of exposure. Emphasize the importance of regular follow-up examinations. Encourage patients to ask questions about the effects of chemotherapy and radiation therapy.

See the Enrichment box for guidelines for protecting the skin against excessive sun exposure, and see Chapter 15 for a discussion of sunburn.

ⓘ *ALERT!*

Tanning Beds

The cancer division of the World Health Organization listed tanning beds as definitive cancer causers. UV radiation emitted from both the sun and tanning beds or sunning devices was identified as a causative agent in cancers, particularly skin cancers. The use of tanning beds has been shown in studies to increase the risk of melanoma.

Abnormal Skin Pigmentation

Description

The skin normally contains special cells called *melanocytes* that produce melanin, a black pigment that gives color to the skin. Several conditions cause the melanocytes to develop abnormally or to be distributed abnormally. Melanocytes sometimes are fewer in number or less active than normal. This results in a pale area of skin that does not tan when exposed to sunlight. When melanocytes are more numerous or more active than normal, it results in a darker area of skin that tans easily. These abnormal conditions include albinism, vitiligo, melasma (chloasma), nevi (moles), seborrheic warts, pityriasis, and abnormal suntan.

Patient Screening

Abnormal skin pigmentation presents a cosmetic problem. For the individual calling for an appointment for these symptoms, the next convenient appointment should be scheduled.

Albinism

ICD-10-CM Code	E70.29 *(Other disorders of tyrosine metabolism)* (E70.20–E70.29 = 3 codes of specificity) E70.30 *(Albinism, unspecified)* (E70.30–E70.39 = 14 codes of specificity) E70.8 *(Other disorders of aromatic amino-acid metabolism)*

Albinism is a rare inherited condition in which the melanocytes are unable to produce melanin. The patient is pale-skinned, with white hair and generally pink or pale blue eyes (Fig. 6.37). A rare disorder occurring in all races, albinism often is accompanied by eye problems. Eye problems may include myopia, hyperopia, astigmatism, nystagmus, strabismus, and photophobia. Patients with albinism must avoid the sun to prevent their eyes and skin from burning. This genetic disorder has no cure, but many of the eye problems can be treated. Counseling may help the child or young adult deal with social problems created by a general lack of understanding about the disorder.

Vitiligo

ICD-10-CM Code	L80 *(Vitiligo)*

Possibly an autoimmune condition, vitiligo produces pale irregular patches of skin, often evenly located on one side of the body (Fig. 6.38). The patches may enlarge, shrink, or stay the same size. Vitiligo can occur on any area of the body and affects all races. Vitiligo often follows a stressful incident. Vitiligo has no cure, but cosmetics may be used to cover the affected skin areas. Patients with vitiligo should be encouraged to use sunscreen.

• **Fig. 6.37** A case of albinism showing lack of pigment in skin, hair, and eyes. (Courtesy Dr. Asra Khumushi, Dermatologist, Cosmetologists and Laser Surgeon, Nagpur.)

Melasma (Chloasma)

ICD-10-CM Code   L81.8 *(Other specified disorders of pigmentation)*
(L81.0–L81.9 = 10 codes of specificity)

Melasma occurs in some females during hormonal changes, such as pregnancy or with oral contraceptive use. Patches of darker skin develop on the face, especially over the cheeks (Fig. 6.39). This condition disappears after childbirth or when oral contraceptive use is discontinued.

Hemangiomas

ICD-10-CM Code   D18.00 *(Hemangioma unspecified site)*
(D18.00–D18.09 = 5 codes of specificity)

Hemangiomas are coded by sites and types. Refer to the physician's diagnosis and then to the current edition of the ICD-10-CM coding manual to ensure the greatest specificity of pathology.

Hemangiomas are benign lesions of proliferating blood vessels in the dermis that produce a red, blue, or purple color. Examples of hemangiomas are the **nevus** flammeus (port wine stain), which is dark red to purple and usually is located on the face (Fig. 6.40A); the strawberry hemangioma, which is bright red and has a protruding, rough surface (see Fig. 6.38B); and the cherry hemangioma, which is red to purple and is a smooth, dome-shaped, small papule that is 2 to 5 mm in diameter (see Fig. 6.40C).

Nevi (Moles)

ICD-10-CM Code   *(Refer to Neoplasm, Skin, Benign in the current edition of the ICD-10-CM coding manual)*

There are many codes for nevus. Refer to the physician's diagnosis and then to the current edition of the ICD-10-CM coding manual to ensure the greatest specificity of pathology.

Moles are small dark areas of skin composed of dense collections of melanocytes (Fig. 6.41); some may contain hair. A mole occasionally may become malignant (see the Malignant Melanoma section).

Pityriasis

ICD-10-CM Code   L30.5 *(Pityriasis alba)*

Pityriasis may be coded according to location or form. Refer to the physician's diagnosis and then to the current edition of the ICD-10-CM coding manual to ensure the greatest specificity of pathology.

Pityriasis is a fungal infection that causes patches of flaky, light, or dark skin to develop on the trunk of the body. This is an uncommon condition. There are many types of pityriasis, with some leaving permanent changes to the skin color.

Abnormal Suntan

ICD-10-CM Code   L57.8 *(Other skin changes due to chronic exposure to nonionizing radiation)*

Abnormal suntan is an unspecified adverse effect resulting from a proper drug, medicinal, or biologic substance properly administered. Some drugs and certain diseases, such as Addison disease, can produce a suntan even without exposure to sunlight.

Etiology
The causes of abnormal skin pigmentation vary, depending on the abnormality.

Diagnosis
Most of these conditions are harmless, and visual examination by a physician confirms the diagnosis. Moles may cause concern, especially if size or shape has changed. The physician may recommend biopsy to rule out a malignancy.

Treatment
When any of these conditions produce skin color variations, nonprescription depigmenting creams may be used to lighten the affected skin. Vitiligo may be improved with UV lamp treatments combined with drug therapy. Pityriasis can be cured with the application of antifungal ointments.

• **Fig. 6.38** Vitiligo. (From Ezzedine K, et al: Vitiligo, *Lancet*, 386(9988):74–84, 2015.)

• **Fig. 6.39** Melasma. (From Micheletti R, James W, Elston D, McMahon A: *Andrews' diseases of the skin clinical atlas*, ed 2, 2023, Elsevier.)

Moles can be removed surgically, and other skin blemishes can be covered by using special cosmetics. Laser surgery may be used to treat hemangiomas.

Prognosis

The prognosis varies, depending on the condition and its extent. When drug therapy and surgical intervention are not appropriate or successful, cosmetics may be used to conceal the pigmentation problem.

Prevention

The etiology varies, so prevention varies as well.

Patient Teaching

Help patients locate and use the available resources for their condition.

Alopecia (Baldness)

Description

Alopecia is the loss or absence of hair, especially on the scalp.

ICD-10-CM Code	L65.9 (*Nonscarring hair loss, unspecified*)
	(L65.0–L65.9 = 5 codes of specificity)

Refer to the physician's diagnosis and then to the current edition of the ICD-10-CM coding manual to ensure the greatest specificity of pathology.

ICD-10-CM Code	L63.2 (*Ophiasis*)
	L63.8 (*Other alopecia areata*)
	L65.0 (*Telogen effluvium*)
	L65.8 (*Other specified nonscarring hair loss*)
	L66.0 (*Pseudopelade*)

• **Fig. 6.40** (A) Port wine stain. (B) Strawberry hemangioma. (C) Cherry hemangioma. (A, From Zitelli BJ, Davis HW: *Atlas of pediatric physical diagnosis*, ed 6, Philadelphia, 2012, Mosby; B and C, From Marks JG, et al: *Lookingbill and Marks' principles of dermatology*, ed 4, Philadelphia, 2006, Saunders.)

L66.2 *(Folliculitis decalvans)*
L66.8 *(Other cicatricial alopecia)*
(L66.0–L66.9 = 7 codes of
 specificity)

Symptoms and Signs

Alopecia can be either temporary or permanent. It can appear gradually, as with aging, or suddenly, occurring all at once or in patchy areas, as with alopecia areata (Fig. 6.42).

Patient Screening

Alopecia is a troublesome and worrisome condition that may also be a sign of an underlying health problem. Schedule an appointment for this patient to be seen when convenient for all involved.

Etiology

In most cases, baldness is a result of the aging process or heredity. It can, however, be a consequence of certain systemic illnesses, such as thyroid diseases, iron deficiency anemia, syphilis, or an autoimmune disease. Certain forms of dermatitis (see the Dermatitis section) also can cause alopecia. Chemotherapy, radiation therapy used to treat cancer, and some other types of medications may lead to thinning and loss of hair. Hair often grows back after treatment has been completed. More often, however, hair loss is not attributed to any specific disease process.

In males, alopecia tends to be part of the aging process and follows a familial pattern on the mother's side. The typical pattern is for the front hairline to recede and for the hair on the top of the head to thin. In some males, these areas eventually meet, leaving hair on only the sides of the head. This pattern of hair loss is called *androgenetic alopecia* (male pattern baldness) (see Fig. 6.42). There are seven stages involved. Most females experience a gradual but slight loss of hair throughout life. Some females experience thinning of hair about 3 months postpartum. This is a fairly common occurrence and corrects itself within a few months.

Loss of hair in oval patches without signs of inflammation is often the result of alopecia areata. It is most commonly seen on the scalp but can affect other hair-bearing areas, such as the eyebrows, beard, arms, or legs. The duration of hair loss is weeks to months and often spontaneous regrowth occurs. It is thought to be an autoimmune disease. A more severe but rare form of alopecia causes permanent hair loss over the entire body, including the eyebrows and eyelashes.

Diagnosis

Visual examination may be all that is needed for the diagnosis, but the cause should also be investigated. Blood and thyroid studies are needed to rule out thyroid disease and anemia. Sometimes punch biopsy is performed if scarring is present.

Treatment

Treatment of alopecia varies, depending on the cause. Effective treatment of any underlying disease usually restores hair growth to normal. To treat male pattern

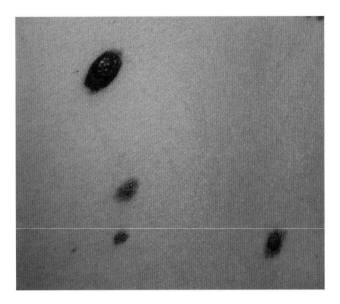

• **Fig. 6.41** Brown and tan nevi showing variation in appearance. (From Marks JG, et al: *Lookingbill* and *Marks' principles of dermatology*, ed 4, Philadelphia, 2006, Saunders.)

• **Fig. 6.42** (A) Alopecia areata: patchy hair loss. The alopecic area is devoid of hairs and the scalp does not present inflammatory changes. (B) Androgenetic alopecia diagram (male pattern baldness). (C) Twenty-six-year-old male with patches of baldness that have been treated with steroids. (A, From Goldman L, Schafer AI: *Goldman's Cecil medicine*, ed 24, Philadelphia, 2012, Saunders; B, From Callen J, et al: *Color atlas of dermatology*, ed 2, Philadelphia, 2000, Saunders; C, Courtesy Margaret Frazier 2019.)

baldness, minoxidil (Rogaine) preparations used topically in cream and spray forms have shown promise. Finasteride (Propecia), is a drug therapy, but it should not be taken by females of child-bearing age because it may have teratogenic effects on their male offspring. Other options include wearing a toupee or wig or undergoing hair transplantation. Transplantation is effective for certain types of hair loss, especially male pattern baldness, but transplantation and the use of minoxidil are expensive and can have side effects. Minoxidil must be continued indefinitely, or hair will begin to fall out again. Alopecia areata can be treated with superpotent topical steroids or intralesional injection of triamcinolone.

Prognosis

The prognosis varies, depending on the cause. Alopecia resulting from the aging process or heredity will not resolve. As previously stated, treatment of an underlying medical cause may result in improvement.

Prevention

No prevention is known for alopecia.

Patient Teaching

Those who have baldness resulting from the aging process or heredity should be encouraged to accept the condition. Offer information about alopecia and permanent or temporary hair replacement.

Corns and Calluses

Description

Corns and calluses are extremely common, localized hyperplastic areas of the stratum corneum layer of the epidermis.

ICD-10-CM Code	L84 *(Corns and callosities)*

Symptoms and Signs

Corns have a glassy core, are small (less than one-fifth of an inch), are more painful than calluses, and develop on the toes. Calluses are larger (up to 1 inch) and commonly develop on the ball of the foot and the palm of the hand. Tenderness and pain over the affected area are the common symptoms.

Patient Screening

Patients with corns and calluses usually report painful feet when requesting an appointment. Schedule the next available appointment that is convenient for all involved.

Etiology

Both conditions may result from pressure or friction caused by ill-fitting shoes, orthopedic deformities, or faulty weight bearing. People who play stringed instruments and manual laborers are prone to calluses caused by repeated trauma to the affected area. In addition, people with impaired circulation in their feet resulting from peripheral neuropathy (sometimes caused by diabetes mellitus) are more prone to corns and calluses.

Diagnosis

It is unusual for corns and calluses to become so painful that the patient needs to consult a physician. When the patient does consult a physician, a physical examination of the affected area and a brief history are sufficient for diagnosis.

Treatment

Relieving pressure and friction points as soon as possible is the goal of treatment. Many self-help measures, such as pads and sponge rings, chemical agents to soften and loosen corns, and pumice stone to rub off dead skin resulting from calluses, are available on the market. If these treatments are ineffective, a physician can trim the corn or callus surgically or with strong chemicals. *Caution:* Patients with diabetes mellitus should not use self-help measures but should seek the help of a podiatrist to treat corns and calluses.

Prognosis

Most corns and calluses resolve with treatment and removal of the offending pressure source.

Prevention

Properly fitting shoes help prevent corns and calluses. Some calluses caused by repeated trauma cannot be prevented.

Patient Teaching

Give patients information about the etiology of corns and calluses. Recommend the wearing of proper footwear. Encourage patients with diabetes and those with impaired circulation to seek professional foot care on a regular basis.

Verrucae (Warts)

Description

Verrucae are elevated growths of the epidermis that result from hyperplasia (Fig. 6.43).

ICD-10-CM Code	B07.9 *(Viral wart, unspecified)* (B07.0–B07.9 = 3 codes of specificity)

Warts have several codes. Refer to the physician's diagnosis and then to the current edition of the ICD-10-CM coding manual to ensure the greatest specificity of pathology.

Symptoms and Signs

Warts are a cutaneous manifestation of human papillomavirus infection. The three most often seen types are common warts, plantar warts, and flat warts. Of the several types of

• **Fig. 6.43** Verruca (common wart). (Courtesy Department of Dermatology, School of Medicine, University of Utah, Salt Lake City, Utah.)

• **Fig. 6.44** Staphylococcal superficial folliculitis. Multiple pustules on a red base. (Reprinted with permission from Morelli JG, Torres-Zegarra C: *Pediatric dermatology*, ed 3, St. Louis, 2021, Elsevier.)

warts, the most common is the common wart, which represents approximately 70% of all cutaneous warts. This wart is a small, hard, white, or pink lump with a cauliflower-like surface. Inside the wart are small, clotted blood vessels that resemble black splinters.

A verruca can develop anywhere on the body but is most likely to appear on the hands or the soles of the feet. For the most part, the wart is painless, but a wart on the sole of a foot (plantar wart) can feel as if there is a stone in the shoe. Pruritus also can accompany a wart. Verrucae are common among teenagers and children, but no serious health risks are associated with these warts.

Etiology

Warts are caused by viruses and are spread by touch or contact with the skin shed from a wart. Each of the types of viruses known to cause warts tends to infect a different part of the body.

Diagnosis

Diagnosis is made on visual examination. There are two types of warts for which a physician should be consulted. One is penile or vulvar warts, and the other is a wart that develops after age 45 years. What looks like a wart actually could be a serious skin condition, such as skin cancer.

Treatment

Most warts disappear naturally over time. Many self-help remedies are available in the form of paints, creams, or plasters. These medications contain chemicals that destroy the abnormal skin cells, but they also damage the surrounding healthy cells. Care must be taken to minimize soreness. Warts located on the face or genitals should not be treated with these chemicals. A physician can remove persistent warts by surgical excision, cryosurgery, or electrodesiccation. Treatment is often painful and prolonged.

Prognosis

With medical intervention, the prognosis for most warts is good. Some warts tend to recur.

Prevention

Warts are contagious, and a wart may shed cells along with the virus when it is touched. The prevention of genital warts is discussed in Chapter 12.

Patient Teaching

Give patients information about warts and how they are spread. Advise them to wear shower shoes when using a public bathing facility.

Folliculitis

Description

Folliculitis is an inflammatory reaction of the hair follicles that produces erythemic, pustular lesions (Fig. 6.44).

ICD-10-CM Code	L66.3 *(Perifolliculitis capitis abscedens)*
	L73.8 *(Other specified follicular disorders)*
	(L73.0–L73.9 = 5 codes of specificity)

Symptoms and Signs

The pustules of folliculitis occur individually and do not combine. They usually are found on the thighs and buttocks but can also occur in the beard area and on the scalp. Some patients may report mild discomfort, mainly because of pruritus, associated with the pustules, but folliculitis is usually asymptomatic.

This is a relatively common condition that affects primarily young adults. It can be chronic or recurrent.

Patient Screening

As with many other skin disorders, folliculitis is a troublesome and worrisome condition. Schedule the next available appointment for the patient.

Etiology

Folliculitis is a bacterial infection usually caused by *S. aureus* or another bacteria on the skin. The bacteria enter the skin through the opening of the hair follicle and cause a low-grade infection within the epidermal layer. Damage to the hair follicle occurs. Shaving, wearing tight clothing, skin rubbing against skin, and touching your skin frequently can damage hair follicles.

Damage to the hair follicle can also occur from using hot tubs or whirlpools.

Diagnosis

The diagnosis of folliculitis is based on the presence of hairs within the pustular lesions. It is confirmed when a culture of the purulent material shows the presence of *S. aureus* or another type of microorganism.

Treatment

There are many types of folliculitis. The treatments may differ depending on the type of folliculitis and the severity of the symptoms. The first step in treatment is to cleanse the skin with an antibacterial cleanser. Topical steroid creams may also be used to treat irritation and itching. In severe cases, oral antibiotics and antifungals may be used to treat persistent or secondary infections.

Folliculitis occasionally results in the development of a furuncle that requires incision and drainage (see the Furuncles and Carbuncles section).

Prognosis

With treatment, the prognosis is good.

Prevention

Try to eliminate the cause of the folliculitis. Shave carefully using a clean razor. Wear loose-fitting clothing during hot and humid months of the year. Maintain hot tubs with accurate levels of chlorine and practice good hygiene.

Patient Teaching

Give patients information about the disorder. Encourage them not to squeeze any pustules.

Deformed or Discolored Nails

Description

Nails with any unusual thickening, shape, or color that deviates from normal are classified as deformed or discolored nails.

ICD-10-CM Code	L60.9 *(Nail disorder, unspecified)* (L60.0–L62 = 9 codes of specificity)

Symptoms and Signs

Any unusual thickening, color variation, and change in the shape of either the fingernails or the toenails can be symptoms of an underlying disease or disorder.

Patient Screening

Patients reporting deformities, odd shapes, or discoloration of nails are usually scheduled for an appointment that fits their convenience.

Etiology

Injury to the nail bed caused by continuous pressure from ill-fitting shoes or poor circulation caused by arteriosclerosis can lead to the thickening of the whole nail. Many disorders can produce nail deformities. Psoriasis, lichen planus, and chronic paronychia can cause the end of the nail to separate from the underlying skin. Bacteria can enter this space and make the nail turn a blackish green. Iron deficiency anemia can cause spooning of the nails. Congenital heart disorders and lung cancer can cause clubbing, or knobby ends of the fingers or toes, and then cause the nails to grow around these ends.

Nail discoloration is caused by many illnesses. With anemia, the nail bed appears pale. A person with chronic hepatic disease has white nail beds. Small, black, splinter-like areas called splinter hemorrhages appear under the nails with infections of the cardiac valves, systemic lupus erythematosus, and dermatomyositis.

Vitamin or mineral deficiencies and injury to a nail may cause one or more white patches to develop in the nail. The nail of the big toe sometimes can curve under at the sides and dig into the skin, causing pain as it grows. This is known as an *ingrown toenail*.

Diagnosis

Examination of the affected nail or nails and a medical history may be all that is needed for a diagnosis. A blood chemistry profile detects any underlying condition or illness.

Treatment

Deformities and discolorations caused by underlying illnesses resolve when the illness is corrected. Nails damaged by injury usually grow back in or grow out again in about 9 months. The patient can practice several self-help measures with an ingrown toenail, such as wearing loose-fitting shoes, keeping the area clean and dry to prevent infection, and cutting the nail straight across the top. If these measures do not help, the patient should see a physician. The physician can remove the ingrowing edge of the nail and the toe's nail fold and apply a chemical to the edge to relieve the discomfort and prevent the edge from growing in again. When the discoloration is caused by a fungus, terbinafine hydrochloride (Lamisil) may be prescribed.

Prognosis

As previously mentioned, deformities and discolorations caused by underlying illnesses usually resolve when the illness is corrected. Nails damaged by injury usually grow back in or grow out again in about 9 months. Treatment for ingrown toenails usually has a positive outcome.

Prevention

Trimming toenails straight across helps prevent ingrown toenails. Malformations of the nails often are the result of injury to the nails or nail beds or the sequela to certain disease processes and cannot be prevented.

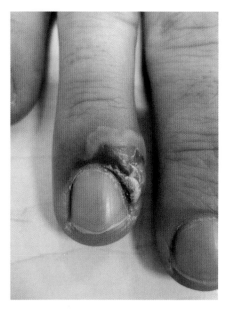

• **Fig. 6.45** Acute paronychia. (From Micheletti RG, et al: *Andrews' diseases of the skin, clinical atlas*, ed 2, Philadelphia, 2023, Elsevier.)

Patient Teaching

Give patients information about proper care and trimming of nails. Encourage those with ingrown toenails to select shoes with sufficient space for the toes.

Paronychia

Description

A paronychia is an infection of the skin around a nail.

ICD-10-CM Code	L03.019 *(Cellulitis of unspecified finger)* (L03.011–L03.019 = 3 codes of specificity)

There are several codes listed for paronychia, so refer to the physician's diagnosis and then to the current edition of the ICD-10-CM coding manual to ensure the greatest specificity of pathology. Additional codes are required to identify the causative organism.

Symptoms and Signs

With acute paronychia, the cuticle or nail fold becomes edematous, red, and painful. If the cuticle lifts away from the base of the nail, purulent material may be expressed from beneath. When the nail fold is affected, a blister of pus called a whitlow develops beside the nail (Fig. 6.45). Chronic infections produce similar symptoms, and often several nails are affected. With the cuticle lifted, the nail roots are no longer protected and become damaged. This produces deformed or discolored nails.

Patient Screening

The patient experiencing paronychia may also feel pain in the hand. If an immediate appointment cannot be scheduled, refer the patient to a medical facility that can provide prompt assessment and treatment.

Etiology

The infection may be caused by bacteria or fungi. Bacteria usually cause acute infections, whereas fungi usually cause chronic infections, which develop slowly and are less painful but also more persistent. Paronychia occurs particularly in people who have their hands in water for long periods.

Diagnosis

A physician can diagnose a paronychia on examination of the affected areas and with a history of the symptoms. A culture of the exudate is needed to identify a bacterial or fungal origin.

Treatment

Antibiotics correct a bacterial infection, and if the infection is chronic, an antifungal cream or paint (ciclopirox [Penlac]) is prescribed.

Prognosis

Drug therapy usually helps resolve the infection. Several months of treatment may be required for the swelling to subside and the raised cuticle to return to normal.

Prevention

Encourage the use of the proper hand-washing technique, along with thorough drying of the hands after washing or being in the water for extended periods.

Patient Teaching

Demonstrate the proper hand-washing technique. Emphasize the importance of drying hands after exposure to water.

Necrotizing Fasciitis

Description

Necrotizing fasciitis is a bacterial infection. The infection spreads systemically and can cause death.

ICD-10-CM Code	M72.6 Necrotizing Fasciitis

Symptoms and Signs

Early symptoms include swollen, red areas of the skin, and severe pain that can radiate from the red area (Fig. 6.46). Swelling is common, and the patient may have a fever. Later symptoms are changes in skin color, blisters, black spots on the skin, ulcers, purulent drainage, fatigue, dizziness, nausea, and diarrhea.

Patient Screening

A break in the skin is usually present and allows bacteria to enter the patient's body. However, in some cases, the pathogen does not enter through a break in the skin.

• **Fig. 6.46** Necrotizing fasciitis. (Courtesy J. H. Brien.)

Etiology
According to the Centers for Disease Control and Prevention (CDC), group A *Streptococcus*, referred to as *flesh-eating bacteria*, is the most common cause of necrotizing fasciitis, but there are other bacteria that can cause the condition.

Diagnosis
Laboratory work to identify the cause of the infection and imaging studies of the affected area are used to diagnose the condition, along with biopsy of the affected tissue to determine the cause.

Treatment
Necrotizing fasciitis is treated with IV antibiotics, and surgery may also be performed to remove affected tissue and prevent the spread of the infection. Prompt treatment is important in preventing death.

Prognosis
Necrotizing fasciitis can lead to serious complications, including loss of limbs as a result of damage and scarring. This can lead to shock, organ failure, and sepsis. One in three people will die as a result of the infection, even with treatment.

Prevention
Cleaning and caring for wounds and keeping the skin free from bacteria are ways to prevent skin infections of all types. Washing with antibacterial soap to remove pathogens is one measure. Covering open wounds with clean bandages helps prevent the spread of bacteria. For a deep wound or puncture, consultation with a physician is recommended. Avoiding swimming in lakes, pools, and rivers when having open wounds is also recommended.

Patient Teaching
Patients should follow up with the physician, take all medications as prescribed, and report any change in the condition of the skin as the wound heals. Bandaging and wound care should be emphasized.

Review Challenge

Answer the following questions:
1. What are the functions of the integumentary system?
2. What is the difference between a macule and a cyst? A plaque and a fissure? A comedo and a pustule?
3. How is cradle cap related to seborrheic dermatitis?
4. What factors might induce the inflammation of contact dermatitis?
5. How is the skin likely to appear in a person diagnosed with atopic dermatitis?
6. What are the general symptoms and signs of urticaria?
7. Where on the body are the lesions of psoriasis most likely to appear?
8. Where does rosacea usually appear?
9. What treatment might the physician prescribe for acne vulgaris?
10. What is the clinical course of herpes zoster?
11. Because impetigo is contagious, what actions may a school decide to take?
12. Describe symptoms and signs of cellulitis, and discuss where the condition usually manifests itself.
13. Are there any conditions considered predisposing to furuncles and carbuncles? If so, what are they?
14. How are dermatophytoses classified?
15. What are the early signs of a decubitus ulcer?
16. What is the comprehensive treatment plan for a human scabies infestation or for lice?
17. What are two of the most common premalignant skin tumors?
18. What is the common cause of actinic keratosis?
19. Name the two nonmelanoma skin cancers.
20. Which skin cancer is the most serious type? What are the characteristics of such a lesion?
21. Which pathology has been associated with the use of tanning beds?
22. Besides the aging process, what are other possible causes of alopecia?
23. What are the ABCDEs of malignant melanoma?
24. What are the special cells that control skin color called?
25. What is the cause of albinism?
26. What is the cause of vitiligo?

27. What is the primary cause of melasma?

28. Describe folliculitis?

29. What is the etiology of warts?

30. Describe the long-term complications of necrotizing fasciitis.

Real-Life Challenge: Shingles

A 57-year-old female has severe pain in the left occipital region, on the left side of her neck, and in the left scapular region. The onset was approximately 36 hours ago. She describes the pain as intermittent, sharp, shooting, and severe. She has been taking ibuprofen for the pain, with little relief. She noticed small blisters forming along the painful areas in the last few hours. She is afebrile and appears quite uncomfortable.

On examination, small blisterlike eruptions are noted along the left side of the neck, left anterior shoulder, and clavicular area. Some eruptions also appear at the base of the skull just in the hairline. These eruptions do not cross the midline on either the front or back of the body.

The patient is diagnosed with shingles, along the C-2, C-3, and C-4 peripheral nerves or the dermatome area. On questioning, the patient confirms having had chickenpox in childhood when she was about 8 years of age.

Medications prescribed include famciclovir (Famvir) 500 mg three times daily for 7 days. Acyclovir (Zovirax) cream also was prescribed for topical application to the affected areas and hydrocodone bitartrate with acetaminophen (Vicodin) for pain.

Questions

1. What is the significance of the previous occurrence of chickenpox?

2. What is the causative agent of chickenpox? Of shingles?

3. Why is the fact that the eruptions do not cross the midline important?

4. Identify other medications that may be prescribed for shingles.

5. What might the patient expect as an outcome of this condition?

6. What is meant by postherpetic neuralgia?

Real-Life Challenge: Malignant Melanoma

A 35-year-old, fair-skinned female has noticed the enlargement of a mole on her right lower arm. The mole has been present for as long as she can remember. In the past month, it appears to have doubled in size and has become darker.

The patient admits to having been exposed to direct sunlight for the past several years. She lives in southern Texas and spends several hours a day in the sun while doing garden work. She has not consistently applied sunscreen to her lower arms and hands.

Visual examination shows a slightly elevated, 7-mm, irregularly shaped, dark, multicolored lesion on the dorsal aspect of the right lower arm, about 3 inches above the wrist. Closer examination shows the lesion to be asymmetric, with a notched border.

Family history reveals that the patient's mother had three lesions removed from her arms and face that were diagnosed as malignant melanoma. In addition, two maternal aunts have had malignant melanomas. One aunt recently died as a result of metastatic cancer. The patient remembers having incurred several sunburns with blistering as a child.

Surgical excision of the lesion is performed, and biopsy confirms the diagnosis of malignant melanoma. The patient is referred to an oncologist for possible chemotherapy.

Questions

1. What characteristics in the patient suggest that she may have malignant melanoma?

2. What symptoms distinguish malignant melanoma from basal cell or squamous cell carcinoma?

3. What is the prognosis for a patient with malignant melanoma, such as this patient?

4. What patient teaching would you offer to patients about extensive exposure to sunlight?

5. What is the importance of a good family history?

6. Why was the patient referred to an oncologist?

7. Would this patient be a candidate for further surgical procedures? If so, what procedures would be performed, and why?

8. List the warning signs of malignant melanoma.

Real-Life Challenge: Rosacea

A 70-year-old male is seen in the office for what he says is a change in his complexion. He presents with a reddened skin color on his face as well as pimples. A significant redness is noted on his cheeks and across the nose. On close examination, the small blood vessels in this area appear enlarged and show through the skin as red lines. The nose appears swollen, showing some small knobby bumps. This male is a businessman in the community, and his wife states that she has heard rumors that he has problems with excessive drinking and that his business is failing because of that. She also states that when he gets flustered or embarrassed, his face gets redder. The patient says that his younger grandchildren are becoming fearful of him.

Questions

1. What characteristics that are common in rosacea does this patient exhibit?
2. What might be the cause of this condition?
3. The grandchildren's mother is concerned that his condition may be contagious. What can be done to ease her concerns?
4. What treatment is available for this condition?
5. What outcome can the patient expect with treatment?
6. What would you advise the patient to avoid?

Internet Assignments

1. Research actinic keratosis at the American Academy of Dermatology, and write a report on its association with squamous cell carcinoma.
2. Research the incidence of malignant melanoma and its treatment at The Melanoma Research Foundation. Investigate the mortality and morbidity rates of this condition.
3. Research the statistics for Group A streptococcus in association with necrotizing fasciitis.
4. Prepare to discuss Critical Thinking case study exercises for this chapter that are posted on Evolve.

Critical Thinking

1. List the functions of the skin.
2. Which layer of the skin gives it strength and elasticity?
3. List manifestations of dermatitis.
4. Discuss the feelings of parents of an infant who had just been diagnosed with "cradle cap."
5. Describe sensitization in relationship to dermatitis.
6. Discuss the psychological effects of eczema and of psoriasis on patients.
7. When can hives become a life-threatening condition?
8. Discuss the possible psychological effects of rosacea experienced by the patient.
9. Discuss some of the options individuals, especially the youth, may attempt to cure or prevent acne.
10. How is herpes zoster cured?
11. Discuss how schools handle the issue of children with impetigo.
12. What is the importance of good hand washing in dermatologic conditions?
13. Discuss the prevention of dermatophytosis.
14. How can decubitus ulcers be prevented?
15. Discuss the contagious state of scabies and pediculosis.
16. Why is it important to have seborrheic keratosis evaluated by a professional?
17. What are the two common types of nonmelanoma skin cancers?
18. Explain differences in melanoma and nonmelanoma skin cancers.
19. Discuss the emotional response of the patient who has just been told of the diagnosis of malignant melanoma.
20. Discuss the various skin pigment disorders.
21. Discuss psychological aspects of alopecia.
22. Explain how you would feel if diagnosed with a skin disorder that affected your appearance.

Credentialing Examination Questions

1. Which type of skin cancer may appear as a fast-growing nodule or bump and may be red, blue, or violet in color?
   A. Basal cell carcinoma
   B. Melanoma
   C. Squamous cell carcinoma
   D. Merkel cell
2. Which type of pediculosis involves burrowing in the skin and moving from one area under the skin to another?
   A. Head lice
   B. Pubic lice
   C. Tick
   D. Scabies
3. Which chronic skin condition is characterized by thick, flaky, red patches of various sizes covered with characteristic white, silvery scales?
   A. Psoriasis
   B. Rosacea
   C. Acne vulgaris
   D. Furuncle
4. Round, gray, scaly lesions on the scalp are an indication of which skin disorder?
   A. Tinea corporis

B. Tinea pedis
C. Tinea capitis
D. Tinea unguium

5. Which diagnosis is caused by several species of fungi that can invade the skin or nails?
   A. Pityriasis
   B. Dermatophytosis
   C. Pediculosis
   D. Verrucae

6. Which statement best describes the appearance of verrucae?
   A. White silver scales
   B. Elevated growth
   C. Red flat area
   D. Dark brown raised area

7. A patient develops acute paronychia. Which class of medication is best for this condition?
   A. Antifungal
   B. Opiod
   C. Diruetic
   D. Antibiotic

8. According to the CDC, which bacteria is believed to be the most common cause of necrotizing fasciitis?
   A. *Staphylococcus aureus*
   B. Group B *Streptococcus*
   C. Group A *Streptococcus*
   D. *Staphylococcus haemolyticus*

9. Which condition is an acute, diffuse, bacterial infection of the skin and subcutaneous tissue?
   A. Cellulitis
   B. Carbuncle
   C. Furuncle
   D. Dermatophytoses

10. In which location of the body is a patient **less** likely to experience a furuncle?
    A. Buttock
    B. Stomach
    C. Neck
    D. Face

7

Diseases and Conditions of the Musculoskeletal System

CHAPTER OUTLINE

LEARNING OBJECTIVES

After studying this chapter, you should be able to:

1. List the functions of the normal skeletal system.
2. Discuss the specifics of a physical examination when fibromyalgia is suspected.
3. Distinguish among the pathologic features of lordosis, kyphosis, and scoliosis.
4. Describe the signs and symptoms of the most common form of arthritis.
5. Explain the importance of early diagnosis and treatment of Lyme disease.
6. Discuss the prevention of bursitis.
7. Describe the clinical picture of osteomyelitis and explain how it is treated.
8. Explain why joint disability results from gout.
9. Describe the treatment of bone tumors, both benign and malignant.
10. Describe the disability that results from advanced osteoporosis.
11. Explain why osteomalacia is termed *a metabolic bone disease*.
12. Distinguish between hallux valgus and hallux rigidus.
13. Explain the causes of fractures (broken bones) and how fractures are classified.
14. Explain what the term *phantom limb* refers to.
15. Differentiate between a strain and a sprain.
16. Explain the importance of proper treatment of dislocations.
17. Recall the medical term for "frozen shoulder."
18. Describe the cause of shin splints.
19. List some factors that contribute to the development of plantar fasciitis.
20. Explain how torn meniscus is treated.
21. Describe the signs and symptoms of rotator cuff tears.

KEY TERMS

avulsion (ah-VUL-shun)

bursae (BURR-see)

calcitonin (kal-sih-TOE-nin)

crepitation (krep-ih-TAY-shun)

fascia (FASH-ee-ah)

hematopoiesis (heem-ah-toe-poy-EE-sis)

meniscus (meh-NIS-kuss)

metatarsophalangeal (met-ah-tar-so-fah-LAN-jee-al)

ossification (oss-ih-fih-KAY-shun)

osteogenesis (oss-tee-oh-JEN-eh-sis)

synovial (sin-OH-vee-al)

tenorrhaphy (teh-NOR-ah-fee)

The Musculoskeletal System

Muscles, bones, ligaments, tendons, cartilage, and the joints they form provide a supportive and functional framework for the body that allows flexibility of movement and protects the internal organs. The tissues of the musculoskeletal system also give shape to the body, act partially as a storage-and-supply area for minerals, and serve as sites for the formation of blood cells.

When the tissues are unable to perform their usual functions because of trauma, rheumatic, inflammatory, or degenerative conditions, a person's physical support, protection, mobility, and ability to perform normal activities are affected. Trauma is a major cause of musculoskeletal disorders; automobile accidents and injuries (strains, sprains, dislocations, and fractures) are the leading causes of disabilities and death.

All muscles are composed of a basic cellular unit called the *muscle fiber*, which is made of protein. Muscles of the skeleton are collections or masses of tissue that cover bones, providing bulk to the body while also helping to hold body parts together and move joints (Fig. 7.1). These skeletal muscles make up approximately 40% of the total body mass.

All movement, including the movement of the body itself and of the internal organs, is performed by muscle tissue. The three types of muscle tissues, defined histologically, are striated (skeletal), nonstriated (smooth), and cardiac (Fig. 7.2). Muscles are also classified as either voluntary or involuntary. Skeletal muscle is voluntary and is under the control of the conscious mind; this includes the muscles used to move the extremities, which are stimulated by nerves at the request of the brain. The point of attachment of a muscle to a stationary bone is referred to as the *origin of the muscle*, and the point of attachment to a bone that is moved by the muscle is referred to as its *insertion* (Fig. 7.3). When a muscle contracts, the insertion moves toward the origin. Smooth muscle and heart muscle are involuntary and function without conscious control or awareness. Examples are the muscles of the intestines, which move food through the bowels, and cardiac muscles, which move blood throughout the chambers of the heart.

The skeletal system is composed of 206 bones. These serve to provide an important support system for the many body parts, enabling a person to assume various body postures (Fig. 7.4). In coordination with muscles and joints, bones assist in body movement.

Some bones encase and protect specific organs (e.g., the skull protects the brain, the rib cage protects the heart and lungs, and the vertebrae protect the spinal cord). Blood cells are formed in bone marrow inside the bones in a process called **hematopoiesis**.

Bones are not lifeless structures but, instead, are structures infused with living cells arranged in a hard framework of minerals (calcium and phosphorus). Bone cells are continuously forming new bone; bone formation is counterbalanced by bone reabsorption or breakdown. Normally the balance of these two processes prevents bones from becoming excessively thick, as in Paget disease of bone, or too thin, as in osteoporosis. This balance also serves to maintain the normal blood level of calcium and phosphorus in the body.

Bones are complete organs; they are composed mainly of connective tissue with a rich supply of blood vessels and nerves. They develop through a process called **osteogenesis**, and the complete skeleton is formed by the end of the third month of fetal age. The fetal skeleton is composed of cartilage tissue, which is replaced gradually by bone cells in a process called **ossification**. Ossification depends on adequate supplies of calcium and phosphorus getting to the bone tissue.

Several different types of bone make up the skeleton. Long bones are strong and have broad ends and large surface areas for muscle attachment. They are found in the humerus (arm), the ulna and radius (forearm), the femur (thigh), and the tibia and fibula (leg). Short bones have small, irregular shapes and include the carpal (wrist) and tarsal (ankle) bones. Flat bones cover soft body parts; they include the scapula (shoulder), ribs, and pelvic bones. Sesamoid bones are small and rounded and are found near joints. The patella (kneecap) is the largest sesamoid bone.

Joints, or articulations, are body structures in which bones are joined or the surfaces of two bones come together for the purpose of creating motion. With the help of ligaments, joints hold bones firmly together yet allow movement between them. Joints are classified by the type of material found between bones: fibrous, cartilaginous, and **synovial**. Joints also are classified according to the degree

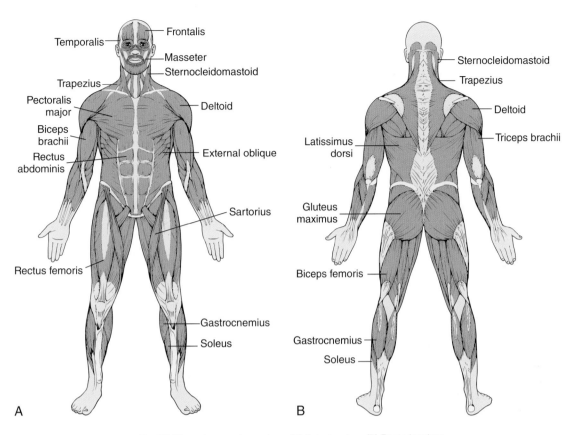

• **Fig. 7.1** Normal muscular system. (A) Anterior view. (B) Posterior view.

• **Fig. 7.2** Types of muscles.

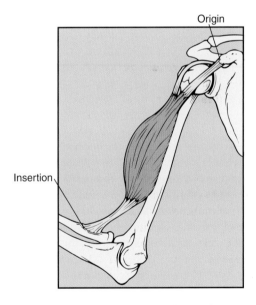

• **Fig. 7.3** Insertion and origin of a muscle.

of movement (Fig. 7.5) they can make. Immovable (synarthrodial) joints (e.g., suture joints between the bones of the skull) are connected by fibrous tissue; slightly movable (amphiarthrodial) joints (e.g., the intervertebral joints and the pubic symphysis) are connected by cartilage; and freely movable (diarthrodial) joints (e.g., the knee and the elbow) are called *synovial joints* because they are lined with the fluid-producing synovial membrane. Also within synovial joints

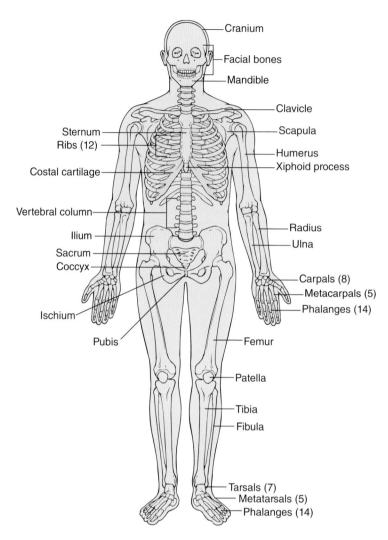

• **Fig. 7.4** Normal skeletal system, anterior view.

are bones; cartilage that covers the ends of bones; ligaments that hold bones together; a joint capsule containing synovial fluid, blood, and lymph vessels; and nerves.

Most joints are of the freely movable type. The amount or degree of movement that a joint has is referred to as its *range of motion* (ROM). Only the freely movable joints can execute a wide range of movements; examples are the shoulder, wrist, and hip.

Ligaments are tough, dense, fibrous bands of connective tissue that hold bones together, either around a joint capsule (e.g., the hip joint) or across a joint (e.g., the knee [Fig. 7.6]). They allow movement in some directions while restricting it in other directions, thereby providing some stability. Injury to ligaments can occur in several ways; they can be overstretched and sustain partial or complete tears (sprains) or be torn completely loose from their attachment to a bone, an injury called **avulsion**. They can also be loosened by the inflammation caused by inflammatory arthritis.

Tendons are tough strands, or cords, of dense connective tissue. They serve to attach muscles to bones and other parts (see Fig. 7.6). Tendons are nonelastic and are capable of withstanding great forces from contracting muscles without sustaining damage. Injury to a tendon is called *strain*.

Fascia is a specialized flat band of tissue located just below the skin that covers and separates underlying tissues, commonly muscle layers. Inflamed or injured fascia is referred to as *fasciitis*.

Cartilage is a semismooth, dense, supporting connective tissue that is found at the ends of bones. It forms a cap over the ends of bones and provides support and protection when bones are engaged in weight-bearing activities. Cartilage absorbs the energy force of weight pressed or thrust against joints to prevent injury to joints, bones, and the cartilage itself; in effect, it functions as a "shock absorber." To remain healthy, cartilage at the joints must receive nutrients from the joint fluid and maintain normal joint movement and weight-bearing activities.

Also necessary for the functioning of the musculoskeletal system are the **bursae**, closed sacs or cavities of synovial fluid lined with a synovial membrane. Positioned between tissues, such as tendons, bones, and ligaments, bursae make it possible for these tissues to glide over each other without

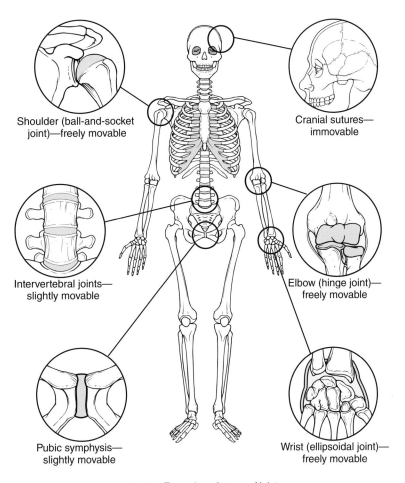

Shoulder (ball-and-socket joint)—freely movable

Cranial sutures— immovable

Intervertebral joints— slightly movable

Elbow (hinge joint)— freely movable

Pubic symphysis— slightly movable

Wrist (ellipsoidal joint)— freely movable

• **Fig. 7.5** Examples of types of joints.

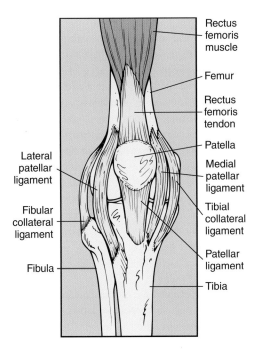

Rectus femoris muscle

Femur

Rectus femoris tendon

Patella

Medial patellar ligament

Tibial collateral ligament

Patellar ligament

Tibia

Lateral patellar ligament

Fibular collateral ligament

Fibula

• **Fig. 7.6** Ligaments and tendons of the knee joint.

creating friction. Bursae are located in the shoulder, elbow, and knee joints.

Another substance found throughout the musculoskeletal system is a fibrous protein called *collagen*. Collagen constitutes 30% of the total body protein and is the major supporting element, or glue, in the connective tissues between the cells that holds them together. In adults, collagen makes up one-third to one-half of the total body protein.

The nervous and muscular systems work together to enable us to perform tasks. Muscle memory, or the way that we remember motor skills and perform them, is involved in tasks performed each day. We perform many tasks each day without "thinking" about what we are doing. Repetitive motions that are involved in typing, exercising, and playing a sport or musical instrument also involve muscle memory as our brains remember how to perform those tasks. If an athlete takes a few months "off" from the sport they play, their body can still perform those same actions such as dribbling a basketball months later. Practicing a sport makes the movements easier to remember over time. Research continues in regard to how muscle memory can potentially impact a person who has cognitive loss, in being able to still perform repetitive motions like playing an instrument.

Fibromyalgia

Description

Fibromyalgia is a chronic pain condition associated with stiffness and tenderness that affects muscles, tendons, and joints throughout the body. Fibromyalgia is also characterized by restless sleep, depression, fatigue, anxiety, and bowel dysfunction.

ICD-10-CM Code	M60.9 *(Myositis, unspecified)*
	(M60.000–M60.19 = 64 codes of specificity; M60.8–M60.9 = 26 codes of specificity)
	M79.1 *(Myalgia)*
	M79.7 *(Fibromyalgia)*

Symptoms and Signs

Fibromyalgia, one of the most common diseases affecting muscles, causes chronic pain in the muscles and soft tissues surrounding joints for at least 3 months. Fatigue is extremely common in patients with this condition. Often, symptoms include diffuse aching or burning in the muscles, stiffness, disturbed sleep patterns, and cognitive problems, including poor concentration and inability to focus on a task. Irritability and depression may also occur. Patients may note extreme tenderness in various areas of the body. Other nonspecific symptoms include headaches, jaw pain, and sensitivity to odors, bright lights, and loud noises. Some patients experience symptoms of irritable bowel syndrome or "spastic colon," including nausea, diarrhea, constipation, or abdominal pain with gas and distention. Urinary symptoms, when present, include urinary urgency or frequency brought on by bladder spasms. Often patients wake up feeling tired, even if they have slept all through the night. Others sleep lightly and wake up during the night due to pain. Females are more likely than males to be diagnosed with fibromyalgia.

Patient Screening

For the patient complaining of persistent fatigue and unexplained muscle pain and tenderness, schedule an appointment at the earliest convenience.

Etiology

The cause of fibromyalgia is not fully known. Patients experience pain in response to stimuli that are normally not perceived as painful. Fibromyalgia appears to be linked to changes in how the brain and spinal cord process pain signals. Genetics, emotional or physical events, and infections may influence whether or not an individual develops the disease. Researchers have found elevated levels of a nerve growth factor and a chemical signal, called *substance P*, in the spinal fluid of patients with fibromyalgia. The amount of serotonin, a chemical produced in the brain that affects nerves, is relatively low in these patients. Furthermore, those with fibromyalgia experience impaired nonrapid eye movement (non-REM) sleep, which likely explains the common feature of waking up feeling fatigued and unrefreshed. The onset of fibromyalgia is sometimes associated with psychological distress, trauma, and infection.

Diagnosis

Many medical conditions can cause pain in multiple areas of the body, thus mimicking fibromyalgia. Blood testing and physical examination are important to *exclude* some conditions, such as hypothyroidism, hypoparathyroidism, other muscle diseases, bone diseases, viral infections, and cancer.

There are no specific laboratory or imaging studies that can be used to diagnose fibromyalgia. The diagnosis of fibromyalgia is made purely on clinical grounds and is based on a thorough history and physical examination and the patient's symptoms.

Historically, fibromyalgia was diagnosed if a patient had widespread tenderness and pain or aching commonly in at least 11 of 18 specific tender points. The problem with these criteria is that the symptoms sometimes come and go. The patient may have 11 symptoms 1 day and then 4 the next day. The American College of Rheumatology no longer uses the tender points as part of the exam. There are now screening tools for chronic widespread pain (Fig. 7.7).

According to the Mayo Clinic, a patient exhibiting widespread pain lasting at least 3 months is a key factor. The patient must have symptoms of pain in four of the following five areas: left or right upper regions, including the jaw, shoulder, or arm. Left or right lower regions, including the leg, hip, or buttock. The patient may also experience pain in the axial area including the chest, neck, back, or abdomen.

Treatment

Although no cure for fibromyalgia is known, treatment can help alleviate symptoms and restore function. Treatment involves patient education, stress reduction, physical activity, and medications. Attempts are made to reduce pain and improve the quality of sleep. Medications that can improve sleep patterns may be prescribed, such as low doses of the antidepressant amitriptyline (Elavil). Other treatments include pregabalin (Lyrica), duloxetine (Cymbalta), and milnacipran (Savella). For muscle and joint soreness, nonsteroidal antiinflammatory drugs (NSAIDs) and/or muscle relaxants can be helpful. Physical and occupational therapy, as well as counseling to learn how to cope with pain, can be helpful. Stress reduction, relaxation techniques, massage therapy, acupressure, and exercise also have been found to be beneficial. Exercises that are helpful in reducing pain include walking, biking, swimming, or water aerobics.

Prognosis

With a good understanding of the concepts of the symptoms and methods of treatment available, patients can generally learn to cope with their illness and the pain involved by using the mechanisms of treatment available to improve their quality of life.

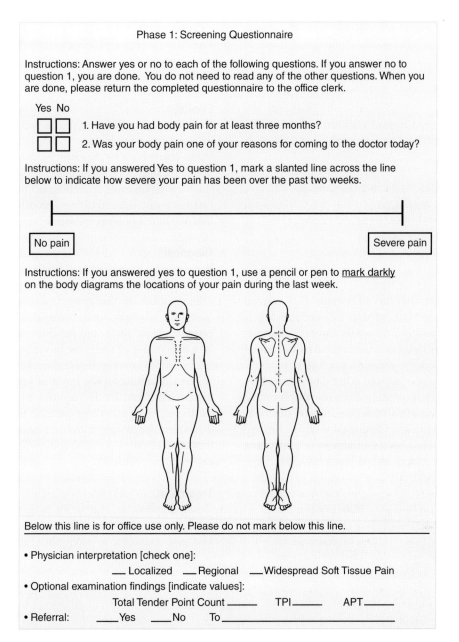

Phase 1: Screening Questionnaire

Instructions: Answer yes or no to each of the following questions. If you answer no to question 1, you are done. You do not need to read any of the other questions. When you are done, please return the completed questionnaire to the office clerk.

Yes No

☐ ☐ 1. Have you had body pain for at least three months?

☐ ☐ 2. Was your body pain one of your reasons for coming to the doctor today?

Instructions: If you answered Yes to question 1, mark a slanted line across the line below to indicate how severe your pain has been over the past two weeks.

No pain   Severe pain

Instructions: If you answered yes to question 1, use a pencil or pen to <u>mark darkly</u> on the body diagrams the locations of your pain during the last week.

Below this line is for office use only. Please do not mark below this line.

• Physician interpretation [check one]:

___ Localized   ___ Regional   ___ Widespread Soft Tissue Pain

• Optional examination findings [indicate values]:

Total Tender Point Count _____   TPI _____   APT _____

• Referral: ___ Yes   ___ No   To _____

• **Fig. 7.7** Screening questionnaire for chronic widespread pain as seen in fibromyalgia syndrome (FM). The findings supportive of FM would be chronic pain from question 1, the relative severity of the pain from question 3, and widespread pain from question 4. Each question could also be applied to other categories of soft tissue pain, and patients with localized or regional musculoskeletal pain, if present, would be identified by the body pain diagram. *APT*; Average pain threshold; *TPI*, tender point index. (From Benzon H, et al: *Practical Management of Pain*, ed 6, 2023, Elsevier.)

Prevention

To prevent symptoms from initiating or worsening, patients should work toward minimizing stressful situations. They should also exercise, eat healthy, and take medications as prescribed to help manage pain symptoms.

Patient Teaching

Optimal management of fibromyalgia involves maximizing the patient's understanding of all known concepts of the illness. The patient and the health care provider then develop the ideal treatment strategy, which is customized for each patient and involves a dynamic balance of patient education, exercise, stress reduction, and medication. Patients should be taught that smoking may worsen symptoms.

Spinal Disorders

The normal curves of the spine are important because they provide a strong supportive structure to the body. Additionally, the spine provides the necessary balance to stand, walk, and even hold the head up straight. The ribs and internal organs are suspended from the spine in the front; the hips and legs are attached to the lower spine.

The following text includes a discussion of three relatively common abnormal curvatures of the spine: lordosis, kyphosis, and scoliosis.

Lordosis

Description

Lordosis is an exaggerated inward curvature of the spine. Lordosis is sometimes referred to as a *swayback* or *saddleback deformity*.

ICD-10-CM Code	M40.40 *(Postural lordosis, site unspecified)* (M40.40–M40.57 = 8 codes of specificity)

Symptoms and Signs

The lumbar spine normally curves inward. This normal anterior curve of the lumbar spine can become exaggerated by a variety of conditions. Excessive inward curvature, or lordosis, occurs as the person compensates for added abdominal girth caused by pregnancy, obesity, or large abdominal tumors. Lordosis also can occur developmentally for unknown reasons. Lordosis may cause no symptoms, or the patient may experience low back pain because of strains on the muscles and ligaments. Compared with the normal spine posture (Fig. 7.8), lordosis results in a protruding abdomen and buttocks and an arched lower back (Fig. 7.9).

Patient Screening

For the patient complaining of persistent low back pain, but no history of injury or symptoms of infection, schedule the first convenient appointment.

Etiology

Excessive abdominal weight gain and mass cause an individual to compensate by unconsciously tightening the muscles in the lower back to maintain balance when standing. One possible cause is rapid skeletal growth that occurs without the necessary natural stretching of the posterior soft tissues. Osteoporosis, with resulting loss of bone mass, may cause lordosis in the older population.

Diagnosis

Patients who have persistent low back pain should be evaluated for degenerative and congenital diseases of the spine, inflammation of the spine (spondylitis), and conditions involving adjacent internal organs, such as the kidneys, prostate gland, aorta, and pancreas.

Observation of the spine in various postures and examination of the lower spine are the primary steps in diagnosis. When the condition is a result of pregnancy, no additional information usually is required to make the diagnosis. Further investigation can include radiographic studies to determine the extent of lordosis, along with a thorough history and physical examination to discover the underlying cause of the condition.

Treatment

When lordosis is caused by pregnancy, delivery usually resolves the condition. When obesity is the cause, weight loss and exercises to strengthen abdominal muscles are

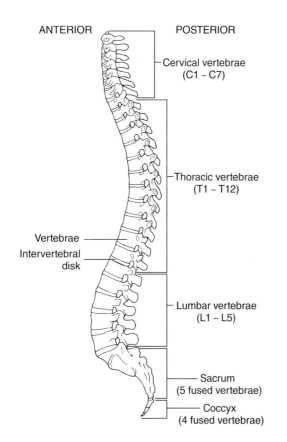

ANTERIOR POSTERIOR

Cervical vertebrae (C1 – C7)

Thoracic vertebrae (T1 – T12)

Vertebrae
Intervertebral disk

Lumbar vertebrae (L1 – L5)

Sacrum (5 fused vertebrae)

Coccyx (4 fused vertebrae)

• **Fig. 7.8** Normal spine.

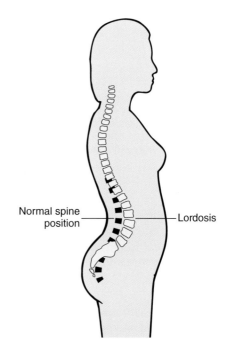

Normal spine position

Lordosis

• **Fig. 7.9** Lordosis.

beneficial. Performing pelvic tilt exercises and maintaining good posture help correct the condition. Progressive untreated lordosis can lead to degenerative lumbar disk disease or ruptured lumbar disks. Additional treatment of the condition can include the use of a brace. For severe lordosis, spinal fusion, and displacement osteotomy are considered. This latter procedure requires the surgical division of a vertebra, with shifting of the bone segments to change the alignment of or alter weight-bearing stress on the spine.

Prognosis

Lordosis may never cause symptoms, but patients who do have symptoms usually respond to conservative management techniques.

Prevention

Optimal prevention measures center on developing ideal posture habits, exercises, and support devices, such as braces and lumbar support when seated.

Patient Teaching

Patients can benefit from a brief review of the normal anatomy of the affected areas, particularly addressing the spine and the paraspinous musculature, as well as specific exercise instructions. Recommendations on proper posturing can be extremely valuable.

Kyphosis

Description

Kyphosis is an abnormal outward curvature of the spine (convexity backward).

ICD-10-CM Code	M40.00 *(Postural kyphosis, site unspecified)* M40.209 *(Unspecified kyphosis, site unspecified)* (M40.00–M40.299 = 19 codes of specificity)

Symptoms and Signs

Kyphosis, an excessive posterior curve of the thoracic spine, often has an insidious onset and is asymptomatic until the hump becomes obvious. As the curve progresses, the patient may begin to experience mild pain, fatigue, tenderness along the spine, and decreasing mobility of the spine. The shoulders appear rounded, and the head protrudes forward.

Patient Screening

For the individual complaining of persistent upper back pain without a history of injury or symptoms of infection, schedule an appointment at the patient's convenience.

Etiology

Kyphosis can be congenital or noticed at birth. It can also result from other causes, including neuromuscular conditions, osteogenesis imperfecta (brittle bone disease), spina

• **Fig. 7.10** Scheuermann disease. (From Ross JS, Moore KR: *Diagnostic imaging*, ed 4, 2020, Elsevier.)

bifida, or poor posture, which is the most common reason for kyphosis to occur.

Adolescent kyphosis usually is related to Scheuermann disease, a degenerative deformity of the thoracic vertebrae where the vertebrae appear to be wedge shaped. (Fig. 7.10). Additional disease processes that contribute to the occurrence of kyphosis include tumors or tuberculosis of the vertebral bodies and ankylosing spondylitis. The collapse of vertebrae from the weakened bone of osteoporosis is often responsible for the hunchback (dowager's hump) that develops in the older person, particularly in postmenopausal females. Wearing away of the anterior portion of the vertebrae in a wedge type of manner (anterior wedging) or deterioration of the vertebrae, from whatever cause, results in excessive curvature with kyphosis.

Diagnosis

Visual inspection of the spine discloses the excessive curve in the thoracic region. Radiographs and imaging confirm the curvature of the thoracic spine and the wedging of the anterior aspect of the vertebral bodies.

Treatment

Exercises to strengthen the muscles and ligaments are prescribed. Back braces also are used to stabilize the condition. The underlying cause must be determined and treated. When other measures fail to produce results and when the respiratory and cardiac systems are compromised, spinal fusion, with instrumentation and temporary immobilization, is performed. Kyphosis, which is caused by a sudden collapse of a vertebra because of osteoporosis, is sometimes treated with a new procedure called *vertebroplasty*, in which bone cement is inserted within the vertebra.

Prognosis

The outlook for patients with kyphosis depends on the cause. Optimal outcome results from accurate diagnosis and early treatment.

Prevention

Optimal prevention measures center on developing ideal posture habits, exercises, and support devices, such as braces and back support when seated. Medications may be needed for osteoporosis, pain, or inflammation of the spine.

Patient Teaching

Patients with kyphosis who are found to have significant osteoporosis should be instructed regarding exercise, calcium and vitamin D supplementation, and prescription medications.

Scoliosis

Description

Scoliosis is lateral (sideways) curvature of the spine. Scoliosis is typically congenital, but some diseases also can cause it.

ICD-10-CM Code	M41.20 (Other idiopathic scoliosis, site unspecified)
	(M41.00–M41.9 = 55 codes of specificity)
	Q67.5 (Congenital deformity of spine)
	Q76.3 (Congenital scoliosis due to congenital bony malformation)
	Q76.425 (Congenital lordosis, thoracolumbar region)
	Q76.426 (Congenital lordosis, lumbar region)
	Q76.427 (Congenital lordosis, lumbosacral region)
	Q76.428 (Congenital lordosis, sacral and sacrococcygeal region)

Symptoms and Signs

Scoliosis, the lateral curvature of the spine, often has an insidious presentation, possibly going unnoticed for years before detection. In females, for example, the first indication is often unequal bra strap lengths. The patient reports back pain, fatigue, and sometimes shortness of breath on exertion. Observation of the back reveals a lateral curve of the spine, one shoulder higher than the other, one scapula more prominent than the other, one hip higher than the other, and when the patient bends over, an enlarged muscle mass on one side of the back.

Patient Screening

Referrals may come from school scoliosis screening programs that have detected possible scoliosis. The state protocol for this may vary from one school system to another.

Etiology

Idiopathic scoliosis is the most common form; however, there are cases where more than one person in a family has scoliosis which suggests that there is a hereditary trait, however as of the writing of this text, there is no single gene identified as causing scoliosis. Researchers continue to identify what happens before birth in the womb. Other suggested causes of scoliosis are deformities of the vertebrae; uneven leg lengths; and muscle degeneration or paralysis from diseases, such as poliomyelitis, cerebral palsy, and muscular dystrophy.

Diagnosis

Patients with scoliosis are evaluated for muscle disease and weakness, congenital conditions, neurologic disorders, and degeneration of the bones and disks of the spine. Diagnosis is made from a visual examination of the back, which reveals uneven shoulder and hip heights, a prominent scapula on one side, an enlarged muscle mass on one side, and a definite torsional curve of the vertebral column. It is important to examine the lengths of the lower limbs, because discrepancy of the leg lengths can lead to spinal curvature. Radiographs not only confirm the diagnosis but also provide the physician with the means to measure the degree of curvature. MRI may also be ordered in some cases to monitor the condition due to decreased radiation exposure throughout the years of monitoring.

Treatment

Treatment depends on the extent and cause of the curvature. Mild scoliosis is treated with exercise to strengthen the weak muscles. Bracing the back may also be necessary along with an exercise program. For moderate scoliosis, bracing may be necessary for 12 to 20 hours a day according to the Boston Children's Hospital, to prevent the degree of curvature from increasing as growth spurts take place. Curves that do not respond to the bracing or that are severe need surgical intervention to decrease the curve and to realign and stabilize the spine. These procedures include fusion of the vertebrae and a newer nonfusion surgery called posterior dynamic distraction which involves one rod instead of two, and the rod can adjust as the patient grows. They can be lengthened every 3 to 6 months using a remote control or surgery. Boston Children's Hospital was the first hospital approved to perform this surgery in 2020. In addition to these treatments, younger children ages 1 to 4 may need scoliosis casting if their curvature is greater than 35 degrees. The other treatments may take place also as the child becomes older. Vertebral body tethering is another treatment. Screws are placed and a flexible strong cord is attached. The cord puts tension on the side of the spine where the curve is, slowing down the curvature as the child grows (Fig. 7.11). This treatment was approved in 2019 by the US Food and Drug Administration for children who did not respond to bracing and who have not reached their full height. The respiratory and cardiac systems may be compromised if the curvature is left untreated.

• **Fig. 7.11** (A) Anterior vertebral body tethering. (B) Before tethering. (C) After tethering. (From *Shriners Hospital for Children Philadelphia Newsletter*, June 18, 2014.)

Prognosis

The outlook for patients with scoliosis depends primarily on the severity of the curvature. Optimal outcome results from accurate diagnosis and early treatment.

Prevention

Prevention measures center on developing ideal posture habits, performing beneficial exercises, and wearing support devices, such as the braces described above.

Patient Teaching

Posture training, regular use of proper bracing, and instructions for avoiding stresses to the affected spine are essential for ideal management. Children should follow the provider's instructions regarding sports, depending upon the severity. Make families and caregivers aware of online support tools.

Osteoarthritis

Description

Osteoarthritis is a type of arthritis that results from the breakdown and eventual loss of the cartilage of one or more joints.

ICD-10-CM Code	M15.9 *(Polyosteoarthritis, unspecified)*
	(M15.0–M15.9 = 7 codes of specificity)
	M19.90 *(Unspecified osteoarthritis, unspecified site)*
	(M19.01–M19.93 = 49 codes of specificity)

Osteoarthritis is coded according to the site affected. Refer to the physician's diagnosis and then to the current edition of the ICD-10-CM coding manual for most accurate specificity.

Symptoms and Signs

Osteoarthritis, also known as *degenerative joint disease* or *degenerative arthritis*, is, by far, the most common form of arthritis. It develops as a result of normal wear and tear on the joints and is most common in older adults. Osteoarthritis occurs mainly in the large weight-bearing joints, especially the knees and hips (Fig. 7.12). There is a tendency for the smallest joints at the ends of the fingers to be affected by spur formation, which leads to the classic bony enlargement referred to as a *Heberden node*. To a lesser degree, involvement of the joints of the fingers at the proximal interphalangeal (PIP) joints (Bouchard nodes; Fig. 7.13), that is, wrists, elbows, and ankles can occur. Degenerative changes in the spinal vertebrae and the joints of the pelvis can lead to abnormal curvature and local pain.

The onset of osteoarthritis is usually insidious, and the symptoms vary with the severity of the disease. Some of the common symptoms are joint soreness, aching, and stiffness, especially in the morning and with changes in the weather; edema; dull pain; and deformity. Stiffness is noted, particularly after the patient has been immobile for a period. Clicking or crackling sounds (**crepitation**) often are heard with joint movement. Decreased ranges of motion, joint instability, and an increase in pain with the use of the joints are also common.

Patient Screening

When a patient develops a persistent joint problem, a thorough history and physical examination are essential. Schedule the first available appointment. Follow office policy for a subsequent referral to a rheumatologist.

Etiology

The exact cause in most osteoarthritis cases is unknown, but it appears to be generally associated with aging. Breakdown

• **Fig. 7.12** Schematic presentation of the pathologic changes in osteoarthritis. Fragmentation and loss of cartilage denude the subchondral bone, which undergoes sclerosis and cystic change. Osteophytes form on the lateral sides and protrude into the adjacent soft tissues, causing irritation, inflammation, and fibrosis. (From Damjanov I: *Pathology for the health professions*, ed 4, St. Louis, 2012, Saunders.)

• **Fig. 7.13** Bouchard nodes. (From Monahan FD, et al: *Phipps' medical-surgical nursing*, ed 8, St. Louis, 2007, Mosby.)

of cartilage between bones occurs. In primary osteoarthritis the joints most frequently affected are those in the hands, knees, spine, hips, and toes. In secondary osteoarthritis, injury, trauma, inflammatory arthritis, or other inflammatory illnesses can cause the changes to occur. The tendency toward developing osteoarthritis is sometimes inherited. In some persons, osteoarthritis may follow injury to the joint or be associated with hormonal disorders or underlying diseases, such as diabetes and obesity.

Diagnosis

Patients must be evaluated to exclude other forms of arthritis, and any underlying diseases or conditions must be detected as well. The diagnostic investigation begins with a physical examination and patient history. Radiographs, computed tomography (CT) scans, and magnetic resonance imaging (MRI) scans confirm the presence and document the severity of osteoarthritis, however plain radiography can be very helpful for excluding other causes of pain in a particular joint. Radiography can also measure the severity of the osteoarthritis and assist in deciding when surgical intervention should be considered.

Treatment

Because osteoarthritis cannot be cured, the goal of treatment is to reduce inflammation, to minimize pain, and to maintain functioning joints. Treatment of osteoarthritis involves physical and drug therapy, nutritional management, and supportive care. Surgery also may be needed in severe cases. Physical therapy includes ROM exercises, alternation of moist heat and cold applications, massage therapy, and the use of elastic bandages and splints for limb support. Drug therapy can include the use of analgesics, muscle relaxants, and NSAIDs. Intraarticular steroid injections may be used for specific or individual joints. Intraarticular hyaluronic acid can be used to reduce pain in affected knee joints. Fish oils have been suggested to have some antiinflammatory properties. Food supplementation with glucosamine and chondroitin may reduce pain and stiffness in some patients. For supportive care, it may be necessary to use a cane, walker, braces, or crutches to lessen the strain on some joints. (Always examine cane tips to be certain that they are not dangerously worn out!) Restricting physical activity or resting the affected joints also may be necessary. Surgery for osteoarthritis may involve total joint replacement. Joint replacement surgery is considered a last resort when other treatments do not improve the severity of pain or quality of life.

Prognosis

The outlook for patients with osteoarthritis depends primarily on the severity and location of the involved joints. Optimal outcome results from accurate diagnosis and early management.

Prevention

Avoiding injury and reinjury to joints is important in preventing osteoarthritis. Persons with flaccid (overstretched) ligaments may require support devices to engage in some activities. Early contact with health care professionals can optimize long-term health. Eliminating risk factors by maintaining a healthy weight, exercising, managing blood glucose and hyperlipidemia levels is beneficial.

Patient Teaching

Providing specific guidance on food supplementation, medications, and proper exercise can significantly improve the quality of life for these patients.

Lyme Disease

Description

Lyme disease is an infectious disease caused by *Borrelia burgdorferi*, a spirochete bacterium. Ticks that bite the skin spread Lyme disease by injecting the bacterium from their gut into the human body when securing a blood meal. Lyme disease can affect the skin, joints, heart, and nervous system.

ICD-10-CM Code	A69.20 *(Lyme disease, unspecified)* (A69.20–A69.29 = 5 codes of specificity)

Symptoms and Signs

Lyme disease, also known as *Lyme arthritis*, was first detected in 1975 in Lyme, Connecticut, in the United States. Lyme disease is more prevalent in the northeast part of the United States, especially New York, New Jersey, Connecticut, District of Columbia, Maine, Maryland, Massachusetts, Minnesota, New Hampshire, Pennsylvania, Rhode Island, Vermont, Virginia, West Virginia, and Wisconsin, where large areas of forests and fields provide a habitat for ticks. The disease has been found throughout the world.

Lyme disease can occur in any age group, and no one is immune to the infection. Approximately half of all patients with Lyme disease have a characteristic red, itchy rash with a red circle center resembling the bull's eye on a target (target lesion) (Fig. 7.14 A) early in the illness. Lyme disease can masquerade as arthritis and cause influenza-like symptoms, such as headache, fever, fatigue, joint pain, and general malaise. If the person does not seek medical attention for the symptoms, late complications of muscle weakness, paralysis, and neurologic conditions (e.g., learning difficulties, excessive

• **Fig. 7.14** (A) Target lesion of Lyme disease. (B) Deer tick attached to skin after spending a day in the woods. Notice the size compared to the penny. (A, From Stone DR, Gorbach SL: *Atlas of infectious diseases*, Philadelphia, 2000, Saunders; B, Courtesy Michael David Fuqua.)

fatigue, and muscle coordination problems) can develop as the bacterium spreads unchecked internally. Encephalitis, gastritis, or carditis may develop in some patients.

Patient Screening

Early detection of Lyme disease is imperative because treatment can eliminate the risk of more significant organ-threatening consequences. In areas where the deer tick is prevalent and/or the patient reports a "target lesion," a visual inspection and diagnostic laboratory tests are necessary. Likewise, if a patient reports flulike symptoms 2 to 4 weeks after sustaining a tick bite, an appointment for prompt diagnostic evaluation is indicated.

Etiology

Lyme disease is caused by *Borrelia burgdorferi*, a spirochete bacterium transmitted to humans by a bite from a small tick (see Fig. 7.14B), which is carried by mice or deer vectors.

Borrelia burgdorferi is prevalent in the United States. *Borrelia mayonii* is the only other bacteria identified in the United States to cause Lyme disease. In Europe, the prevalent bacterium is *Borrelia afzelii or Borrelia garinii* which also causes Lyme disease. The disease is usually transmitted to humans while they are camping or hiking in the woods, fields, or other areas that ticks inhabit. After infiltrating the skin, the bacterium can infect internal organs of the body, causing a variety of symptoms, which often leads to delays in making the correct diagnosis.

Diagnosis
The evaluation of patients with the nonspecific symptoms of early Lyme disease, such as headache, fever, fatigue, joint pain, and general malaise can be exhaustive. A complete history, physical examination, and laboratory tests are important for excluding other infectious diseases, forms of arthritis, immune diseases, muscle diseases, and even cancer.

The diagnosis of Lyme disease can be based on physical examination (the discovery of a tick on the skin), the presence of the classic target lesion, and the patient's history. Confirmation is made on the basis of positive test results for the Lyme antibodies or by directly identifying the bacterium in the infected skin via biopsy, if necessary.

Treatment
Treatment of Lyme disease begins with the removal of the tick if it is found on the skin or clothing. Early treatment is imperative because treatment in the early stages of disease leads to a complete cure with simple oral antibiotics. The drug of choice for Lyme disease is doxycycline. Alternatively, the Centers for Disease Control and Prevention also recommends amoxicillin or cefuroxime. Lyme disease in the later stages requires intravenous antibiotics, such as ceftriaxone or penicillin, to cure the disease. Antipyretics are given for headaches and fever. Bed rest is necessary if neurologic symptoms are present, and physical therapy is prescribed for impaired musculoskeletal mobility. Joint symptoms are often treated with antiinflammatory medications and hydroxychloroquine.

Prognosis
Lyme disease is curable with antibiotics. The outlook for patients with Lyme disease depends on how early it is detected. Early-stage Lyme disease involves a minor skin rash with muscle aches that easily resolve with antibiotics. Later-stage Lyme disease can cause residual damage to the joints, heart, or nervous system. Optimal outcome results from accurate diagnosis and early treatment.

Prevention
Avoiding tick bites is the best prevention against Lyme disease. In locations known to harbor ticks, one should wear long clothing to protect the skin. All clothing first and then the entire body, including the scalp, should be carefully examined to detect the presence of ticks after being in high-risk areas. Close inspection of children and pets is especially important. Ticks can be removed gently with tweezers and saved in a jar in case identification is needed later. Bathing the skin and scalp and washing clothes after possible exposure to ticks may prevent not only the bite but also the subsequent transmission of the disease. Vaccines were once available, but these have been removed from the market. Further studies of vaccines are needed.

Patient Teaching
Community awareness of tick avoidance measures is essential for prevention. Patients who develop Lyme disease should be instructed to closely follow the specific instructions regarding therapeutic medications provided by their qualified health care professionals.

Bursitis

Description
Bursitis is inflammation of a bursa. A bursa is a tiny fluid-filled sac that functions as a gliding surface to reduce friction between tissues of the body. Bursae are found between muscles and tendons and cover bony prominences to facilitate movement. They can become inflamed, infected, or traumatized. The major bursae are located adjacent to the tendons of the large joints, such as the shoulders, elbows, hips, and knees.

ICD-10-CM Code	M71.50 (*Other bursitis, not elsewhere classified, unspecified site*) (M71.10–M71.19 = 24 codes of specificity; M71.50–M71.58 = 20 codes of specificity) M70.039 (*Crepitant synovitis [acute] [chronic], unspecified wrist*) (M70.031–M70.049 = 6 codes of specificity) M70.30 (*Other bursitis of elbow, unspecified elbow*) (M70.30–M70.32 = 3 codes of specificity) M70.40 (*Prepatellar bursitis, unspecified knee*) (M70.40–M70.52 = 6 codes of specificity)

Symptoms and Signs
The classic symptoms of bursitis are tenderness, pain when moving the affected part, flexion and extension limitation, and edema at the site of inflammation. The most frequently affected bursae are those of the shoulder (Fig. 7.15), elbow, knee, hip, and between the tendons and muscles of the tibia. Point tenderness may be present, in which case the patient actually can point to the spot of greatest tenderness. If bursae are continually or chronically irritated and inflamed, calcifications can develop. In addition, adhesions can occur around an affected bursa, which limits the movement of the tendons.

• **Fig. 7.15** Bursae of the shoulder.

Patient Screening

Pain, swelling, or limitation of motion in any joint, with or without previous injury, requires an appointment for diagnostic evaluation. Early treatment and relief from pain are important measures.

Etiology

Bursitis can result from continual or excessive friction between the bursae and the surrounding musculoskeletal tissues. Systemic diseases (e.g., gout and rheumatoid arthritis) and infection can lead to the development of bursitis. In addition, repeated trauma from overuse of a joint can cause bursitis.

Diagnosis

Bursitis is generally a straightforward diagnosis that can be made after evaluating information gained from the history and physical examination. However, in patients with bursitis that is not associated with injury, possible underlying gout or arthritis should be considered. In patients with abrasion or puncture wounds of the overlying skin, infection also must be considered. Range of motion may be impaired, and the pain is acute. MRI indicates an enlarged bursa, and radiographs may show calcified deposits at the affected site when the bursitis is chronic. Aspiration of fluid from an inflamed bursa can assist in diagnosing gouty or infectious bursitis (septic bursitis).

Treatment

The treatment for traumatic bursitis may include avoidance of activities until acute pain subsides, the application of moist heat, immobilization of the affected part, the use of aspirin or acetaminophen for pain, the administration of NSAIDs (e.g., ibuprofen and indomethacin), and local injection of a corticosteroid. If infection is present, drainage of the inflamed bursa and the use of antibiotics specific to the infectious microbe are critical. Active ROM exercises to prevent adhesions and to maintain or regain motion are needed after the

acute pain subsides. Surgical excision of the bursa and any accompanying calcified deposits can be required for either chronic noninfectious or infectious bursitis.

Prognosis

Bursitis is curable. With treatment and proper attention to any underlying cause, the outlook is excellent.

Prevention

Actions that initiate or promote tissue inflammation, such as repetition of a throwing motion in the case of shoulder bursitis, prolonged leaning on the elbow in the case of elbow bursitis, or prolonged kneeling in the case of knee bursitis should be avoided.

Patient Teaching

Patients can benefit from specific information regarding the cause of the inflamed bursa and instructions regarding aggravating factors to avoid. It is important to help the patient understand that the bursitis problem is adjacent to but not involving the joint. The joint should otherwise be unharmed. For any recurrent inflammation, patients should be instructed to immediately apply ice packs to the area so that inflammation can be minimized. Those with past infectious bursitis should notify their physician's office.

Osteomyelitis

Description

Osteomyelitis (Fig. 7.16) is a serious infection of bone that requires aggressive antibiotic treatment.

ICD-10-CM Code	M86.9 (Osteomyelitis, unspecified) (M86.00–M86.9 = 189 codes of specificity)

Refer to the physician's diagnosis and then the current edition of the ICD-10-CM coding manual for greatest specificity of site and stage (acute or chronic) of bone infection.

Symptoms and Signs

Inflammation, swelling, localized heat, redness, pain, and local tenderness over and around the affected bone are characteristic signs of osteomyelitis. Other symptoms of osteomyelitis include chills, fever, sweating, and malaise. As the infection progresses, a purulent material called a *subperiosteal abscess* may develop, causing pressure and eventual fracturing of small pieces of the bone. These fractured, dead pieces of bone may, in turn, become surrounded by the purulent material and form a sequestrum.

The most commonly involved bones in osteomyelitic infections are the upper ends of the humerus and tibia, the lower end of the femur, and occasionally the vertebrae.

Osteomyelitis most often begins as an acute infection; however, it can remain undetected for months or years and

• **Fig. 7.16** Osteomyelitis. (From Cooke RA, Stewart B: *Colour atlas of anatomical pathology*, ed 3, London, 2003, Churchill Livingstone.)

evolve into a chronic condition. Both the acute and chronic forms can present the same clinical picture.

Patient Screening

Patients with localized bone inflammation and pain must be evaluated for possible fractures and bone tumors before the diagnosis of osteomyelitis can be ascertained.

Etiology

Staphylococcus aureus is the bacterial organism responsible for most cases of osteomyelitic infections but other bacteria such as streptococcal bacteria can also cause this infection. Rarely, viruses and fungi have also been known to cause osteomyelitis. Osteomyelitis can develop when bloodborne pathogens are deposited in the metaphyseal area of a bone after physical trauma or surgery.

Diabetes mellitus or peripheral vascular disease may predispose individuals to the development of osteomyelitis, as can the presence of prosthetic hardware (e.g., rods,

screws, and plates within bone) and total joint replacement. Osteomyelitis in infants and children develops as a secondary infection from streptococcal pharyngitis (strep throat). Persons with sickle cell disease, immunodeficiency, or malignancies are also at increased risk for the development of osteomyelitis.

The possible development of osteomyelitis must be the concern of any person who has an open wound, sore (strep) throat, or a systemic infection that could be transmitted to the bones.

Diagnosis

Aspiration and culture of material taken from the site of the infection are essential to isolating the causative organisms. Blood culture, white blood cell count, and erythrocyte sedimentation rate (ESR) are also helpful for determining diagnosis and monitoring treatment. MRI, CT, or bone scanning aid in determining the site and extent of acute or chronic infection.

Treatment

Osteomyelitis usually requires extensive, long-term antibiotic treatment with follow-up care to prevent recurrent infections. Parenteral or locally administered antibiotics (e.g., aqueous penicillin, cephalosporin, and ampicillin), at a dosage specific to the patient's age and the pathogenic organism involved, are needed. Additional measures include increased intake of proteins and vitamins A, B, and C to promote cell regeneration; bed rest, as needed, to conserve energy; control of chronic conditions (e.g., diabetes); immobilization of the affected part to prevent fracture of weakened bones; and analgesics. Surgical drainage to remove purulent material and sequestrum also may be necessary, along with bone grafting. Hyperbaric oxygen treatments may prove beneficial as well. Intravenous antibiotic treatments may also be needed at home in some instances when there is a concern for recurring infection after the initial infection.

Prognosis

Osteomyelitis is curable. The long-term outcome depends on the amount of bone and/or joint damage as a result of the infection. Damaged bone can lead to deformity and impaired function, especially if growth plates are affected in children. Chronic cases of osteomyelitis will also affect the prognosis.

Prevention

For most patients, osteomyelitis cannot be prevented because it occurs randomly. However, patients with diabetes mellitus, sickle cell disease, or impaired immune systems should be particularly diligent about reporting any signs of infection to their doctors.

Patient Teaching

Patients must be instructed on the specific details and importance of their antibiotic management. Long-term antibiotic treatments administered intravenously can require special catheters, such as a peripherally inserted central catheter (PICC), which must be cared for according to specific guidelines. Caregivers sometimes administer the antibiotics at home, through the PICC line after training,

Gout

Description

Gout is a chronic disorder of uric acid metabolism that manifests as an acute, episodic form of arthritis; chronic deposits of uric acid forming hard nodules in tissues; and/or kidney impairment or stones.

ICD-10-CM Code	M10.9 *(Gout, unspecified)*
	(M1a.00–M10.9 = 243
	codes of specificity)

Gout is coded according to site and type of pathologic involvement. Refer to the physician's diagnosis and then to the current edition of the ICD-10-CM manual for greatest specificity.

Symptoms and Signs

Gout involves an overproduction or decreased excretion of uric acid and urate salts. When purines in food are metabolized, uric acid is the end result. A diet high in purines leads to high levels of uric acid in the blood and also in the synovial fluid of joints. Deposits of other urate compounds can be found in and around the joints of extremities, often leading to joint deformity and disability (Fig. 7.17A).

Typically, gout affects the first metatarsal joint of the great toe (podagra), causing severe to excruciating pain when an attack occurs. The joints of the feet, ankles, knees, and even hands also can be affected. Pain usually peaks after several hours and then subsides gradually. A slight fever, chills, headache, or nausea may accompany an acute attack. Between attacks, the person is characteristically free from any symptoms. Gout also is characterized by renal dysfunction, hyperuricemia, and renal calculi (kidney stones).

The disease is uncommon in children; gout generally appears in males after puberty. Males are affected more often compared with females. In females, gout generally appears after menopause. Gout also can develop secondary to cell breakdown resulting from drug therapy, especially with chemotherapy for malignant diseases (e.g., leukemia).

Patient Screening

The patient with gout may complain of severe, acute joint pain and possibly mild systemic symptoms. Schedule an urgent appointment (especially if acute gouty arthritis is present) so that treatment can begin and medication that will relieve the pain can be prescribed.

Etiology

The cause of this disorder is most often an inherited abnormality of metabolism. It may result from a deficiency of enzymes needed to completely metabolize purines in foods

for excretion from the kidneys. This incomplete metabolism leads to the buildup of uric acid in the tissues of the body. Uric acid is a breakdown product of purines that are digested in foods. Renal gout is caused by some forms of kidney dysfunction. The body may produce levels of uric acid that are normal, but kidney function is insufficient to remove the product from the blood. Excessive weight gain, leukemias and lymphomas, and certain drugs, including diuretics and tuberculosis medications, also can precipitate gout. Chronic or untreated conditions such as diabetes, heart disease, hypertension, metabolic syndrome, and obesity can also increase the risk of gout.

Diagnosis

Patients with new-onset joint inflammation are evaluated to exclude many types of arthritis, such as rheumatoid arthritis, spondylitis, reactive arthritis, and joint infection. Microscopic examination of aspirated synovial joint fluid or material from soft tissue uric acid deposits (called *tophi*) demonstrates the presence of urate crystals (see Fig. 7.17B) and proves the diagnosis. A serum uric acid test can indicate hyperuricemia, though up to one-third of patients with acute gout will have a normal uric acid level. Radiographs may be used to assess the amount of damage to the affected joints.

Treatment

General treatment of an acute attack of gout can involve bed rest to lessen pressure on affected joints, immobilization of the affected limb, and the application of cold packs to the inflamed joints, if the patient is able to tolerate the pressure of an ice bag. An NSAID, colchicine (Colcrys), or corticosteroids taken orally or injected into the gouty area are options that can reduce inflammation. Dietary modifications include a low-purine diet and adequate fluid intake. Dairy products have been shown to reduce the frequency of attacks of gouty arthritis. For chronic gout, after the acute attack has subsided, the patient may be given antihyperuricemic medications, such as probenecid (Benemid), allopurinol (Zyloprim), febuxostat (Uloric). Gradual weight reduction can be helpful for those patients who are overweight.

Prognosis

With proper management, potential damage to bones and joints can be avoided. Chronic gouty deposits of uric acid (tophi) can be difficult to treat, so if the tophi do not shrink with medication, they can be surgically resected.

Prevention

Limiting alcohol intake, avoiding dehydration, and eating a proper (low-purine, high-dairy) diet are keys to the prevention of gout attacks.

Patient Teaching

Patients should understand that early measures to treat inflammation, such as ice packs and antiinflammatory medication,

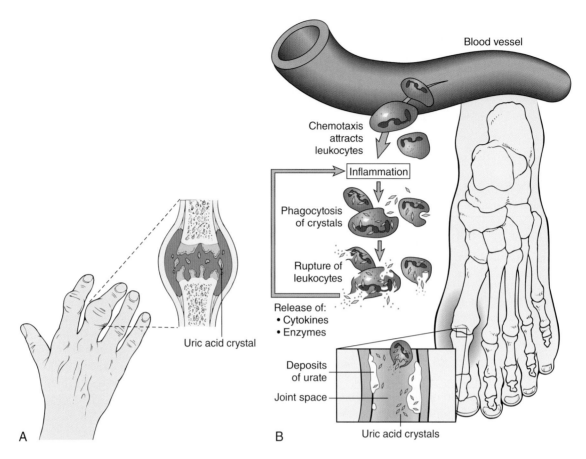

• **Fig. 7.17** (A) Gout. (B) Gouty arthritis. Deposits of uric acid crystals in the connective tissue have a chemotactic effect and cause exudation of leukocytes into the joint. The inflammation most often affects the metatarsophalangeal joint. (From Damjanov I: *Pathology for the health professions*, ed 4, St. Louis, 2012, Saunders.)

may help them avoid prolonged pain and dysfunction. Any patient with gout should be given specific dietary instructions, including which foods are low in purines.

Paget Disease (Osteitis Deformans)

Description
Paget disease is a chronic bone disorder that typically results in enlarged, deformed bones resulting from irregular breakdown and formation of bone tissue. Paget disease can cause bones to weaken and may result in bone pain, arthritis, bone deformities, and fractures. Paget disease is also known as *osteitis deformans*.

ICD-10-CM Code	M88.9 *(Osteitis deformans of unspecified bone)* (M88.0–M88.9 = 27 codes of specificity)

Symptoms and Signs
In patients with Paget disease, affected areas of bone produce new bone tissue faster than the old bone can be broken down. Paget disease occurs characteristically in two stages.

The initial stage is called the *vascular stage*. Bone tissue is broken down, but the spaces left are filled with blood vessels and fibrous tissue instead of new strong bone. In the second, or *sclerotic*, stage, the highly vascular fibrous tissue hardens and becomes similar to bone, but it is fragile instead of being strong (Fig. 7.18). This can lead to pathologic fractures.

This disease can occur in a part of one bone, all of one bone, or many bones throughout the skeletal system. The most common sites of the disease are the pelvis and the tibia. Other sites often affected are the femur, spine, skull, and clavicle. Paget disease usually affects individuals older than 40 years of age and becomes increasingly more common with advancing age.

Paget disease often causes no symptoms. When symptoms do occur, they usually include local bone pain. The pain can become disabling. Aching is almost continuous and is often worse at night. Some patients may have edema or deformity in one of the bones or may notice that they need a larger hat size because the bones of the skull have enlarged. If the ossicles of the ear are involved, hearing loss or deafness may occur. Weakness and tingling in an extremity may be noticed in some cases. Complications of Paget disease can include frequent fractures, spinal cord injuries, hypercalcemia, renal calculi, and rarely, bone sarcoma, a serious form of cancer.

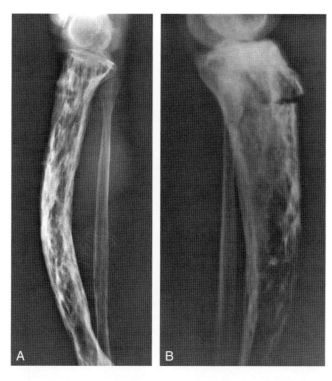

• **Fig. 7.18** Paget disease of bone: radiographic features. (A and B) Lateral radiographs of two examples of Paget disease involving tibia. Note anterior bowing deformity and coarse trabecular pattern with obscured corticomedullary demarcation in both radiographs. Incomplete transverse fracture is seen in proximal tibial shaft in part (B). (From Czerniak B: *Dorfman and Czerniak's Bone Tumors*, ed 2, 2016, Elsevier.)

Patient Screening

A patient with bone pain must be evaluated for fracture and infection of bone along with blood calcium and alkaline phosphatase levels.

Etiology

The full cause of Paget disease is not known. Environmental and genetic factors have been identified as playing a role in the incidence of the disease. The children of a person who has been diagnosed with Paget disease are seven times more likely to be diagnosed with the disease.

Diagnosis

A physical examination and history of the patient's symptoms are needed. The physician then orders several tests and blood work. Radiographic imaging, bone scanning, and possibly bone marrow biopsy assist in the diagnosis. Blood analysis will indicate an elevated serum concentration of alkaline phosphatase, and special urine tests reveal elevated hydroxyproline concentration. Both these findings are produced by the high rate of bone production.

Treatment

Patients with Paget disease who have no symptoms require no treatment. With symptoms, treatment options include analgesics, antiinflammatory drugs, cytotoxic agents, or injections of a hormone called **calcitonin**. Calcitonin is produced naturally by the thyroid gland and works with parathyroid hormone (parathormone) and vitamin D to regulate the level of calcium in the blood. Increased amounts of calcitonin can reduce pain for some patients and prevent bone loss. Eating a high-protein, high-calcium diet, with vitamin D supplementation, may be advised as well. Newer treatments include bisphosphonate medications, such as alendronate (Fosamax), risedronate (Actonel), pamidronate (Aredia), and zoledronic acid (Reclast).

Prognosis

In most patients with Paget disease, few, if any, symptoms are noted. If needed, medications can relieve persistent bone pain. Complications including hypercalcemia, fractures, heart failure, gout, and bone cancer (sarcoma) can lead to increased morbidity.

Prevention

Patients with Paget disease should receive 1000 to 1500 mg of calcium, adequate exposure to sunshine, and at least 400 units of vitamin D daily. This is especially important for patients being treated with bisphosphonates. Patients with a history of kidney stones should discuss calcium and vitamin D intake with their physician. A healthy diet and exercise programs are beneficial, according to the provider's recommendation.

Patient Teaching

Exercise is an important part of maintaining skeletal health, as is avoiding weight gain and maintaining joint mobility. Because undue stress on affected bones should be avoided, patients should discuss any planned exercise program with their physician before beginning. Taking precautions to prevent falls at home should be discussed.

Marfan Syndrome

Description
Marfan syndrome is a group of inherited conditions featuring abnormal connective tissue, weakness of blood vessels, and excessive length and flexibility of the extremities (Fig. 7.19).

ICD-10-CM Code	Q87.40 *(Marfan syndrome, unspecified)* (Q87.40–Q87.43 = 5 codes of specificity)

Symptoms and Signs
Marfan syndrome is characterized by abnormally long extremities and digits. Additional deformities include subluxation of the lens of the eyes and heart and vascular anomalies. This condition may go undetected until harmful complications are precipitated. The person with Marfan syndrome is tall and slender and has long, narrow digits. An asymmetry of the skull may be noted. Visual difficulties are encountered when lens dissociation occurs. Scoliosis is another manifestation. Joints can be hyperextensible in those with Marfan syndrome. Mitral valve prolapse, thickening of the heart valves, and aortic aneurysm may be present but frequently go undetected (see the Valvular Heart Disease section in Chapter 10). Often the first indication of the syndrome occurs during exercise that precipitates rupture of an aortic aneurysm, with catastrophic results.

Patient Screening
A patient diagnosed with Marfan syndrome may develop serious complications of the eyes or cardiovascular system requiring immediate medical attention. Defer to the health care professional for direction.

• **Fig. 7.19** (A and B) This young male has prominent arachnodactyly of both fingers and toes. Note the clubbing due to associated cardiopulmonary problems and the flattening of the arch of his foot. He also has severe pectus carinatum (C) and significant kyphosis and joint contractures (D). Also note his long arms. (From McIntire S, et al: *Zitelli and Davis' Atlas of Pediatric Physical Diagnosis*, ed 8, 2023, Elsevier.)

Etiology

This syndrome is an autosomal dominant genetic disorder. The affected gene is on the long arm of chromosome 15. The defective gene can be inherited as follows: The child of a person who has Marfan syndrome has a 50% chance of inheriting the gene. The defective gene determines the structure of fibrillin, a protein that is an important component of connective tissue. Although everyone with Marfan syndrome has the same defective gene, not everyone experiences the same symptoms. This is referred to as *variable expression* of the gene.

Diagnosis

Patients with Marfan syndrome may sometimes be confused with those who have homocystinuria (an amino acid disorder) because connective tissue abnormalities and abnormal movement of the lens of the eye are present in both conditions. A person with Marfan syndrome is born with the disorder, although it may not be diagnosed until later in life. Genetic testing can confirm the diagnosis, but the family history and physical examination findings may lead to that testing. Abnormal length of the limbs and lens abnormality in the eye, and results of tests of the heart and blood vessels. Diagnosis of the syndrome in early childhood is possible when the lens dissociation and mitral valve prolapse anomalies are detected. The clinical picture of a rapid growth spurt and scoliosis, coupled with the visual disturbance and mitral valve prolapse, leads to further investigation. Echocardiographic measurements of the aortic diameter aid in detecting potential aortic dissection. Patients at risk for impending aortic dissection may be asymptomatic or may experience chest pain that is tearing in nature and radiates to the neck, back, and arms. Other family members may have genetic testing before symptoms occur, in order to have an early diagnosis.

Treatment

Treatment involves controlling excessive height with hormones before puberty, preventing glaucoma, controlling blood pressure, and preventing aortic dissection. Ophthalmic examinations should be conducted on a routine basis to detect any problem at an early stage. Monitoring blood pressure and maintaining it at a normal level is essential. Close observation of aortic status is necessary, and surgical replacement of diseased portions may be indicated. Aortic and mitral valves may need to be replaced surgically. Echocardiography is used on a regular basis to assess the status of the aorta.

Prognosis

The major risk to life is the rupture of blood vessels, particularly the aorta. Patients can be disabled because of severe spine abnormalities and joint dislocations.

Patient Teaching

Patients should be educated about the anomalies in their own anatomy and physiology so that they understand the need to minimize high-risk activities and report any signs of problems to their health care providers. Following the physician's advice and monitoring the condition is important. Genetic counseling may be helpful.

Prevention

The key measures to prevent complications include avoiding elevated blood pressure and trauma that could cause bleeding or bone and joint injury. Evaluation and monitoring of the status of the aorta and heart valves by echocardiography is essential.

Musculoskeletal Tumors

Description

Musculoskeletal tumors are abnormal growths, whether benign or malignant, within muscles or bones. Benign neoplasms are much more common than malignant tumors.

Bone Tumors

Description

The term *bone tumor* describes any abnormal growth, whether benign or malignant, in bone. The definition includes chondrogenic (from cartilage), osteogenic (from bone), and fibrogenic (from fibrous tissue) tumors.

ICD-10-CM Code	*(Refer to the Neoplasm table in the current edition of the ICD-10-CM coding manual.)*

Neoplasms of the bone are coded according to anatomic site, classified as benign or malignant, or designated as unspecified. Refer to the physician's diagnosis and then to the current edition of the ICD-10-CM coding manual for greatest specificity.

Symptoms and Signs

With bone tumors, pain is the most common presenting complaint. It is often worse at night or with exercise. A parent may notice a child beginning to limp or curtailing physical activity. Painful soft tissue swelling may be evident as the neoplasm enlarges. Patients with Ewing sarcoma often have systemic symptoms, such as fever, fatigue, and pallor caused by anemia.

Sometimes bone tumors produce no symptoms and are detected incidentally when radiographic imaging is performed for some other reason. Radiographic studies can reveal osteonecrosis or increased ossification and calcification. Different types of malignant tumors have characteristic radiographic findings. Osteosarcoma has a "sunburst" appearance on the radiograph. The Ewing sarcoma lesion has an "onion skin" appearance. Chondrosarcomas have a lobular pattern.

The bone tumor weakens the bone and makes it susceptible to fracture when subjected to the slightest strain. This is called a *pathologic fracture* (see Fig. 7.25I). A pathologic fracture is often one of the first indications of the presence of metastases to bones, and it commonly occurs in the acetabulum or the proximal femur.

Patient Screening

Bone pain, with or without local swelling, requires a timely medical evaluation. Systemic symptoms also may be present and indicate the need for the earliest possible appointment.

Etiology

Malignant tumors may be primary or secondary in origin. Primary tumors are most commonly found in adolescents, often during the adolescent growth spurt. Males are affected more often than females. Metastatic, or secondary, tumors in bones occur more often than primary tumors and are more common in older age groups. Cancers that commonly metastasize to bones include breast, lung, prostate, thyroid, and kidney cancers. The bones affected most often are the pelvis, vertebrae, ribs, hip, femur, and humerus. Risk factors for primary bone tumors include prior chemotherapy, radiation therapy, or a history of Paget disease or other benign bone lesions.

Osteosarcoma is the most common type of primary bone neoplasm (Fig. 7.20). Osteosarcoma develops most often in the distal femur, followed by the proximal tibia and the humerus. Metastasis to the lung within 2 years of treatment is common. Ewing sarcoma most often involves the pelvis and the lower extremity and can extend into soft tissues. Both often metastasize to the lungs. Metastases in the lungs and other bones occur early in the disease. Chondrosarcoma often arises in the pelvis and proximal femur. It primarily affects individuals who are middle-aged or older adults, but it can occur at any age. Chondrosarcoma grows more slowly compared with other malignant tumors of the bone and is locally invasive.

Diagnosis

The diagnosis is made on the basis of findings from a complete patient history, physical examination, laboratory studies, and diagnostic procedures. Many studies, including radiography, radionuclide bone scanning or positron emission tomography, CT, and MRI greatly aid in determining the diagnosis and in evaluating the extent of disease. For Ewing sarcoma, bone marrow aspiration is performed to check for metastasis to bone marrow. Other markers may be useful in the identification of tumor type. Osteosarcomas generally have an elevated serum alkaline phosphatase level, whereas in Ewing sarcoma, the level of lactate dehydrogenase (LDH) can be elevated. Biopsy is necessary for definitive diagnosis and for staging purposes. Bone cancers are often staged by using a system based on the tumor grade, tumor site, and presence of metastases.

Treatment

Bone tumors, whether benign or malignant, are treated with surgical excision. The surrounding muscle, bone, and other tissue are often removed also, and bone grafting may be needed. The goal is to perform limb-sparing surgery,

• **Fig. 7.20** Osteosarcoma. (From Kumar V, et al: *Robbins basic pathology*, ed 8, Philadelphia, 2008, Saunders.)

but tumor location and extent may necessitate amputation. Isolated metastases to the lungs may be amenable to surgical resection as well. Surgery alone is enough to treat benign tumors, whereas treatment of malignant neoplasms usually includes the administration of chemotherapy and/or radiation therapy. Treatment choice depends on tumor type. For example, Ewing sarcoma is usually chemosensitive, whereas chondrosarcomas are generally chemoresistant.

Prognosis

The prognosis depends largely on tumor type, extent of disease at presentation, and anatomic location. Poor prognostic indicators are a high-grade tumor, large tumor size, and presence of metastasis. A high LDH level at diagnosis often correlates with a poor prognosis in Ewing sarcoma.

Prevention

Prevention is difficult because few risk factors have been identified. Bone pain and masses should be evaluated promptly to reduce the risk of complications, such as fractures, deformity, and need for amputation. No type of routine screening is recommended, even for those with risk factors for bone tumors, such as Paget disease or prior radiation therapy.

Patient Teaching

Patients and families require specific instructions regarding the use and rehabilitation of the involved extremities. Managing the timing and intensity of weight bearing with leg involvement, for example, is crucial for avoiding injury.

Muscle Tumors

Description

Neoplasms of muscle include benign tumors or malignant sarcomas that may arise at any site in the body. The most commonly affected areas are the buttocks, groin, extremities, head and neck region, trunk, and retroperitoneum.

| ICD-10-CM Code | *(Refer to the Neoplasm table in the current edition of the ICD-10-CM coding manual.)* |

Neoplasms of the muscle are coded according to anatomic site, classified as benign or malignant, or designated as unspecified. Refer to the physician's diagnosis and then to the current edition of the ICD-10-CM coding manual for greatest specificity.

Symptoms and Signs

Skeletal muscle tumors often present as a painless lump with a duration of a few weeks or months, often with erythema of the overlying skin. In some instances, pain and tenderness may be present secondary to pressure effects on a nerve from the mass. Smooth muscle tumors often cause pain in and/or bleeding from the organ affected. For example, a uterine leiomyoma may cause abnormal uterine bleeding. At times, benign tumors are asymptomatic and are discovered incidentally on physical or radiographic examinations.

Patient Screening

A child or adult with a lump or painless swelling in a muscle should be scheduled for a visual inspection and medical evaluation.

Etiology

Muscle neoplasms are often benign and not life threatening (e.g., leiomyomas [tumors of smooth muscle] and rhabdomyomas [tumors of striated muscle]). Malignant tumors (e.g., leiomyosarcomas and rhabdomyosarcomas) often grow and metastasize rapidly. Malignant muscle tumors grow by local extension and infiltration along tissue planes. In contrast to primary bone tumors, muscle sarcomas occur most often in patients older than 50 years of age. The exception is the small peak of incidence of rhabdomyosarcoma in early childhood. Risk factors include radiation treatment for previous cancer and exposure to carcinogenic chemicals.

Diagnosis

MRI is the most effective imaging technique for muscle tumors. Radiography or CT of the chest is performed to look for metastasis to the lungs. Biopsy (usually core-needle biopsy) can compromise subsequent treatment and should be carefully planned by using the information from imaging studies. Bone marrow aspiration is performed if a malignant tumor is present. The most common staging system used is a variation of the TNM (tumor-node-metastasis) system that also incorporates grade and tumor depth into the stage grouping. See Chapter 1 for information about the staging and grading systems used to assess malignant neoplasms.

Treatment

Surgical resection of the tumor is performed for all tumors, benign or malignant. For benign tumors, complete surgical resection is usually all that is required for treatment. For sarcomas, surgery is often combined with radiation therapy. Chemotherapy is used as an adjunct to surgery in children with rhabdomyosarcoma. Resection of pulmonary metastases may offer survival benefit and possible cure. Because lung metastasis can be clinically silent, follow-up imaging studies are indicated for all patients after initial treatment.

Prognosis

The prognosis worsens significantly with increasing tumor grade. Other poor prognostic indicators include deep anatomic tumor location, large tumor size, and presence of metastases. The 5-year survival rate for malignant tumors varies widely, depending on tumor subtype and grade.

Prevention

No methods of prevention are known.

Patient Teaching

Explain the scheduled diagnostic procedures to the patient, and describe what is normally experienced during the tests. Tell the patient when to expect the results. If surgery is necessary, explain the preoperative and postoperative procedures. Address patient concerns if the tumor is malignant, within the guidelines suggested by the physician. Give a full explanation of the radiation and chemotherapy regimens and what side effects may occur. Offer sensitive support to parents when the patient is a child, and make appropriate referrals for additional support.

Osteoporosis

Description

Osteoporosis is a condition characterized by loss of normal bone density. Osteoporosis leads to literally porous bone that can be described as being compressible, like a sponge, rather than being dense, like a brick (Fig. 7.21).

| ICD-10-CM Code | M81.0 *(Age-related osteoporosis without current pathological fracture)* |

Osteoporosis may be coded according to cause or onset. Refer to the current edition of the ICD-10-CM coding manual for greatest specificity.

Symptoms and Signs

Osteoporosis is a condition in which there is wasting or deterioration of bone mass and density. It occurs more often in females, especially postmenopausal females, than in males. Females who are small boned, who are of northern European

• **Fig. 7.21** (A) Normal metacarpal bone. (B) Osteoporotic metacarpal bone. (From Long BW, et al: *Radiography essentials for limited practice*, ed 4, St. Louis, 2013, Elsevier.)

or Asian descent, who smoke, and who have a family history of the disease have the greatest risk for osteoporosis.

Unless it occurs in the vertebrae or the weight-bearing bones, osteoporosis usually does not produce symptoms. Osteoporosis is a silent disease until a bone break causes pain. Spontaneous fractures, especially in the vertebrae of the mid-to-lower thoracic spine, and loss of height are the most common signs.

Patient Screening
Patients with risk factors should undergo bone density testing. Unrecognized osteoporosis may be first discovered when the patient sustains a fracture. Emergency care is required for breathing difficulty, severe pain, protrusion of bone through the skin, or numbness in a limb.

Etiology
Osteoporosis is the most common metabolic bone disease. It is caused by the imbalance between the breakdown of old bone tissue and the production of new bone. Metabolic bone diseases primarily originate from hormonal or dietary factors or disuse, but trauma also may cause the development of this condition. Osteoporosis can be caused by radiation treatments, malabsorption, smoking, alcohol abuse, calcium-wasting nephropathy, immobility, and chronic disease, such as rheumatoid arthritis. Senile and postmenopausal osteoporosis, usually resulting from a lack of estrogen, are the most common forms. Osteoporosis can also result from the use of medications, such as heparin,

phenytoin, and the cortisone medications prednisone and prednisolone. Males with a low testosterone level are at risk for osteoporosis.

Diagnosis
Patients with spontaneous bone fracture are screened for cancer in the involved bone by using radiographic testing. When osteoporosis is detected, patients are further evaluated for hormone imbalances, kidney disease, diet inadequacy, intestinal malabsorption, and use of certain medications, including cortisone medications, such as prednisone and prednisolone.

The diagnosis of osteoporosis is based on the results of blood serum studies, radiography, urinalysis, CT, and bone scanning. The best test for osteoporosis is dual-energy x-ray absorptiometry. If more specific diagnostic data are needed, a bone biopsy may be ordered.

Treatment
Osteoporosis can cause permanent disability if not arrested, and treatment varies, depending on the cause. Increased dietary intake of calcium, calcium carbonate, calcium carbonate with sodium fluoride, phosphate supplements, and vitamins, especially vitamin D, may be prescribed. Estrogen replacement therapy may be used for postmenopausal osteoporosis. Alternatives to estrogen replacement therapy are bisphosphonate medications, such as alendronate sodium (Fosamax), risedronate (Actonel), ibandronate (Boniva), or zoledronate (Reclast). Calcitonin (Miacalcin) nasal spray and parathyroid hormone (Forteo) are other options in certain situations. Exercise can help minimize osteoporosis by slowing the loss of calcium. Moderate exercise in the form of walking, swimming, or use of a stationary bicycle is best. Physical therapy exercises for persons who are immobilized or paralyzed are necessary. If, however, the bones have become brittle, exercise of any type may be limited. To alleviate pain and muscle spasms, analgesics and muscle relaxants may be prescribed.

Prognosis
The outlook for patients with osteoporosis depends on many factors, including age and mobility, severity of bone loss, underlying causes, and complications related to fractures. The prognosis improves when the underlying causes are identified and treatment is provided.

Prevention
Prevention is absolutely the key to osteoporosis management. Bone density testing should be performed in all females older than 65 years of age, in all postmenopausal females with risk factors for osteoporosis, and postmenopausal females who sustain fractures. Females should consult their clinicians regarding adequate calcium intake and regular exercise programs.

Patient Teaching
Patients must be instructed regarding diets that promote bone health, smoking cessation, calcium and vitamin D

intake, and exercise programs. Fall risk education can prevent fractures.

Osteomalacia and Rickets

Description

Osteomalacia is a bone disease characterized by defective mineralization.

ICD-10-CM Code	M83.9 *(Adult osteomalacia, unspecified)*
	(M83.0–M83.9 = 8 codes of specificity)

Additional codes may be required to identify the nature or cause of osteomalacia. Refer to the physician's diagnosis and then to the current edition of the ICD-10-CM coding manual for greatest specificity.

Symptoms and Signs

Osteomalacia causes bones to become increasingly soft, flexible, and deformed. When the disorder occurs in children, it impacts the growing skeleton and is called *rickets* (Fig. 7.22). In adults, it usually is referred to as *osteomalacia*.

Early symptoms may include general fatigue; progressive stiffness; tender, painful bones; backaches; muscle twitches and cramps; and difficulty standing up. As the disease progresses, the patient may experience fractures, bowing of the legs, chest deformity, and shortening of the spine leading to an overall reduction in height.

Patient Screening

The early symptoms mentioned above require an appointment for a medical assessment.

Etiology

Osteomalacia is a metabolic bone disease resulting from deficiency or ineffective use of vitamin D, which is essential for proper bone formation. Without adequate vitamin D, the body cannot absorb and use the bone-building minerals (calcium and phosphorus).

Other causes of this disorder may include inadequate exposure to sunlight, which prevents the body from synthesizing its own vitamin D; intestinal malabsorption of vitamin D; and chronic renal diseases.

Diagnosis

Children with skeletal abnormalities suggestive of rickets are evaluated for genetic disorders and disease of the kidneys and bowels. Adults with osteomalacia are screened for metabolism disorders, as well as kidney and bowel disease.

The diagnosis of osteomalacia can involve a series of blood tests (e.g., serum calcium, serum alkaline phosphatase, vitamin D levels, and ESR), radiographic studies, bone scanning, and possibly bone biopsy.

• **Fig. 7.22** Rickets. (From Kumar V: *Robbins basic pathology*, ed 9, Philadelphia, 2013, Saunders.)

Treatment

Treatment involves vitamin D supplementation and adding dietary vitamin D, calcium, and calcitonin. Exposure to sunlight increases vitamin D metabolism and absorption, especially in older persons. Any underlying disorder causing the deficiency, such as kidney or bowel disease, must be treated.

Prognosis

The outlook for patients with osteomalacia depends, to a great extent, on how early the condition is detected. The severity of the disorder, underlying causes, and complications, such as fractures, are all important factors affecting the long-term outlook.

Prevention

Prevention focuses on early diagnosis and prevention of bone injury.

Patient Teaching

Patients are instructed regarding vitamin D and calcium metabolism, dietary requirements, and the role of ultraviolet radiation in sunlight for producing natural vitamin D within the body.

Hallux Valgus (Bunion)

Description

A bunion is a localized area of enlargement of the inner portion of the first metatarsophalangeal (MTP) joint at the base of the big toe (Fig. 7.23).

ICD-10-CM Code	(M20.10–M20.12 = 3 codes of specificity)

Symptoms and Signs

Bunions cause progressive enlargement of the inner aspect of the first MTP joint. This can be associated with local inflammation and pain. If an adjacent inflamed bursa develops, secondary to pressure and inflammation at the joint, it can become even more painful. At times, the great toe may override or undercut the second toe. This causes crowding of the other toes and the possible development of hammer, claw, or mallet toes. Bunion development is more common in females and adolescent girls.

Patient Screening

Schedule an appointment for a visual examination for a patient complaining of a painful large toe.

Etiology

A bunion is often the result of a foot disorder known as *hallux valgus*, in which the great toe is positioned toward the midline of the body. The condition has been associated with rheumatoid arthritis. A flatfoot also contributes to hallux valgus and the development of a bunion because of the fallen, or dropped, longitudinal arch of the foot. The wearing of improperly fitting or high-heeled shoes aggravates hallux valgus. There is also a familial tendency for developing this condition. Bunions are common in ballet dancers.

Metatarsophalangeal joint

• **Fig. 7.23** Bunion (hallux valgus).

Diagnosis

Patients with bunions are evaluated for underlying forms of arthritis, particularly osteoarthritis, rheumatoid arthritis, and gout. Footwear should be closely scrutinized. Physical examination of the foot, along with a history of the symptoms, may be sufficient for the diagnosis. Radiographic studies confirm the lateral displacement of the great toe and any degenerative arthritic joint changes.

Treatment

Management of a bunion can include wearing shoes with a roomy "toe box" to avoid crowding the toes together; wearing shoes with lower heels; using padding between the toes or around the bunion to relieve pressure; applying ice to the bunion to reduce the inflammation and lessen the pain; and resting the affected joints.

Analgesic medications (e.g., aspirin and acetaminophen) are given for pain. Intraarticular (joint) injections of a corticosteroid may be helpful as well.

There are many different surgical procedures for the treatment or correction of hallux valgus. Bunionectomy, osteotomy, and arthroplasty are the more common procedures.

Prognosis

With proper footwear, bunions often can be tolerated without surgical intervention. For those with persistent pain, surgical treatments can be curative.

Prevention

Proper footwear to minimize trauma to the toe and MTP joint is essential for the best outcome.

Patient Teaching

Patients can benefit by learning about the anatomy of the foot and the affected joint. They should be alerted to the risk for secondary infection if the bunion is abraded by footwear; if such is the case, antibiotics are instituted, if needed.

Hallux Rigidus

Description

Hallux rigidus is a stiff big toe that develops as a result of degeneration of the cartilage of the first MTP joint.

ICD-10-CM Code	(M20.20–M20.22 = 3 codes of specificity)

Symptoms and Signs

Hallux rigidus causes pain and loss of motion in the joint. The MTP joint becomes painful, stiff, and swollen. The onset may be insidious, with the limitation of movement being gradual.

Patient Screening

An appointment for visual inspection and possibly radiographic studies are indicated for a patient complaining of pain in the large toe.

Etiology

Degeneration of the MTP joint can occur as a result of injury or underlying arthritis, such as osteoarthritis. Over time, constant wear or repetitive minor trauma to the joint causes the articular cartilage to degenerate, resulting in raw bone surface rubbing against raw bone surface. This degenerative arthritic-type process allows for the formation of bone spurs or osteophytes in the joint space that restrict joint motion.

Diagnosis

Diagnosis is made from a history of pain, either continuous or when walking, and restriction of motion of the MTP joint of the great toe. Physical examination usually reveals a straight hallux with an enlarged and tender joint with limited dorsiflexion. Radiographic studies confirm the degenerative process and the joint space is diminished. Advanced conditions may cause chips of the cartilage in the joint space, which may eventually calcify.

Treatment

Conservative treatment includes drug therapy with antiinflammatory medications and wearing shoes with thick, hard soles and low heels. When surgical intervention is indicated, cheilectomy to remove bone spurs and degenerative changes of the joint is considered. During cheilectomy, a portion of the dorsal aspect of the metatarsal head also is removed. This is followed by rehabilitation with ROM exercises. When the progression of the condition is extensive, arthrodesis, or fusion of the joint, may be the only method of pain relief. Some surgeons may perform arthroplasty to replace the destroyed joint with a plastic prosthesis or an artificial joint. The problem with this procedure is that the lifetime of the joint usually is limited, possibly necessitating future procedures.

Prognosis

With proper footwear and medication to relieve intermittent pain, hallux rigidus often can be tolerated without surgical intervention. For those with persistent pain, surgical treatments can be curative.

Prevention

Proper footwear to minimize trauma to the toe and MTP joint is essential for the best outcome.

Patient Teaching

Patients can benefit by learning about the anatomy of the foot and the affected joint. Repeated impact loading of the affected joint can lead to progressive worsening.

Hammer Toe (Mallet Toe)

Description

Hammer toe is a condition in which the toe bends upward like a claw because of an abnormal flexion of the PIP joint; it can occur in any one of the four lesser toes (Fig. 7.24).

• **Fig. 7.24** (A) Hammer toe. (B) Hammer toe of second lesser toe, right foot.

ICD-10-CM Code	M20.40 *(Other hammer toe(s) [acquired], unspecified foot)* (M20.40–M20.42 = 3 codes of specificity)

Symptoms and Signs

Hammer toe most often occurs in the second toe and with hyperextension of the MTP joint. This deformity can be painful and often causes abrasion and inflammation where the flexed toe rubs against footwear. It can lead to the formation of a corn on the top of the affected toe and callus formation on the sole of the foot and tip of the involved toe. Mallet toe is an unusual bend in the joint of the toe nearest the toenail.

Patient Screening

Patients with hammer toe are evaluated for underlying forms of arthritis, such as rheumatoid arthritis and psoriatic arthritis.

Etiology

Many factors may contribute to the occurrence of hammer toe. Although a congenital tendency of a long second metatarsal bone may exist, often shoes that are too short and have pointed toes or high heels may be the contributing factor. Nerves supplying the muscles of the toe are subjected to repeated insult, resulting in muscle imbalance in the foot and the development of hammer toe. Underlying arthritis from such diseases as rheumatoid arthritis and psoriatic arthritis can lead to the formation of hammer toes.

Diagnosis

A history of pain in the affected toe along with visual inspection is usually sufficient for determining diagnosis. Imaging studies confirm the diagnosis and rule out certain forms of arthritis.

Treatment

If the patient comes in early in the onset of symptoms, often switching to shoes that fit properly and allow enough space for the second toe can reverse the process, and the toe will eventually straighten. Splinting the affected toe and performing therapeutic exercises can be helpful. Orthotic shoe inserts may also be recommended for pain and to take pressure off the toe. The more advanced conditions when a contracture exists require surgical arthroplasty and possible fusion of the PIP joint.

Prognosis

Proper footwear and monitoring for secondary infection improve the outcome. For those with persistent pain and irritation, surgical treatments can be curative.

Prevention

Proper footwear to minimize trauma to the toe is essential for the best outcome. Box-toed shoes can be very helpful.

Patient Teaching

Patients can benefit from learning about the anatomy of the foot and the affected toe. They should be instructed on the care of the foot and toenails and monitoring for signs of secondary infection. Using recommended orthotics as directed.

Traumatic and Sports Injuries

Fractures

Description

Fractures, or broken bones, are caused by stress on the bone resulting from a traumatic insult to the musculoskeletal system, severe muscle spasm, or bone disease. They can occur in any bone in the body and are classified by the nature of the fracture, which is the result of the mechanism of injury (Fig. 7.25A–O).

ICD-10-CM Code   S codes that require 7 digits

Fractures are classified and coded according to site, type, multiple fractures of sites, and cause of injury, and subclassified by factors such as the occurrence of complications and late effects. Refer to the physician's diagnosis and then the current edition of the ICD-10-CM coding manual for greatest specificity.

Fractures are described by specific names or by location:

- Colles fracture is fracture of the distal head of the radius, with possible involvement of the ulnar styloid. Colles fractures usually result from a fall in which the person attempts to break the fall with an extended arm and open hand. Pain and swelling are experienced. Treatment includes closed reduction of the fracture and immobilization of the arm, including the elbow, with a cast.
- Fracture of the humerus involves an obvious displacement of the bone of the upper arm along with shortening of the extremity and abnormal mobility of the upper arm. Closed reduction of the fracture is followed by immobilization in a hanging arm cast, sling, and swathe.
- Fracture of the pelvis is usually the result of severe trauma, such as from a motor vehicle accident or a fall, but can occur spontaneously in patients with osteoporosis. Complications of this fracture include lacerated colon, paralytic ileus, bladder, and urethral injury, and intrapelvic hemorrhage. Treatment includes bed rest, possible immobilization with a pelvic sling or skeletal traction, and open reduction and repair.
- A fractured hip is usually the result of a fall. It can also occur because of an underlying condition such as osteoporosis. An outward rotation along with a shortening of the affected extremity is noted and there is severe pain. Weight bearing on the affected side is not possible. Repair is accomplished with surgery that involves the insertion of a prosthesis, pins, or both.
- Fracture of the femoral shaft is more common in young adults and usually is the result of a severe direct impact related to motor vehicle accidents or severe trauma. A notable angulation deformity and shortening of the affected leg are present. The patient is unable to move the knee or hip. The fracture is stabilized by skeletal traction or internal fixation with a rod or plate and screws.
- A fracture of the tibia results from a strong force exerted on the lower leg that causes soft tissue damage in addition to the fracture. Open or closed reduction is employed, followed by immobilization with a cast.
- Vertebral fracture in the neck can be the result of acceleration–deceleration trauma. Immediate immobilization is imperative to prevent spinal cord damage and resulting paralysis. Thoracic and lumbar vertebrae can be fractured often as a result of a fall and landing directly on the buttocks or may be associated with osteoporosis. Immobilization may be followed by surgical repair and possible insertion of surgical hardware (rods, plates) for stabilization.
- In some cases, a less invasive orthopedic procedure called *vertebroplasty* can be used to repair fractured and compressed vertebrae. Bone cement is injected into the area of compression to seal and stabilize the fracture.
- A basilar skull fracture is a fracture of the floor of the cranial vault. It is usually the result of massive trauma to the head caused by a motor vehicle accident.
- LeFort fracture, a bilateral horizontal fracture of the maxilla, often results when the face is forced against the steering wheel in a motor vehicle accident.
- In Pott fracture, the lower part of the fibula is fractured. The lower tibial articulation sustains serious injury.

• **Fig. 7.25** Types of fractures. (A) Closed or simple. The overlying skin is intact. (B) Open or compound. The skin overlying the bone ends is not intact. (C) Longitudinal. The fracture extends along the length of the bone. (D) Transverse. The fracture is at right angles to the axis of the bone. (E) Oblique. The fracture extends in an oblique direction. (F) Greenstick. The fracture is on one side of the bone; the other side is bent. (G) Comminuted. The bone is splintered or crushed. (H) Impacted. The fractured ends of the bone are driven into each other. (I) Pathologic. The fracture results from the weakening of the bone by disease. (J) Nondisplaced. The bone ends remain in alignment. (K) Displaced. The bone ends are out of alignment. (L) Spiral. The fracture results from a twisting mechanism, causing the break to wind around the bone in a spiral. (M) Compression. Excessive pressure causes the bone to collapse. (N) Avulsion. The tearing away of a muscle or a ligament is accompanied by the tearing away of a bone fragment. (O) Depression. Bone fragments of the skull are driven inward.

• A clavicular fracture is a fracture of the clavicle (collar bone). It is a common sports injury, commonly occurring in bicycling accidents and often in children of all ages.

Symptoms and Signs

Pain accompanies most fractures. Edema, tenderness, discoloration, and inability to move the affected part follow. In some instances, deformity of the affected part is noted. The location of the fracture and the type of the fracture are determining factors in the symptoms and signs. There may be intense bruising of the skin, especially in patients taking blood thinners, which can lead to excessive blood loss.

Patient Screening

Severe pain, deformity, inability to move an extremity, bone protruding through the skin, numbness or tingling in a joint, or difficulty breathing are indications for emergency care.

Etiology

Any force, external or internal, that disrupts the continuity of the bone causes a fracture. Diseases such as neoplasms, tuberculosis of bone, Paget disease, and osteoporosis cause pathologic fractures, which occur without significant external trauma.

Diagnosis

The major issues in assessing patients' injuries include defining the extent and location of the fracture and any complications resulting from the fracture and also detecting any underlying disease of bone. A complete history and physical examination are followed by radiographic studies of the affected structure. Bone scanning and MRI aid in determining diagnosis. Any underlying pathologic change is investigated and diagnosed; sometimes this requires bone biopsy. Patients who fall and are unable to walk or get up, need to call emergency services to come and assist.

Treatment

Treatment depends on the location, severity, type, and cause of the fracture, as described earlier. Simple fractures of the long bones are reduced and immobilized. Compound fractures are cleaned, débrided, reduced, and immobilized (tetanus status must be checked in the case of a compound fracture). Immobilization is accomplished by splinting (including the use of posterior splints), casting, taping, and external or internal fixation. Internal fixation (open reduction) includes the use of surgically implanted pins, wires, rods, plates, screws, or other devices. Some fractures are placed in traction to hold the ends of the bones in proper alignment until healing takes place.

Prognosis

The outlook depends on the location severity of the fracture, complications, and the presence of an underlying disease. Fractures that damage the epiphyseal plate (growth plate) in the child may have long-term residual effects, such as stunted growth or osteoarthritis. Physical and occupational therapy may be needed to restore full use of range of motion in some cases. Rehabilitative services may be needed for some patients after fractures at an inpatient facility.

Complications of fractures include compartment syndrome, in which circulation to the area is compromised because of edema; nonunion and malunion of bones; infection; necrosis; fat emboli; and pulmonary emboli.

Prevention

Wearing protective gear when playing contact sports and engaging in conditioning exercises can decrease the risk of fractures. Seatbelts and airbags have been proven to decrease injuries when involved in a motor vehicle accident.

Patient Teaching

Patient education should be focused on appropriate conditioning programs to prevent future fractures. After a fracture, instructions to the patient regarding cast or brace care, activity limitations, and gradual rehabilitation exercises are essential.

To ensure optimal rehabilitation of the involved body areas, explain the exact condition and the long-term goals to the patient.

Strains and Sprains

Description

A strain is an injury of a tendon, muscle, or other tissue resulting from overuse, overstretching, or excessive forcible stretching of the tissue beyond its functional capacity.

A sprain is an acute tear of a ligament (Fig. 7.27). Sprains are classified as first-, second-, or third-degree, or -grade, sprains.

ICD-10-CM Code	S codes that require 7 digits

Strains and sprains are classified and coded according to such factors as site, occurrence of injury, and involvement of adjacent structures. Refer to the physician's diagnosis and then the current edition of the ICD-10-CM coding manual for greatest specificity.

◆ ENRICHMENT

Amputation

Most limb amputations involve the legs and are necessary because of peripheral vascular disease caused by atherosclerosis and consequent gangrene. Trauma, malignancy, and congenital defects are additional reasons for amputation of limbs and digits. Those in the military have traumatic injuries that, at times, result in amputation. Amputations can also be necessitated by crushing injuries, open fractures, frostbite, and thermal or electrical burns. Infection and malignancy also may necessitate amputations. The extent of the amputation can range from the removal of a portion of a digit to complete disarticulation at the hip or shoulder.

Rehabilitation is important and is attempted as soon as possible to afford the patient independence. Many customized prostheses are available for both upper and lower extremities. Technological advances have given individuals with amputations their mobility and independence with prosthesis, which are as "life-like" as possible. Robotics and 3D imaging are giving hope to individuals who have suffered amputation (Fig. 7.26).

• **Fig. 7.26** Pediatric patient performing a bimanual coordination assessment using a transradial 3D-printed prosthesis. The device was manufactured at the Department of Biomechanics, University of Nebraska Omaha. (From Stergiou N: *Biomechanics and Gait Analysis*, ed 1, 2020, Elsevier.)

Phantom Limb and Phantom Limb Pain

Phantom limb sensation is an unpleasant complication that sometimes follows an amputation, especially of a leg, and is difficult to treat. It is the feeling that the limb still is attached. Phantom limb pain of the leg can present as a burning sensation of the foot or as a feeling of having the toes stepped on, even though no limb exists.

Both conditions usually disappear with time and with the realization that the limb is gone. Phantom limb pain may necessitate injection or removal of troublesome nerve endings that are located in the stump.

• **Fig. 7.27** Ankle sprain.

Symptoms and Signs

Strains and sprains can be acute injuries or can be the result of chronic overuse (cumulative trauma). Symptoms may include localized pain, weakness, numbness, and possibly edema around the site of the injury. With both strain and sprain injuries, using, moving, or bearing weight on the affected limb or part is difficult or sometimes nearly impossible for the patient. Sprains may include damage to blood vessels and nerves; edema; ecchymosis; and sharp, transient pain. When sprains and strains are caused by chronic overuse, they typically cause stiffness, tenderness, and soreness.

Patient Screening

Ankle injury accompanied by obvious deformity, bone protruding through the skin, or bleeding requires emergency care. Schedule a same-day appointment for an individual with a painful ankle injury that involves inability to bear weight or walk.

Etiology

Strains and sprains can be caused by acute trauma (e.g., sports injury or automobile accidents) or cumulative trauma (e.g., overuse, as in occupational or sports-related injuries).

Diagnosis

A physical examination and medical history of a recent injury resulting from physical activity, an accident, or repetitive overuse may suggest the diagnosis. Sometimes the patient will describe feeling or hearing a "pop" when the injury occurs. Patients with obvious significant physical trauma should be evaluated for possible associated fractures. Bruising, swelling, and limited movement are indicators the patient needs tests to determine the severity of the injury. Radiographic studies are ordered to rule out the possibility of a fracture. MRI may be also ordered.

Treatment

The treatment of both strains and sprains is similar and depends on the degree or grade of the injury. The sprain, being the more serious injury, requires more intense treatment. Treatment of sprains and strains includes elevation and rest of the affected limb and the application of a cold pack or ice to control edema. Immobilization of the limb with an elastic bandage, soft cast, or splint may be necessary. Analgesics and antiinflammatory agents are used to control pain and inflammation. Surgery may be indicated if the injury involves a large tear or if it heals improperly.

Prognosis

Healing of a strain or sprain usually takes 2 to 4 weeks or longer, with the more serious degrees of strain or sprain. The outlook is best when the patient participates in a progressive rehabilitation program.

Prevention

Recognizing personal physical limitations, following safety precautions, and taking time to warm up the muscles with slow, easy stretching before engaging in exercise or physical activity all help prevent sprains and strains. Sometimes support bracing is necessary when engaging in strenuous activities after incurring one of these injuries.

Patient Teaching

Encourage compliance with the treatment plan and rehabilitation program. Discuss the importance of the preventive measures mentioned above to avoid reinjury.

Dislocations

Description

A dislocation is the forcible displacement of a bone from its joint, thereby causing loss of joint function (Fig. 7.28).

ICD-10-CM Code	S codes that require 7 digits

Dislocations are coded according to site, type (e.g., open or closed), occurrence of injury, and nature (e.g., congenital, pathologic, recurrent). Refer to the physician's diagnosis and then the current edition of the ICD-10-CM coding manual for greatest specificity.

Symptoms and Signs

A dislocated joint appears misshapen, is extremely painful, and rapidly becomes edematous, ecchymotic, and

Normal position of humerus   Clavicle

Humerus   Scapula

• **Fig. 7.28** Dislocation of the shoulder.

immovable. Injury to the ligaments and capsule of the joint is present. Other symptoms are a function of the extent of damage to the surrounding tissues, nerves, and blood vessels.

Dislocation of spinal vertebrae can result in damage to the entire spinal cord and cause numbness, tingling, or paralysis below the injured area. A dislocation of a shoulder or hip can damage the nerve supply and cause paralysis of the limb. Some joints that have been dislocated tend to be susceptible to developing osteoarthritis in later years.

Patient Screening

Traumatic dislocations require *immediate* emergency medical care.

Etiology

The cause of a dislocation is usually a severe injury (e.g., a fall, automobile accident, or sports-related trauma) that exerts force great enough to tear the joint ligaments. Occasionally the injury that causes the dislocation also causes a fracture.

Dislocations not caused by injury may result from congenital weakness of the joint structures or from a complication of arthritis. They can happen repeatedly, without apparent cause, to a joint already weakened by an earlier injury. Jaw and shoulder joints are especially susceptible to recurring dislocations.

The elbow is an area on a young child that sometimes becomes partially dislocated. This condition is referred to as *"nursemaids elbow."* A parent or caregiver may be holding a child's hand and the child may try to run, be going to fall, or intentionally become "dead weight," which results in jerking the arm. This also may happen if one is swinging a small child by their arms. The elbow will have an abnormal appearance and the child will be in pain and cry. The elbow can be manipulated back into a normal position by the pediatrician or provider, but once a dislocation has occurred once, there is more likelihood that it will happen again. Avoiding similar types of movements will prevent the dislocation from happening again.

A rare congenital cause of recurrent dislocations is the inherited connective tissue disorder Ehlers-Danlos syndrome, which is characterized by joint hypermobility and skin laxity.

Diagnosis

The obvious abnormal appearance of the affected joint, the history of the injury, and a physical examination may be all that is necessary to determine the diagnosis. A radiographic study can confirm whether a dislocation has occurred and whether any fractures are present. Patients also must be evaluated for nerve and blood vessel injuries.

Treatment

An untrained individual never should attempt to reduce a dislocation; doing so may cause extensive damage to blood vessels and nerves. A physician should be seen immediately for proper repositioning of the joint. After that time, a dislocated joint may be so edematous and painful that reduction may have to be performed with the patient under general anesthesia. If dislocation is a recurring problem, patients may be taught how to reposition the joint themselves.

Surgery is sometimes necessary to achieve satisfactory reduction. If a joint has become weakened from repeated dislocation, surgery to tighten the ligaments that hold the adjoining bones may be recommended.

Prognosis

The outlook for a dislocated joint depends on the amount of damage to the tissues of the joint and the overall strength of the adjacent muscles. Surgical procedures can stabilize the joint but sometimes limit ROM.

Prevention

Persons who have suffered a dislocation to a joint may require use of stabilization splints when engaging in activities. Repeated dislocation is potentially damaging to the joint. Avoiding what caused the initial dislocation may be helpful.

Patient Teaching

Teaching the proper use of splinting devices and proper timing of the resumption of activities is essential for the optimal outcome. Advise parents of which actions should be avoided when holding a child's hand.

Adhesive Capsulitis (Frozen Shoulder)
Description

Adhesive capsulitis is a condition in which a shoulder is significantly limited in its ROM as a result of inflammation, scarring, thickening, and shrinkage of the capsule that surrounds the normal shoulder joint. Adhesive capsulitis is commonly called *frozen shoulder*.

ICD-10-CM Code	M75.00 *(Adhesive capsulitis of unspecified shoulder)* (M75.00–M75.02 = 3 codes of specificity)

Symptoms and Signs

Adhesive capsulitis presents as a shoulder that has become stiff and painful, making normal movement impossible. The pain can be either localized in the shoulder itself or spread out, encompassing the upper arm or neck. It is often severe enough to disrupt sleep. Symptoms become gradually worse during the first few months after injury and then remain at a constant degree of discomfort for a couple more months, and finally a period of gradual improvement begins. With time, the pain subsides, but the mobility of the shoulder often remains permanently impaired, or frozen.

Patient Screening

Regular follow-up appointments are important for patients undergoing treatment for adhesive capsulitis.

Etiology

Adhesive capsulitis is caused by inflammation of the capsule of the joint with secondary scarring. It usually begins after a slight injury or minor problem, such as bursitis or tendinitis, which prevents normal use of the joint. Disuse of the shoulder leads to increasing stiffness and disuse. It can also happen after a broken bone or surgery if the shoulder has to be kept still. Adhesive capsulitis may occur more frequently in patients with diabetes, Parkinson disease, thyroid dysfunction, and cardiovascular disease.

Diagnosis

The symptoms alone are usually enough to identify this condition. However, a review of the patient's history may indicate a recent injury that precipitated bursitis or tendonitis. Patients with adhesive capsulitis are evaluated for underlying arthritis, injury, and diabetes.

Radiographic tests can be helpful for detecting underlying problems in the shoulder and can demonstrate calcification that would indicate past chronic inflammation. Ultrasound and MRI images, in addition to radiographs, can also help determine if there are other underlying problems contributing to the symptoms the patient is experiencing.

Treatment

A stiff shoulder must be kept in motion as much as possible to prevent permanent immobility. A physical or occupational therapist may be needed to teach and assist the patient with ROM exercises. Analgesics, antiinflammatory agents, and often an injection of steroid medication into the joint is needed. If adhesive capsulitis is severe and persistent, the physician may suggest shoulder manipulation under general anesthesia to increase mobility. Exercise as indicated by the provider after surgery or stroke can help maintain joint mobility.

Prognosis

The outlook for a patient with adhesive capsulitis depends on the severity and duration of the condition and the presence of underlying joint disorders. Longstanding adhesive capsulitis tends to be less responsive to treatments.

Prevention

Persons who have had surgery should perform upper body exercises to minimize the risk of developing adhesive capsulitis, according to their surgeons recommendation.

Patient Teaching

Patients are instructed on the details and importance of ROM exercises to restore joint function. Avoiding reinjury to the shoulder is key to an optimal outcome.

Severed Tendon

Description

Tendons are long, fibrous cords that connect muscles to bones (e.g., the Achilles tendon connects the gastrocnemius muscle to the calcaneus bone at the back of the heel). A severed tendon is torn completely into two sections and thus prevents the muscle from performing its function of moving a body part.

ICD-10-CM Code   T14.90 *(Injury, unspecified)*

Note: This code is for use only when no documentation is available that identifies the specific injury. This code is not for use in the inpatient setting.

Symptoms and Signs

A severed tendon produces immediate, severe pain, swelling, inflammation, and immobility of the affected parts (Fig. 7.29). A "pop" may also be heard or felt by the patient. Tendons can be torn in almost any part of the body and will require repair.

Patient Screening

Injury followed by pain and immobility of the affected area requires urgent medical care.

Etiology

The cause of a severed tendon is an injury or laceration. The injury may extend partially or completely through one or more tendons.

Diagnosis

Physical examination of the injured site and the patient's inability to move the affected parts are indications that a tendon is torn. A radiographic study can be used to detect an accompanying bone fracture and ultrasound imaging may also be ordered. An MRI can confirm the severity of the tear and show other tissues that may also be damaged. A person with a severed tendon must be closely evaluated for possible infection and foreign objects or materials in the wound site.

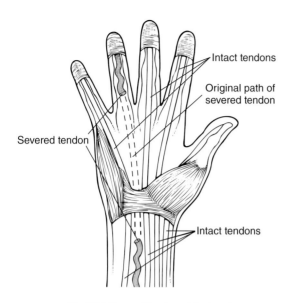

• **Fig. 7.29** Severed tendon of the hand.

Treatment

Tendons are under tension, so if they become severed, the two ends snap away from each other and are difficult to retrieve. A surgeon may suture the two ends of the tendon together (**tenorrhaphy**) immediately or may wait for the injury to heal, depending on the extent of the injury. A large incision may be necessary to locate the ends of the tendon to expose and retrieve the tendon before the tenorrhaphy can be attempted. A tendon transfer may be necessary in some cases based on the severity of the damage to the existing tendon. A tendon from another area of the body is moved to the damaged site and attached. The outcome of tendon repair is usually satisfactory. However, in some cases, the affected parts may be stiff and have less mobility after the surgery than before the injury. Physical therapy ensures as much mobility as possible. Scar tissue may also develop after tendon repair and need to be released surgically when exercise and other modalities do not solve stiffness.

Prognosis

The prognosis depends on the tendon involved and the results of surgery. Infection complicates the outcome. Permanent muscle atrophy can result from tendon damage.

Prevention

Persons with lacerated tendons should receive tetanus vaccination.

Patient Teaching

Patients are instructed on the details of rehabilitation and progressive exercise, beginning with gentle ROM exercises.

Shin Splints (Medical tibial stress syndrome)

Description

Shin splints are a painful condition involving inflammation of the periosteum, the extensor muscles in the lower leg, and the surrounding tissues.

ICD-10-CM Code	S83.90XA *(Sprain of unspecified site of unspecified knee, initial encounter)* (S83.001(A)(D)(S)–S83.92XX(A)(D)(S) = 118 codes of specificity) S86.919A *(Strain of unspecified muscle(s) and tendon(s) at lower leg level, unspecified leg, initial encounter)* (S86.101(A)(D)(S)–S86.999(A)(D)(S) = 60 codes of specificity)

Symptoms and Signs

Inflammation, edema, pain, and tenderness along the inner aspect of the tibia are common symptoms of shin splints. The pain worsens with exercise and then disappears with rest. Shin splints occur most commonly during the first weeks of a new exercise program or after a sudden increase in the amount of exercise in an ongoing program. Dancers and runners are examples of individuals who may develop shin splints.

This disorder is especially common in sports and fitness enthusiasts who jog, run, or engage in high-impact aerobics and is most often bilateral.

Patient Screening

A physical examination is required to evaluate the cause of pain and identify tenderness along the tibia.

Etiology

Overuse and overpronation are the most common factors that predispose an individual to shin splints. Repetitive stress of connective tissue attached to the tibia is involved. Pronation of the foot is an inward rotation of the ankle that causes the inner arch of the foot to sag and the ankle joint to tip upward (Fig. 7.30). All people pronate when they walk to some degree; however, excessive pronation places abnormal stress on the calf muscles. This leads to the development of shin splints and tendon and ligament strain around the ankles and knees.

Improper conditioning and running on hard surfaces also can contribute to the development of shin splints.

Diagnosis

The diagnosis is based on physical examination and a history of pain that worsens with exercise and disappears after rest. A patient with symptoms of shin splints can also have a stress fracture of the tibia bone. This can be detected with bone scanning and is considered when pain and tenderness are severe and persistent. Other imaging studies may be ordered to rule out other problems.

Treatment

The key to successful treatment of shin splints is rest. Applications of ice four or more times a day for at least 15 to 20 minutes may be helpful. Over-the-counter pain medication such as acetaminophen and NSAIDs will help alleviate pain. Prescription NSAIDs may be ordered to relieve

• **Fig. 7.30** Excessive pronation of the foot. (From Seidel HM, et al: *Mosby's guide to physical examination*, ed 7, St. Louis, 2003, Mosby.)

the pain and to reduce inflammation if the over-the-counter medications are not successful in providing relief. Gradually, physical therapy with specific stretching exercises can be helpful. Specially designed shoes to correct overpronation or the use of an orthotic device in existing shoes may be recommended.

Prognosis
The prognosis is generally very good for complete recovery, although this can sometimes be prolonged for serious athletes. Shin splints are painful but not dangerous, unless they are ignored and consequently result in stress fractures.

Prevention
Proper conditioning and gradual stretching of the legs before exercise, jogging or running on grass or other soft surfaces, performing aerobic exercises on mats, and ensuring that exercise shoes are well padded for arch support can help prevent this condition.

Patient Teaching
Patient education is focused on proper footwear and conditioning and gradual return to exercise while incorporating a stretching and strengthening program.

Plantar Fasciitis (Calcaneal Spur)

Description
Plantar fasciitis, also known as *calcaneal* or *heel spur syndrome*, is an inflammatory response at the bottom of the heel bone (calcaneus). There the flat tissue (fascia) that acts like a bowstring for the arch of the foot attaches to the bottom of the heel.

ICD-10-CM Code	M72.2 *(Plantar fascial fibromatosis)*

Symptoms and Signs
Plantar fasciitis is a common problem among people who are active in sports, especially runners. Symptoms begin with dull, intermittent pain on the bottom of the foot and

can progress to a sharp, persistent pain. The pain is worse after getting out of bed and taking the first few steps in the morning, after sitting for a time, after standing or walking, and when beginning a sporting activity. Plantar fascia injury can also occur at the midsole or near the toes.

The plantar fascia is a thick, fibrous material on the bottom of the foot. It is attached to the calcaneus, fans toward the toes, and acts like a bowstring to maintain the arch of the foot.

Patient Screening
Patients complaining of significant foot or heel pain (usually not associated with trauma) require the first available appointment to determine the cause and begin treatment as soon as possible.

Etiology
Plantar fasciitis usually occurs when part of the inflexible fascia is repeatedly placed under tension (e.g., when running). This constant tension causes an inflammatory response, usually at the point where the fascia is attached to the calcaneus. The result is pain and the development of the spur.

Factors contributing to the development of plantar fasciitis include:
• Flat (pronated) feet
• High-arched, rigid feet
• Toe running or hill running
• Running on soft terrain (e.g., sand)
• Poor shoe support
• Sudden increase in activity level
• Sudden weight increase
• Increasing age
• Familial tendency
• Possible underlying disease

The inflammatory response at the calcaneus can produce spike-like projections of new bone called *calcaneal* (heel) *spurs* (Fig. 7.31A). They do not cause the initial pain or initial problem; they are a result of the problem.

Diagnosis
Physical examination and the patient history of symptoms usually provide sufficient information for making the diagnosis. The bottom of the foot is typically very tender, typically at the heel. Radiographs sometimes show the spur (see Fig. 7.31B). Patients with plantar fasciitis are evaluated for possible reactive arthritis, inflammatory bowel disease, ankylosing spondylitis, and diffuse idiopathic skeletal hyperostosis.

Treatment
The initial treatment of heel spurs consists of resting, applying ice to the sore area, taking antiinflammatory or analgesic medication, using heel pads (doughnut-shaped pads that equalize and absorb the shock on the heel and ease pressure on the plantar fascia), and wearing a shoe with good arch support. Sometimes local cortisone injection can reduce inflamed tissues. In addition, the physician may tape the

A   Heel spur   Plantar fascia

B

• **Fig. 7.31** (A) Calcaneal (heel) spur. (B) Radiographic appearance.

• **Fig. 7.32** Typical appearance of a dorsal wrist ganglion cyst arising from the dorsal scapholunate ligament region. (From Beredjiklian P, et al: *Review of Hand Surgery*, ed 2, 2022, Elsevier.)

foot to maintain the arch and help take some of the tension off the plantar fascia. Shoe inserts called *orthotics* also may be prescribed. Shock wave therapy may also be used to cause the healing process to take place.

After the inflammation has subsided, physical therapy to strengthen the small muscles of the foot can begin. If done regularly, this helps prevent reinjury. Surgery rarely is required for the correction of heel spurs. It is considered only if all forms of more conservative treatment fail and the pain still is incapacitating after several months of treatment. When performed, surgery involves removing the bone spur and releasing the plantar fascia.

Prognosis

The prognosis is generally very good in response to conservative management. Surgical procedures are usually not required.

Prevention

The key to prevention is the use of proper footwear. Any underlying associated medical condition should be optimally managed.

Patient Teaching

Understanding the anatomy of the foot and what causes the condition can benefit affected individuals as they undertake measures to promote healing.

Ganglion

Description

A ganglion is a benign saclike swelling or cyst that is filled with a colorless, jellylike fluid. A ganglion is formed from the tissue that lines a joint or tendon.

ICD-10-CM Code   M67.40 *(Ganglion, unspecified site)*
                   (M67.40–M67.49 = 24 codes of
                   specificity)

Symptoms and Signs

A ganglion most commonly develops on the back of the wrist as a single smooth lump, just under the surface of the skin (Fig. 7.32). It can, however, develop near other joints, such as around the ankle joint, behind the knee, and on the fingers. Ganglia may appear as multiples or in clusters. Most are about the size of a pea, but others may grow as large as an inch or more in diameter. Ganglia may be soft to the touch or firm, and they are usually either painless or only somewhat bothersome. Pain may occur when moving the wrist from a wrist ganglion, especially if the growth is large or inflamed.

Patient Screening

A visual examination by the health care provider is indicated for cystic swelling on a joint. Imagining tests may be needed to rule out a tumor or other pathology.

Etiology

Although sometimes ganglia are caused by repetitive minor injuries, the underlying cause usually is unknown. A ganglion is sometimes a sign of arthritis of the adjacent joint. Whatever triggers the ganglion's development, it usually arises either in the joint capsule or in a tendon sheath.

Diagnosis

The primary concern in evaluating a patient with a ganglion is whether or not underlying arthritis is present. A ganglion can usually be diagnosed by palpation and observation of the appearance of the lump and the characteristic site. If in

• **Fig. 7.33** Torn meniscus.

doubt, the physician can perform needle aspiration to withdraw some of the fluid for laboratory analysis.

Treatment
If the ganglion does not cause pain and is not large enough to cause disfigurement or to interfere with wrist function, treatment is unnecessary. However, if the ganglion is causing pain, disfigurement, or impairment of the ROM, several options are available. The physician may try to rupture the ganglion by applying firm pressure. Needle aspiration may be used to remove as much fluid as possible, followed by instillation of a steroid, such as cortisone, or a sclerosing solution that helps prevent recurrences. Limiting movement by using a brace may also help keep the ganglion cyst from getting larger. The physician may recommend a surgical procedure called *ganglionectomy* to remove the ganglion.

Ganglia that originate in the wrist joint may be difficult to remove completely and therefore tend to recur. Even after surgical excision, a cyst may recur. Over a period of months, ganglia often disappear spontaneously.

Prognosis
Ganglia are usually harmless and do not impair function.

Prevention
The key to prevention is the identification of underlying arthritis.

Patient Teaching
Simple reassurance that the condition can be resolved, along with an explanation of the nature of the ganglion, is generally helpful to patients.

Torn Meniscus
Description
A **meniscus** is a semilunar cartilage found in the knee joint. There are two menisci within the joint, a medial and a lateral

(Fig. 7.33). A tear of the meniscus is a crack or fissure that is usually a result of wear or injury.

ICD-10-CM Code	S83.209 A *(Unspecified tear of unspecified meniscus, current injury, unspecified knee, initial encounter)*
	S83.30XA *(Tear of articular cartilage of unspecified knee, current, initial encounter)*

Symptoms and Signs
A person with a torn meniscus has acute pain when putting full weight on the affected leg and knee. The person may report that the knee "locks" or "gives way." Snapping or clicking sounds (crepitus) may be heard on flexion or extension. Full flexion of the affected knee may be difficult, and pain increases with full extension.

Patient Screening
Patients experiencing acute knee pain should be seen by a health care professional as soon as possible.

Etiology
Most torn menisci are related to some type of sports injury; however, they can happen to anyone. Participants in football, baseball, soccer, dance, skiing or other activities are at risk. Tears can also occur when someone is not exercising or playing a sport. Tears in the meniscus usually result from sudden twisting or external rotation of the leg while the knee is flexed.

Diagnosis
Patients with symptoms suggestive of a meniscal tear are evaluated for ligament injury and arthritis of the affected joint. Physical examination of the knee indicates the limitation of movement. Radiographic studies and MRI, which

is the preferred procedure, are ordered; MRI may show the exact injury to the meniscus and, if any, to the ligaments.

Treatment

The injured knee should be immobilized immediately and elevated, with ice applied to slow bleeding and edema. No weight bearing should be allowed, and the physician should be seen as soon as possible. Antiinflammatory or analgesic medications are often needed.

The treatment of a torn meniscus might only require physical therapy. Surgical repair can be done arthroscopically with the patient under anesthetic, unless injury to the cruciate ligaments has also occurred. Ligament tears require more extensive surgery to expose and repair them. Total excision or partial excision of the torn meniscus is called *meniscectomy*. Physical therapy may be indicated to help strengthen muscles in the legs and around the knee joint.

Prognosis

Meniscal tears respond very well to surgical treatments when indicated.

Prevention

The key to prevention is the early care of the underlying problem. Seeking medical treatment when pain symptoms occur is important in preventing further damage.

Patient Teaching

A customized, extensive, progressive exercise rehabilitation program begins after the immediate postoperative period and continues over the subsequent months.

Rotator Cuff Tears

Description

The four tendons of the rotator cuff, formed by the muscles of the shoulder, partially surround the head of the humerus and stabilize it in the glenoid cavity or socket (Fig. 7.34). The infraspinatus muscle rotates the humerus externally, and the subscapularis muscle rotates the humerus internally. Other muscles with tendons that form the rotator cuff are

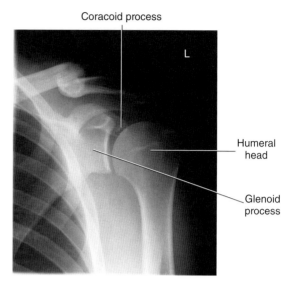

• **Fig. 7.34** Structures of the shoulder. (From Long BW, Frank ED, Ehrlich RA: *Radiography essentials for limited practice*, ed 4, St. Louis, 2013, Elsevier.)

the supraspinatus and the teres minor. Tears in any of the rotator cuff tendons limit the function of the shoulder.

ICD-10-CM Code	S43.429 A *(Sprain of unspecified rotator cuff capsule, initial encounter)* (S43.421–S43.429 = 3 codes of specificity)

Symptoms and Signs

Tears in the tendons of the rotator cuff muscles can produce an immediate snapping sound and acute pain. The person may be unable to abduct the arm. ROM becomes limited to varying degrees, depending on the severity of the particular tear.

Patient Screening

Patients with acute shoulder pain and limited mobility require medical attention as soon as possible.

◆ **ENRICHMENT**

Arthroscopy

Arthroscopy is a surgical procedure used to examine the structures within a joint by using a tubelike viewing instrument called an *arthroscope*. The arthroscope is a small tube that contains optical fibers and lenses and is passed through tiny incisions in the skin into the joint to be examined. The arthroscope is connected to a video camera that allows the interior of the joint to be seen on a display monitor. The size of the arthroscope varies with the size of the joint being examined.

Arthroscopy can be used for diagnosis and/or treatment. When procedures are performed in addition to examining the joint with the arthroscope, this is referred to as *arthroscopic surgery*. A number of procedures are done in this fashion. When a procedure can be done arthroscopically instead of using traditional open surgical methods, it usually causes less tissue trauma and therefore results in less pain. This tends to promote a quicker recovery.

Arthroscopy is performed by orthopedic surgeons, typically in an outpatient setting. After the procedure, patients usually can return home and begin a reabilitation program.

Etiology

Tears can result from acute trauma injuries or from degenerative changes with age. Because of the degenerative changes, calcium deposits may develop in the insertion sites, predisposing the tendons to tears or rupture. Steroid injections into the tendon areas can also predispose them to tears or rupture.

Diagnosis

The diagnosis is based on physical examination findings and patient history. The shoulder may have limited and painful ROM. An arthrogram or an MRI scan confirms the diagnosis. Patients are screened for bursitis and arthritis of the shoulder.

Treatment

Acute pain is managed with pain-relieving medications. Acetaminophen is given for moderate pain, and antiinflammatory medications are given for inflammation. With rest and conservative therapy, minor tears can heal with restoration of function.

Significant acute tendon tears are surgically repaired immediately to preserve the strength of the muscles and restore motion of the shoulder. After surgery, the affected arm is placed in a shoulder immobilizer or abduction splint and physical therapy is ordered during healing.

Prognosis

Minor tears can heal in response to conservative measures. Major tears require surgical repair and intense physical therapy after surgery.

Prevention

Conditioning and stretching exercises are the best prevention for rotator cuff tears.

Patient Teaching

Rubber band shoulder exercises and stretching are keys to long-term rehabilitation of the rotator cuff. A customized, extensive, progressive exercise program begins after the immediate postoperative period and continues over the subsequent few months. A sling is also necessary for a few weeks after surgery to prevent injury by overuse until healing takes place.

Review Challenge

Answer the following questions:

1. What are the functions of the normal skeletal system?
2. What procedures are employed in diagnosing scoliosis?
3. What pathology is characteristic of osteoarthritis?
4. The symptoms of Lyme disease mimic which disease?
5. Are any preventive measures recommended for Lyme disease?
6. What is the clinical picture of a patient with osteomyelitis?
7. What metabolite forms crystals in the joints in gout?
8. Which disease is characterized by irregular breakdown and formation of bone tissue?
9. What would the treatment plan for a patient with osteoporosis include?
10. How is vitamin D deficiency related to osteomalacia?
11. What specific findings from a physical examination are typical of fibromyalgia?
12. What causative factors contribute to hallux valgus (bunion)? Hallux rigidus? Hammer toe?
13. How are fractures classified?
14. How would you describe a Colles fracture?
15. What is meant by the term *phantom limb?*
16. What methods are used to immobilize fractures?
17. Why is a sprain considered more serious than a strain?
18. What joints are more susceptible to dislocation?
19. What conditions result in adhesive capsulitis ("frozen shoulder")?
20. What is the relationship of overpronation to shin splints?
21. Under what conditions might plantar fasciitis (spur syndrome) develop?
22. What acute symptoms is a person with torn meniscus likely to describe? A person with rotator cuff tear?

Real-Life Challenge: Osteoporosis

A 72-year-old female recently experienced bandlike, midthoracic back pain after a minor fall. Imaging studies confirmed fractures of T-7 and T-8 vertebrae. Measurements in this small-boned female revealed a loss of 1 inch in height, with the current measurement being 5 feet 1 inch compared with 5 feet 2 inches at the last physical examination 14 months ago. Serum calcium is elevated. The computed tomography (CT) scan indicates osteoporosis.

According to history, the patient does not include many dairy products in her diet and takes no dietary supplements. In addition, she has never taken any form of estrogen replacement and does not exercise regularly.

Questions

1. In what type of individual would you expect to find the greatest incidence of osteoporosis?
2. What bones other than vertebrae are prone to fractures in osteoporosis?
3. Why would serum calcium be elevated in osteoporosis?
4. What is meant by the description of osteoporosis as a metabolic bone disease?
5. What should be included in a diet to prevent or slow the onset of osteoporosis?
6. Why is daily exercise important in preventing osteoporosis?
7. What type of drug therapy may be prescribed for the patient?

Real-Life Challenge: Lyme Disease

A 27-year-old male has been experiencing flulike symptoms for four days. He reports headache, fatigue, joint pain, and "just not feeling well." Vital signs are temperature of 102.28°F, pulse of 96, respirations of 20, and blood pressure of 132/86 mm Hg. Physical examination reveals two areas on the left lower leg that have a fading red rash in a circle type of pattern. The center of each circle is pale, and there is a possible spot at the center of each.

Questioning discloses that the patient was deer hunting five days ago, walking through tall grass. He remembers experiencing itching on the lower left leg. Lyme disease is suspected. A blood test to detect antibodies to the spirochete *Borrelia burgdorferi* is ordered. Antibiotics and acetaminophen for the fever, pain, and aches are prescribed. The patient is encouraged to rest and return for a recheck in a few days.

Questions

1. In what region of the United States would you expect this patient to live?
2. What precautions should be taken by people who will be out walking in tall grass?
3. What should individuals who think they have been bitten by a tick do as soon as they discover the bite?
4. If Lyme disease is not diagnosed in its early stages, what complications may develop?
5. What is the causative agent of Lyme disease?
6. Discuss the prevention of Lyme disease.

Real-Life Challenge: Fibromyalgia

A 23-year-old female has been diagnosed with fibromyalgia. She complained of chronic pain in the muscles and soft tissue surrounding joints. Additionally she mentioned feeling fatigued most of the time and a diffuse aching or burning in the muscles along with stiffness. She also experienced headaches, some jaw pain, and sensitivity to odors, bright lights, and loud noises. Disturbances in sleep patterns were experienced on a regular basis.

1. Along with the chronic muscle pain and restless sleep, what other symptoms may the patient experience?
2. Although the cause of fibromyalgia is unknown, what might be a possible cause?
3. How is rapid eye movement (REM) sleep affected?
4. What is a key factor in the diagnosis of fibromyalgia?
5. State some beneficial options other than drug therapy that may help this patient.
6. What may help provide a more positive outcome for the patient?

Internet Assignments

1. Visit the American Lyme Disease Foundation website to research the latest statistics on Lyme disease; also gather information on other tickborne diseases.
2. Research the "News and Events" page on the National Osteoporosis Foundation website, and report on the recent findings.

Critical Thinking

1. How would you approach discussing bursitis, possible causes, and the treatment plan as prescribed by the physician with a patient just diagnosed with the condition?
2. Gout is a disease known to be extremely painful. In an acute attack, the treatment can be extensive. What does the treatment typically involve? Explain the importance of empathy and patience during the patient teaching phase.
3. Why should a patient with a chronic arthritic condition be strongly encouraged to comply with the treatment plan and keep all follow-up appointments?

4. Discuss the kinds of muscle tumors and the variety of diagnostic procedures used to determine the type and extent of the treatment required.
5. What are the differences between an ankle strain and an ankle sprain? Describe some prevention measures.

6. What is a necessary assessment of patients with open injuries?
   Prepare to discuss Critical Thinking case study exercises for this chapter that are posted on Evolve.

Credentialing Examination Questions

1. Which condition affects the joint of the toe nearest the nail?
   A. Hammer toe
   B. Mallet toe
   C. Hallux bunion
   D. Hallux valgus
2. Which area of the body is affected when a person is diagnosed with adhesive capsulitis?
   A. Ankle
   B. Knee
   C. Shoulder
   D. Elbow
3. What statement best describes the way fibromyalgia is diagnosed, in addition to blood testing?
   A. Pain in 4 of 5 areas of the body over a 1-month period of time
   B. Pain in 2 of 5 areas over a 3-month period of time
   C. Pain in 4 of 5 areas over a 3-month period of time
   D. Pain in tender points 11 of 18
4. Which abnormal curvature of the spine involves a sideways curve?
   A. Lordosis
   B. Kyphosis
   C. Scoliosis
   D. Ankylosis
5. Which condition is an excessive posterior curve of the thoracic spine?
   A. Lordosis
   B. Kyphosis
   C. Scoliosis
   D. Ankylosis
6. Which abnormal curvature of the spine involves a sideways curve?
   A. Scoliosis
   B. Lordosis
   C. Kyphosis
   D. Ankylosis

7. Which fracture is evident by the end of the bone sticking through the skin?
   A. Greenstick
   B. Compound
   C. Transverse
   D. Pathologic
8. Which fracture results in the bone being splintered or crushed?
   A. Greenstick
   B. Transverse
   C. Displaced
   D. Comminuted
9. Which condition is a metabolic bone disease resulting from deficiency or ineffective use of vitamin D?
   A. Rickets
   B. Hallux valgus
   C. Ewing sarcoma
   D. Hallux rigidus
10. Which condition results from a loss of normal bone density and is common in postmenopausal females?
    A. Osteomalacia
    B. Bunion
    C. Hallux rigidus
    D. Osteoporosis
11. A patient develops compartment syndrome. Which option best describes the cause of this condition?
    A. Results from bone demineralization
    B. Osteomyelitis
    C. Occurs after a fracture due to Loss of circulation from swelling
    D. Amputation

8

Diseases and Conditions of the Digestive System

CHAPTER OUTLINE

LEARNING OBJECTIVES

After studying this chapter, you should be able to:

1. Explain the process of normal digestion and absorption.
2. Discuss the importance of normal teeth and a normal bite.
3. Describe the presenting symptoms of temporomandibular joint disorder.
4. Compare the etiology of herpes simplex with the etiology of thrush.
5. Describe the treatment of oral leukoplakia.
6. Describe the treatment of gastroesophageal reflux disease.
7. Explain the clinical significance of Barrett esophagus.
8. Name a serious complication of esophageal varices.
9. Describe the pathology of peptic ulcers and identify the etiology.
10. Explain the diagnosis of gastric cancer.
11. List the symptoms a patient with appendicitis may experience.
12. Describe hiatal hernia.
13. Distinguish the types of abdominal hernias.
14. Explain the differences between the pathology of Crohn's disease and that of ulcerative colitis.
15. Describe the etiology of gastroenteritis.
16. Discuss the pathologic conditions that may result in intestinal obstruction.
17. Explain the difference between a mechanical obstruction and a functional obstruction of the bowel.
18. Distinguish between diverticulosis and diverticulitis.
19. Discuss the screening program for and the treatment of colorectal cancer.
20. Explain the relationship between broad-spectrum antibiotics and pseudomembranous enterocolitis.
21. Explain the preventive measures for *Clostridioides difficile* infection.
22. List the causes of inflammation of the peritoneum.
23. Explain the pathologic symptoms and signs of cirrhosis of the liver.
24. Contrast the causes and preventive measures of hepatitis A and hepatitis C. Explain how health care providers are at special risk for hepatitis B.
25. Name the most important etiologic factor for hepatocellular carcinoma and other additional risk factors.
26. Name the most common bloodborne infection in the United States.
27. Describe the clinical picture of an individual with (1) biliary colic and (2) acute pancreatitis.
28. State the prognosis of pancreatic cancer.
29. State the components of a successful weight loss program.
30. Describe the clinical manifestations of malnutrition and malabsorption.
31. Explain the diagnostic criteria for celiac disease.
32. List some ways to lower the risk of food poisoning.
33. Distinguish between the clinical picture of the patient with anorexia and bulimia.

KEY TERMS

adenocarcinoma (ad-ih-no-kar-sin-OH-ma)

anastomosis (ah-nas-toh-MOH-sis)

antiemetic (an-tih-ee-MET-ik)

aphthous (AF-thus)

ascites (ah-SIGH-teez)

cholinergic (ko-lin-ER-jik)

endoscopy (en-DOS-ko-pee)

fistula (FIS-tew-lah)

fulminant (FUL-mih-nant)

gastroscopy (gas-TROS-koh-pee)

gingivitis (jin-jih-VIE-tis)

hematemesis (hem-ah-TEM-eh-sis)

hepatomegaly (hep-ah-toh-MEG-ah-lee)

hypokalemia (high-poh-ka-LEE-me-ah)

inguinal (ING-gwih-nal)

intussusception (in-tah-sus-SEP-shun)

periodontitis (per-ee-oh-don-TIE-tis)

peritonitis (per-ih-toh-NIE-tis)

proctoscopy (prock-TAHS-ko-pee)

pseudomembranous (soo-doe-MEM-brah-nus)

sigmoidoscopy (sig-moy-DOS-ko-pee)

temporomandibular (tem-poh-roh-man-DIHB-you-lar)

varices (VAR-ih-seez)

Orderly Function of the Digestive System

The digestive system comprises the alimentary canal, or digestive tract, and the accessory organs of digestion (Fig. 8.1). Each unit, or organ, of the system must be normal in structure and function to regulate the ingestion, digestion, and absorption of nutrients. The alimentary canal processes and transports the products of digestion. The accessory organs, located outside the gastrointestinal (GI) tract, manufacture and secrete endocrine and exocrine enzymes—secretions that are essential to the breakdown, digestion, and absorption of nutrients.

Diseases of the GI tract negatively affect health and threaten life because they interfere with the critical functions of ingestion and digestion of food, absorption of nutrients for metabolism, and elimination of wastes. General

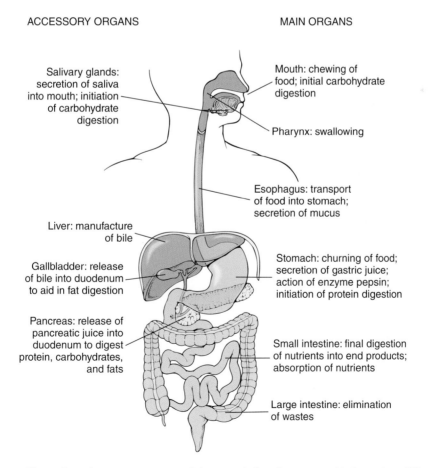

ACCESSORY ORGANS

MAIN ORGANS

Salivary glands: secretion of saliva into mouth; initiation of carbohydrate digestion

Mouth: chewing of food; initial carbohydrate digestion

Pharynx: swallowing

Esophagus: transport of food into stomach; secretion of mucus

Liver: manufacture of bile

Gallbladder: release of bile into duodenum to aid in fat digestion

Stomach: churning of food; secretion of gastric juice; action of enzyme pepsin; initiation of protein digestion

Pancreas: release of pancreatic juice into duodenum to digest protein, carbohydrates, and fats

Small intestine: final digestion of nutrients into end products; absorption of nutrients

Large intestine: elimination of wastes

• **Fig. 8.1** The main and accessory organs of the normal digestive system. (Redrawn from Miller M: *Pathophysiology: principles of disease*, Philadelphia, 1983, Saunders.)

categories of diseases and conditions of the digestive system include erosion of tissue, inflammation, infection, benign and malignant tumors, obstruction, interference with blood or nerve supply, malnutrition, and malabsorption syndromes.

Disorderly Function of the Digestive System

Diseases and Conditions of the Oral Cavity and Jaws

The function of the teeth is mastication (chewing) to break down food into pieces that can be swallowed and digested easily (Fig. 8.2). Hindrance of the chewing function caused by decay, infection of the teeth or gums, malocclusion, or missing teeth can interfere with this phase of the digestive process. A decrease in saliva production, called *xerostomia*, can adversely affect the digestive process. Xerostomia may be caused by dehydration, medications, either prescription or over-the-counter (OTC) ones, or less often by an autoimmune condition called *Sjögren disease*. Research has identified the interrelationship between oral health and general health. For instance, there can be a connection between oral infections and cardiovascular diseases, respiratory diseases, or diabetes. Periodontal disease (gum disease) and the increase in systemic cross-reactive protein have been recognized as risk factors for cardiovascular disease (arteriosclerosis), diabetes, and pancreatic cancer. An example of the serious nature of gum disease is seen in premature and low birthweight babies born to females who have periodontal disease.

Most treatments for oral disease are simple and effective. The dentist performs screening examinations for any lump or change in the mouth or on the tongue as part of a routine oral examination. Patients should report any oral lesions with different-colored pigmentation (white, red, or blue) or lumps in any part of the mouth that persist.

Missing Teeth

Description
Permanent teeth are missing.

ICD-10-CM Code	K08.109 *(Complete loss of teeth, unspecified cause, unspecified class)*
	(K08.101–K08.199 = 25 codes of specificity)

Loss of teeth is coded by causative factors. Refer to the physician's diagnosis and then to the current edition of the ICD-10-CM coding manual to ensure the greatest specificity.

Symptoms and Signs
The loss of permanent teeth after the loss of primary teeth can cause serious dental problems later in life (Fig. 8.3). Missing teeth, for any reason, can alter the bite or how the teeth come together (occlusion). Malocclusion eventually leads to jaw pain, called ***temporomandibular*** *joint disorder*

US Tooth Numbering

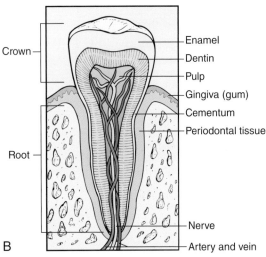

• **Fig. 8.2** (A) Thirty-two permanent teeth. (B) Structure of a tooth.

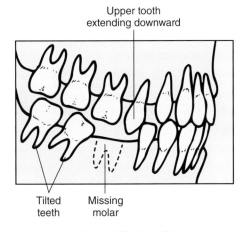

• **Fig. 8.3** Missing molar.

(see the Temporomandibular Joint Disorder section), if not corrected. Missing teeth can cause bolting (inadequate chewing) of food. Digestive disturbances (i.e., gastritis or constipation) and loss of the nutrient value of food may result. Patients may express cosmetic concerns with tooth loss and experience low self-esteem.

Patient Screening
Schedule an appointment for the patient for an evaluation by the dentist.

Etiology
The most common cause of tooth loss results from dental decay in all age groups but is most commonly caused by periodontal disease in adults. Tooth loss increases with age or may be a result of dental injury. Teeth may also be congenitally missing, or they may be impacted and prevented from erupting by the root of an adjacent tooth.

Diagnosis
Diagnosing missing teeth may be as simple as performing an oral examination and obtaining radiographs to determine whether the tooth is absent or impacted.

Treatment
Treatment is aimed at restoring the occlusion. This is accomplished by placement of a permanent or removable prosthesis (false tooth) with orthodontics or by placing a dental implant.

Prognosis
The prognosis is good when a prosthesis or a dental implant provides replacement. The patient with low self-esteem prior to the tooth replacement will also feel more confident with their cosmetic appearance.

Prevention
Regular dental hygiene is the only method to prevent tooth decay and tooth loss.

Patient Teaching
Emphasize the importance of complying with the individualized treatment plan. When the patient has a dental appliance in place, teach the proper cleaning technique to prevent tooth decay.

Impacted Third Molars
Description
An impacted third molar is malpositioned, thereby preventing normal eruption.

ICD-10-CM Code	K00.6 *(Disturbances in tooth eruption)*
	K01.0 *(Embedded teeth)*
	K01.1 *(Impacted teeth)*

Symptoms and Signs
Third molars, also known as *wisdom teeth*, are the last teeth in the back of the mouth and can become impacted (pressed together) and cause pain. They begin developing between ages 8 and 10 years and emerge or erupt (through the gums) between ages 17 and 21 years. In some people, one or more of these teeth never erupt. There are usually no symptoms until these teeth begin to emerge and if they do develop normally they are hard to clean.

Patient Screening
Schedule an initial consultation with the dentist for diagnostic evaluation.

Etiology
Third molars become impacted when they do not have enough room to erupt because of bone structure or because adjacent teeth block eruption (Fig. 8.4). Sometimes they erupt at an angle, creating a space in which food can become trapped. This can lead to pericoronitis around the tooth, which, in turn, causes pain when biting and a foul taste in the mouth.

Diagnosis
Radiographic studies are needed to determine the position of the tooth if it has not erupted completely. An examination also is performed to look for any infection.

Treatment
The dentist is likely to prescribe an antibiotic (penicillin or amoxicillin) to clear up any infection that is present and an analgesic to relieve pain temporarily. After the infection clears up and pain has lessened, the impacted tooth must be extracted to prevent recurrence of infection. The patient is typically referred to an oral surgeon for this procedure due to the need for IV sedation and possibility of complications, in addition to patient comfort during the extraction.

Prognosis
Treatment of the infection and extraction of the impacted tooth solve the problem.

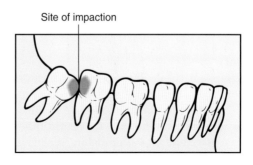

Site of impaction

• **Fig. 8.4** Impacted wisdom tooth.

Prevention

No prevention is known.

Patient Teaching

Emphasize the importance of following the dentist and oral surgeon's instructions.

Dental Caries

Description

Dental caries is considered an infection resulting in erosion of the tooth surface.

ICD-10-CM Code	K02.9 *(Dental caries, unspecified)*
	(K02.51–K02.9 = 8 codes of
	specificity)

Symptoms and Signs

Dental decay, also known as *dental caries*, first manifests as white spots on the tooth surface. The major symptom in the early stage of dental caries is a mild toothache, with hypersensitivity to sweets and temperature extremes in foods or beverages. An unpleasant taste in the mouth results from the accumulation of food and bacteria in the cavity area. Some patients say they feel a stabbing pain in the jaw. As the tooth continues to decay, an abscess may form (see the Tooth Abscesses section).

Patient Screening

Schedule an appointment for the patient for an immediate dental examination.

Etiology

Dental caries occurs when bacteria in the mouth break down the sugars present in foods, converting them into acid plaque. The acid plaque erodes the calcium in the tooth's enamel (demineralization), causing the formation of a cavity (Fig. 8.5). In addition to this plaque in the mouth, other disorders, such as stomach acid from gastroesophageal reflux disease (GERD) or episodes of purging in bulimia, may contribute to tooth decay.

Diagnosis

The dentist examines the patient's teeth for signs of cavity formation and may obtain radiographs to determine the extent of the decay.

Treatment

In early treatment, the dentist removes the diseased portion of the tooth enamel and pulp and fills the cavity to prevent further decay and to restore the tooth's size and shape. If the decay has advanced into the pulp, the dentist may perform a root canal procedure. In this procedure, the infected pulp tissue is removed, and then the canals in the roots of the tooth are filled, treated with antibiotics, and sealed. Tooth extraction may be necessary if the tooth is not salvageable or

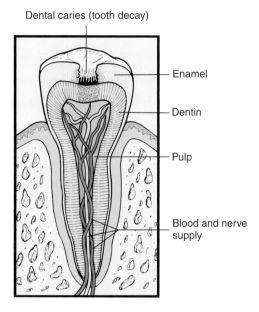

Dental caries (tooth decay)

Enamel

Dentin

Pulp

Blood and nerve supply

• **Fig. 8.5** Dental caries (tooth decay).

• **Fig. 8.6** Dental implant. (From Christensen GJ: *A consumer's guide to dentistry*, ed 2, St. Louis, 2002, Mosby.)

if root canal therapy fails. In this case, a dental implant (an artificial tooth root) may be inserted to support restorations that resemble a tooth or group of teeth (Fig. 8.6).

Prognosis

The prognosis is good with prompt treatment. The bacteria that cause decay can be transmitted via saliva, enter the bloodstream, and damage to other major organs may occur. When the cavity is allowed to erode and damage the inner pulp of the tooth, infection and tooth abscess can result.

Prevention

Caries may be prevented with good oral hygiene, including brushing, flossing, and using an effective antibacterial mouthwash after eating, and biannual professional cleaning of the teeth. Braces should also be brushed after each meal or snack including the gum line to prevent caries at the bottom of the tooth near the gum. Limiting ingestion of sweets, simple carbohydrates, and between-meal snacks is suggested. Some dentists prescribe the use of oral fluorides. Dental sealants may be placed by dentist as a barrier.

Patient Teaching

Discuss good brushing, flossing, and rinsing with antibacterial mouthwash techniques. Explain what causes dental caries. Professional cleaning of teeth and biannual dental examinations should be strongly recommended. Children should be taught at a young age to brush their teeth as a part of their daily routine to promote good oral health for life.

Discolored Teeth

Description

In this condition, teeth are discolored.

ICD-10-CM Code	K03.7 *(Posteruptive color changes of dental hard tissues)*

Symptoms and Signs

Symptoms of discolored teeth are obvious, and colors may range from a slight yellow to brown and gray. Some teeth may have brown spots, patches, and dark lines in or on them.

Patient Screening

Schedule an appointment for the patient for a dental consultation.

Etiology

Aging causes slight yellowing of teeth; smoking turns teeth surfaces brown; and a dead tooth often turns gray. Red wine, coffee, tea, and foods such as blueberries can stain teeth. Certain drugs (e.g., tetracyclines) taken in large quantities during childhood can cause the formation of defective, discolored enamel (Fig. 8.7). Use of certain illegal drugs may also cause tooth discoloration and tooth loss.

Diagnosis

The dentist performs an oral examination. A pertinent history includes recent illnesses, medications, and trauma to teeth. Hereditary factors are also considered.

Treatment

The extent of treatment varies, depending on the discoloration being superficial or deep within the enamel. Superficial discoloration can be removed or reduced by polishing. Deeper discolorations can be treated by dentist-provided bleaching procedures or by capping, crowning, or bonding a synthetic veneer to the tooth. There are also OTC products to whiten teeth, however the patient may want to see which ones are recommended as safe by the dentist.

Prognosis

Resolution of discoloration is possible with a range of treatments. Those who abuse drugs such as methamphetamine do not have a positive prognosis and experience tooth loss as a result.

Prevention

Dental hygienists suggest avoiding smoking and drinking coffee, tea, or red wine to prevent staining of teeth.

Patient Teaching

In addition to the preventive measures mentioned previously, the dentist may suggest treatment for deeper discoloration to whiten teeth. Consultation with a dentist is advised before beginning the use of an at-home whitening system.

Gingivitis

Description

Gingivitis is inflammation and swelling of the gums (Fig. 8.8).

ICD-10-CM Code	K05.00 *(Acute gingivitis, plaque induced)*
	(K05.00–K05.01 = 2 codes of specificity)
	K05.10 *(Chronic gingivitis, plaque induced)*
	(K05.10–K05.11 = 2 codes of specificity)

Symptoms and Signs

Gums that are normally pale pink and firm become red, soft, and shiny. They bleed easily, even with gentle tooth

• **Fig. 8.7** Discolored teeth. (From Christensen GJ: *A consumer's guide to dentistry*, ed 2, St. Louis, 2002, Mosby.)

• **Fig. 8.8** Gingivitis. (From Murray PR, et al: *Medical microbiology*, ed 6, Philadelphia, 2009, Mosby.)

brushing. The disease can be painless and therefore be discovered after it has progressed. If gingivitis is not treated, it leads to the destruction of the gums and bone disease called **periodontitis** (see the Periodontitis section). Advanced cases of gingivitis can cause loss of healthy teeth.

Patient Screening

Schedule an appointment for the patient for a dental examination and consultation.

Etiology

Approximately half of US adults have some areas of gingivitis, and it is the second most common cause of toothache. The most common cause of gingivitis is plaque. Plaque is a sticky deposit of mucus, food particles, and bacteria that builds up around the base of teeth as a result of inadequate or incorrect technique when brushing or flossing. As the gums become inflamed and swollen, the plaque causes a pocket to form between gums and teeth, and that space becomes a food trap. Other causes of gingivitis include vitamin deficiencies, glandular disorders, blood diseases, viral infections, and the use of certain medications. Pregnant females and patients with diabetes are particularly susceptible to gingivitis as a result of vascular and hormonal changes.

Diagnosis

If symptoms develop, a dentist should be seen as soon as possible to confirm gingivitis and to begin treatment to prevent complications.

Treatment

Treatment includes the removal of plaque and calculus by a professional dental hygienist. In advanced cases of gingivitis, the dentist may prescribe an antibacterial mouthwash, such as chlorhexidine (Peridex), to clear up the infection.

In some cases, a local anesthesia may be used to thoroughly clean teeth and exposed tooth roots, in a procedure called *root planing* and *subgingival curettage*. Oral antibiotics may follow to treat gum infection or abscess. Follow-up treatment is required for loosened teeth or when there is bone destruction.

Prognosis

It has been estimated that 80% of adults will suffer from some type of gum (periodontal) disease during their lifetime. Identifying and treating underlying causes offers the best outcome

Prevention

Prophylaxis includes good oral hygiene and removal of plaque at the gum line. Toothbrush trauma caused by brushing teeth incorrectly and excessively should be avoided. Excessive use of abrasives (teeth whitening products) is contraindicated.

Patient Teaching

See the preventive measures listed earlier. Encourage the patient to have regular dental examinations and keep follow-up appointments. Discuss symptoms to report to the dentist if the patient is on antibacterial therapy. Share research findings that support the strong correlation between cardiac disease, plaque, and poor dental status in patients.

Periodontitis

Description

Periodontitis, also called *periodontal disease*, is a destructive gum and bone disease around one or more teeth (Fig. 8.9).

ICD-10-CM Code	K05.20 *(Aggressive periodontitis, unspecified)* (K05.20–K05.22 = 3 codes of specificity) K05.30 *(Chronic periodontitis, unspecified)* (K05.30–K05.32 = 3 codes of specificity)

Symptoms and Signs

Periodontitis is the end result of gingivitis (see the Gingivitis section) that was treated too late or not at all. The pockets that form between teeth and gums in gingivitis gradually deepen, exposing the root. Plaque develops in this area, causing an unpleasant taste in the mouth and offensive breath (halitosis). As more root is exposed, one or more teeth become extremely sensitive to temperature extremes in foods, and pain may be experienced when chewing. Abscesses can form (see the Tooth Abscesses section), and eventually, a tooth or several teeth become loose and possibly fall out.

• **Fig. 8.9** Advanced periodontitis. (From Murray PR, et al: *Medical microbiology*, ed 6, Philadelphia, 2009, Mosby.)

Patient Screening

Schedule a complete dental examination and consultation immediately. If uninsured, some patients may need assistance in finding resources for those without dental insurance, which may prevent them from following up with a dentist as instructed by the health care provider.

Etiology

The cause of periodontitis is plaque biofilm and unchecked gingivitis. This commonly results from poor oral hygiene and a lack of professional dental periodontal care. Over time, the bacteria in plaque destroy the bone surrounding and supporting teeth. Contributing factors include smoking, certain medications, chemotherapy, diabetes, and human immunodeficiency virus (HIV) infection. Stress, poor nutrition, hormonal medications, and pregnancy may also contribute to periodontitis.

Diagnosis

To determine the stage of the periodontal disease, the dentist measures the depth of the pockets and obtains radiographs. Radiographs reveal the condition of the underlying bone, and this knowledge aids the dentist in deciding how to treat the disease.

Treatment

Conservative treatment includes a thorough cleaning of the root surfaces of teeth, a procedure called *scaling and root planing* and *curettage*. Multiple daily sessions of brushing and flossing of teeth are required. An oral or local application of a sub-antimicrobial dose of an antibiotic may be prescribed. Periodontal surgery may be required if the pockets have become deep and nonresponsive to more conservative therapy. The procedure, called *respective periodontal surgery*, requires the dentist to trim the gums to reduce the depth of the pockets and to remove any damaged bone. In certain situations, the dentist may graft bone and/or gum tissue to resolve the periodontal condition.

Prognosis

The prognosis varies with the extent of the disease process, the presence of complications, and the effectiveness of treatment.

Prevention

Adherence to a schedule for professional cleaning and examination of teeth by a dentist is of primary importance.

Patient Teaching

Reinforce the education provided by the dentist regarding an ongoing dental care plan. Emphasize the long-term advantages of early detection and treatment to save teeth, because a history of periodontal disease predisposes the patient to rapid progression of the disease. Education for patients with diabetes should include adherence to periodontal therapy, and good oral hygiene may enhance diabetic control.

Oral Tumors

Description

Oral tumors, or neoplasms, are classified as benign or malignant and localized or invasive.

> ICD-10-CM Code   D10.0 *(Benign neoplasm of lip)*
> *Benign oral tumors have code modifiers according to location. Refer to the physician's diagnosis and then to the current edition of the ICD-10-CM coding manual to ensure the greatest specificity. See oral cancer for coding of malignant oral tumors.*

Symptoms and Signs

Tumors can develop anywhere in or on the surface of the mouth, gums, cheeks, or palate but not on teeth. They begin as single, small, pale lumps, in or on the mouth, which may or may not bleed easily and may or may not cause pain. There are two types of tumors: benign (or noncancerous) and malignant (or cancerous). Benign tumors grow slowly over several years, do not metastasize (spread to other areas), and are not usually life threatening. Malignant tumors are generally not painful until they reach advanced stages (see the Oral Cancer section).

Patient Screening

The lesion(s) or lumps should be evaluated by a dentist without delay. Patients may describe a lesion as being red, blue, or white. A biopsy of the lesion may be required.

Etiology

The cause of benign and malignant oral tumors is unknown, although certain factors, such as tobacco use, seem to cause the tumor to develop into a malignancy.

Diagnosis

An oral surgeon or a physician should be consulted if the patient has a lump, ulcer, or color change in or on the surface of the mouth that does not clear up within a few days. If a tumor is discovered, biopsy is needed to determine whether it is benign or malignant.

Treatment

If the tumor has been determined to be benign, it should be observed periodically by a medical professional to ensure that it has not become malignant. Benign tumors will be assessed and may be excised if they are subject to chronic irritation or interfere with the fit of a denture, implant, crown, and so on. See the Oral Cancer section for a discussion about malignant oral tumors.

Prognosis

Benign tumors are usually curable with excision.

Prevention

Avoid chronic irritation to the lips and the mouth. This includes excessive brushing, tongue probing, and so on.

Any mouth lesion that does not heal must be evaluated and treated to avoid potential invasive disease.

Patient Teaching
Educate the patient regarding the causes of lesions that result from chronic irritation. Review the course of action prescribed to promote healing.

Malocclusion
Description
Malocclusion describes specific angles of malposition and contact of the maxillary and mandibular teeth.

ICD-10-CM Code	M26.4 *(Malocclusion, unspecified)*

Symptoms and Signs
The relationship of the upper and lower teeth when the mouth is closed is called *occlusion*, or bite; a faulty bite is called *malocclusion* (Fig. 8.10). Signs of malocclusion include protrusion or recession of the jaws and teeth that are turned or twisted out of position because of crowding. The patient may or may not experience some degree of difficulty with mastication or chewing.

Patient Screening
Schedule an appointment for dental examination and consultation. Inform the patient that radiographic studies may be indicated.

Normal teeth

Protruding upper teeth

Receding upper teeth

• **Fig. 8.10** Malocclusion.

Etiology
Malocclusion generally results from genetic factors. It is a rarity to have perfectly aligned teeth. Heredity is not the only cause of malocclusion; crowding can result from the early loss of primary teeth or from oral habits, such as thumb/finger sucking. Thumb/finger sucking often causes orthopedic (skeletal) changes and dental crowding. Airway problems (deviated septae, enlarged tonsils, or allergies) can affect the normal growth and development of the facial skeleton and dentition. Other teeth may shift to fill the space left by this loss of teeth, causing the loss of space where the permanent tooth normally would erupt.

Diagnosis
A visual examination and radiographic studies clearly identify the malocclusion.

Treatment
Several treatments are used to correct this problem. These include the application of braces for a minor problem, extraction of one or more teeth, or surgical removal of portions of the jaw in situations of protrusion and recession of the jaw. Additional treatment includes combining crowns or bridges to replace the missing teeth.

Prognosis
The prognosis is favorable with treatment.

Prevention
If caused by genetics, there is no prevention. Parents are reminded to discourage thumb/finger sucking, and they are encouraged to seek professional dental advice to curtail the behavior in the child. Airway problems need to be addressed when major skeletal development begins at age 6 to 8 years. Professional dental evaluation can help decrease costly orthodontic/orthopedic treatment in the future.

Patient Teaching
Special care is needed to avoid the development of caries while wearing corrective dental appliances. The patient should practice thorough, regular cleaning of teeth and avoid eating candy and gum. Often use of alternative flossing instruments, such as a water device, may be advised to reach tooth areas that are not accessible with a standard brush.

Temporomandibular Joint Disorder
Description
Temporomandibular joint disorder (TMD) is a symptom complex related to inflammation, disease, or dysfunction of the temporomandibular joint.

ICD-10-CM Code	M26.60 *(Temporomandibular joint disorder, unspecified)*
	M26.69 *(Other specified disorders of temporomandibular joint)*
	(M26.60–M26.69 = 5 codes of specificity)

Symptoms and Signs

The synovial joints between the condyles of the mandible and the temporal bones of the skull are known as *temporomandibular joints*. When these joints are inflamed or diseased, jaw movement is markedly limited. The patient reports hearing clicking sounds during chewing, or they experience severe pain or aching in or around the ears and jaw joints, and the pain is worse with chewing. This pain and limitation of movement can be unilateral but is usually bilateral, with one side markedly more painful than the other. Headache, dizziness, a feeling of pressure, tinnitus, or a draining sensation may be present in one or both ears; deafness may be experienced. Patients often complain of sinus pain, which is, in reality, muscle pain from the superior or deep masseters.

Patient Screening

Significant pain usually prompts a request for medical treatment. Complete medical and dental assessments may be necessary.

Etiology

Temporomandibular disorders result from unbalanced activity of the jaw muscles caused by a number of conditions, including bruxism (grinding of teeth, an action emanating from the central pattern generator in the brain); malocclusion; poorly fitting dentures; rheumatoid, degenerative, or traumatic arthritis; and neoplastic diseases. Emotional stress, with accompanying clenching and grinding of teeth, and habitual gum chewing are also contributing factors.

Diagnosis

The diagnosis of TMD is made through oral examination, patient history, and radiographic studies, including computed tomography (CT) and magnetic resonance imaging (MRI), to analyze the hard and soft tissues of the temporomandibular complex. There may be a history of previous trauma to the jaws or fractured facial bones. An assessment for domestic violence or child or elder abuse may be indicated. In the case of a neoplasm, a biopsy would rule out malignancy.

Treatment

Treatment is aimed at the cause of the condition or disease. Symptoms of rheumatoid or traumatic arthritis often subside after 3 to 5 days of immobilization of the mandible. In cases where inflammation causes TMD, nonsteroidal antiinflammatory drugs (NSAIDs) often are used to treat the condition. Some patients wear special appliances to prevent them from grinding their teeth. If TMD is caused by jaw misalignment, a plastic bite plate, called a *splint*, may be used to better align the jaw. The splint is worn over teeth and establishes proper alignment, which can eliminate jaw locking, pain, and clicking sensations associated with TMD. Intraarticular injections of hydrocortisone may be needed in more severe cases of rheumatoid or degenerative arthritis. When teeth experience premature contact, the dentist adjusts the occlusion by grinding the surfaces of the teeth. More complex dental conditions, such as worn or broken teeth or restorations, may require orthodontic and/or comprehensive restorative dental care. Physical therapy, stress counseling, and the use of muscle relaxants may be prescribed. As a last resort, Arthroscopy, joint restructuring, and joint replacement are considered.

Prognosis

Mild cases respond well to resting of the joint. More complicated chronic cases require extended treatment of the underlying cause.

Prevention

Regular dental checkups can identify the underlying conditions. Treatment of these conditions can prevent the onset of TMD. Assessment for domestic violence and child or elder abuse may reveal physical trauma that can be prevented with appropriate interventions.

Patient Teaching

When the dentist prescribes an appliance, tell the patient what kind of initial discomfort he or she may expect. The patient is encouraged to use the appliance exactly as directed and is urged to report any unusual discomfort during treatment. Referrals appropriate to the cause are made.

Tooth Abscesses

Description

A tooth abscess is a pus-filled sac that develops in the tissue surrounding the base of the root.

ICD-10-CM Code	K04.7 *(Periapical abscess without sinus)* (K04.6–K04.7 = 2 codes of specificity)

Symptoms and Signs

An abscessed tooth that aches or throbs persistently and can be extremely painful when biting and chewing food. Glands in the neck and face on the affected side may become swollen and tender. Fever also can develop, along with a feeling of general malaise.

Patient Screening

Tooth abscesses require prompt medical attention.

Etiology

An abscess forms when a tooth is decayed or dying or when the tooth structure loss (i.e., from aggressive brushing, traumatic fracture, or acid erosion) exposes the dental nerve to bacteria from the mouth. Severely receding gums, which expose the root, are a risk factor. The dead pulp, along with invading bacteria, can infect the surrounding tissues and the jaws, even after a root canal procedure, and form an abscess.

Diagnosis

If any of the symptoms or signs are present, the patient should see the dentist immediately. Swelling in the neck or face must be treated immediately to prevent spreading of the infection.

Treatment

Antibiotic therapy is prescribed to treat the infection and relieve pain and acute swelling. The definitive treatment is root canal therapy, which entails the removal of the infected dental pulp and the cleansing, shaping, and definitive filling of the root canal system of the tooth. Restorative procedures, such as a dental crown or sometimes a filling, are required to seal the root canal system from the oral environment. If a lesion is a longstanding one, is large, or does not heal after a period, an apicectomy may be necessary. In this procedure, the dentist or the oral surgeon makes an incision into the gum and removes the bone that covers the tip of the root and the infected tissue as well. If this fails to clear the infection, the tooth must be extracted.

Prognosis

A positive outcome is likely with early intervention and a favorable response to antibiotic therapy.

Prevention

Prophylaxis includes good oral hygiene and regular dental checkups.

Patient Teaching

Educate patients that neglect of a tooth abscess may cause serious complications resulting from the spread of infection to the bone. If untreated, this becomes systemic and life threatening.

Mouth Ulcers

Description

An ulcer in the mouth is a lesion on the mucous membrane, exposing the underlying sensitive tissue.

ICD-10-CM Code	K13.70 *(Unspecified lesions of oral mucosa)* K13.79 *(Other lesions of oral mucosa)*

Symptoms and Signs

Mouth ulcers (sometimes called *canker sores*) are common and look alike but vary considerably in their causes and degrees of seriousness. The two most common types of ulcers are **aphthous** ulcers (Fig. 8.11), which occur during stress or illness, and traumatic ulcers, which result from injury and are caused by burns by hot foods, rough dentures, or even toothbrushes. Ulcers appear as pale-yellow spots with red borders. Aphthous ulcers usually occur in clusters and last for 3 or 4 days. Traumatic ulcers are usually single and larger and last for a week or longer.

• **Fig. 8.11** Mouth ulcers. (From Stevens A, et al: *Core pathology*, ed 3, London, 2010, Mosby.)

Patient Screening

Ulcers that do not heal within 10 days require a physician's or health care provider's attention. Any mouth ulcer that is not caused by trauma from mechanical devices (braces) or brushing must be assessed irrespective of duration.

Etiology

A viral cause for aphthous ulcers has not been established. Acute ulcerations are usually the result of mechanical trauma (braces, excessive brushing, and so on), viral and bacterial infections, stress (inducement of hormonal changes), illness, or certain medications used in chemotherapy. Certain health issues, such as autoimmune diseases, may put a person at higher risk for developing mouth ulcers. In rare instances, an ulcer may be the first sign of a tumor in the mouth, anemia, or leukemia.

Diagnosis

If an ulcer does not heal within a few days or recurs, the patient should consult a medical professional. Blood tests and a biopsy of the ulcer are needed to determine the cause. When the ulcer results from trauma, it does not heal until it is diagnosed and treated.

Treatment

Self-treatment of ulcers includes using antiseptic mouthwashes, rinsing with warm salt water, and avoiding spicy or acidic foods and hot foods or drinks. Topical analgesics, such as benzocaine, and soothing agents can be used to reduce painful irritation. The medical professional may prescribe a steroid mouthwash and topical or oral antiviral agents to promote healing.

Prognosis

Most ulcers heal spontaneously in less than 10 days.

Prevention

No specific prevention is known, except when the ulcer is attributed to mechanical trauma or improper brushing. Avoidance of gum chewing may lessen the risk of an ulcer resulting from accidentally biting the cheek.

Patient Teaching

Educate the patient regarding the self-help measures listed previously under the Treatment section.

Herpes Simplex (Cold Sores)

Description

Herpes simplex is a contagious, recurrent viral infection that affects the skin and mucous membranes. Herpes type 1 commonly produces cold sores and fever blisters (Fig. 8.12).

ICD-10-CM Code	B00.9 *(Herpes viral infection, unspecified)*

Symptoms and Signs

Herpes simplex (cold sore) blisters can develop on the lips and inside the mouth, producing painful ulcers that last a few hours or days. Exposure to strong sun, wind, stress, nicotine, and stimulants (caffeine and chocolate) is associated with the onset of recurrent oral-facial herpes simplex. Injury to the skin is also another predisposing condition. These ulcers also can form on the gums, causing them to become red and swollen. Tingling and numbness around the mouth precede their appearance. This is called the *prodrome*. Untreated, the prodrome is followed by the appearance of the vesicles (blisters), their rupture and scabbing, and finally healing of the scabs; this pathogenesis can often last 14 days or more. Although most infections are subclinical, constitutional symptoms can occur.

Patient Screening

Lesions near the eye are considered more serious. A patient having generalized symptoms, such as fever, anorexia, and lymphadenopathy, should be seen by the physician or health care provider immediately, especially if the patient is pregnant.

• **Fig. 8.12** Primary herpes simplex of the oral cavity. Numerous painful ulcers occur on the lower lip mucosa and indicate a florid herpes simplex infection. (From Dinulos JG: *Habif's clinical dermatology: a color guide to diagnosis and therapy*, ed 7, 2021, Elsevier.)

Etiology

The vesicles are caused by the herpes simplex virus type 1 (HSV-1) and are common. They tend to recur because the virus can lie dormant. Exposure to sunshine or wind or the presence of another infection, such as a common cold, can reactivate the virus. Once patients develop extraoral and/or intraoral herpes, they can have recurrent attacks throughout their lives. Patients may anticipate an outbreak of herpes with symptoms of the prodrome (burning tingling sensation in the soon-to-be affected area). Patients with weakened immune systems from chemotherapy or antirejection drugs after a transplant may experience these types of lesions.

Diagnosis

An oral examination is usually sufficient for the diagnosis. Isolating HSV-1 from local lesions can confirm the cause of the infection. The HSV-2 causes a similar lesion in the oral cavity.

Treatment

Currently, no cure is known. If the infection is mild, no treatment is necessary, but severe cases require medical attention. Herpes simplex usually does not cause serious health risks, but rubbing the eyes after touching the ulcer could cause the formation of a herpetic corneal ulcer, and the infection can produce severe illness in an immunocompromised patient. A physician or health care provider may advise using an antiviral ointment or capsules, such as acyclovir or penciclovir, to arrest or shorten the duration of the episode. Immediate attention to the symptoms and the use of an antiviral ointment are the most conservative and comfortable measures for the treatment of extraoral herpes. Intraoral herpes benefits from a prescription of an antiviral, such as acyclovir (Zovirax). Comfort measures include resting, taking aspirin, and using an anesthetic mouthwash and a topical cream to relieve the pain and heal the sores. Creams such as docosanol (Abreva) can be used to shorten the duration of herpes sores and speed the healing of cold sores. A single-day dosage of antiviral medication (acyclovir, famciclovir, or valacyclovir), beginning at the very onset of symptoms, has been proven to shorten the severity of cold sores. Avoiding triggers is also recommended.

Prognosis

Cold sores usually clear up uneventfully in 7 to 14 days. Lesions tend to recur when reactivated by trauma or stress. Serious complications can result from lesions close to the eye. Secondary bacterial infection of the skin may occur.

Prevention

Early treatment with an antiviral medication controls the outbreak and reduces the risk of transmission. Direct contact with cold sores from associates with the patient should be avoided. Gentle cleansing with antiseptic soap may help prevent the spreading of infection or secondary bacterial infection.

Patient Teaching

Recommend that close contact between the patient and his or her partner be avoided. This includes kissing of any part of the body of the infected person, because the virus may remain in saliva after the vesicle has healed. Personal items (cups, eating utensils, towels, razors, and so on) should not be shared between an infected individual and others. Touching the affected vesicles as they appear should be avoided, because a break in the skin of the finger can result in a *whitlow finger* (extremely painful herpetic infection of the finger). When the patient has multiple lesions in the oral cavity, the use of anesthetic mouthwashes helps reduce pain, enabling the patient to eat and drink. Avoidance of proper nutrition may result in dehydration or vitamin deficiencies.

Thrush

Description

Thrush is candidiasis of the oral mucosa and involves the mouth, tongue, palate, and gums.

ICD-10-CM Code	B37.0 *(Candidal stomatitis)*
	B37.83 *(Candidal cheilitis)*
	(B37.0–B37.9 = 16 codes of specificity)

Symptoms and Signs

Thrush is a fungal infection of a relatively short duration that produces sore, slightly raised, pale-yellow patches in the mouth and sometimes the throat. These lesions cause a burning sensation in the mouth and become painful when rubbed by dentures, toothbrushes, or food when eating; light bleeding may occur. Some patients suffering from severe cases of thrush have the smell of yeast in their breath. Thrush most often develops in young children, in immunodeficient individuals, and in older adults, but it can occur at any age.

Patient Screening

If the patient also complains of fever or other systemic symptoms, he or she should see a health care provider immediately.

Etiology

The fungus *Candida albicans* causes most cases of thrush. Normally present in the mouth in small numbers, the fungus can multiply out of control. This may occur during lowered resistance or as a result of prolonged treatment with antibiotics, which upsets the normal number of protective microbes. Other predisposing factors are cancer chemotherapy, diabetes, or glucocorticoid therapy. It is also very common in patients with removable dental prostheses, such as complete or partial dentures. The infection rarely becomes systemic or infectious. This same fungus can cause vaginitis.

Diagnosis

Diagnosis is made by the dentist, physician, or health care provider through an oral examination and laboratory analysis of a sample taken from a lesion. Blood tests may rule out a serious underlying disease, such as iron deficiency anemia or early HIV infection.

Treatment

Thrush is treated successfully with an antifungal medication for 14 days. The antifungals used most often are nystatin, an antifungal suspension that is swished and then swallowed, and fluconazole (Diflucan), available as a suspension or an oral tablet. After diagnosis of thrush, patients with removable dental prostheses are advised to soak their prostheses in a cup of water with a few drops of household bleach (5% sodium hypochlorite) for a few hours to disinfect them and to subsequently use an OTC denture cleaner on a daily basis to prevent reinfection.

Prognosis

The infection tends to recur in some patients. In all cases, treatment must begin immediately after a confirmed diagnosis, because thrush can extend into the esophagus, causing esophagitis. Thrush can spread to other parts of the body in those with weakened immune systems.

Prevention

Patients who have had treatment with antibiotics should report any signs of thrush. Those using inhaled corticosteroids should rinse their mouths thoroughly after use to avoid the development of thrush.

Patient Teaching

Palliative care includes a soft diet, the use of a nonirritating mouthwash, and a soft toothbrush for oral hygiene. Foods containing sugar or yeast should be limited. Good oral hygiene is encouraged. The patient is advised to quit smoking and vaping. See the procedure for disinfection of dental prostheses earlier in the Treatment section.

Necrotizing Periodontal Disease

Description

Necrotizing periodontal disease (formerly called *acute necrotizing ulcerative gingivitis* [trench mouth]) is a common infection affecting gums and the anchoring structure of teeth.

ICD-10-CM Code	A69.0 *(Necrotizing ulcerative stomatitis)*
	A69.1 *(Other Vincent's infections)*

Symptoms and Signs

Necrotizing periodontal disease is a rare, painful ulceration and disease of the gums, particularly between teeth, and is sometimes called *Vincent angina*. The primary symptom is

• **Fig. 8.13** Necrotizing periodontal disease. (From Stevens A, et al: *Core pathology*, ed 3, London, 2010, Mosby.)

painful, red, swollen gums with ulcers that bleed. Gums also can appear grayish in areas of decomposing tissue. The patient may also report a metallic taste in the mouth and bad breath (Fig. 8.13). Mild systemic symptoms include fever and enlarged lymph nodes.

Patient Screening

Prompt medical treatment is advised. An oral examination by a dentist or appropriate physician or health care provider is needed as soon as possible.

Etiology

Anaerobic opportunistic bacteria cause necrotizing periodontal disease. It results from poor oral hygiene and bacterial infection secondary to gingivitis (see the Gingivitis section). The infection is most often seen in association immune disorders. Stress, poor nutrition, throat infections, smoking, and serious illnesses, such as leukemia, are also contributing factors. Some cases have been linked to the use of oral contraceptives. Vaping can cause the mouth to dry out, which results in less saliva which contributes to periodontal problems.

Diagnosis

Throat culture and blood work may be necessary to rule out serious illness.

Treatment

The patient receives antibiotics and hydrogen peroxide mouthwash to relieve pain and inflammation. After the disease has been halted, teeth and gums must be professionally cleaned. A minor surgery on the gums, called *gingivectomy*, may be advised.

Prognosis

With treatment, improvement can be expected within days.

Prevention

Prophylactic professional cleaning of teeth, good oral hygiene, and avoidance of the contributing factors, such as smoking and poor diet, are recommended.

• **Fig. 8.14** Leukoplakia. (From Kumar V, et al: *Robbins basic pathology*, ed 10, Philadelphia, 2018, Saunders.)

Patient Teaching

Emphasize prevention as described earlier. Explain that particular medications and systemic diseases can aggravate periodontal disease.

Oral Leukoplakia

Description

Leukoplakia is hyperkeratosis or epidermal thickening of the buccal mucosa, palate, or lower lip.

ICD-10-CM Code	K13.21 (*Leukoplakia of oral mucosa, including tongue*)

Symptoms and Signs

Leukoplakia, or white plaque, is the thickening and hardening of a part of the mucous membrane in the mouth (Fig. 8.14). It develops over several weeks and can vary in size. At first, the patient is asymptomatic, but as the leukoplakia progresses, the mucous membrane becomes rough, hard, and whitish-gray and is sensitive to hot or highly seasoned foods. Small bumps may also be present. There are two types and subtypes of leukoplakia. Homogeneous is typically noncancerous or benign and may be ridged, smooth, or wrinkled. Nonhomogeneous is more likely to become malignant than homogeneous leukoplakia and has a white or red color, with irregularly shaped borders. Subtypes are proliferative verrucous leukoplakia and oral hairy leukoplakia.

Patient Screening

Schedule an appointment for the patient for an oral examination.

Etiology

Leukoplakia may develop at any age, but it is more common in older adults. It usually results from chronic irritation, such as friction caused by habitual cheek biting, dentures, or a rough tooth that rubs an area raw. Leukoplakia may also be a reaction to the heat from tobacco smoke or local irritation from chewing tobacco.

Diagnosis

An oral examination is needed. If the condition does not improve a biopsy may be indicated.

Treatment

The treatment of leukoplakia consists of eliminating the source of irritation. A rough tooth or denture may be smoothed, and giving up smoking may be advised. These measures are usually all that is needed to correct the condition. Until proven otherwise, the leukoplakia is considered precancerous.

Prognosis

The lesions require monitoring because of the risk of malignant transformation.

Prevention

Although the cause is not always known, the patient is urged to eliminate tobacco and avoid exposure to persistent irritants.

Patient Teaching

Advise patients to avoid common potentiating influences, including consumption of alcohol and tobacco (especially chewing tobacco); ill-fitting dentures; and frequent eating of spicy foods.

Oral Cancer

Description

Oral cancer includes squamous cell carcinoma (SCC) or **adenocarcinoma** of the lips, cheek mucosa, anterior tongue, floor of the mouth, hard palate, and upper and lower gingivae.

ICD-10-CM Code	C06.9 *(Malignant neoplasm of mouth, unspecified)* (C06.8–C06.9 = 3 codes of specificity)

Refer to the physician's diagnosis and then to the current edition of the ICD-10-CM coding manual for malignant neoplasm of other parts of the mouth to ensure the greatest specificity.

Symptoms and Signs

Oral cancer usually appears as a white, patchy lesion or an oral ulcer that fails to heal. If the cancer is on the lip or the tongue, the ulcer is likely to be associated with pain. However, for most other locations of oral cancer, pain occurs very late in the disease process, which often leads to delays in seeking medical treatment. Associated symptoms may include dysphagia, odynophagia, weight loss, bleeding, or referred pain in the ear or jaw. The patient may also experience loose teeth or dentures.

Patient Screening

Follow office policy for new referrals or oncology follow-ups.

Etiology

Greater than 90% of oral cancers are SCCs. The lip is the most common location of oral cancer because it has the risk factor of sun exposure. Those who smoke and drink have 15 times higher incidence of oral cancer compared with those who do not. Use of alcohol and tobacco, especially cigarette smoking and snuff dipping, accounts for a large percentage of cases of oral cancer. The combined effect of alcohol and smoking is multiplicative. Betel nut chewing, a practice common in Southeast Asia and Micronesia, also presents increased risk, as does infection with human papillomavirus (HPV), poor oral hygiene, and periodontal disease. HPV-16 infection is specifically of concern because of an increase in its prevalence and because it leads to oral cancer. Tobacco use decline is affecting statistics, which are being monitored.

According to the American Cancer Society: "More than half of all head and neck cancers have mutations of the PIK3CA oncogene. This can cause cells to grow out of control which can lead to cancer. Drugs that target the protein, called PI3K, made by the abnormal PIK3CA gene are already approved for use to treat other cancers, such as breast cancer. Studies are being done to see if similar targeted therapy drugs will work in head and neck cancer, especially HPV-positive cancers because they tend to make too many copies of the PIK3CA oncogene." Mutations in the TP53 gene have been identified. This gene produces a protein that normally secretes a protein that is involved in the destruction of cells that are beyond repair.

Oral leukoplakia (see Fig. 8.14), a reactive process that presents as a white patch on the oral mucosa, and erythrodysplasia, a red patch on the mucosa, can progress to oral cancer in some individuals, so patients with these lesions require close monitoring.

Diagnosis

Although the patient often notices the oral lesion, he or she often ignores it because the lesion is usually painless. Therefore the diagnosis of oral cancer is most often made in a dental office. The diagnosis is confirmed via fine-needle aspiration biopsy. Staging of oral cancer is performed via contrast-enhanced CT, MRI, or positron emission tomography (PET) to determine the extent of tumor infiltration. The lung, liver, and bone are the most common sites for metastasis, so chest x-rays and measurements of serum alkaline phosphatase and liver function tests are usually performed. Oral tumors are classified and staged according to the TNM classification system proposed by the American Joint Committee on Cancer (AJCC). See Chapter 1 for information about the staging and grading systems used to assess malignant neoplasms.

Treatment

The treatment for oral cancer depends on the stage. Early oral cancers are treated with surgery, with or without radiotherapy, although the use of laser therapy in the excision of early-stage oral cancers has been increasing. Neck dissection may be performed at the time of surgery to detect nodal metastases. Patients may undergo extensive and long (8 hours or longer) surgery to remove the teeth, lymph nodes, and even the bone of the jaw when the cancer has spread. This approach is referred to as *"Jaw in a Day Surgery."* Bone, tissue, and skin may be removed from another part of the body and used in the reconstruction process to replace parts or all of the jaw. For example, bone and tissue from the wrist may be used in the jaw reconstruction, and then skin or tissue from the thigh or hip is used to cover the wrist. Use of 3D model imaging and printing has changed the landscape for successfully making the jaw functional after bone tumor removal. In some cases, teeth may be reimplanted or teeth dental implants may be placed.

Radiation therapy is often used for advanced tumors and may be required in addition to surgery. Regular follow-up is needed to evaluate for recurrences after tumor removal. Speech and swallowing rehabilitation may be needed after treatment.

Prognosis

Patients with large tumors or nodal metastases have a worse prognosis compared with patients with small, localized tumors. Survival percentages increase in patients who stop smoking or using smokeless tobacco such as dip or snuff.

Prevention

Oral examination to detect premalignant or early malignant lesions should be performed during routine visits to the dentist. Abstinence from tobacco and alcohol is recommended. Immunization with the HPV vaccine decreases the risk of HPV-associated oral cancer. After treatment, close follow-up is needed, because many of these cancers recur.

Patient Teaching

Review information about the treatment plan, and encourage questions. Ensure that the patient understands the plan for controlling the pain and side effects of any therapeutic intervention. Educate treated patients on the symptoms of recurrence, such as hoarseness, pain, and lymphadenopathy. The patient who undergoes extensive surgery and jaw reconstruction will need to be educated on tube feedings, which are necessary for nutrition and speech therapy may be necessary for swallow training and learning how to speak clearly with the new anatomy of the jaw and mouth.

Diseases of the Gastrointestinal Tract

The alimentary canal, or GI tract, is a hollow continuous tube that extends from the mouth to the anus. It propels the products of digestion by peristalsis, a coordinated, wavelike muscular motion that forces food along the alimentary canal. It is also the site of the processes of mechanical and chemical breakdown of food. As the food passes through the tract, it is broken down into molecules that can be absorbed through the intestinal wall for distribution to body cells for metabolism via the bloodstream.

Water and electrolytes are absorbed in the proximal colon; waste material is stored in the rectum, and indigestible wastes are voluntarily evacuated through the anus.

Gastroesophageal Reflux Disease

Description

GERD refers to clinical manifestations of regurgitation of the stomach and duodenal contents into the esophagus, frequently occurring at night (Fig. 8.15A). Mild episodes may be described as heartburn by the patient. Most people may experience acid reflux occasionally but if the acid reflux is persistent then GERD may result.

ICD-10-CM Code	K21.9 *(Gastroesophageal reflux disease without esophagitis)* (K21.0–K21.9 = 2 codes of specificity)

Symptoms and Signs

The patient typically experiences belching, with a burning sensation in the chest and mouth. A coughing spell and wheezing caused by irritation to the oropharynx or respiratory tree may follow. Vomitus may regurgitate into the mouth. Chronic and frequent GERD may lead to dysphagia and erosive esophagitis with bleeding. Acid gastric fluid (pH < 4) is extremely caustic to the esophageal mucosa and is the major injurious agent in the majority of cases. In some patients, reflux of bile or alkaline pancreatic secretions may be contributory. Tooth enamel may become eroded, leading to dental caries. Other complications include esophageal stricture caused by scar tissue, ulceration of the mucosa, and pulmonary aspiration. A subtype of GERD is laryngopharyngeal reflux, which may present as a chronic nonproductive cough, hoarseness, or frequent clearing of the throat.

A

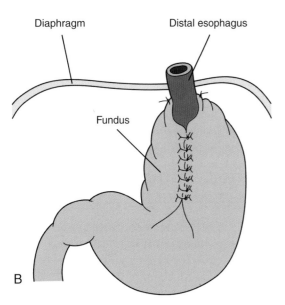

B

• **Fig. 8.15** (A) Gastroesophageal reflux disease (GERD). (B) Nissen fundoplication surgery for hiatal hernia or to treat GERD. (A, From Thompson T, Williamson P, Patton KT, Bell F: *The human body in health & disease*, ed 8, 2024.)

Patient Screening

The patient may have symptoms that mimic angina pectoris or may report blood in sputum. These are indications for prompt evaluation by the appropriate health care professional.

Etiology

Reflux can result from overeating, pregnancy, or weight gain. GERD that causes pathology frequently is associated with relaxation of the lower esophageal sphincter (LES) or an increase in intraabdominal pressure. Patients with hiatal hernia frequently experience GERD. Certain medications, including theophylline, calcium channel blockers, alendronate, and meperidine, can contribute to GERD. Some foods, coffee, and alcohol can aggravate the condition. Some medications, such as birth control pills, antihistamines, antispasmodics, and some asthma drugs, can reduce the strength of the esophageal sphincter, causing the symptoms of GERD. Genetic or DNA factors can predispose one to develop GERD or GERD-related disorders.

Diagnosis

The history and clinical evidence of GERD are most important in establishing a diagnosis. A radiographic test called *Barium swallow* may help diagnose gross changes, such as strictures or ulcerations. Esophagoscopy or esophagogastroduodenoscopy (EGD) is a superior diagnostic method, which may include a biopsy of any abnormality or dilation of strictures. Esophageal pH monitoring and scanning tests are other methods of diagnosis.

Treatment

When symptoms are mild and of short duration, simple measures to eliminate episodes of reflux may be employed. These include elevating the head of the bed about 6 inches, using multiple pillows to maintain the nonsupine position, ingesting a light evening meal no less than 4 hours before bedtime, and using antacids. Weight loss is indicated if the person is obese. Strict limitation or elimination of alcohol ingestion and smoking is recommended. Should these interventions fail, systemic medical management is initiated. Use of a histamine-2 (H_2) receptor antagonist, such as ranitidine or famotidine, or a proton pump inhibitor (PPI; omeprazole, lansoprazole, rabeprazole, or esomeprazole), inhibits acid secretion and allows for healing of the esophagus. Nissen fundoplication is a surgical method used to reinforce the esophageal sphincter. The top of the stomach is wrapped around the lower esophagus to help prevent acid from backing up into the esophagus (Fig. 8.15B). Symptomatic complications of chronic GERD are treated as needed.

Prognosis

When simple interventions fail and the condition is chronic, symptoms typically improve with drug therapy. Complications include ulceration and strictures of the esophagus, asthma, and Barrett esophagus, a precancerous condition.

Prevention

Preventive measures are directed at managing the causes that can be controlled.

Patient Teaching

Explain how positional therapy uses gravity to reduce the onset of reflux. Instruct the patient not to recline until 4 hours after eating. List the warning signs of complications, such as dysphagia, odynophagia, pulmonary symptoms, an

Digestive Distress Signals

- A hiccup is an involuntary spasmodic contraction of the diaphragm in which the beginning of an inspiration is suddenly checked by the closure of the glottis, resulting in the characteristic sound. It is usually transient.
- *Indigestion* is a term frequently used to denote vague abdominal discomfort after meals. Indigestion and eructation (belching) are common symptoms of upper GI tract disease.
- Heartburn is a sensation of retrosternal warmth or burning that occurs in waves and tends to rise upward toward the neck; it may be accompanied by the reflux of fluid into the mouth (regurgitation).
- Nausea is an unpleasant sensation in the epigastrium. It often culminates in vomiting.
- Vomiting is the forcible expulsion of the contents of the stomach through the mouth.
- Colic is acute visceral pain caused by spasm, torsion, or obstruction of a hollow organ.
- Flatulence is the presence of extensive amounts of air or gases in the stomach or intestines, leading to distention of the organs.
- Diarrhea is an abnormally frequent passage of loose stools.
- Constipation is a condition of infrequent bowel evacuation. It may have functional or organic causes.
- Fecal incontinence is an inability to control defecation.

increase in esophageal burning, bleeding, or unexplained weight loss and dehydration. Explain the importance of follow-up appointments with the physician or health care provider to monitor the treatment plan. All medications should be taken as prescribed.

Esophageal Varices

Description
Esophageal varices are dilated submucosal veins that develop in patients with underlying portal hypertension and may result in serious upper GI bleeding.

ICD-10-CM Code	I85.00 (*Esophageal varices without bleeding*)
	I85.01 (*Esophageal varices with bleeding*)
	(I85.0–I85.11 = 4 codes of specificity)

Symptoms and Signs
The superficial veins lining the esophagus become dilated and twisted at the distal end of the esophagus (Fig. 8.16). In some cases, there may be preceding retching or dyspepsia attributable to alcoholic gastritis or withdrawal. Varices may be asymptomatic until a rupture causes a massive hemorrhage. With rupture, the patient experiences hematemesis or melena, and signs of hypovolemic shock may develop.

Patient Screening
Variceal hemorrhage can be life threatening and is a medical emergency.

Etiology
Varices result from increased pressure within the veins. This pressure develops when the venous return to the liver is impeded. Esophageal varices occur in some patients with serious liver disease or cirrhosis of the liver which is often associated with alcoholic cirrhosis. Esophageal varices are a common complication of cirrhosis of the liver because the destruction of hepatic tissue interferes with emptying of the portal vein, resulting in portal hypertension. All patients who have varices will not develop serious bleeding. Other causes are blood clots in the portal or splenic veins. A parasitic infection called schistosomiasis can also result in varices. These parasites are found in South America, Africa, the Middle East, East Asia, and the Caribbean. The parasite can cause problems with the liver and other organs too.

Diagnosis
Diagnosis is based on the clinical picture and a history of hepatic disease, specifically cirrhosis. Radiographic examination is indicated to study any obstruction of blood flow that causes back pressure in the esophageal vessels. Esophageal varices can be noted during endoscopic examination. They are graded I to IV depending on size. Patients with cirrhosis are prone to varices and should be screened with endoscopy so that preventive measures can be instituted.

Treatment
The principal treatment of a patient with bleeding esophageal varices is the same as that for any patient with gross GI bleeding: replacing the blood volume and maintaining the fluid and electrolyte balance to restore homeostasis. Interventions to control and prevent recurrences of bleeding include endoscopic sclerotherapy and ligation of bleeding varices. Beta blockers may be indicated to lower the pressure in the portal vessels. In patients with variceal bleeding that cannot be controlled with pharmacologic or endoscopic therapy, emergency portal decompression may be considered.

Prognosis
Bleeding esophageal varices have a significant morbidity and mortality rate. The long-term prognosis is somewhat guarded because of the tendency to hemorrhage. Forty percent of patients die during the first episode of massive hemorrhage. Of those who survive, recurrent bleeding frequently occurs within 1 year, with a similar mortality rate for each episode.

Prevention
Esophageal varices are often associated with hepatic disease, which may or may not be preventable.

• **Fig. 8.16** Esophageal varices. (From Kumar V, et al: *Robbins basic pathology,* ed 10, Philadelphia, 2018, Saunders.)

Patient Teaching

Illustrate how obstruction of blood flow causes back pressure in the esophageal vessels. Teach the patient how to monitor for overt signs of upper GI bleeding. When intervention is required to control bleeding, explain the procedure and its purpose.

Esophagitis

Description

Esophagitis is inflammation and tissue injury of the esophagus.

ICD-10-CM Code   K20.9 *(Esophagitis, unspecified)*
(K20.0–K20.9 = 3 codes of specificity)
Esophagitis is coded according to types and causes. Refer to the physician's diagnosis and then to the current edition of the ICD-10-CM coding manual to ensure the greatest specificity.

Symptoms and Signs

The main symptom that the patient experiences is burning chest pain (heartburn), which can make the patient believe

• **Fig. 8.17** Corrosive esophagitis. (Endoscopic image Courtesy Dr. Ira Hanan, The University of Chicago, Chicago, Illinois.)

that he or she is having a heart attack. The onset of pain typically follows eating or drinking. Some patients will have sores in the mouth and nausea and vomiting. The patient even may have some vomiting of blood (hematemesis).

Corrosive esophagitis is severe inflammation of the esophagus resulting from ingestion of a caustic chemical (alkali or acid) that causes tissue damage (Fig. 8.17). In children, ingestion is usually accidental; in adults, chemical ingestion often is a suicide attempt. The degree of damage to the esophageal tissue ranges from pain and inability to swallow and speak to perforation and even destruction of the esophagus.

Patient Screening
Acute cases caused by ingestion of a caustic chemical require emergency care.

Etiology
The most common cause of esophagitis is reflux of the acid contents of the stomach resulting from a defect of the LES. The stomach acids irritate the esophageal lining and may cause an inflammatory response. Persistent or chronic vomiting, infection, radiation treatments, and other allergies, and infections can result in esophagitis. Erosive esophagitis may occur after taking antiinflammatory medications, and antibiotics, such as tetracycline, without drinking adequate amounts of water. Chemical injury may also be a cause. Esophagitis also can appear as a GI manifestation of HIV infection.

Diagnosis
Assessment begins with patient history and radiography of the upper GI tract (esophagoscopy) to confirm diagnosis and determine the extent of inflammation and tissue damage. A history of chemical ingestion, the presence of redness, and oropharyngeal burn point to caustic esophagitis.

Treatment
The treatment of esophagitis is determined by etiology. In mild cases of reflux esophagitis, treatment may include a bland diet and a course of antacids. Underlying causes of reflux, such as hiatal hernia, are addressed in the treatment plan. Medications to reduce gastric acid production, such as cimetidine (Tagamet) or omeprazole (Prilosec), are effective. Sucralfate (Carafate) suspension sometimes is prescribed to relieve discomfort and to promote healing. Meals should be small and frequent. Alcohol must be avoided. Esophageal stricture may require dilation; esophageal perforation requires emergency endoscopic or surgical repair.

Prognosis
The prognosis for esophagitis is good if the patient adheres to treatments prescribed by the health care professional. Complications of chronic or caustic esophagitis include scarring and stricture of the esophagus. Caustic ingestions increase the risk of esophageal cancer throughout the patient's lifetime.

Prevention
There is no known prevention for esophagitis, but avoiding alcohol, spicy foods, and caffeine helps relieve the symptoms.

Patient Teaching
Advise the patient that close monitoring of the condition is required during the treatment and the healing process.

Assess the need for psychological counseling when chemical ingestions result from suicide attempts or any nonaccidental causes. Follow instructions regarding timing of medication and eating when taking Carafate, since the coating may affect absorption of other medications.

Esophageal Cancer

Description

Esophageal cancer occurs in two main forms. The esophagus is lined for most of its length with squamous epithelium, which can give rise to SCC (Fig. 8.18). Adenocarcinoma may develop in the columnar epithelium near the esophagogastric junction.

ICD-10-CM Code	C15.9 *(Malignant neoplasm of esophagus, unspecified)* (C15.3–C15.9 = 5 codes of specificity)

Esophageal cancer is coded according to the site of the lesion. Refer to the physician's diagnosis and then to the current edition of the ICD-10-CM coding manual to ensure the greatest specificity.

Symptoms and Signs

Symptoms may include dysphagia, weight loss, and retrosternal discomfort or a burning sensation. Iron deficiency anemia may result from chronic esophageal blood loss. The patient may not experience symptoms in the early stage. If the tumor involves the laryngeal nerve, hoarseness may result. A tracheoesophageal fistula may develop during the late stages of the disease, with coughing or frequent pneumonias occurring when saliva, liquid, or food spills into the lungs.

• **Fig. 8.18** Carcinoma of the esophagus. (A) Esophageal adenocarcinoma. (B) Esophageal squamous cell carcinoma. (From Kumar V, et al: *Robbins basic pathology*, ed 10, Philadelphia, 2018, Saunders.)

Patient Screening

A health care professional must be contacted for patient referrals to appropriate specialists who treat this type of cancer.

Etiology

Mutations in the DNA of cells in the esophagus take place. The incidence of SCC of the esophagus varies, with the highest rates being found in Asia, Africa, and Iran. Risk factors for SCC include cigarette smoking, alcohol consumption, betel nut chewing (a practice common in some Asian countries), drinking very hot beverages (greater than 149°F [65°C]); eating foods containing *N*-nitroso compounds (e.g., pickled vegetables); a diet low in fruit and vegetables; a history of head and neck cancer; and underlying esophageal disease, such as achalasia or caustic strictures. Adenocarcinoma predominantly affects Caucasians and males. The major risk factors are Barrett esophagus (see the Enrichment box about Barrett Esophagus) and chronic GERD. The risk of adenocarcinoma is greater in patients who smoke or those who are obese.

Diagnosis

Physicians and other health care providers detect most esophageal cancers during evaluation of symptomatic patients or incidentally during screening of high-risk individuals with endoscopic examination. Among patients who have symptoms suggestive of esophageal cancer, a barium study may be used for the initial assessment. An endoscopic biopsy is necessary to confirm the diagnosis.

After the initial patient evaluation, diagnosis includes assessment of the operative risk and staging. Esophageal tumors are staged according to the TNM classification system proposed by the AJCC. SCCs and adenocarcinomas have different staging groups. Staging involves CT, PET, and endoscopic ultrasonography (EUS) to evaluate for metastatic disease and to determine whether surgical resection of the tumor is a realistic option. Bronchoscopy is another test used for determining if the cancer has spread to lung tissue. The most common sites of metastasis are the lung, liver, bone, and adrenal gland. At times, a diagnostic laparoscopy is required for complete staging.

Treatment

Accurate staging is critical to selecting a treatment method. Patients with clinically localized cancer often undergo chemoradiotherapy either before or after surgery. EUS is used to detect recurrence of the disease after successful tumor excision. For patients with advanced, unresectable disease, the therapeutic goal is to maintain the ability to swallow. Nonoperative measures may be used to palliate symptoms. Radiation, with or without chemotherapy, and endoscopic stent placement are used to treat dysphagia by shrinking the tumor and dilating the esophagus, respectively. These methods also reduce the risk of aspiration and weight loss but rarely improve the survival of the patient. There is little doubt that SCC and adenocarcinoma represent different disease processes, but it is unknown whether or how they should be treated differently. Surgical options include removal of the esophagus. Targeted drug therapy with chemotherapy is also one method of treatment. Immunotherapy is also used in cases of esophageal cancer.

Prognosis

The prognosis is highly associated with the stage but is generally poor because esophageal cancer of both types has a high propensity for metastasis even in the earliest stages. The overall 5-year survival rate is approximately 20%, for all esophageal cancers. Esophageal cancer which is diagnosed in early stages has a higher 5-year survival rate.

❖ ENRICHMENT

Barrett Esophagus

One of the most severe consequences of chronic gastroesophageal reflux disease (GERD) is the replacement of the normal stratified squamous epithelium of the distal esophagus by abnormal columnar epithelium. This condition is known as *Barrett esophagus*. In one sense, it is a protective metaplastic change produced because the columnar epithelium is more resistant to acid damage compared with the original stratified squamous epithelium, but at the same time, this adaptation predisposes the individual to the development of adenocarcinoma of the esophagus and of the proximal stomach.

Barrett esophagus is usually diagnosed during an endoscopic examination of middle-aged and older adults (Fig. 8.19). The metaplasia itself causes no symptoms, and the condition is usually discovered when patients are being seen for symptoms of GERD, such as heartburn, regurgitation, and dysphagia. Endoscopic screening of patients with GERD is only recommended if the patient has multiple other risk factors for adenocarcinoma, such as obesity, age greater than 50 years, male gender, or a history of hiatal hernia.

The gene-related changes leading from the development of Barrett esophagus to adenocarcinoma are not completely understood. We do know that before the cells acquire enough DNA damage to become malignant, dysplastic morphologic changes appear. The use of acid-suppressive medications has been shown to slow the progression of dysplasia.

Although no management strategy has been proven to prolong life, there are several options currently in use: treatment of GERD, endoscopic surveillance to detect dysplasia, and treatment of the dysplasia. GERD is usually treated with PPI medications. For patients found to have diffuse low-grade dysplasia on endoscopic examination, the frequency of endoscopic examination often is 1 year, 2 years, and 4 years after remission. In patients with high-grade dysplasia, progress to adenocarcinoma is much more common but still varies. Because of this risk, however, the American Gastroenterological Association now recommends endoscopic eradication of the dysplastic tissue by using radiofrequency ablation, photodynamic therapy, or resection.

• **Fig. 8.19** Barrett esophagus. (Endoscopic image Courtesy Dr. Ira Hanan, The University of Chicago, Chicago, Illinois.)

Prevention

Those with Barrett esophagus usually undergo endoscopies to screen for progression to adenocarcinoma. In addition, the patient should avoid practices associated with increased risk, such as the use of alcohol and tobacco. Research on the effects of vaping continues to be expanded to fully understand if vaping is a risk factor.

Patient Teaching

Assess the patient's comprehension of the diagnosis and the treatment plan. Discuss the possible side effects of radiation, chemotherapy, or surgery, as appropriate. Encourage the patient to ask questions and discuss his or her anxiety. Provide a list of local cancer support groups and other appropriate referrals.

Gastric and Duodenal Peptic Ulcers

Description

Should the protective mucous membrane of the stomach or upper intestinal tract break down, the lining is prone to ulceration. These internal surface lesions can be acute or chronic, clustered or singular, and shallow or deep. Deep sores develop within the deep muscle layer of tissue (Fig. 8.20).

ICD-10-CM Code	K25.9 *(Gastric ulcer, unspecified as acute or chronic, without hemorrhage or perforation)* (K25.0–K25.9 = 9 codes of specificity) K26.9 *(Duodenal ulcer, unspecified as acute or chronic, without hemorrhage or perforation)* (K26.0–K26.9 = 9 codes of specificity) K27.9 *(Peptic ulcer, site unspecified, unspecified as acute or chronic, without hemorrhage or perforation)* (K27.0–K27.9 = 9 codes of specificity)

Gastric, duodenal, and peptic ulcers are coded according to the pathology involved. Refer to the physician's diagnosis and then to the current edition of the ICD-10-CM coding manual to ensure the greatest specificity.

Symptoms and Signs

When the peptic ulcer occurs in the stomach (gastric ulcer), often the patient is asymptomatic, particularly if it is caused by ingestion of antiinflammatory agents, such as NSAIDs (e.g., ibuprofen [Motrin]). However, the patient may report heartburn or indigestion and epigastric pain that is described as gnawing, dull, aching, or "hungerlike." Some patients experience pain or a feeling of uncomfortable fullness after eating, causing them to avoid eating, and this results in loss of weight and predisposition to dehydration.

The most common type of peptic ulcer is the duodenal ulcer (an ulcer of the first part of the small intestine), which causes symptoms that range from subtle midepigastric pain and heartburn to intense pain in the upper abdomen with nausea and vomiting. The patient may be observed guarding the painful area by clutching the stomach, assuming a crouching position, or sitting with the knees drawn up to the chest. Some patients have reported that frequent eating helps relieve discomfort; attacks of the most intense pain may erupt 2 hours after a meal. Some ulcers cause nocturnal pain that awakes the patient at night.

If these ulcers bleed internally, occult (hidden) or frank (obvious) blood is found in the vomitus or stool. The situation is more serious if the lesion invades deeply and perforates, causing hemorrhage and leakage of the contents of the stomach or intestine into the abdominal cavity. A change from a patient's typical rhythmic discomfort to constant or radiating pain may indicate penetration or perforation.

• **Fig. 8.20** Peptic ulcer. (Endoscopic image Courtesy Dr. Ira Hanan, The University of Chicago, Chicago, Illinois.)

Patient Screening

Sudden onset of pain and vomiting with overt signs of bleeding present an urgent need for medical care.

Etiology

Although the cause is not always clear, an area of breakdown of the mucous membrane precipitates ulceration of the epithelial lining of the stomach or the intestine. A crucial causal factor of peptic ulcers is *Helicobacter pylori* infection, which is thought to be the most common worldwide human bacterial infection (Fig. 8.21). When present, it produces inflammation in the mucous membrane of the GI tract. The second most common form of ulcer is related to the use of NSAIDs (e.g., ibuprofen [Motrin]). The less common gastric ulcers follow chronic gastritis, in which the gastric mucosa becomes less able to defend itself against erosion. Some of the known contributing catalysts are the ingestion of gastric irritants; the use of ulcerogenic drugs, such as alcohol, aspirin, and other antiinflammatory agents; smoking; and the presence of a bacterial infection *(H. pylori)*. Gastric ulcers are most common in middle-aged males.

Duodenal ulcers are associated with an increase of acid and gastric juice (pepsin). Predisposing factors include the presence of *H. pylori* infection, drinking alcohol, and use of NSAIDs. Other less common causes are Zollinger-Ellison syndrome and severe physiological stress from severe illness, burn, or injury. Zollinger-Ellison syndrome is rare, yet in those cases the stomach makes too much gastric acid. Physiological stress ulcers form more rapidly than ulcers caused from other conditions. An approximate 400,000 cases are diagnosed each year in the United States, and it is estimated that 1 out of 10 people will be diagnosed with ulcers at some time throughout their life.

Diagnosis

The patient report of an illness can help distinguish between a gastric ulcer and a duodenal ulcer. The diagnosis of a peptic ulcer can be suspected on the basis of the patient's history and physical examination findings. The diagnosis may be confirmed with barium radiography of the upper GI tract to detect abnormal appearance and function, or the ulcer may be visualized through upper GI tract endoscopy referred to as an esophagogastroduodenoscopy (EGD) (Fig. 8.22). Diagnostic studies are available to identify *H. pylori*. Gastric contents are sometimes collected and analyzed for the level of acidity or the presence of blood in the secretions. The patient's stool also is analyzed for evidence of blood. Blood tests indicating reduced hemoglobin (Hgb) concentration and reduced hematocrit (Hct) may confirm a bleeding ulcer. Biopsy, with microscopic study of the tissue specimen, rules out or confirms the presence of cancer. Serum albumin and transferrin levels may be reduced if the patient has weight loss and malnutrition. Abdominal radiographic studies are performed to investigate the possibility of perforation or other abdominal conditions.

Treatment

The management of peptic ulcers requires rest, medication, changes in the diet, and adjustments in lifestyle, especially for stress reduction. Surgery may be indicated in severe cases. If the etiology is confirmed (e.g., use of an ulcerogenic drug, such as aspirin; NSAIDs; and alcohol), the identified agent must be eliminated. Drug therapy includes one or more of the following: H_2 receptor blocking agents to control gastric secretion (e.g., nizatidine [Axid], famotidine

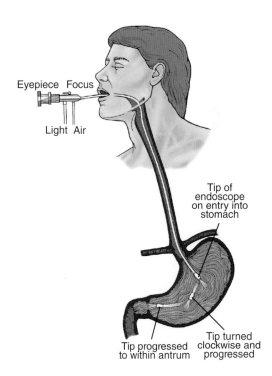

• **Fig. 8.22** Upper gastrointestinal (GI) tract endoscopy is a procedure that allows direct visualization of the interior of upper GI structures resulting in an accurate and sensitive evaluation of mucosal lesions; it is possible to obtain biopsy specimens, to perform superficial operative procedures, or to make an assessment of the course of a disease. The endoscope, a thin flexible tube equipped with a camera and a light source, is inserted through the mouth and guided by the camera. (From *Mosby's dictionary of medicine, nursing and health professions*, ed 8, St. Louis, 2009, Mosby.)

• **Fig. 8.21** *Helicobacter pylori*. (From Cotran R, et al: *Robbins pathologic basis of disease*, ed 6, Philadelphia, 1999, Saunders.)

[Pepcid], cimetidine [Tagamet], and ranitidine [Zantac]); antacids (e.g., magnesium hydroxide-aluminum hydroxide [Maalox]) to reduce gastric acidity; coating agents (e.g., sucralfate) to protect the mucosa; and PPIs (e.g., omeprazole [Prilosec], esomeprazole [Nexium], pantoprazole [Protonix], and lansoprazole [Prevacid]) to suppress the secretion of gastric acid. When *H. pylori* is identified as the cause, antibiotic therapy, such as clarithromycin (Biaxin) with amoxicillin, combined with a PPI, may be prescribed. Small, frequent meals of soft, bland foods are better tolerated.

All of these measures attempt to relieve symptoms and encourage the healing process. Significant bleeding or perforation of the ulcer calls for more aggressive measures, such as surgical intervention, the administration of intravenous (IV) fluids, and blood replacement.

Prognosis
Peptic ulcers can heal. Patients are instructed to follow the recommended preventive measures even after healing, because peptic ulcer disease tends to recur. Any nonhealing ulcer, and all gastric ulcers should be evaluated via endoscopy to rule out cancer.

Prevention
Avoid alcohol ingestion and smoking. NSAIDs and aspirin must be used appropriately.

Patient Teaching
Referral to a registered dietitian (RD) for nutritional consultation may be helpful. Have the patient eliminate caffeine, alcohol, smoking, and any other identified irritants. Reinforce the importance of strict adherence to a bland diet high in vitamin K. Instruct the patient to take prescribed analgesics or antiemetics 1 hour before meals to help control pain or nausea. Warn the patient to report any signs of hematemesis and any occurrence of black or bloody stools. Credible online medical patient resources should also be shared with the patient.

Gastritis
Description
Gastritis is inflammation of the lining of the stomach; the acute form is a common disorder.

ICD-10-CM Code	K29.70 (Gastritis, unspecified, without bleeding)
	K29.90 (Gastroduodenitis, unspecified, without bleeding)
	(K29.00–K29.91 = 18 codes of specificity)

Gastritis is coded according to the pathology involved. Refer to the physician's diagnosis and then to the current edition of the ICD-10-CM coding manual to ensure the greatest specificity.

Symptoms and Signs
The mucosal layer of the stomach normally acts as a physical barrier to protect against injury, inflammation, and erosion. When the stomach lining becomes inflamed, the patient experiences epigastric pain, indigestion, and a feeling of fullness after meals. Other discomforts, such as nausea, belching, and fatty food intolerance, cause the patient to lose his or her appetite. When the gastric mucosa is inflamed and swollen, it can bleed, and blood can be seen and detected in the patient's vomitus and stool. Chronic gastritis is more common in older adults.

Patient Screening
Sudden onset of pain and hematemesis requires emergency medical care.

Etiology
Similar to symptoms of peptic ulcers, the main cause of gastritis is inflammation associated with *H. pylori*. Many agents damage the gastric lining, including common medications, such as aspirin and other antiinflammatory drugs, poisons, alcohol, smoking tobacco or other substances, infectious diseases, stress, and mechanical injury resulting from the swallowing of a foreign object (Fig. 8.23). The repeated ingestion of irritating foods or allergic reaction to foods irritates the gastric mucosa.

Chronic gastritis is associated with peptic ulcer disease and recurring exposure to irritating substances. It can also occur in patients with a history of chronic disease, such as pernicious anemia. Those with inflammatory conditions or autoimmune disease such as ulcerative colitis are at higher risk for gastritis. A substantial number of patients have idiopathic gastritis. Paradoxically, gastritis also can result from the lack of production of gastric acids, which is sometimes associated with a condition caused by vitamin B_{12} deficiency called *pernicious anemia*.

Diagnosis
Gastroscopy allows for visualization of the interior of the stomach, and radiography helps rule out other structural

• **Fig. 8.23** Chemical gastritis caused by aspirin. (From Damjanov I, Linder J: *Pathology: a color atlas*, St. Louis, 1999, Mosby.)

abnormalities. Biopsy specimens are obtained to determine the cause and extent of disease. Blood counts and serum tests offer additional findings. Fecal occult blood test results may be positive because of gastric bleeding.

Treatment

Curing *H. pylori* infection with antibiotic therapy often rapidly resolves superficial gastritis. If any other source of irritation is known, it is eliminated or controlled. Gastric discomfort is relieved with the use of antacids and medications, such as cimetidine (Tagamet), ranitidine hydrochloride (Zantac), famotidine (Pepcid), omeprazole (Prilosec), or pantoprazole (Protonix) to reduce the secretion of gastric acid. If the patient has bleeding, it is monitored and treated with medicines that constrict blood vessels. Antibiotics are given for *H. pylori* infection, and antiemetics are given to help control nausea and vomiting. The patient is given a bland diet as tolerated, with vitamin and mineral supplements as needed. If the patient has vitamin B_{12} deficiency, injections of vitamin B_{12} must be administered each month for an indefinite period.

Prognosis

Acute mild cases of gastritis improve with conservative treatment and elimination of the known irritant. Chronic gastritis is monitored for complications.

Prevention

Preventive measures are the same as those for gastric and duodenal ulcers.

Patient Teaching

It is essential to refer patients to a psychologist for extreme stress resulting from experiencing a serious illness. Teaching the patient about the relationship between gastritis and the contributing lifestyle factors can promote healing and prevent recurrences (see Patient Teaching in the Gastric and Duodenal Peptic Ulcers section).

Gastric Cancer

Description

Gastric cancer occurs in the stomach, the organ located in the upper abdomen that connects the esophagus and the small intestine (Fig. 8.24).

ICD-10-CM Code	C16.9 *(Malignant neoplasm of stomach, unspecified)* (C16.0–C16.9 = 9 codes of specificity)

Gastric cancer is coded according to the site of the lesion. Refer to the physician's diagnosis and then to the current edition of the ICD-10-CM coding manual to ensure the greatest specificity.

Symptoms and Signs

The patient with early carcinoma of the stomach is frequently asymptomatic. As the disease progresses, the most

• **Fig. 8.24** Ulcerative gastric carcinoma. (From Cotran R, et al: *Robbins pathologic basis of disease*, ed 8, Philadelphia, 2007, Saunders.)

common symptoms at initial presentation are weight loss and persistent abdominal pain, although nausea, dysphagia, melena, and anorexia are also seen. Anorexia is present more often with gastric cancer than with ulcers. The most common physical finding is a palpable abdominal mass, which usually indicates advanced disease. Left supraclavicular adenopathy (Virchow node) is commonly found in metastatic disease.

Patient Screening

The patient being treated for gastric cancer may experience a variety of complications resulting from surgery, chemotherapy, or radiation. Symptoms of GI obstruction or malnutrition may be present. Physicians and other health care providers often give priority attention to these patients.

Etiology

Japan has the highest incidence of gastric cancer in the world. *H. pylori* is a known carcinogen and can cause gastric cancer, usually in the distal stomach. Barrett esophagus is the main risk factor for the development of gastric cancer in the proximal stomach. A diet high in salt, smoking, previous gastric surgery, and prior abdominal radiation exposure are known risk factors. There can be a genetic predisposition (e.g., family history of gastric cancer and blood type A). Twenty-five percent of patients have a history of gastric ulcer. A diet rich in fruits and vegetables can be protective.

Diagnosis

When gastric cancer is suspected, an upper GI endoscopy with a biopsy of any suspicious lesion is used for diagnosis. If a biopsy of an ulcer proves it to be benign, a follow-up endoscopy is recommended in 8 to 12 weeks to verify the healing of the ulcer detected on the initial test. Gastric cancer is staged by using the TNM classification system proposed by the AJCC. Staging is performed on the basis of findings from the physical examination; CT of the chest, abdomen, and pelvis to detect metastases; and EUS to assess the depth of tumor invasion. For patients with significant tumor depth, laparoscopy may also be used to directly visualize the surface of the liver, peritoneum, and local lymph nodes, which are the most likely sites of metastasis. See Chapter 1 for information about the staging and grading systems used to assess malignant neoplasms.

Treatment

The treatment regimen is identified after accurate tumor staging. All patients should be tested for *H. pylori* infection and, if infected, treated with antibiotics. Gastric resection, often followed by combined chemoradiotherapy, offers the best chance of long-term survival for patients with localized disease. Total gastrectomy is performed for lesions of the proximal stomach (upper third), and subtotal gastrectomy with resection of adjacent nodal tissue is usually sufficient for distal gastric cancer. Chemoradiotherapy is often added for more advanced diseases. Palliation is an important part of the care for patients with gastric cancer because the majority have advanced disease at the time of diagnosis and because of the high rate of recurrence after surgical resection.

Prognosis

The prognosis of gastric cancer has improved only slightly over the last few decades despite surgical advances and a decline in incidence. Most patients will develop metastases at some point during the course of their illness. Localized distal gastric cancer has a rate of cure at approximately 50%. Advanced, incurable cancer is present in other patients at initial presentation. Even those who undergo potentially curative surgery have high rates of local and distant recurrences.

Prevention

The high mortality rate of gastric cancer largely results from the advanced stage of the disease at presentation. Therefore detection at an early stage is very important to improve survival. The cost-effectiveness of screening asymptomatic patients remains controversial, but in Japan, Venezuela, and Chile, this practice has rendered positive outcomes with early detection of gastric cancer. In the United States, with a relatively low incidence of gastric cancer, screening is limited to those who are identified as "high risk" (those with gastric adenomas, pernicious anemia, partial gastrectomy, or familial colon cancer syndromes). These patients should receive screening endoscopy as recommended by their health care provider, depending on their underlying conditions. *H. pylori* infection should be eradicated to reduce the risk of progression to gastric cancer.

Patient Teaching

Assess the patient's knowledge of the disease process and the medical management prescribed by the physician, usually an oncologist. Address any related impairment to eating and nutrition. Encourage the patient to ask questions and express any feelings of anxiety. Discuss the side effects of chemotherapy or surgery. Ensure that the patient understands all of the palliative measures provided and the warning signs to report to a physician or health care provider. Provide information regarding cancer support groups which meet in person or online.

Acute Appendicitis

Description

Appendicitis is inflammation of the appendix, a narrow pouch that is about 3.5 inches long and extends from the first part of the large intestine (cecum) (Fig. 8.25).

ICD-10-CM Code	K35.2 (Acute appendicitis with generalized peritonitis) (K35.2–K38.9 = 12 codes of specificity)

Appendicitis is coded according to the pathology involved. Refer to the physician's diagnosis and then to the current edition of the ICD-10-CM coding manual to ensure the greatest specificity.

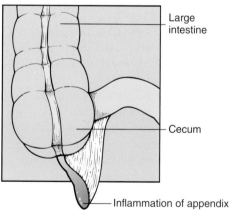

Large intestine

Cecum

Inflammation of appendix

• **Fig. 8.25** Acute appendicitis. (From Cotran R, et al: *Robbins pathologic basis of disease*, ed 6, Philadelphia, 1999, Saunders.)

Symptoms and Signs

The appendix has no known function in humans. Classic symptoms of appendicitis include abdominal pain that usually starts as vague discomfort around the navel and, within a few hours, localizes in the right lower quadrant. As the condition worsens, the patient becomes nauseated and may vomit, run a fever, and have diarrhea or constipation.

Patient Screening

Clinical signs vary but usually follow a sequence, as described previously. A patient with lower abdominal pain, fever, nausea, and vomiting requires immediate medical attention.

Etiology

Obstruction of the narrow appendiceal lumen initiates the clinical illness of acute appendicitis. Obstruction has multiple causes, including lymphoid hyperplasia (related to viral illnesses, including upper respiratory infection, mononucleosis, and gastroenteritis), fecaliths, parasites, foreign bodies, Crohn's disease, and primary or metastatic cancer. Whatever the cause, the pathophysiology of the disease is the same. As bacteria multiply, they invade the wall of the appendix, and eventually the circulation to the appendix is compromised. Appendicitis is most common in the 20- to 40-year-old age group.

Diagnosis

The physician or health care provider makes a differential diagnosis to rule out other causes of right lower abdominal pain and acute abdomen. Appendicitis generally can be diagnosed on the basis of physical examination findings and reported symptoms; one significant diagnostic indicator is maximal tenderness of the abdomen at the McBurney point. Rebound tenderness on the opposite side may be a sign of peritoneal irritation. Complete blood count (CBC) and urinalysis are performed and possibly repeated during hospital observation. Laboratory findings indicate an elevation in the white blood cell (WBC) count (leukocytosis). The WBC count is elevated in adults in 80% to 85% of all cases of acute appendicitis. It should be noted that the WBC count is also elevated in patients with other causes of right lower abdominal pain. Serial WBC measurements (over 4–8 hours) in suspected cases may increase the specificity because the WBC count often increases in acute appendicitis. The usual signs and symptoms of appendicitis in older patients are diminished, atypical, or absent and remain unrecognized, leading to a higher rate of perforation.

Treatment

Surgical removal of the appendix (appendectomy) is the indicated treatment and is performed on confirmation of appendicitis. Broad-spectrum antibiotic therapy is initiated before surgery. If appendicitis is left untreated, necrosis and rupture of the appendix can result in peritonitis, a life-threatening complication. Factors that increase the rate of perforation are delayed presentation to medical care, age extremes (the very young and the very old), and the hidden location of the appendix.

Prognosis

Complete recovery is expected with prompt medical and surgical intervention. Laparoscopic appendectomy allows for expedited recovery.

Prevention

No prevention is known, but the appendix may be removed during unrelated abdominal surgery as a prophylactic measure.

Patient Teaching

Local application of heat to the abdomen is contraindicated in the presence of the characteristic clinical symptoms of appendicitis. Postsurgical instructions include deep breathing and early ambulation, a little at a time, over the course of the first couple of weeks to prevent pneumonia and constipation. Heavy lifting should be avoided until the physician approves for the patient to do so. Review all postoperative instructions. Encourage the patient to notify the physician or health care provider about any signs of infection at the incision site.

Hiatal Hernia

Description

A hiatal hernia is a defect in the diaphragm that causes a segment of the stomach to slide into the thoracic cavity.

ICD-10-CM Code	K44.9 *(Diaphragmatic hernia without obstruction or gangrene)* (K44.0–K44.9 = 3 codes of specificity)

Symptoms and Signs

Hiatal hernia is a condition in which the upper part of the stomach protrudes through the esophageal opening of the diaphragm and into the thoracic cavity (Fig. 8.26). As a consequence, the LES muscle at the junction of the esophagus and stomach malfunctions, allowing the contents of the stomach to be regurgitated into the esophagus. This esophageal reflux (see the Gastroesophageal Reflux Disease section) can irritate the lining of the esophagus. The patient reports heartburn, which is usually worse when reclining or after a large meal. Symptoms of chest pain and difficulty swallowing may suggest that a large portion of the stomach has slipped into the opening. Respiratory complications can develop as a result of aspiration.

Some hiatal hernias are asymptomatic.

Patient Screening

When patients report heartburn, excessive belching, or distention of the stomach, a routine appointment is scheduled. If the patient has substernal chest pain, dysphagia, or bleeding, he or she should be seen as soon as possible.

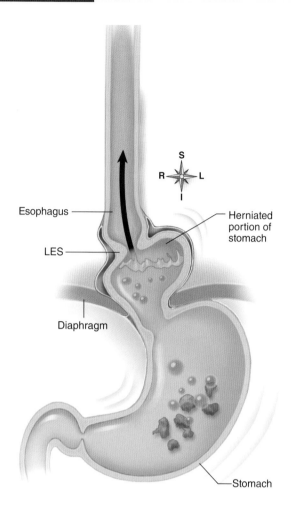

• **Fig. 8.26** Hiatal hernia. *LES,* Lower esophageal sphincter. (From Patton KT, Thibodeau GA: *The human body in health & disease,* ed 6, Maryland Heights, 2014, Elsevier.)

> ❖ **NOTE**
>
> Cardiac ischemia may present as chest discomfort, nausea, or belching, which may be mistaken as symptoms of reflux or hiatal hernia.

Etiology

Hiatal hernia, a common condition, can be caused by a congenital defect in the diaphragm or a weakness that develops in the diaphragm, causing part of the stomach to protrude into the thoracic cavity. The weakening of the muscle can result from obesity, old age, trauma, or intraabdominal pressure; sometimes the exact cause is uncertain.

Diagnosis

Large hiatal hernias may be seen on a chest radiograph. The diagnosis is based on barium radiographic studies of the esophagus and the stomach. Endoscopy confirms the diagnosis and differentiates the condition from other diseases, such as peptic ulcers and malignant tumors. Additional diagnostic studies include measuring reflux pH and examining the reflux contents for the presence of blood.

Treatment

Initial treatment identifies the symptoms and prevents complications. This includes dietary modifications (smaller, more frequent meals of bland food). The patient is advised to minimize activities that increase intraabdominal pressure, such as straining and coughing. The obese patient is advised to lose weight.

Antacids and medications that control acid secretions in the stomach, such as H_2 blockers or PPIs are given. Drug therapy may include a cholinergic agent, which helps control the episodes of reflux by strengthening the LES. Smoking is discouraged because it aggravates heartburn. Because gravity plays a role in hiatal hernia, the patient is advised to avoid lying down for 4 hours after a meal; elevating the head of the bed on blocks also helps.

If these measures fail to provide symptom relief or if the hernia becomes strangulated, surgical repair of the hiatus is the treatment of choice. Patients may also undergo a Nissen fundoplication (Fig. 8.15B) procedure to correct the problem.

Prognosis

Compliance with conservative measures may result in the control of symptoms. Should complications occur, antireflux surgical repair may be required.

Prevention

Prevention is not possible when the condition results from congenital weakness or aging.

Patient Teaching

Encourage the patient to follow the conservative measures listed earlier to control symptoms. Suggest ways to manage obesity and avoid any physical exertion that increases intraabdominal pressure.

Abdominal Hernia

Description

Abdominal hernia is a condition in which an organ protrudes through an abnormal opening in the abdominal wall.

ICD-9-CM Code	553.9 *(Unspecified site)*
ICD-10-CM Code	K46.9 *(Unspecified abdominal hernia without obstruction or gangrene)*
	(K46.0–K46.9 = 3 codes of specificity)

Symptoms and Signs

An abdominal hernia results from a weakness in the muscles and membranes of the abdominal wall that allows an organ or part of an organ to break through the wall (herniate) or protrude. This can occur to an individual of either sex and at any age. The signs and symptoms of abdominal hernias vary with the site and the size of the hernia.

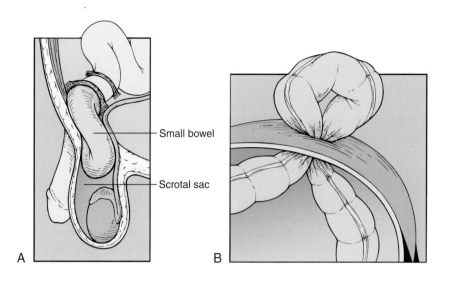

Small bowel

Scrotal sac

A

B

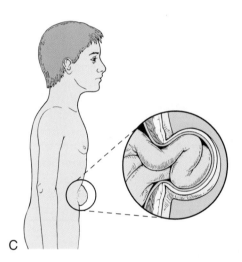

C

• **Fig. 8.27** Abdominal hernias. (A) Inguinal hernia. (B) Strangulated hernia. (C) Umbilical hernia.

The **inguinal** canal is a common site for hernias. A loop of bowel protrudes into the inguinal canal and, in a male, may progress to fill the scrotal sac (Fig. 8.27A). The patient notices a lump or bulge in the inguinal area and may discover that pressing on the hernia to push it back into the abdomen can reduce it. A sharp pain in the groin is continuous or made worse when standing or straining.

Complaints of severe pain usually indicate the hernia may be trapped or strangulated (see Fig. 8.27B). This means that the blood flow to the herniated organ or bowel has been stopped, and gangrene, a serious condition, can set in. The umbilicus is another common site of herniation (see Fig. 8.27C), as are surgical incisions.

Patient Screening

A patient complaining of extreme pain and an unusual lump or bulge in these areas needs to be scheduled as soon as possible. In children, the hernia may be noticed if the child is upset or crying.

Etiology

An abdominal hernia begins when an abnormal opening develops in a weak area or when a congenital malformation exists in the containing structures of the abdominal cavity. Trauma or increased intraabdominal pressure resulting from heavy lifting or pregnancy also can cause a hernia. A hernia occasionally develops near the weakened site of a previous surgical scar.

Diagnosis

A visible hernia can be assessed by palpation for size, with the patient standing or supine. The physician or health care provider listens for bowel sounds. An inguinal hernia can be detected in the male by asking him to perform the Valsalva maneuver. The medical assessment also might include radiographic studies of the abdomen and WBC count.

Treatment

Therapeutic measures vary with the type of hernia and are dependent on the age and physical condition of the patient. If the hernia is uncomplicated and the hernial sac can be reduced back into the abdominal cavity, the patient can wear a device called a *truss*. If this measure keeps the patient comfortable and there are no signs of strangulation, surgical intervention may be avoided. Surgical repair of the hernia (herniorrhaphy) is the treatment of choice in children and healthy adults.

Prognosis

In uncomplicated cases, the prognosis is good. An incarcerated or strangulated hernia requires prompt surgical repair and a variable postoperative recovery time.

Prevention

When the patient has a known weakness in the abdominal wall, heavy lifting and trauma should be avoided. Coughing may contribute to hernias. Encourage patients to stop smoking.

Patient Teaching

Provide patient education on how to apply a truss, which is a device that is often recommended to reduce a hernia. Discuss any activity restrictions or permissions. When surgical repair (herniorrhaphy) is planned, review the preoperative and postoperative procedures, and discuss the warning signs of complications.

Crohn's Disease (Regional Enteritis)

Description

Crohn's disease is a chronic inflammatory disorder of the GI tract that affects up to 480,000 persons in the United States. It is also called *regional enteritis*.

ICD-10-CM Code	K50.90 *(Crohn's disease, unspecified, without complications)* (K50.00–K50.919 = 28 codes of specificity)

Symptoms and Signs

Crohn's disease is a chronic inflammatory disorder of the alimentary canal in which all layers of the bowel wall are edematous and inflamed (Fig. 8.28). Any portion of the GI tract from the mouth to the anus can be affected. Patients with Crohn's disease may have chronic diarrhea or crampy, intermittent abdominal pain, often in the right lower quadrant of the abdomen. They may also experience weight loss, malaise, nausea, anorexia, fever, and abdominal fullness. If obstruction develops, patients have symptoms of an acute abdomen. The abdomen is tender and distended, and patients may vomit, and there may be blood in the stools. However, symptoms of Crohn's disease are often insidious. Patients may have intermittent symptoms, with varying periods of remission. Over time, symptomatic periods may increase in frequency and severity. If the condition is chronic, signs and symptoms of malnutrition begin to manifest; perianal *fissures* and fistulas usually develop. Complications associated with chronic inflammation include deep ulcerations, symptoms of bowel obstruction, adhesions, and abscesses. Symptoms may mimic those of small intestine bacterial overgrowth. In this condition, abdominal pain, bloating, and diarrhea result from an abnormally high level of normal small-intestinal bacteria. After treatment, relapse may occur, with symptoms reemerging.

Patient Screening

The acute symptoms of Crohn's disease can mimic those of appendicitis and require prompt medical investigation.

Etiology

The cause remains unknown despite major research endeavors. Immunologic factors play a role; autoimmune factors, allergies, and genetic causes have also been investigated. There is a familial tendency.

• **Fig. 8.28** Gross pathology of Crohn's disease. (A) Small-intestinal stricture. (B) Linear mucosal ulcers and thickened intestinal wall. (C) Creeping fat. (From Kumar V, et al: *Robbins basic pathology*, ed 10, Philadelphia, 2018, Saunders.)

Sigmoid colon

• **Fig. 8.29** Colonoscopy. A lighted fiberoptic endoscope is inserted through the anus to allow direct examination of the colon. This method is useful in differential diagnosis of bowel disease to obtain a biopsy and in minor surgery, such as polypectomy.

Diagnosis

Diagnosis is based on symptoms, radiographic studies of the small and large intestines, colonoscopy (Fig. 8.29), and enteroscopy. The small intestine can be visualized with an endoscope or a pill-sized camera which transmits images as the pill travels throughout the gastrointestinal system. Radiographs reveal the diseased segments (strictures) separated by normal bowel in a characteristic distribution called *skip lesions*. Direct examination with endoscopy shows characteristic ulcerations; biopsy confirms the diagnosis. Anemia, leukocytosis, and hypoalbuminemia may be detected in blood tests. Electrolyte abnormalities reflect the severity of diarrhea. CT may help identify abscesses and other complications. The differential diagnosis includes also small bowel obstruction, ulcerative colitis, irritable bowel syndrome (IBS), malabsorption syndromes, infectious or ischemic colitis, neoplasia, hemorrhoids, and diverticular disease.

Treatment

Crohn's disease is considered a medically incurable condition. Therapy has two goals: to treat acute disease flare-ups and to maintain remission. General medical management includes nutritional support and control of symptoms by controlling inflammation. The patient may require dietary supplements of vitamins, minerals, protein, and calories. In cases of severe and prolonged bouts of diarrhea, IV nutrition may be necessary to avoid dehydration and electrolyte imbalance. Medication therapy is determined by the phase of the disease: acute or chronic. Acute therapy may include antibiotics or steroids. Chronic therapy may include azathioprine, methotrexate, infliximab, adalimumab, certolizumab, or natalizumab. Drug therapy with anticholinergics and narcotic agents relieves cramping and diarrhea, but its use should be limited. If the disease is complicated by infection, the physician prescribes antibiotics. Mesalamine is an effective agent for mild infections. Corticosteroid therapy controls inflammation, but duration of use should be limited because of side effects.

Immunosuppressive drugs are also used to decrease underlying inflammation and promote healing. Administration of antibodies to tumor necrosis factor (TNF) is effective and used in moderate to severe cases. When there is blood loss, attempts are made to detect the site of bleeding. If bowel obstruction, uncontrolled GI hemorrhage, or perforation develops, surgery to remove the affected portion of the intestine may be indicated. Abscesses can be drained by the placement of a percutaneous catheter. Poorly controlled disease or strictures may require surgical resection.

Prognosis

Crohn's disease has a high rate of recurrence and requires continuous treatment. The course of the disease varies. High stress levels cause exacerbations as a result of changes in the body's hormone balance as a reaction to stress. A slightly increased risk for colon cancer exists, possibly because of constant inflammatory injury to the GI tract.

Prevention

Because the cause is uncertain, prevention is directed toward avoiding complications, with careful monitoring of the patient.

Patient Teaching

The clinician is challenged to address the many physical and psychological implications of this type of chronic disease. Teaching includes compliance with medications to prevent the progression of the disease, good nutrition, a diet that is tolerated, lifestyle modifications, and coping with altered body image. Educate the patient that signs of intestinal bleeding or fever associated with increased abdominal tenderness must be reported to the physician. Because this disease is chronic in nature, patients may benefit from counseling, participation in a support group, and physical rest. Low-impact exercise programs also have been shown to improve patients' quality of life. Websites with accurate patient information may also be helpful in patient teaching.

Ulcerative Colitis

Description

Ulcerative colitis is a chronic inflammatory bowel disease (IBD) affecting the mucosa and submucosa of the rectum and colon (Fig. 8.30A and B).

ICD-10-CM Code	K51.90 *(Ulcerative colitis, unspecified, without complications)* (K51.00–K51.919 = 49 codes of specificity)

Symptoms and Signs

Ulcerative colitis, a common cause of serious bowel disease, does not discriminate for age or gender but usually occurs between ages 15 and 30 years, and less frequently between ages 50 and 70 years. A higher incidence of ulcerative colitis is seen in white people and those of Jewish descent. The symptoms result from a chronic, diffuse, continuous inflammation of the mucosa of the rectum and colon. The patient reports intermittent episodes of bloody diarrhea, abdominal cramping, urgency to defecate, and mucoid stools. As the disease progresses, the stools become looser and more frequent (10–20 per day), with cramping and rectal pressure; the patient also experiences weight loss, fever, and malaise. Some patients report tenesmus, which is mistaken for constipation. The watery stools contain blood, mucus, and pus resulting from mucosal ulceration of the bowel. If the disease is fulminant, major complications result from severe diarrhea, massive bleeding, and perforation.

Patient Screening

The hallmark sign is frequent and bloody diarrhea. A prompt evaluation by a physician or health care provider is warranted.

Etiology

The cause is unknown. Current thinking suggests an association with autoimmune response. Having a family member with ulcerative colitis increases the risk of developing the condition, which also supports a genetic relationship to the disorder.

Diagnosis

The diagnosis is based on the clinical symptoms, examination of the stool for blood, and laboratory values. Findings could include a reduced Hgb level and leukocytosis. Electrolyte abnormalities may be noted when the diarrhea is severe. Stool cultures are needed to rule out pathogenic bacteria or parasites. Barium enema studies and colonoscopy are performed to confirm the diagnosis. Colonoscopy with biopsy shows typical inflammatory changes in the mucosa.

Treatment

The patient is encouraged to consume a well-balanced diet devoid of foods that are irritating to the stomach. The goal of drug therapy is to induce and maintain remission and to improve the quality of life for people with ulcerative colitis. Anticholinergic drugs and occasionally antidiarrheal agents are prescribed. Mesalamine and sulfasalazine are used for mild to moderate cases. Corticosteroid therapy is used in more severe cases, but the duration is limited because of side effects. Anti-TNF medications such as adalimumab (Humira) is effective in severe disease. Surgical removal of the diseased colon is indicated for severe hemorrhage or perforation. Surgery to remove the colon and rectum, known as *proctocolectomy*, is followed by ileostomy or ileoanal anastomosis. The patient is examined annually because chronic ulcerative colitis is associated with an increased risk of colon cancer.

Prognosis

The severity varies from mild to severe. The risk for colon cancer increases with the duration of the disease and how much the colon has been damaged.

Prevention

As in other types of IBDs, the etiology may be uncertain. The medical approach is to prevent and manage recurrent attacks and complications.

• **Fig. 8.30** Ulcerative colitis, endoscopic appearance. (A) The entire colonic mucosa is inflamed, friable, and granular with obvious exudate and bleeding. (B) Transition zone with erythematous mucosa (left) transitioning to normal appearing colon (right). (From McIntire S, et al: *Zitelli and Davis' Atlas of pediatric physical diagnosis*, ed 8, 2023, Elsevier.)

Patient Teaching

A multidisciplinary health care team approach is important to address multiple aspects of care. During an acute phase, encourage the patient to identify emotional or physical stressors. Discuss the results that the patient can expect from the prescribed regimen of diet, rest, and medication. Advise patients regarding dehydration and GI bleeding. Uncontrolled disease, despite maximal medical therapy, requires surgical intervention.

Gastroenteritis

Description

Gastroenteritis is a general term for acute inflammation of the lining of the stomach and intestines.

ICD-10-CM Code	K52.89 *(Other specified noninfective gastroenteritis and colitis)* K52.9 *(Noninfective gastroenteritis and colitis, unspecified)* (K52.0–K52.9 = 7 codes of specificity)

Symptoms and Signs

The patient experiences increased intestinal motility, sometimes with mucus, pus, and blood in the stool. The body may lose fluids too rapidly, causing dehydration with a disturbance in the body's electrolyte balance.

A common syndrome of gastroenteritis called *traveler's diarrhea* is characterized by varying degrees of anorexia, abdominal cramping, frequent loose stools, nausea, and profuse vomiting. The same symptoms occur with viral gastroenteritis, which is referred to as *stomach flu*; food or chemical poisoning; allergic reactions to food; and some drug reactions.

Patient Screening

Weakness, dizziness, reduced urine output, and mental confusion are indications of dehydration. A patient who experiences acute vomiting and hematemesis or reports ingestion of a poisonous or corrosive agent should be treated as a medical emergency.

Etiology

Ingestion of disease-causing bacteria or parasites from contaminated food or water is the primary cause of traveler's diarrhea, whereas viral gastroenteritis is the result of a virus. Some bacteria produce toxins in food that cause food poisoning when ingested (see the Food Poisoning section). Ingestion of the poison in certain foods (e.g., poisonous mushrooms) or chemicals (e.g., arsenic) causes gastroenteritis. Other causes are chronic ingestion of spicy or irritating food, alcohol, caffeine, aspirin, and antiinflammatory agents. Gastroenteritis may be a complication of acute illness.

Diagnosis

The first important step in identifying the cause is to consider the medical history. Laboratory analysis and culture of the stool reveal the signs and the actual causes of infection or poisoning. The stool is inspected by microscopy for leukocytes, erythrocytes, and ova and parasites (O&P). The clinical evaluation includes blood studies for causative organisms, the presence of antibodies, abnormal blood cell counts, and serum electrolyte values. Endoscopy may also be indicated.

Treatment

The treatment varies with the cause, the severity of the disease, and the age and general health of the patient. Children, older adults, and the chronically ill are most vulnerable to serious complications from electrolyte imbalance resulting from dehydration.

The goal of treatment is to control symptoms and to maintain a normal fluid and electrolyte balance. Direct management of the cause as diagnosed accomplishes this; the subsequent treatment includes the use of antiemetics, antibiotics, antacids, and either oral or IV rehydration solutions. The patient should rest and eat as tolerated. Antidiarrheal agents should not be used for the treatment of traveler's diarrhea because they delay the body's elimination of the offending organisms, thus increasing the duration of symptoms.

Prognosis

Simple gastroenteritis is self-limiting.

Prevention

Education directed at eliminating the cause helps prevent recurrences. Excellent preventive measures for the most common causes of gastroenteritis include frequent and thorough hand washing and avoidance of food that has not been well refrigerated and well cooked.

Patient Teaching

Teach infection control measures. Advise the patient that when traveling, well-cooked foods, rather than raw foods, and purified bottled water should be consumed.

Intestinal Obstruction

Description

Intestinal obstruction is a mechanical or functional blockage of the intestines.

ICD-10-CM Code	K56.60 *(Unspecified intestinal obstruction)* (K56.60–K56.69 = 2 codes of specificity)

Mechanical obstructions of the intestines are coded according to the nature of the obstruction. Refer to the physician's diagnosis and then to the current edition of the ICD-10-CM coding manual to ensure the greatest specificity.

Symptoms and Signs

Intestinal obstruction occurs when the contents of the intestine cannot move forward because of a partial or complete blockage of the bowel. Although the cause and nature of the obstruction can vary, the patient's discomfort and the signs of blockage are characteristic and include severe pain, nausea, vomiting, and a bloated and painful abdomen without the passage of stool or gas. Symptoms also include an electrolyte imbalance and an elevated WBC count. The bowel sounds can be hyperactive or absent, depending on the nature of the obstruction. This condition is more common in middle-aged and older people but can also occur in all age groups.

Patient Screening
The level of intestinal obstruction dictates the severity of the symptoms. A sudden increase in symptoms or an acute onset of symptoms requires urgent medical care.

Etiology
Mechanical blockage of the bowel narrows the normal lumen and prevents the flow of intestinal contents. Mechanical causes of intestinal obstruction are many and include:
- Neoplasm (benign or malignant)
- Foreign bodies
- Fecal impaction
- Strictures, from Crohn's disease
- Compression of the bowel
- Volvulus (a twisting of the bowel on itself) (Fig. 8.31)
- Intussusception (in which the bowel telescopes into itself; see Fig. 8.31)
- Strangulated hernia (see Fig. 8.31)
- Adhesions that form tight bands of scar tissue on the bowel (see Fig. 8.31)

In some cases of mechanical obstruction, the blood supply to the affected area of the intestine is blocked, resulting in tissue death, which leads to perforation and peritonitis from intestinal contents being outside the intestine. This becomes a toxic condition that endangers the patient.

A paralytic condition of the small bowel, called *ileus*, can occur after abdominal surgery when peristalsis and bowel sounds are absent. Normal peristalsis also can be inhibited by the use of certain medications (e.g., codeine and aluminum-containing antacids) or disease conditions, such as peritonitis. The motility of the bowel often returns spontaneously.

Diagnosis
Radiographic studies of the abdomen show the point of obstruction of the bowel. CBC shows an elevated WBC count; the patient also has electrolyte imbalances and acid-base disturbances.

Treatment
When the obstruction is mechanical and does not resolve with conservative measures, surgery is performed to remove the cause of the blockage. If necessary, the diseased bowel is resected. An ostomy may be needed. A second surgical procedure is often required to reverse the ostomy and rejoin the bowel. When this is not possible, the patient retains a permanent ostomy.

In a nonmechanical or functional obstruction (ileus), the patient is not given anything by mouth and is fed intravenously until peristalsis has returned. A nasogastric tube is

Herniation

Adhesions

Intussusception

Volvulus

• **Fig. 8.31** Schematic of intestinal obstructions. (From Cotran R, et al: *Robbins pathologic basis of disease*, ed 6, Philadelphia, 1999, Saunders.)

inserted to relieve distention and vomiting of gastric juices. The gastric juices come out of the stomach through a tube which leads to a collection container. Surgery is not usually indicated for a functional obstruction. In cases of fecal impaction, manual disimpaction or enemas are used in treatment.

Prognosis
The prognosis generally is good for mechanical obstructive bowel conditions treated promptly. The outcome, however, is guarded with malignant tumors.

Prevention
Screening tests for colorectal cancer permit early detection and treatment of malignant tumors of the colon. Laxative therapy, especially for older adults or bedridden persons, helps prevent fecal impaction.

Patient Teaching
Review the physician's explanations, and discuss any anticipated surgical procedure or need for nasogastric tube. Ensure that the patient has a list of signs and symptoms that need to be reported to a doctor, such as any change in bowel habits or sign of GI bleeding. Review any diet restrictions, and urge adequate fluid intake. Obtain referrals for home health care, as needed and instructions for ostomy care when appropriate.

Diverticulosis (Diverticular Disease)

Description
Diverticulosis is a progressive condition, common with age, characterized by defects in the muscular wall of the large bowel (Fig. 8.32).

ICD-10-CM Code	K57.30 *(Diverticulosis of large intestine without perforation or abscess without bleeding)*
	K57.31 *(Diverticulosis of large intestine without perforation or abscess with bleeding)*
	(K57.30–K57.93 = 16 codes of specificity)

Symptoms and Signs
Diverticulosis is a condition in which outpouches (diverticula) of the mucosa penetrate the weak points in the muscular layer of the large intestine. Colonic diverticula may vary in size, from a few millimeters to several centimeters, and in number, from one to several dozen. Diverticulosis occurs particularly in the distal part of the colon, the sigmoid colon, because intraluminal pressures are higher in this region (see Fig. 8.32). Diverticulosis usually causes no symptoms or inflammation. Occasionally the patient reports nonspecific abdominal distress, such as pain and flatulence, and difficulty in defecation. The patient may

• **Fig. 8.32** Sigmoid diverticular disease. (A) Endoscopic view of two sigmoid diverticula. Compare with B. (B) Gross examination of a resected sigmoid colon shows regularly spaced stool-filled diverticula. (C) Cross-section showing the outpouching of mucosa beneath the muscularis propria. (D) Low-power photomicrograph of a sigmoid diverticulum showing protrusion of the mucosa and submucosa through the muscularis propria. (Endoscopic image Courtesy Dr. Ira Hanan, The University of Chicago, Chicago, Illinois.)

experience alternating constipation and diarrhea and even blood in the stool.

Patient Screening
Vague symptoms of intermittent abdominal pain and constipation are typical. Schedule a consultation with the health care provider.

Etiology
The causes are not clear. A diet that contains inadequate roughage and excessive amounts of highly refined food is thought to contribute to diverticulosis. Lack of roughage produces small-caliber, drier stools, which fail to distend the bowel lumen. The small volume of stool causes higher intraluminal pressure during peristalsis and defecation, which, in turn, contributes to the small herniations or pouches through the mucosa of the muscular wall of the intestine. Colonic diverticulosis increases with age.

Diagnosis

Diagnosis is based on the clinical picture and an air-contrast barium enema radiographic study or colonoscopy.

Treatment

A diet that includes adequate fluids and roughage is indicated to produce soft, formed stools daily. Fiber supplements and stool softeners are helpful.

Prognosis

The prognosis is positive unless the condition progresses to diverticulitis.

Prevention

Adequate hydration and a high-fiber diet rich in fruits and vegetables help prevent constipation and straining during defecation which may decrease risks.

Patient Teaching

Instruct the patient to follow the preventive measures mentioned earlier. Inform the patient to report rectal bleeding or symptoms of colon obstruction to the physician.

Diverticulitis

Description

Diverticulitis is an infection of one or more diverticula.

ICD-10-CM Code	K57.32 (Diverticulitis of large intestine without perforation or abscess without bleeding)
	K57.33 (Diverticulitis of large intestine without perforation or abscess with bleeding)

Symptoms and Signs

When fecal matter becomes trapped in one or more diverticula, inflammation and infection can ensue, causing diverticulitis (see Fig. 8.32C). The patient has abdominal pain or tenderness, usually in the left lower quadrant. The patient may or may not have a fever. A palpable mass may be felt, and the patient reports changes in bowel function. Constipation or loose stools may present. The pain sometimes appears in the right lower quadrant or in the suprapubic area. Blood in the stools indicates small hemorrhages. Perforation into the abdominal cavity can produce symptoms of peritonitis, intestinal obstruction, and sepsis. Recurrent diverticulitis can cause complications, such as the formation of adhesions, abscesses, and fistulas. Fistula formation may involve the bladder, ureter, vagina, uterus, bowel, and abdominal wall.

Patient Screening

A patient previously diagnosed with diverticulitis can develop acute symptoms that require prompt medical attention. Warning signs may include persistent abdominal pain, fever, and changes in bowel habits. Because diverticulitis carries the risk of bowel perforation and peritonitis, the condition may progress to a medical emergency.

Etiology

Diverticulitis, which is not nearly as common as diverticulosis, can develop when one or more diverticula become inflamed and infected. Lack of dietary bulk, inadequate fluid intake, and constipation are thought to contribute. Fecal plugs in the diverticula can predispose patients to infection of the diverticula by colonic bacteria.

Diagnosis

The patient is assessed through history and physical examination with attention to signs of inflammation at the location of the patient's symptoms, usually pain or tenderness. Blood tests may show leukocytosis, low Hgb level, and low Hct. CT will confirm the diagnosis. Colonoscopy or barium enema should not be performed in acute diverticulitis but can be helpful after treatment with antibiotics.

Treatment

Antibiotics may be prescribed for infection. Stool softeners may be indicated, and a liquid diet is often encouraged. If the symptoms are severe or if the bowel is perforated, hospitalization is indicated. Surgical intervention to remove the diseased portion of the colon may be necessary. Small perforations can be treated without surgery with IV antibiotics, nutritional support, and percutaneous drainage if an abscess develops.

Prognosis

In mild cases, the disease is self-limiting. Recovery becomes more complicated when surgery is required or an abscess is present, but the final outcome is usually favorable. Diverticulitis recurs in one-third of patients treated with medical management. Multiple recurrent attacks warrant elective surgical resection, which carries lower morbidity and mortality risks compared with emergency surgery.

Prevention

Regular elimination of soft-formed stools is recommended, especially in a patient with diverticulosis.

Patient Teaching

Explain diverticulosis, the underlying contributing condition. Surgical patients who have had a colon resection need to understand the progression to a normal diet and the schedule for antibiotic therapy. Those who have had a colon resection with a diverting colostomy can be referred to an enterostomy nurse for ostomy care and education (Fig. 8.33). Assess for signs of depression after surgery.

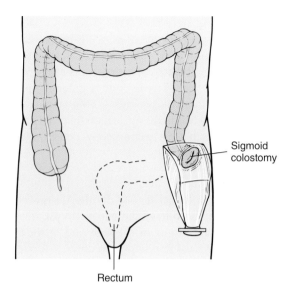

Sigmoid
colostomy

Rectum

• **Fig. 8.33** Colostomy. Colostomy is a surgical procedure that creates an opening for feces to pass through the abdominal wall. The opening in the colon is brought to the surface of the skin to divert feces into an external pouch worn by the patient. The colostomy may be **temporary to** promote healing or permanent if the distal bowel has been removed because of malignancy or other disease.

• **Fig. 8.34** Adenocarcinoma of distal rectum. (From Doughty DB, Jackson DB: Gastrointestinal disorders—Mosby's clinical nursing series, St. Louis, 1993, Mosby.)

Colorectal Cancer

Description

Colorectal cancer is a cancer that arises in any part of the colon or the rectum (Fig. 8.34). According to the American Cancer Society, it is the third most common site in new cases of cancer and the third most common cause of cancer death.

ICD-10-CM Code	C19 *(Malignant neoplasm of rectosigmoid junction)*

Colorectal cancer is coded according to the site of the lesion. Refer to the physician's diagnosis and then to the current edition of the ICD-10-CM coding manual to ensure the greatest specificity.

• **Fig. 8.35** Abdominal bloating in ascites. (From Swartz MH: *Textbook of physical diagnosis*, ed 6, Philadelphia, 2010, Saunders.)

Symptoms and Signs

Although symptoms in the early stages are often vague and nonspecific, most patients with colorectal cancer have one or more of the following symptoms at presentation: abdominal pain, change in bowel habits (diarrhea, constipation), bloody stools, weakness, weight loss, or symptoms related to iron deficiency anemia. Colon cancer should be considered in any older patient who develops iron deficiency anemia or stool positive for occult blood. Later symptoms include abdominal distention, pallor, **ascites** (Fig. 8.35), cachexia, lymphadenopathy, and **hepatomegaly**.

Patient Screening

Follow office policy for referrals and follow-up appointments.

Etiology

The risk of developing colon cancer increases with age. Greater than 90% of cases occur after age 50 years. The rare genetic disorders of familial adenomatous polyposis and hereditary nonpolyposis colorectal cancer predispose affected individuals to the early development of colorectal cancer. Risk factors also include a history of large adenomatous polyps, diabetes mellitus, ulcerative colitis, or Crohn's disease; a first-degree relative with colorectal cancer; cigarette smoking; and obesity. Several dietary factors may be protective against colorectal cancer, such as a higher intake of fruits and vegetables. Aspirin and NSAIDs may also offer a protective effect. The highest incidences are in Western Europe and North America, possibly because of the higher average dietary fat intake in those living in countries of these regions.

Adenomatous polyps of the colon are the precursor lesion of colorectal cancer. Adenomas are composed of dysplastic epithelium that has proliferated to form a mass. Most colorectal carcinomas arise from adenomas over an average time frame of 7 to 10 years. Most adenomas, however, do not develop into carcinoma.

Diagnosis

Many early-stage cases of colorectal cancer are detected with prevention screening tests, such as colonoscopy or the fecal occult blood test, along with a double-contrast barium enema. Colonoscopy is the best test to use in symptomatic patients and for screening because it allows the physician to visualize, sample, and remove lesions throughout the colon. The differential diagnosis of a colonic mass includes many benign and malignant disorders, so histologic evaluation is necessary for the diagnosis of cancer.

Although several staging systems have been proposed for colorectal cancer, physicians now prefer to use the TNM classification system proposed by the AJCC. In the case of colorectal cancer, however, "T" reflects the depth of penetration by the tumor into or through the bowel wall rather than the size of the lesion. Clinical staging is determined through physical examination and CT of the chest, abdomen, and pelvis. For rectal cancers, EUS may also be performed. The level of carcinoembryonic antigen (CEA) can be obtained for postoperative follow-up purposes but should not be used for screening or diagnosis of colorectal cancer. The most common sites for distant metastases are the liver and lungs.

Treatment
Surgical resection of the affected part of the colon or rectum and any affected lymph nodes is the mainstay of treatment. A colostomy may be indicated should surgical intervention be unable to reconnect the parts of the colon (see Fig. 8.33). Locally advanced colon cancer is treated with chemotherapy. Radiation therapy can be helpful if the cancer is confined to the rectum. Although treatment for metastatic colorectal cancer is still aimed at palliation of symptoms, advances have been made in the use of chemotherapy that can prolong overall survival. Metastatic colon cancer can also be treated with surgery if the metastatic tumor (usually in the liver) can be removed as well.

Prognosis
The pathologic stage at diagnosis remains the best prognostic indicator. In addition, patients with preoperative serum levels of CEA greater than 5 ng/mL have a worse prognosis, stage for stage, compared with those with lower levels. Elevated CEA levels that do not become normal after surgery indicate persistent disease. The survival rate for rectal cancer is a little lower than that for colon cancer.

Prevention
Relatively simple improvements in nutrition and physical activity and the use of available screening procedures may help prevent many cases of colorectal cancer and resulting deaths. A diet high in fruits and vegetables, regular exercise, and maintenance of a healthy weight reduce the risk of colorectal cancer. Screening for colorectal cancer has two functions: It enables the discovery and removal of adenomas to prevent the incidence of cancer, and it detects cancer in the earlier, more curable stages. First, the patient's relative risk of developing colorectal cancer must be determined. A person is considered to be at high risk for colorectal cancer if he or she has hereditary nonpolyposis

colon cancer, familial adenomatous polyposis, a previous history of colon cancer or polyps, a history of IBD, or a first-degree relative with colorectal cancer or adenoma. People at average risk for colorectal cancer are urged to start screening at age 45 years with a colonoscopy then every 10 years. High-risk patients should start screening by age 40 years. Health care providers may recommend high-risk patients have a colonoscopy every 5 years in some cases.

Patient Teaching
Assess the patient's knowledge of the disease process and the medical plan. Encourage the patient to ask questions and discuss any anxiety he or she feels and provide emotional support. Discuss tests and procedures, side effects of surgery, chemotherapy, or intraoperative radiation therapy, and potential complications as applicable. Explain familial tendencies and relay that members of the family may need screening as deemed appropriate by their health care provider.

Pseudomembranous Enterocolitis
Description
Pseudomembranous enterocolitis is acute inflammation with a plaque-like necrotic debris and mucus adhered to the damaged superficial mucosa of the small and large intestines.

ICD-10-CM Code	A04.7 *(Enterocolitis due to Clostridioides difficile)* (A04.0-A04.9 = 10 codes of specificity)

Symptoms and Signs
Enterocolitis, in which bowel mucosa has a membranous appearance, is a disease marked by mild to severe greenish, foul-smelling watery diarrhea (up to 30 stools per day). The patient may have a fever and weakness and report abdominal cramping and tenderness. Some patients experience nausea and vomiting. A patient with severe diarrhea will exhibit signs of dehydration, including dry mouth, lightheadedness, and dizziness. The urine is concentrated, and the skin displays decreased *turgor*. Irritation develops around the anal area as a result of frequent and watery stools; fecal incontinence can be a problem. Blood and mucus in stools may be reported.

Patient Screening
A patient who has been on antibiotics during the preceding 6 weeks, is currently on antibiotics, has a history of long-term use of PPIs, and complains of sudden onset of copious watery diarrhea, abdominal pain, and fever should seek the advice of the physician who prescribed the antibiotics.

Etiology
Pseudomembranous enterocolitis often is related to the use of broad-spectrum antibiotics; the patient either is taking the antibiotics or has been undergoing antibiotic therapy

• **Fig. 8.36** Pseudomembranous colitis. (From Kumar V, et al: Robbins basic pathology, ed 8, Philadelphia, 2008, Saunders.)

during the previous 6 weeks. Although almost all antibiotics have been implicated, colitis most commonly develops after the use of ampicillin, clindamycin, third-generation cephalosporins, and fluoroquinolones. Changes in the natural intestinal flora from antibiotics or chemotherapy drugs allow the development of a bacterial infection with *Clostridioides difficile*. This organism, a cytotoxic-producing strain of a normal gut organism, produces powerful toxins that cause the bowel wall to become inflamed, ulcerated, and necrotic (Fig. 8.36). The products of inflammation and dead tissue form a coating that is called a *pseudomembrane*. Pseudomembranous enterocolitis is more common in health care facilities, including skilled nursing facilities, where fecal contamination is more likely. Hospitalized patients are most at risk, especially those who are severely ill, malnourished, or receiving chemotherapy. Most infections occur as a result of fecal-oral transmission. Those who have had abdominal surgery and those older than age 65 years of age are more susceptible. Asymptomatic patients with colonization by *C. difficile* can be a source of contamination. Long-term use of PPIs increases the risk of *C. difficile* infections. An even more aggressive form, which is more difficult to manage, has been identified and is not associated with antibiotic use in some individuals.

Diagnosis

Pseudomembranous enterocolitis is diagnosed when *C. difficile* toxin is found in the stool or rectal biopsy confirms pseudomembranous enterocolitis. The WBC count is elevated as a result of the immune response to the infection. In severe cases, blood protein (serum albumin) levels are reduced, the serum electrolyte levels are abnormal; abdominal radiographs may show a distended colon.

Treatment

Treatment is initiated by discontinuing the broad-spectrum antibiotic and substituting it with metronidazole or vancomycin to fight the infection. Cholestyramine (Questran) may be given to bind the toxins produced by the causative bacteria.

Fecal transplantation is also called fecal microbiota transplantation, stool transplant, fecal bacteriotherapy or intestinal microbiota transplant is another treatment method for patients who have recurrent infections. Healthy bacteria from a screened donor is introduced into the colon of the patient. The donor stool may be taken from a family member and introduced through colonoscopy or through endoscopy.

The general management of the patient includes monitoring the fluid and electrolyte balance, with oral or IV supplements as needed. Careful hand washing with antibacterial soap and water, using gloves with all patient interaction, isolation, and decontamination measures are encouraged to prevent cross-infection.

Prognosis

Some cases may require more than one course of autoinfection therapy, however treatment is successful in most cases.

Prevention

Prevention includes infection control in health care facilities and caution in prescribing broad-spectrum antibiotics to patients who have had abdominal surgery. *C. difficile* bacteria and spores are easily transmitted from infected patients to the hands of health care workers, and the spores are hard to kill. All health care providers should be educated about the precautions to avoid transmitting *C. difficile* to other patients. Public swimming pools can be a source of bacteria, but well-maintained pools with appropriate levels of chemicals pose lower risks than other swimming options.

Patient Teaching

It is important to note that alcohol-based hand sanitizers are ineffective against *C. difficile*. Thorough hand washing with soap and water is stressed. Additionally, inform the patient with pseudomembranous enterocolitis that drugs that slow peristalsis are contraindicated. Patients should not swim in public pools until they are completely well.

Short Bowel Syndrome

Description

In short bowel syndrome, the small bowel fails to absorb nutrients because of an inadequate absorptive surface.

ICD-10-CM Code	K91.2 *(Postsurgical malabsorption, not elsewhere classified)*

Symptoms and Signs

Short bowel syndrome is the result of an insufficient amount of functioning small bowel to absorb the nutrients, fluids, vitamins, and minerals that the body needs. Depending on the amount of missing or damaged bowel, significant signs of malnutrition, including pathologic changes in other organs and body systems, are noted. Diarrhea and abnormal stools occur. The patient loses weight and feels weak, tired, and dizzy. As the malnutrition continues, the hair and nails become brittle, and rashes develop.

Patient Screening

After bowel surgery, patients may require frequent follow-up appointments with their physician or health care provider. Nutritional status assessment is a priority.

Etiology

Crohn's disease, intestinal infarction, radiation enteritis, volvulus, tumor resection, and trauma are conditions that may cause extensive resection of the small intestine. This loss of functioning small bowel interferes with the digestion and absorption of needed nutrients. The type and degree of malabsorption depend on the length and site of the resection and the degree of adaptation of the remaining bowel.

Diagnosis

The patient history initially may indicate the presence of bowel disease, with or without surgical intervention that has reduced the length or function of part of the small bowel. In short bowel syndrome, the results of blood tests reflect abnormal electrolyte levels, pH disturbance, and anemia. Stool studies show an increased amount of fat.

Treatment

The treatment plan depends on the cause of the syndrome and the particular manifestations of malnutrition. Medical management includes prescription drugs for infection, diarrhea, vitamin and mineral deficiency, and pain, as required. Food supplements are administered orally or intravenously, as needed. Surgery may be performed to correct the underlying condition or to reconstruct the bowel. Postoperative parenteral hyperalimentation is required for weeks or until the remaining gut adapts and becomes functional, at which time oral feeding is gradually introduced.

Prognosis

Many patients recover without difficulties, even with extensive resection, as the remaining bowel adapts to increased nutrient absorption.

Prevention

After surgical resection of the small bowel, the patient is monitored closely for manifestations of malnutrition, dehydration, or weight loss.

Patient Teaching

After surgery, the patient needs nutritional counseling as oral food is gradually reintroduced. Give instructions for controlling diarrhea with the prescribed agents.

Irritable Bowel Syndrome

Description

IBS is a *functional* bowel disorder characterized by chronic abdominal pain or discomfort, bloating, and erratic dysfunction of bowel habits.

ICD-10-CM Code | K58.0 *(Irritable bowel syndrome with diarrhea)*
K58.9 *(Irritable bowel syndrome without diarrhea)*

Symptoms and Signs

Classic symptoms of IBS include episodes of cramping or aching abdominal pain typically relieved by defecation. A key feature of IBS is a change of bowel habits with predominant diarrhea or constipation, or an alternation between the two. Bloating and abdominal distention are commonly experienced, and the patient may complain of tenesmus (a feeling of incomplete or ineffectual straining). Some patients report gastroesophageal reflux, nausea, and the feeling of a lump in the throat.

Patient Screening

A patient requesting an appointment for recurrent abdominal pain and changes in bowel habits should be seen as soon as possible by a physician or a health care provider.

Etiology

The exact cause of IBS is unknown. The incidence of developing IBS increases after acute GI infection; this may suggest an immune or neuroimmune contribution. Many patients report other chronic pain disorders, such as fibromyalgia, lactose intolerance, back pain, urinary symptoms, anxiety, and depression. In the United States IBS is diagnosed more frequently in female patients. Stressful events may precipitate the onset of symptoms.

Diagnosis

A positive clinical diagnosis of IBS begins with history, physical examination, and tests to exclude organic disease. The diagnosis depends largely on physical symptoms based on abnormal GI motility. Diagnosis of IBS involves excluding other conditions with similar symptoms, such as parasitic infections, lactose intolerance, Crohn's disease, and other IBDs. Older patients (age >50 years) with recent onset of symptoms require colonoscopy or a double-contrast barium enema with sigmoidoscopy.

Treatment

There is no cure for IBS. There are treatments to relieve and manage symptoms. Treatment is determined according to the type of IBS. Medications may include soluble fiber supplements (e.g., psyllium), stool softeners, and laxatives in constipation-dominant IBS (IBS-C); for diarrhea-dominant IBS (IBS-D), an antidiarrheal medication (e.g., loperamide) may provide relief. Ondansetron has been shown to block 5-hydroxytryptamine (5-HT3) receptors in the gut and may also be used. Antispasmodic drugs (dicyclomine and hyoscyamine) for postprandial pain are available. Tricyclic antidepressants are useful for chronic pain for their anticholinergic effects. The probiotic *Bifidobacterium* has been shown to reduce pain and bloating. Nonabsorbed antibiotics have alleviated the symptoms in some patients with IBS-D. A new class of medications, guanylate cyclase-c agonists (Trulance, Linzess, Amitiza), have shown promise for patients with IBS-C.

A multidisciplinary team approach to the treatment plan, including referral for relaxation therapy, cognitive behavioral therapy, or psychotherapy, may be indicated. Dietary modifications may be included.

Prognosis

IBS does not usually lead to more serious conditions, but it can affect the quality of life of the patient. IBS does not affect life expectancy, and prolonged remissions are possible.

Prevention

Because the exact cause is not known, there is no prevention.

Patient Teaching

Encourage patients to follow specified dietary recommendations and follow the medical therapy prescribed by their health care provider for the best outcome. IBS support group referrals may benefit chronic sufferers.

Peritonitis

Description

Peritonitis, inflammation of the peritoneum, can be acute or chronic and local or generalized.

ICD-10-CM Code	K67 *(Disorders of peritoneum in infectious diseases classified elsewhere)*

Peritonitis is coded by etiology. Refer to the physician's diagnosis and then to the current edition of the ICD-10-CM coding manual to ensure the greatest specificity.

Symptoms and Signs

The large serous membrane that lines the abdominal cavity and folds over the visceral organs is normally transparent and sterile. When it is irritated or infected, the peritoneum becomes *hyperemic* and edematous as fluid accumulates in the peritoneal space. The inflammatory process of peritonitis has the potential to cause abscesses and adhesions to form in the abdominal cavity (Fig. 8.37).

The patient reports abdominal pain, nausea and vomiting, weakness, and profuse sweating. Abdominal pain may be so severe that the patient may prefer not to move. Symptoms include fever, abdominal tenderness, and distention. Occasionally a paralytic ileus is present and the patient may not have bowel movements. Examination of the abdomen reveals tenderness to direct touch and rebound (or percussion), indicating peritoneal inflammation. In a fulminating case of peritonitis, the bacteria or bacterial endotoxins enter the circulation, leading to septicemia, shock, and death.

• **Fig. 8.37** Peritonitis.

Patient Screening

A patient having sudden, severe, and diffuse abdominal pain, fever, weakness, nausea, and vomiting requires emergency medical attention.

Etiology

Peritonitis can occur as a primary infection caused by bloodborne organisms or organisms originating in the GI or genital tract. The infection is considered secondary if the source of infection is contamination by GI secretions resulting from a perforation of the GI tract or intraabdominal organs. For example, bacterial invasion could occur after surgery as a result of a breakdown of anastomoses, allowing contaminated intestinal contents to spill into the abdominal cavity. Causes of secondary bacterial peritonitis include appendicitis, diverticulitis, perforated peptic ulcer, and perforated gallbladder. A penetrating wound to the abdomen is another common cause. Systemic lupus erythematosus also can cause bouts of peritonitis as a result of continuous inflammation.

Noninfective secretions (e.g., bile from a ruptured, inflamed gallbladder) can cause aseptic peritonitis resulting from chemical irritation of the membrane. Eventually there is bacterial invasion. The organisms most often involved include *Escherichia coli, Klebsiella pneumoniae, Enterococcus* species, anaerobic streptococci, and *Pseudomonas aeruginosa*.

Diagnosis

Diagnostic findings include an elevated WBC count, abnormal serum electrolyte levels (e.g., altered levels of sodium, potassium, and chloride), and gaseous distention of the bowel evident on radiographic examination of the abdomen. Radiographic studies or CT may also reveal perforation of an abdominal organ evidenced by air in the abdominal cavity. Aspiration of peritoneal fluid shows cloudy peritoneal fluid and allows for a culture and sensitivity study to identify the causative organism.

Treatment

The clinical manifestations of peritonitis must be assessed and the source of the irritation or infection identified as quickly as possible. The patient is promptly and aggressively treated with broad-spectrum antibiotics, analgesics, and antiemetics. The patient is not given anything by mouth, and fluid and electrolyte losses are replaced parenterally. If there is a perforation, surgery is required to correct the source of infection and to drain the spilled contents.

Prognosis

Without prompt and aggressive medical intervention, including antibiotics, peritonitis is life threatening.

Prevention

Many of the underlying causes are not easily predicted.

Patient Teaching

After the patient has been stabilized with medical interventions, emphasize special instructions about activity, medications, surgical wound care, and follow-up visits.

Hemorrhoids

Description

Hemorrhoids are varicose dilations of a vein in the anal canal or the anorectal area.

ICD-10-CM Code	K64.8 *(Other hemorrhoids)*
	(K64.0–K64.9 = 8 codes of specificity)

The codes vary by the location and complications. Refer to the physician's diagnosis and then to the current edition of the ICD-10-CM coding manual to ensure the greatest specificity.

Symptoms and Signs

Hemorrhoids are tumorlike lesions in the anal area caused by dilated veins; hemorrhoids often are painless. When hemorrhoids are symptomatic, the patient experiences rectal pain, itching, protrusion, or bleeding, especially after defecation. The patient may also experience a mucous discharge from the rectum, a sensation of incomplete evacuation, and difficulty cleaning the anal area. A painful anal lump may indicate thrombosis of an external hemorrhoid that requires medical attention.

Patient Screening

The patient reporting frequent, unrelieved urge to defecate, severe constipation, or bright red rectal bleeding needs a consultation with the physician.

Etiology

The veins in the rectal and anal area become varicose, swollen, and tender as a result of blockage. If they are located within the rectum above the junction of skin and rectal mucosa, these swollen and twisted varicosities are considered internal hemorrhoids; varicosities lower in the anal area covered by skin are considered external hemorrhoids (Fig. 8.38). A large, firm subcutaneous lump indicates thrombosis of the external hemorrhoids. Constipation, straining, pregnancy, and any condition that increases pressure on the veins often exacerbate this condition. Obesity can also put one at higher risk for hemorrhoids.

Diagnosis

The diagnosis is based on visual inspection of the anal area and proctoscopy to visualize internal hemorrhoids of the rectum. The patient's Hgb level and red blood cell (RBC) count may be below normal if the patient has experienced significant bleeding.

Treatment

Conservative treatment consists of measures to correct constipation and prevent straining. Stool softeners and a diet high in fruits, vegetables, and whole-grain cereals are recommended. If the patient is symptomatic, warm sitz baths may be prescribed, along with a topical anesthetic ointment or witch hazel compresses. Products, such as hydrocortisone acetate or pramoxine hydrochloride (ProctoCream-HC), may be applied locally to reduce inflammation. If these measures do not help, sclerotherapy

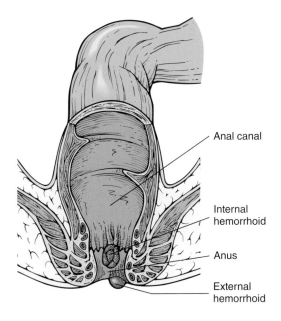

• **Fig. 8.38** Hemorrhoids.

injections may be used to induce scar formation and reduce prolapse. The hemorrhoids can be destroyed by band ligation or by cryosurgery, a procedure that uses a probe to expose the hemorrhoids to extreme cold. Photocoagulation using an infrared device also is effective. Electrocoagulation and thermocoagulation are other alternatives. When bleeding and other symptoms are severe, hemorrhoidectomy is the best treatment. *Stapled hemorrhoidopexy* is sometimes used for internal hemorrhoids but has some risks of infection, recurrence, and rectal prolapse when compared with traditional hemorrhoidectomy.

Prognosis
The procedures used to treat hemorrhoids produce positive outcomes. Complications are uncommon, and recurrences are unusual.

Prevention
To prevent exacerbation of the condition, the patient should avoid constipation, straining during defecation, and heavy lifting. A high-bulk diet is recommended to promote regular bowel habits.

Patient Teaching
Reinforce the preventive measures listed earlier. Encourage adequate fluid intake. Urge good anal hygiene with gentle wiping after stools along with the other comfort measures listed in the Treatment section. Give special consideration during pregnancy to minimize discomfort.

Diseases of the Liver, Biliary Tract, and Pancreas

The liver, gallbladder, and pancreas are accessory digestive organs that introduce digestive hormones and enzymes into the alimentary canal. This ensures that the nutrients critical to life can be absorbed selectively by the small intestines into the bloodstream.

Cirrhosis of the Liver

Description
Cirrhosis of the liver is a chronic degenerative disease that is irreversible. It brings slow deterioration of the liver, resulting in the replacement of normal liver cells with hard, fibrous scar tissue, known as *hobnail liver*.

ICD-10-CM Code	K70.30 *(Alcoholic cirrhosis of liver without ascites)* (K70.30–K70.31 = 2 codes of specificity) K74.0 *(Hepatic fibrosis)* K74.60 *(Unspecified cirrhosis of liver)* K74.69 *(Other cirrhosis of liver)* (K74.0–K74.69 = 8 codes of specificity)

Symptoms and Signs
In the early stages of the disease, the symptoms are vague and mild. As the liver is destroyed, the patient experiences loss of appetite and weight, nausea and vomiting, indigestion, abdominal distention (caused by ascites), and edema. The patient tends to bleed and bruise more easily, and frequent nosebleeds are common. The skin appears *jaundiced* and is dry with pruritus. Small, red, spidery marks (spider nevi) may appear on the face and body. Changes in the endocrine system cause testicular atrophy, gynecomastia, and loss of chest hair in the male (Fig. 8.39).

As the cirrhosis advances, memory is impaired, and confusion and drowsiness occur and intensify. If cirrhosis is left untreated, hepatic failure and death eventually follow.

Patient Screening
The medical history determines the urgency to see the physician or health care provider. The following changes in a patient diagnosed with cirrhosis should be reported to the provider immediately: changes in behavior or intellectual function, increased ascites, edema, shortness of breath, or GI bleeding.

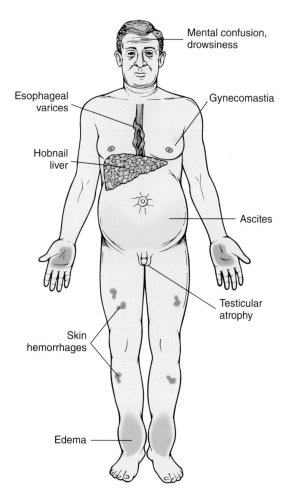

• **Fig. 8.39** Cirrhosis of the liver (in the male).

Etiology

The causes of cirrhosis are many. Alcoholism, malnutrition, hepatitis (see the Hepatitis B and Hepatitis C sections), parasites, toxic (poisonous) chemicals, and congestive heart failure are other possible causes of this disease. Inherited disorders, such as Wilson disease and *hemochromatosis*, can be predisposing conditions leading to cirrhosis of the liver. Cirrhosis may also be idiopathic.

Diagnosis

On physical examination, the liver appears enlarged, firm to hard; palpable blunt edge; abdominal radiographs show this enlargement. Blood studies may reveal elevated liver enzyme and bilirubin levels. CT, ultrasonography, and needle biopsy of the liver are helpful in determining the type and extent of fibrosis.

Treatment

Treatment is directed at the cause of the disease in an attempt to prevent further damage to the liver. Regardless of the underlying cause, alcohol intake is prohibited. Malnutrition must be prevented, and adequate rest is essential. Vitamin and mineral supplements, along with antacids, are given. Diuretics reduce the excessive fluid (edema) that accumulates in the abdomen (ascites) and ankles. With significant ascites, it is sometimes necessary to drain the accumulated fluid by inserting a large needle into the peritoneal cavity (paracentesis). Paracentesis alleviates the discomfort from all of the fluid causing edema, but it also carries a risk of infection. In other cases, fluid accumulates in tissues, and paracentesis is not indicated. When the disease progresses to liver failure, liver transplantation is a viable option.

Prognosis

Some early liver damage can be reversed. Patients with cirrhosis are at risk for the development of hepatocellular carcinoma (HCC). Liver transplantation has greatly improved the outlook for patients who are acceptable candidates and are referred early for evaluation.

Prevention

Early diagnosis of the cause of the patient's abnormal liver function tests and the institution of appropriate treatment can prevent the progression to cirrhosis. Drinking alcohol in moderation, avoiding chemical toxins, such as arsenic and carbon tetrachloride are helpful. Exposure to infections known to damage the liver, such as those that cause hepatitis must be avoided. Caution must be exercised when taking medications known to be damaging to the liver and routine labwork to check liver enzymes.

Patient Teaching

Because the cause and progression of symptoms vary, patient teaching is highly customized. Give the patient a written schedule explaining how to take prescribed medications. Advise the patient to inform any other health care professional, including the dentist, about the cirrhotic liver disease because of the resulting reduction in medication tolerance. Explain the importance of a low-sodium, highly nutritious diet, and give the patient a list of food and alcohol restrictions.

Viral Hepatitis

Description

Viral hepatitis is a systemic infection causing symptoms ranging from mild inflammation of the liver to severe involvement with the destruction of hepatic cells. Viral hepatitis, a common cause of acute hepatitis, is endemic in much of the world. Most cases are caused by one of several viral agents described by the letters of the alphabet. The transmission of the disease varies with the type of virus: Hepatitis A virus (HAV) moves through the fecal-oral route; hepatitis B virus (HBV) and hepatitis C virus (HCV) are bloodborne. Similar symptoms occur with all forms of viral hepatitis. The differential diagnosis is based on the results of laboratory tests. Treatment is symptomatic in acute cases; some chronic cases respond to antiviral agents.

Patient Screening

When the patient complains of an abrupt onset of fatigue, fever, jaundice, malaise, dark urine, and/or yellowing of the sclera of the eyes, prompt medical evaluation is indicated.

Symptoms and Signs

Many patients, especially children, are asymptomatic. Clinical manifestations of viral hepatitis can range from mild to chronic or severe. Many cases are self-limiting, with complete recovery. Severe viral hepatitis can be life threatening when liver function is destroyed and waste products accumulate in the blood. Because the liver has many functions, many abnormal findings are possible on blood and urine tests. The specific type of hepatitis can be established through laboratory tests that look for antibody and antigen markers.

Common symptoms in all forms of hepatitis include abrupt onset of headache, anorexia, malaise, fever, nausea, dark urine, and clay-colored stools. Jaundice and yellowing of the sclera of the eyes are evident in most patients. The patient may complain of abdominal discomfort and myalgia. Liver enlargement may be noted during physical examination.

Hepatitis A

Description

Hepatitis A is highly contagious and results in mild acute liver infection. The incubation period varies from 15 to 50 days. Symptoms can be mild to severe. In most cases, the infection is self-limiting, liver function is fully recovered, and lifelong immunity to HAV is conferred. Hepatitis A is the only viral hepatitis causing spiking fevers.

ICD-10-CM Code	B15.9 *(Hepatitis A without hepatic coma)* (B15.0–B15.9 = 2 codes of specificity)

Etiology

The causative virus, HAV, is highly contagious and is transmitted by the fecal-oral route from contaminated food (including shellfish and contaminated raw fruit and vegetables), water, and stools. HAV is present in the stool before symptoms are evident. This form of hepatitis is sometimes known as *epidemic* or *infectious hepatitis* because it frequently occurs at schools, camps, or institutions.

Diagnosis

A hepatitis profile is performed to identify the antibody and antigen markers and thereby establish the causative virus. Liver function studies are used to support the diagnosis. Blood tests show elevated serum levels of alanine aminotransaminase (ALT) and aspartate aminotransaminase (AST), usually found in the liver. The prothrombin time (PT) is prolonged, and the serum bilirubin level is elevated. Urine tests show bilirubinuria. The presence of antibody to HAV in serum or a positive RNA nucleic acid amplification test (such as polymerase chain reaction or genotyping) for hepatitis A virus.

Treatment

General medical management includes rest and symptom control. Intramuscular administration of immune globulin is recommended within 2 weeks of exposure. The patient is isolated, and care is taken to prevent cross-infection. Medications to control nausea and pain are given, as needed. Other measures taken while the liver heals are a low-fat, high-carbohydrate diet and restriction of physical activity. Alcohol should be avoided.

Prognosis

In adult patients, the disease can be severe during the acute stage and lasts 4 to 8 weeks. Recovery is usually complete. Chronic hepatitis A does not occur, and there is no carrier state. Clinical illness is more severe in adults; children may not present symptoms.

Prevention

Vaccination against hepatitis A is recommended before travel into areas where hepatitis A is prevalent and where sanitation is poor. The vaccine should be received at least 2 weeks before potential exposure. One dose is sufficient for primary immunization, and a booster dose is given 6 to 12 months later. The duration of immunity has not been established. Vaccination is recommended for anyone with close contact with an infected person.

Prevention includes education about proper sanitation, hand washing, food preparation, and immunizations.

Patient Teaching

Preventive measures and immunization are recommended. The patient should habitually practice proper hand washing, careful food preparation, cooking, and storage. The patient should dispose of fecal matter, including soiled diapers,

properly. Person-to-person contamination is common in such places as daycare centers, among family members, and spread to customers in eating places. Inform the patient that the virus can be spread until recovery is complete.

Hepatitis B

ICD-10-CM Code	B16.9 *(Acute hepatitis B without delta-agent and without hepatic coma)* (B16.0–B16.9 = 4 codes of specificity) B19.10 *(Unspecified viral hepatitis B without hepatic coma)* (B19.10–B19.11 = 2 codes of specificity)

Symptoms and Signs

The symptoms and signs of hepatitis B, or serum hepatitis, can mimic flu and are similar to those mentioned previously. The onset of hepatitis B is more insidious and the aminotransferase levels are higher than in HAV infection. Liver inflammation causes the destruction of liver cells and necrosis. These changes can be detected in abnormal results of liver profile studies.

Etiology

HBV is transmitted primarily through the percutaneous and permucosal routes. When the virus enters the body, it multiplies quickly and destroys liver cells. The mode of transmission includes contact with blood, semen, vaginal secretions, and saliva. Many infections result from sexual contact or blood exchange from the sharing of contaminated needles. Health care providers are at risk of infection from "needlesticks"; therefore all patients must be considered potential sources of infection, and standard precautions must be maintained. An infected mother can transmit the virus to her infant during birth.

Diagnosis

Patient history indicates both the mode of transmission and source of infection. The detection of hepatitis B surface antigen (HBsAg) in blood confirms the diagnosis. When HBsAg is detected in blood for more than 6 months, chronic hepatitis is present. While the hepatitis B antigen is present in blood, the disease is highly transmissible with exposure to the blood and body fluids of the infected individual.

Treatment

Some cases are self-limiting; general medical management is the same as that described previously for hepatitis A virus. Oral antiviral therapy may be employed in chronic cases when effective results are long lasting without relapses. Interferon can be effective; younger patients may prefer it because of its shorter duration of therapy. Hepatitis B immune globulin is given to create passive immunity and is given to the exposed, nonimmune individual. Such exposure may occur through needlesticks or sexual relations with an infected person.

Prognosis

Because HBV infection can be acute or chronic, the prognosis varies. Some people become chronic carriers because the virus remains in the blood. In most cases, however, the liver heals and regenerates, but this takes time, perhaps several months. Later in life, patients with chronic hepatitis are prone to cirrhosis and cancer of the liver. Some patients may require liver transplantation.

Prevention

Employers are required by the Occupational Safety and Health Administration to make the hepatitis B vaccine available to workers in high-risk occupations, such as staff at hemodialysis centers, physicians, dentists, nurses, physical therapists, and personnel working in clinical and pathology laboratories and blood banks. Initially, hepatitis may not cause symptoms, so it is important that high-risk individuals be screened for the disease. Among the general population, IV drug users, those who have multiple sexual partners, and homosexual or bisexual males are at high risk. Other transmissions of the disease may occur through mother-to-newborn, blood transfusions, nonsterile tools during acupuncture, tattoos, and body piercings. Hepatitis B is not transmitted through casual contact. The vaccine for hepatitis B is recommended for all children and for individuals at high risk of contracting the disease. Cases of HBV must be reported to the appropriate county or state health department.

Patient Teaching

Compliance with medical treatment and follow-up care improve outcome. Safe practices are taught for procedures that involve blood or body fluids to avoid transmission of HBV. High-risk behaviors and high-risk occupations should be discussed, as indicated by the medical history or as needed. Not everyone who is infected with hepatitis is symptomatic, so it can be transmitted unknowingly. This makes awareness of safe practices very important.

Hepatitis C

ICD-10-CM Code	B17.10 (Acute hepatitis C without hepatic coma) (B17.10–B17.11 = 2 codes of specificity) B18.2 (Chronic viral hepatitis C) (B18.2; B19.20–B19.21 = 3 codes of specificity)

Symptoms and Signs

HCV infection, considered a widespread epidemic, is the most common bloodborne infection in the United States. Many of those infected by HCV, often young adults, are asymptomatic and may unknowingly infect others. When present, symptoms resemble those of hepatitis A but are typically less severe and sometimes without jaundice.

• **Fig. 8.40** Cirrhosis of the liver resulting from hepatitis C. (From Cotran R, et al: *Robbins pathologic basis of disease*, ed 6, Philadelphia, 1999, Saunders.)

Chronic HCV infection results in gradual, insidious liver disease. Over a period of years, the infection causes necrosis, fibrosis, and cirrhosis of the liver (Fig. 8.40).

Abnormal laboratory findings may include elevated serum levels of liver enzymes and bilirubin, although this evidence is inconclusive without a positive blood test for anti-HCV antibodies. Physical assessment may find liver tenderness and enlargement.

Etiology

Hepatitis C is caused by HCV, which is transmitted via blood and body fluids. Hepatitis C infections can be caused by different genotypes. Exposure may be traced to blood transfusions, especially those performed before 1990, when blood bank procedures became rigorous; kidney dialysis; organ transplantations before 1990; or behaviors involving contact with the blood of an infected person. Other risk factors include working in the health care environment, injecting illegal drugs, sexual transmission, or sharing articles of personal hygiene (i.e., razor) with an infected person. When a person infected with HIV becomes infected with HCV, a more rapid progression to end-stage liver disease is likely and may necessitate liver transplantation. In many cases, the source of infection is not discovered.

Diagnosis

A clinical history of possible exposure to HCV accompanied by symptoms of hepatitis may point to the diagnosis. Ultrasonography of the liver may rule out other causes of liver disease. Laboratory findings include elevated serum levels of liver enzymes, elevated serum bilirubin, and bilirubinuria. HCV ribonucleic acid (RNA) serum tests detect circulating virus in the blood, however it can take approximately 8 to 11 weeks for the HCV test to be positive. Most people will show a positive result by the sixth month following exposure. A nucleic acid test, which can detect HCV RNA, can provide results within 1 to 2 weeks after exposure. A positive blood test result for the presence of anti-HCV antibodies indicates infection, past or present. A liver biopsy confirms the diagnosis.

Treatment

Sofosbuvir (Sovaldi) administered with ribarvin was the first FDA all oral medication therapy approved to treat hepatitis C. It may also be used in conjunction with peginterferon. Sofosbuvir may be effective on genotypes 1, 2, and 4 with a 12-week regimen. Genotype 3 may be treated with a 24-week regimen. Sofosbuvir can cause birth defects and death in neonates. It should not be used with certain prescription medications or St. John wort. Other medications indicated for the treatment of hepatitis C include glecaprevir/pibrentasvir (Mavyret), sofosbuvir/velpatasvir/voxilaprevir (Vosevi), sofosbuvir/velpatasvir (Epclusa), elbasvir/grazoprevir (Zepatier), and ledipasvir/sofosbuvir (Harvoni).

Standard treatment is typically aimed at control of symptoms and improving long-term liver function. Glucocorticoids may be given to reduce inflammation. Supportive measures include rest and a well-balanced diet. The increase in HCV infection (particularly when coinfection with HIV is present) has contributed to a high demand for liver transplants in the United States.

Prognosis

Patients may recover completely, however in some patients, cirrhosis of the liver eventually occurs because many people are not aware of their HCV status until they start having symptoms. As mentioned previously, coinfection with HIV presents a more complicated prognosis. Chronic hepatitis carries an increased risk of liver cancer and may result in patients succumbing to liver failure.

Prevention

Standard universal precautions must be enforced. Avoiding known risk factors is important. There is currently no vaccine for hepatitis C.

Patient Teaching

The patient is taught the importance of diet and rest during the acute stage of infection by HCV. In the case of known infection, one should emphasize precautions to prevent transmission of the virus. Risk factors should be clearly identified. Patients addicted to alcohol or actively using IV drugs should delay treatment until these addictions are under control. When drug therapy is begun, the patient should be taught the possible side effects. Patients should discuss becoming pregnant with the health care provider as there is a small risk of transmitting the virus. Breastfeeding is not known to be a method of transmission from mother to infant.

Cancer of the Liver Description

HCC is a primary tumor of the liver that usually arises in the setting of chronic liver disease. Hepatoblastoma is a childhood cancer that arises in an otherwise normal liver.

ICD-10-CM Code	C22.0 *(Liver cell carcinoma)*
	C22.2 *(Hepatoblastoma)*
	C22.7 *(Other specified carcinomas of liver)*
	C22.8 *(Malignant neoplasm of liver, primary, unspecified as to type)*
	(C22.0–C22.9 = 8 codes of specificity)

Symptoms and Signs

Patients who develop HCC often have no symptoms other than those associated with their chronic liver disease. Symptoms of HCC or hepatoblastoma may include upper abdominal pain, weight loss, early satiety, and a palpable abdominal mass. Physical findings may include ascites, hepatomegaly, splenomegaly, and jaundice. Laboratory tests may reveal thrombocytopenia, elevated bilirubin, low albumin, and electrolyte abnormalities. Serum alpha-fetoprotein (AFP), a protein secreted by neoplastic liver cells, is usually elevated.

Patient Screening

Schedule a prompt appointment, on request, for a patient with a history of cirrhosis.

Etiology

Chronic Hepatitis (B and C) are primary risk factors. Other risk factors include hereditary hemochromatosis, cirrhosis resulting from any cause, and exposure to aflatoxins (toxins produced by molds that may contaminate food supplies, such as corn, soybeans, and peanuts). Hepatoblastoma is more common in children with a history of prematurity or with certain genetic syndromes, such as Beckwith-Wiedemann syndrome or familial colonic polyposis.

Diagnosis

The diagnosis of HCC should be suspected in a patient with cirrhosis whose condition suddenly deteriorates. An increase in AFP level to greater than 500 g/L (normal value 10–20 g/L) in a high-risk patient is diagnostic of HCC, although any AFP elevation should arouse suspicion. In any patient with an elevated AFP level, ultrasonography, CT, or MRI of the liver is the next diagnostic procedure. A liver biopsy can help make a definitive diagnosis, but it may be risky in patients with cirrhosis. Therefore it is attempted only in these patients when the result will affect disease management. Common sites of metastatic spread include bone, lungs, brain, peritoneum, and adrenal glands. A biopsy is typically necessary for hepatoblastoma diagnosis.

Treatment

Surgical resection (partial hepatectomy) of the liver is the treatment of choice for HCC, but many patients are not eligible because of tumor extent or underlying liver disease. For patients with no extrahepatic spread, liver transplantation is an option. Nonsurgical options for nonmetastatic disease are radiofrequency ablation or percutaneous ethanol injection. in some patients with unresectable disease, systemic therapy with sorafenib has shown benefits. Research into other molecularly targeted therapies for HCC is currently underway. Unlike HCC, hepatoblastoma is often sensitive to chemotherapy. Surgical resection or liver transplantation can be curative.

Prognosis

The most important factors predicting survival are tumor size, severity of underlying liver disease, and presence of metastatic disease. Because HCC often is detected late, the median survival after diagnosis is 6 to 20 months. Patients living in high-incidence regions and those with higher AFP levels often have a worse prognosis. For hepatoblastoma, a low AFP level is also associated with a poor prognosis. The 5-year overall survival for hepatoblastoma is around 70%.

Prevention

Immunization to prevent hepatitis B, and eliminating risks for HCV can be beneficial. Avoiding excessive alcohol consumption and maintaining a healthy weight are other prevention measures. Children with genetic conditions associated with hepatoblastoma should get regular ultrasound screening.

Patient Teaching

Explain the need for special diet restrictions and total abstinence from alcohol. The treatment plan will be highly customized, depending on the therapies employed and the stage of the cancer. Give written and oral directions.

Cholelithiasis (Gallstones)

Description

Cholelithiasis is a common condition in which there is an abnormal presence of calculi or gallstones that form in the bile.

ICD-10-CM Code	K80.20 *(Calculus of gallbladder without cholecystitis without obstruction)* (K80.00-K81.9 = 44 codes of specificity)

 ENRICHMENT

Nonalcoholic Fatty Liver Disease

There are patients who drink little or no alcohol but are diagnosed with various liver conditions that fall under the diagnosis of nonalcoholic fatty liver disease (NAFLD). Patients with NAFLD have one thing in common: too much fat stored in the cells of the liver. The incidence rates of NAFLD are increasing around the world, and in the United States, this is the most frequently seen form of chronic liver disease. About 25% of the population is affected. Those who have NAFLD are at risk of developing nonalcoholic steatohepatitis (NASH). NASH causes liver inflammation and can advance to cirrhosis of the liver and liver failure. Liver damage is similar to that with heavy alcohol use. Obesity is one thing that puts a patient at a higher risk for developing NAFLD and NASH. Patients diagnosed with NAFLD can reverse the process toward scarring and potential liver damage by losing 10% of their body weight in the first year after diagnosis. A healthy diet and moderate approach to losing weight and regular exercise are recommended as part of the treatment protocol.

Symptoms and Signs

The patient with cholelithiasis (gallstones) may be asymptomatic until the bile ducts become obstructed by the stones (Fig. 8.41). Colicky pain, or biliary colic, signals the obstruction of the cystic duct or the common bile duct by one or more stones. The pain is in the epigastric region or the right upper quadrant of the abdomen, often radiating to the right upper back in the area of the scapula. Nausea and vomiting accompany the typically severe pain. The patient may report flatulence and clay-colored stools. If the obstruction is prolonged, jaundice may appear. Laboratory tests may show elevations of bilirubin, alkaline phosphate, AST, and ALT.

Patient Screening

The patient may describe URQ pain as "gripping or stabbing pain." The patient should be asked about nausea and vomiting and the presence of jaundice noted.

• **Fig. 8.41** (A) Cholelithiasis. (B) Cholesterol gallstones. (From Kumar V, et al: *Robbins basic pathology*, ed 8, Philadelphia, 2008, Saunders.)

• **Fig. 8.42** Oral cholecystogram. (From Doughty DB, Jackson DB: *Gastrointestinal disorders—Mosby's clinical nursing series*, St. Louis, 1993, Mosby.)

Etiology

Gallstones form in the gallbladder from insoluble cholesterol and bile salts; they vary in size and number. Gallstones are more common with increasing age, high-calorie cholesterol diet associated with obesity, and in the female population. Other risk factors are oral contraceptive use and ileal disease. People with alcoholic cirrhosis, biliary tract infection, and diabetes mellitus are also susceptible.

Diagnosis

The clinical picture and ultrasonography of the gallbladder and biliary ducts are highly accurate in confirming the presence of cholelithiasis. One can estimate the size and type of stones with some accuracy through test results (Fig. 8.42). The serum bilirubin level is elevated with obstruction of the common bile duct.

Treatment

Asymptomatic gallstones are usually left alone. Fatty intake should be controlled through dietary changes. If the patient experiences recurring pain, surgical removal of the gallbladder (cholecystectomy) is indicated. Endoscopic retrograde cholangiopancreatography (ERCP) is used to identify and remove stones in the common bile duct. The use of oral preparations such as Ursodiol to dissolve the gallstones may be indicated for some patients. Another nonsurgical treatment is called *extracorporeal shock wave lithotripsy*.

Prognosis

In mild cases, diet modifications may resolve symptoms, but a cholecystectomy provides the best prognosis by eliminating recurrences. Recovery varies with the method of

• **Fig. 8.43** Cholecystitis. (From Damjanov I, Linder J: *Pathology: a color atlas*, St. Louis, 1999, Mosby.)

treatment. Nonsurgical interventions require more time to achieve results and have a limited role.

Prevention

Maintaining a healthy weight and consuming a healthy diet is recommended. Avoiding added sugar and foods that are high in saturated fats can also be beneficial.

Patient Teaching

Explain the risk factors, including a high-fat, high-calorie diet; hormone replacement therapy; obesity; diabetes; and liver disease. Emphasize the importance of a healthy diet and the purpose of the prescribed medication.

Cholecystitis

Description

Cholecystitis is an acute or chronic inflammation of the gallbladder, usually associated with obstruction of the cystic duct.

ICD-10-CM Code	K81.2 (*Acute cholecystitis with chronic cholecystitis*) (K81.0–K81.9 = 4 codes of specificity)

Refer to the physician's diagnosis and then to the current edition of the ICD-10-CM coding manual to ensure the greatest specificity.

Symptoms and Signs

Cholecystitis, or inflammation of the gallbladder, usually is associated with cholelithiasis; infection often follows the inflammation (Fig. 8.43). The condition can become chronic.

The patient experiences acute colicky pain, which localizes in the URQ of the abdomen and becomes more severe when radiating around to the right lower scapular region. In addition, the patient may experience nausea and vomiting, followed by guarding of the URQ muscles and shallow respirations. A fever may ensue. Other signs are jaundice, clay-colored stools, dark urine, and pruritus. In some cases, the acutely inflamed gallbladder ruptures, causing peritonitis.

Patient Screening

Acute onset of biliary colic with nausea, vomiting, chills, fever, and jaundice requires a prompt medical evaluation.

Etiology

Most cholecystitis results from an obstruction of the gallbladder caused by gallstones. However, trauma or other insult to the gallbladder, including infection, occasionally causes it.

Diagnosis

The diagnosis is based on the clinical picture and ultrasonography of the gallbladder and biliary ducts. A radioisotope gallbladder study (hepatobiliary iminodiacetic acid scan) that indicates a nonvisualized gallbladder points to acute gallbladder disease. Other findings include an elevated WBC count and an increased serum bilirubin level.

Treatment

Treatment in uncomplicated cases consists of dietary modification with the elimination of fatty foods. The acutely ill patient with persistent vomiting is given nothing by mouth, and a nasogastric tube might be inserted. IV solution is given to replace fluids and electrolytes. When the patient is stabilized, surgical intervention to remove the gallbladder (cholecystectomy) is indicated. Medical management may include the administration of antibiotics, analgesics, and antiemetics while the patient is awaiting surgery.

Prognosis

Mild and uncomplicated cases have a positive prognosis. Acute complications include gangrene of the gallbladder, gallbladder perforation, emphysematous cholecystitis (secondary infection with a gas-forming organism), and empyema.

Prevention

Early medical attention and dietary modifications at onset of symptoms related to inflammation of the gallbladder are the initial attempts to control the stages and complications of chronic gallbladder disease.

Patient Teaching

Explain the relationship between a high-calorie, high-fat diet and the onset of gallstone disease that can, in turn, predispose to inflammation of the gallbladder. If a patient undergoes a cholecystectomy, explain that the liver will continue to produce bile for fat digestion.

Acute and Chronic Pancreatitis

Description

Pancreatitis is an acute or chronic inflammation of the pancreas with variable involvement of adjacent and remote organs. (Fig. 8.44).

ICD-10-CM Code	K85.9 (*Acute pancreatitis, unspecified*)
	(K85.0–K85.9 = 6 codes of specificity)
	K86.1 (*Other chronic pancreatitis*)
	(K86.0–K86.9 = 6 codes of specificity)

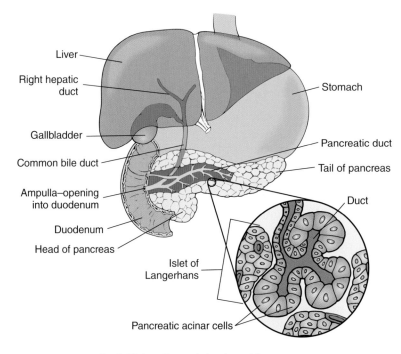

• **Fig. 8.44** Location and structure of the pancreas.

Liver
Right hepatic duct
Gallbladder
Common bile duct
Ampulla–opening into duodenum
Duodenum
Head of pancreas
Stomach
Pancreatic duct
Tail of pancreas
Duct
Islet of Langerhans
Pancreatic acinar cells

• **Fig. 8.45** Acute pancreatitis. (From Cotran R, et al: *Robbins pathologic basis of disease*, ed 6, Philadelphia, 1999, Saunders.)

Symptoms and Signs

In pancreatitis, the pancreas becomes inflamed, edematous, hemorrhagic, and necrotic (Fig. 8.45). The patient with acute pancreatitis has a sudden onset of severe abdominal pain that radiates to the back and nausea and vomiting. Epigastric pain is often worsened by walking and lying supine or improved by sitting and leaning forward. In acute pancreatitis, the patient appears acutely ill, diaphoretic, and tachycardic, with shallow, rapid respirations. Blood pressure falls, and body temperature rises. The abdomen is tender mainly in the upper quadrants, most often without guarding and rigidity. Bowel sounds are reduced. Mild jaundice is common. Many local and systemic complications (e.g., pancreatic abscess, necrotizing pancreatitis, and pneumonia) are possible. Chronic pancreatitis can present a vague clinical picture. Anorexia, nausea, vomiting, constipation, flatulence, and weight loss are common. Psychiatric disturbances, including depression and anxiety, have been reported.

Patient Screening

Acute pancreatitis is a life-threatening emergency requiring medical intervention.

Etiology

Pancreatic enzymes that are released prior to leaving the pancreas, alcoholism, biliary tract disease, trauma, infection, structural anomalies, greatly elevated calcium levels in the blood, hemorrhage, hyperlipidemia, or drugs may cause pancreatitis. Gallstones are often the cause of pancreatitis in nonalcoholic individuals. Less often, the cause is a metabolic or endocrine disorder. Some cases are idiopathic. Smoking may increase the risk of alcoholic and idiopathic pancreatitis.

Diagnosis

The diagnosis is based on the clinical picture, with dramatically elevated serum amylase and lipase levels on the first day of the attack. The WBC count and Hct are usually elevated. Hyperglycemia is commonly present. Radiography and ultrasonography may reveal stones in the biliary tract or dilation of the common bile duct, and the bilirubin level may be elevated. CT, with oral or IV contrast material, identifies pancreatic changes and complications.

Treatment

Treatment includes general supportive care for mild cases in addition to monitoring in the hospital. In contrast, acute pancreatitis may require emergency treatment consisting of IV fluid and electrolyte replacement. The patient is given nothing by mouth; and in some cases, a nasogastric suction tube is introduced with intermittent suction. Pain medication, usually a narcotic, is given per health care provider's order. Laboratory blood values are monitored. The development of a pancreatic abscess is an indication for prompt percutaneous or surgical drainage.

In chronic pancreatitis, the patient also must be monitored closely for malabsorption, steatorrhea, and impaired glucose tolerance indicating diabetes mellitus. If the underlying cause of pancreatitis is an obstructed pancreatic duct, then surgery may be necessary to remove the obstruction.

Prognosis

The prognosis is good in most cases. Severe cases with systemic complications or pancreatic necrosis face a variable outcome. Recurrences are common in alcoholic pancreatitis.

Prevention

Preventive measures are based on the many clinical conditions, medications, and toxins associated with acute pancreatitis.

Patient Teaching

Explain the measures needed to reduce recurrent episodes including carefully managing gallstone disease. Avoidance of alcohol consumption if caused by alcohol use.

Pancreatic Cancer

Description

Cancer of the pancreas is a neoplasm, usually an adenocarcinoma, and occurs more often in the head of the pancreas.

ICD-10-CM Code	C25.9 *(Malignant neoplasm of pancreas, unspecified)* (C25.0–C25.9 = 8 codes of specificity)

Symptoms and Signs

Most patients with pancreatic cancer experience abdominal pain, weight loss, or jaundice. Nausea, vomiting, acholic (without bile) stools, and steatorrhea are also common. On examination, the patient may have ascites, abdominal tenderness, or a palpable gallbladder. As pancreatic tissue is infiltrated and destroyed, the patient can experience glucose intolerance, increasing weakness, fatigue, and diarrhea. Laboratory studies may reveal elevated bilirubin and alkaline phosphatase concentrations.

Patient Screening

The patient often reports feeling generally quite ill and experiencing the symptoms listed previously; a prompt appointment is indicated.

Etiology

Risk factors for pancreatic cancer include cigarette smoking, obesity, a history of chronic pancreatitis or diabetes, and a family history of pancreatic cancer. Mutations in the cancer susceptibility genes (*BRCA1, BRCA2, STK11, PALB2, CDKN2A, ATM, TP53, STK11, MLH1, MSH2, MSH6, PMS2, and EPCAM*) are also associated with an increased risk of pancreatic cancer.

Diagnosis

Because of the retroperitoneal location of the pancreas, carcinoma is difficult to detect. The diagnosis of pancreatic cancer is typically made radiographically and histologically. The initial study in a patient with suspected pancreatic cancer is either abdominal ultrasonography or CT. ERCP may be done. Cancer is suggested by dilated bile ducts or a mass in the pancreas. An elevated level of the serum tumor marker CA19-9 suggests the presence of cancer and very high levels correlate with a poor prognosis.

If cancer is suspected or a mass lesion is present, a tissue diagnosis by EUS fine-needle aspiration biopsy of the mass and lymph nodes is necessary to guide treatment. If EUS is not available, a staging laparoscopy may be performed. The patient may be a candidate for surgery if the patient shows no evidence of distant metastases and no involvement of the major vessels.

Treatment

Surgical resection is the only potentially curative treatment for pancreatic cancer. It is a viable option only for patients with disease confined to the pancreas and peripancreatic nodes. Because of late detection of the disease, only a small percent of patients are candidates for surgery. For palliative treatment of advanced pancreatic cancer, chemotherapy with or without radiation therapy is the current standard of care. Stents can be placed to relieve bile duct obstruction or gastric outlet obstruction.

Prognosis

The prognosis is poor for pancreatic cancer.

Prevention

There is no way to prevent most pancreatic cancers. Healthier lifestyles, including cessation of cigarette smoking, avoidance of alcohol, and maintaining a healthy weight, may be of some benefit.

Patient Teaching

Give the patient and his or her family both written and verbal instructions, as indicated, about surgery, pain management, and chemotherapy. Assist with at-home services as needed.

Disorders of Nutrient Intake and Absorption

Proper nutrition is needed to enable the regulation and function of all processes to ensure that the human body is healthy and has the energy and nutrients to build and repair tissues. Nutritional deficiencies, excesses, or imbalances can affect the body's homeostasis. Any inability of the GI tract to digest or absorb nutrients can cause forms of malnutrition, even with adequate intake of food. Prolonged malnutrition or malabsorption results in anatomic lesions or disease entities.

Malnutrition

Description

Malnutrition is a disorder of nutrition caused by primary deprivation of protein-energy (seen in poverty or self-imposed starvation) or secondary to deficiency diseases (e.g., cancer or diabetes).

ICD-10-CM Code	E46 *(Unspecified protein-calorie malnutrition)*

Symptoms and Signs

Disturbances in nutrition can result from eating too much or too little food or from having an imbalanced diet. When a body cannot absorb or use food properly, malnutrition will result, even with sufficient nutritional intake. Malnutrition disrupts the body's metabolic processes, disturbing normal physical structure and biologic function.

Malnourishment can cause many specific disease conditions, such as abnormal growth, with physical and intellectual impairment. A human body deprived of adequate nutrition cannot maintain health. The appetite may decrease or increase, resulting in emaciation or obesity. Signs and symptoms of malnutrition include loss of energy, diarrhea, drastic weight change, skin lesions, loss of hair, poor nails, and generalized edema; delayed healing and greasy stools may result from loss of fat. More advanced signs may include muscle wasting (most noticeably in the temporalis and interosseus muscles), enlarged glands, and hepatomegaly. Many abnormal findings of blood and urine tests are possible.

Patient Screening

A patient with a recent, unintended, or unexplainable weight loss of 10 lb or greater should be scheduled for a complete physical examination.

Etiology

Protein-energy malnutrition has been described as two distinct syndromes. Kwashiorkor, caused by a deficiency of protein in the presence of adequate energy, is typically seen in weaning infants at the birth of a sibling in areas where food containing protein is insufficiently abundant. Marasmus (extreme malnutrition and emaciation), caused by combined protein and energy deficiency, is most commonly seen where adequate quantities of food are not available (Fig. 8.46).

• **Fig. 8.46** Protein-energy malnutrition. (From Morgan SL, Weinsier RL: *Fundamentals of clinical nutrition*, ed 2, St. Louis, 1998, Mosby.)

In industrialized societies, protein-energy malnutrition is most often secondary to other disease. Kwashiorkor-like secondary protein-energy malnutrition occurs primarily in association with increased metabolic acute illnesses, such as trauma, burns, and sepsis. Marasmus-like secondary protein-energy malnutrition typically results from chronic diseases, such as chronic obstructive pulmonary disease, congestive heart failure, cancer, or AIDS.

In both syndromes, protein-energy malnutrition is caused either by decreased intake of energy and protein, increased nutrient losses, or increased nutrient requirements dictated by the underlying disease. For example, diminished oral intake may result from poor dentition or various GI disorders. Loss of nutrients results from malabsorption, diarrhea, and glycosuria. Nutrient requirements are increased by fever, surgery, neoplasia, and burns.

Diagnosis

Clinical evaluation of the patient includes a complete physical examination with special attention to weight and measurements of body fat and muscle mass. Laboratory diagnostic findings vary, depending on the cause and type of malnutrition. Laboratory tests include blood protein level, CBC, and a 24-hour urine test for urea nitrogen. The tests may show evidence of mineral deficiency, anemia, abnormal protein metabolism, and other changes in metabolism related to malnourishment.

Treatment

The treatment of malnutrition is based on the underlying cause. After the patient's nutritional needs are assessed, nutritional supplements and replacement begin with appropriate oral and IV feedings. Certain pathologic conditions may necessitate feedings through a nasogastric tube. Treatment may include a combination of dietary modifications with appropriate supplements of proteins, vitamins, and minerals. Diarrhea and infections are controlled with medications.

Surgery may be indicated when lesions of the GI tract cause malnutrition. Patients with eating disorders require special counseling or psychiatric interventions in addition to medical treatment. Vulnerable populations, such as those in poverty or older adults, may require community services that make healthy nutrition available on a daily basis.

Prognosis

The prognosis varies with the nature and severity of malnutrition. Severe cases have a high morbidity and mortality rate. Loss of 35% to 40% of body weight usually results in death.

Prevention

Address the underlying cause to correct nutritional deficiencies, restore weight, and prevent complications.

◆ ENRICHMENT

Hypervitaminosis

- Hypervitaminosis is a condition of toxicity resulting from an excess of any vitamin, but especially the fat-soluble vitamins A and D.
- The four fat (lipid)–soluble vitamins A, D, E, and K are stored in fat tissue.
- Symptoms of vitamin A toxicity include irritability, loss of hair, anorexia, enlargement of the liver and spleen, jaundice, skin changes, and psychiatric disorders. Vitamin A excess can be toxic to a developing fetus. Chronic toxicity in infants and children can cause increased pressure in the brain, tinnitus, pruritus, swelling of the optic nerve, and abnormal bone growth.
- Vitamin D is considered highly toxic, especially in infants and children. It can cause calcification of soft tissue, poor appetite, weakness, kidney damage, excessive thirst and urination, and mental changes. Note: The tolerable upper level for adults has been set at 2000 international units (IU; 50 mcg). 4000 IU is the new upper limit recommendation for ages 8 years or greater.
- Very high doses of vitamin E may interfere with the blood-clotting action of vitamin K.
- Vitamin K toxicity is uncommon. Rapid infusion causes dyspnea, flushing, cardiovascular complications, red blood cell (RBC) hemolysis, jaundice, and brain damage.
- Water-soluble vitamin C taken in excess causes nausea, diarrhea, and acidification of urine; niacin (B_3) may cause flushing, hyperglycemia, and liver damage; vitamin B_6 may cause photosensitivity and peripheral nerve damage.
- An overload of nutritional trace elements also produces toxicity.

Facts about Obesity

- Overweight and obesity are identified objectively by the use of the body mass index (BMI). The formula is weight-adjusted for height. For instance, the calculation is weight in pounds, divided by (height in inches)^2 and multiplied by 703. A number greater than 25.0 defines overweight, and a BMI of 30.0 or higher is classified as morbid obesity. A BMI of 40.0 or higher defines extreme obesity.
- In the United States, more than two of three people are overweight or obese. Adult obesity is an epidemic in the country despite the popularity of fad diets and sugar-free and fat-free products that are presented as antidotes to overweight and obesity.
- More females are obese compared with males, especially as they age.
- The causes of obesity are complex, but a major correlation has been made with greater energy intake than output.
- Fatness and the regional distribution of fat have a strong genetic component.
- Factors that may contribute to obesity include overeating (sometimes linked to psychological stress or environment), a low rate of energy expenditure, inactivity, and more rarely, endocrine disorders.
- Obesity contributes to severe health problems, such as diabetes mellitus, hypertension, cardiovascular disease, sleep apnea, blood lipid abnormalities, orthopedic problems, and skin problems. Obesity has been associated with metabolic syndrome. Being overweight when younger than 45 years of age is more dangerous.
- Obesity can make a person feel self-conscious and can impair social relationships; overweight people sometimes experience prejudice and discrimination. Obese children are often bullied.
- Treatment goals are (1) to lose as much nonessential fat as possible while minimizing the loss of lean body mass and (2) to maintain a balance between energy intake and energy expenditure.
- Important elements in successful weight loss are active patient self control; a supportive physician; a reduced-calorie, nutritionally adequate diet; and increased physical activity. Portion control alone has proven to be successful in weight loss.
- Other controversial treatment modalities that have known risks or lack proven long-term success include extremely low-calorie diets, anorectic drugs, and surgical procedures. Newer medications given to aid in weight loss include orlistat (Xenical) and rimonabant (Acomplia).
- The study of overweight people is called *bariatrics*. Some bariatric surgery centers are gaining recognition for their favorable outcomes. Bariatric surgery requires a lifetime commitment to lifestyle changes to prevent nutrient deficiencies.
- Many patients have great difficulty maintaining their reduced body weight. Lifestyle changes, including exercise and control of food intake through behavioral modification, remain important.
- Consultation with a health care provider is recommended before a patient starts on a substantial weight loss program.

Patient Teaching

After contributing factors have been identified, one can explain the treatment plan and the goals of therapy. Nutritional status is monitored, and the therapeutic diet is adjusted to allow for the patient's preferences. Address the psychological problems associated with eating disorders by making referrals for counseling and support.

Malabsorption Syndrome

Description

Malabsorption syndrome refers to a group of disorders in which intestinal absorption of dietary nutrients is impaired.

ICD-10-CM Code	K90.9 (Intestinal malabsorption, unspecified) (K90.4–K90.9 = 4 codes of specificity)

Symptoms and Signs

A person with malabsorption syndrome has impaired digestion and is unable to absorb fat or certain other components of the diet. Symptoms include abdominal discomfort, bloating, chronic diarrhea, and abnormal bowel movements. Stools may appear yellowish gray and may be greasy looking. The stools tend to float because of their high-fat content. Over time, untreated malabsorption leads to weight loss, anemia, shortness of breath, and symptoms of vitamin and mineral deficiencies.

Patient Screening

The patient with malabsorption syndrome needs regular appointments for follow-up care until stable.

Etiology

The main cause of malabsorption syndrome is defective mucosal cells in the small intestine. A diseased pancreas or a blocked pancreatic duct, which deprives the small intestine of amylase and lipase, may cause secondary malabsorption syndrome. Reduced secretion of bile, caused by hepatic disease or a bile duct obstruction, also prevents lipid (fat) digestion. Metabolic or endocrine disorders, such as hyperparathyroidism and diabetes mellitus, are other possible causes of the syndrome. Severe parasitic and worm infestations, more common in developing countries, can cause malabsorption.

Diagnosis

The health care provider usually orders several blood tests to determine the levels of proteins, fats, and minerals in the patient's bloodstream. A laboratory analysis of a stool sample may also be performed. A biopsy of the small bowel may reveal a primary condition responsible for malabsorption.

Treatment

The main task for the physician or health care provider is to discover the underlying cause and to choose the course of treatment. Diet is controlled carefully. A high-protein, high-calorie diet with vitamin and mineral supplements, such as the fat-soluble vitamins A, D, E, and K, which are not being absorbed, aids the recovery.

Prognosis

Improvement can be expected when the underlying causes are identified and successfully treated. When areas of the intestines are damaged or resected, the remaining bowel can adapt to absorb nutrients.

Prevention

Many specific and nonspecific therapies are available for malabsorption.

Patient Teaching

Refer the patient to a dietitian for a nutrient-specific therapeutic diet.

Celiac Disease (Gluten Enteropathy)

Description

Celiac disease (celiac sprue), a disease of the small intestine, is characterized by malabsorption, gluten intolerance, and damage to the lining of the intestine.

ICD-10-CM Code   K90.0 (Celiac disease)

Symptoms and Signs

Celiac disease has multisystem effects that can produce serious health problems. Symptoms include weight loss, anorexia, abdominal cramping, diarrhea, flatulence (gas), abdominal distention, intestinal bleeding, weakness, muscle wasting, dermatitis herpetiformis, and the characteristically large, pale, greasy, foul-smelling stools. The end result of celiac disease is malabsorption and malnutrition.

Patient Screening

Assess the severity of symptoms to determine the patient's level of urgency to be seen by the health care provider.

Etiology

The cause of this disease may be either a toxic or an immunologic reaction to a component of gluten (a protein that is found in wheat and wheat products, barley, and rye). The majority of individuals with celiac disease have a gene mutation associated with HLA-DQ2 or HLA-DQ8. It is most frequently seen in those who are assigned female at birth.

Diagnosis

Celiac disease is often difficult to diagnose and differentiate from other intestinal diseases and disorders. Biopsy and laboratory testing, which may include genetic testing are performed.

Treatment

The patient must strictly adhere to a lifelong gluten-free diet; eliminating gluten allows the bowel to heal and reverses malabsorption.

Prognosis

A lifelong gluten-free diet usually leads to gradual recovery and a good prognosis.

Prevention

No prevention for celiac disease is known. Delayed recognition and treatment expose the affected individuals to long-term complications.

Patient Teaching

Provide education about the disease process. Refer the patient to a dietitian for counseling.

Food Poisoning

Description

Food poisoning is an illness resulting from eating food that contains bacterial toxins and viral, chemical, or toxic substances. The Centers for Disease Control and Prevention estimates that up to 48 million cases of food poisoning occur in the United States each year.

ICD-10-CM   A05.9 (Bacterial foodborne
Code   intoxication, unspecified)
              (A05.0-A05.9 = 8 codes of
                specificity)

Symptoms and Signs

The symptoms of food poisoning are determined, in part, by the cause. The onset is sudden, with rumbling stomach sounds, nausea, vomiting, diarrhea with abdominal pain and cramps, malaise, and fever. The symptoms usually disappear within 24 to 48 hours. If an extreme case of food poisoning persists, the situation becomes life threatening due to dehydration and electrolyte imbalances that can affect the cardiac system.

Patient Screening

Screen the patient for severity of symptoms and signs of dehydration, mindful that the very young and the very old are more prone to dehydration. It is appropriate to inquire about skin turgor, dry tongue, sunken eyes, and/or parched lips.

Etiology

True food poisoning includes poisoning from cheese, mushrooms, shellfish, food contaminated by poisonous insecticides, and toxic substances, such as lead and mercury. In addition, poisoning results from eating food that has undergone putrefaction or decomposition and food contaminated with bacteria or toxins (Table 8.1).

TABLE 8.1 — Bacterial Causes of Food Poisoning

Organism	Major Food Source(s)	Pathophysiologic Mechanism	
		Toxin in Food	Ingestion of Bacteria
Staphylococcus aureus	Cooked meat, cheese, pasta, cream buns, custard pies	Yes	No
Clostridium perfringens type A	Cooked meat, vegetable soup (prepared in bulk)	No	Yes (bacteria release enterotoxin in intestine)
Clostridium botulinum	Uneviscerated cured fish, preserved or fermented meat, home-preserved vegetables	Yes	No
Salmonella enteritidis/Salmonella typhimurium	Raw eggs, mayonnaise, incompletely cooked meat and poultry	No	Yes
Salmonella dublin	Raw milk, unpasteurized cheese	No	Yes
Salmonella typhi/Salmonella paratyphi	Food contamination by infected food handlers	No	Yes
Vibrio cholerae O1	Raw seafood	No	Yes
Vibrio cholerae non-O1	Raw oysters	No	Yes
Vibrio parahaemolyticus	Raw seafood	No	Yes
Vibrio vulnificus	Raw seafood (especially oysters)	No	Yes
Listeria monocytogenes	Soft cheese	No	Yes
Shigella species	Food contamination during preparation	No	Yes
Escherichia coli O157:H7	Ground beef	No	Yes
Campylobacter jejuni/Campylobacter coli	Incompletely cooked poultry and other meats, raw milk	No	Yes
Bacillus cereus	Fried rice	Yes	No
Heat-stable toxin Enterotoxin	Meat products	Yes	No
Yersinia enterocolitica	Pork, raw milk	No	Yes

From Goldman L, Schafer AI: *Goldman's Cecil medicine*, ed 24, Philadelphia, 2012, Elsevier/Saunders.

Diagnosis

The patient's history is important to diagnosis and can point to the cause. A stool or blood culture reveals the presence of any parasites or bacteria. The actual contaminated food may also be cultured.

Treatment

Most treatment is symptomatic, controlling vomiting and diarrhea. Bed rest is beneficial. To prevent or minimize fluid and electrolyte imbalances, nutritional support and fluid replacement are essential. If the patient becomes dehydrated, these may have to be given intravenously.

Prognosis

The prognosis for this condition varies with the cause. The prognosis generally is good if the cause has been determined and the treatment has begun. The earlier the diagnosis is made and treatment is begun, the better the chances for a successful recovery.

Prevention

Food poisoning can be prevented by the fastidious practice of infection control techniques as primary prevention. Careful hand washing to prevent oral-fecal transmission of disease-causing organisms is especially important in restaurants, daycare centers for children or elders, and health care institutions. Avoid swimming in contaminated water and drinking untreated water. Careful handling of food, eating of well-cooked food, and proper refrigeration of food reduces the risk.

Patient Teaching

Emphasize the preventive measures listed earlier. Patients who are stabilized after a severe episode are given a diet as tolerated and are advised to rest and rehydrate.

Anorexia Nervosa

Description

Anorexia nervosa, an eating disorder, is linked to a psychological disturbance in which hunger is denied by self-imposed starvation, resulting from a distorted body image and a compulsion to be thin (Fig. 8.47).

ICDTH_TSH-10-CM Code	F50.00 (Anorexia nervosa, unspecified)
	(F50.00–F50.02 = 3 codes of specificity)

Refer to the current edition of the ICD-10-CM coding manual for exclusions.

Symptoms and Signs

The patient with anorexia is one of the most difficult to treat. The patient does not eat a normal diet and is concerned with body image and being thin. The patient concentrates on losing weight, has a distorted perception of their appearance, and becomes malnourished. Signs of malnutrition include thinning hair, poor wound healing, and dental changes. Both females and males can become anorexic, but males may fail to seek help. The patient with anorexia usually is hyperactive and overexercises, is hypotensive, and experiences bradycardia and hypothermia. Feelings of sadness, insomnia, and withdrawal from friends and family may occur. Bulimia, which includes purging and binging, may occur concurrently.

Patient Screening

A parent or responsible party may be the first to report concern about a person's weight loss, anorexia, behavioral changes, and malnutrition-related health problems; the patient frequently denies the condition until it is more advanced. Recommend a physical examination and

• **Fig. 8.47** Anorexia nervosa. Persons with anorexia overestimate their body width, insisting that they are too fat despite profound weight loss.

consultation with the physician or health care provider as soon as possible.

Etiology

The etiology is unknown, although it is believed that family and social factors may precipitate the condition. Stress hormones are biologic factors, which have been linked to the onset in some people. Research continues to identify genes that are responsible for the likelihood of becoming anorexic if other members of the family suffer from anorexia.

Diagnosis

The diagnosis is based on the clinical picture and history: The patient has lost significant weight and may appear emaciated, has intense fear of weight gain, and, if female, has absent or irregular menstruation. Assessment of vital signs may reveal hypotension and bradycardia. The nutritional status and the electrolyte balance are evaluated through laboratory tests, including blood tests, urinalysis, and electrocardiography. Other organic causes and psychiatric disorders that cause physical wasting are ruled out.

Treatment

The goal of treatment is to promote normal weight and to restore nutrition. A team approach combining medical management, psychotherapy, behavior modification, family counseling, and nutritional counseling works best. The patient often is hospitalized to provide fluid and electrolyte replacement, to remove the patient from the home environment, and to place the patient in a controlled environment. Long-term emotional support is needed, and long-term psychiatric counseling often is indicated to correct any underlying dysfunction.

Prognosis

The outcome is more favorable when the patient seeks help willingly. Without medical intervention, life-threatening complications, such as cardiac arrest, are possible. Recovery is usually slow, and some patients become suicidal. Long-term health complications include anemia, osteoporosis, loss of kidney function, and heart failure. There is a high incidence of recurrence of the disease. Complications can lead to death.

Prevention

Until the causes and risk factors are better understood, there is no certain prevention. Because of the high incidence of anorexia in the United States, clinicians suggest prevention programs and media-based awareness campaigns are essential. Some health experts suggest that an educational shift from valuing people for body size and shape to valuing people for positive inner qualities and personality is needed.

Patient Teaching

It is important to build trust and sensitivity in presenting the plan for recovery to the patient. Establish a target weight. Give the patient as much control as possible over his or her preferred food and drink while beginning an adequate diet. A referral for psychological evaluation may be indicated.

Bulimia

Description
Bulimia is a behavioral disorder characterized by recurring episodes of binge eating followed by self-induced vomiting or purging, usually in secret.

ICD-10-CM Code   F50.2 *(Bulimia nervosa)*

Symptoms and Signs
The binge-purge eating pattern of bulimia is fueled by a morbid fear of becoming fat. Vomiting can result in poor dentition, pharyngitis, esophagitis, aspiration, and electrolyte abnormalities. Gastric dilatation and pancreatitis have been reported after binges. The patients also abuse laxatives and diuretics by using them excessively. Other signs are compulsive exercise, swollen salivary glands, and broken blood vessels in the eye.

Patient Screening
Be alert to recognize the shame and denial associated with the disease. The patient may admit only to depression and resist medical intervention.

Etiology
Although the etiologic factors are similar to those of anorexia nervosa, the exact cause is uncertain. Psychosocial factors, depression, control issues, and conflict frequently are identified. Characteristic perfectionist personality traits are identified, as in anorexia nervosa. The condition is associated with depression and, in some cases, compulsion.

Diagnosis
The diagnostic approach is similar to that for anorexia nervosa. Increased loss of electrolytes and metabolic acidosis are noted on laboratory tests. The patient exhibits a loss of muscle mass, cardiac irregularities, and dehydration. Anger and denial are part of the emotional state. Sudden death can result from hypokalemia and resulting cardiac arrhythmias.

Treatment
Treatment is similar to that of anorexia nervosa, with a multidimensional approach, including the administration of antidepressant drugs and participation in a support group.

Prognosis
Treatment may continue for years, because recovery may be a slow process. After the patient has discontinued the bulimic behavior, she or he should be taught proper nutrition in the form of a balanced diet.

Prevention
No prevention is known.

Patient Teaching
Encourage the patient's efforts to comply with medical management, psychotherapy, and provider instructions. Praise the patient for reaching goals in weight gain and behavior modification.

Motion Sickness

Description
Motion sickness is a loss of equilibrium experienced during motion.

ICD-10-CM Code   T75.3XXA *(Motion sickness, initial encounter)*

Symptoms and Signs
During an episode of motion sickness, the patient experiences nausea and vomiting when riding in a motor vehicle, boat, airplane, or other means of transportation. Air hunger, excessive salivation, pallor, sweating, dizziness, or headache may precede nausea and vomiting.

Patient Screening
A person susceptible to motion sickness may require medication before an airplane flight, car trip, or boating excursion. Some OTC medications are available.

Etiology
Motion sickness results from a disturbance in the sense of balance. The fluid in the semicircular canals of the ears becomes dislocated because of the motion. In addition, repetitive acceleration and deceleration and angular and linear motions cause excessive stimulation of the vestibular apparatus in the inner ear.

Diagnosis
The diagnosis is based on the clinical picture.

Treatment
The patient is encouraged to sit in the vehicle in the position that has the least amount of motion and where he or she can see the horizon. The patient is urged to avoid food and liquid before travel. If the patient must eat, only small amounts of food should be eaten.

Prognosis
The prognosis is good with prophylactic medication.

Prevention
Good results can be expected from taking an antiemetic in anticipation of a motion event. Sit toward the front when traveling by bus, or in the front seat of a vehicle. Window seats are best when flying or traveling by train. Prophylaxis with dermal patches of scopolamine (Transderm-Scop) or dimenhydrinate (Dramamine) is helpful, but should only be used as directed by the provider.

Patient Teaching
Warn the patient about any possible adverse effects associated with the medication.

Review Challenge

Answer the following questions:

1. What are the accessory organs of digestion and their functions?
2. How does malocclusion lead to complications?
3. What problem may result from untreated gingivitis?
4. How would you describe the symptoms of temporo-mandibular joint disorder?
5. What is the difference between an aphthous mouth ulcer and a "cold sore?"
6. What causes gastroesophageal reflux disease? How is it treated?
7. How does *Helicobacter pylori* relate to peptic ulcers and gastritis?
8. What is a serious possible complication of esophageal varices?
9. How are peptic ulcers treated?
10. What is the diagnostic value of (1) endoscopy and (2) colonoscopy?
11. Is pain usually the initial symptom of gastric cancer?
12. What is the diagnostic significance of the McBurney point?
13. What is strangulated hernia?
14. What is the difference between ulcerative colitis and Crohn's disease?
15. What is the goal in the treatment of gastroenteritis?
16. What is the difference between functional and mechanical intestinal obstructions? Give an example of each.
17. How would you compare the pathology of diverticulosis with that of diverticulitis?
18. How is colorectal cancer detected?
19. What causes pseudomembranous enterocolitis?
20. If a person has peritonitis, what serious complications may occur?
21. What are the signs and symptoms of cirrhosis of the liver?
22. How do hepatitis A and hepatitis C compare in etiology? What are the preventive measures for each disease?
23. What are the presenting symptoms of a patient with (1) biliary colic and (2) acute pancreatitis?
24. What are the causes of pancreatitis?
25. What are some examples of disorders of nutrition caused by deficiencies and excesses?
26. In what ways do pathogens cause food poisoning?
27. What are the three diagnostic criteria for celiac disease?
28. What are the similarities and differences between anorexia nervosa and bulimia?
29. What is the leading cause of liver transplantation in the United States?
30. What is the third most common site of cancer incidence in males and females?
31. What are the recommendations for patients diagnosed with nonalcoholic fatty liver disease and nonalcoholic steatohepatitis?

Real-Life Challenge: Cholelithiasis

A 43-year-old female is experiencing an intermittent colicky type of pain in the upper right quadrant (URQ) of the abdomen, radiating to the right scapular region. The onset was approximately 1 week ago. In the past few days, she has had nausea and vomiting, increasing in the past 24 hours. The pain is more severe today, and the emesis is bile colored. Vital signs are temperature, 99.68°F; pulse, 96 beats per minute; respirations, 26 breaths per minute; and blood pressure, 144/92 mm Hg. Her skin is warm, dry, and slightly jaundiced. The patient is somewhat obese and has been on oral contraceptives for 15 years.

Cholelithiasis is suspected. CT of the gallbladder confirms the presence of stones in the gallbladder and also in the common bile duct. Serum bilirubin is elevated. The patient is scheduled for laparoscopic surgery.

Questions

1. When would a patient with gallstones be asymptomatic?
2. How do gallstones develop?
3. Which type of person would be most likely to have gallstones?
4. Which diagnostic imaging studies would be ordered when gallstones are suspected?
5. Which blood studies would be ordered when gallstones are suspected?
6. What is the usual treatment for asymptomatic gallstones?
7. What is the treatment for symptomatic gallstones?
8. What is the difference between cholelithiasis and cholecystitis?

Real-Life Challenge: Ulcers

A 50-year-old male is experiencing midepigastric pain and heartburn along with nausea and vomiting, with the onset occurring approximately 1 week ago. The patient says that the pain is better after eating and more severe 2 hours after eating. The patient is observed sitting slightly bent over with knees drawn up. Vital signs are temperature, 99.88°F; pulse,

104 beats per minute; respirations, 24 breaths per minute; and blood pressure, 136/88 mm Hg. His skin is warm, dry, and pale. The physician suspects a duodenal ulcer. The abdomen is slightly distended and tender to palpation.

Diagnostic investigation include hemoglobin (Hgb), hematocrit (Hct), gastric analysis, stool examination for occult blood, upper gastrointestinal (GI) series, and gastroscopy. Drug therapy includes antacid, histamine (H_2) blockers, and an antibiotic. The patient is instructed to adhere to a bland diet, with small and more frequent meals.

Questions

1. What population is most prone to ulcers?
2. Compare gastric, duodenal, and peptic ulcers.
3. Why would symptoms of gastric and duodenal ulcers vary?
4. Discuss theories of the cause of ulcers. Compare theories of ulcerogenic drugs versus bacterial origin.
5. What warnings should be given to patients taking nonsteroidal antiinflammatory drugs?
6. Explain the complications of perforation.
7. Discuss the various forms of drug therapy available to treat ulcers.
8. What side effects might a patient on H_2 blockers experience?
9. What would a positive guaiac test indicate?

Internet Assignments

1. Explore the American Dental Association website, and report the latest news about the call for early detection of oral cancer. What do the relevant statistics suggest about oral cancer?
2. Visit the website of the National Eating Disorders Association, and report on a relevant headline article.

For example, what is being done to reach preteen children with a positive message about body image to prevent tragic deaths resulting from eating disorders?
3. Research the latest approaches to the treatment of hepatitis C by searching the American Liver Foundation website and related links.

Critical Thinking

1. Discuss the relationship between neglecting oral infections, such as dental decay, gingivitis, or periodontal disease, and the risk of damage to major organs including the heart.
2. Discuss the possible damage to the oral cavity, the larynx, the esophagus, and respiratory tree that can be caused by frequent and chronic gastroesophageal reflux disease (GERD). Explain the interventions a patient can use to help control GERD.
3. Why is it important for a patient to understand how to take a prescription for nonsteroidal antiinflammatory drugs (NSAIDs)?
4. A patient being treated for gastritis benefits from understanding the many agents that damage the gastric lining. Explain them as you would to a patient.
5. The symptoms experienced by a person suffering from irritable bowel syndrome (IBS) can be unpredictable and cause embarrassment with social interaction. How would you address the psychological and emotional concerns of the patient?
6. Discuss the advantages of screening for early detection and prevention of colorectal cancer.
7. Discuss how the distorted body image and self-imposed starvation of a patient with anorexia nervosa affect family members she or he lives with. What are some ways the family may try to reinforce the treatment plan?
8. Discuss the lifestyle changes recommended to lower the risk of oral cancer.
9. What measures can be taken to help prevent food poisoning in daycare centers and institutions?

Prepare to discuss Critical Thinking case study exercises for this chapter that are posted on Evolve.

Credentialing Examination Questions

1. If dental caries advances into the pulp of the tooth, which procedure may be necessary first?
    A. Sealant
    B. Filling
    C. Crown
    D. Root canal
2. How many hours can a person expect the "jaw in a day" surgery to last?
    A. 6 or less
    B. 8 or more
    C. 14 maximum
    D. 10 maximum

3. Which organ may be compromised when a patient has esophageal varices?
   A. Kidney
   B. Stomach
   C. Liver
   D. Heart
4. Which bacteria is associated with peptic ulcers?
   A. *Helicobacter pylori*
   B. *Clostridium difficile*
   C. *Staphylococcus*
   D. *Streptococcus*
5. Which organ protrudes through the esophageal opening of the diaphragm and into the thoracic cavity resulting in a diagnosis of hiatal hernia?
   A. Stomach
   B. Large Intestine
   C. Small intestine
   D. Pancreas
6. Which disease or condition is a chronic inflammatory disorder of the alimentary canal in which all layers of the bowel wall are edematous and inflamed?
   A. Ulcerative colitis
   B. Crohn's disease
   C. Diverticula
   D. Gastroenteritis

7. What is one initial treatment for a paralytic ileus?
   A. Pepcid
   B. Nasogastric tube
   C. Ostomy
   D. Bowel resection
8. A physician sees multiple outpouches or pockets within the large intestine while performing sigmoidoscopy on a patient? Which term refers to this condition?
   A. Polyp
   B. Ulcer
   C. Diverticula
   D. Hernia
9. A patient presents with irritable bowel syndrome. Which symptom or symptom is associated with this condition?
   A. Diarrhea
   B. Constipation
   C. Cramping
   D. All the above may be experienced
10. A patient experiences a ruptured appendix. Which condition will result if emergent care is not sought quickly?
    A. Diarrhea
    B. Peritonitis
    C. Colitis
    D. Biliary colic

9

Diseases and Conditions of the Respiratory System

CHAPTER OUTLINE

LEARNING OBJECTIVES

After studying this chapter, you should be able to:

1. Explain the process of respiration.
2. Discuss the causes and medical treatment for (1) the common cold, (2) sinusitis, and (3) pharyngitis.
3. Name the treatment of choice for nasal polyps.
4. Name some systemic disorders that might cause epistaxis.
5. Discuss the prognosis of cancer of the larynx.
6. Define atelectasis and discuss some possible causes.
7. Compare the clinical pictures of (1) a patient with pulmonary embolism and (2) one with pneumonia.
8. List some health hazards of common molds.
9. List some possible causes of a pulmonary abscess.
10. Compare legionnaires disease with Pontiac fever.
11. Explain who is at greatest risk for (1) respiratory syncytial virus pneumonia and (2) histoplasmosis.
12. List the groups recommended to receive prophylactic use of influenza vaccines.
13. Recall what the acronym COPD stands for.
14. Contrast the pathologic course of acute bronchitis with that of chronic bronchitis.
15. Compare the pathology involved in bronchiectasis with that of pulmonary emphysema.
16. Name and describe three causes of pneumoconiosis.
17. Describe the presenting symptoms of pleurisy.
18. Explain the difference between pneumothorax and hemothorax.

19. Describe the cause of the instability of the chest wall in a patient with flail chest.
20. Discuss contributing factors to, and concern about, the rising prevalence of pulmonary tuberculosis.
21. Describe the clinical course of infectious mononucleosis.
22. Explain the pathologic changes in the lungs in adult respiratory distress syndrome.
23. Explain what determines the prognosis of sarcoidosis.
24. Name the leading cause of cancer deaths worldwide for both males and females.
25. Explain the possible health consequences of smoking tobacco.
26. What are the potential health risks for individuals who use tobacco-free nicotine delivery devices, such as electronic cigarettes and atomizers?
27. Describe signs and symptoms of COVID-19, including "long-term COVID."

KEY TERMS

anosmia (an-OZ-me-ah)
anthracosis (an-thrah-KOE-sis)
aphonia (ah-FOE-nee-ah)
asbestosis (as-beh-STOH-sis)
aspiration (as-pih-RAY-shun)
circumoral cyanosis (sir-kum-OH-ral sigh-an-OH-sis)
dysphonia (dis-FOE-nee-ah)
epistaxis (ep-ih-STAK-sis)
exsanguination (eck-sang-win-AY-shun)
hemoptysis (he-MOP-tih-sis)

laryngectomy (lar-in-JECK-toh-me)
lymphadenitis (limf-ad-eh-NIGH-tis)
lymphadenopathy (limf-ad-eh-NOP-ah-thee)
pneumoconiosis (nu-moh-koh-nee-OH-sis)
rhonchi (RONG-ki)
silicosis (sill-ih-KO-sis)
sinusotomy (sigh-nus-OT-oh-me)
stridor (STRY-dor)
syncytial virus (sin-SIGH-shal virus)
tachypnea (tach-ip-NEE-ah)

Orderly Function of the Respiratory System

The primary functions of the pulmonary system are ventilation and respiration. Respiration maintains life by supplying oxygen to organs, tissues, and cells and by allowing for the removal of carbon dioxide (a waste product of metabolism). This process is made possible by ventilation (the bellows-like action of the chest) and healthy lung tissue that is adequately perfused with blood. Breathing is controlled by the central nervous system (CNS); nerve stimulation of breathing begins in the medulla oblongata and the pons. Pulmonary circulation is composed of pulmonary arteries, which carry deoxygenated venous blood from the heart to the lungs; pulmonary capillaries, in which gas exchange occurs; and pulmonary veins, which return freshly oxygenated blood to the heart for systemic circulation. The lung tissue itself is supplied with oxygen and nutrients by the blood supply that is carried to it by the bronchial arteries.

The lungs, along with the kidneys, have a major metabolic function: the maintenance of acid-base (pH) balance of blood. Lack of oxygen with hypercapnia (increased carbon dioxide in the blood) causes respiratory acidosis; hyperventilation may produce hypocapnia (a decreased amount of carbon dioxide in blood), causing respiratory alkalosis. In both conditions, arterial blood gases are abnormal. The kidneys work to adjust bicarbonate in blood in response to carbon dioxide.

In the lungs, oxygen inhaled from the air is exchanged with carbon dioxide from blood; this process is called *external respiration*. *Internal respiration* refers to the exchange of gases between blood and tissue cells. Carbon dioxide is then exhaled as a waste product. Inhaled air and exhaled air pass through the respiratory tract, which includes the nose, pharynx, larynx, and trachea (Fig. 9.1).

In the chest, the trachea bifurcates into bronchi. Each bronchus enters a lung, where it further divides into increasingly smaller air passages called *bronchioles*. At the end of each bronchiole is a saclike cavity called an *alveolus*. There are approximately 300 million alveoli in each lung, and this is where the exchange of carbon dioxide for oxygen takes place.

A muscular, dome-shaped partition, called the *diaphragm*, attaches to the lower ribs and separates the thoracic cavity from the abdominal cavity. On inspiration, the diaphragm contracts, pulling downward and causing air to be sucked into the lungs. During expiration, the diaphragm relaxes, pushing upward and forcing air out of the lungs (Fig. 9.2). Expansion of the chest cavity and diaphragmatic contraction are active, energy-requiring processes. Exhalation occurs as the stretched chest cavity springs back to its resting state along with the relaxation of the diaphragm. This is a passive process.

A membrane called the *visceral pleura* encases the lungs, and the *parietal pleura* line the inside of the chest or thoracic cavity. The potential space between the visceral and parietal pleura is called the *pleural cavity*. Depending on the body size, approximately 10 to 20 mL of pleural fluid is contained in the space between the pleurae, preventing friction and allowing the pleurae to slide easily on each other. Between the lungs is the mediastinum, where the heart, great vessels, trachea, esophagus, and lymph nodes are located.

Respiratory failure can result from the impairment of alveolar-arterial gas exchange (hypoxia), which results in a

• **Fig. 9.1** The structural plan of the respiratory system. (From Patton KT, Thibodeau GA: *The human body in health & disease*, ed 6, Maryland Heights, 2014, Elsevier.)

decrease of oxygen in blood. Additionally, respiratory failure can be caused by the inability to ventilate, which results in an increasing buildup of carbon dioxide. Diseases of the respiratory system result from infection, circulatory disorders, tumors, trauma, immune diseases, congenital defects, CNS damage or diseases, inflammatory disturbances, or environmental conditions.

The chief symptoms indicating respiratory tract disorders that should receive medical attention include:
- Chest pain
- Dyspnea (difficulty in breathing), shortness of breath
- Productive or nonproductive cough that is acute or chronic
- hemoptysis (spitting up blood)
- dysphonia (hoarseness)
- Chills

- Low- or high-grade fever
- Wheezing
- Fatigue

Common Cold/Upper Respiratory Tract Infection

Description

The common cold, also referred to as an *upper respiratory infection* (URI), is an acute inflammatory process that affects the mucous membrane that lines the upper respiratory tract.

| ICD-10-CM Code | J00 (*Acute nasopharyngitis [common cold]*) |

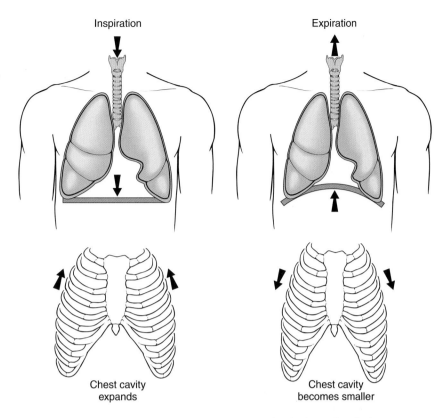

• **Fig. 9.2** Diaphragm and chest movement on inspiration and expiration.

Symptoms and Signs

Although the common, or "head," cold is confined to the nose and the pharynx, the same viruses can infect the larynx (see the Laryngitis section) and various areas of the lungs (see the Acute and Chronic Bronchitis section). The suffix -*itis* is added to the anatomic location where most of the inflammation occurs (i.e., pharyngitis, laryngitis, tracheitis, or bronchitis). The symptoms of a cold tend to be subjective and, to some extent, depend on which virus is responsible; the symptoms include nasal congestion and discharge, sneezing, watery eyes, sore throat, hoarseness of the voice, and coughing. When this highly contagious inflammatory process first begins, the nasal discharge is usually clear and thin. In adults, the symptoms usually abate in 7 to 10 days without antibiotic therapy. In some cases, the cold progresses, and the discharge becomes greenish-yellow and thick. Headache, slight fever, and chills often accompany a cold. A high fever and malaise, however, are more likely to be symptoms of influenza (see the Influenza section).

Patient Screening

Symptoms of a cold that are prolonged or accompanied by fever, chest pain, chest congestion, earache, severe headache, stiff neck, decreased urine, or other complications indicate the need for medical care within 24 hours.

Etiology

The common cold is a group of minor illnesses that can be caused by almost 200 different viruses. Cold viruses are not part of normal body flora; thus viruses that cause a cold are passed from one human to another. Colds are frequent diseases and a common cause of absenteeism from work and school. Rhinoviruses cause about one-half of the colds in adults. (Some colds may result from *Mycoplasma* and other atypical organisms that are more like bacteria than viruses. These are also transmitted by airborne respiratory droplets.) Viral infections sometimes are followed by bacterial infections of the pharynx, middle ear, sinuses, larynx, or lungs. General poor health, lack of exercise, and poor nutrition predispose a person to the common cold.

Diagnosis

Diagnosis is made from the symptoms described by the patient. To rule out a more serious disease, cultures of the nasal discharge and sputum, along with a complete blood count (CBC), may be needed.

Treatment

An ordinary cold should clear up in 7 to 10 days. Persistent cough or nasal congestion may suggest the presence of another process, such as allergies or asthma. There is no cure for a cold. Resting, drinking plenty of fluids, using a vaporizer, and taking over-the-counter antihistamines, decongestants, cough suppressants, and mild analgesics can give temporary relief of symptoms.

Mechanism of Action. Antihistamines are drugs that inhibit the action of or inhibit the formation of histamine in the body. Antihistamines help dry up nasal secretions,

> ⚡ *NOTE*
>
> Aspirin is contraindicated in infants and children; acetaminophen is the drug of choice.

diminish itchy or watery eyes, and decrease flare-ups of allergic reactions. Antihistamines may cause drowsiness.

Decongestants are drugs that stimulate adrenergic receptors and induce vasoconstriction of blood vessels in the nose, throat, and sinuses. Stimulation of the alpha-adrenergic receptors decreases the swelling of the nasal tissue and reduces mucus formation.

Expectorants (mucolytics) are medications that help dissolve mucus and reduce the viscosity of mucous secretions.

Cough suppressants are medications used to treat or lessen cough.

All medication should be approved by a child's physician before being administered.

Prognosis

The common cold is usually benign and self-limiting. Patients who are immunocompromised may be more susceptible to developing frequent colds and complications. Possible complications include secondary bacterial infections, as listed previously under the Etiology section.

Prevention

The mechanisms of cold-virus transmission are not always clearly defined. In many cases, the mode of transmission is airborne respiratory droplets and hand-to-hand contact, so prevention is difficult.

Patient Teaching

Colds are more common in children than in adults and are a frequent cause of absenteeism. Once infected, children can easily transmit new strains to family members. Frequent, thorough hand washing and isolation during the acute stage of illness are commonsense measures that can help control transmission. Stress to the patient that antibiotics do not cure the common cold. Instruct the patient to avoid overuse of drugs, such as nasal sprays, and to take all medications only as instructed. List the warning signs of complications that should be reported to the health care provider (i.e., shortness of breath, severe headache, chest pain, high fever, and symptoms of dehydration or stiff neck).

Sinusitis

Description

Sinusitis is an acute or chronic inflammation of the mucous membranes of the paranasal sinuses.

ICD-10-CM Code	J01.90 *(Acute sinusitis, unspecified)*
	(J01.90–J01.91 = 2 codes of specificity)
	J32.9 *(Chronic sinusitis, unspecified)*
	(J32.0–J32.9 = 7 codes of specificity)

Sinusitis is classified by location, type, and extent of pathology. Refer to the physician's diagnosis and then to the current edition of the ICD-10-CM coding manual for greatest specificity.

Symptoms and Signs

The sinuses, which are cavities behind the facial bones that shape the nose, cheeks, and eye sockets, are normally air filled. In sinusitis, the frontal sinuses (located in the forehead above the eyes) and the maxillary sinuses (located under the maxillary bones in the face) are the most commonly involved sinuses (Fig. 9.3). When the frontal sinuses

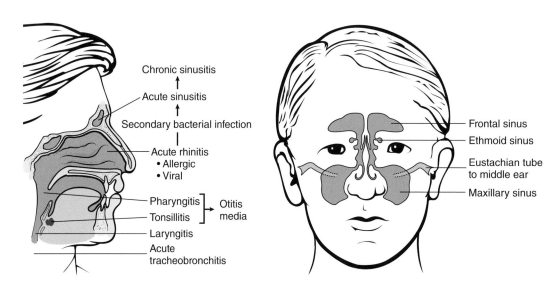

• **Fig. 9.3** Sinusitis. (From Damjanov I: *Pathology for the health-related professions*, ed 4, St. Louis, 2011, Saunders/Elsevier.)

are affected, a headache is common over one or both eyes, especially on waking in the morning. Pain and tenderness, which are felt just above the eyes and usually intensify when bending over, are also common symptoms. Pain in the cheeks and upper teeth is a symptom of sinusitis in the maxillary sinuses. If present, drainage will be a thick, greenish-yellow, mucopurulent liquid. The course of acute sinusitis is 3 to 4 weeks.

Patient Screening

Individuals with symptoms of acute sinusitis (fever, sinus congestion, facial tenderness and pain, and severe headache) are encouraged to seek medical attention as soon as possible.

Etiology

Sinusitis can be caused by viral, fungal, or, more commonly, bacterial infections that travel to the sinuses from the nose, often after the patient has been infected by a common cold. This occurs easily because the mucous membranes that line the nasal cavity extend into and also line the sinuses. One is predisposed to sinusitis by any condition that blocks sinus drainage and ventilation (e.g., a deviated nasal septum or nasal polyps). Sinusitis also may result from swimming or diving, tooth extractions, tooth abscess, or allergies that affect the nasal passages. The cause of chronic sinusitis may never be determined; however, a common variable immunodeficiency disease may be involved (see Chapter 3).

Diagnosis

The diagnosis of sinusitis is made by evaluating the findings from the physical examination, patient history, sinus radiographic studies, computed tomography (CT), and endoscopic sinoscopy. Sinuses that are air filled appear as dark patches on a radiograph, whereas fluid-filled sinuses appear as white areas. Bedside transillumination can suggest the presence of sinusitis. Additionally, a specimen of nasal secretions may be taken for culture to identify or rule out bacterial agents.

Treatment

Treatment of sinusitis can include saline nasal spray, corticosteroid nasal sprays, broad-spectrum antibiotics, oral corticosteroids, antihistamines, and decongestants. Decongestants alleviate symptoms by shrinking the swollen mucous membranes and drying up the nasal discharge to expand the airway and ease breathing. Oral and topical corticosteroids decrease the inflammation of the affected area and decrease sensitivity to aggravating stimuli. Oral antibiotics are used if bacterial infection is present and may include amoxicillin, doxycycline, sulfamethoxazole-trimethoprim, or cephalosporins. Other antibiotics may be used, depending on the infecting organism. Determination of allergic sinusitis may include allergy testing followed by appropriate desensitization with immunotherapy and corticosteroids. If the inflammation persists, a minor surgery called sinusotomy may be advised by the physician.

Prognosis

The prognosis for uncomplicated acute sinusitis is good. Chronic sinusitis may require more prolonged medical treatment with antibiotics.

Prevention

The management of conditions that predispose an individual to sinusitis may help prevent chronic sinusitis.

Patient Teaching

Emphasize the importance of complying with the treatment plan and returning for follow-up appointments. List the warning signs of complications, such as chills, fever, facial edema, severe headache, stiff neck, lethargy, or confusion. Prepare the patient for diagnostic testing or surgery by explaining each procedure and what to expect in terms of preparation and postprocedure care.

Pharyngitis

Description

Pharyngitis (sore throat) is acute or chronic inflammation or infection of the pharynx.

ICD-10-CM Code	J02.9 (Acute pharyngitis, unspecified) (J02.0–J02.9 = 3 codes of specificity)

Symptoms and Signs

Pharyngitis may be acute or chronic and often involves inflammation of the tonsils, uvula, and palate. A sore throat with dryness, a burning sensation, or the sensation of a lump in the throat is common. Clinical manifestations vary with the type of pharyngitis. Generally chills, fever, dysphonia, dysphagia, and cervical lymphadenopathy are common. On examination of the throat, the mucosa of the pharynx is found to be red and swollen, with or without tonsillar exudate, depending on the causative organism.

Patient Screening

An individual complaining of a persistent sore throat with systemic symptoms should be seen by a physician within 24 hours. The patient should be advised not to initiate antibiotic therapy before the appointment because this can impede the accuracy of diagnostic testing.

Etiology

The most common cause of pharyngitis is a viral infection; tonsillitis is the most important cause. In children, it is often an extension of streptococcal infection from the tonsils, adenoids, nose, or sinuses. Persistent infection, or chronic pharyngitis, occurs when an infection (respiratory, sinus, or oral disease) spreads to the pharynx and remains. Acute pharyngitis may be secondary to systemic viral infections, such as chickenpox and measles, whereas chronic pharyngitis may accompany other diseases, such as syphilis and tuberculosis (TB). Gonococcal pharyngitis may result from oral-genital sexual activity with an infected partner. Pharyngitis also can be caused by irritation and inflammation without infection. Breathing in excessively heated air or chemical irritants and swallowing sharp objects (e.g., a large ice chip or hard candy) also can cause trauma. Seasonal allergies may induce pharyngitis.

Diagnosis

Physical examination usually shows red, swollen mucous membranes. For chronic pharyngitis, the physician needs to identify and locate the primary source of the infection or irritation. Further examination of the nasopharyngeal area, throat culture or strep test, and a CBC may be necessary.

Treatment

Home treatment with the use of lozenges, mouthwashes, salt water gargles, an ice collar, and antiinflammatory medication may be helpful in viral infections. When symptoms persist for longer than a few days, a physician should be consulted. Because most cases of pharyngitis are viral in origin, antibiotics are not prescribed. However, acute bacterial infections necessitate the systemic administration of antibiotics. Documented streptococcal pharyngitis is treated with a 7- to 10-day course of antibiotics. Chronic tonsillitis, adenoiditis, and adenoid hypertrophy may be treated with surgical excision. Bed rest and copious amounts of fluids may be advised.

> **‡ NOTE**
> Aspirin is not given to children because of the threat of Reye syndrome.

Prognosis

Uncomplicated pharyngitis resolves within a few days. Bacterial causes are cured with appropriate antibiotics. Chronic cases may require eliminating the underlying cause, such as smoking or allergens, before improvement can be achieved. A potential complication of streptococcal pharyngitis is peritonsillar abscess. This is a pocket of infection that occurs behind the tonsil (usually unilateral) and can compromise the airway. This is an emergent issue and needs to be addressed the same day.

Prevention

Prevention measures include maintaining general good health, avoiding infections, evading known irritants, and controlling allergies.

Patient Teaching

Instruct the patient to take the entire course of antibiotic therapy and keep follow-up appointments to ensure a complete cure and prevent complications. Provide a list of comfort measures, such as safe use of analgesics, warm saline gargles, adequate fluid intake, and a soft diet.

Nasopharyngeal Carcinoma

Description

Nasopharyngeal tumors arise in the area of the pharynx that opens into the nasal cavity anteriorly and the oropharynx inferiorly. They are unique among head and neck cancers in that they are not as strongly linked to tobacco use. Instead, they are often linked to dietary intake or Epstein-Barr virus (EBV) infection.

ICD-10-CM Code	C11.9 *(Malignant neoplasm of nasopharynx, unspecified)* (C11.0–C11.9 = 6 codes of specificity)

Symptoms and Signs

Because of the anatomic location of the nasopharyngeal tumor, patients are often asymptomatic during the early stages of the disease. The classic clinical triad of symptoms is neck mass, nasal obstruction with epistaxis, and serous otitis media. Although it is rare to find all three symptoms in a patient, the individual symptoms occur frequently. Other symptoms include headache, hearing loss, tinnitus, pain, and impaired function of the cranial nerves.

Patient Screening

Provide the first available appointment to the individual reporting neck mass or related symptoms.

Etiology

Although nasopharyngeal carcinoma is a rare disease in the United States and Western Europe, several subpopulations do have a relatively high incidence. These include people from southern China, areas around the Mediterranean Sea, Southeast Asia, and the Arctic. Several known risk factors in the high-risk areas include consumption of salted fish as a diet standard, foods with high levels of nitrates (e.g., processed meats), and Chinese herbs; infection by EBV; and having a first-degree relative with nasopharyngeal carcinoma. The use of alcohol and tobacco is a risk factor in low-risk areas.

Diagnosis

Diagnosis is made after a full clinical examination of the head and neck and an endoscopic examination of the nasopharynx with a biopsy of suspicious lesions. Testing for EBV should also be performed. Staging is determined according to the tumor-node-metastasis (TNM) system. Magnetic resonance imaging (MRI) of the head and neck, bone scanning, and a CT or positron emission tomography (PET) are used for staging.

Treatment

Because of the anatomic constraints of the nasopharynx, surgery is usually not performed. Nasopharyngeal carcinoma is commonly quite radiosensitive, and most patients with early-stage cancer are treated with radiation therapy, with or without adjuvant chemotherapy. Close follow-up is important after completion of therapy to monitor for recurrence.

Prognosis

Because early neoplasms rarely cause symptoms, most patients present with advanced carcinoma, and many already have distant metastases to bones, the lungs, or the liver. If the tumor has extended to involve one of the cranial nerves or has metastasized to the cervical lymph nodes, the prognosis is worse. In addition, the presence of high plasma levels of EBV deoxyribonucleic acid (DNA) at the time of diagnosis or after treatment is correlated with a poorer outcome.

Prevention

There is no prevention. Living a healthy lifestyle by avoiding smoking and exercising may lower your risk of getting cancer.

Patient Teaching

Prepare the patient for diagnostic testing by providing information about an endoscopy of the nasopharynx and a biopsy of any lesion in the nasopharynx. Encourage the patient to ask questions, and defer to the physician for revealing the prognosis.

Laryngitis

Description

Inflammation of the larynx (hoarseness), including the vocal cords, is called *laryngitis*.

ICD-10-CM Code   J04.0 *(Acute laryngitis)*

Laryngitis coding includes modifiers that specify causative agents and factors, such as obstruction. Refer to the physician's diagnosis and then to the current edition of the ICD-10-CM coding manual for the appropriate modifiers.

Symptoms and Signs

Because the opening of the larynx is narrow, inflammation of the larynx sometimes interferes with breathing. Symptoms vary with the severity of the inflammation, but the main symptom of laryngitis is hoarseness, which causes aphonia. Fever, malaise, a painful throat, dysphagia, and other symptoms associated with influenza occur in more severe infections.

Patient Screening

Laryngitis associated with recent trauma requires immediate medical attention. A sensation of swelling in the throat, difficulty breathing, and laryngitis indicate a medical emergency, especially if the patient feels like their air is being restricted.

Etiology

The cause of laryngitis can be either viral or bacterial infection, and the condition can be either chronic or acute. URIs, such as the common cold, tonsillitis, pharyngitis, and sinusitis, are the most common causes of inflammation of the larynx. Laryngitis also occurs with bronchitis, pertussis, influenza, pneumonia, measles, mononucleosis, diphtheria, syphilis, and TB. Occasionally, laryngitis is caused by irritation without infection. Reflux laryngitis may result from repeated attacks of acid reflux. Inclement weather, tobacco smoking, alcohol consumption, inhalation of irritating materials, and excessive use of the voice (i.e., yelling at a concert or sports event) are all predisposing factors, especially in the case of chronic laryngitis. Hoarseness can also be caused by benign or malignant lesions of the larynx. In most cases, the pathology is benign, but malignancy must be ruled out.

Diagnosis

Laryngoscopic examination reveals mildly or highly inflamed mucosa, and vocal cord movement may be limited. If no inflammation is present, laryngitis is not the cause of dysphonia, and further diagnostic tests are needed to determine the underlying condition.

Treatment

Treatment of viral laryngitis includes the following palliative measures: absolute voice rest, bed rest in a well-humidified room, liberal fluid intake, no tobacco or alcohol consumption, and the use of lozenges and cough syrup. Improvement should be seen in 4 or 5 days. Antibiotic administration gives good results when laryngitis occurs in conjunction with a bacterial infection. Corticosteroids may be used to decrease inflammation when symptoms are more severe. When hoarseness persists for longer than 1 week, the condition may be chronic. Treatment of chronic laryngitis is based on the elimination, as much as possible, of the causative factors.

Prognosis

Recovery is generally complete within 1 week.

Prevention

Known irritants that cause laryngitis are avoided or treated, if possible. Infections are difficult to prevent. Avoid speaking when at all possible.

Patient Teaching

Explain the importance of resting the voice and taking medications as prescribed, along with drinking plenty of fluids. Avoid irritants.

Deviated Septum

Description

A crooked nasal septum (the cartilage partition between the nostrils) is called a *deviated septum* (Fig. 9.4).

ICD-10-CM Code   J34.2 *(Deviated nasal septum)*

Symptoms and Signs

A deviated septum causes narrowing and obstruction of the air passage, making breathing somewhat difficult. Other than mild breathing problems or a slightly increased tendency to develop sinusitis, no significant symptoms are associated with a deviated septum.

Patient Screening

The deviation may be found by chance during a routine physical examination. The condition may be of no consequence until aggravated by trauma to the nose. In that case, schedule the first available appointment for evaluation.

Etiology

Congenital anomaly is usually the cause of minor deviation of the septum. Substantial septal deviation is uncommon and is usually the result of trauma to the nose.

Diagnosis

Patient history and the amount of obstruction aid the physician in determining the diagnosis and treatment of this condition.

• **Fig. 9.4** Deviated septum. (From Monahan FD, Neighbors M: *Medical-surgical nursing: foundations for clinical practice*, ed 2, Philadelphia, 1998, Saunders.)

Treatment

Treatment is not usually necessary unless a compromise of the air passage is noted. The septum can be straightened surgically to repair a significant obstruction or for cosmetic reasons. Straightening a deviated septum involves removing the cartilage (rhinoplasty or septoplasty), and reshaping or repositioning the nose structure.

Prognosis

This fairly common condition has a good prognosis.

Prevention

The only possible prevention is to avoid trauma to the nose.

Patient Teaching

If surgical correction is scheduled, tell the patient what to expect after surgery, such as the use of nasal packing to control bleeding, nasal splints, and analgesics for pain.

Nasal Polyps

Description

Nasal polyps are benign growths that form as a consequence of distended mucous membranes protruding into the nasal cavity (Fig. 9.5).

ICD-10-CM Code	J33.9 *(Nasal polyp, unspecified)*
	(J33.0–33.9 = 4 codes of specificity)

Nasal polyps are coded by anatomic site and underlying pathology. Refer to the physician's diagnosis and then to the current edition of the ICD-10-CM coding manual for greatest specificity.

Symptoms and Signs

Nasal polyps are not harmful but can become large enough to obstruct the nasal airway, making breathing difficult.

• **Fig. 9.5** Nasal polyps. (From Jarvis C: *Physical examination & health assessment*, ed 5, St. Louis, 2008, Saunders.)

Polyps often affect or impair the sense of smell. When polyps obstruct one of the sinuses, symptoms of sinusitis are present.

Patient Screening
Nasal polyps may be found in a patient exhibiting symptoms of allergic rhinitis and/or sinusitis. The degree of urgency for an appointment is based on the severity of symptoms.

Etiology
Polyps are caused by the overproduction of fluid in the cells of the mucous membrane. They are hyperplastic. This overproduction is often the result of a condition called *allergic rhinitis.* Some aspirin-sensitive people have the triad of nasal polyps, asthma, and urticaria (hives).

Diagnosis
The physician examines the inside of the nose using an instrument called a *nasal speculum,* or they can be viewed by a nasal endoscope. Polyps appear as pearly gray lumps along the nasal passage.

Treatment
Nasal corticosteroid spray may be used as an initial treatment to shrink the polyps. Oral corticosteroids may also be prescribed. Endoscopic surgery may become necessary if the medications do not achieve a positive outcome in shrinking the polyps.

Prognosis
The prognosis is good, although nasal polyps tend to recur.

Prevention
No specific preventive measures are known. Management of allergic rhinitis is beneficial.

Patient Teaching
Instructions given to the patient are related to the treatment of choice. When appropriate, explain the relationship of allergic rhinitis to nasal polyps.

Anosmia

Description
Anosmia is the impairment or loss of the sense of smell.

ICD-10-CM Code	R43.0 *(Anosmia)*
	R43.1 *(Parosmia)*
	R43.2 *(Parageusia)*
	(R43.0–R43.9 = 5 codes of specificity)

Symptoms and Signs
The loss of smell that continues without an obvious cause is termed *anosmia.* The ability to taste liquids and food is also impaired or lost.

Patient Screening
The patient complaining of prolonged, unexplained loss of the sense of smell is scheduled for a diagnostic evaluation.

Etiology
Chronic conditions, such as nasal polyps and allergic rhinitis, are the most common causes of anosmia. Intranasal swelling accompanying an upper respiratory condition causes temporary anosmia. Sometimes a phobia concerning a particular odor accounts for a psychological basis for anosmia. It may, however, be the result of damage to the olfactory nerves caused by a head injury or, rarely, a symptom of a brain tumor. COVID-19 and other viral illnesses can also cause symptoms of anosmia, sometimes lasting months after the patient is better.

Diagnosis
If the physician does not find any physical abnormality on examination or the patient's history does not reveal recent head trauma or an allergic condition, a neurologist may be consulted. Additional diagnostic tests may be needed to provide a definitive diagnosis.

Treatment
Treatment is aimed at the cause of the condition. When polyps are found, they are treated or removed. Topical or oral steroids may be used for olfactory dysfunction. For allergic rhinitis, a series of injections containing increasingly stronger concentrations of the offending allergen is used to desensitize the patient. Olfactory training is another technique that may be of benefit in cases such as those caused by COVID-19. Four different scents are sniffed for several seconds two times a day while focusing on what the scent smells like. This is repeated every day for approximately 3 months, then four new smells are introduced.

Prognosis
Anosmia is often related to a URI and is thus a temporary condition. Anosmia resulting from nerve damage is permanent.

Prevention
Avoid toxic chemicals and environments, and head injury.

Patient Teaching
Patients may benefit from an explanation of how the olfactory nerve normally functions, and how it is affected by the determined cause of anosmia.

Epistaxis (Nosebleed)

Description
Epistaxis is hemorrhage from the nose.

| ICD-10-CM Code | R04.0 *(Epistaxis)* |

Symptoms and Signs

Hemorrhage from the nose, known as *epistaxis*, is a common, sudden emergency. Bleeding usually occurs from only one nostril, and often no apparent explanation for the bleeding is known.

Patient Screening

Hemorrhage from the nose that persists for 10 minutes or more after constant pressure is applied is considered severe and requires immediate emergency care. If the patient reports a severe headache at the onset of epistaxis or is experiencing sequential nosebleeds, an immediate appointment should be arranged.

Etiology

Common causes of epistaxis are colds and infections, such as rhinitis, sinusitis, and nasopharyngitis. Direct trauma to the nose, picking the nose, and the presence of a foreign body can also result in epistaxis. Nasal hemorrhage also has been encountered in relation to many systemic disorders, such as measles, scarlet fever, pertussis, rheumatic fever, hypertension, congestive heart failure, and chronic renal disease. Epistaxis may be the foremost symptom of some blood disorders or systemic diseases and should be investigated if it is frequent and unexplained.

Diagnosis

The diagnosis of epistaxis is made on the basis of the patient's history regarding the frequency of the nosebleeds, whether an injury has occurred, or whether the symptoms indicate that systemic disease may be present. All medications, dietary supplements, and herbal preparations taken by the patient are noted to identify contributing offenders.

Treatment

Mild hemorrhage may be controlled by applying constant direct pressure on either side of the bridge of the nose for 5 to 10 minutes. An internal compression device, such as Rhino Rocket or Rapid Rhino may be used. Persistent bleeding can be treated with local application of epinephrine, followed by cauterization with silver nitrate or laser cauterization. If bleeding continues, a posterior nasal packing left in place for 1 to 3 days may be necessary. A mild sclerosing agent also may be injected into a bleeding vessel if it can be visualized by the physician.

Prognosis

The prognosis is generally good.

Prevention

Specific treatment of the underlying disease, if present, is of prime importance. Prevention includes instructing patients on how to avoid recurrences.

Patient Teaching

Demonstrate first-aid measures for controlling epistaxis, sitting with the head tilted forward while applying constant local pressure by compressing the side of the nose against the septum. Tell the patient to report repeated or severe nosebleeds immediately to the health care provider.

Tumors of the Larynx

Description

Growths or tumors on the larynx may be benign or malignant.

ICD-10-CM Code	C00-D49

The above general codes represent the broad category of neoplasms that are classified by such diagnostic criteria as malignant or benign, as primary or secondary, or according to site, function, and morphology. Refer to the physician's diagnosis and then to the current edition of the ICD-10-CM coding manual to ensure the greatest specificity of pathology.

Symptoms and Signs

Dysphonia is usually the only symptom of a tumor in the larynx. No influenza-like symptoms occur as with laryngitis (see the Laryngitis section), but when the tumor is malignant, dysphagia may be experienced. In children with tumors, a high-pitched crowing sound, called stridor, is present because of the small airways. Hoarseness caused by a benign tumor is usually intermittent, whereas hoarseness caused by cancer is continuous and gradually becomes worse. Neither type of laryngeal tumor is common, but malignant tumors are more common in males than in females.

Patient Screening

Unexplained, persistent hoarseness lasting longer than 3 weeks requires prompt medical evaluation. Schedule an appointment as soon as possible.

Etiology

There are two types of benign tumors: papillomas, which usually appear in multiples, and polyps, which usually appear as single lesions (Fig. 9.6). These tumors are caused by misuse or overuse of the vocal cords, although smoking and acid reflux are contributing factors. Malignant tumors occur more often in those who indulge in heavy tobacco use.

Diagnosis

The physician or otolaryngologist thoroughly examines the larynx and vocal cords. When a tumor or tumors are found, a biopsy is done to determine whether a malignancy is present. Cancer of the larynx can almost always be cured if it is diagnosed early.

Treatment

Benign growths, whether papillomas or polyps, may be treated with correction of the vocal strain, management

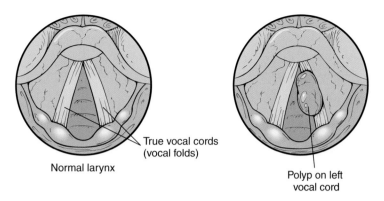

True vocal cords
(vocal folds)

Normal larynx

Polyp on left
vocal cord

• **Fig. 9.6** Vocal cord polyp.

of acid reflux, and smoking cessation. The growths may also be excised under local anesthesia. Malignant tumors, if discovered early, are often treated and cured by radiation therapy. When the cancer has metastasized, **laryngectomy** may be needed. After a laryngectomy, the patient needs extensive speech therapy to learn a substitute form of speech.

Prognosis
The prognosis depends on the type of tumor.

Prevention
Avoidance of smoking or any chronic irritation of the larynx is recommended.

Patient Teaching
Give the patient preoperative instructions, and encourage the patient to express any concerns about treatment. When laryngectomy is necessary, provide every avenue of psychological support available to the family and the patient. Help the patient plan alternative means of communication during speech rehabilitation.

Laryngeal Cancer

Description
Laryngeal cancer describes a neoplasm of the larynx, the part of the respiratory tract between the pharynx and the trachea that houses the vocal cords. It is the most common site for head and neck tumors. Most laryngeal tumors are squamous cell carcinomas.

ICD-10-CM Code	C32.9 *(Malignant neoplasm of larynx, unspecified)* (C32.0–C32.9 = 6 codes of specificity)

The above code is a nonspecific code and may be valid as a principal diagnosis, except for Medicare. Refer to the physician's diagnosis and then to the current edition of the ICD-10-CM coding manual to ensure the greatest specificity.

Symptoms and Signs
If the tumor involves the vocal cord area of the larynx, persistent hoarseness tends to occur early in the disease process and is the most common initial complaint. Hoarseness related to benign causes, such as a vocal cord polyp or nodule caused by chronic irritation or overuse, is usually intermittent, whereas that caused by a malignant neoplasm is continuous and gradually becomes worse over time. Other symptoms may include dysphagia, hemoptysis, chronic cough, referred pain to the ear, and stridor (a high-pitched crowing sound). Airway obstruction also may occur, depending on the tumor location.

Patient Screening
Unexplained, persistent hoarseness lasting longer than 3 weeks requires medical evaluation. Other symptoms related to the throat also may be present.

Etiology
The major risk factors for the development of laryngeal cancer include tobacco and alcohol use, gastroesophageal reflux, viral infections, diet, radiation, and individual predisposition. Other risk factors include infection with human papillomavirus (HPV)-16 or HPV-18, occupational exposure to carcinogenic agents, such as perchloroethylene (a dry cleaning agent) or asbestos, and having a first-degree relative with laryngeal cancer.

Diagnosis
Laryngeal cancer is often diagnosed at an earlier stage compared with other head and neck cancers because hoarseness usually occurs early in the disease process. Flexible fiberoptic endoscopy allows visualization of the larynx, assessment of vocal cord mobility, and biopsy. Staging is done by using the TNM system. CT or MRI is performed to evaluate the depth and extent of tumor invasion and to look for nodal metastasis. A panendoscopy (laryngoscopy, esophagoscopy, and bronchoscopy) is also generally done to look for other areas of tumor growth because tobacco and alcohol use often have widespread toxic effects on the aerodigestive tract. PET can be done to look for distant metastases.

Treatment

For early-stage cancer, often the physician will explain the risks and benefits of surgery and radiation therapy, both of which have similar outcomes, and will let the patient decide on the therapy. Surgical options include partial laryngectomy, total laryngectomy, and endoscopic laser resection. The choice largely depends on the tumor stage. Treatment of later-stage (III and IV) cancer is more difficult. For patients with resectable tumors, treatment usually consists of surgery followed by radiation therapy or radiation alone. Chemoradiotherapy may be tried in patients choosing an organ-sparing approach. For patients who do undergo laryngectomy, follow-up care generally requires the services of a speech therapist for speech therapy and swallowing therapy.

Prognosis

Because of the early manifestation of symptoms, laryngeal cancer is often diagnosed at a stage in which a cure is possible. The most significant prognostic indicator is the status of the cervical lymph nodes.

Prevention

Cessation of smoking and reducing alcohol consumption are highly recommended. Periodic panendoscopy may be used to detect primary cancers occurring after treatment for laryngeal cancer.

Patient Teaching

Encourage the patient to express any concerns about the diagnostic procedures or the course of treatment chosen. Provide every venue of psychological support available to the patient and the family. Give specifics about the postoperative care after laryngectomy, as appropriate. Help the patient plan for alternative means of communication during speech rehabilitation.

Hemoptysis

Description

Hemoptysis is the coughing or spitting up of blood from the respiratory tract.

ICD-10-CM Code	R04.2 *(Hemoptysis)*
	P26.9 *(Pulmonary hemorrhage originating in the perinatal period)*
	(P26.0–P26.9 = 4 codes of specificity)
	A15.0 *(Tuberculosis of lung)*
	A15.7 *(Primary respiratory tuberculosis)*

Symptoms and Signs

Sputum streaked or spotted with blood can be present in minor infections. Hemoptysis can be massive, indicating a serious underlying condition. The patient expectorates bright or dark blood-streaked sputum or dark red clots from the pulmonary or bronchial circulation. Profuse bleeding is present in severe lung infections (i.e., aspergillus infection with angioinvasion), a respiratory malignancy, or erosion of a pulmonary vessel.

Patient Screening

Blood of unknown origin in the sputum is a symptom that requires medical evaluation. If the bleeding is slight and associated with a known respiratory infection, an appointment should be scheduled within 24 hours. Advise the patient experiencing profuse bleeding to seek emergency care, and inform the physician immediately.

Etiology

Trauma, erosion of a vessel, calcification, or tumors can cause bronchial bleeding, as can inflammatory conditions, such as bronchitis or bronchiectasis; chronic infection can result in damaged and irregularly shaped airways. Pulmonary arterial hypertension (often associated with right-sided heart failure) and, at times, pulmonary venous hypertension (associated with left-sided heart failure) may precipitate bleeding from pulmonary vessels. Additional origins of the bleeding can be fungal infections, pulmonary infarcts, tumors or ulcerations of the larynx or pharynx, and coagulation (clotting) defects.

Diagnosis

Of primary importance is determining the source of bleeding. This is accomplished by visual examination of the mouth and the nasopharynx; visualization of the larynx, trachea, and bronchi with endoscopy; and inspection of the lung fields with radiographic studies. Pulmonary angiography can be used for diagnosis and therapeutic embolization.

Blood coagulation studies ascertain whether the problem is caused by a clotting deficiency. The patient is tested for TB. If the previously mentioned investigations are inconclusive, lung scanning, CT of the chest, and/or pulmonary angiography may be indicated.

Treatment

After the location and cause of the bleeding are determined, the source is treated. When the bleeding is severe, ligation or surgical removal or repair of the involved vessels is indicated. Measures are implemented to prevent asphyxiation by clotted blood in the air passages; to prevent obstruction of the bronchial tree by clots, with resulting lung collapse; and to prevent exsanguination of the patient. If minor bleeding occurs or the cause is uncertain, antibiotics and cough suppressant therapy are often prescribed.

Prognosis

The prognosis is good with treatment, but guarded if associated with a serious underlying illness.

Prevention

Hemoptysis is generally considered a symptom, so there is no direct prevention.

Patient Teaching

Steps are taken to allay any fear and anxiety that the patient might be experiencing. Explain the diagnostic procedures and when to expect the results. Reassure the patient that hemoptysis may occur after endoscopy. Reinforce information about the treatment regimen and encourage the patient to voice any concerns. It is also necessary to advise the patient to seek medical attention on an emergent basis if the amount of hemoptysis increases significantly.

Atelectasis

Description

Atelectasis is an airless or collapsed state of the pulmonary tissue.

ICD-10-CM Code   J98.11 (Atelectasis)
                 J98.19 (Other pulmonary collapse)

Symptoms and Signs

Atelectasis occurs when the lungs cannot inflate properly, resulting in oxygen deprivation to blood, tissues, and organs. The patient has difficulty breathing and the lungs can collapse. Substernal retraction and cyanosis may be seen on physical examination, and diminished breath sounds over the affected area are noted on auscultation. Chest radiographs may indicate a mediastinal shift toward the side of collapse. Additionally, the patient experiences anxiety, diaphoresis, and tachycardia. Fever may be present because collapsed lung tissue is prone to infection. Atelectasis also can occur with incomplete expansion of the lungs at birth.

Patient Screening

The patient experiencing dyspnea requires prompt medical attention for evaluation. Severe dyspnea with or without a history of previous atelectasis is a medical emergency; instruct the patient and the family to call an ambulance. The physician should be notified immediately.

Etiology

Atelectasis is caused by an obstruction in the bronchial tree; this can be a mucous plug, foreign body, or bronchogenic cancer. Compression atelectasis results when a tumor exerts pressure on the lung and does not allow air to enter that part. Inflammatory pulmonary disease can result in the accumulation of fluid in the pleural cavity (pleural effusion) and induce atelectasis. Any condition that makes deep breathing difficult can lead to atelectasis (Fig. 9.7). Failure to breathe deeply postoperatively or prolonged inactivity also can induce the collapse of pulmonary tissues. In the newborn, causes include prematurity, hyaline membrane disease, decreased stimulus to breathe, narcotics that cross the placental barrier during labor, and obstruction of the bronchus by a mucous plug. Any condition that decreases the amount of surfactant (a lubricating fluid in the air sacs) can lead to the collapse of these air sacs and, hence, atelectasis.

Diagnosis

Chest radiography, a thorough history, and a physical examination play important roles in the diagnosis. CT of the chest may be necessary to detect subtle changes. Oxygen saturation level will be measured. Breath sounds are diminished over the affected area, and percussion is dull. Bronchoscopy may be indicated to evaluate obstruction by a foreign body or a neoplasm.

Treatment

Because postsurgical patients are at high risk for atelectasis, they are encouraged to ambulate as soon as possible, breathe deeply, and cough periodically; an incentive spirometer is often used to encourage deep breathing. Percussion is used to loosen mucus. Postural drainage by lowering the head lower than the lungs may be used. Other therapeutic measures include suctioning of the airway to remove any obstruction, spirometry, and the use of antibiotics to treat accompanying infection. Analgesics are given for chest pain. Surgical drainage of pleural effusion (abnormal fluid accumulation in the intrapleural spaces of the lungs) may be indicated to reduce intrathoracic pressure.

Suctioning the trachea of the newborn is indicated to remove mucus and facilitate a patent airway. Suctioning usually is followed by the administration of oxygen.

Prognosis

The outcome depends on the treatment of the primary cause. Mild cases may resolve spontaneously. More severe cases are prone to complications, such as pneumonia. Individuals with obesity, upper abdominal or chest surgery, neuromuscular weakness, or pulmonary disease are at higher risk.

Prevention

Early ambulation and good ventilation therapy after surgery or for any condition that causes prolonged immobility are important. Individuals with lung disease are strongly advised not to smoke or breathe irritants.

Patient Teaching

Discuss the diagnostic and therapeutic procedures. Explain the importance of postoperative ambulation and ventilation therapy. Tell the patient to seek prompt medical care for respiratory infections.

Pulmonary Embolism

Description

A pulmonary embolism occurs when a blood clot or other material (e.g., foreign body or tumor) lodges in and occludes an artery in the pulmonary circulation (Fig. 9.8).

ICD-10-CM   I26.99 (Other pulmonary embolism
Code   without acute cor pulmonale)
              (I26.90-I26.99 = 3 codes of
                   specificity)

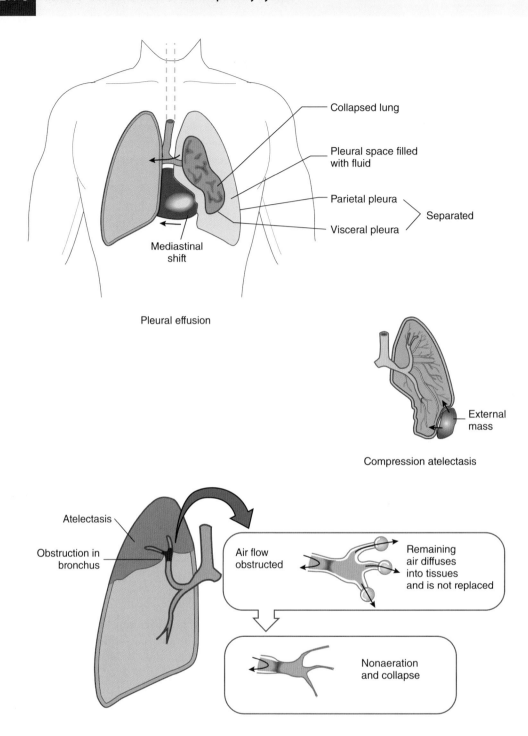

Pleural effusion

Compression atelectasis

Obstructive atelectasis – Absorption atelectasis

• **Fig. 9.7** Atelectasis. (From Gould B: *Pathophysiology for the health professions,* ed 3, Philadelphia, 2006, Saunders.)

Symptoms and Signs

The size and location of the embolism, coupled with the general physical condition of the patient, determine the resulting symptoms and signs. The most common symptom of acute pulmonary embolism is the sudden onset of dyspnea when taking a deep breath. The patient may think they are experiencing a heart attack. Apprehension is common. The patient with a small, uncomplicated embolism experiences a cough, chest pain, and a low-grade fever. The patient with a more extensive infarction experiences dyspnea, tachypnea (with a respiratory rate of at least 20 breaths per minute), chest pain, and occasionally hemoptysis. Massive embolism

• **Fig. 9.8** Pulmonary embolism. (A) Drawing depicting pulmonary embolism. (B) Lung with pulmonary embolism. (B, From Kumar V, et al: *Robbins basic pathology*, ed 10, Philadelphia, 2018, Saunders.)

leads to the sudden onset of cyanosis, shock, and death. Shortness of breath that appears suddenly, chest pain that may become worse when breathing, dizziness, lightheadedness, fainting, leg pain or swelling, back pain, blue nails or lips, and sweating.

Patient Screening

Patients experiencing chest pain need emergent care. An ambulance should be called immediately for emergent care. Individuals with milder symptoms of chest pain, fever, and dyspnea should be given prompt medical attention, with a quick appointment scheduled.

Etiology

Although most emboli are thrombi (blood clots) that have broken loose from a deep vein in the legs or the pelvis, emboli also may be composed of air, fat globules, a small piece of tissue, or a cluster of bacteria. The mass moves through the venous circulation and is pumped by the right side of the heart to the pulmonary circulation, where it becomes lodged in a vessel, usually at a division of an artery where it narrows.

Stasis of blood flow from immobility, injury to a vessel, predisposition to clot formation, thrombophlebitis, cardiovascular disease, smoking, or pulmonary disease increases the risk of embolism formation. In pregnancy, multiple factors predispose individuals to venous thrombosis. Oral contraceptives high in estrogen, diabetes mellitus, and myocardial infarction are considered contributing factors.

Diagnosis

The clinical picture, along with a history of physical immobility or other risk factors, leads to further investigation of respiratory status. CT angiography, D-dimer, pulmonary V/Q (ventilation perfusion) scan, electrocardiogram, echocardiogram, and pulmonary angiography are some of the diagnostic tests. MRI may be used in cases where the patient cannot tolerate dye used in other procedures. Auscultation

often reveals rales and pleural rubs in the area of the embolism. Arterial blood gas determination shows reduced partial pressure of oxygen and carbon dioxide. Studies performed to find residual thrombi in the veins of the lower extremities are helpful because the vast majority of pulmonary emboli originate there.

Treatment

Primary treatment is aimed at preventing a potentially fatal episode and maintaining cardiopulmonary integrity and adequate ventilation and perfusion. Oxygen therapy and anticoagulant administration are used to meet these goals. Drugs of choice include apixaban (Eliquis), rivaroxaban (Xarelto), and dabigatran (Pradaxa). They do not require laboratory tests for monitoring the levels in the blood and have fewer drug and food interactions compared with drugs previously used. Additionally, when there are hemodynamic compromises (shock and right-sided heart failure), thrombolytic drugs sometimes are administered to dissolve a clot, especially when low blood pressure or cardiac arrest occurs.

Prognosis

Mild cases can have a positive outcome with treatment. Mortality is high in cases of massive pulmonary embolism.

Prevention

Management of risk factors, such as long-term immobility, can prevent the formation of emboli that can potentially obstruct pulmonary circulation. Postoperative prophylactic measures include early ambulation, low-dose anticoagulant agents, and the use of a variety of stockings, such as thromboembolic deterrent stockings or sequential stockings that intermittently pump the legs. Optimal management of systemic diseases, such as myocardial infarction, thrombophlebitis, and atrial fibrillation, is beneficial. An inferior vena cava filter may be used to prevent clots from traveling from the legs to the lungs.

Patient Teaching

Explain anticoagulation therapy and the importance of following the provider's instructions. Make the patient aware of the side effects that should be reported to the health care provider, such as nosebleeds, blood in the stool, or spontaneous bruising under the skin. Explain the postoperative measures prescribed to prevent venostasis, such as antiembolism stockings. Avoid extended sitting and move around frequently.

Pneumonia

Description

Pneumonia is infective inflammation of the lungs.

ICD-10-CM Code	J18.9 (*Pneumonia, unspecified organism*) (J12.0–J18.9 = 29 codes of specificity)

Symptoms and Signs

Pneumonia is not only a condition but also a general term applied to several types of inflammation of the lungs. The inflammation may be either unilateral or bilateral and involve all or only a portion of an infected lung (Fig. 9.9). The symptoms of pneumonia vary. The patient may have a cough, fever, shortness of breath even while at rest, chills, sweating, chest pains, cyanosis, and blood in the sputum. The infant or child exhibits "panting" or shallow, rapid respirations. The larger the area of the lung affected, the more severe the symptoms are. How quickly the symptoms develop and which symptoms are most evident vary with the cause.

Aspiration pneumonia results from the aspiration of liquids or other materials into the tracheobronchial tree. It tends to occur in patients who have serious problems with swallowing; it is commonly seen in older adults, especially those weakened by cancer or those with neurological problems, such as stroke or Parkinson disease. Individuals with a suppressed gag reflex from alcohol or drugs are also at risk.

Patient Screening

Cough, fever, and shortness of breath are symptoms that require a prompt, same-day appointment for medical evaluation. Parents of infants may report that the child exhibits symptoms of a cold with fever and fast respirations.

Etiology

Pneumonia usually is caused by viral bacterial infections. Fungal infections can also result in pneumonia. Organisms commonly causing bacterial pneumonia are pneumococci, staphylococci, group A hemolytic streptococci, *Haemophilus influenzae* type B, *Klebsiella pneumoniae* types 1 and 2, and other gram-negative organisms. A syndrome referred to as *atypical pneumonia*, previously

• **Fig. 9.9** Appearance of pneumonia. (From Long BW, Frank ED, Ehrlich RA: *Radiography essentials for limited practice*, ed 4, St. Louis, 2013, Elsevier.)

referred to as *walking pneumonia*, often demonstrates marked abnormalities on the chest radiograph, yet the patient does not appear significantly ill. The organisms most commonly identified with this syndrome include *Legionella, Mycoplasma,* and *Chlamydia*. Viruses, such as adenoviruses, influenza viruses, the COVID-19 virus, and respiratory syncytial viruses (RSVs), also can produce pneumonia. It also may be caused by damage to the lungs from the inhalation of poisonous gas, such as chlorine, or by the aspiration of foreign matter. Pneumonia can range from a mild complication of URI to a life-threatening illness. Bacterial pneumonia can be community acquired by patients living independently in the community, or it may arise in a hospital setting associated with health care or with the use of a ventilator.

Diagnosis

The diagnostic evaluation begins with a physical examination, patient history, and chest radiography to evaluate the pulmonary system. Further tests, such as arterial blood gas, bronchoscopy, and sputum and blood cultures, are also done.

Treatment

Treatment is based on the underlying cause of the pneumonia. Organism-specific antibiotics are prescribed for bacterial pneumonia. Medications such as azithromycin and amoxicillin are commonly used as first-line treatments. Tetracycline drugs, clarithromycin, doxycycline, and sulfonamides may also be administered. *Mycoplasma* infections may be treated with broad-spectrum antibiotics. Fungal infections require the use of various antifungal medications, whereas viral infections are treated with specific antiviral agents. The use of analgesics, such as aspirin, helps relieve chest pain, and oxygen therapy may be necessary for shortness of breath. Bed rest, increased fluid intake, a high-calorie diet, and postural drainage also prove beneficial.

Prognosis

The prognosis is good for otherwise healthy individuals. Those with multiple health issues may have a longer recovery of weeks and months.

Prevention

Vaccines are available for adults, children, and certain groups. Anyone can contact their health care provider to find out if they should be vaccinated to prevent pneumococcal and other types of pneumonia.

Antibiotic therapy for URIs determined to be caused by bacteria, such as *Streptococcus* or *Staphylococcus*, can prevent pneumonia. Prophylactic measures against aspiration in patients with stroke or those in an altered state of consciousness are prudent.

Patient Teaching

Instruct the patient to take the full course of antibiotics and other medications as prescribed and to follow up as instructed. Stress the importance of rest, plenty of fluid intake, and coughing to clear secretions. Counsel the patient to avoid smoking and of contraindications in using alcohol with some medications. Tell the patient to seek prompt medical care for signs of respiratory infection in the future, to avoid known persons with infections, and to take seasonal influenza vaccines as recommended by the provider.

Pulmonary Abscess

Description

A cavity of infectious material contained in the lung is known as a *pulmonary abscess* (Fig. 9.10).

ICD-10-CM Code	J85.0 *(Gangrene and necrosis of lung)*
	J85.1 *(Abscess of lung with pneumonia)*
	J85.2 *(Abscess of lung without pneumonia)*

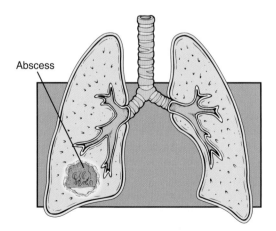

• **Fig. 9.10** Pulmonary abscess.

Abscess

Symptoms and Signs

Abscesses are more common in the lower portions of the lungs and in the right lung because of its more vertical bronchus. The main symptoms are alternating chills and fever. Chest pain and a productive cough accompanied by purulent, bloody, or foul-smelling sputum and foul-smelling breath may also be present.

Patient Screening

Fever, bloody and/or foul-smelling sputum, and chest discomfort indicate a serious respiratory infection that requires immediate medical care. The patient may report "a turn for the worse" while under treatment for pneumonia. Generalized fatigue, weight loss, and persistent fever may be the only symptoms.

Etiology

Lung abscesses are often a complication of pneumonia caused by bacteria from the oral cavity or the aspiration of food due to unconsciousness. A pulmonary abscess also may develop when a septic embolism is carried to the lung via the pulmonary circulation. Immune deficiency, poor oral hygiene, altered level of consciousness resulting from drug or alcohol abuse, or neurological disorders such as seizure, sedation, and anesthesia may predispose one to develop this type of infection.

Diagnosis

Decreased breath sounds are revealed on chest auscultation. Chest radiography, CT of the chest, and bronchoscopy may be used to diagnose this condition.

Treatment

The treatment of choice for an abscess is antibiotics for a fairly long duration or until the abscess is gone. Surgical resection of the abscess and a portion of the affected lung may be required if the antibiotic therapy is not successful.

Prognosis

An otherwise healthy individual who responds favorably to treatment has a good prognosis. Prognosis is guarded for the very young, older adults, the immunocompromised, or the chronically ill.

Prevention

Precautions should be taken to minimize aspiration by elevating the head, especially for those at high risk. Proper treatment of dental infections and early treatment of pneumonia minimize the risk of bacterial lung abscesses. Some individuals (e.g., older patients) benefit from taking vaccines.

Patient Teaching

Explain to the patient the importance of taking medications exactly as prescribed, especially the entire course of antibiotics. Stress the importance of follow-up care until the condition is completely resolved.

Legionellosis (Legionnaires Disease and Pontiac Fever)

Description

Legionellosis is a type of pneumonia caused by the bacterium *Legionella pneumophila*.

ICD-10-CM Code	A48.1 *(Legionnaires disease)*
	(A48.1–A48.2 = 2 codes of specificity)

Symptoms and Signs

This infection can take two forms: the more severe legionnaires disease and the milder Pontiac fever.

Typical symptoms include general malaise, headache, and productive cough. These are followed rapidly by the onset of chills, fever, chest pain, dyspnea, myalgia, GI disturbances, including anorexia. The symptoms often mimic those of pneumonia. The incubation period for legionnaires disease is 2 to 10 days after exposure to Legionella bacteria. The symptoms of Pontiac fever are less severe and include a high fever and muscle aches, with a duration of 2 to 5 days. The incubation period for Pontiac fever is much shorter than that for legionnaires disease, and it does not usually affect the lungs.

Patient Screening

Initially the patient may experience malaise, fatigue, and flulike symptoms that progress to be more severe: headache, chills, high fever, dyspnea, restlessness, confusion, nausea, and vomiting. A prompt medical evaluation should be scheduled. Hospitalization may be required.

Etiology

Both disorders are caused by *L. pneumophila* and are not contagious. These bacteria thrive in warm aquatic environments and are inhaled from contaminated aerosolized water droplets. Air conditioning systems, cooling towers, whirlpool spas, showers, and the hot water plumbing of buildings in which the temperature is kept at optimal growth for bacteria permit the reproduction of the bacterium. Predisposing factors include smoking, physical debilitation, especially among patients with chronic obstructive pulmonary disease (COPD), immunosuppression, and alcoholism. Pontiac fever usually occurs in otherwise healthy individuals.

Diagnosis

Complete physical examination and patient history, along with chest radiographic studies and testing of blood samples, are performed. Laboratory analysis of blood indicates elevated white blood cell (WBC) count, liver enzyme level, and erythrocyte sedimentation rate (ESR). A culture from the sputum to isolate the *Legionella* bacterium is necessary for confirmation of legionnaires disease. The detection of the presence of bacteria in a urine sample indicates the disease. Evaluating convalescent serum samples to detect antibodies is the best diagnostic tool.

Treatment

Typically antibiotic therapy is initiated before confirmation of the diagnosis is made because the response to treatment is usually slow. The antibiotics of choice are azithromycin or levofloxacin, except for mild cases, when erythromycin or doxycycline is prescribed. Rifampin may be added when the response to the antibiotic is not adequate. Oxygen may be used for the dyspnea; antipyretics, antiemetics, and analgesics are also helpful.

Pontiac fever usually resolves itself in a few days, requiring no specific treatment. Legionellosis occurs worldwide. The National Center for Infectious Diseases monitors the incidence of legionellosis in the United States. Attempts are made to identify the sources of disease transmission, and recommendations for prevention and control measures are made.

Prognosis

Improvement of symptoms occurs in 2 to 4 days with specific antimicrobial therapy and without complications. Septic shock, respiratory failure, and acute renal failure may result if left untreated, especially in those in a high-risk population.

Prevention

Prevention can be accomplished by the appropriate design of facilities to prevent stagnant water. The temperature of the water in cooling towers and air conditioning units must be maintained below 77°F (45°C). Closed-circuit systems provide less chance of bacterial growth. Adequate chlorination to kill the *Legionella* bacillus is required. Monitoring the chlorine content of whirlpool baths and spas is a necessary obligation of the owners.

Patient Teaching

Urge the patient to take the entire course of antibiotics as prescribed. Give instructions to call the office if symptoms persist or worsen.

Respiratory Syncytial Virus Pneumonia

Description

RSV pneumonia, an inflammatory and infectious condition of the lungs, is most common in infants, young children, and older adults.

ICD-10-CM Code	J12.1 *(Respiratory syncytial virus pneumonia)*

Symptoms and Signs

RSV causes cold-like symptoms, including nasal congestion, otitis media, and coughing, in the mild upper respiratory tract form of infection. As the virus progresses downward to the lower respiratory tract, the patient experiences fever, malaise, lethargy, more frequent coughing, wheezing, and dyspnea. The symptoms may not all occur at once.

Patient Screening

Infants with symptoms of a lower respiratory tract infection require prompt medical attention and close monitoring thereafter until well. Older adults, especially those in nursing homes, are considered to be at high risk. In young adults, symptoms consist of nasal discharge, pharyngitis, and low-grade fever.

Etiology

RSV is the causative agent of RSV pneumonia. The greatest occurrence of these annual epidemic infections is during the fall through early spring. RSV can be more complicated in infants, children, and adults with predisposing upper respiratory conditions. RSV can live on hard surfaces and can be transmitted by touching surfaces other than the face. Most

people have experienced several RSV URIs in their lifetimes, and most cases of mild RSV infection are self-limiting.

RSV is spread by contact with the secretions of an infected person. Thorough hand washing, hand sanitization, sanitizing hard surfaces, and the use of disposable tissues for nasal secretions can prevent the spread of this disease

Diagnosis

Clinical findings, a thorough physical examination, nasal or oral swabs for RSV testing, blood laboratory tests, and imaging studies, in some cases, assist in diagnosis of RSV.

Treatment

Most cases of RSV infection involving the upper respiratory tract are self-limiting. Antipyretics are prescribed for fever, and antibiotics are given for otitis media. When the infection invades the lower respiratory tract of an infant or a young child, treatment may involve inhalation therapy. Inhalation of 3% hypertonic saline is frequently used to treat RSV. Beyfortus (nirsevimab) and Synagis (palivizumab) are monoclonal antibody injections that are administered to provide patients with passive immunity to RSV. Hospitalization may be required for oxygen therapy and hydration.

Prognosis

The prognosis is generally good. Infants are prone to otitis media as a complication.

Prevention

RSV vaccination in individuals who are at least 60 years old is recommended. Anyone sick should not expose infants to illness. Strict hand washing and sanitization are prudent because the virus is transmitted by respiratory secretions. Antibacterial wipes should be used to wipe down surfaces exposed to droplets spread by coughing and sneezing.

Patient Teaching

Infants are sometimes hospitalized so that supportive therapy can be provided; thus parents need reassurance and support. Inform the parents that the head of the crib or bed is elevated to prevent aspiration of secretions and aid respiration.

Histoplasmosis
Description

Histoplasmosis is a fungal disease originating in the lungs and is caused by inhalation of dust containing *Histoplasma capsulatum*.

ICD-10-CM Code	B39.9 *(Histoplasmosis, unspecified)* (B39.0–B39.9 = 7 codes of specificity)

Symptoms and Signs

Many patients with histoplasmosis are *asymptomatic* at the onset of the disease; it is not contagious. As the fungus disseminates throughout the pulmonary tissue, the patient reports dyspnea and loss of energy to the point of incapacitation. The patient becomes febrile. The spleen and lymph nodes become enlarged. In patients with weakened immune systems, histoplasmosis may become severe.

Patient Screening
The patient with the above-mentioned symptoms should be seen for medical evaluation within 24 hours.

Etiology
Histoplasmosis is caused by the fungus *H. capsulatum*, which is carried by dust and is inhaled. It is the most common endemic mycosis in the United States and may also be found in South and Central America and in Africa. Often the fungus is found in soil contaminated by droppings from birds or bats specific to the area, which may be a source of the airborne fungus. Infections are associated with the disruption of the soil, cleaning attics or barns, and tearing down old structures.

> **NOTE**
>
> Blastomycosis (also called *Gilchrist disease*) is a fungal infection caused by inhaling the fungus *Blastomyces dermatitidis*, which grows as a mold in moist soil and wood. It is found in specific endemic areas in North America and has the greatest prevalence in the upper Midwest and southward along the Mississippi and Ohio riverbeds. In the Southwest, coccidioidomycosis is caused by the fungus *Coccidioides immitis*, which produces spores that live in the soil. This is the agent that causes the disease known as San Joaquin Valley fever. The disease is contracted when dry soil is picked up by wind and the spores are breathed in; it is not communicable.

Diagnosis
Diagnosis is made by evaluating the clinical findings, a positive skin test result, blood serologic findings specific to the fungus, or the identification of the fungus in pus, sputum, or tissue specimens. Chest radiographs may be normal or may reveal patchy infiltrates and diffuse opacities.

Treatment
When the disease is self-limiting, no antifungal therapy is necessary. The antifungal drugs itraconazole, fluconazole, and amphotericin B are used to treat more severe or progressive diseases. In severe cases, corticosteroid use may be beneficial.

Prognosis
Spontaneous recovery is usual. Secondary infections may occur. Reinfection is possible, especially in a setting of high exposure. Small calcifications remain in the lungs after infection. Progressive histoplasmosis can be fatal. Infection confers immunity.

Prevention
It is prudent to teach safety practices to workers in high-risk jobs that expose them to contaminated soil.

Patient Teaching
Review appropriate prevention measures with individuals at risk because of poor health. Advise the patient to avoid contact with soil contaminated with bat or bird droppings. Use available computer-based health education on how to avoid histoplasmosis infection.

Influenza

Description
Influenza is a generalized, highly contagious, acute viral disease that occurs in annual outbreaks.

ICD-10-CM Code   J10.1 *(Influenza due to other influenza virus with other respiratory manifestations)*
(J10.0–J10.89 = 9 codes of specificity)

The above codes are nonspecific and may be valid as a principal diagnosis, except for Medicare. Refer to the physician's diagnosis and then to the current edition of the ICD-10-CM coding manual to ensure the greatest specificity.

Symptoms and Signs
Influenza is characterized by inflammation of the upper and lower respiratory tract mucous membranes, a severe protracted cough, fever, headache, sore throat, and generalized malaise. The onset is usually sudden and marked by chills and a feverish feeling. Acute symptoms usually subside rapidly with a decreasing fever. The weakness, sweating, and fatigue may continue for a few days to a few weeks; malaise may persist for several days before full recovery.

Fever, cough, and other respiratory symptoms persisting for longer than 5 days may indicate secondary bacterial pneumonia. Possible complications of influenza are bronchitis, sinusitis, otitis media, and cervical **lymphadenitis**.

Patient Screening
During a known epidemic, the health care provider may give the telephone screener(s) guidelines for addressing callers with typical influenza symptoms.

Individuals with severe symptoms or those who are at high risk for complications (i.e., the very young, older adults, or those chronically ill) are given a prompt appointment for close medical monitoring.

Etiology
Known viruses that cause influenza are designated as orthomyxovirus types A, B, and C. However, many mutant strains also reproduce in both humans and animals. An acute uncomplicated influenza with recovery is the most frequently encountered type of this disease. Secondary bacterial pneumonia after influenza is most often caused by hemolytic *Streptococcus, Staphylococcus,* or *Pneumococcus*.

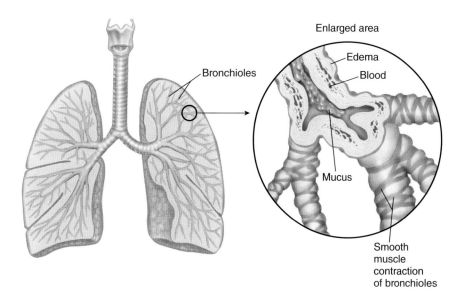

• **Fig. 9.11** Influenza. (From Seidel HM, et al: *Mosby's guide to physical examination*, ed 5, St. Louis, 2003, Mosby/Elsevier.)

Influenza outbreaks may be sporadic or epidemic. Transmission is from person to person by inhalation of the virus in airborne mucus discharge. Fatalities can occur in as short a time as 48 hours after the onset of symptoms.

Diagnosis

Clinically, influenza (Fig. 9.11) may be indistinguishable from the common cold. When differentiating influenza from other respiratory tract infections, consideration should be given to the amount of time passed since onset, the presence of an epidemic in the community, and the severity of the patient's symptoms. Frequent recurrences of influenza-like syndromes may make the physician suspect TB (see the Pulmonary Tuberculosis section). A complicating pneumonia may be present if the patient has dyspnea, cyanosis, hemoptysis, or rales in the lungs. The WBC count may indicate leukopenia with relative lymphocytosis. Confirmation of the influenza diagnosis is made by the isolation of the virus from nasopharyngeal culture. A sputum culture isolates bacteria in secondary infections.

Treatment

Treatment is symptomatic; vaccines are useless after the disease is established. Bed rest, increased fluid intake, a light diet, and the use of antipyretic and analgesic drugs, when needed, are helpful. Oseltamivir may be used for influenza A or B and is only effective if administered within the first 48 hours of symptoms, usually when the disease is known to be present in the community. In less severe cases, treatment of respiratory tract symptoms may not be necessary; however, warm salt water gargles, steam inhalation, and the use of cough syrups may be comforting. Antibiotics are effective against bacterial pneumonia and other less serious complications, such as sinusitis, otitis media, and lymphadenitis.

Prognosis

Recovery is usually complete; however, complications, such as pneumonia, can occur. Those at highest risk are the very young, older adults, and the chronically ill. Epidemics can cause substantial morbidity, financial loss, and even death. During seasonal influenza, the vast majority of deaths occur in people aged 65 years and older.

Prevention

The prophylactic use of vaccines against influenza is effective in reducing the occurrence of the disease, especially in older adults or those at high risk for complications. Because immunity from vaccination lasts only 1 year, annual booster doses are needed for optimal protection. After vaccination, it takes 10 to 14 days for immunity to develop.

Patient Teaching

Reinforce the use of comfort measures, including antipyretics and analgesics as prescribed. Advise the patient to rest and take adequate fluids. Infection control, such as thorough and frequent hand washing, is prudent to reduce the spread of the virus. Educate individuals at high risk about annual influenza immunizations.

Chronic Obstructive Pulmonary Disease

COPD is a condition of slow and irreversible progressive airway obstruction. It encompasses several obstructive diseases of the lungs, including chronic bronchitis, bronchiectasis, asthma, emphysema, cystic fibrosis, and pneumoconiosis. Although the mechanism of the obstruction can vary, the consequence is the same: the patient with COPD is unable to ventilate the lungs freely, which results in an ineffective exchange of respiratory gases. This causes the patient's normal respiratory response to elevated carbon dioxide levels to become diminished.

Acute and Chronic Bronchitis

Description
Bronchitis is inflammation of the mucous membrane lining the bronchi.

ICD-10-CM Code	J40 *(Bronchitis, not specified as acute or chronic)*
	J41.8 *(Mixed simple and mucopurulent chronic bronchitis)*
	(J40–J42 = 5 codes of specificity)

Symptoms and Signs
In acute bronchitis, a deep, persistent, productive cough is the main symptom. The patient has thick, yellow-to-gray sputum. Other symptoms include shortness of breath, wheezing, a slightly elevated temperature, and pain in the upper chest, which is aggravated by the cough. Acute symptoms subside within a week, but the cough may continue for 2 to 3 weeks. Physical signs within the lungs are few or absent if the bronchitis is uncomplicated. Scattered or occasional rales are often heard on auscultation. There is no clinical or radiologic evidence of pneumonia.

Chronic bronchitis is similar to acute bronchitis, except that the inflammation persists and becomes worse for at least 3 months of the year for 2 consecutive years. Mild forms may exist for many years, with the patient having only a slight cough in the mornings. Then the condition becomes aggravated when the patient contracts acute URIs. Obstructive and asthmatic symptoms and dyspnea appear as the condition progresses. Chest expansion becomes diminished, and scattered rales and wheezing are often heard. In the beginning stages of the disease, flare-ups of chronic bronchitis are likely to occur after the patient has experienced severe colds or influenza. In later stages, even a minor head cold can cause a severe attack. During the final stages, coughing, shortness of breath, and wheezing occur almost continuously. Prolonged, recurrent attacks cause gradual deterioration of the lungs.

For both acute and chronic bronchitis, symptoms appear more troublesome during the winter months. Living or working in a cold, damp environment or in a polluted atmosphere can aggravate the condition.

Patient Screening
An individual complaining of a persistent, productive cough is advised to seek medical care if there has been no improvement. When the cough is described as chronic, with purulent sputum, and fever and/or wheezing present, the patient should be examined by a health care professional within 24 hours. Persons known to have chronic bronchitis should be seen promptly to be examined for suspected infections or sudden worsening of symptoms.

Etiology
Acute bronchitis is part of a general URI. It begins after a common cold or other viral infections of the nasopharynx and pharynx or occurs as a complication of bacterial infections. Recurring attacks in adults may indicate a focus of infection, such as chronic sinusitis, bronchiectasis, and pneumonia. In children, hypertrophied tonsils and adenoids may be the source of acute bronchitis. Allergens are also frequently predisposing factors. The same bacteria known to cause pneumonia may be responsible for chronic bronchitis. Progressive and irreversible changes in the bronchi can result from constant irritation.

Diagnosis
Acute or chronic bronchitis can be suspected on the basis of the patient's symptoms and history. The presence of other diseases or their complications must be ruled out, especially if the symptoms are serious or prolonged. Diagnostic tests include chest radiographic studies, pulmonary function tests, arterial blood gases, and other blood and sputum analyses.

Treatment
Because acute bronchitis is usually caused by a viral infection, no specific treatment is prescribed except for those measures that will relieve the symptoms. Increased fluid intake, along with the use of a vaporizer and humidifier, helps clear the nasal passages and bronchi. The physician may prescribe the use of a bronchodilator aerosol inhaler for wheezing and shortness of breath and a cough suppressant if the chest is sore from coughing. If a secondary bacterial infection is suspected, an antibiotic is prescribed.

The treatment of chronic bronchitis is based on the stage of the disease at the time the patient consults professional help. Prompt treatment of acute infections is of primary importance. Low-flow oxygen therapy may be administered, as needed, for hypoxemia. Postural drainage and percussion are techniques used to help loosen and expectorate thick mucus. Aerosolized corticosteroids may be ordered to control inflammation. The patient is advised to give up smoking, vaping, and to avoid smoke-filled rooms or irritants.

Prognosis
Acute bronchitis resolves completely within a few days; however, a residual cough can remain for 2 to 3 weeks or longer in some cases. Chronic bronchitis has a guarded prognosis because it may be progressive and involves airway obstruction and general debilitation. Bronchitis may also lead to pneumonia.

Prevention
It is important for the patient to avoid the primary causative factors: smoking, chronic exposure to pollutants in the air, and recurrent respiratory infections.

Patient Teaching
For acute bronchitis, advise the patient to rest and take any palliative medications as prescribed. Advise patients with

chronic bronchitis not to smoke, vape, or expose themselves to known respiratory irritants. Demonstrate methods of chest physiotherapy. Explain the use of home equipment designed for oxygen therapy or inhalation therapy.

Bronchiectasis

Description
Bronchiectasis is the permanent, irreversible dilation or distortion of one or more of the bronchi, resulting from the destruction of muscular and elastic portions of the bronchial walls (Fig. 9.12).

ICD-10-CM Code	J47.9 (Bronchiectasis, uncomplicated) (J47.0–J47.9 = 3 codes of specificity)

Symptoms and Signs
Bronchiectasis, a condition that takes many years to develop, is usually bilateral and involves the lower lobes of the lungs. A chronic cough producing large quantities of purulent, foul-smelling sputum is the main symptom of bronchiectasis. Hemoptysis, dyspnea, wheezing, fever, and general malaise develop as the condition progresses. The patient also may experience chronic halitosis.

Patient Screening
Schedule the patient with a chronic, highly productive cough for a clinical examination at his or her earliest convenience.

Etiology
Bronchiectasis may be caused by repeated damage to the bronchial wall caused by recurrent airway infections. It also can result from pneumonia, TB, bronchial obstruction, or the inhalation of a corrosive gas. This condition is a common life-threatening complication of cystic fibrosis or other childhood infections, such as measles and pertussis (whooping cough), and may also result from immune deficiency (e.g., hypogammaglobulinemia).

Diagnosis
Initially, when symptoms are vague, determining the diagnosis of bronchiectasis may be difficult. Physical examination, history of symptoms, chest radiography, high-resolution CT of the chest, bronchoscopy, sputum culture, and pulmonary function tests are of the utmost value in making the diagnosis.

Treatment
Antibiotics and bronchodilators are prescribed, and postural drainage is encouraged. Sputum removal management is very important and can be accomplished with vibratory devices. Avoiding environmental irritants, such as smoke, fumes, and large amounts of dust, is important. If the patient has a great deal of hemoptysis, surgery to remove the affected part of the lung may be advised.

• **Fig. 9.12** Bronchiectasis. (From Cross S: *Underwood's pathology: a clinical approach*, ed 7, Philadelphia, 2019, Elsevier.)

Prognosis
The prognosis varies with the underlying cause. Serious respiratory and cardiac complications, such as pulmonary hypertension and cor pulmonale, develop with advanced bronchiectasis.

Prevention
Childhood immunizations and early treatment of respiratory infections are recommended for prevention, as is the avoidance of smoking, vaping, and exposure to any other respiratory irritants.

Patient Teaching
Explain the medical management regimen and demonstrate how to use home equipment for oxygen therapy and/or inhalation therapy. Teach the patient proper techniques for postural drainage and percussion, and how to properly discard secretions. Use demonstration videos or print-on-demand electronic materials to teach the proper technique for postural drainage. Smoking/vaping cessation materials can be shared.

Asthma

Adult-onset asthma manifests for the first time in middle-aged or older individuals, with the usual moderate to severe symptoms of asthma: wheezing, productive cough, and difficulty breathing. During an attack, airway narrowing can be severe and result in airway closure and severe anxiety in the patient. This condition, called *status asthmaticus*, requires emergency hospitalization for treatment. There are many common asthma triggers, and the causes can be intrinsic or extrinsic. Both environmental and genetic factors are important in the etiology of asthma. Medical management includes pharmacologic therapy with antiinflammatory drugs and bronchodilators. Both quick-relief medications and long-term medications are given to treat and prevent asthma attacks. Patient education is crucial for obtaining the maximum benefit from the treatment plan. See Fig. 9.13 for the effects of smoking.

Pulmonary Emphysema

Description

Pulmonary emphysema is a chronic obstructive pulmonary disorder characterized by destructive changes in the alveolar walls and irreversible enlargement of alveolar air spaces.

ICD-10-CM Code	J43.9 (*Emphysema, unspecified*) (J43.0–J43.9 = 5 codes of specificity)

The above codes are nonspecific codes and may be valid as a principal diagnosis, except for Medicare. Refer to the physician's diagnosis and then to the current edition of the ICD-10-CM coding manuals to ensure the greatest specificity.

Symptoms and Signs

Pulmonary emphysema, a destructive disease of the alveolar septa, interferes with both the breathing process and gas exchange in the lungs. Alveoli become enlarged, which precipitates destruction of the alveolar walls and damage to the adjacent capillary walls. As a result of the decreased area for gas exchange and the trapped air, the patient experiences dyspnea. The onset of symptoms is insidious, with gradually increasing difficulty breathing, dyspnea, tachypnea, and wheezing. Cough can be a minor component or absent in patients with emphysema. The inability to exhale carbon dioxide in the normal manner requires the patient with emphysema to use accessory muscles to force out air trapped in the alveoli, resulting in the characteristic barrel chest (Fig. 9.14). Shortness of breath and dyspnea increase, and the patient purses the lips to assist in exhaling. As the disease progresses, the patient develops **circumoral cyanosis**, symptoms of right ventricular heart failure, and digital clubbing.

Patient Screening

The patient who complains of an insidious onset of difficulty breathing, wheezing, and/or persistent coughing should be given the first available appointment within 24 hours for clinical evaluation.

Etiology

Although the etiology of pulmonary emphysema is not completely understood, long-term cigarette smoking appears to

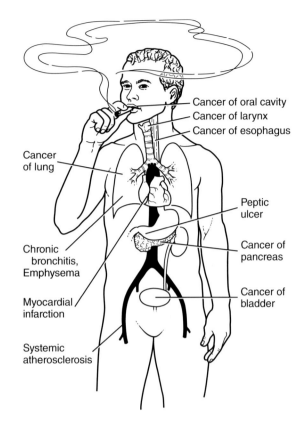

• **Fig. 9.13** Effects of smoking. (From Kumar V, Cotran R, Robbins S: *Robbins basic pathology*, ed 8, Philadelphia, 2008, Saunders.)

• **Fig. 9.14** Note the barrel chest and bluish discoloration around mouth in a patient with emphysema.

be a contributing factor. Repeated respiratory tract infections beginning in childhood and continuing throughout adulthood may also contribute to the increased occurrence of the disease. Additionally, irritants, such as ozone, sulfur dioxide, and nitrogen oxides, are thought to play a role in the etiology. The possibility of a familial tendency is supported by the increased frequency of the disease in families who experience an enzyme deficiency (alpha$_1$-antitrypsin).

Diagnosis

Diagnosis is based on a clinical examination and a thorough patient history, which usually show prolonged exposure to possible respiratory irritants, especially cigarette smoking. Pulmonary function studies indicate increased tidal volume and residual volume, along with decreased vital capacity and expiratory maneuver volumes. Radiographic chest studies show translucent-appearing lungs and a depressed or flattened diaphragm. The patient exhibits tachypnea, tachycardia, hypertension, polycythemia, diminished breath sounds, and wheezing or rhonchi. Blood gas determinations in the advanced stages indicate decreased arterial oxygen tension and increased carbon dioxide.

Treatment

The patient is instructed and encouraged to avoid the inhalation of irritating substances, particularly cigarette smoke. Patients with pulmonary emphysema should take care to avoid exposure to possible respiratory tract infections and should receive influenza virus vaccination annually. Supplemental low concentrations of oxygen may help as well.

Drug therapy includes beta$_2$-adrenergic sympathomimetic drugs alone or in combination with inhaled corticosteroids. Drugs used in treatment may include albuterol (Ventolin and Proventil) and terbutaline sulfate (Brethine) for bronchodilation and antispasmodic activity; theophylline (rarely); expectorants; and antibiotics. Other medications may include treatments for gastroesophageal reflux disease to prevent tracheal and/or bronchial irritation from gastric reflux. Oxygen therapy is also used when necessary. Pulmonary rehabilitation, a program of education and progressive exercise training, is essential to improving the quality of life for these patients. In some special circumstances, surgery may be an option to improve the serious air trapping seen in severe emphysema.

Prognosis

The prognosis for long-term disease is poor; in the United States, emphysema is the most common cause of death from respiratory disease.

Prevention

Education about the possible health consequences of long-term smoking is imperative. It is helpful for patients to avoid exposure to respiratory irritants and to guard against repeated respiratory infections.

Patient Teaching

Provide strong advice to the patient who smokes to cease smoking; offer a referral to a smoking cessation support group. Explain the medical management regimen and demonstrate how to use home equipment for oxygen therapy and/or inhalation therapy. Demonstrate appropriate breathing techniques that maximize expiration and ventilation.

Pneumoconiosis

Description

Pneumoconiosis is any disease of the lung caused by long-term mineral dust inhalation.

ICD-10-CM Code	J64 (Unspecified pneumoconiosis)

Symptoms and Signs

Pneumoconiosis means the presence of dust in the lungs, which results in interstitial lung disease. It refers to a number of occupational diseases that cause progressive, chronic inflammation, fibrosis, and infection in the lungs. The onset of symptoms can be insidious, with dyspnea on exertion being the first symptom. In all types of dust-related diseases, a dry cough, which later turns productive and becomes similar to the cough of chronic bronchitis, is typical. The patient may report that increasing effort is required for inspiration. Pulmonary hypertension, tachypnea, general malaise, and recurrent respiratory tract infections are common. Other symptoms may be associated with TB of the lungs. Family members are also at risk for pneumoconiosis if they are constantly exposed to the dust particles in the worker's clothing.

Patient Screening

Persistent cough over a period of weeks or months and dyspnea are symptoms that require clinical evaluation; schedule the first available appointment. Inform the patient to call back for an immediate appointment if signs of infection occur or symptoms worsen.

Etiology

Pneumoconiosis is considered an occupational disease caused by inhaling inorganic dust particles over a prolonged period. It usually takes at least several years to develop.

Asbestosis is a form of dust disease caused by exposure to asbestos fibers. It is characterized by a slow and progressively diffuse fibrosis of the lungs. Asbestosis is the most commonly occurring type of pneumoconiosis.

Another form of pneumoconiosis is anthracosis, also known as *black lung* or *coal miner's lung*. Anthracosis is caused by the accumulation of carbon deposits in the lungs, resulting from inhaling smoke or coal dust (Fig. 9.15).

Silicosis, another type of dust disease, affects stone masons, metal grinders, and those who work in quarries. Silicosis develops as a result of inhaling silica (quartz) dust and causes dense fibrosis of the lungs and emphysema with respiratory impairment.

Other workers who are also susceptible to dust diseases are those who work with aluminum, beryllium, iron, cotton, sugar cane, and a number of synthetic fibers.

Diagnosis

A thorough patient history and a complete physical examination are essential for making the diagnosis. Chest x-ray, CT scan, pulmonary function tests, and arterial blood gas determination confirm the diagnosis.

• **Fig. 9.15** Pneumoconiosis. (From Damjanov I, Linder J: *Pathology: a color atlas*, St. Louis, 1999, Mosby.)

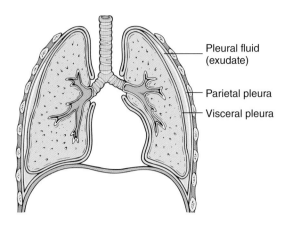

Pleural fluid (exudate)

Parietal pleura

Visceral pleura

• **Fig. 9.16** Pleurisy.

Treatment

The treatment of all pneumoconioses is directed toward relieving symptoms. Typically this includes administering bronchodilators, oxygen therapy, chest physical therapy to help remove secretions, and the use of short-term corticosteroid drugs. Lung transplantation may be considered in some patients. TB, a common complication, must be treated aggressively. Cessation of smoking and breathing dust is strongly advised.

Prognosis

The damage to lung tissue is irreversible, and infections are common. There is an increased risk for lung cancer, especially in those with asbestosis.

Prevention

Pneumoconiosis is considered an environmental disease; thus reducing or ceasing exposure to dust in the workplace is essential. Smoking worsens the condition, and embedded asbestos fibers increase the risk of lung cancer.

Patient Teaching

Stress the importance of prompt treatment of infections. Advise the patient to avoid exposure to the offending dust particles. Explain the medication dosage schedule and demonstrate the proper use of the inhaler and/or home oxygen therapy equipment.

Pleuritis

Description

Pleurisy is inflammation of the membranes surrounding the lungs and lining the pleural cavity (Fig. 9.16).

ICD-10-CM Code   R09.1 *(Pleurisy)*

Symptoms and Signs

The patient reports generally unilateral sharp, needle-like pain, which increases with inspiration and coughing. Additionally, the patient experiences a cough, fever, and chills. Inspirations are shallow, rapid, and restricted. Pain may radiate to the shoulder or the abdomen.

Patient Screening

Usually significant pain with inspiration prompts the call for medical intervention. Schedule the first available appointment as soon as possible.

Etiology

Pleurisy is usually secondary to other diseases or infections. The inflammation also may result from injury or the presence of a tumor.

Two types of pleurisy exist: wet and dry. When extra pleural fluid (effusion) is present between the two layers of the plural membranes that cover the lungs, the increased volume causes compression of the pulmonary tissue and dyspnea. Dry pleurisy occurs when the pleural fluid decreases in volume, resulting in dryness between the pleura; the layers rub together and become congested and edematous.

Diagnosis

Diagnosis is made from the symptoms, history, and physical examination. A pleural rub can be heard on the auscultation of the lungs. Radiography or CT may indicate the presence of pleural effusion and/or underlying pulmonary disease. An ultrasound may be ordered. Labwork may be performed to identify if the etiology is bacterial, or viral and if there is an autoimmune disease. An ECG may be ordered to rule out cardiac causes, which would explain the severe pain.

Treatment

Treatment is directed at the underlying cause. Antibiotic therapy and analgesics to control the pain may be given. Splinting of the chest and deep breathing exercises help promote good ventilation. A therapeutic thoracostomy may be performed.

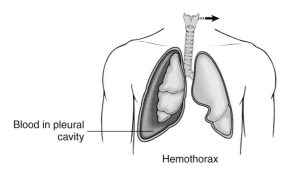

• **Fig. 9.17** Pneumothorax and hemothorax.

Prognosis

Recovery is usually complete. In some cases, permanent adhesions may restrict lung expansion.

Prevention

No specific prevention is known.

Patient Teaching

Explain to the patient the importance of deep breathing exercises and demonstrate proper splinting for adequate lung expansion. Stress the importance of taking medications as prescribed.

Pneumothorax

Description

Pneumothorax is a collection of air or gas in the pleural cavity that results in a collapsed or partially collapsed lung (Fig. 9.17).

ICD-10-CM Code	J93.9 *(Pneumothorax, unspecified)*
	(J93.0–J39.9 = 4 codes of specificity)
	P25.1 *(Pneumothorax originating in the perinatal period)*
	(P25.1–P25.3 = 3 codes of specificity)
	J95.81 *(Post procedural pneumothorax)*
	J93.8 *(Other pneumothorax)*

(J93.0–J93.9 = 7 codes of specificity)
S27.0 *(Traumatic pneumothorax [7 digits required])*

Symptoms and Signs

Collapse of a lung causes severe shortness of breath, sudden and sharp chest pain, falling blood pressure, rapid weak pulse, and shallow and weak respirations. The patient may be cyanotic and appear anxious. Increased air pressure on the affected side causes a mediastinal shift to the unaffected side.

Patient Screening

The patient experiencing the crisis, as described earlier, requires urgent care and immediate transport to the emergency room.

Etiology

Pneumothorax can be spontaneous or traumatic. Spontaneous pneumothorax occurs when an opening occurs on the surface of a lung. Causative factors can be the erosion of alveoli from a tumor or disease, increased pressure from within the respiratory system (too great a force with artificial ventilation), or a spontaneous tear in the tissue. Traumatic pneumothorax occurs when the integrity of the pleural cavity is breached from the outside as the result of trauma, such as a gunshot wound, stab wound, or crushing type of wound to the chest. The object (possibly the patient's own rib) penetrates the chest cavity, allowing air to enter from the atmosphere. Gas or an accumulation of pus in the pleural space generated by microorganisms can result in a pneumothorax.

Diagnosis

Diagnosis is made after evaluating the history, the clinical findings, and radiographic studies. Radiographs will show the air in the pleural cavity, the collapsed portion of the lung, and the mediastinal shift. Breath sounds are diminished, and sucking air sounds are heard at the wound site. The patient is in acute distress.

Treatment

The patient is more comfortable in the Fowler or semi-Fowler position and may require oxygen. An occlusive dressing is placed over any sucking wound to seal the portal of entry and prevent additional air from entering the chest cavity. A thoracostomy is performed to withdraw air from the cavity. A closed drainage system is established if air continues to leak into the pleural space. This allows expansion and healing of the lungs.

Prognosis

Recovery depends on the degree of lung collapse, the cause, and prompt medical intervention.

Prevention

No specific measures for prevention are known.

Patient Teaching

Throughout emergency care and after the patient is medically stable, offer support to the individual and family. Encourage patients receiving conservative therapy to rest during a period of close monitoring. Provide teaching about treatments used to expand the lungs to more severe cases or those that result from trauma.

Hemothorax

Description

Hemothorax is the accumulation of blood and fluid in the pleural cavity (see Fig. 9.17).

ICD-10-CM Code	J94.2 *(Hemothorax)*
	P54.8 *(Other specified neonatal hemorrhages)*
	S27.1 *(Traumatic hemothorax)*
	A15.6 *(Tuberculous pleurisy)*

Symptoms and Signs

The patient experiences symptoms similar to those of a pneumothorax. Signs of hemorrhage include pale and clammy skin, a weak and thready pulse, and falling blood pressure. The patient may experience chest pain, and respirations are labored and shallow or gasping.

Patient Screening

A hemothorax is a life-threatening condition that requires emergency medical care.

Etiology

Blood enters the pleural space as a result of trauma, erosion of a pulmonary vessel, or hematologic disorders, causing the lung to collapse.

Diagnosis

Breath sounds are diminished or absent on the affected side, as is chest wall movement. Radiographs show blood in the pleural space. Blood tests indicate hemorrhage; arterial blood gas analysis reflects respiratory failure. The patient is in acute distress.

Treatment

The treatment employed is similar to that for a pneumothorax. The lung must be reexpanded, usually by performing a thoracostomy, with closed drainage to evacuate the blood. The underlying cause, once discovered, is treated, often necessitating surgical intervention to repair the wound. Vital signs are monitored, and blood loss is replaced.

Prognosis

The prognosis for a hemothorax is guarded, depending on the cause and the availability of effective treatment.

Prevention

No specific prevention measures are known.

Patient Teaching

Make every effort to reassure the patient while emergency and diagnostic measures are taking place. Once the patient is stabilized, explain the purpose of therapeutic procedures, such as chest tube drainage and thoracentesis. Use available visual aids to demonstrate the therapeutic procedures.

Flail Chest

Description

Flail chest is a condition of instability in the chest wall caused by multiple rib fractures; the sternum also may be fractured.

ICD-10-CM Code	S22.5XXA *(Flail chest, initial encounter for closed fracture)*
	S22.5XXB *(Flail chest, initial encounter for open fracture)*
	S22.5 *(Flail chest, 7 digits required)*
	(S22.5XXA–S22.5XXS = 6 codes of specificity)

Symptoms and Signs

The patient with flail chest, a double fracture of three or more adjacent ribs, experiences severe pain and dyspnea and is cyanotic and extremely anxious. The segment of the chest involved moves inward during inspiration and outward during expiration; this is termed *paradoxical breathing*.

Patient Screening

Flail chest is a medical emergency and may be a life-threatening condition.

Etiology

Direct trauma to the chest wall that fractures three or more adjacent ribs is the cause of flail chest. This trauma may be from direct compression by a heavy object, a motor vehicle accident (especially injury caused by the steering wheel), a hard fall onto a solid object, or an industrial accident. The paradoxical movement and instability of the chest wall occur when three or more adjacent ribs are broken in two places or break loose from the sternum while also being broken at another site (Fig. 9.18).

Diagnosis

Diagnosis is made by noting the history of chest trauma and observing the paradoxical movement of the chest wall. Chest radiography will confirm the diagnosis.

Treatment

First responder emergency care employs measures to stabilize the chest wall until surgical repair is possible. The treatment of flail chest involves allowing the rib fractures to heal while maintaining respiratory integrity. This may entail

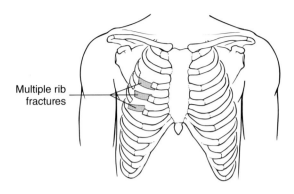

• **Fig. 9.18** Flail chest.

• **Fig. 9.19** Tuberculosis. (From Kumar V, Cotran R, Robbins S: *Robbins basic pathology*, ed 8, Philadelphia, 2008, Saunders.)

mechanical ventilation and sedation of the patient with an endotracheal tube in place. Pain medications are administered to keep the patient comfortable. Additionally, supplemental oxygen is administered. Rib fixation can be done to facilitate healing and pain relief.

Prognosis
Emergency medical care and transport to the hospital as soon as possible help achieve a positive outcome. Delayed medical intervention and complications resulting from trauma can worsen the chances for recovery.

Prevention
The use of safety measures, such as wearing seat belts that protect the chest from trauma, is prudent.

Patient Teaching
Make every effort to dispel the patient's anxiety during emergency measures to stabilize the chest wall. Advise the patient of all procedures necessary to achieve respiratory integrity.

Pulmonary Tuberculosis

Description
Pulmonary TB is a chronic, acute, or subacute infection of the lungs by *Mycobacterium tuberculosis.*

ICD-10-CM Code	A15.0 *(Tuberculosis of lung [includes: infections due to* Mycobacterium tuberculosis *and* Mycobacterium bovis])*

Symptoms and Signs
Pulmonary TB, an infectious and inflammatory disease of the lungs, is acquired by inhaling dried droplet nuclei that contain the tubercle bacillus. These droplet nuclei may remain suspended in room air for many hours. The patient with a primary TB infection is often asymptomatic initially. When the infection is secondary, the patient experiences vague symptoms, such as weight loss, reduced appetite, listlessness, vague chest pain, dry cough, loss of energy, and fever. As the disease progresses, the patient has a productive

cough with purulent sputum, the appearance of blood streaking or hemoptysis, fever, and night sweats.

Patient Screening
Schedule a prompt appointment for the patient complaining of a persistent cough with blood-tinged or purulent sputum. Constitutional symptoms, such as fatigue, fever, and night sweats, may also exist.

Etiology
The tubercle bacillus *M. tuberculosis* causes TB and is spread by droplet nuclei. The primary lesion usually is located in the lungs. The bacteria can survive in their dried form for months if not exposed to sunlight. Any tissue of the body can be affected; however, the lung is their typical site (Fig. 9.19).

The infection begins with a primary lesion. As the body's defense mechanisms respond to the bacterial invasion, antigens that cause necrosis are produced, followed by fibrosis and calcification of the affected tissue. The infection may then be arrested, and the disease becomes inactive, remaining so for years. If the infection is not arrested, the patient will experience progressive primary TB.

The patient's resistance to secondary TB depends on general health and environment. Malnutrition, poor health, an unsanitary and crowded living environment, and the presence of other illnesses tend to lower resistance to reinfection. The source of a secondary exacerbation of TB can be a reactivation of the previous primary infection or another infected person. TB is a very serious condition and a public health risk worldwide.

Diagnosis
The Mantoux test (purified protein derivative test) is a standard intradermal test used to detect the presence of tuberculin antibodies. The test result is available in 48 to 72 hours; an induration of 8 to 10 mm indicates sensitivity to the bacillus and is considered a positive result. The positive test result is followed by chest radiographic studies, examination of gastric washings, fiberoptic bronchoscopy, and sputum cultures. The typical walled-off lesions (tubercles) can be seen on chest radiographs. Apical pulmonary infiltrates

with cavities are present in patients with TB. Final confirmation is a positive result on the culture of the sputum for the tubercle bacillus.

Treatment

Persons with communicable TB should be quarantined until cleared by their physician, after taking the prescribed medication. The treatment will continue, but the person is no longer contagious. New cases must be reported to the local health department.

Treatment is dependent on whether the TB is latent or active. Latent TB is generally treated with isoniazid (INH). Therapy can last upward of 6 to 9 months. Active TB consists of drug therapy with multiple antituberculosis agents. INH is administered with rifampin, ethambutol, or pyrazinamide. Drug-resistant TB is treated more aggressively with various combinations of medications.

Prognosis

Early and complete treatment affords an excellent prognosis. Drug therapy may continue for several months to a year. The prognosis is not as good for individuals infected with strains that are drug resistant. Risk factors exist for reactivation of infection.

Prevention

All those who come in contact with infected patients are advised to have the tuberculin skin test, chest radiography, and prophylactic treatment with INH. As of the writing of this text, research trials are being conducted for a new vaccine M72/AS01.

Patient Teaching

TB is considered infectious and is reportable to the local public health department; therefore thorough, consistent hand washing techniques and respiratory precautions must be practiced. Patient and family education about sources of contagion and transmission is indicated. A nutritious diet and sanitary living conditions are important for recovery. Provide information on adverse drug effects to report to the health care provider. Stress the importance of regular follow-up care, and that the provider will let the patient know when they are no longer contagious.

Infectious Mononucleosis: Epstein-Barr Virus Infection

Description

Infectious mononucleosis is an acute Epstein-Barr Virus infection.

• **Fig. 9.20** Tonsils coated with debris during infection of mononucleosis. (From Sigler B: *Ear, nose, and throat disorders—Mosby's clinical nursing series*, St. Louis, 1994, Mosby.)

ICD-10-CM Code — B27.90 (*Infectious mononucleosis, unspecified without complication*) (B27.90–B27.99 = 4 codes of specificity)

Symptoms and Signs

The two main symptoms of this infection are lymphadenopathy and fever, which typically peaks in the afternoon. Initially, symptoms are vague. They include general malaise, anorexia, and chills. As the infection progresses, symptoms include sore throat, fever, headache, fatigue, and cervical and generalized lymphadenopathy; the tonsils may appear coated with debris (Fig. 9.20). The syndrome causes mild, transient hepatitis and atypical lymphocytosis. The incubation period ranges from 4 to 6 weeks after exposure. This disease affects primarily adolescents and young adults. Infection is rare after the age of 35 years.

Patient Screening

Schedule a prompt appointment for a patient complaining of fever, sore throat, fatigue, and swollen glands.

Etiology

Mononucleosis is caused by EBV, a herpes virus. The virus is carried in the saliva of previously infected individuals and may be transmitted through the oral pharyngeal route (e.g., during kissing), through blood transfusions, or organ donation. After it is inside the body, the virus infects a type of WBC found in lymph, blood, and connective tissue. EBV infection is not highly contagious but is lifelong. The virus is shed asymptomatically in oropharyngeal secretions.

Diagnosis

A thorough patient history and physical examination are essential to rule out hepatitis and other lymphomatous disorders, such as leukemia, Hodgkin lymphoma, and lymphosarcoma. Two procedures of prime diagnostic importance are blood smear examination and immunologic study of blood serum. Laboratory tests include the infectious mononucleosis blood screening test, antinuclear antibody, total serum bilirubin, liver function tests, and EBV serology.

Treatment

Treatment is based almost entirely on symptoms. During the acute phase of fever and malaise, bed rest should be enforced. Fluid intake should be forced orally, or with a high fever, intravenous fluids are given if needed. Antipyretic medications, such as acetaminophen, are needed when the temperature rises.

Prevention

Prevention is difficult because infectious mononucleosis can be transmitted by infected people before they have developed any symptoms. Carriers exist among the general population. No vaccine is available.

Prognosis

Barring complications, recovery is complete within 3 to 4 months. Infection confers permanent immunity.

Patient Teaching

Stress the importance of bed rest to prevent serious complications affecting the liver or the spleen. A soft, bland diet is often better tolerated. Advise the patient and the caregiver that although the disease is not highly infectious, strep throat also may be present; it is prudent to practice infection control during the recovery period. Another important patient teaching point is to report any abdominal pain immediately to their health care provider. Although rare, spontaneous splenic rupture may occur and is a medical emergency. Contact sports should be avoided.

Adult Respiratory Distress Syndrome

Description

Adult respiratory distress syndrome (ARDS) is a type of acute lung injury, characterized by severe pulmonary congestion, acute respiratory distress, and hypoxemia.

ICD-10-CM Code	J95.3 (Chronic pulmonary insufficiency following surgery)

Symptoms and Signs

The sudden onset of severe hypoxemia, progressive hypercapnia, and acidosis are present. The patient experiences shortness of breath, tiredness, confusion, tachypnea, and hypotension.

Patient Screening

The sudden onset of respiratory distress is a medical emergency. The patient is directed to call an ambulance for immediate transport to an emergency care facility. The physician is notified.

Etiology

ARDS occurs many times after another extreme illness or injury, such as sepsis, severe pneumonia, breathing chemicals, aspiration, brain injury, or COVID-19. The alveoli fill with fluid, which affects the gas exchange that normally takes place. Consequently, low pulmonary compliance, pulmonary hypertension, decreased functional residual capacity, and hypoxemia result.

Diagnosis

Arterial blood gas determinations indicate reduced perfusion and increased pH. Chest radiographs are performed. The physical examination is abnormal, and the provider may rule out other problems which can cause the same symptoms. The *Berlin criteria definition* is used to determine whether or not the patient meets the criteria for a diagnosis of ARDS.

Treatment

No cure for ARDS is known; therefore the patient receives supportive care only. Efforts are made to correct the underlying cause of ARDS. When ventilation cannot be maintained with supportive measures such as high-flow nasal oxygen, mechanical ventilation is attempted with the addition of positive end-expiratory pressure. Nutritional status and cautious hydration are maintained intravenously. The patient is observed for signs of renal failure and superinfection. Arterial blood gases, blood pressure, and urine output are monitored.

Prognosis

The prognosis is guarded, depending on the cause and severity of lung damage.

Prevention

There is no single way to prevent ARDS; however, seeking medical attention when experiencing symptoms and cessation of smoking and vaping are ways to lessen the risk. This is especially true for populations of people with preexisting health conditions.

Patient Teaching

Follow all instructions given by the provider, and call if symptoms persist.

Sarcoidosis

Description

Sarcoidosis is a multisystem granulomatous (small lesions of inflamed cells) disorder most commonly detected in the lungs.

ICD-10-CM Code	D86.9 (Sarcoidosis, unspecified) (D86.0–D86.9 = 13 codes of specificity)

Symptoms and Signs

Patients may have no complaints or mild to severe symptoms, depending on the site of the lesions and the degree of involvement. In pulmonary sarcoidosis, patients may have a dry cough, shortness of breath, or mild chest pain resulting from loss of lung volume and abnormal lung stiffness. Other symptoms are fatigue, fever, weight loss, swollen ankles, and joint pain. Organ-specific symptoms can occur in chronic, multisystem cases. Typical epithelioid lesions can also affect the skin, eyes, musculoskeletal system, and other internal organs.

Granulomas in the lungs are often found incidentally when chest radiography or CT is performed for some other reason. Lesions may also be found in the walls of the bronchioles, the alveoli, and the lymph nodes of the chest.

Patient Screening

In most cases, the disease is insidious and can have a range of symptoms. Acute onset or worsening of respiratory symptoms always requires immediate attention by a physician. Follow office policy for a possible referral to a pulmonary specialist.

Etiology

The exact cause is not clear. The disorder is thought to be a malfunction of the immune system or caused by a virus. Some scientists suspect exposure to toxins in the environment or other insults can trigger it. Although the disease is found throughout the world, in the United States, it occurs more commonly in young adults between the ages of 25 and 40 years and in black individuals. Genetic factors are suspected.

Diagnosis

Sarcoidosis can be difficult to detect. Sometimes symptoms and signs are uncovered through a complete medical evaluation, which includes history, physical examination, and chest radiography. Laboratory tests and pulmonary function studies are also helpful. When possible, a biopsy of the affected tissue is essential to confirm the diagnosis.

Treatment

In many cases, sarcoidosis resolves spontaneously. Treatment is not necessarily indicated when there are no symptoms or mild symptoms, regardless of radiologic abnormalities. Corticosteroid therapy, such as prednisone, helps relieve severe symptoms. The immunosuppressant drug methotrexate is also used to treat widespread diseases, such as disfiguring skin lesions and cardiac or CNS involvement. A few newer treatments are available as well. These include monoclonal antibody immunosuppressants such as infliximab (Remicade) and adalimumab (Humira).

Prognosis

Serious disability is rare with sarcoidosis, and most people can live normally. The prognosis varies for people with pulmonary sarcoidosis if the lungs become scarred and fibrotic or if other organ damage exists. Relapses can occur after cessation of immunosuppressive drugs. The disease is rarely fatal.

Prevention

Because the cause remains uncertain, there is no known prevention.

Patient Teaching

Review the doctor's instructions, including the medication schedule and possible side effects, such as insomnia and irritability. Advise the patient not to smoke or vape. Explain the importance of follow-up visits with the doctor to monitor the treatment.

Coronovirus *Disease (COVID-19)*
Coronavirus disease 2019 (COVID-19) (U07.1)

Description

COVID-19 is an infectious disease that spreads rapidly from one person to another and affects the respiratory system as well as other body systems, depending on the variant. In March 2020, the World Health Organization (WHO) declared COVID-19 a global pandemic. Everyone except essential personnel were told to stay home and businesses closed their doors. Schools and colleges moved to remote learning for several months.

Signs and Symptoms

Upper respiratory symptoms include cough, congestion, rhinitis, and sneezing. Fever may accompany symptoms. Fatigue, headache, and general malaise can accompany other symptoms. Low oxygen saturation is common in some cases and patients may develop pneumonia. In addition to respiratory symptoms, COVID-19 can cause symptoms in other body systems.

Etiology

Coronavirus is caused by the SARS-CoV-2 virus.

Diagnosis

Diagnosis is made from patient symptoms and positive nasopharyngeal swab or by COVID-19 quick test, which provides results in a few minutes. If one member in a family tests positive and other members present with upper respiratory symptoms, the provider will determine whether or not testing of other family members is necessary. There are also COVID-19 tests that can be purchased over the counter for at-home use.

Treatment

Supportive treatment is directed toward alleviating symptoms. Over-the-counter medications for fever, muscle ache, cough, and rhinitis may be taken. The US Food and Drug Administration (FDA) has approved several medications for treating COVID. Paxlovid (nirmatrelvir/ritonavir) is used for the treatment of mild to moderate COVID-19. Veklury (remdesivir) may be used for hospitalized patients or ambulatory patients with mild to moderate COVID-19, who are at a high risk of progression to severe COVID-19. Actemra (tocilizumab) and Olumiant (baricitinib) are indicated for the treatment of hospitalized patients with COVID-19 who may be receiving supplemental oxygen therapy or are on mechanical ventilation.

There are also emergency-use drugs the FDA can allow under specific conditions. These may be unapproved medications or medications that are approved but have a different indication.

Prognosis

Mild to moderate cases of COVID-19 have a positive outlook. Severe cases of COVID-19 are known to have lasting side effects. COVID "brain" has been diagnosed in some patients and is responsible for affecting memory and causing individuals to have confusion. COVID-19 has the potential to shrink the brain tissue. Individuals with other preexisting conditions are more likely to have a less positive outcome. According to the WHO at the time of the authoring of this text, 6,957,216 people have died from COVID-19, or COVID-related illness.

Prevention

There are current COVID-19 vaccinations available. Avoiding contact with individuals who have tested positive for COVID-19 is advised. N95 masks are helpful in protecting oneself from exposure to other people known to be positive for COVID-19.

Patient Teaching

Practice good hygiene and hand sanitization. Sanitize hard surfaces with antibacterial wipes to prevent the spread. Cover mouth and nose when coughing or sneezing. Stay home unless you are going to a medical facility or a physician. Do not use public transportation. Avoid interaction with others in the household and isolate yourself from them as much as possible. Check oxygen saturation with pulse oximeter and if the oxygen level goes below 90%, seek medical attention.

Lung Cancer

Description

Lung cancer is the most common cause of cancer-related deaths worldwide among both males and females. It is usually caused by repeated carcinogenic irritation to the bronchial epithelium, leading to increased rates of cell division (Fig. 9.21).

ICD-10-CM Code	C34.0 *(Malignant neoplasm of main bronchus)* (C34.0–C34.92 = 16 codes of specificity)

The above code is a nonspecific code and may be valid as a principal diagnosis, except for Medicare. Refer to the physician's diagnosis and then to the current edition of the ICD-10-CM coding manual to ensure the greatest specificity of pathology and any appropriate modifiers.

Symptoms and Signs

The most common symptom is cough with or without sputum production. Because many patients diagnosed with lung cancer have coexisting COPD with a chronic cough, it is important to note any changes in the character of the cough. Other symptoms may include dyspnea, hemoptysis, chest pain (usually dull, intermittent pain on the side of the tumor), and weight loss. The brain is a common site for metastasis for some types of lung cancer. Symptoms of brain metastasis include headache, weakness, change in mental status, and seizures. Other common sites of metastasis are the liver, bone, and brain.

Patient Screening

A patient complaining of a chronic cough, chest pain, or dyspnea is scheduled for medical evaluation at the first available appointment.

Etiology

Lung cancers are subdivided into two main types by histology: nonsmall cell lung cancer (NSCLC) and small cell lung cancer (SCLC). The distinction is important because it relates to staging, treatment, and prognosis. Approximately

• **Fig. 9.21** Examples of lung carcinomas. (A) Centrally located tumor attached to bronchus. (B) Mesothelioma on pleural surface. (From Damjanov I: *Pathology for the health-related professions*, ed 4, St. Louis, 2011, Saunders.)

• **Fig. 9.22** Examples of neoplastic lung disease. (From Long BW, Frank ED, Ehrlich RA: *Radiography essentials for limited practice*, ed 4, St. Louis, 2013, Elsevier.)

80% of all lung cancers are NSCLCs. SCLC occurs almost exclusively in smokers, has a rapid growth rate, and metastasizes early in the disease process.

Diagnosis

Many patients are symptomatic at the time of diagnosis, although some may be diagnosed incidentally by a chest radiograph (Fig. 9.22) or during imaging being performed for another health problem. A tissue biopsy specimen is required for a definitive diagnosis. It can be obtained through bronchoscopy, mediastinoscopy, or CT-guided fine-needle aspiration. CT of the chest, abdomen, and head and bone scanning are done to look for metastases. Laboratory tests are done to check for abnormalities caused by metastatic disease (Fig. 9.23). Testing is also done to look for specific biomarkers, such as gene mutations in epidermal growth factor receptor (EGFR) or anaplastic lymphoma kinase, which may affect the treatment choice. SCLC and NSCLC are staged differently. NSCLC is staged by using the TNM system. SCLC staging involves distinguishing between disease that is confined to one side of the chest ("limited") and disease that has spread to encompass the other lung or other parts of the body ("extensive").

Treatment

Treatment decisions are based on the type of tumor (SCLC or NSCLC) and the stage of the tumor. For early-stage NSCLC, surgical resection, with or without radiation or chemotherapy, is the preferred option and offers the best chances for survival. Surgery usually involves lobectomy, which is the removal of the portion of the lung affected by the tumor, or pneumonectomy, which is the removal of the entire affected lung. Later-stage NSCLC is generally not treatable by surgical resection alone. A combined modality approach is used, including chemotherapy, radiotherapy, surgery, and/or palliative therapy for symptom control. Because SCLC often metastasizes early in the disease

> ### ❖ ENRICHMENT
>
> #### Vaping and Electronic Cigarettes
>
> Electronic cigarettes (e-cigarettes) deliver nicotine through a device and are used by people of all ages. According to the CDC, e-cigarettes are sometimes called *e-cigs*, *vapes*, *e-hookahs*, *vape pens*, and *electronic nicotine delivery systems*. Some e-cigarettes look like regular cigarettes, cigars, or pipes. Some look like USB (Universal Serial Bus) flash drives, pens, and other everyday items.
>
> Vaping has become quite common, particularly among teenagers and young individuals. The use of nicotine while the brain is still developing, which occurs into the mid-20s, can cause problems with brain development and function. The liquid used in e-cigarettes and vape devices can also contain other harmful substances. The battery-operated devices used for this type of nicotine delivery heat the liquid substance that contains nicotine and produce an aerosol that is inhaled. Users of e-cigarettes and parents need to be aware of the risks of this habit. The long-term effects of vaping during the teenage period or young adulthood are still being studied.

process, it is usually treated by using systemic chemotherapy along with radiation therapy rather than surgery, even in the limited disease stage.

There have been many recent advances in the use of targeted therapy or immunotherapy in the treatment of lung cancer. For example, patients with EGFR mutations may respond well to treatment with EGFR tyrosine kinase inhibitors. Much research is currently being done in this field, and many clinical trials are underway.

Prognosis

The prognosis for patients with lung cancer is generally poor. The 5-year survival rate for all stages and types combined is

• **Fig. 9.23** Metastatic lung disease. Hematogenous (spread via blood) metastases are well-defined lesions scattered throughout the lungs. (From Long BW, Frank ED, Ehrlich RA: *Radiography essentials for limited practice*, ed 4, St. Louis, 2013, Elsevier.)

just 15%. Some factors that have been shown to affect the prognosis are the stage at the time of diagnosis, the histologic tumor type, the degree of differentiation of the tumor, the presence or absence of symptoms at diagnosis, and the presence and degree of weight loss.

Prevention

The US Preventative Services Task Force now recommends lung cancer screening for high-risk individuals with an annual low-dose chest CT. *High risk* is defined as people aged 55 to 80 years with at least a smoking history of 30 packs per year and who are current smokers or have quit within the past 15 years. Screening should be discontinued if more than 15 years have elapsed since smoking cessation or if there is a limited life expectancy.

The importance of smoking cessation cannot be stressed enough, and reducing exposure to secondhand smoke is recommended. It is important to emphasize the benefits of smoking cessation even for patients who already have lung cancer, especially those with limited SCLC disease. If patients survive their lung cancer, relapse is much more likely in patients who continue to smoke.

Patient Teaching

Explain the diagnostic procedures, their purposes, and when to expect results. Encourage the patient to express concerns and offer to supply answers to any specific questions. After diagnosis, the patient benefits from explanation and clarification of the treatment regimen through verbal and written instructions. Offer referrals to community support groups and information agencies, such as the American Cancer Society and the American Lung Association. Provide information on smoking cessation programs, when appropriate. Stress the importance of follow-up care.

Review Challenge

Answer the following questions:
1. What are the physical and chemical dynamics of normal respiration?
2. Why is the common cold so common?
3. How is sinusitis treated?
4. What are the possible causes of nasal polyps?
5. How is severe epistaxis treated?
6. What is the prognosis for malignant tumors of the larynx?
7. What are some causes of and risk factors for (1) atelectasis and (2) pulmonary embolism?
8. What determines the treatment of pneumonia?
9. Why does the patient with a pulmonary abscess exhibit foul-smelling sputum?
10. Where does the causative organism of legionnaires disease thrive?
11. What is the profile of individuals vulnerable to respiratory syncytial virus pneumonia?
12. How is histoplasmosis contracted?
13. Who would benefit from influenza immunization?
14. Why is influenza considered a serious infection?
15. What does the abbreviation *COPD* refer to?
16. How is chronic bronchitis associated with other pulmonary conditions?

17. Are emphysema and bronchiectasis reversible? What are some causes of both conditions?
18. Why is pneumoconiosis considered an occupational disease?
19. What is the treatment for a hemothorax and a pneumothorax?
20. Why is pulmonary tuberculosis more prevalent and difficult to treat today?
21. How would you describe the pathology of a patient with adult respiratory distress syndrome?
22. What steps are recommended to prevent lung cancer?
23. What effect may electronic cigarettes have on the brain?

Real-Life Challenge: Sinusitis

A 45-year-old male is experiencing a headache over both eyes on awakening. The patient says he also experiences pain above the eyes when bending over. Tenderness above the eyes in the frontal area of the forehead and also in both cheeks is noted on palpation. A thick greenish-yellow mucous drainage is present. Sinus radiographs show cloudiness in the region of the maxillary and frontal sinuses.

Vital signs are temperature, 99.88°F; pulse, 90 beats per minute; respirations, 26 breaths per minute; and blood pressure, 136/88 mm Hg. Mouth breathing is noted.

Questions

1. Compare the symptoms and signs of sinusitis and those of an upper respiratory tract infection.
2. What are the causes of sinusitis?
3. Discuss the correlation between allergies and sinusitis.
4. What drug therapy might be prescribed for the treatment of sinusitis?
5. What is the principle behind the use of decongestants for sinusitis?
6. How would air-filled sinuses appear on radiographs?

Real-Life Challenge: Acute Bronchitis

A 39-year-old female is experiencing a deep cough that produces thick, yellow sputum. She is complaining of shortness of breath and pain in the upper chest. Audible wheezing is heard without a stethoscope. Vital signs are temperature, 100.2°F; pulse, 102 beats per minute; respirations, 32 breaths per minute; and blood pressure, 134/88 mm Hg. Auscultation of the chest confirms the presence of bilateral wheezing and scattered rales.

The patient has a history of an URI infection 2 weeks before the onset of coughing 3 days ago. Her husband is a cigarette smoker. Diagnostic studies ordered include chest radiography, pulmonary studies, sputum analysis, CBC, and ESR. The patient is diagnosed with acute bacterial bronchitis.

Questions

1. Why is increased fluid intake recommended?
2. Which treatment would be recommended to relieve wheezing?
3. Which treatment would be recommended to relieve coughing?
4. Compare the symptoms and signs of chronic bronchitis with those of acute bronchitis.
5. Compare the etiology of chronic bronchitis versus acute bronchitis.
6. How significant is the exposure to primary or secondary smoke to patients with acute or chronic bronchitis?
7. What is this patient's risk for developing chronic bronchitis?

Real-Life Challenge: Epistaxis

A 60-year-old female has called the office stating that she is experiencing a severe nosebleed. She says her nose started bleeding last night and has been bleeding off and on since then. The blood is bright red and seems to be coming from the left side of her nose. On questioning, she reports that she has a few periods of feeling lightheaded. She is advised to apply pressure to the left nostril and to sit down. The provider is not in the office. The patient's son is with her and is able to transport her to an emergency facility. She is instructed to take along her current medication. After talking with her son, you suggest that he take his mother to a nearby facility. You also tell him that you will call the facility so they will be expecting her arrival.

Questions

1. On looking at the patient's chart, you see that she is taking Plavix. Why is that important?
2. Should you also advise the son to assist her to his vehicle?
3. Will the emergency facility inquire about her health status?
4. What might be significant about her medical history?
5. What is the significance of the patient feeling lightheaded?
6. Which treatment protocols do you anticipate the patient will receive at the facility?
7. What would you do if the son were not with the patient?

Internet Assignments

1. Research the American Lung Association website (www.lung.org) for an update on a respiratory condition of your interest.
2. Visit the American Lung Association website. Search for "Work" and report on some of the work-related illnesses.
3. Explore the National Institute of Allergies and Infectious Diseases (NIAID) website at https://www.niaid.nih.gov. Search for "asthma," and answer the following questions:
   a. Why is the study of asthma a priority for NIAID?
   b. How is NIAID addressing this critical topic?
4. Perform an Internet search on "vaping statistics," and report on your findings on teenagers and their use of electronic delivery devices.

Critical Thinking

1. Discuss how smoking affects the tissues and structures of the respiratory system.
2. Cancer of the lung and bronchus is the number one cause of cancer-related death. What help is available to those who want to stop smoking?
3. How would you respond to a person choking in a restaurant and obviously unable to dislodge the obstruction? Demonstrate the Heimlich maneuver. What if that person is a child? How would you adjust the procedure?
4. How would you come to the aid of a person experiencing a severe nosebleed (epistaxis)? When should emergency treatment be obtained?
5. Explore how chronic respiratory diseases can present a daily challenge to keep the patient's airway open, to allow for ventilation and respiration. What are some ways anxiety enters into each day of the patient's life?
6. Compensation for lung disease may require the patient to regularly take medication, breathing treatments, and perhaps even different levels of oxygen therapy. In some cases, tracheostomy and an intermittent positive-pressure breathing machine may be used to improve ventilation of the lungs. How can these interventions change a person's life, depending on age and occupation?
7. What makes sputum removal management vitally important for the patient with bronchiectasis?
8. How would you respond to a person who suddenly complains of shortness of breath and chest pain? What possible pathologic conditions come to mind?

Prepare to discuss Critical Thinking case study exercises for this chapter that are posted on Evolve.

Credentialing Examination Questions

1. For what length of time can the bacteria *M. tuberculosis* survive in its dried form, if not exposed to sunlight?
   A. Less than 24 hours
   B. Days
   C. Weeks
   D. Months
2. Which sign is present when a patient experiences a flailing chest?
   A. High oxygen saturation
   B. Double fracture of three or more ribs
   C. Single fracture of one rib
   D. Normal breathing
3. Which activity should be avoided for a few weeks when diagnosed with mononucleosis?
   A. Reading
   B. Attending a concert
   C. Contact sports
   D. Attending school or college
4. Which acronym stands for the type of lung cancer that metastasizes early in the disease process?
   A. SCLC
   B. NSCLC
   C. SC
   D. GC
5. Which serious long-term side effects are associated with COVID brain?
   A. Confusion
   B. Memory loss
   C. Poor concentration
   D. All of the above

6. Which pulmonary disorder has symptoms which include pursing of the lips when exhaling, barrel chest, and circumoral cyanosis?
   A. Pneumonia
   B. Bronchitis
   C. Pneumothorax
   D. Emphysema

7. Which condition is the most common endemic mycosis in the United States and may also be found in South and Central America and in Africa?
   A. Histoplasmosis
   B. Blastomycosis
   C. Mononucleosis
   D. Coccidioidomycosis

8. Which diagnosis is a type of acute lung injury, characterized by severe pulmonary congestion, acute respiratory distress, and hypoxemia
   A. Small cell lung cancer
   B. Acute respiratory distress syndrome
   C. Pneumonia
   D. Sarcoidosis

9. Which condition describes a collection of air or gas in the pleural cavity that results in a collapsed or partially collapsed lung?
   A. Bronchitis
   B. Pneumonia
   C. Pneumothorax
   D. Hemothorax

10. Which condition results from the accumulation of blood and fluid in the pleural cavity?
    A. Hemothorax
    B. Bronchitis
    C. Pneumonia
    D. Pneumothorax

10

Diseases and Conditions of the Circulatory System

CHAPTER OUTLINE

LEARNING OBJECTIVES

After studying this chapter you should be able to:

1. Discuss the anatomy and physiology of the heart.
2. Name the common presenting symptoms in patients with cardiovascular disease.
3. Describe the pathology of coronary artery disease (CAD).
4. Name the contributing factors for CAD.
5. Explain what causes the pain of angina pectoris.
6. Explain the difference between angina pectoris and myocardial infarction (MI).
7. Describe the treatment of MI and cardiac arrest.
8. Name and describe the symptoms of the most prevalent cardiovascular disorder in the United States.
9. Explain what happens when the pumping action of the heart fails.
10. Compare left-sided heart failure with right-sided heart failure.
11. Name some causes of cardiomyopathy.
12. Distinguish among pericarditis, myocarditis, and endocarditis.
13. Explain why rheumatic fever is considered a systemic disease.
14. Recall the cardiac manifestations of rheumatic heart disease.
15. Explain the pathophysiology of valvular heart disease.
16. Name the causes of cardiac arrhythmias.
17. Discuss treatment options for cardiac arrhythmias.
18. Describe the signs and symptoms of shock.
19. Discuss cardiac tamponade.
20. Explain the possible consequences of emboli.
21. Compare arteriosclerosis with atherosclerosis.
22. Describe *aneurysm* and explain how it is diagnosed.

23. Explain the treatment for (1) thrombophlebitis and (2) varicose veins.
24. Describe the vascular pathology of Raynaud disease.
25. Define *anemia* and list the presenting symptoms.
26. Describe how anemias are classified and give some examples.
27. State the causes of agranulocytosis.
28. Describe the typical symptoms in all types of leukemias.
29. Distinguish between lymphedema and lymphangitis.
30. Explain the diagnostic significance of Reed-Sternberg cells in lymphoma.
31. Name the signs and symptoms of transfusion incompatibility reaction.
32. Explain the cause of classic hemophilia.
33. Describe disseminated intravascular coagulation.

KEY TERMS

agglutination (ah-glue-tih-NAY-shun)
aggregation (ag-reh-GAY-shun)
angioplasty (AN-jee-oh-plas-tee)
arteriosclerosis (ar-tee-ree-oh-skleh-ROW-sis)
asystole (a-SIS-toh-lee)
atherosclerosis (ath-er-oh-skleh-ROW-sis)
bradycardia (brady-KAR-dee-ah)
bruit (BREW-ee)
cardiomegaly (car-dee-oh-MEG-ah-lee)
cardiomyopathy (car-dee-oh-my-OP-ah-thee)
cellulitis (sell-u-LIE-tis)
dyscrasia (dis-CRAY-zee-ah)
ecchymosis (ech-ih-MO-sis)
embolism (EM-boh-lizm)
hematopoiesis (hem-ah-toh-poy-EE-sis)

hemolytic (hem-oh-LIT-ik)
hypovolemia (high-poh-voh-LEE-mee-ah)
hypoxia (high-POX-see-ah)
ischemia (is-KEY-mee-ah)
orthopnea (or-THOP-nee-ah)
perfusion (per-FYOU-zhun)
petechiae (pee-TEE-kee-ee)
phlebotomy (phleh-BOT-oh-mee)
plaque (PLACK)
purpura (PUR-pu-rah)
syncope (SIN-ko-pee)
tachycardia (tack-ee-CAR-dee-ah)
tamponade (tam-pon-ADE)
thrombus (THROM-bus)

Orderly Function of the Circulatory System

The circulation of blood to the organs and tissues of the body is the primary function of the circulatory system. The heart is at the center of the circulatory system (Figs. 10.1 and 10.2). Its steady beating pumps about 5 quarts of blood through a complete vascular circuit of the body every minute in an adult. This circuit comprises a network of vessels: the arteries, veins, and capillaries (Fig. 10.3).

The heart consists of two side-by-side pumps, each divided into two chambers: two upper chambers called *atria* and two lower chambers called *ventricles*. As venous blood returns to the heart from the body, it enters the right atrium, passes through the tricuspid valve, and, with atrial contraction, enters the right ventricle. Heart valves prevent blood from flowing backward. From the right ventricle, blood is pumped through the pulmonary valve and, with ventricular contraction, into the pulmonary arteries and on to the lungs. In the lungs, carbon dioxide is removed and oxygen is added to the blood. Freshly oxygenated blood then returns to the heart via the pulmonary veins. Blood enters the left atrium, moves through the mitral (bicuspid) valve with atrial contraction, and enters the left ventricle. As the left ventricle contracts, blood is forced through the aortic valve, into the aorta, and on to the rest of the body. This process is called the *cardiac cycle*.

The heart is enclosed by the double-layered pericardium, which is composed of an inner serous layer (visceral pericardium, or epicardium) and an outer fibrous layer (parietal pericardium). Between these layers in the pericardial cavity is a small amount of serous fluid that reduces friction during cardiac movements. Cardiac muscle tissue, or myocardium, is composed of striated muscle cells that can contract rhythmically on their own and characteristically are both voluntary and involuntary responses. Inside the cavities of the heart is a smooth serous lining called *endocardium*. The conduction system of the heart coordinates the contraction and relaxation (cardiac cycle) of the heart by initiating impulses and distributing the impulses throughout the myocardium. Coronary arteries and a network of vessels continuously supply cardiac muscle tissue with oxygen.

Cardiovascular Diseases

There are many and varied disorders of the heart and circulatory system. In some disorders, the rhythm of the heartbeat becomes irregular, may enter tachycardia (become abnormally fast), or may enter bradycardia (become abnormally slow). Disorders of cardiac rhythm are called *arrhythmias* or *dysrhythmias*.

Approximately 20% of all deaths in the United States are attributed to heart disease, according to the Centers for Disease Control and Prevention (CDC). Most of these

• **Fig. 10.1** The heart and great vessels, anterior view. (From Patton KT, Thibodeau GA: *Anatomy and physiology*, ed 9, St. Louis, 2016, Mosby.)

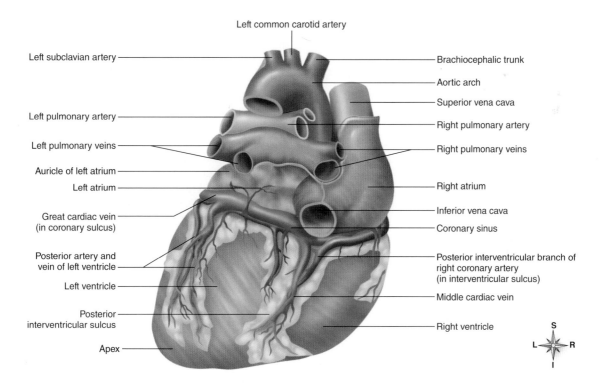

• **Fig. 10.2** The heart and great vessels, posterior view. (From Patton KT, Thibodeau GA: *Anatomy and physiology*, ed 9, St. Louis, 2016, Mosby.)

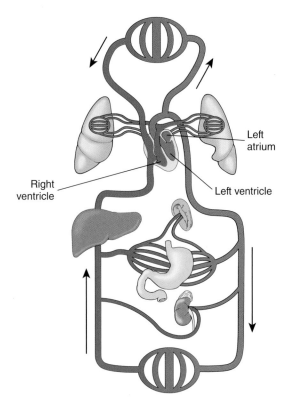

• **Fig. 10.3** Circulation through the body.

Left atrium

Right ventricle

Left ventricle

deaths are caused by coronary artery disease (CAD) and hypertension. Cardiovascular disorders, such as angina pectoris, myocardial infarction (MI), congestive heart failure (CHF), cardiac arrest, shock, and cardiac tamponade also can result in death. Other diseases of the cardiovascular system include rheumatic fever, pericarditis, myocarditis, endocarditis, thromboangiitis obliterans (Buerger disease), Raynaud disease, and vascular (blood vessel) diseases.

Important presenting symptoms that tend to recur in patients with cardiovascular disease and need further investigation include:

- Chest pain
- Dyspnea (difficulty in breathing) on exertion
- Tachypnea (rapid breathing)
- Palpitations (rapid fluttering of the heart)
- Cyanosis (slight blue color)
- Edema
- Fatigue
- Syncope (fainting)

Coronary Artery Disease

Description

CAD is a condition involving the arteries supplying the myocardium. The arteries become narrowed because of atherosclerotic deposits over time, causing temporary cardiac ischemia and eventually MI (or heart attack).

ICD-10-CM Code | I25.10 (Atherosclerotic heart disease of native coronary artery without angina pectoris) (I25.10–I25.119 = 5 codes of specificity)

Codes for coronary vascular disease are classified by location and type. Refer to the physician's diagnosis and then to the current edition of the ICD-10-CM coding manual to ensure the greatest specificity.

Symptoms and Signs

Patients are asymptomatic initially. The first symptoms may be the pain of angina pectoris (see the Angina Pectoris section) or even an extreme shortness of breath or tiredness. In advanced disease, the severe pain of MI is described as burning, squeezing, crushing, and radiating to the arm, neck, or jaw and results from diminished blood flow and lower oxygen saturation. Nausea, vomiting, and weakness also can be experienced. Changes are often, but not always, recognized on the patient's electrocardiogram (ECG). Many patients may be asymptomatic until an MI or sudden death event; this is why noninvasive screening of high-risk patients is imperative.

Patient Screening

Severe chest pain of sudden onset, with or without a previous diagnosis of angina, is considered to be a cardiac event and has the potential to be catastrophic; therefore the patient should immediately be entered into the emergency medical system.

Etiology

Deposits of fat-containing substances, called plaque, in the lumen of the coronary arteries result in atherosclerosis and subsequent narrowing of the lumen of the arteries. The myocardium must have a good blood supply to function. The coronary arteries supply the cardiac muscle with blood but become constricted by atherosclerosis (Fig. 10.4), which can also cause other systemic problems.

Arteriosclerosis, commonly called *hardening of the arteries*, is associated with older adults and patients with diabetes. The arteries eventually lose elasticity and become hard and narrow, resulting in cardiac ischemia. Replacement scar tissue forms, interfering with the heart's ability to pump, resulting in heart failure.

Factors contributing to increased risk of the disease include family history, history of smoking, hypertension, diabetes, chronic kidney disease, obesity, and a history of elevated serum cholesterol or reduced serum high-density lipoprotein (HDL) levels. Lack of exercise, unhealthy diet, and stress are additional risk factors.

Diagnosis

ECG shows ischemia (caused by lack of blood supply) and possibly arrhythmias. Treadmill testing, thallium or Cardiolite scanning, computed tomography (CT), stress echocardiography, cardiac catheterization, and angiography are other tools of cardiac status evaluation used to detect insufficient oxygen supply and to confirm the diagnosis. Electron beam computerized testing, a noninvasive assessment for identifying calcium buildup in arteries, is another means of risk evaluation.

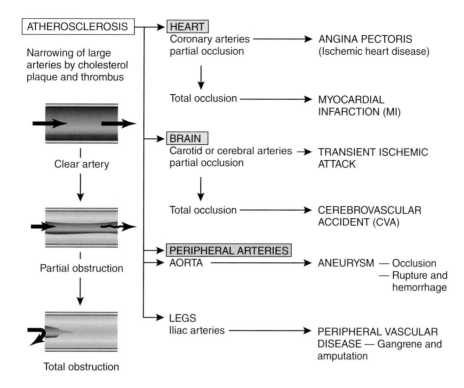

ATHEROSCLEROSIS

Narrowing of large arteries by cholesterol plaque and thrombus

Clear artery

Partial obstruction

Total obstruction

HEART
Coronary arteries partial occlusion → ANGINA PECTORIS (Ischemic heart disease)

Total occlusion → MYOCARDIAL INFARCTION (MI)

BRAIN
Carotid or cerebral arteries partial occlusion → TRANSIENT ISCHEMIC ATTACK

Total occlusion → CEREBROVASCULAR ACCIDENT (CVA)

PERIPHERAL ARTERIES
AORTA → ANEURYSM — Occlusion — Rupture and hemorrhage

LEGS
Iliac arteries → PERIPHERAL VASCULAR DISEASE — Gangrene and amputation

• **Fig. 10.4** Possible consequences of atherosclerosis. (From Gould B: *Pathophysiology for the health professions*, ed 3, Philadelphia, 2006, Saunders/Elsevier.)

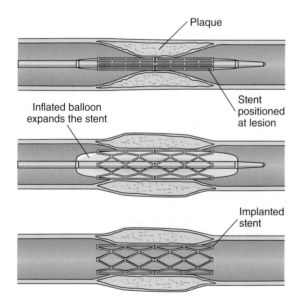

• **Fig. 10.5** Coronary artery stent. (From *Mosby's dictionary of medicine, nursing and health professions*, ed 7, St. Louis, 2010, Mosby/Elsevier.)

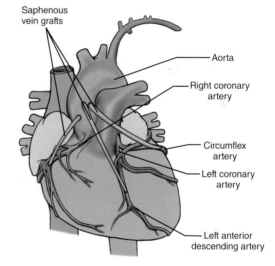

• **Fig. 10.6** Coronary bypass graft. (From *Mosby's dictionary of medicine, nursing and health professions,* ed 7, St. Louis, 2010, Mosby/Elsevier.)

Treatment

Treatment consists of measures to restore adequate blood flow to the myocardium. Vasodilators and other types of medicines are prescribed. Angioplasty with a balloon and stenting is attempted in some instances to open the constricted arteries (Fig. 10.5). First-line drug therapy for the prevention of CAD may include angiotensin-converting enzyme (ACE) inhibitors, angiotensin receptor blockers (ARBs), calcium channel blockers (CCBs), thiazide diuretics, or vasodilators. Beta-blockers and anticoagulants are used to prevent blood clots from breaking off and lodging in the cerebral arteries. When the blockage is severe or does not respond to drug therapy or angioplasty, coronary artery bypass surgery (CABG) may be indicated to restore circulation to the affected myocardium (Fig. 10.6). Research at Mayo Clinic includes cardiac regenerative medicine which involves stem cell treatment to help restore function to damaged heart tissue cells. This is an emerging technology with a promising future that's being used in several areas of heart condition treatment.

Prognosis

The prognosis varies, depending on the patient's response to the treatment, whether drug therapy, angioplasty, or CABG. Smoking also has an effect on prognosis.

Prevention

Measures to prevent CAD include a healthy diet that is low in salt, fat, and cholesterol, in addition to exercise. Patients are encouraged to reduce stress and, if they smoke, to stop or reduce smoking.

Patient Teaching

Give patients information about symptoms of impending MI, and encourage them to seek immediate emergency medical care at the first sign of any related symptoms. Emphasize the importance of a nutritious low-fat diet, weight control, exercise, and smoking cessation.

Angina Pectoris

Description

Angina pectoris, which is chest pain caused by ischemia during or shortly after exertion, is the result of reduced oxygen supply to the myocardium.

ICD-10-CM   I20.8 *(Other forms of angina pectoris)*
Code   I20.9 *(Angina pectoris, unspecified)*
             (I20.0–I20.9 = 4 codes of specificity)
Codes for angina pectoris are classified by type. Refer to the physician's diagnosis and then to the current edition of the ICD-10-CM coding manual to ensure the greatest specificity.

Symptoms and Signs

The patient experiences a sudden onset of left-sided chest pain during or shortly after exertion. The pain may radiate to the left arm or back (Fig. 10.7). The pain may also occur at the neck, rather than at the chest. The patient also may experience dyspnea. Blood pressure may increase during the attack, and arrhythmias may occur.

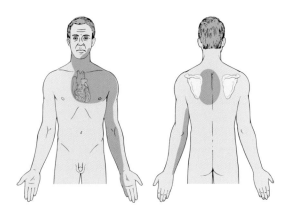

• **Fig. 10.7** Common sites of pain in angina pectoris.

Patient Screening

Patients experiencing symptoms of angina for the first time require immediate assessment. Acute MI must be ruled out. Those who have been diagnosed with angina pectoris and in whom cessation of activity and use of vasodilating medications does not provide relief from the pain within 20 minutes need to seek immediate medical intervention through the emergency medical system.

Etiology

Atherosclerosis causes narrowing of the coronary arteries, compromising the blood flow to the myocardium. Blood vessels cannot supply oxygen appropriately. Severe prolonged tachycardia, anemia, and respiratory disease also can cause cardiac ischemia.

Diagnosis

The patient's history reveals previous exertional chest pain or extreme tiredness or fatigue, especially after even simple activities. ECG performed during the anginal episode may show ischemia. It is important to realize that a normal result on ECG does not preclude the diagnosis of angina. Other diagnostic measures, such as those described for CAD, are performed.

Treatment

Treatment consists of cessation of the strenuous activity and placing of nitroglycerin tablets or spray under the tongue. When angina persists after treatment or for longer than 20 minutes, immediate medical attention is indicated.

Prognosis

The prognosis varies, depending on the extent of the arterial involvement. When patients can stop the pain by ceasing strenuous activities and using vasodilating medications, the angina usually will diminish or disappear. The patient's ability to modify his or her lifestyle may improve the prognosis.

Prevention

Preventive measures are similar to those recommended for CAD. Recommendations focus on lifestyle modification, including appropriate exercise; a diet low in fat, cholesterol, and salt; control of hypertension; weight loss; and smoking cessation. Patients are encouraged to reduce stress. Transdermal nitroglycerin patches help to prevent angina associated with this condition.

Patient Teaching

Emphasize the importance of compliance with prescribed drug therapy and diet.

Patients should be instructed to carry the nitroglycerin with them at all times. Additionally, patients and their families should be instructed to use nitroglycerin as directed.

Myocardial Infarction

Description

MI is the death of myocardial tissue caused by the development of ischemia.

ICD-10-CM Code	I21.0 *(fifth digit required) (ST elevation [STEMI] myocardial infarction of anterior wall)*
	(I21.01–I21.4 = 9 codes of specificity)

Acute myocardial infarction has many codes according to episode and location. The code can include a fifth-digit subclassification according to episode. Codes for location are as follows:

ICD-10-CM Code	I21.09 *(ST elevation [STEMI] myocardial infarction involving other coronary artery of anterior wall)*
	I21.19 *(ST elevation [STEMI] myocardial infarction involving other coronary artery of inferior wall)*
	I21.11 *(ST elevation [STEMI] myocardial infarction involving right coronary artery)*
	I21.29 *(ST elevation [STEMI] myocardial infarction involving other sites)*
	I21.4 *(Non-ST elevation [NSTEMI] myocardial infarction)*
	I21.3 *(ST elevation [STEMI] myocardial infarction of unspecified site)*

Note: The physician must designate the area of the infarction before a code is applied to the episode. Refer to the physician's diagnosis and then to the current edition of the ICD-10-CM coding manual to ensure the greatest specificity.

Symptoms and Signs

Occlusion of a coronary artery resulting in ischemia and infarct (death) of the myocardium (Fig. 10.8) causes sudden, severe substernal or left-sided chest pain. The pain may be crushing, causing a feeling of massive constriction of the chest, may be burning, or may just be a vague discomfort. This pain may radiate to the left or right arm, back, or jaw (Fig. 10.9) and is not relieved by rest or the administration of nitroglycerin. Irregular heartbeat, dyspnea, diaphoresis, anxiety and nausea may accompany the pain, MI occasionally is clinically silent, especially in patients with diabetes.

Patient Screening

Early and immediate intervention improves the chances of survival and minimizes irreversible injury to the myocardium. Emergency (911) intervention must be initiated immediately to control pain, stabilize heart rhythm, and minimize damage to the heart muscle. Automated external defibrillators (AEDs), if available, provide auditory instructions to the rescuer.

Etiology

MI results from insufficient oxygen supply, as occurs when a coronary artery is occluded by atherosclerotic plaque, thrombus, or myocardial muscle spasm. The pain is caused by ischemia which causes the cardiac muscle to die.

Left of sternum or entire upper chest

Mid-chest, neck, and jaw

Mid-chest and inside arms (left more than right)

Upper abdomen

Chest, neck, jaw, and inside arms

Center of lower neck to both sides of upper neck and all of jaw

Inside right arm to below elbow, shoulder, and inside left arm to waist (left side more often than right)

Between shoulder blades

• **Fig. 10.9** Locations of pain from myocardial infarction. (From *Mosby's dictionary of medicine, nursing and health professions*, ed 7, St. Louis, 2010, Mosby/Elsevier.)

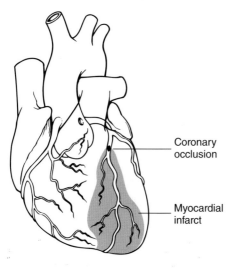

Coronary occlusion

Myocardial infarct

• **Fig. 10.8** Myocardial infarction.

Diagnosis

The diagnosis includes a thorough history, ECG, chest radiographic studies, and laboratory tests for cardiac troponin I and troponin T enzyme levels. Changes in the enzyme levels indicate the death of cardiac tissue. Troponin levels will rise in cases of myocardial infarction within 3 to 24 hours after cardiac muscle is compromised. ECG changes in the P-R and QRS complexes and in the ST segment correspond to the ischemic areas. Diagnostic confirmation is assisted by elevated cardiac enzyme levels and altered CPK isoenzyme levels identified through blood tests.

Treatment

Oxygen is administered, and morphine is given for pain. Aspirin is given as soon as possible to reduce the risk of additional damage to the heart and cardiac tissue caused by ischemia. Recent recommendations include calling 911 for entry into the emergency medical system and chewing one 5-grain/325-mg aspirin tablet. Vasodilation is attempted by administering a nitroglycerin drip. Lidocaine or amiodarone given by an intravenous (IV) drip, after a loading bolus, helps control arrhythmias. Thrombolytic drugs, including tissue plasminogen activator (tPA), streptokinase, or alteplase (Activase) may be administered as soon as possible after the diagnosis, unless there are contraindications. An attempt may be made to open the occlusion and to restore blood flow to the area through angioplasty with stent placement, the administration of thrombolytic drugs, or CABG.

Prognosis

The prognosis of MI is determined by the amount of damage to heart tissue.

Prevention

Preventive measures are similar to those recommended for CAD. Recommendations focus on lifestyle modification, including appropriate exercise; a diet low in fat, cholesterol, and salt; control of hypertension; weight loss; and smoking cessation. Patients are encouraged to reduce stress. Those surviving MI are urged to take a daily aspirin dose and a beta-blocker or ACE inhibitor for life. Lipid-lowering medications are also recommended.

Patient Teaching

Emphasize the importance of compliance with prescribed drug therapy, dietary needs, and cardiac rehabilitation.

Cardiac Arrest

Description

Cardiac arrest is the sudden, unexpected cessation of cardiac activity.

ICD-10-CM I46.9 *(Cardiac arrest, cause unspecified)*
Code (I46.2–I46.9 = 3 codes of specificity)

Symptoms and Signs

The patient is unresponsive, with no respiratory effort and no palpable pulse.

Patient Screening

Cardiac arrest is a true life-threatening emergency. The American Heart Association (AHA) or American Red Cross protocol for caregivers in the field requires immediate contact with the emergency medical system by calling 911. Inpatient facilities use codes such as "code blue" to alert hospital personnel.

Etiology

Cardiac arrest results from anoxia (absence of oxygen to the tissue) or interruption of electrical stimuli to the heart. It can be caused by respiratory arrest, arrhythmia, or MI. Electrocution, drowning, severe trauma, massive hemorrhage, or drug overdose also can cause cardiac arrest.

Diagnosis

The diagnosis is based on the absence of respiratory effort and lack of palpable pulse. ECG shows ventricular fibrillation or asystole.

Treatment

Immediate intervention with instantaneous initiation of cardiopulmonary resuscitation (CPR) and defibrillation by means of an AED may successfully restore contraction of the heart (Fig. 10.10). Ambulance or other medical personnel administer cardiac drugs, including epinephrine and isoproterenol or dobutamine to stimulate the heart. Antiarrhythmic drugs, including lidocaine and amiodarone may also be administered.

Prognosis

The prognosis varies, depending on the length of time the individual has been in cardiac arrest, and how quickly CPR is initiated. The earlier CPR and defibrillation are instituted, the greater the possibility of survival. The general health and age of the patient and the cause of the arrest also play a part in the final outcome.

• **Fig. 10.10** Photo of an automated external defibrillator. (Courtesy David Frazier, 2011, in cooperation with St. Johns County Sheriff's Office, St Augustine, Florida.)

Prevention

Prevention of the catastrophic event of cardiac arrest is difficult. Controlling blood pressure and a healthy lifestyle are beneficial and can reduce risk. One cannot predict near-drowning or electrical shock accidents, but most individuals will try to avoid situations that carry this risk. In high-risk patients with a history of abnormal heart rhythms or weak cardiac muscle, the implanting of defibrillators has been shown to decrease the risk of sudden cardiac death. Another option is a vest those high at risk can wear the LifeVest. This is a wearable defibrillator that can deliver a shock if there is an abnormal rhythm or absence of a heartbeat.

Patient Teaching

Encourage survivors of cardiac arrest to comply with the provider's instructions, prescribed regimen of drug therapy, testing, and lifestyle modifications.

Broken Heart Syndrome (Takotsubo Cardiomyopathy)

Description

Broken heart syndrome can occur when the heart's pumping function is abnormal. This can result from a temporary problem in a single area or region of the heart.

ICD-10-CM Diagnosis Code I51.81 (Takotsubo syndrome)

Symptoms and Signs

The individual experiences chest pain and shortness of breath. Symptoms are very similar to myocardial infarction.

Patient Screening

Sudden onset of chest pain and shortness of breath requires calling 911 for emergency assistance.

Etiology

The exact cause is unclear, however, it is believed that a surge of stress hormones may be responsible. There is a physiological change that takes place and causes the overall heart function to change. The syndrome occurs after a physical event such as major surgery, broken bone, trauma, or accident. Emotionally stressful events can also cause this problem to occur. Some examples include the death of a loved one, divorce, loss of a job, argument, a surprise party, winning the lottery, or a happy event.

Diagnosis

There is not one specific test used to diagnose this condition. Cardiac enzymes may be high leading to a cardiac workup. The arteries are not obstructed. Blood flow may be reduced. A chest x-ray may or may not show an abnormal size or shape of the heart. ECG is performed, and echocardiography may also be performed. ECG may show changes from normal rhythm. Echocardiography may show an enlarged left ventricle. Coronary angiography is performed to rule out arterial blockages. The lungs will be evaluated for pulmonary edema. Blood pressure is monitored.

Treatment

Treatment is the same as that for a coronary obstruction until it is ruled out. Usually the patient will remain in the hospital for a few days. The patient may be put on medications to reduce the workload of the heart. Medications may include beta-blockers, ACE inhibitors, and/or diuretics. LifeVest, a wearable defibrillator may be indicated for at-home use.

Prognosis

Many patients will recover within 1 to 2 months.

Prevention

The only prevention is avoidance of stressful situations.

Patient Teaching

Explain the importance of following all the provider's instructions, using medications as directed, and wearing the external defibrillator Lifevest as instructed.

Hypertensive Heart Disease

Hypertensive heart disease is the result of chronically elevated pressure throughout the vascular system. Atherosclerosis, arteriosclerosis, renal disease, and any condition that creates increased vascular pressure cause the heart to work harder as it pumps against the increased resistance.

Essential Hypertension

Description

Essential, or primary, hypertension, a condition of abnormally high blood pressure in the arterial system, has an insidious onset, with the patient exhibiting few, if any, symptoms until permanent damage has occurred.

ICD-10-CM Code   I10 (Essential [primary] hypertension)

Essential hypertension is listed under hypertensive heart disease in several ways. Other mentions of hypertension are listed under hypertensive heart disease, hypertensive renal disease, hypertensive heart and renal disease, and secondary hypertension. Refer to the physician's diagnosis and then to the current edition of the ICD-10-CM coding manual to ensure the greatest specificity.

Symptoms and Signs

The patient may experience headaches, epistaxis, lightheadedness, or syncope. Hypertension is usually detected when blood pressure is taken during a physical examination or a screening process.

Patient Screening

Many patients with essential hypertension have no indication of the condition. They may seek an appointment for a headache and should be scheduled for the next available appointment. Others may have had a blood pressure reading at a recent health screening or other event and have been advised to see their physician to report the elevated reading.

For these patients also, the next available appointment should be scheduled, preferably on the day of or the day after the call.

Etiology
The etiology is unknown, but many factors are thought to contribute to the condition. Stress is considered a major factor in hypertension. Age, heredity, smoking, obesity, sedentary lifestyle, poor dietary habits, and hyperactive personality or type A personality are possible causative factors in essential hypertension.

Diagnosis
Elevated blood pressure readings are the first indication of hypertension. According to the American College of Cardiology and the American Heart Association, blood pressure can be categorized. Normal is considered systolic less than 120 and diastolic less than 80. Elevated blood pressure is a systolic of 120 to 129 and diastolic less than 80. Stage 1 hypertension readings are 130 to 139 systolic and 80 to 89 diastolic. Stage 2 hypertension readings are measured at 140 or higher systolic and 90 or higher diastolic. The diagnosis is based on a series of blood pressure readings in which elevated values are obtained several times. A careful, complete medical history, physical examination, and laboratory evaluation should be performed before the diagnosis is confirmed and therapy is initiated.

Treatment
Drug therapy used in the treatment of hypertension includes diuretics (to reduce circulating blood volume), ACE inhibitors (to produce vasodilation and to increase renal blood flow), ARBs (to produce vasodilation and to increase renal blood flow), CCBs (to slow the heartbeat and to dilate vessels), and beta-blockers (to slow the heartbeat). These drugs may be prescribed singly or in combination. Additional modes of therapy include limitation of sodium intake, dietary management, weight reduction, exercise, reduction of stressful situations, and cessation of smoking.

Prognosis
The prognosis varies, depending on the patient's response to prescribed drug therapy and lifestyle modifications.

Prevention
Because the etiology is unknown, one cannot always prevent essential hypertension. The patient may be able to alter contributing lifestyle factors.

Patient Teaching
Teaching the patient that this condition is not cured but only controlled by drug therapy is essential. Education reinforces the need to monitor blood pressure on a regular basis and the need to continue drug therapy and maintain a healthy lifestyle.

Malignant Hypertension
Description
Malignant hypertension, a life-threatening condition, is a severe form of hypertension. It may also be referred to as a hypertensive crisis.

ICD-10-CM Code	I10 *(Essential [primary] hypertension)*

Malignant hypertension is listed in several ways under hypertensive heart disease. Other mentions of malignant hypertension are listed under hypertensive heart disease, hypertensive renal disease, hypertensive heart and renal disease, and secondary hypertension. Refer to the physician's diagnosis and then to the current edition of the ICD-10-CM coding manual to ensure the greatest specificity of pathology.

Symptoms and Signs
Severe headache, blurred vision, and dyspnea are symptoms that suggest the condition. The onset of symptoms may be sudden.

Patient Screening
Previously diagnosed patients with essential hypertension may complain of the sudden onset of symptoms. These patients are at risk for a cerebrovascular accident (CVA) and require prompt emergency intervention by calling 911.

Etiology
Uncontrolled hypertension, kidney damage, and endocrine disorders can result in malignant hypertension.

Diagnosis
Notable blood pressure elevation is considered malignant hypertension. In severe cases, the systolic pressure reading may be greater than 180 mm Hg and the diastolic pressure reading greater than 120 mm Hg.

Treatment
IV vasodilators, such as nitroprusside and labetalol, should be administered. After the condition is under control, blood pressure should be monitored on a regular basis and drug therapy continued for life.

Prognosis
The prognosis varies, depending on the patient's response to drug therapy. Patients who do not respond to drug therapy have worse outcomes, especially if the episode is accompanied by damage to organs.

Prevention
When one has essential hypertension, following the provider's instructions, as well as dietary and lifestyle modifications, may help prevent an episode of malignant hypertension.

Patient Teaching

Emphasize the importance of complying with drug therapy to patients and their families. Encourage patients to modify lifestyles as instructed by the provider, including maintaining a healthy weight and participating in activities/exercises according to their needs.

Congestive Heart Failure

Description

CHF is the acute or chronic inability of the heart to pump enough blood throughout the body to meet the demands of homeostasis.

> ICD-10-CM Code   I50.9 *(Heart failure, unspecified)*
> (150.1–I50.9 = 14 codes of
> specificity)
> *Refer to the physician's diagnosis and then to the current edition of the ICD-10-CM coding manual to ensure the greatest specificity.*

Symptoms and Signs

CHF usually has an insidious onset, with the patient experiencing gradually increasing dyspnea. Cardiac and respiratory rates increase, and the patient becomes anxious. As the condition progresses, the neck veins distend, and edema is noted in the ankles. When the right side of the heart fails, the liver and spleen enlarge, and peripheral edema is more prominent. (Fig. 10.11) Left-sided CHF causes increased pulmonary congestion and more pronounced respiratory difficulties (Fig. 10.12).

Patient Screening

Patients reporting unexplained chest discomfort, shortness of breath, or swelling of limbs require prompt medical assessment.

Etiology

Underlying conditions can compromise the pumping action of the heart, resulting in heart failure and inadequate perfusion. Genetic heart diseases can also put one at higher risk of developing heart failure. A common cause of acute CHF is MI. Some other causes of chronic CHF are coronary artery disease (CAD), hypertension, chronic obstructive pulmonary disease, cardiac valve damage, arrhythmias (dysrhythmias), and cardiomyopathy.

Diagnosis

The diagnosis is made after a thorough history and physical examination. Breath sounds are diminished, and radiographs indicate the presence of fluid in the lungs. ECG is used to discover the underlying causes. Echocardiography helps evaluate cardiac chamber size, ventricular function, and disease of the myocardium, valves, cardiac structures (walls, septum, and papillary muscles), and pericardium (the covering of the heart). Catheterization can be used to monitor the pressures in the circulation.

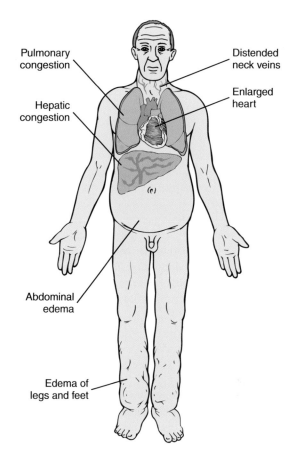

• **Fig. 10.11** Signs of congestive heart failure.

• **Fig. 10.12** Radiograph: congestive heart failure. (From Long BW, Frank ED, Ehrlich RA: *Radiography essentials for limited practice,* ed 4, St. Louis, 2013, Elsevier.)

Treatment

Treatment is directed at reducing the heart's workload and increasing its efficiency. ACE inhibitors and ARBs are used in the treatment of CHF, primarily to increase blood flow. Diuretics help reduce the volume of fluid in the body, and vasodilators help reduce vascular pressure. Digoxin may also be prescribed in specific cases to strengthen and slow the heartbeat. Fluid and sodium intake is restricted. Some patients with severe CHF may require special pacemakers, defibrillators, or, in extreme cases, heart transplantation.

Prognosis

The prognosis varies according to the cause. Acute CHF usually responds well to medical interventions and therefore has a positive outcome. The patient with chronic CHF is vulnerable to major organ impairment and resulting complications.

Prevention

Early medical intervention for CHF is important to prevent multiple organ complications.

Patient Teaching

A primary goal is promoting good patient compliance with the medical treatment plan. Explain that many patients experience quick alleviation of symptoms when they take medications as prescribed, follow dietary instructions, and modify activities to allow required rest and avoid fatigue. The use of diuretics requires patients to monitor their weight on a daily basis.

Cor Pulmonale

Description

Cor pulmonale, also known as *right-sided heart disease*, results in enlargement of the right ventricle as a sequela of primary lung disease.

ICD-10-CM	I27.81 *(Cor pulmonale [chronic])*
Code	I27.9 *(Pulmonary heart disease, unspecified)*
	(I27.0–I27.9 = 7 codes of specificity)

Symptoms and Signs

Cor pulmonale causes the patient to experience dyspnea, distended neck veins, fainting, fatigue, and edema of the extremities.

Patient Screening

Patients reporting unexplained chest discomfort, shortness of breath, or swelling of limbs require prompt medical assessment.

Etiology

Right-sided heart failure is an outcome of acute or chronic pulmonary disease and pulmonary hypertension. The diseased pulmonary blood vessels impair the flow of blood to pulmonary tissue. The increased pulmonary blood pressure increases the workload of the right side of the heart, causing the right ventricle to hypertrophy and thus to become less effective in pumping blood to the lungs. Chronic conditions causing cor pulmonale include emphysema and fibrotic pulmonary lesions, and the primary acute causative factor is pulmonary emboli. Chronic hypoxemia stimulates bone marrow in an adaptive response to produce an increased number of red blood cells (RBCs) to carry additional oxygen. This condition of abnormally high levels of RBCs (polycythemia) increases the viscosity of blood.

Diagnosis

The diagnosis is based on a history of pulmonary disease and hypoxia. The patient's respiratory status and cardiac status are assessed for neck vein distention and peripheral edema. Chest radiographic studies and echocardiography reveal pulmonary congestion and right-sided heart enlargement, and ECG frequently shows arrhythmias. CT angiogram, heart MRI, and lung scintigraphy may also be ordered. If polycythemia is present, the RBC count is elevated.

Treatment

Treatment entails relieving the causative factors in the pulmonary system and reducing hypoxemia. Bronchodilators are administered. Supplemental oxygen provides additional comfort to the patient. Bed rest is encouraged, and digitalis preparations are administered to strengthen and slow the heartbeat. Diuretics are prescribed when edema is present. Anticoagulants are given to avoid the risk of thromboembolisms. Phlebotomy, a surgical puncture of a vein to withdraw blood, may be used when polycythemia is a problem.

Prognosis

The outcome depends on the patient's response to treatment of the many possible disorders that predispose to cor pulmonale.

Prevention

No direct prevention of this condition is known. Many of the predisposing factors have no preventive measures to be taken.

Patient Teaching

Emphasize the instructions given by the physician. Explain the dosage schedule, and encourage compliance with drug therapy. Give patients information on possible side effects. Advise patients to report any adverse effects of medications.

Pulmonary Edema

Description

Pulmonary edema is a condition of fluid shift into the extravascular spaces of the lungs.

ICD-10-CM Code	J81.0 *(Acute pulmonary edema)*
	(J81.0–J81.1 = 2 codes of specificity)
	I50.1 *(Left ventricular failure)*
	J18.2 *(Hypostatic pneumonia, unspecified organism)*
	(J18.0–J18.9 = 5 codes of specificity)
	J81.1 *(Chronic pulmonary edema)*

Refer to the physician's diagnosis and then to the current edition of the ICD-10-CM coding manual to ensure the greatest specificity.

Symptoms and Signs

Pulmonary edema causes patients to experience dyspnea and coughing; orthopnea, a condition in which breathing becomes easier in the upright standing or sitting position; increased cardiac and respiratory rates; and often bloody, frothy sputum. Blood pressure may fall, and the skin becomes cold and clammy. The symptoms often occur at night after the patient lies down.

Patient Screening

Patients complaining of shortness of breath, typically when lying down, should be instructed to seek emergency care.

Etiology

Pulmonary edema is caused by left-sided heart failure, mitral valve disease, pulmonary embolus, systemic hypertension, arrhythmias, and renal failure. Head trauma, drug overdose, and exposure to high altitudes are other causes. Excessive fluid accumulates in the pulmonary tissue and air spaces of the lungs. The pulmonary circulation is overloaded with an excessive volume of blood.

Diagnosis

The clinical picture of dyspnea, orthopnea, and bloody, frothy sputum leads to further investigation. Breath sounds are diminished, with the presence of rales, rhonchi, and wheezing. Arterial blood gas measurement shows reduced oxygen saturation, increased carbon dioxide retention, increased bicarbonate levels, and decreased pH of the blood. Chest radiographs show increased opacity of the pulmonary tissue, an enlarged heart, and prominent pulmonary vessels. CT scan, B-type natriuretic peptide blood test, and other labwork may be ordered in addition to an echocardiogram, ultrasound of lungs, and cardiac catheterization if indicated.

Treatment

The patient is placed in the Fowler position (sitting), and oxygen therapy is administered. Drug therapy includes diuretics to improve fluid excretion; vasodilators, such as nitroglycerine or nitroprusside; morphine sulfate to induce venous dilation; and beta$_2$-adrenergic drugs to dilate the bronchioles and to control bronchial spasms. Severe cases may require mechanical ventilation.

Prognosis

Pulmonary edema is a life-threatening condition and is considered a medical emergency. The prognosis varies, depending on the severity of the pulmonary edema and the patient's response to intervention.

Prevention

Certain causes are controlled by the prevention of heart disease and avoidance of risk factors, such as drug overdose.

Patient Teaching

Encourage compliance with drug therapy and follow-up care. Patients taking diuretics are instructed about the importance of monitoring weight on a daily basis.

Cardiomyopathy

Description

Cardiomyopathy is a noninflammatory disease of the cardiac muscle resulting in enlargement of the myocardium and ventricular dysfunction.

ICD-10-CM Code	I42.3 (Endomyocardial [eosinophilic] disease)

Cardiomyopathy is coded according to type. Refer to the physician's diagnosis and then to the current edition of the ICD-10-CM coding manual to ensure the greatest specificity.

Symptoms and Signs

Cardiomyopathy causes the patient to experience symptoms of CHF, including dyspnea, fatigue, tachycardia, palpitations, and occasionally chest pain. Peripheral edema and hepatic congestion also may be present. Syncope and cardiac murmurs may occur. The symptoms and signs vary with the type and cause of this condition.

Patient Screening

Patients reporting dyspnea, fatigue, tachycardia, palpitations, and occasional chest pain require prompt assessment by a physician.

Etiology

The primary causes are mostly unknown. Cardiomyopathies are divided into three groups: dilated, hypertrophic, and restrictive. Dilated cardiomyopathy can be the result of infections, diabetes, hypertension arrhythmia, obesity, valvular dysfunction, hemochromatosis, complications of late-stage pregnancy, excessive iron, alcohol misuse, toxins, cancer medications, illegal drug use. Regardless of the cause, dilated cardiomyopathies result in diffuse degeneration of the myocardial fibers. This is followed by a decrease in contractile effort.

Hypertrophic cardiomyopathies are thought to be caused from mutations in genes. The left ventricular wall hypertrophies, as does the interventricular septum, resulting in a small and elongated left ventricle and possible obstruction of the aortic valve.

Restrictive cardiomyopathy is a rare condition in which any infiltrative process of the heart causes fibrosis and thickening of the myocardium, resulting in stiffened ventricle walls.

The walls are usually normal in size or only slightly thickened. The stiff muscle that does not relax normally results in the chamber not filling properly with blood. Thus it is harder for the ventricles to fill with adequate blood. The rigidity of the walls does not permit the ventricular muscles to pump correctly, resulting in reduced amounts of blood being pumped from the ventricles. The inability of the heart to pump blood properly may lead to heart failure.

Diagnosis

The diagnosis includes a thorough patient history and a complete physical examination. Cardiomegaly at various stages is present, along with assorted cardiac murmurs. Chest radiographs confirm the presence of cardiomegaly, and ECG reveals rate and rhythm abnormalities. Echocardiography and cardiac catheterization may help identify the type of cardiomyopathy and the extent of the condition. A biopsy may be required.

Treatment

Treatment is determined by the type of cardiomyopathy. Therapy for dilated cardiomyopathies is aimed at appropriate control of CHF by means of the measures previously described. Antiarrhythmic agents, digoxin, and anticoagulant drugs are prescribed. Activities are limited, with some patients restricted to bed rest. Treatment of hypertrophic cardiomyopathies also is aimed at reducing the workload of the heart. Beta-blockers, such as propranolol reduce myocardial contractility, heart rate, and conductivity, thus preventing arrhythmias. CCBs are prescribed to help reduce blood pressure and relax the heart muscle. ACE inhibitors are used to help relax blood vessels and reduce the heart's workload. Treatment of restrictive cardiomyopathies also includes reducing the workload of the heart. The changes in the cardiac muscle caused by the infiltrates are irreversible, making the prognosis poor for these patients.

Prognosis

Medication improves the survival of these patients. Some conditions can be fatal, with the only hope for survival being offered by heart transplantation.

Prevention

In many cases, these conditions are idiopathic. Prevention is nonspecific, depending on the original underlying causative factor.

Patient Teaching

Focus on improving the patient's compliance with the medical treatment plan. Encourage patients to avoid alcohol and to limit salt intake. Provide information about support groups for people living with chronic disease.

Pericarditis

Description

Pericarditis is an acute or chronic inflammation of the pericardium (serosa), the sac enclosing and protecting the heart (Fig. 10.13).

ICD-10-CM Code	I31.9 *(Disease of pericardium, unspecified)*
	(I30.0-I32 = 12 codes of specificity)

Pericarditis is coded by type. Refer to the physician's diagnosis and then to the current edition of the ICD-10-CM coding manual to ensure the greatest specificity.

• **Fig. 10.13** Pericarditis. (From Damjanov I: *Pathology for the health professions*, ed 5, St. Louis, 2017, Elsevier.)

Symptoms and Signs

The space between the outer parietal layer of pericardium and the inner visceral layer of epicardium (heart wall) is normally filled with a small amount of thin, lubricating serous fluid. When blood or inflammatory exudate is released into the pericardial sac, or pericardial space, friction and irritation between the layers result in pericarditis. Associated manifestations include fever, malaise, chest pain that fluctuates with inspiration or heartbeat, dyspnea, and chills. The patient may feel anxious and report a "pounding heart." A detectable friction rub, or grating sound, in phase with the heartbeat can be heard on auscultation with a stethoscope. Tachycardia may be present. Pericarditis can occur in different forms. It can be a benign or isolated process or can be secondary to infection elsewhere in the body, so the clinical signs vary.

Patient Screening

Patients complaining of chest pain are advised to seek immediate medical attention.

Etiology

Pericarditis is idiopathic or a consequence of inflammation or infection elsewhere in the body. Causative agents include viruses such as COVID-19, bacteria (producing suppurative pericarditis), trauma, rheumatic fever, inflammatory disorders, and malignant neoplastic disease. The condition may occur secondary to MI and result from injury to the chest or heart. Acute inflammation of the pericardium can cause adhesions (scarring) to form between the pericardium and the heart, or it can cause a loss of elasticity, producing constrictive pericarditis. Conversely, chronic pericarditis can incite fibrous calcification of the visceral membrane, which comes in direct contact with the myocardium. A scarred and rigid pericardium interferes with the heart's ability to contract normally, with a subsequent drop in cardiac output.

Diagnosis

Blood studies may lead to the identification of a causative organism. They may also reveal elevated white blood cell (WBC) count, erythrocyte sedimentation rate (ESR), and cardiac enzyme levels. Changes are noted on ECG. Echocardiography may confirm the presence of pericardial fluid and reveal a thickened pericardium. In constrictive pericarditis, cardiac catheterization shows elevated pressures in the cardiac chambers.

Treatment

Treatment is directed at managing the underlying systemic disease and at reducing inflammation and pain. Therapy for infectious pericarditis requires treatment with antibiotic drugs and possibly surgical drainage or aspiration. Complete bed rest and the administration of analgesics, antipyretics, and nonsteroidal antiinflammatory drugs (NSAIDs) are prescribed. Corticosteroids may be prescribed.

Prognosis

Acute pericarditis usually resolves with complete recovery. Extensive adhesions or calcification resulting from chronic pericarditis may necessitate resection of the pericardium.

Prevention

Prompt treatment of infections is a preventive measure for pericarditis.

Patient Teaching

Encourage the patient to seek prompt treatment for infections. Emphasize the importance of completing the antibiotic regimen.

Myocarditis

Description

Myocarditis is inflammation of the muscular walls of the heart.

ICD-10-CM Code	I51.4 (Myocarditis, unspecified)

Symptoms and Signs

Myocarditis involves damage to the myocardium by pathogenic invasion or toxic insult. The condition may be acute or chronic, may involve a small part of the myocardium or be diffuse and can occur at any age. The patient may report palpitations, fatigue, and dyspnea. Physical examination may reveal fever, arrhythmia, and tenderness in the chest.

Patient Screening

Patients complaining of dyspnea and palpitations are advised to seek immediate medical attention.

Etiology

Myocarditis is frequently a viral, bacterial, fungal, or protozoal infection or a complication of other diseases, such as influenza, diphtheria, mumps, and, most significantly, rheumatic fever; it is occasionally idiopathic. It also may be associated with MI. Exposure to certain toxic agents through lithium use, chronic use of cocaine, chronic alcoholism, radiation, and chemical poisoning can cause inflammation of the myocardium. In addition, it may be a complication of a collagen disease.

Diagnosis

Diagnostic findings may include an elevated WBC count, increased ESR, elevated cardiac enzyme levels, ventricular enlargement noted on chest radiographs, and an abnormal ECG reading. Myocardial biopsy confirms the inflammation of cardiac muscle tissue and may identify the cause.

Treatment

When infection is the underlying cause, appropriate antiinfective agents are given. The patient is advised to rest and to reduce the heart's workload. Medications such as quinidine and procainamide, digoxin, and diuretics may be required to stabilize arrhythmia. Analgesics, antiinflammatory agents, ACE inhibitors, and oxygen are also prescribed.

Prognosis

The prognosis for complete recovery is favorable unless the condition is chronic and causes damage to the cardiac muscle.

Prevention

Depending on the underlying cause, prevention is not always possible. In some cases, early treatment of infections with a complete course of antimicrobial agents can prevent the onset of myocarditis.

Patient Teaching

Emphasize the importance of rest and close monitoring by the physician through follow-up appointments during the recovery process. Give the patient a list of the complications that should be reported to the physician, such as difficulty breathing, weakness, and accumulation of fluid in the extremities.

Endocarditis

Description

Endocarditis is inflammation of the lining and the valves of the heart (Fig. 10.14).

ICD-10-CM Code	I38 (Endocarditis, valve unspecified)

Endocarditis is coded by type and site. Refer to the physician's diagnosis and then to the current edition of the ICD-10-CM coding manual to ensure the greatest specificity.

Symptoms and Signs

The patient may have vague to pronounced symptoms of infection, including fever, chills, night sweats, weakness, anorexia, and fatigue.

The condition is characterized by vegetative growths on the cardiac valves that may be released into the bloodstream in the form of emboli. These emboli can lodge in vessels and cause symptoms of ischemia. The sites of ischemia may be

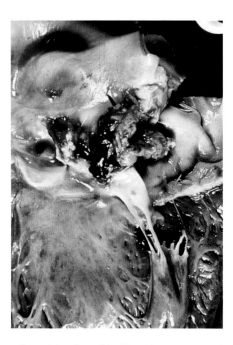

• **Fig. 10.14** Bacterial endocarditis. The valves are covered with extensive vegetations. (From Damjanov I: *Pathology for the health professions*, ed 5, St. Louis, 2017, Elsevier.)

the heart, lungs, kidneys, brain, or extremities. Dysfunction of the valves, which may not close effectively, disrupts or obstructs blood flow through the chambers of the heart; this dysfunction of the valves usually produces a cardiac murmur heard on auscultation. Serious obstruction or regurgitation of blood flow through the heart affects the pumping effectiveness of the heart and causes complications.

Patient Screening

A patient complaining of persistent fatigue, night sweats, and/or fever requires prompt assessment by a physician.

Etiology

Endocarditis is usually secondary to infection elsewhere in the body (Fig. 10.15), the result of preexisting heart disease, or the consequence of an abnormal immunologic reaction. Bacteremia, or the presence of infectious agents in the bloodstream, can lead to endocarditis. Common infecting organisms include *Staphylococcus aureus*, group A beta-hemolytic streptococci, and *Escherichia coli*. IV drug users are at high risk for fungal endocarditis. Patients with damaged cardiac valves as a result of rheumatic disease are more prone to endocarditis. Septic emboli from endocarditis can be carried by the arterial circulation and then embedded in major organs, resulting in infarcts and new places of bacterial infections.

Diagnosis

A complete blood count (CBC) may indicate leukocytosis and an elevated ESR may be present. Blood cultures may reveal the causative organism. Echocardiography shows valve involvement with vegetation or abscesses. ECG may indicate arrhythmia and conduction defects.

Treatment

Identification of the causative organism dictates the anti-infective therapy (usually IV antibiotics), which continues for several weeks. Other medications include antipyretics,

Respiratory tract infection

Dental infection

Urinary tract infection

Skin infection

• **Fig. 10.15** Causative factors in endocarditis.

anticoagulants, and drugs indicated to treat any complications. Bed rest is recommended during the acute phase. Damaged cardiac valves may need surgical repair or replacement.

Prognosis
Early diagnosis and treatment with antibiotics usually bring complete recovery. Untreated patients can have a poor prognosis.

Prevention
Antibiotic prophylaxis is recommended for dental procedures that involve manipulation of the gingival tissue or the periapical region of teeth or perforation of the oral mucosa. Current guidelines should always be checked for updates.

Patient Teaching
Instruct the patient to take the full course of antibiotics and to obtain plenty of rest.

Rheumatic Fever

Description
Rheumatic fever is a systemic inflammatory and autoimmune disease involving the joints and the cardiac tissue.

ICD-10-CM Code	I00 (Rheumatic fever without heart involvement)

Rheumatic fever is coded according to mention of heart involvement. Refer to the physician's diagnosis and then to the current edition of the ICD-10-CM coding manual to ensure the greatest specificity of pathology.

Symptoms and Signs
Rheumatic fever follows a sore throat caused by group A beta-hemolytic *Streptococcus*. The patient, usually a child, experiences a fever and polyarthritis, including joint pain, edema, redness, and limited range of motion. Joints frequently involved include the finger, knee, and ankle joints, with transient inflammation in these joints. In addition, the patient experiences carditis, cardiac murmurs, cardiomegaly, and even CHF. Other symptoms include weakness, malaise, anorexia, weight loss, a rash on the trunk, abdominal pain, and the development of small nodules on the tendon sheaths in the knees, knuckles, and elbows.

Patient Screening
Patients with vague symptoms of fatigue, joint pain, and fever after an episode of upper respiratory infection and sore throat require prompt assessment by a physician.

Etiology
After a sore throat caused by group A beta-hemolytic *Streptococcus*, antibodies against the bacteria develop and cross-react with normal tissue. This autoimmune disease causes the antibodies to attack the body's own cells and initiate an inflammatory reaction. The antibodies migrate to

the endocardium and the mitral and sometimes the aortic valves, where vegetations form on the tissue. Carditis usually follows joint pain and fever and can affect all layers of the heart (Fig. 10.16).

Diagnosis
A history of an upper respiratory tract infection in the preceding few weeks suggests rheumatic fever. No single diagnostic feature identifies the condition. The presence of carditis and polyarthritis adds to the evidence for the disease. The streptococcal antibody level, antistreptolysin O titer, is elevated in a series of tests. Increases in cardiac enzyme levels, WBC count, and ESR aid in the diagnosis.

Treatment
After the diagnosis of streptococcal pharyngitis (strep throat), which precedes rheumatic fever, treatment with a complete course of antibiotics prevents the onset of the fever

• **Fig. 10.16** Pathogenesis of rheumatic fever. After infection (with strep throat), an immune response elicited by the streptococci acts on the heart and several other organs, most notably the joints, skin, and central nervous system. In the heart, it causes endocarditis, myocarditis, and pericarditis. (From Damjanov I: *Pathology for the health professions*, ed 5, St. Louis, 2017, Elsevier.)

and subsequent rheumatic heart disease. The administration of antibiotics is necessary to eradicate the streptococcal infection. Antipyretics are given for fever, and antiinflammatory agents are given for relief of the arthritic symptoms. Bed rest is indicated, as is prophylactic administration of antibiotics.

The completion of the full course of antibiotic therapy is essential. Pediatric autoimmune neuropsychiatric disorders associated with streptococcal infections (PANDAS; an obsessive-compulsive disorder) can be the result of untreated or undertreated beta-hemolytic streptococcal infections.

Prognosis
The prognosis is good with treatment.

Prevention
Prevention is through prophylactic administration of antibiotics after strep throat has been diagnosed.

Patient Teaching
Emphasize the importance of completing the full course of antibiotic therapy. Reassure the parents of the child with rheumatic fever that recovery usually occurs after medical treatment.

Rheumatic Heart Disease

Description
Rheumatic heart disease refers to cardiac manifestations that occur after rheumatic fever.

> ICD-10-CM Code   I01.0 *(Acute rheumatic pericarditis)*
> (I01.0–I01.9 = 5 codes of specificity)
> *Rheumatic heart disease is coded according to type and tissue involvement. Refer to the physician's diagnosis and then to the current edition of the ICD-10-CM coding manual to ensure the greatest specificity of pathology.*

Symptoms and Signs
Acute endocarditis, which leads to chronic cardiac involvement, includes valvular damage because vegetations cause stenosis of the valves, particularly the mitral and aortic valves (Fig. 10.17). Rheumatic heart disease causes dyspnea, tachycardia, edema, a nonproductive cough, and cardiac murmurs.

Patient Screening
Patients with vague symptoms of fatigue, joint pain, and fever after an episode of upper respiratory infection and sore throat require prompt assessment by a physician.

Etiology
After rheumatic fever, the vegetations may become enlarged or the valves may become scarred, causing stenosis of the openings. The frequency of rheumatic heart disease is decreasing as a result of prompt diagnosis and aggressive antibiotic treatment of streptococcal pharyngitis (strep throat). Patients who experienced rheumatic fever and rheumatic heart disease before the advent of penicillin may have damaged cardiac valves (Fig. 10.18).

Diagnosis
The diagnosis is based on a history of rheumatic fever and cardiac murmurs. Echocardiography shows vegetations or resulting damage to the valves.

Treatment
Treatment is aimed at reducing stenosis of the valves and preventing further damage. Surgery to relieve stenosis or to replace the valve may be necessary. Good dental hygiene is important to prevent gingival infection, which would cause further bloodborne infection and damage the valves. Prophylactic antibiotics are given to the patient before any dental procedures.

Prognosis
The prognosis varies, depending on the extent of damage to the valves. Recurrences are likely. Valve replacement may result in a better outlook.

Prevention
The prevention is prophylactic administration of antibiotics for a diagnosed episode of strep throat.

Patient Teaching
Emphasize the importance of completing the full course of antibiotic therapy. PANDAS (an obsessive-compulsive disorder) can be the result of untreated or undertreated beta-hemolytic streptococcal infections.

Encourage the parents of a child with a sore throat to seek medical attention, including beta-hemolytic strep screening. Give information on incision care to patients who have had valve replacement surgery. Encourage the patient to comply with prescribed rehabilitation therapy and activity level.

Valvular Heart Disease

Valvular heart disease is an acquired or congenital disorder that can involve any of the four valves of the heart. This condition can occur in the form of either insufficiency or stenosis. Insufficiency, the failure of the valves to close completely, allows blood to be forced back into the previous chamber as the heart contracts. This exerts added pressure on that chamber and increases the heart's workload. Stenosis, the hardening of the cusps of the valves that prevents complete opening of the valves, impedes the blood flow into the next chamber (Fig. 10.19). The mitral valve is involved most often. The diagnosis of valvular heart disease requires ECG, chest radiographic studies, echocardiography, and cardiac catheterization. Treatment entails the administration of digitalis or quinidine for arrhythmias and antibiotic prophylaxis.

• **Fig. 10.17** (A) Cardiac valves. (B) Artificial valve. (B, From Damjanov I: *Pathology for the health professions*, ed 5, St. Louis, 2017, Elsevier.)

• **Fig. 10.18** Chronic rheumatic endocarditis of the aortic valve. The valves are deformed, and the orifice is stenosed. (From Damjanov I, Linder J: *Pathology: a color atlas*, St. Louis, 1999, Mosby/Elsevier.)

Mitral Stenosis

Description

Mitral stenosis is a hardening of the cusps of the mitral valve that prevents complete and normal opening of the valve for the passage of blood from the left atrium into the left ventricle.

ICD-10-CM Code   I05.0 *(Rheumatic mitral stenosis)*

Symptoms and Signs

The mitral, or bicuspid, valve lies between the left atrium and the left ventricle. Mitral stenosis causes patients to have exertional dyspnea and fatigue. In addition, they may experience cough and palpitations, followed by hemoptysis. In severe cases, patients may become cyanotic.

NORMAL VALVE

Blood flows freely forward   No backflow of blood

STENOSIS

Less blood flows through   No backflow of blood
narrowed opening

INCOMPETENT VALVE

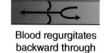

Blood flows freely forward   Blood regurgitates
backward through
"leaky" valve

EFFECT OF AORTIC STENOSIS

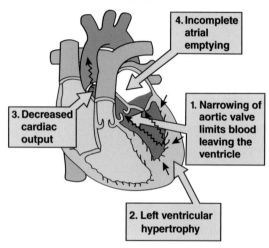

4. Incomplete atrial emptying

3. Decreased cardiac output

1. Narrowing of aortic valve limits blood leaving the ventricle

2. Left ventricular hypertrophy

• **Fig. 10.19** Effects of heart valve defects. (From Gould B: *Pathophysiology for the health professions*, ed 3, Philadelphia, 2006, Saunders/Elsevier.)

Patient Screening

Patients reporting exertional dyspnea and fatigue that may be accompanied by palpitations require prompt assessment by a physician.

Etiology

Rheumatic heart disease is the cause of most cases of mitral stenosis. Group A beta-hemolytic *Streptococcus* stimulates antibody production, and the antibodies often attack the body tissues in an autoimmune response.

Diagnosis

The onset of symptoms of mitral stenosis may be insidious or acute. A cardiac murmur, including a diastolic murmur, is heard. Echocardiography confirms diagnostic suspicions.

Treatment

Limitation of sodium intake, along with the administration of diuretics, helps reduce the workload on the heart. Anticoagulants prevent the formation of thrombi. If atrial fibrillation results from stenosis, digoxin is often given to slow the rapid heart rate. Surgical intervention in the form of

a commissurotomy may be needed to free up the valve and allow adequate blood flow; this can also be done nonsurgically with balloon valvuloplasty. Valve replacement is a final option.

Prognosis

The prognosis improves with corrective intervention.

Prevention

Prevention of rheumatic fever and subsequent rheumatic heart disease is a major factor in preventing mitral stenosis.

Patient Teaching

When possible, use visual aids to demonstrate the effect that valvular disease has on blood circulation through the heart. Explain the medical regimen and how medications can improve the condition. Explain the procedure for surgical reconstruction of the valve, if appropriate.

Mitral Insufficiency

Description

In mitral valve insufficiency, the mitral valve fails to close completely and allows blood from the left ventricle to flow back into the left atrium.

ICD-10-CM Code	I05.1 *(Rheumatic mitral insufficiency)* I05.2 *(Rheumatic mitral stenosis with insufficiency)* (I05.0–I05.9 = 5 codes of specificity)

Symptoms and Signs

The patient with mitral insufficiency experiences dyspnea, shortness of breath and fatigue. A heart murmur can be heard as blood leaks back into the left atrium as a result of the valve's failure to close completely. Fluid may accumulate in the lungs and swelling of the lower extremities may occur.

Patient Screening

Patients with mitral insufficiency often call reporting that they are simply very tired and having some difficulty breathing. Anyone complaining of difficulty breathing requires prompt assessment by a physician. For those complaining of generalized fatigue, the next available appointment should be scheduled.

Etiology

The valve may fail to close because of scar tissue resulting from inflammation and vegetations (a consequence of endocarditis), rheumatic fever, mitral valve prolapse (MVP), CAD, or MI or from cardiac dilation.

Diagnosis

The diagnosis is based on a thorough patient history, especially a history of sore throat or rheumatic fever. Physical examination reveals a murmur, and echocardiography discloses the insufficiency. The cardiac status can be assessed with ECG, chest radiography, cardiac MRI, and cardiac catheterization.

Treatment

Treatment includes bed rest, oxygen therapy, and administration of antibiotics for any infectious process. When severe, surgical repair or replacement of the valve may be necessary.

Prognosis

The prognosis generally is good, but the condition can lead to CHF.

Prevention

Preventing rheumatic fever and the resulting scarring of the mitral valve helps prevent mitral insufficiency.

Patient Teaching

When possible, use visual aids to demonstrate the effect that valvular disease has on blood circulation through the heart. Explain the medical regimen and how medications can improve the condition. Explain the procedure for surgical reconstruction of the valve, if appropriate.

Mitral Valve Prolapse

Description

MVP, usually a benign condition, occurs when one or more of the cusps of the mitral valve protrude back into the left atrium during ventricular contraction.

ICD-10-CM Code	I34.0 *(Nonrheumatic mitral [valve] insufficiency)*
	I34.8 *(Other nonrheumatic mitral valve disorders)*
	(I34.0–I34.9 = 5 codes of specificity)

Symptoms and Signs

MVP, usually a benign condition, occurs when the valve cusps do not close completely (see Fig. 10.17B). Most patients are asymptomatic, and the condition is usually discovered during a routine examination. The few patients who experience symptoms report chest pain, dyspnea, dizziness, fatigue, racing heartbeat and syncope. These patients may experience severe anxiety. This fairly common condition can affect all age groups.

Patient Screening

Most individuals with MVP are unaware of any problem. The condition is usually diagnosed incidentally during physical examination. Those who report chest pain require prompt assessment by a physician.

Etiology

Damaged chordae tendineae may be the cause of the valve's inability to close properly. MVP can be inherited and associated with other conditions.

Diagnosis

The typical click-murmur syndrome is heard on auscultation of the heart. Echocardiography confirms the failure of

the valve to close. The premature ventricular contractions (PVCs) detected on ECG are not considered harmful and are not an indication of insult to the myocardium.

Treatment

Treatment generally is not required for asymptomatic patients. Those who experience discomfort and anxiety often are treated with beta-blockers, and they are advised to avoid caffeine and smoking.

Prognosis

The prognosis is good.

Prevention

No prevention is known for this condition.

Patient Teaching

Reassure patients that this is usually a benign condition. Emphasize the importance of avoiding caffeine and when to call the provider if symptoms begin.

Arrhythmias

Description

Cardiac arrhythmias are any deviation from the normal heartbeat, that is, the normal sinus rhythm. They are often called *irregular heartbeats*.

ICD-10-CM Code	I47.1 *(Supraventricular tachycardia)*
	(I47.1–I47.9 = 3 codes of specificity)

Arrhythmias or dysrhythmias are coded by type and point of origin. Refer to the physician's diagnosis and then to the current edition of the ICD-10-CM coding manual to ensure the greatest specificity.

Symptoms and Signs

Arrhythmias result when there is interference with the conduction system of the heart, resulting in an abnormality of the heartbeat. Symptoms include palpitations, rapid heartbeat (tachycardia), skipped heartbeats, slow heart rate (bradycardia), syncope, and fatigue.

Patient Screening

Patients who report feeling abnormal heartbeats, usually as missed beats, palpitation, or rapid heartbeats, require prompt assessment by a physician.

Etiology

Arrhythmias can arise from disturbances in the normal conduction system of the heart, including the pacemaker (the sinoatrial [SA] node), the atrioventricular (AV) node, the bundle branches, and the Purkinje fibers (Fig. 10.20). Ischemia and drugs cause many arrhythmias. Failure of the SA node may be responsible. Table 10.1 lists the causes of arrhythmias. Heart block occurs when the impulses from the SA node become slow or irregular at or below the AV node.

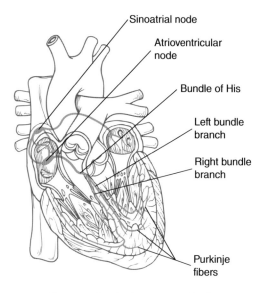

- **Fig. 10.20** Conduction system of the heart.

Labels: Sinoatrial node; Atrioventricular node; Bundle of His; Left bundle branch; Right bundle branch; Purkinje fibers.

Diagnosis

The diagnosis is made with the use of 12-lead ECG. Various arrhythmias are evident to the physician. Echocardiography may help confirm a particular arrhythmia. The patient may wear a Holter monitor (ambulatory ECG) to capture any arrhythmic event.

Treatment

Treatment depends on the cause (see Table 10.1). Drug-induced arrhythmias usually resolve with cessation of the drug administration. Anticoagulants, especially warfarin (Coumadin), are given to prevent thromboembolism. Ischemia should respond to oxygen administration and increased blood flow to the tissue. If the arrhythmia is unstable, cardioversion may be performed by electric shock to the heart to restore normal heart rhythm. This mild shock interrupts the arrhythmia pattern by resetting the heart's rhythm and may enable the patient's heart to be

TABLE 10.1 Arrhythmias

Types	Symptoms and Signs	Etiology	Diagnosis	Treatment
Normal sinus rhythm	Rate of 60–100 bpm, regular, P wave uniform	Impulse originates in SA node, conduction normal	Normal	None indicated
Sinus tachycardia	Rate >100 bpm, regular, P wave uniform	Rapid impulse originates in SA node, conduction normal	Rapid rate	Beta-blockers, CCBs; may be candidate for ICD
Sinus bradycardia	Rate <60 bpm, regular, P wave uniform	Slow impulse originates in SA node, conduction normal	Slow rate	Atropine
Premature atrial contraction	Rate depends on underlying rhythm, usually normal P wave, different morphology from other P waves	Irritable atrium, single ectopic beat that arises prematurely, conduction through ventricle normal	Irregular heartbeat, diagnosis with ECG	Treatment usually unnecessary; if needed, antiarrhythmic drugs
Atrial tachycardia	Rate of 150–250 bpm, rhythm normal, sudden onset	Irritable atrium, firing at rapid rates, normal conduction	Rapid rate with atrial and ventricular rates identical, diagnosis with ECG	Reflex vagal stimulation, CCBs (verapamil), cardioversion; may be candidate for ICD or ablation
Atrial fibrillation	Atrial rate > 350 bpm, ventricular rate < 100 bpm (controlled) or > 100 bpm (rapid ventricular response)	Atrial ectopic foci discharging at too rapid and chaotic a rate for muscles to respond and contract, resulting in quivering of atrium; AV node blocks some impulses and ventricle responds irregularly	ECG shows no P waves, grossly irregular ventricular rate	IV verapamil; if unsuccessful, procainamide; if unsuccessful, cardioversion; may be candidate for ICD or ablation
First-degree heart block	Rate depends on rate of underlying rhythm, P-R interval > 0.20 second	Delay at AV node, impulse eventually conducted	ECG shows P-R interval > 0.20 second	Atropine; if unsuccessful, artificial pacemaker insertion

TABLE 10.1   Arrhythmias—cont'd

Types	Symptoms and Signs	Etiology	Diagnosis	Treatment
Second-degree heart block, Wenckebach heart block	Intermittent block with progressively longer delay in conduction until one beat is blocked; atrial rate normal, ventricular rate slower than normal, rhythm irregular	SA node initiates impulse, conduction through AV node is blocked intermittently	ECG shows normal P waves, some P waves not followed by QRS complex; P-R interval progressively longer, followed by block of impulse	Mild forms, no treatment; severe, insertion of artificial pacemaker
Classic second-degree heart block	Ventricular rate slow (½, ½, or ¼ of atrial rate)—rhythm, regular; P waves normal, QRS complex dropped every second, third, or fourth beat	SA node initiates impulse, conduction through AV node is blocked	ECG shows P waves present, QRS complex blocked every second, third, or fourth impulse	Artificial pacemaker is inserted
Third-degree heart block	Atrial rate normal, ventricular rate 20–40 or 40–60 bpm; no relationship between P wave and QRS complex	SA node initiates impulse, which is completely blocked from conduction, causing atria and ventricles to beat independently	ECG shows P waves and QRS complexes with no relationship to each other, rhythms are regular but independent of each other	Insertion of artificial pacemaker is necessary
Premature ventricular contraction (single focus)	Single ectopic beat, arising from ventricle, followed by compensatory pause	Ectopic beat originates in irritable ventricle	ECG shows a wide, bizarre QRS complex > 0.12 second usually followed by a compensatory pause	Usually no treatment if <6/min and single focus; may be candidate for ICD or ablation
• Multifocal arrhythmia • Coupling, two in a row • Bigeminy, every other beat • Trigeminy, every third beat • Quadrigeminy, every fourth beat	Rate dependent on underlying rhythm; rhythm regular or irregular; P wave absent before ectopic beat	Same as single focus (above)	Same as single focus (above)	Same as single focus (above); may be candidate for ICD or ablation
Ventricular tachycardia	Rate of 150–250 bpm, rhythm usually regular; focus of pacemaker normally single, patient experiences palpitations, dyspnea, and anxiety followed by chest pain	Four or more consecutive PVCs at a rapid rate caused by advanced irritability of myocardium, indicating ventricular command of heart rate	ECG shows runs of four or more PVCs, P wave buried in QRS complex	Often forerunner of ventricular fibrillation; immediate intervention necessary— IV lidocaine; if unsuccessful, follow by cardioversion; procainamide or bretylium may be used; this is a candidate for ICD or ablation
Ventricular fibrillation (a lethal arrhythmia)	Patient loses consciousness immediately after onset; no peripheral pulses palpable, no heart sounds, no blood pressure	Ventricular fibers twitch rather than contract, reason unknown	Pulseless, unconscious patient; ECG shows rapid, repetitive, chaotic waves originating in ventricle	Recognize and terminate rhythm; precordial shock (defibrillation); survivors become candidates for ICD or ablation

AV, Atrioventricular; *bpm*, beats per minute; *CCB*, calcium channel blocker; *ECG*, electrocardiography; *ICD*, implantable cardioverter-defibrillator; *IV*, intravenous; *PVCs*, premature ventricular contractions; *SA*, sinoatrial.

normal enough to allow discontinuation of antiarrhythmic medications. Occasionally the heart rhythm does not stabilize, and the arrhythmia can be fatal. Some arrhythmias can be treated with cardiac ablation (radiofrequency ablation) techniques with catheters. Bradycardic heart rates may be treated by the insertion of a pacemaker to maintain a rate at or greater than 60 beats per minute. Implantable cardioverter-defibrillators (ICDs) may be used for those with tachycardic heart rates or ventricular arrhythmias. Refer to Table 10.1 for pacemaker application, ICD application, and ablation procedures. Refer to the Enrichment box about Pacemakers and Implantable Cardioverter-Defibrillators and the Enrichment box about Cardiac Ablation procedures for additional information. Common terms for ablation include *cardiac catheter ablation, radiofrequency ablation, cardiac ablation,* or simply *ablation.*

Prognosis
The prognosis varies, depending on the type and cause of the arrhythmia.

Prevention
Preventing drug-induced arrhythmias requires stopping the use of the offending drug substances. Avoiding the identified causative activities helps prevent certain arrhythmias. There is no prevention for certain types of arrhythmias.

Patient Teaching
Give patients information about the causes of arrhythmias. Emphasize the importance of complying with prescribed drug therapy. Encourage patients to comply with the scheduled appointments. Emphasize the symptoms that require prompt medical intervention.

 ENRICHMENT

Pacemakers and Implantable Cardioverter-Defibrillators

Implantable electronic cardiac assist devices have extended the lives of those with cardiac arrhythmias. They are surgically implanted for the regulation of heart rate and for correcting arrhythmias. In an emergent situation, a temporary pacemaker may be used until a permanent pacemaker or an implantable cardioverter-defibrillator (ICD) can be implanted.

Assisting the heart's natural pacemaker, the sinoatrial (SA) node, and, when necessary, the rest of the impulse conduction system, artificial pacemakers can be external (a temporary intervention) or implanted. These devices are used to treat arrhythmias, heart block, and sick sinus syndrome. ICDs are implanted when ventricular tachycardia has the potential to become irregular and unstable, progressing to ventricular fibrillation and even to cardiac arrest.

The artificial pacemaker helps relieve symptoms of heart rhythm bradycardic disturbances. As the normal heart rate and rhythm are restored, circulation of blood returns to normal, and symptoms of dizziness, shortness of breath, and fatigue typical of bradycardia usually abate. The pacemaker also provides treatment for sick sinus syndrome.

ICDs are used to treat tachyarrhythmias, rapid heartbeats that usually result from heart diseases, including coronary artery disease (CAD), myocardial infarction (MI), and cardiomyopathy. The rapid rates originating in the ventricle result in the chambers of the heart not filling adequately, resulting in less blood reaching the brain; pounding heart; and faintness or dizziness. When this rhythm becomes irregular and unstable, the ventricle beats in a disorganized manner, resulting in no blood being pumped out of the heart. This is very rapidly followed by cardiac arrest. The ICD contains an internal defibrillator that will automatically pace or shock the heart out of the dangerous or lethal rhythm. An additional feature of the ICD is that it also is responsive to slow heart rates and at the interpretation of bradycardia, the ICD will act as a pacemaker.

Pacemakers and ICDs are small electronic battery-powered units that are implanted usually just under the skin of either side of the chest wall. The lead that transmits impulses from the pacemaker or ICD to the wall of the heart is threaded through the subclavian vein, the superior vena cava, into the right atrium of the heart, where it is attached to the wall of the right atrium. When a block of impulses exists, as in a heart block, a dual-chamber pacemaker with two lead wires is implanted. The second lead is threaded along with the first into the right atrium, then into the right ventricle,

where it is attached to the wall of that chamber. The single-chamber pacemaker sends impulses to initiate the heartbeat in the atrium. When there is a block, either at or below the atrioventricular (AV) node, the second lead will transmit impulses to stimulate the contraction of the right ventricle. Most pacemakers have a rate-responsive feature to adjust the rate of pacing according to the activity of the individual's body. Sensors in the unit monitor changes in the body and adjust the rate according to the body's need for adequate perfusion. The leads for the ICD run through the right chambers of the heart and end in the apex of the right ventricle.

Pacemakers and ICDs contain small microprocessors, batteries, and electronic circuitry. Both store the history of the heart's and the device's activities, which are retrieved at the pacemaker clinic. This information is reviewed by the physician, and any changes may be made to the settings of the devices. Regular pacemaker checks are conducted according to an established schedule. A programming head is placed over the pacemaker. Electrocardiography (ECG) leads remain on the arms and chest, allowing the clinician to view information collected and stored in the recording device in the pacemaker. The computers in the office make a recording of the activity since the last check. Current pacemaker settings are viewed and reset if required. The condition of the battery is checked, including predicted end-of-service date or estimated battery life. Precautions are necessary for patients with implanted pacemakers and ICDs. Technology has emerged with MRI-compatible pacemakers and lead systems. Individuals with the devices should avoid magnetic or electronic security scanning and identify themselves (using a pacemaker or ICD identification card) as individuals with implantable pacemakers and request a "patdown" or hand-held screening. Cellular phones and smart watches may present a problem when held within 6 inches of the unit. Individuals with implantable cardiac assist devices should always keep the phone on the ear on the opposite side of the implant site. Other precautions include avoiding arc welding with the cables draped over the neck, not working with a demagnetizer, and not using a gas-powered chainsaw. All of these activities may create an electromagnetic field that can disturb the settings of the unit.

It is important that the patient and the family receive instructions on pacemaker or ICD restrictions. These devices have allowed many with cardiac arrhythmias to live normal lives.

ⓘ *ALERT!*

Caution During Procedures That Use Electrical Activity

Individuals with pacemakers and/or implantable cardioverter-defibrillators (ICDs) should inform all healthcare providers that they have these devices. Any procedure that uses electrical activity may cause the devices to fail. Pacemakers interpret the electrical activity as the heart beats and will stop pacing. The impact of the electrical activity depends on its duration and its proximity to the pacemaker. The defibrillator will interpret the electrical activity as ventricular fibrillation and shock the individual.

Any procedure involving electrical activity should be performed in an outpatient setting at a hospital-type setting, where a special magnet can be placed over the device. The magnet prevents the electrical activity from reaching the device.

◆ ENRICHMENT

Cardiac Ablation

Patients with abnormal heart rhythms may be candidates for cardiac ablation. Drug therapy is usually attempted to correct the arrhythmia. When there is little or no response, cardiac ablation may be attempted.

Cardiac ablation is a nonsurgical procedure in which catheters are inserted into the chambers of the heart to administer energy to destroy the small amount of tissue that causes electrical rhythm disturbances in the cardiac conduction system.

The procedure is performed by an electrophysiologist after he or she completes "mapping" of the heart's electrical system. The electrophysiologist watches the procedure with the aid of fluoroscopy, inserting an electrode catheter usually through a vein (sometimes an artery) and threading it into the heart chambers. The electrode catheters sense the electrical activity in various areas of the heart and measure the speed of the impulses. Should it be necessary during the procedure, the electrodes can pace the heart (cause it to beat). This study, using several electrode catheters, helps isolate where the aberrant pathway is located.

The ablating catheter is introduced into the heart close to the abnormal electrical pathway. Radiofrequency energy is passed through the catheter, heating the tip. The area of the heart containing the abnormal pathway is destroyed. A scar that cannot conduct the electrical impulse results and the abnormal pathway can no longer cause the arrhythmia.

Ablation is used to treat both atrial and ventricular tachycardias. The idea is to obliterate the focus that is firing too rapidly and prevent the impulse from spreading through the heart. Other common terms for this procedure are *cardiac catheter ablation, radiofrequency ablation, cardiac ablation,* or simply *ablation.*

Shock

Description

Shock is the collapse of the cardiovascular system, including vasodilation and fluid shift, accompanied by inefficient cardiac output.

ICD-10-CM Code	R57.9 *(Shock, unspecified)*
	R57.0 *(Cardiogenic shock)*
	R57.1 *(Hypovolemic shock)*
	R57.8 *(Other shock)*

Refer to the physician's diagnosis and then to the current edition of the ICD-10-CM coding manual to ensure the greatest specificity.

Symptoms and Signs

Shock causes inadequate perfusion of organs and tissues. The patient has pale, cold, and clammy skin; rapid, weak, and thready pulse; rapid breathing; and altered level of consciousness. Blood pressure drops, and the patient may be anxious, irritable, or restless and often express a feeling of impending doom. The patient may experience dizziness, extreme thirst, and profuse sweating. In late stages, the pupils dilate, the eyes become dull and lusterless, and the patient experiences shaking and trembling.

Patient Screening

Shock is a life-threatening condition requiring the patient's immediate entry into the emergency medical system. The caller should be assisted in contacting the EMS.

Etiology

This life-threatening emergency can be caused by anaphylaxis, hemorrhage, sepsis, respiratory distress, heart failure, neurologic failure, emotional catastrophe, or severe metabolic insult. Regardless of the cause, the amount of blood that is effectively circulating in the body is reduced. The final effect is that vital organs (heart, brain, lungs, and kidneys) do not receive sufficient oxygen and nutrients to sustain life. Rapid blood loss or significant fluid loss with subsequent hypovolemia precipitates shock. Failure of the heart to pump adequately is another cause of shock. Vascular collapse with subsequent massive dilation or constriction of the vessels can cause blood to pool away from vital areas. Insufficient oxygen supply to the circulating system can generate shock (Fig. 10.21).

Diagnosis

The clinical picture, along with a history of a precipitating event, leads to the diagnosis of shock resulting from inadequate cellular perfusion. An altered level of consciousness and respiratory distress suggest shock. Immediate intervention is needed to halt the progression of the condition.

Treatment

Because of the severity and rapid progression of the condition, aggressive intervention is undertaken at the earliest possible opportunity. The CABs (compressions, airway, and breathing) of emergency care require maintaining an open airway and establishing ventilation to supply vital organs

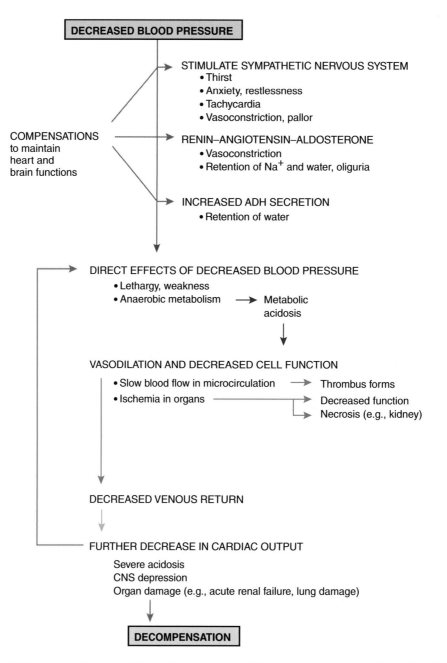

• **Fig. 10.21** Progress of shock. *ADH*, Antidiuretic hormone; *CNS*, central nervous system. (From Gould B: *Pathophysiology for the health professions*, ed 3, Philadelphia, 2006, Saunders/Elsevier.)

with oxygen. Any visible bleeding is controlled, and surgical intervention may be needed to halt internal bleeding. The patient should be placed in the supine position, with feet and legs elevated, and should be kept warm but not overheated. If the patient is not in an inpatient facility, contacting the EMS for immediate transport to an emergency facility is indicated. Vital signs are monitored, and volume replacement is instituted with IV fluids. Supplemental oxygen is administered, when available.

Prognosis
Immediate assessment and intervention improve the prognosis for complete or near-complete recovery. When the condition is not addressed promptly, shock may become

unstoppable, and the consequences may be irreversible, resulting in a fatal outcome.

Prevention
Most occurrences of shock are not preventable. Immediate intervention helps prevent rapid progression of the condition to a fatal outcome.

Patient Teaching
Give patients and their family members information about causes and emergency intervention measures for patients with known allergic reactions. Encourage community education in first aid and CPR to help reduce the damaging outcomes of shock.

Cardiogenic Shock

Description

Cardiogenic shock is the inadequate output of blood by the heart.

ICD-10-CM Code   R57.0 *(Cardiogenic shock)*

Symptoms and Signs

In cardiogenic shock (shock resulting from inadequate cardiac output), the myocardium fails to pump effectively. The patient exhibits the previously mentioned symptoms and signs of shock. The event usually is preceded by MI or severe heart failure, certain arrhythmias, or acute valve failure.

Patient Screening

These patients have a life-threatening condition. They should be entered promptly into the emergency medical system.

Etiology

Any insult that disturbs the heart's ability to pump blood can cause cardiogenic shock. MI, severe heart failure, certain arrhythmias, or valve failure can lead to cardiogenic shock (Fig. 10.22).

Diagnosis

The clinical picture and a history of a major cardiac insult lead to the suspicion of cardiogenic shock. ECG is another

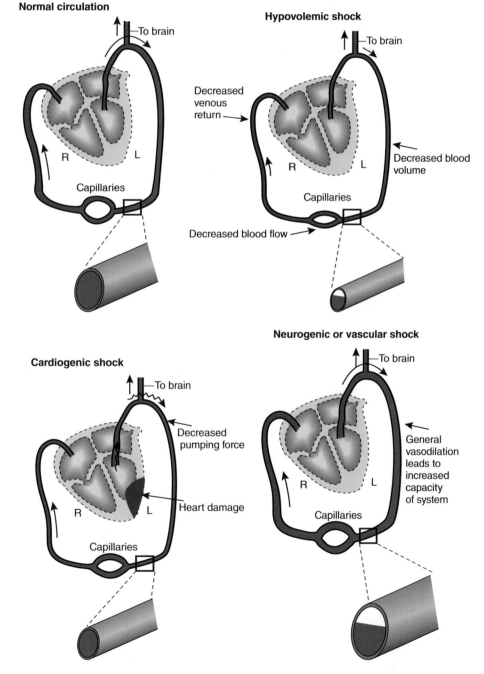

• **Fig. 10.22** Causes of shock. (From Gould B: *Pathophysiology for the health professions*, ed 3, Philadelphia, 2006, Saunders/Elsevier.)

diagnostic tool, as are chest radiographic studies. A hypotensive state that continues to worsen also indicates the diagnosis.

Treatment

Treatment consists of general measures for shock, along with the administration of medications that increase the efficiency of the myocardium and/or affect the blood vessels. Blood supply to vital organs must be improved, and the oxygen demands of myocardial tissue must be reduced. Blood volume assessment determines whether drugs are given to dilate or constrict cardiac vessels. Sometimes an intraaortic balloon pump may be inserted.

Prognosis

The prognosis varies but, in many cases, is poor.

Prevention

Prevention, in most cases, is unlikely. An important factor in preventing a fatal outcome is immediate assessment and intervention when symptoms and signs are identified.

Patient Teaching

Emphasize the importance of immediate emergency intervention when symptoms are detected. Promote community awareness of the benefits of first aid and CPR training in increasing survival rates in the community.

Cardiac Tamponade

Description

Cardiac tamponade is the compression of the heart muscle and restriction of heart movement caused by blood or fluid trapped in the pericardial sac. It may be called *cardiac compression.*

ICD-10-CM Code	I31.4 *(Cardiac tamponade)*

Symptoms and Signs

Cardiac tamponade occurs when a coronary, epicardial, or pericardial vessel breaks and blood is trapped in the pericardial sac. In addition, the myocardium may rupture, also sending blood into the pericardial sac. The blood constricts the heart, thus restricting heart movement, and less blood can enter the heart chambers per beat. The patient with cardiac tamponade experiences sudden severe dyspnea and rapidly falling blood pressure. The pulse becomes weak, thready, and rapid. The patient is in shock and becomes cyanotic above the nipple line. The level of consciousness falls.

Patient Screening

These patients have a life-threatening condition and should be entered promptly into the emergency medical system.

Etiology

Cardiac tamponade may result from an insult to the integrity of a vessel in the pericardium, allowing blood to fill the pericardial space. The pressure of the blood causes the heart to beat inappropriately, leading to cardiac arrest. Cardiac tamponade may also occur in patients with certain cancers, chronic kidney failure, and other medical conditions, such as hypothyroidism or lupus.

Diagnosis

The diagnosis is based on the clinical picture and a history of a traumatic event. Heart sounds become muffled or distant, but breath sounds remain normal.

Treatment

Treatment consists of periocardiocentesis (inserting a needle into the pericardial space and withdrawing the offending blood). Surgery usually is indicated to repair the leak.

Prognosis

The prognosis varies, depending on the causative factor, the success of the intervention, and the health status of the patient. Surgical repair usually has a positive outcome.

Prevention

Because of the etiology of this condition, prevention usually is not possible.

Patient Teaching

Give the patient information about the mechanism and results of the insult. Explain care of the incision and emphasize the importance of following postoperative orders.

Vascular Conditions

The vascular system, a closed transport system composed of arteries, arterioles, capillaries, venules, and veins, is responsible for supplying tissues with blood containing oxygen and nutrients. This system also conveys waste products and carbon dioxide to the appropriate organs for excretion. Arteries carry blood away from the heart (Fig. 10.23A), veins transport blood back to the heart (see Fig. 10.23B), and capillaries are the point of exchange at the cellular level (see Fig. 10.23C).

Blood vessel walls, other than one-cell-walled capillaries, are composed of three layers: the tunica intima, the tunica media, and the tunica externa (Fig. 10.24). The lining of the vessel lumen, the tunica intima, is composed of smooth, thin endothelium, allowing minimal friction with the flowing blood. The middle portion, the tunica media, is composed of smooth muscle and elastic tissue that are under the control of the sympathetic nervous system. This innervation allows constriction or dilation of the vessel walls and changes in blood pressure. Connective tissue composes the outermost layer, the tunica externa, creating support and protection for the vessels.

Arterial walls are much thicker than venous walls. The tunica media is heavier in arteries to compensate for the stronger blood pressure under which the arteries must function. Veins, with their lower blood pressure, contain valves

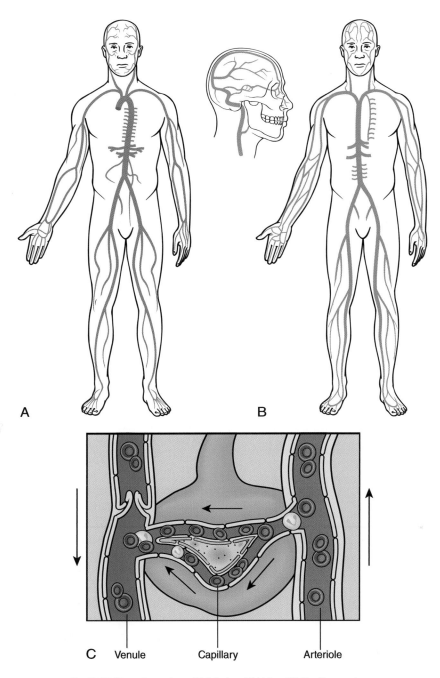

• **Fig. 10.23** Vascular system. (A) Arteries. (B) Veins. (C) Capillary exchange.

to prevent backflow and to assist in the return of blood to the heart (Fig. 10.25).

Vascular conditions include emboli, arteriosclerosis, atherosclerosis, aneurysms, phlebitis, thrombophlebitis, varicose veins, thromboangiitis obliterans (Buerger disease), and Raynaud disease.

Emboli

Description
Emboli are clots of aggregated material (usually blood). They can lodge in a blood vessel and inhibit the blood flow.

ICD-10-CM Code	I74.0 *(Embolism and thrombosis of abdominal aorta)*

(I74.0–I75.89 = 20 codes of specificity)

Emboli are coded according to location of involvement in the arterial system. Refer to the physician's diagnosis for the location of arterial involvement and then to the current edition of the ICD-10-CM coding manual to ensure the greatest specificity.

Symptoms and Signs
Symptoms of emboli depend on the location of the occluded vessel and the magnitude of the area of tissue served by the vessel. The initial symptom is severe pain in the area of the embolus. Emboli lodging in arteries of the extremities can cause the area to become pale, numb, and cold to the touch.

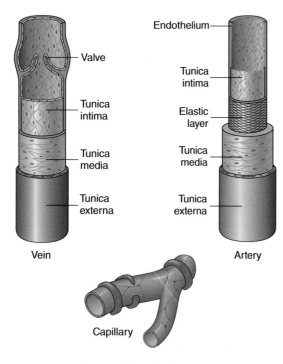

• **Fig. 10.24** Vessel wall structure.

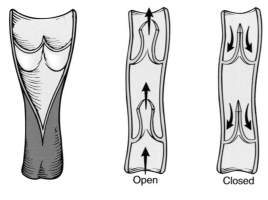

• **Fig. 10.25** Venous valves.

In addition, arterial pulses are absent below the occlusion if it is arterial. When a large artery is involved, the patient also experiences nausea, vomiting, fainting, and eventually shock.

Patient Screening

A patient reporting severe pain in an extremity that is accompanied by paleness, numbness, and coolness in the area requires prompt assessment by a physician. In addition, those experiencing nausea, vomiting, fainting, and shock are in an emergency state and require immediate entry into the emergency medical system.

Etiology

Emboli are usually blood clots, but the offending embolus may also be composed of air bubbles, fat globules, bacterial clumps, or pieces of tissue, including the placenta. The most common offender is a venous thrombus, a blood clot

that has formed in the deep veins of the legs as a result of venous stasis (Figs. 10.26, 10.27, and 10.28). A portion of the thrombus breaks loose from the clot and travels through the venous system until it becomes lodged in a vessel that is too narrow to allow passage, often in the lungs. Cardiac arrhythmias also can cause thrombi to form in the heart. Those that travel from the left ventricle can enter the coronary arteries, resulting in MI, or can enter the carotid and cerebral arteries, compromising blood supply and resulting in CVAs.

Diagnosis

The clinical picture and a history of bed rest, physical inactivity, heart failure, arrhythmias, and any condition that has put pressure on or decreased flow in the veins of the legs or pelvis alert the physician to the possibility of an embolus. Pain in the calf of the leg in a patient who has any of the aforementioned predispositions is another clue.

Treatment

Treatment depends on the area of involvement. Treatment of pulmonary embolism is aggressive and immediate to ensure patient survival. The treatment of a patient with an arterial embolus in an extremity is also aggressive and immediate to prevent the death of tissue and eventual gangrene. Blood flow is reestablished to the affected part by lowering the limb, wrapping it to maintain warmth in the area, and treating any constriction of blood vessels. Heparin or enoxaparin (Lovenox) are administered to prevent further clot formation, and antispasmodic drugs are given for vascular spasms. If this therapy is not successful, surgical intervention may be indicated to remove the obstruction and restore circulation. In another option, a thrombolytic drug (e.g., urokinase, tPA, tenecteplase, alteplase, reteplase, or streptokinase) can be administered via a central catheter directly into the spot of the coronary embolism to break down the emboli. Apixaban (Eliquis) is prescribed for patients diagnosed with atrial fibrillation.

Prognosis

The prognosis varies depending on the location of the emboli. When the embolus is in an extremity, aggressive treatment and surgical intervention are usually successful.

Prevention

Stand up and move around periodically when sitting or traveling. Moving extremities and stretching, compression stockings (TED) hosiery if you have a procedure or surgery to help move the blood back up the legs are recommended. Drinking plenty of water and following all the provider's advice are beneficial.

Patient Teaching

Encourage those who will be traveling and sitting for long periods to get up and walk every hour for a few minutes. If that is not possible, suggest exercises that stimulate the contraction of the calf muscles.

Carotid and cerebral arteries (E)

Coronary arteries (D)

Aortic atherosclerosis (C)
Aortic aneurysm

Valvular thrombi (vegetations) (B)

Thrombus over myocardial infarct

Varicose veins (A)

• **Fig. 10.26** Common sites of thrombus formation. (From Damjanov I: *Pathology for the health-related professions*, ed 4, St. Louis, 2011, Saunders/Elsevier.)

Arteriosclerosis

Description

Arteriosclerosis is a group of diseases characterized by hardening of the arteries. Arteriosclerosis has three forms: atherosclerosis, Mönckeberg arteriosclerosis, and arteriolosclerosis. Atherosclerosis occurs when plaques of fatty deposits form within the arterial tunica intima. Mönckeberg arteriosclerosis, medial calcific sclerosis, involves the arterial tunica media; there is the destruction of muscle and elastic fibers along with calcium deposits. Arteriolosclerosis occurs when the walls of the arterioles thicken, resulting in loss of elasticity and contractility.

Atherosclerosis

Description

Atherosclerosis, thickening and hardening of the arteries, occurs when plaques of cholesterol and lipids form in the arterial tunica intima.

ICD-10-CM Code   I70.0 *(Atherosclerosis of aorta)*

Atherosclerosis is coded according to the site. Refer to the physician's diagnosis and then to the current edition of the ICD-10-CM coding manual to ensure the greatest specificity.

Symptoms and Signs

Atherosclerosis is responsible for most MIs and cerebral infarctions. The patient with atherosclerosis often is asymptomatic. The first symptoms may be angina pectoris, dizziness, elevated blood pressure, and shortness of breath.

Patient Screening

Patients reporting symptoms of angina pectoris, dizziness, elevated blood pressure, and shortness of breath require prompt assessment by a physician. Those who are asymptomatic may report just not feeling well; after careful questioning, an appointment should be scheduled as soon as possible, or since the patient is experiencing angina, referred to emergency services.

Venous embolism

Arterial embolism

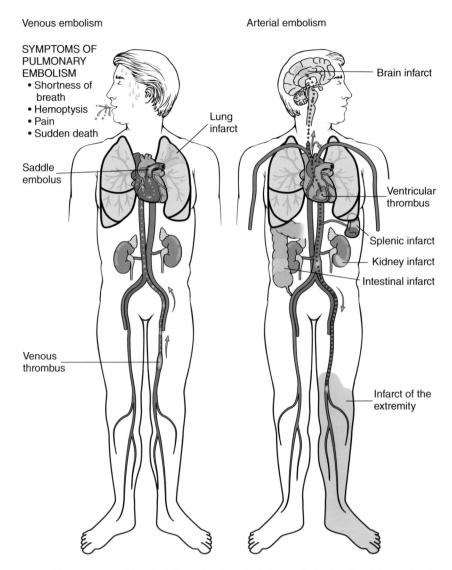

SYMPTOMS OF
PULMONARY
EMBOLISM
- Shortness of
  breath
- Hemoptysis
- Pain
- Sudden death

Saddle
embolus

Lung
infarct

Brain infarct

Ventricular
thrombus

Splenic infarct

Kidney infarct

Intestinal infarct

Venous
thrombus

Infarct of the
extremity

• **Fig. 10.27** Venous and arterial emboli. (From Damjanov I: *Pathology for the health-related professions*, ed 4, St. Louis, 2011, Saunders/Elsevier.)

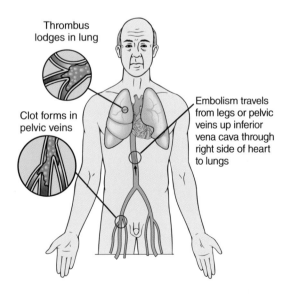

Thrombus
lodges in lung

Clot forms in
pelvic veins

Embolism travels
from legs or pelvic
veins up inferior
vena cava through
right side of heart
to lungs

• **Fig. 10.28** Venous thrombosis.

Etiology

The etiology of atherosclerosis is not fully understood, but there are factors that appear to increase the risk of development of the condition. Heredity seems to increase the occurrence, as do a sedentary lifestyle, a diet rich in lipids and cholesterol-producing foods, cigarette smoking, diabetes mellitus, hypertension, and obesity. The lipids and cholesterol in blood form thick, stiff, and hardened lesions in the medium- and large-size arteries. The lesions are eccentric and eventually expand to occlude the artery (Fig. 10.29). A fatty streak forms in the arterial wall and migrates to the tunica intima. Plaque forms and thickens the arterial wall. A sequela is an ulcer, crack, or fissure in the plaque, where platelets can aggregate and form a thrombus. Ischemia results from reduced blood supply to the dependent tissue, with resulting pain. Infarct occurs with advanced occlusion of the artery and is followed by tissue necrosis.

Normal arterial lumen

Atherosclerotic plaque deposit

Advanced arterial atherosclerotic disease

• **Fig. 10.29** Atherosclerosis.

Diagnosis

The diagnosis often is made during a routine physical examination or screening process. Blood studies indicate elevated cholesterol, triglyceride, and lipid levels. Hypertension may be noted. Doppler studies of major vessels show reduced blood flow.

Treatment

Treatment consists of decreasing the risk factors including dietary changes to reduce saturated fats and foods high in cholesterol and lipids. Cigarette smokers are encouraged to stop smoking. Hypertension and diabetes mellitus are treated and controlled. Hyperlipidemic drugs, such as lovastatin, simvastatin, pravastatin, rosuvastatin, or atorvastatin, are prescribed. Other therapies include cholestyramine, colesevelam, colestipol, or omega-3 ethyl esters. Research is being conducted to confirm claims that hyperlipidemic drug therapy can bring about regression of the condition and actually reverse the plaque buildup.

Prognosis

The prognosis varies, depending on the patient's compliance with prescribed drug therapy, exercise, and dietary changes. With good compliance, it is possible to prevent the progression of the disease.

Prevention

Education about risk factors and changes in lifestyle can lower the occurrence.

Patient Teaching

Emphasize the importance of following dietary and exercise recommendations. If the patient has diabetes, explain the need to keep blood glucose levels within the normal range. Inform smokers of the dangers that smoking poses to their health.

Aneurysms

Description

An aneurysm is a weakening and resulting local dilation of the wall of an artery (Fig. 10.30).

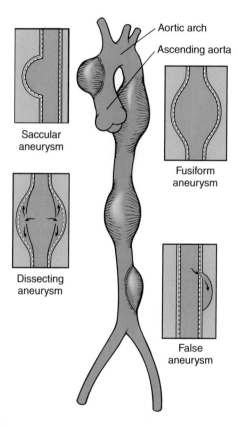

Aortic arch

Ascending aorta

Saccular aneurysm

Fusiform aneurysm

Dissecting aneurysm

False aneurysm

• **Fig. 10.30** Types of aortic aneurysms.

ICD-10-CM Code	I72.9 *(Aneurysm of unspecified site)* (I72.0–I72.9 = 7 codes of specificity)

Aneurysms are coded according to site and type.
   Refer to the physician's diagnosis for site and type of aneurysm and then to the current edition of the ICD-10-CM coding manual to ensure the greatest specificity.

Symptoms and Signs

The onset of the symptoms of an aneurysm may be either insidious or sudden and acute. Symptoms depend on the location and size of the aneurysm and the extent of the dilation. An abdominal aortic aneurysm is the most common form; however, they can occur in other areas, such as the brain. An asymptomatic aneurysm of the aorta often is discovered during a routine physical examination when the abdomen is being palpated or as the result of an abdominal radiographic study conducted for another reason. As the aortic aneurysm enlarges, the patient may experience abdominal or back pain, and a pulsating mass is observed in the abdomen. A complication of any aneurysm is leakage from the wall of the artery or sudden rupture of the weak area. When this occurs, the patient exhibits symptoms and signs of hemorrhagic shock. Signs of rupture of a cerebral aneurysm mimic those of a CVA, with unilateral neurologic deficits being noted.

Patient Screening

Patients reporting a pulsating mass in the abdomen require prompt physician assessment. Those with symptoms of impending or evolving rupture require immediate entry into the emergency medical system.

Etiology

A common cause of aneurysms is a buildup of atherosclerotic plaque that weakens the vessel wall. Trauma, infection or inflammation, and congenital tendencies are additional causative factors. A family history of aneurysms also puts an individual at higher risk.

Diagnosis

The aortic mass is noted in the midabdomen, and pulsation is observed. A bruit heard on auscultation is another sign of the arterial dilation. Cerebral aneurysms are usually discovered when they rupture with catastrophic consequences. Radiographic studies, ultrasonography, CT, and MRI all help confirm the diagnosis. A ruptured aneurysm precipitates symptoms and signs of shock.

Treatment

Treatment depends on the size, location, and likelihood of rupture of the defect. Most diagnosed aortic aneurysms will be treated with surgical repair before they leak or rupture. Catheter-based stent grafts are now available for many patients as an alternative to surgery. After the integrity of the aortic wall has been breached, immediate surgical intervention is required to repair the rupture, usually with a synthetic graft, to ensure patient survival. Watchful waiting is often employed when the aneurysm itself is small or is located in a small vessel.

Prognosis

The prognosis varies, depending on the location and extent of the aneurysm. Surgical intervention before rupture or severe leakage of the vessel creates a better prognosis than when the aneurysm has ruptured or is leaking large amounts of blood. The speed of emergency intervention also affects the prognosis.

Prevention

Absolute prevention is not possible because the condition is the result of many uncontrollable factors, but controlling known risk factors and following a healthy lifestyle regimen may lower the risk.

Patient Teaching

Instruct those who have had surgery about postoperative care of the incision. Encourage compliance with any prescribed drug therapy, dietary modifications, and exercise regimens.

Phlebitis

Description

Phlebitis, inflammation of a vein, occurs most often in the lower legs, but any vein, including the cranial veins, may be affected.

> ICD-10-CM   I80.9 *(Phlebitis and thrombophlebitis*
> Code   *of unspecified site)*
> *Phlebitis is coded by site. Refer to the physician's*
> *diagnosis for location of phlebitis and then to the current*
> *edition of the ICD-10-CM coding manual to ensure the*
> *greatest specificity.*

Symptoms and Signs

Superficial vein involvement results in pain and tenderness in the affected area, which becomes more severe as the condition progresses. Swelling, redness, and warmth are noted, followed by the development of a tender, cordlike mass under the skin.

Deep venous inflammation affects the tunica intima, resulting in the formation of clots (thrombophlebitis).

Patient Screening

Patients reporting swelling, redness, warmth, and pain in a limb require prompt assessment by a physician.

Etiology

The cause is uncertain, and the condition may occur for no apparent reason. Possible causes include venous stasis, obesity, blood disorders, injury, and surgery. Superficial phlebitis can occur after having blood drawn which results in a bruise.

Diagnosis

The clinical picture and history of a preceding event help establish the diagnosis.

Treatment

The treatment of superficial phlebitis is symptomatic, with analgesics given for pain. Caution must be taken not to massage the affected tender area because this manipulation may stimulate the formation of clots or the release of formed clots as emboli.

Prognosis
The prognosis is usually good with treatment.

Prevention
Because the cause is uncertain, prevention is not possible.

Patient Teaching
Warn patients and family members about not massaging the affected area.

Thrombophlebitis

Description
Thrombophlebitis is the result of inflammation of a vein with the formation of a thrombus on the vessel wall.

ICD-10-CM Code	I80.00 *(Phlebitis and thrombophlebitis of superficial vessels of unspecified lower extremity)*

(I80.00–I80.9 = 31 codes of specificity)
Thrombophlebitis is coded by site. Refer to the physician's diagnosis for location of phlebitis and then to the current edition of the ICD-10-CM coding manual to ensure the greatest specificity of pathology.

Symptoms and Signs
Thrombophlebitis causes interference in the blood flow, resulting in edema. As with phlebitis, the patient experiences pain, swelling, heaviness, and warmth in the affected area, along with chills and fever. The involved area is tender to palpation.

Patient Screening
Patients reporting swelling, redness, warmth, and pain in a limb require prompt assessment by a physician.

Etiology
Venous stasis, blood disorders that cause a hypercoagulable state, and injury to the venous wall play important roles in the occurrence of thrombophlebitis. The deep venous inflammation in phlebitis affects the tunica intima, resulting in the formation of clots (thrombophlebitis).

Diagnosis
The clinical picture of gross edema in one leg resulting in a measurable difference in the circumference of the legs suggests thrombophlebitis. The affected area is tender to palpation. Imaging of the vessel with radiographic venography and ultrasonography confirms the diagnosis.

Treatment
Immediate intervention is necessary. The affected part is immobilized to prevent the thrombus from spreading and dislodging to become an embolus. Heparin is administered to prevent the clot from enlarging, and antibiotics are given to prevent infection.

Prognosis
Prompt intervention usually leads to a positive outcome. The condition usually resolves, and no further treatment is indicated. If the condition does not resolve, surgical intervention may be needed to ligate the affected vessel. Collateral circulation develops. As with emboli, preventing DVT during periods of immobilization or reduced physical activity is essential.

Prevention
The prevention of thrombophlebitis includes implementing activities that encourage the movement of legs during long periods of sitting, such as on long flights or automobile trips. If the individual is unable to walk around during this time, he or she must exercise the leg muscles regularly to encourage blood to flow back to the heart and to prevent the formation of blood clots. Individuals who will be sitting for extended periods are encouraged to drink plenty of fluids to prevent dehydration.

Females using oral contraceptives are encouraged not to smoke while taking the medications because smoking increases the risk of the formation of blood clots that may become thrombi.

Patient Teaching
Encourage those who will be traveling and sitting for long periods to get up and walk every hour for a few minutes or perform leg exercises.

Varicose Veins

Description
Varicose veins are swollen, tortuous, and knotted veins that usually occur in the lower legs (Fig. 10.31).

• **Fig. 10.31** Varicose veins.

ICD-10-CM Code	I83.009 *(Varicose veins of unspecified lower extremity with ulcer of unspecified site)*
	I83.019 *(Varicose veins of right lower extremity with ulcer of unspecified site)*
	I83.029 *(Varicose veins of left lower extremity with ulcer of unspecified site)*
	(I83.001–I83.93 = 57 codes of specificity)

Varicose veins are coded by type. Refer to the physician's diagnosis for specific site and then to the current edition of the ICD-10-CM coding manual to ensure the greatest specificity.

Symptoms and Signs

Symptoms of varicose veins develop gradually, beginning with a feeling of fatigue in the legs, which is followed by a continuous dull ache. Leg cramps may be experienced at night, and the ankles may swell. As the condition progresses, the veins thicken and feel hard to the touch. The pain worsens and can have a dull or stabbing quality.

Patient Screening

These patients usually are not in acute distress, and the next available appointment can be scheduled for them. Should they report swelling accompanied by pain and redness in the area, prompt assessment by a physician is recommended.

Etiology

Varicose veins have no clearly identifiable cause. However, defective or absent valves in the veins may be suspected. Prolonged standing or sitting causes pressure on the valves in the superficial veins of the lower legs. Normal movement of the legs causes the muscles to contract and relax, thus "milking" the blood upward. When the person stands or sits for extended periods, gravity pushes blood downward, with resulting pressure on the valves. Without the normal muscular contractions, the venous walls distend, reaching a point at which they and the valves are no longer competent. Stasis of blood follows, causing swelling of the veins. The enlarging uterus during pregnancy increases pressure on the leg veins and pelvic veins, compromising the free flow of venous blood.

Diagnosis

The presence of the twisted, swollen, knotted veins of the lower legs on clinical inspection and a history of prolonged standing, prolonged sitting, or pregnancy is usually all that is needed to make the diagnosis. Advanced varicosities cause the skin around the affected areas to take on a brown discoloration.

Treatment

Rest periods throughout the day, with the patient lying down and elevating the feet higher than the heart, afford relief in mild cases. Engaging in exercise and submerging the legs in warm water increases the flow of blood. The patient may wear support or compression stockings that promote the return flow of blood. Compression stockings apply different amounts of compression to increase blood flow from the lower extremities back to the heart. Low-compression stockings provide less than 20 mm Hg of pressure to the leg. Medium-compression stockings provide 20 to 30 mm Hg of pressure to the leg. There are also stockings that provide 30 mm Hg or higher pressure. Individuals who have to stand for long periods are instructed to move their legs at frequent intervals to stimulate the muscular milking of the veins.

Painful, twisted, and swollen veins that have progressed beyond treatment with rest and exercise usually require surgical intervention in the form of ligation and stripping of veins or injection of sclerosing solutions that harden and eventually atrophy the affected veins. Collateral circulation develops to augment the return of blood to the heart. Some patients have incompetent valves in their veins that do not function accurately or have varicose veins. This causes venous distention and leg swelling, in addition to pain. This can be treated by destroying the incompetent veins through an endovenous laser ablation procedure. The vein is identified by using ultrasonography, and then injections of an anesthetic and a tissue-protecting agent are deposited near the vein down the entire length of the leg. Then a small incision is made, a catheter is inserted into the vein, and sections of the vein are heated to destroy it. The catheter is advanced until the entire vein is destroyed.

Prognosis

Treatment with venous ligation or injection of sclerosing solutions usually relieves the symptoms and resolves the condition.

Prevention

Wearing support stockings and moving the legs during long periods of standing help prevent this condition. Some individuals, however, may be predisposed to the condition, especially during pregnancy. Weight loss to relieve abdominal pressure also helps. Support hosiery can be worn on a routine basis.

Patient Teaching

Give patients information about preventing blood flow stasis in the legs and caring for postoperative incisions.

Thromboangiitis Obliterans (Buerger Disease)

Description

Thromboangiitis obliterans (Buerger disease) is inflammation of the peripheral arteries and veins of the extremities, along with clot formation.

ICD-10-CM Code	I73.1 *(Thromboangiitis Obliterans [Buerger Disease])*

Symptoms and Signs

When walking, the patient experiences intense pain in the affected area, usually the legs, ankle, or foot. Changes in skin color may be evident. If the condition is not resolved and circulation to the affected area is not restored, atrophy, ulcers, and even gangrene can develop.

Patient Screening

When patients report intense limb pain that is aggravated by exercise and relieved by rest, usually the next available appointment is scheduled for them. Those complaining of a breakdown of skin tissue require prompt assessment by a physician.

Etiology

Buerger disease is linked to long-term tobacco use.

Diagnosis

Arteriography and other studies, such as ultrasonography, identify the site of the clot or the obliteration. Ulcers on the skin are another indication of the disease and its severity. A history of long-term use of tobacco products suggests the diagnosis.

Treatment

The first step in treatment is immediate and complete cessation of nicotine use. This often reduces inflammation and restores partial circulation to the area. Several medications, such as clopidogrel, may improve circulation. Buerger-Allen exercises also help improve circulation in the area. In these exercises, the patient elevates the legs by 45 to 90 degrees until the skin blanches and then lowers the legs to a level below the rest of the body until the skin reddens. The patient then rests in the supine position. Surgical intervention to establish blood flow may be necessary. Amputation of gangrenous tissue is imperative.

Prognosis

No cure is known for this condition, but cessation of nicotine use is needed to help alleviate symptoms. When treatments fail, amputation may be necessary.

Prevention

Prevention requires smoking and nicotine use cessation.

Patient Teaching

Give information about the care of foot injuries and instructions on avoiding constrictions around the affected limb.

Raynaud Disease

Description

Raynaud disease is a vasospastic condition of the fingers, hands, or feet. It causes pain, numbness, and sometimes discoloration in these areas.

ICD-10-CM Code	I73.00 *(Raynaud syndrome without gangrene)*
	(I73.00–I73.01 = 2 codes of specificity)

Symptoms and Signs

This bilateral condition is precipitated by cold and causes white discoloration (blanching), followed by blue discoloration as venous blood remains, and finally, red or purple discoloration when circulation is restored. The attacks occasionally are triggered by stressful events. Raynaud disease is much more common in females than in males. The primary disorder is called *Raynaud disease;* when it is secondary to another disease, it is called *Raynaud phenomenon*. In severe cases of Raynaud phenomenon, the digits may ulcerate and become very painful. In most cases, the prognosis is good.

Patient Screening

Those who have been diagnosed usually know they need to warm the area gently. Those experiencing the condition for the first time and experiencing severe pain require prompt intervention.

Etiology

There is no known cause for primary Raynaud disease. Secondary Raynaud disease results from another condition, disease, lifestyle characteristic, or medication.

Diagnosis

The diagnosis is based on the clinical picture and a history of numbness and paleness in the areas. Normal arterial pulses are present. Laboratory test such as antinuclear antibody(ANA) and erythrocyte sedimentation rate (ESR) may be performed to determine if there is an autoimmune condition or connective tissue disorder. In severe cases, the compromise in circulation can lead to tissue necrosis and even amputation in Raynaud phenomenon.

Treatment

Treatment of the episode involves the application of warmth to the affected areas. Patients are encouraged to stop all use of nicotine products, avoid exposure to cold, and avoid stressful situations that bring on the attacks. Drug therapy to dilate the vessels and increase the blood flow includes vasodilators, alpha blockers, and CCBs. The side effects of these drugs may limit their use in treating the condition.

Prognosis

The painful event resolves with application of warmth to the affected area. The condition will continue to recur, however, with exposure to cold.

Prevention

Preventing the attacks requires avoiding exposure to cold and wearing gloves, heavy socks, and shoes for protection from extreme cold. Cessation of nicotine use also helps prevent recurrences of the condition because nicotine constricts blood vessels. Avoiding stress is also helpful.

Patient Teaching

Encourage the patient to avoid direct skin exposure to extreme cold and to wear gloves, heavy socks, and warm shoes to protect the fingers, hands, feet, and toes. Advise avoiding products that contain nicotine.

Blood Dyscrasias

Blood is composed of formed elements, RBCs (erythrocytes), WBCs (leukocytes), platelets (thrombocytes), and a liquid portion (plasma). Blood is responsible for transporting vital elements, including oxygen, nutrients, and hormones, to the body cells. It also plays a part in the removal of waste products, in the inflammatory response, and in the function of the immune system. In addition, blood helps maintain homeostasis, acid-base and fluid balance, and body temperature.

Blood is synthesized by the hematopoietic system in bone marrow (myeloid) and the lymphoid tissue found in the lymph nodes, spleen, thymus, bone marrow, and gastrointestinal (GI) tract (Fig. 10.32). The reticuloendothelial system is found in the spleen, liver, lymph nodes, and bone marrow. It is responsible for removing worn-out blood cells from the bloodstream and breaking down

blood cell components for recycling or elimination from the body.

Stem cells in bone marrow form blast cells, including erythroblasts (rubriblasts), which eventually become erythrocytes, and myeloblasts, which eventually become leukocytes.

Deviation or malfunctioning in this system results in various blood dyscrasias, either because of impairment in the formation of the blood components or because of unusual destruction of cells. Dyscrasias involving erythrocytes and platelets are anemia, thrombocytosis, thrombocytopenia, and polycythemia. Leukocyte dyscrasias include leukemia, lymphoma, and leukopenia. Bleeding and clotting problems arise from alterations affecting thrombocytes and plasma-clotting factors. Normal values of blood components are measured by performing specific laboratory tests.

Anemias

Description

Anemia is defined as a condition in which there is a reduction in the quantity of either RBCs or hemoglobin in a measured volume of blood, reducing the blood's ability to carry oxygen to cells.

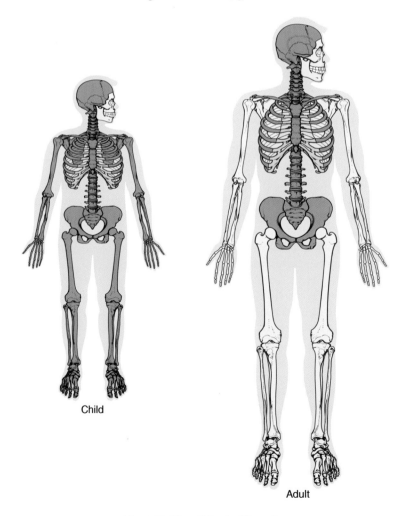

Child

Adult

• **Fig. 10.32** Sites of blood cell formation.

Depending on the severity of anemia, one or many symptoms, including pallor, fatigue, dizziness, shortness of breath, and irregular heartbeats, may occur. Treatment varies, depending on the cause. Several possible causes are acute or chronic blood loss, impaired production of RBCs (including aplastic anemia, iron deficiency anemia, anemias of chronic disease, or megaloblastic anemia), inherited or acquired hemolytic conditions, anorexia nervosa, and hemolytic-hemoglobin disorders. Hemoglobin in RBCs is necessary to transport oxygen to all cells, and any condition that reduces the amount of hemoglobin results in anemia. Iron and other components are needed to synthesize hemoglobin.

Types of anemias include iron deficiency, folic acid deficiency, pernicious, aplastic, sickle cell, hemorrhagic, and hemolytic anemias.

Important presenting symptoms that tend to recur in patients with anemia and need further investigation include:
- Fatigue
- Dyspnea (difficulty breathing)
- Headache
- Loss of appetite
- Heartburn
- Edema, especially of the ankles
- Numbness and tingling sensations
- Syncope (fainting)
- Pallor

ICD-10-CM Code	
D50.0	(Iron deficiency anemia secondary to blood loss [chronic])
D51.0	(Vitamin B12 deficiency anemia due to intrinsic factor deficiency)
D58.0	(Hereditary spherocytosis)
D59.0–D59.1	(Autoimmune hemolytic anemia)
D64.0–D64.3	(Sideroblastic anemia)
D66	(Hereditary factor VIII deficiency)
D69.0	(Allergic purpura)
D70.9	(Neutropenia, unspecified)
D75.1	(Secondary polycythemia)

Anemias are coded by type. Refer to the physician's diagnosis for specific type of anemia and then to the current edition of the ICD-10-CM coding manual to ensure the greatest specificity of pathology.

Symptoms and Signs

Irrespective of the cause, patients with anemia experience fatigue. Most appear pale. As the disease progresses, the symptoms become more pronounced, and the patient may experience dyspnea, tachycardia, and pounding of the heart. Pallor is noted on the palmar surface of the hands and in the nail beds, the conjunctiva, and the mucous membranes of the mouth.

Patient Screening

Anemias often are diagnosed incidentally during a physical examination or during evaluation for other disorders. The individual reporting dyspnea, tachycardia, and a pounding heart require prompt assessment by a physician. For those reporting they are pale and "just plain tired," the next available appointment should be scheduled.

Etiology

Anemias are classified by the color of the RBC as hypochromic, normochromic, or hyperchromic (spherocytosis), and by size as microcytic, normocytic, or macrocytic (Fig. 10.33). Anemias also are classified by causative factor, as previously mentioned.

Iron deficiency anemia may be secondary to blood loss through hemorrhage; a slow insidious bleed, such as bleeding hemorrhoids; and even heavy menstrual flow or because of insufficient intake of dietary iron.

Folic acid deficiency anemia results when insufficient amounts of folic acid are available for DNA synthesis, thus preventing the maturation of blood cells. This can be the consequence of a dietary deficiency and is clinically similar to pernicious anemia.

Pernicious anemia is considered a macrocytic anemia, in which immature RBCs are larger than normal. The hemoglobin volume is reduced, with a subsequent reduction in oxygen-carrying capacity. Autoimmune hemolytic anemia is also considered an autoimmune response.

Aplastic anemia results from an insult to the hematopoietic cells (stem cells) in bone marrow. Erythrocyte, leukocyte, and thrombocyte production are reduced because

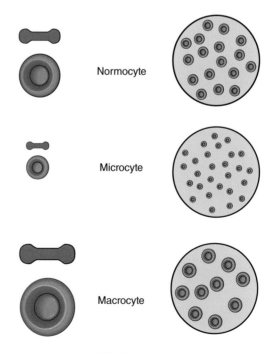

• **Fig. 10.33** Sizes of erythrocytes.

of exposure to myelotoxins, such as benzene, alkylating agents, antimetabolites, certain drugs and insecticides, and radiation.

Sickle cell anemia is a chronic hereditary hemolytic form of anemia, diagnosed most frequently in the African American population, and the Hispanic American population. A person may also have the sickle cell trait. The true number of people living with sickle cell anemia is unknown. Research includes projects to identify people living with the disease to understand the impact on the individual and find treatments to improve health. The presence of hemoglobin S along with hemoglobin A is noted in erythrocytes, causing them to acquire a sickle or elongated shape on deoxygenation (Fig. 10.34). These rigid, misshapen cells obstruct capillary flow and lead to tissue hypoxia and further sickling; this, in turn, causes further obstruction and, eventually, infarction. When the sickling causes obstruction in the blood flow, the individual experiences severe pain. When the sickled cells are reoxygenated, they resume the natural round disk shape of normal erythrocytes. In addition, hemoglobin S has reduced oxygen-carrying capacity.

Hemorrhagic anemia results from a large decline in blood volume (hypovolemia) in a short time.

Hemolytic anemia is caused by abnormal destruction of RBCs. Heredity plays a role in some hemolytic anemias, but exposure to chemical toxins and certain bacterial toxins or autoimmunity also may be the cause.

Diagnosis

Blood studies show reduced RBC numbers, reduced hemoglobin levels and hematocrit, and changes in the morphology of the corpuscles (Table 10.2). Bone marrow studies may be ordered to detect any aberrations.

Treatment

Treatment is directed at the cause of anemia. Dietary or supplemental iron administration is beneficial in iron deficiency anemia. If anemia is the result of a slow insidious bleed, the underlying cause must be found and treated. Folic acid replacement is indicated in folic acid deficiency anemia. Vitamin B_{12} injections are the treatment of choice for pernicious anemia. The causative factor must be uncovered in hemolytic and aplastic anemias and, if possible, eliminated. Currently, sickle cell anemia is treated with blood transfusion, antibiotics for infection, and bone marrow transplant if there is a match. Rest, increased fluid intake, and the administration of analgesics are helpful. Medications such as **hydroxyurea, l-glutamine (Endari), and crizanlizumab** (Adakveo) can be used to manage the frequency of pain symptoms. When the condition is exacerbated, the patient requires hospitalization for oxygen administration, IV therapy, the use of narcotic analgesics, and transfusion of packed RBCs.

In all forms of anemia, blood replacement may be needed when other measures fail to restore the RBC numbers and hemoglobin levels.

Prognosis

The prognosis varies, depending on the cause and type of anemia and the patient's response to prescribed therapy.

Prevention

Prevention depends on the type and cause of anemia. Most types of anemia are not preventable. Proper nutrition may play a role in preventing anemia caused by low iron intake.

Patient Teaching

Give patients information about proper nutrition. Emphasize the importance of complying with the prescribed drug therapy.

Agranulocytosis

Description

Agranulocytosis (also called *neutropenia*) is a blood dyscrasia in which leukocyte levels become extremely low.

ICD-10-CM Code	D70.9 *(Neutropenia, unspecified)*
	(D70.0–D70.9 = 7 codes of specificity)

Symptoms and Signs

The onset of this condition can be rapid. The patient experiences severe fatigue and weakness, followed by a sore throat, ulcerations on the oral mucosa, dysphagia, elevated body temperature, weak and rapid pulse, and chills.

Patient Screening

Patients reporting severe fatigue and weakness, followed by a sore throat, ulcerations on the oral mucosa, dysphagia, an elevated body temperature, weak and rapid pulse, and chills, require prompt assessment by a physician.

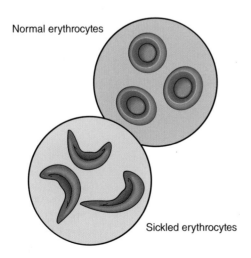

Normal erythrocytes

Sickled erythrocytes

• **Fig. 10.34** Sickled erythrocytes.

TABLE 10.2 Blood Values in Anemia

	Red Blood Cell (per mm³)	Hemoglobin (g/dL)	Hematocrit (%)	Mean Corpuscular Volume (per mm³)	Mean Corpuscular Hemoglobin (pg)	Mean Corpuscular Hemoglobin Concentration (g/dL)	White Blood Cell (per mm³)	Reticulocyte Count (per mm³)	Platelet Count (per mm³)
Normal	Male: 4.7–6.1; female: 4.2–5.4	Male: 14–18; female: 12–16	Male: 42–52; female: 37–47	80–90	27–31	32–36	5000–10,000	0.5–2	150,000–400,000
Acute hemorrhagic anemia	Initial increase, latent decrease	Initial decrease, latent decrease	Normal initially, latent decrease	Increase	Decrease	Normal	Increase	Increase	Decrease
Chronic hemorrhagic anemia	Decrease	Decrease	Decrease	Slight decrease	Slight decrease	Slight decrease	Normal	Decrease	Normal
Iron deficiency anemia	Decrease	Decrease	Decrease	Decrease	Decrease	Decrease	Normal	Decrease	Normal to increase
Aplastic anemia	Gross decrease	Gross decrease	Gross decrease	Moderate decrease	Gross decrease	Gross decrease	Gross decrease	Decrease	Gross decrease
Pernicious anemia	Decrease	Gross decrease	Gross decrease	Increase	Increase	Increase	Slight decrease	Decrease	Slight decrease
Folic acid deficiency anemia	Decrease	Gross decrease	Gross decrease	Increase	Increase	Increase	Slight decrease	Decrease	Slight decrease
Sickle cell anemia	Decrease	Decrease	Decrease	Decrease	Normal	Normal	Increase	Increase	Normal
Hemolytic anemia	Decrease	Decrease	Decrease	Increase	Slight decrease	Normal	Normal	Increase	Normal to increase

Etiology

Agranulocytosis usually is caused by drug toxicity or hypersensitivity. Agranulocytosis can also be inherited or congenital and occurs due to a genetic disorder that affects white blood cell production. For example, cancer chemotherapy with chemotoxic agents can be a cause. Benzene is another chemical agent that causes neutropenia. Agranulocytosis, or neutropenia, is an acute insult to the body's immune system and drastically reduces the body's response to bacterial infection. The infectious agents usually invade the body through the oral or pharyngeal mucosa and often are already present but are no longer held in check by the now-absent granulocytes. Patients occasionally are sensitive to a particular drug, such as chlorpromazine, propylthiouracil, phenytoin, chloramphenicol, and phenylbutazone. Agranulocytosis also can accompany aplastic or megaloblastic anemia, tuberculosis, uremia, or malaria. This condition occurs a little more often in people assigned female at birth.

Diagnosis

Blood studies show leukopenia, with a substantial decrease in the number of polymorphonuclear cells, less than 100 per microliter. Bone marrow studies reveal a lack of granulocytes, and the developing WBCs are not mature and are reduced in number. History may reveal exposure to the offending infectious agents; blood, urine, and oral cultures may be positive for bacteria; and toxins may be present. Genetic testing may also be recommended.

Treatment

The primary thrust of treatment is to eliminate any offending microorganism through aggressive antimicrobial therapy. Cultures are repeated several times and are monitored for the growth of microbes. If the cause of the toxicity is identified as a drug or chemical, exposure to the toxic agent must be halted. Aggressive therapy is indicated because the condition can be fatal. Immunosuppressants may be prescribed if the condition results from an autoimmune disease. Granulocyte colony-stimulating factor drugs such as filgrastim (Neupogen), and pegfilgrastim (Neulasta) are also available and used in some cases to help the body make neutrophil blood cells faster.

Prognosis

The prognosis varies, depending on the etiology of the condition. Cessation of exposure to a toxic substance often results in improvement. As previously mentioned, in some cases, this condition, if left untreated, may be fatal within a week.

Prevention

Prevention involves avoiding the toxic substance after it has been identified. Individuals taking medications that lower neutrophil levels will need to have routine labwork to monitor levels of neutrophils. Prevention is not always possible.

Patient Teaching

Give the patient information about follow-up labwork, and avoiding exposure to the toxic substance.

Polycythemia

Description

Polycythemia (polycythemia vera) is an abnormal increase in the amount of hemoglobin, the RBC count, or the hematocrit, causing an absolute increase in RBC mass.

| ICD-10-CM Code | D45 *(Polycythemia vera)* |

Symptoms and Signs

The symptoms of polycythemia are related to the increased RBC mass and include headaches, itching, dyspnea, irritability, mental sluggishness, dizziness, syncope, night sweats, and weight loss. Circulatory stagnation, thrombus, and increased blood viscosity may be noted. Splenomegaly, clubbing of fingers, and cyanosis may be observed.

Patient Screening

Patients reporting headaches, dyspnea, irritability, mental sluggishness, dizziness, syncope, night sweats, and weight loss require prompt assessment. Schedule an appointment as soon as possible. If a prompt appointment is not possible, refer the patient to a facility where assessment can be performed quickly.

Etiology

Mutations in the gene Janus kinase-2 (JAK2) have been identified in approximately 90% of individuals diagnosed with polycythemia vera, but it is not understood why the mutation takes place. JAK2 has also been associated with other types of cancer. It is not known why a sustained increase in the hematopoiesis of bone marrow causes absolute or primary polycythemia. Relative polycythemia results when plasma volume is reduced by dehydration, plasma loss, fluid and electrolyte imbalances, or burns. Reduced oxygen supply to the tissues results in compensation by the body as it manufactures additional hemoglobin to carry additional oxygen. The body uses this compensatory process when patients have chronic pulmonary and cardiac diseases or live at high altitudes, where the oxygen concentration is reduced.

Diagnosis

An abnormal increase in RBC numbers, hemoglobin levels, and hematocrit suggests the condition. Leukocyte and thrombocyte counts also are elevated, and the spleen may be enlarged. Blood tests, bone marrow biopsy and genetic testing are used to aid in the diagnosis.

Treatment

Periodic phlebotomy is employed to reduce the blood volume. Myelosuppressive drugs and radiation also improve the blood count. Hydroxyruea, Interferon alfa-2b (Intron

A), Ruxolitinib (Jakafi), and Busulfan (Busulfex, Myleran) are drugs that reduce the number of red blood cells. Medications for itching may also be prescribed if the patient exhibits that symptom.

Prognosis

The prognosis is good if the patient adheres and responds to treatment, however this is a fatal disease if not managed.

Prevention

Primary polycythemia vera cannot be prevented. Avoiding activities that result in oxygen depletion may be helpful in preventing secondary PV.

Patient Teaching

Emphasize the importance of routine blood cell counts and the need for continued phlebotomy. Encourage patients to keep appointments and to follow medication regimens, if applicable.

Thrombocytopenia

Idiopathic thrombocytopenic purpura is considered an autoimmune response. This dyscrasia involves a reduction in the clotting capability of blood and is discussed in Chapter 3.

Leukemias

Leukemias are malignant neoplasms of the blood-forming organs (bone marrow, spleen, and lymph nodes) and produce an abnormal, uncontrolled, clonal proliferation of one specific type of blood cell in the lymphoid or myeloid cell lines. The large number of leukemic cells leads to bone marrow overcrowding, resulting in the reduced production and function of normal blood cells. The reduced numbers of functional neutrophils, erythrocytes, and platelets result in frequent infections, anemia, and clotting problems.

Leukemias are classified by cell type and degree of differentiation of the neoplastic cells. In acute leukemias, immature-appearing, large hematopoietic cells (blasts) are present. In chronic leukemias, the cells are more mature appearing yet hypofunctional. Acute disease has a rapid progression and can be quickly fatal, whereas chronic leukemias have a slower progression that is measured in years rather than months. Common types of leukemia include acute lymphocytic leukemia (ALL), chronic lymphocytic leukemia (CLL), acute myelogenous leukemia (AML), and chronic myelogenous leukemia (CML).

Acute Lymphocytic Leukemia

Description

ALL is characterized by the overproduction of immature lymphoid cells (lymphoblasts) in the bone marrow and lymph nodes. It is generally classified into two subtypes, depending on the type of cells affected: B-cell ALL or T-cell ALL.

ICD-10-CM Code	C91.00 *(Acute lymphoblastic leukemia not having achieved remission)*
	(C91.00–C91.02 = 3 codes of specificity)

Refer to the physician's diagnosis for specific type of lymphoid leukemia and then to the current edition of the ICD-10-CM coding manual to ensure the greatest specificity of pathology.

Symptoms and Signs

The patient appears pale and may report bone pain, weight loss, sore throat, fatigue, fever, night sweats, and weakness. There is a tendency toward increased bruising and bleeding. As the leukemic cells infiltrate the spleen, liver, lymph nodes, and nervous system, they interfere with the normal functioning of these organs. Lymphadenopathy and splenomegaly are common at presentation. Symptoms of central nervous system (CNS) involvement include headache, blurred vision, nausea, vomiting, and cranial nerve palsies. A mediastinal mass can be found in many patients with the T-cell ALL.

Patient Screening

Patients complaining of bone pain, weight loss, fatigue, night sweats, weakness, persistent fevers, a tendency toward increased bruising and bleeding, recurrent infections, headache, blurred vision, and/or cranial nerve palsies require prompt assessment by a physician.

Etiology

ALL accounts for some adult leukemias and is the most common childhood leukemia. Childhood ALL is covered in more detail in Chapter 2. The exact cause is unknown. Prolonged exposure to radiation, certain chemicals and drugs, smoking, viruses, and genetic factors (certain chromosomal abnormalities) are considered contributing factors.

Diagnosis

Peripheral blood smear analysis shows increased numbers of immature lymphocytes and reduced numbers of erythrocytes and platelets. Microscopic examination of a bone marrow aspiration or biopsy specimen is necessary for definitive diagnosis. Blast cells are counted to diagnose ALL. Cerebrospinal fluid (CSF) should be withdrawn and examined for leukemic cells. Karyotyping is performed to look for any abnormalities that may help determine prognosis and treatment options.

Treatment

Treatment regimens for ALL involve aggressive chemotherapy for 2 to 3 years, consisting of three phases: induction, consolidation, and maintenance. Because CNS invasion is common in ALL, the CNS is treated with intrathecally administered chemotherapy even if blasts are not noted in CSF. Those with the Philadelphia chromosome are often treated with tyrosine inhibitors. Hematopoietic stem cell transplantation (HSCT) is an option for patients who have relapsed or for adults with poor prognostic features.

Prognosis

Children generally have a better prognosis than adults. Approximately 98% of children are in remission after a few weeks of treatment. About 90% of children are cured. Adults often have cytogenetic abnormalities that carry a worse prognosis than the ones found in children. In addition, children often can tolerate relatively higher doses of the drugs currently used to treat ALL than adults can.

Prevention

No prevention methods are known for ALL.

Patient Teaching

Give patients and caregivers information about chemotherapy and treatments. Help them find and contact community support groups.

Chronic Lymphocytic Leukemia

Description

CLL is a neoplasm that involves lymphocytes. It is a slowly progressing disease that results in the accumulation of mature-appearing but hypofunctional lymphocytes.

> ICD-10-CM   C91.10 *(Chronic lymphocytic leukemia*
> Code   *of B-cell type not having achieved*
>   *remission)*
>   (C91.10–C91.12 = 3 codes of specificity)
> *Refer to the physician's diagnosis for specific type of*
> *lymphoid leukemia and then to the current edition of*
> *the ICD-10-CM coding manual to ensure the greatest*
> *specificity of pathology.*

Symptoms and Signs

Patients often have no symptoms when a routine CBC reveals lymphocytosis, thrombocytopenia, or anemia. Symptoms may include weight loss, fever, night sweats, extreme fatigue, splenomegaly, hepatomegaly, and painless swelling of cervical, supraclavicular, or axillary lymph nodes that spontaneously waxes and wanes. Patients are susceptible to frequent viral and fungal infections.

Patient Screening

Patients complaining of weight loss, fever, night sweats, extreme fatigue, and noticeable swelling of the cervical, supraclavicular, or axillary lymph nodes require prompt assessment by a physician.

Etiology

CLL is the most common leukemia in adults. The median age at diagnosis is 70 years, and there is a slight male predominance. Having a first-degree relative with CLL increases the risk for CLL.

Diagnosis

The majority of cases are discovered incidentally during routine blood work. Peripheral blood smear analysis, with or without bone marrow studies, is performed and reveals an increased number of mature-appearing lymphocytes. In most cases of CLL, the absolute lymphocyte count is greater than 5000/µL. Because CLL most often involves B lymphocytes, screening for the presence of certain B-cell markers is performed. Karyotyping and testing for certain genetic mutations are performed.

Many staging systems for CLL have been proposed, but the Rai system is the most commonly used one in the United States. The stage of the disease is important in determining the appropriate treatment and prognosis. The Rai system stratifies patients into risk groups according to their symptoms and assigns average survival times to those groups. Patients usually move through the risk groups during the course of their disease.

Treatment

Treatment often is withheld until the patient is symptomatic and has evidence of hemolytic anemia, painful lymphadenopathy, symptomatic organomegaly, cytopenia, prolonged fever, chills, or weight loss. CLL is usually treated with chemotherapy. Radiation therapy can be used to reduce the symptoms caused by lymphadenopathy and splenomegaly. Other therapies include the use of monoclonal antibodies directed against B-lymphocyte surface antigens; these agents include rituximab (Rituxan) (directed against CD20) or alemtuzumab (Campath) (directed against CD52). Other medication therapies may include chlorambucil, pentostatin, prednisone, or cladribine; transplantation is generally not an option for patients with CLL, although the newly developed nonmyeloablative transplants show promise as a potential treatment for CLL.

Prognosis

CLL has a variable natural course. Survival times from diagnosis are different based on different factors with some living 20 years after diagnosis. The overall 5-year survival rate for those 20 years and older is currently 87%. Poor prognostic indicators are low platelet count and low hemoglobin level at the time of diagnosis. Certain genetic aberrations have prognostic implications as well. During the initial asymptomatic phase, patients often can maintain their normal lifestyle, but performance levels during the terminal phase are poor, and frequent causes of death include systemic infection, bleeding, and cachexia.

Prevention

No methods for the prevention of CLL are known.

Patient Teaching

Give patients and caregivers of affected children information about chemotherapy and how to follow the plan of treatment. Support group referrals may be helpful.

Acute Myelogenous Leukemia

Description

AML (also known as *acute myeloid, myelocytic,* or *granulocytic leukemia*) is a rapidly progressive neoplasm of cells committed to the myeloid line of development. Leukemic cells accumulate in bone marrow, peripheral blood, and other tissues.

ICD-10-CM Code	C92.00 *(Acute myeloblastic leukemia, not having achieved remission)* (C92.00–C92.02 = 3 codes of specificity) C92.40 *(Acute promyelocytic leukemia, not having achieved remission)* (C92.40–C92.42 = 3 codes of specificity) C92.50 *(Acute myelomonocytic leukemia, not having achieved remission)* (C92.50–92.52 = 3 codes of specificity)

Refer to the physician's diagnosis for specific type of myeloid leukemia and then to the current edition of the ICD-10-CM coding manual to ensure the greatest specificity of pathology.

Symptoms and Signs

A rapid accumulation of myeloblasts (myeloid precursors) leads to pancytopenia and the resulting symptoms of anemia, easy bleeding and bruising, and increased risk of infection. Bleeding symptoms include gingival bleeding, epistaxis, and menorrhagia. Weight loss, fatigue, and pallor are common. Lymphadenopathy and organomegaly are rare.

Etiology

AML accounts for 80% of acute adult leukemia. Risk factors include a positive family history of AML or other leukemias; prior therapeutic treatment with ionizing radiation; prior aggressive chemotherapy treatment for Hodgkin disease, non-Hodgkin lymphoma (NHL), ovarian cancer, or breast cancer; chronic exposure to benzene (a toxic liquid found in gasoline, rubber cement, and cleaning solvents); and smoking.

Diagnosis

The diagnosis is suggested by the clinical picture and the results of peripheral blood smear analysis. Half the patients have an Auer rod (abnormal lysosomal granules) visible inside the leukemic cell. Bone marrow aspiration and biopsy are needed for definitive diagnosis.

Treatment

Chemotherapy is the first approach to treating AML. Drug treatment depends on the subtype of AML. Cytarabine (cytosine arabinoside or ara-C), and an anthracycline drug regimen, such as daunorubicin, or idarubicin may be used.

Prognosis

The overall 5-year survival rate for AML is highly dependent on the prognostic indicators. The 5-year survival rate for patients who are 20 years of age or older is approximately 28%. Patients who are younger than 20 years of age have a 5-year survival rate of 69%. Adverse prognostic indicators are advanced age, history of a prior hematologic disorder, and poor performance status at diagnosis.

Prevention

No methods of preventing AML are known.

Patient Teaching

Give patients and caregivers of affected children information about chemotherapy, side effects, and methods of chemotherapy delivery.

Chronic Myelogenous Leukemia

Description

CML (also known as *chronic myeloid* or *myelocytic leukemia*) is a slowly progressing neoplasm that arises in a hematopoietic stem cell or early progenitor cell, resulting in an excess of mature-appearing but hypofunctional neutrophils.

ICD-10-CM Code	C92.10 *(Chronic myeloid leukemia, BCR/ABL-positive, not having achieved remission)* (C92.10–C92.22 = 6 codes of specificity)

Refer to the physician's diagnosis for specific type of myeloid leukemia and then to the current edition of the ICD-10-CM coding manual to ensure the greatest specificity of pathology.

Symptoms and Signs

The disease has a triphasic course: a chronic phase, an accelerated phase, and a blast crisis. Most patients are diagnosed in the chronic phase, where abnormal proliferation of WBCs has begun. These patients are usually asymptomatic at the time of diagnosis, with the disease being suspected on the basis of abnormalities, such as leukocytosis and thrombocytosis, on routine blood tests. Splenomegaly is common, but the symptoms are mild. In the accelerated phase, leukocytosis increases, and neutrophil differentiation becomes further impaired. The patient may experience bone pain, fever, night sweats, and other systemic symptoms. The blast crisis resembles AML and is defined by the presence of 30% or greater blasts in the peripheral blood or bone marrow.

Etiology

CML is almost invariably associated with an abnormal chromosome 22 which is called the Philadelphia chromosome. A section of chromosome 9 switches places with part of chromosome 22, making the chromosome 9 longer than usual and chromosome 22 shorter than usual.

Hematopoietic Stem Cell Transplantation

Many patients with leukemias and lymphomas cannot be cured with conventional chemotherapy treatments alone. The very large doses of chemotherapy or radiation that would be required to fully destroy all the neoplastic cells in patients with relapsed disease or disease refractory to conventional treatment make people very sick and destroy bone marrow. Few people are able to withstand this severe treatment.

Hematopoietic stem cell transplantation (HSCT), also known as *bone marrow transplantation* (BMT), was developed to treat such patients. In the traditional BMT protocol, the patient first receives high-dose chemotherapy and/or radiation therapy to eradicate all malignant cells in the body and suppress the body's immune system so that it is less likely to attack the donor marrow. Next stem cells obtained from a donor's bone marrow are infused into the recipient. The stem cells find their way into the marrow space of the recipient and restore marrow functioning in 2 to 4 weeks.

A newer method of HSCT has been developed. Studies have shown that stem cells may be harvested directly from the donor's peripheral blood after hematopoietic growth factors have been administered to the donor to mobilize stem cells from bone marrow to the bloodstream. The stem cells are collected by using a pheresis machine and then infused into the recipient. These peripheral blood cells can restore neutrophil and platelet production several days faster than stem cells derived from bone marrow. This peripheral blood stem cell transplantation is preferred over the traditional HSCT for many patients.

Nonmyeloablative transplantation, or "mini transplantation," uses mild chemotherapy and low-dose radiation before transplantation of the donor stem cells. The donor cells gradually replace the host marrow and kill neoplastic cells by an immunologic "graft-versus-tumor" effect.

All of these transplantations carry the risk of severe infections and bleeding, serious damage to vital organs caused by the initial chemotherapy and radiation therapy, and graft rejection by the host's cells. Graft-versus-host disease, an immunologic reaction in which the donor T lymphocytes see host tissues, especially the skin, liver, and GI tract, as foreign and attack it, is not uncommon. Relapse may also occur and is seen most often in patients with ALL and CML who received transplantations during blast crisis.

Definitions of some terms commonly used in conjunction with BMT are:

- *Autologous transplantation:* Transplantation in which the patient serves as their own donor for stem cells.
- *Allogeneic transplantation:* Transplantation in which the donor is a human leukocyte antigen (HLA) identical to the patient (usually a sibling).
- *Haploidentical transplantation:* Transplantation in which the donor is a relative only half-matched to the recipient (usually a parent).
- *HLA type:* The identity of the leukocyte surface antigens, the HLAs, is determined for the patient and donor to define the degree of compatibility. The closer the match is, the lower the risk of transplantation-related complications.
- *Syngeneic transplantation:* Transplantation in which the patient's identical twin serves as the stem cell donor.
- *Unrelated donor/mismatched transplantation:* Transplantation in which the donor does not match all of the key HLA antigens. This type of transplantation is associated with the greatest risk of complications.

Diagnosis

The diagnosis is suggested by the clinical picture and blood and bone marrow studies. CBC reveals anemia, leukocytosis, and thrombocytosis. Bone marrow biopsy shows hyperplasia, but the cells appear more mature than the leukemic cells in AML. Definitive diagnosis requires demonstrating the presence of the Philadelphia chromosome or the *BCR/ABL* fusion gene product with cytogenetic analysis, fluorescence in situ hybridization, or polymerase chain reaction (PCR). The presence of the Philadelphia chromosome distinguishes CML from other disorders that may resemble CML clinically.

Treatment

Cure can only be achieved via HSCT (see the Enrichment box about Hematopoietic Stem Cell Transplantation). However, HSCT is not a viable option for all patients. Initial treatment is with drugs that specifically inhibit the BCR/ABL tyrosine kinase, known as *tyrosine kinase inhibitors* (TKIs). Their use is aimed at achieving long-term control of the disease, although they do not cure the disease. With TKIs, many patients can obtain complete remission, which can be sustained for years. *Complete remission* is defined as ablation of the Philadelphia chromosome and its gene product.

Prognosis

The overall 5-year survival rate has increased in the past few years. Indicators of poorer prognosis include a large spleen size, older age of the patient, a higher percentage of blast cells, and a platelet count greater than 700,000/μL.

Prevention

No methods are known to prevent CML.

Patient Teaching

Give patients and parents of affected children information about chemotherapy. Help them find and contact community support groups.

Lymphatic Diseases

The lymphatic system is composed of lymphatic vessels, lymphatic tissue (lymph nodes, tonsils, thymus, and spleen), and lymph. The lymphatic vessels originate at the capillary level and, along with the venous system, progress to empty into the right and left subclavian veins. This system has no pump. Lymph nodes, collections of lymphatic tissue, filter foreign material (e.g., bacteria and viruses) from the lymphatic circulation (Fig. 10.35). Lymphocytes are produced mainly in the lymph nodes as part of the body's defense mechanism. The lymphatic vessels are thin-walled, and the larger vessels contain valves. As in the case of the venous system, the muscles exert intermittent pressure on the vessels, causing the lymph to flow by a milking action. Smooth muscle in the vessel wall contracts to aid the return of lymph to the cardiovascular system. Swollen lymph nodes or glands may indicate the trapping of microbes during an infectious process.

Lymphedema

Description
Lymphedema is an abnormal collection of lymph, usually in the extremities.

ICD-10-CM Code	I89.0 *(Lymphedema, not elsewhere classified)*
	I97.2 *(Postmastectomy lymphedema syndrome)*

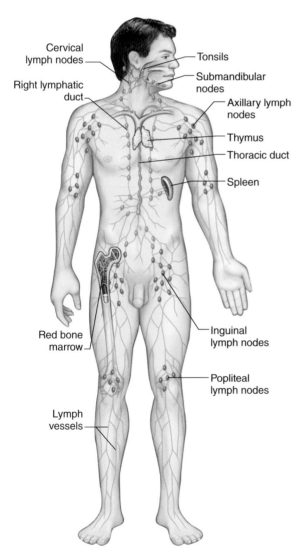

• **Fig. 10.35** The lymphatic system. The bean-shaped structures shown in green are lymph nodes. (Modified from Patton KT, Thibodeau GA: *The human body in health and disease*, ed 7, St. Louis, 2018, Elsevier.)

Symptoms and Signs
Lymphedema results in swelling of the extremities. Most patients experience no pain, although in severe cases, lymphedema can cause pain and limit movement. The affected extremity becomes swollen and grossly distended (Fig. 10.36).

Patient Screening
Patients reporting unilateral limb swelling require prompt assessment. Schedule an appointment for these patients to be seen as soon as possible, or refer them to a facility where they can be assessed quickly.

Etiology
The obstruction of the lymph vessel or node may be inflammatory or mechanical. If lymphedema is left untreated, the connective tissues lose their elasticity, and the edema becomes permanent. The lymphatic circulation may be compromised by an infection, neoplasm, or thrombus. Allergic reactions also may be implicated, along with trauma or surgery involving the affected part. Tight clothing that constricts the lymphatic vessels can cause temporary lymphedema. Removing the constriction usually resolves the swelling. Females who have had mastectomies may experience lymphedema in the adjacent arm. Prolonged lymphedema rarely is associated with the development of lymphosarcoma (a cancer).

Diagnosis
Painless swelling in an extremity suggests lymphedema. Imaging procedures, including lymphangiography and radioactive isotope studies, are means of confirming the diagnosis and ascertaining the site of obstruction.

• **Fig. 10.36** A patient with left leg lymphedema. (From Cheng M, Chang DW, Patel KM: *Principles and practice of lymphedema surgery*, ed 2, 2022, Elsevier.)

Treatment

Treatment is aimed at reducing the swelling. The affected limb is elevated to a level above the heart to encourage drainage of the lymph. Elastic bandages or stockings are applied when the affected part is elevated to compress the area, also encouraging lymph drainage. Diuretics may be administered to reduce fluid volume. In severe cases, surgical intervention is also an option when conservative methods are not successful. Radical debulking and liposuction procedures are successful in some cases in improving quality of life. Antibiotics may be administered if infection is present.

Prognosis

The prognosis varies, depending on the cause of the lymphedema and the patient's response to therapeutic intervention. Surgical intervention to remove the cause of the obstruction usually has a positive outcome. When lymphedema is left untreated connective tissues can lose their elasticity, resulting in the edema becoming permanent.

Lymphedema is not in itself life threatening, but it carries the danger of uncontrolled infection developing in the affected tissue. The essentially stagnant interstitial fluids are a breeding ground for infections and their resulting toxins.

Prevention

Many cases are not preventable. Wearing tight clothing that can restrict lymphatic flow should be discouraged.

Patient Teaching

Give patients information about their treatment plan. Encourage postmastectomy patients to follow the prescribed rehabilitation exercises that help reduce the incidence of lymphedema.

Lymphangitis

Description

Lymphangitis is an inflammation of the lymph vessels.

| ICD-10-CM Code | I89.1 *(Lymphangitis)* |
| | (I89.0–I89.9 = 4 codes of specificity) |

Symptoms and Signs

Lymphangitis usually manifests as a red streak at the site of entry of the infective organism. The redness extends to the regional lymph node, which is swollen and tender. Cellulitis may develop in the surrounding tissue. Manifestations of generalized infection, including fever, chills, and malaise, are present.

Patient Screening

Patients reporting fever, chills, and generalized malaise, accompanied by tenderness and redness in the region of a lymph node, require prompt assessment by a physician.

Etiology

Bacterial invasion into the lymph vessels at the site of local trauma or ulceration is a frequent cause of lymphangitis. Occasionally no portal of entry is detectable.

Diagnosis

Visual inspection of the involved area and observance of typical systemic manifestations of bacterial invasion are usually sufficient for diagnosis. Blood studies indicate leukocytosis. Final confirmation is made from cultures of the infected tissue.

Treatment

Treatment includes the administration of systemic antibiotics. The affected area is elevated, rested, and warm, and wet dressings are applied locally. Surgical drainage of purulent material is indicated.

Prognosis

The prognosis varies, depending on the amount of tissue involved and the nature of the causative organism. The patient's response to antibiotics also plays a role in recovery. Surgical intervention usually contributes to a more positive outcome.

Prevention

This condition usually cannot be prevented.

Patient Teaching

Give patients information about postoperative care of incision sites. Emphasize the importance of complying with and completing any prescribed antibiotic therapy.

Lymphoma

Lymphomas are malignant neoplasms that arise from uncontrolled proliferation of the cellular components of the lymph system. The dysfunctional cells may be B cells, T cells, or, rarely, both. The neoplastic lymphocytes are migratory and can be found not only in the lymph structures but also in the bloodstream, bone marrow, and, later in the disease, nonlymph organs (e.g., liver or lung). Lymphomas are divided into two main categories: Hodgkin lymphoma (HL) and other types that are grouped as NHL.

Treatment selection is determined by the cell type and the stage of the disease. Both kinds of lymphoma are staged by using the Ann Arbor-Cotswolds staging system and its modification the Lugano Classification. The Ann Arbor staging system and its modification, the Lugano Classification, are used for staging HL and NHL. Neoplastic involvement of lymph structures (lymph nodes, spleen, and thymus), extranodal tumor sites, and the presence or absence of the systemic "B" symptoms of lymphoma (unexplained weight loss of greater than 10% of body weight in the past 6 months, persistent or recurrent fevers with temperatures greater than 38°C during the previous month, and recurrent, drenching night sweats during the previous month).

- Stage I: A single lymph structure or region is involved.
- Stage II: Two or more lymph structures are involved, with the involvement being on the same side of the diaphragm.
- Stage III: Lymph regions on both sides of the diaphragm, or above the diaphragm and spleen are involved.
- Stage IV: There is widespread involvement of extranodal tissue above and below the diaphragm, lymph nodes, bone marrow and other organ involvement.

Each stage designation carries either an "A", "B" or "X" after the stage number, indicating whether any of the "B" symptoms are absent (A) or present (B), and if the lymphoma is more than 10 cm wide (X).

Hodgkin Lymphoma

Description

Hodgkin lymphoma is a cancer of the body's lymphatic system, in which the involved cells proliferate and interfere with normal functioning by collecting in masses in various parts of the body. Tumors arise in the tissue of the lymph nodes and spread to other lymph nodes, the spleen, the liver, and bone marrow.

ICD-10-CM Code	C81.90 (Hodgkin lymphoma, unspecified, unspecified site)
	C81.99 (Hodgkin lymphoma, unspecified, extranodal and solid organ sites)
	(C81.00–C81.99 = 70 codes of specificity)

Hodgkin disease is coded by type. Refer to the physician's diagnosis and then to the current edition of the ICD-10-CM coding manual to ensure the greatest specificity of pathology.

Symptoms and Signs

The initial symptoms of HL are painless enlargement of the lymph nodes in the neck or the mediastinum, fatigue, and pruritus (Fig. 10.37). As the disease progresses, the patient may experience systemic "B" symptoms, such as fever, night sweats, and weight loss. Hodgkin disease is differentiated from other lymphomas by the presence in the lymphatic tissue of a Reed-Sternberg cell, a large cell with two or more mirror-image nuclei, each with a single nucleolus.

Patient Screening

For patients reporting a painless enlargement of cervical lymph nodes, fatigue, and pruritus, fever, night sweats, and weight loss, prompt assessment by a physician is required.

Etiology

The cause is not fully understood. Risk factors identified as putting one at higher risk include

previous history of malignancy, prior treatment with chemotherapy or radiation therapy, family history of lymphoma, immunosuppression or taking immunosuppressant drugs, and exposure to Epstein-Barr virus (EBV) or similar viruses. Those of the male sex have a higher incidence.

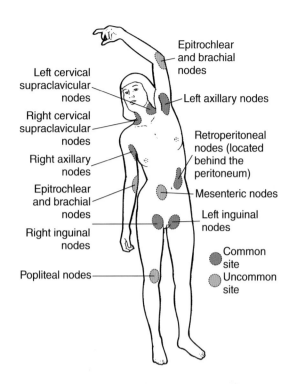

• **Fig. 10.37** Lymph node sites for Hodgkin disease. (From Huether SE, McCance KL: *Understanding pathophysiology*, ed 4, St. Louis, 2008, Mosby/Elsevier.)

Diagnosis

A history of painless lymphadenopathy and the typical symptoms of HL lead to an excisional lymph node biopsy for a definitive diagnosis. The node biopsy shows the presence of Reed-Sternberg cells. Immunophenotyping of the tissue for certain markers is very helpful in making the diagnosis. Blood studies indicate mild normochromic, normocytic anemia; neutrophilic leukocytosis; lymphopenia; and eosinophilia. The ESR is elevated, as is the serum alkaline phosphatase level. Bone marrow biopsy is performed only on select patients and may show abnormal cells. CT scans of the chest, abdomen, and pelvis help evaluate the extent of the disease. Liver and kidney function tests are performed.

Treatment

Combined chemoradiotherapy is preferred for patients in stages I and II and some patients in stage III. Patients in stage IIIB and stage IV often are treated with chemotherapy alone. The preferred regimen is ABVD (doxorubicin, bleomycin, vinblastine, dacarbazine) therapy. Other medication therapies may include chlorambucil, pentostatin, prednisone, or cladribine. Relapses usually are treated with additional chemotherapy. HSCT may be used to treat patients with multiple relapses.

Prognosis

HL is one of the most treatable forms of cancer and can be cured. The overall 5-year survival rate approaches 93%. Death may result from HL itself or from secondary cancers or cardiovascular disease, side effects of treatment that often are not apparent until years after therapy. Important indicators of poor prognosis include the presence of B symptoms, low serum albumin and hemoglobin levels, male sex, age greater than 45 years, anemia, leukocytosis, and a high ESR.

Prevention
No ways of preventing HL are known.

Patient Teaching
Give patients information about chemotherapy, radiation therapy, and their treatment plan.

Non-Hodgkin Lymphoma
Description
NHL describes a number of heterogeneous neoplasms of the lymphoid cells that exhibit a wide variety of clinical signs and symptoms, ranging from slow, indolent growth to rapidly fatal progression.

ICD-10-CM Code	C85.80 *(Other specified types of non-Hodgkin lymphoma, unspecified site)* C85.89 *(Other specified types of non-Hodgkin lymphoma, extranodal and solid organ sites)* *(C85.10-C85.99 = 40 codes of specificity)*

Symptoms and Signs
Symptoms include painless lymphadenopathy, fatigue, pruritus, bone pain, and GI symptoms. Lymphatic tissue, such as tonsils and adenoids, may be enlarged and the patient can experience "B" symptoms, including fever, night sweats, and weight loss.

Patient Screening
For patients reporting painless enlargement of the cervical lymph nodes, fatigue, pruritus, fever, night sweats, and weight loss, prompt assessment by a physician is required.

Etiology
White blood cells proliferate and cause tumors. The reason is not fully understood, as with HL, but the risk factors are very similar.

Diagnosis
The patient evaluation must include the determination of the histologic subtype, the extent of the disease, and the performance status of the patient because treatment and prognosis greatly depend on this information. All potentially involved lymphoid sites should be physically examined. An excisional biopsy of an intact, involved lymph node is necessary for accurate histopathologic identification of the disease. Immunologic, cytogenetic, and molecular studies may be performed to further aid in therapeutic decisions and in the determination of the prognosis. Bone marrow aspiration and biopsy are performed to determine the extent of the disease. If bone marrow is involved, the patient is placed at stage IV. Laboratory tests after diagnosis generally include CBC, peripheral blood smear analysis, and studies of kidney and liver functions. Chest radiography and CT of the abdomen, chest, and pelvis are performed to determine the extent of the disease. PET is a useful adjunct. GI endoscopy may detect GI involvement. MRI of the CNS may be performed if neurologic signs are present.

Treatment
The treatment plan includes chemotherapy, radiation, or targeted therapy. The more aggressive lymphomas have rapid progression but may be cured with appropriate treatment. They are commonly treated with CHOP (cyclophosphamide, doxorubicin, vincristine, and prednisone) chemotherapy regimen. When rituximab is added to the therapy, it is referred to as R-CHOP. Relapses may be treated with high-dose chemotherapy followed by HSCT or with chemotherapy alone.

Prognosis
Histopathology is the most important prognostic indicator, followed by age, presence of extranodal disease, presence of B symptoms, and stage at the time of diagnosis. Indolent lymphomas generally are associated with a survival measured in years even if left untreated but they generally are not curable even with treatment. In contrast, the aggressive lymphomas are curable but are rapidly fatal if left untreated or if unresponsive to therapy.

Prevention
No methods of prevention of NHL are known.

Patient Teaching
Give patients information about chemotherapy, radiation therapy, and their treatment plan.

Transfusion Incompatibility Reaction
Description
Transfusion incompatibility results when the blood or blood product transfused has antibodies to the recipient's RBCs or the recipient has antibodies to the donor's RBCs.

ICD-10-CM Code	T80.30X(A)(D)(S) *(ABO incompatibility reaction due to transfusion of blood or blood products, unspecified)* T80.40X(A)(D)(S) *(Rh incompatibility reaction due to transfusion of blood or blood products, unspecified)* T80.92X(A)(D)(S) *(Unspecified transfusion reaction)*

Symptoms and Signs

This hypersensitivity reaction can range from mild to fatal. Most severe transfusion reactions are incompatibility related and are characterized by hemolysis or agglutination. Other forms include bacterial, allergic, and circulatory-overload transfusion reactions. The severity of the reaction depends on the amount of incompatible blood that is transfused and prior transfusion reactions of the patient.

The patient who has an incompatibility reaction and is receiving a blood transfusion experiences chills, fever, and tachycardia. The patient with a more severe reaction has severe back pain, vomiting, diarrhea, hives or rash, a substernal tightness, and dyspnea. The patient becomes hypotensive and progresses to a state of circulatory collapse. As the condition worsens, there is bleeding from the puncture site, blood in urine, and eventually renal failure.

The most frequent transfusion reaction is associated with WBCs or WBC remnants in donor blood. It is febrile and short lived, ceasing when the transfusion is halted and there is no hemolysis or allergic response.

The patient experiencing an allergic reaction exhibits hives and itching and possibly bronchial spasms and anaphylaxis.

Patient Screening

Patients receiving blood transfusions will be in a clinic or hospital environment. The trained professionals observing the patient will immediately institute intervention and care to reverse or modify the reaction

Etiology

ABO- and Rh-incompatible blood and antigens that screening does not reveal cause an antigen-antibody reaction that produces hemolysis (destruction of RBCs) or agglutination (clumping of RBCs that obstructs the flow of blood through capillaries). Histamine and serotonin are released from mast cells and platelets. DIC usually is triggered (see the Disseminated Intravascular Coagulation section) with resulting coagulation problems (Fig. 10.38).

Diagnosis

Any sign of chills, fever, hives, back pain, or dyspnea during the transfusion alerts the healthcare professional attending the patient to a possible reaction. Blood and urine specimens are examined to confirm the incompatibility and the presence of hemolysis or activated coagulation.

Treatment

Transfusion protocol mandates that a set of baseline patient vital signs be taken before the start of a transfusion. During the first 15 minutes, the patient is observed closely, and the assessment of vital signs is repeated. This monitoring of vital signs and observation of the patient continues at designated intervals until the procedure is completed. At the first indication of any symptoms or signs of reaction, the blood transfusion is stopped immediately. Blood and urine samples are obtained from the patient and sent to the laboratory, along with the remaining untransfused blood. Mild reactions are treated with antihistamines, and anaphylaxis is treated aggressively according to institutional protocol.

Prognosis

The prognosis varies, depending on the amount of blood infused, the cause of the reaction, and the speed of the intervention.

Prevention

Prevention is the best form of treatment. Careful typing and crossmatching of the blood product is mandatory. Two attendants must compare the patient's information with that on the blood bag and the physician's orders before starting the transfusion.

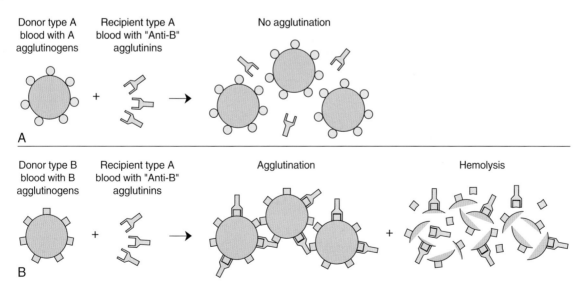

• **Fig. 10.38** Illustration showing agglutination of red blood cells during blood transfusion incompatibility reaction. (From Applegate E: *The anatomy and physiology learning system*, ed 4, St. Louis, 2011, Saunders/Elsevier.)

Patient Teaching

Instruct the patient to report any symptoms or unusual sensations during the transfusion process immediately, especially early in the transfusion.

Clotting Disorders

Classic Hemophilia (Hemophilia A)

Description

Classic hemophilia is a hereditary bleeding disorder resulting from a deficiency of clotting factors.

ICD-10-CM Code	D66 *(Hereditary factor VIII deficiency)*

Symptoms and Signs

The condition can be mild, moderate, or severe. Any unusually prolonged bleeding episode, easy bruising, hematomas, or excessive nosebleeds in a male child suggest hemophilia. Females can also have hemophilia, but it is much rarer. The first sign of hemophilia may be ecchymosis at birth, irritability, bleeding resulting from circumcision. Joint swelling and pain suggest bleeding in the joints.

Patient Screening

When parents report that an infant, toddler, or child has experienced unexplained prolonged bleeding, noticeable hematomas, easy bruising, and/or excessive nosebleeds, the physician should promptly assess the child. The condition is often diagnosed during the neonatal period of hospitalization. It can also occur or be discovered later in life. Schedule the next available appointment for the patient as soon as possible.

Etiology

Hemophilia is an X-linked genetic disorder that typically affects males and those assigned male at birth. In rare cases, hemophilia can affect females or those assigned female at birth. Hemophilia is transmitted by the asymptomatic carrier to the child. Factor VIII, a clotting factor in the intrinsic clotting cascade, is functionally inactive. Any minor trauma can initiate the bleeding episode.

Diagnosis

The diagnosis is based on the clinical picture and a thorough history. Clotting studies indicate normal platelet count, bleeding time, and prothrombin time (PT); prolonged partial thromboplastin time (PTT); and a very low factor VIII assay.

Treatment

Hemophilia cannot be cured, but treatment is available. Concentrated factor VIII (antihemophilic factor [AHF]) is administered to stop the bleeding by replacing the missing clotting factor. Transfusions of whole blood may be necessary. Patients are encouraged to avoid situations that initiate

bleeding episodes. Gene therapy is also being investigated to determine if the condition can be treated by using this treatment or gene replacement therapy.

Prognosis

No cure for hemophilia is known, however an individual can live a normal lifespan with treatment.

Prevention

No prevention is known for this condition. Genetic counseling may help explore the probability of the disorder being transferred to offspring.

Patient Teaching

Give parents or the patient if an adult, information about X-linked genetic disorders.

Disseminated Intravascular Coagulation

Description

DIC is a condition of simultaneous hemorrhage and thrombosis. It is a syndrome that occurs secondary to other diseases or dramatic events.

ICD-10-CM Code	D65 *(Disseminated intravascular coagulation [defibrination syndrome])*

Refer to the physician's diagnosis and then to the current edition of the ICD-10-CM coding manual to ensure the greatest specificity of pathology.

Symptoms and Signs

Oozing of blood from needle puncture sites, mucous membranes, or incisions may be noted, as may bleeding

---

◆ ENRICHMENT

Lupus Anticoagulant (Antiphospholipid syndrome)

The patient with lupus anticoagulant (LA) usually does not have lupus erythematosus; however, some may progress to the disease with joint pain, dermatologic problems, or renal involvement.

Many individuals with LA are asymptomatic, however others will have symptoms which include abnormal bleeding of nose or gums, atypical bruising, abnormal menstrual cycles, multiple miscarriages, blood clots in the legs (DVT) or in the lungs (pulmonary embolism), strokes, and heart attacks.

Blood tests for the anticoagulant antibody are performed. When a positive result is obtained, the tests are repeated. Some individuals with positive test results do not require any treatment. Others require ongoing treatment with anticoagulant medications, including heparin or warfarin (Coumadin). Some may be instructed to take aspirin. Many require anticoagulant drug therapy along with routine blood tests for their lifetime. These individuals are at risk for blood clots that may lead to pulmonary embolism, stroke, or heart attack.

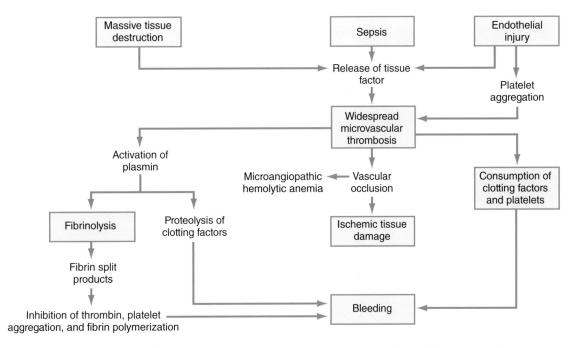

• **Fig. 10.39** Pathophysiology of disseminated intravascular coagulation. (From Kumar V, Cotran R, Robbins S: *Robbins basic pathology*, ed 8, Philadelphia, 2008, Saunders/Elsevier.)

in the form of purpura, wound hematomas, or petechiae. Hematemesis, hematuria, and bloody stools may be present. The patient is weak, reports headaches, and experiences air hunger and tachycardia. Low blood pressure may also be experienced. DIC follows a major event, such as obstetric complications, septicemia, trauma, burns, hypothermia, and extensive tissue destruction.

Patient Screening
Most of these individuals are usually in an inpatient facility, and immediate intervention is indicated. If they suffer the condition at home after a major precipitating event, they must be entered into the emergency medical system for prompt assessment.

Etiology
Thrombin activates the production of fibrin, causing clots to form where they are not needed (i.e., in the microcirculation). The thrombin also causes platelet aggregation, forming more clots. In addition, the fibrinolytic system is activated by the presence of thrombin in plasma; thrombin causes excessive fibrinolysis and additional bleeding. Predisposing factors include hypotension, hypoxemia, acidosis, and stasis of capillary blood. Any of these factors may be the result of the aforementioned major precipitating events (Fig. 10.39).

Diagnosis
The diagnosis is based on the clinical picture; a thorough history, including a probable precipitating event; and laboratory studies. Platelet count and fibrinogen levels are reduced, whereas PT is prolonged. Positive D-dimer test indicates clot formation.

Treatment
The administration of IV heparin inhibits the formation of additional microthrombi and prevents the aggregation of platelets. Platelet replacement and plasma-clotting factors are administered when serious hemorrhage is present. The condition is life threatening and often fatal.

Prognosis
The prognosis is guarded due to organ failure resulting in death if not treated immediately.

Prevention
Because this condition is a sequela to a major systemic insult, prevention is unlikely.

Patient Teaching
If the patient survives the event, teaching may include an explanation of the incident. Help family members find and contact support groups in the community.

Review Challenge

Answer the following questions:
1. What are the common symptoms of cardiovascular disease?
2. How would you describe the pathology of CAD?
3. How is the patient likely to describe the pain in angina pectoris?
4. How do the symptoms of MI differ from those of angina pectoris?

5. List and discuss possible stress factors contributing to the onset of broken heart syndrome.
6. Why is angioplasty used for MI?
7. What conditions can cause cardiac arrest? What is the time frame in which CPR may be successfully initiated?
8. What are the diagnostic criteria for essential hypertension?
9. What happens when the pumping action of the heart is inadequate? How can CHF be treated?
10. Which conditions may lead to cor pulmonale?
11. How is pulmonary edema treated?
12. What does cardiomyopathy refer to, and how is it treated?
13. How does endocarditis affect the cardiac valves?
14. Discuss the importance of completing a drug regimen for an infection caused by beta-hemolytic *Streptococcus*.
15. Why is rheumatic fever described as a systemic disease? What infection often precedes it?
16. Explain the relationship between rheumatic fever and valvular heart disease?
17. What are the sources of cardiac arrhythmias? How are they diagnosed?
18. Which methods may be used to treat cardiac arrhythmias?
19. Why is shock considered a life-threatening emergency? What are the signs and symptoms?
20. What is cardiac tamponade?
21. What is the relationship between venous thrombosis and pulmonary emboli?
22. What is the difference between arteriosclerosis and atherosclerosis? Why are both conditions a health threat?
23. How might an aneurysm be detected? When are they a serious threat?
24. What is the relationship of phlebitis to thrombophlebitis? Why should the clinician avoid massaging the affected area?
25. What medical intervention is available for severe varicose veins?
26. Which conditions may precipitate an episode of Raynaud disease?
27. What are the presenting symptoms of anemia?
28. What are some possible causes of anemia?
29. How are the following anemias differentiated: aplastic, sickle cell, hemolytic, iron deficiency, hemorrhagic, and pernicious?
30. What are some usual causes of agranulocytosis?
31. What are the typical symptoms in all types of leukemia?
32. Which leukemia is considered more a disease of later life?
33. How does lymphedema differ from lymphangitis?
34. Which lymphoma is characterized by the presence of Reed-Sternberg cells in lymphatic tissue?
35. Discuss the recently identified possible cause of NHL.
36. What symptoms does a patient experience with a transfusion incompatibility reaction?
37. How is classic hemophilia A treated?
38. Referring to the AHA's website, list the AHA-recommended dietary guidelines for a healthy diet that is suggested as a weapon to fight cardiovascular disease.

Real-Life Challenge: Essential Hypertension

A 46-year-old male reports intermittent headaches and lightheadedness for about 3 months. In the past 2 weeks, he has had several episodes of epistaxis. Vital signs are temperature, 98.6°F; pulse, 106 beats per minute; respirations, 20 breaths per minute; and blood pressure, 168/98 mm Hg. His weight is 265 lb, and his height is 5 feet, 11 inches.

Patient history reveals that he has a highly stressful job requiring extensive travel with overnight stays. He regards himself as a high achiever. His family history reveals that his father died at age 53 years as a result of a CVA and that his mother, age 69 years, has CHF and hypertension. His brother has a history of hypertension, and his two sisters are alive and well. The patient has been smoking one pack of cigarettes a day for the past 30 years.

The patient is advised to stop smoking or at least reduce the number of cigarettes smoked per day. In addition, he is advised to begin a weight-reduction and exercise program and to reduce his sodium intake. He is also told that he should avoid stressful situations, if possible. The medications ordered are a beta-blocker, atenolol, and an ACE inhibitor, ramipril. The patient is instructed to return in 1 week for reevaluation. Essential hypertension is a suspected diagnosis.

Questions

1. What factors contribute to the symptoms and signs of essential hypertension that this patient is experiencing?
2. Why would his onset of symptoms be considered insidious?
3. Why could the diagnosis of essential hypertension not be confirmed on the initial encounter?
4. Why might a diuretic be ordered?
5. What is the significance of the family history?
6. What is the action of calcium channel blockers (CCBs) in the treatment of essential hypertension?
7. If essential hypertension is not controlled, what complications may evolve from the condition?
8. How important was the symptom of epistaxis in the diagnosis?

Real-Life Challenge: Anemia

A 32-year-old female reports feeling tired all the time, having an excessively fast heartbeat, having difficulty catching her breath, and experiencing some lightheadedness. She appears quite pale. Vital signs are: temperature, 98.4°F; pulse, 118 beats per minute; respirations, 26 breaths per minute; and blood pressure, 100/69 mm Hg.

The patient is married, has three children ages 7 years, 4 years, and 6 months, and is employed outside the home. She says she can barely get out of bed in the morning and make it through the day. She has had four episodes of syncope in the past week. Menstrual periods have been regular but heavy. She denies experiencing any observable blood in her urine or stools. CBC with differential is ordered. The RBC count is below normal and normocytic; hemoglobin is 9, hematocrit is 27, and WBC and platelet counts are normal. The patient is diagnosed with iron deficiency anemia and encouraged to rest and increase her dietary intake of red meat, liver, and egg yolks. Supplementary iron is prescribed in the form of ferrous sulfate tablets, and the patient is instructed to return to the office in 1 week for follow-up.

Questions

1. What might have been the cause of the iron deficiency anemia in this patient?
2. What causes RBCs to be microcytic? Macrocytic?
3. What is the importance of the absence of blood in the stool and urine?
4. What might be the connection with the previous pregnancy?
5. What type of food, in addition to the red meat, liver, and egg yolks, would help increase the hemoglobin?
6. What might blood tests show if this was sickle cell anemia?
7. Compare hemolytic anemia with iron deficiency anemia.
8. As the hemoglobin improves, what changes might be expected in the vital signs?

Real-Life Challenge: Abdominal Aortic Aneurysms

A 75-year-old female patient with diabetes was diagnosed with two small abdominal aortic aneurysms. She also had a history of elevated blood pressure, 150/90 mm Hg. Lisinopril had been prescribed to maintain an acceptable level. The physician had suggested that the course of treatment could be watchful waiting. A surgeon had been consulted, and after reviewing laboratory values and CT scans of the abdomen and abdominal aorta, the surgeon recommended not pursuing a surgical course at the time of the tests.

Follow-up appointments every 3 months were scheduled. The first 3-month examination revealed no significant change. The second 3-month examination showed that the aneurysm had started to increase in size. The course of watchful waiting was to continue. The patient was instructed to monitor her blood pressure closely and not to lift anything heavier than 10 pounds. Additionally she was advised not to stretch or reach out.

The surgeon preferred to schedule a procedure to install a stent into the abdominal aorta. The patient began to experience severe muscle spasms in the muscles of the lower legs. She also was unsure about the proposed procedure and asked what would happen if she did not have the procedure.

Questions

1. What might be the cause of the aneurysms?
2. Why is controlling blood pressure important?
3. Why would the surgeon want to adopt a wait-and-see approach at first?
4. What is the significance of cramping in the legs?
5. Why would the patient be instructed not to lift or stretch?
6. What would be the outcome if the aneurysm began to leak?
7. What would be the chances of survival if the aneurysm ruptured?

Internet Assignments

1. Research by the AHA has suggested treatment interventions for CHF. In particular, research and list drug interventions and patient teaching about the administration of these drugs.
2. Research by the AHA has suggested treatment interventions for cardiac arrhythmias. Use the arrhythmia chart in the chapter to identify the arrhythmias that are considered potentially lethal arrhythmias. Record your findings from the website about treatment interventions.
3. Research the incidence of hypertension at the AHA website. Record the ages and sexes of patients and the seriousness of their conditions. Verify and record any drug therapy suggested.
4. Research the incidence of hemophilia in the US population in the past 10 years at the National Hemophilia Association website. Also research suggested drug treatments and their side effects.

Critical Thinking

1. As a review of the anatomy of the heart, list the four chambers and the four valves.
2. Identify the structures of the conduction system.
3. After reviewing the AHA website, discuss the AHA Healthy Heart Recommendations.
4. Locate AEDs in your educational or work facility, and describe how you would use an AED. Discuss situations when you would use an AED.
5. List and discuss the dangers of malignant hypertension.
6. Discuss the importance of compliance with the prescribed drug regimen in the treatment of hypertension and malignant hypertension.
7. Review the interventions that may offer some relief to the patient with congestive heart failure.
8. Discuss the feelings that patients may experience as CHF progresses and there is increasing difficulty breathing.
9. How would you explain the differences between cor pulmonale and CHF?
10. Discuss the feelings of patients experiencing dyspnea.
11. A patient is experiencing the symptoms of cardiomyopathy. Discuss his or her response to dyspnea, fatigue, tachycardia, palpitations, and occasional chest pain.
12. What infectious processes in the body might be the cause of pericarditis?
13. Discuss causative agents, including infections in the body that may be the cause of myocarditis and/or endocarditis.
14. Discuss the psychological effects of an asymptomatic patient being diagnosed with mitral valve prolapse.
15. Explain what you think arrhythmias might feel like, including both atrial and ventricular types.
16. Research and report on interventions for mitral stenosis.
17. Explain the importance of diagnosis and treatment for strep throat.
18. What is the importance of completing the antibiotic regimen prescribed for the treatment of strep throat?
19. Patients with pacemakers usually have to wait until the battery reaches the "end of service" before the battery or pacemaker can be replaced. Discuss the psychological aspects of waiting for the "end of service" message to be obtained.
20. Explain some of the precautionary measures that might be taken by travelers or those with sedentary lifestyles to avoid developing a thrombus in the legs.
21. Discuss the psychological effects of an individual being diagnosed with an abdominal aortic aneurysm when a "watch and wait" attitude versus surgical intervention is chosen by the healthcare provider. Research various methods of treatment, and then discuss treatment options.
22. List the components that make up blood.
23. List various types of anemias, and identify their causes.
24. Discuss the effects of the diagnosis of leukemia on the patient and his or her family, workplace, and community.
25. What might be the psychological effects of postmastectomy lymphedema?
26. Discuss hematopoietic stem cell transplantation (HSCT).
27. Prepare to discuss Critical Thinking case study exercises for this chapter that are posted on Evolve.

Credentialing Examination Questions

1. Into how many chambers is the heart divided?
   A. One
   B. Two
   C. Three
   D. Four
2. A patient experiences angina pectoris. Which key symptom is associated with this condition?
   A. Headache
   B. Palpitations
   C. Chest pain
   D. Muscle weakness
3. Which term causes narrowing of the coronary arteries which compromises blood flow to the myocardium?
   A. Arteriosclerosis
   B. Atherosclerosis
   C. Tachycardia
   D. Bradycardia
4. Which blood pressure reading is considered a "normal" value according to the American College of Cardiology and the American Heart Association?
   A. 112/78
   B. 130/85
   C. 148/88
   D. 168/98
5. A patient has endocarditis. Which other problem can put the patient at a higher risk for this condition?
   A. Hypertension
   B. Bradycardia
   C. Rheumatic heart disease
   D. Mitral valve prolapse
6. Which class of medication is used to treat a thrombus?
   A. Antibiotic
   B. Beta-blocker
   C. Anticoagulant
   D. Stimulant

7. Which description best describes an aneurysm?
   A. Hardening of a vessel wall.
   B. Weakening of a vessel wall.
   C. Blood clot inside the brain.
   D. Blood clot inside a coronary artery.
8. Which vasospastic condition of the fingers, hands, or feet is precipitated by cold and causes white discoloration (blanching), which progresses to blue and red or purple discoloration?
   A. Stroke
   B. Raynaud disease
   C. Hemophilia
   D. Anemia
9. Which prognosis best describes untreated DIC?
   A. Fatal due to organ failure
   B. 50% mortality rate
   C. Good
   D. 100% recovery
10. Which diagnostic test is used to diagnose mitral valve prolapse?
    A. ECG
    B. Cardiac catheterization
    C. Holter monitor
    D. Echocardiography

11

Diseases and Conditions of the Urinary System

CHAPTER OUTLINE

LEARNING OBJECTIVES

After studying this chapter, you should be able to:

1. Explain the structure and function of the normal urinary system.
2. Explain how pathologic conditions of the urinary system threaten homeostasis and result in illness.
3. Explain the diagnostic value of urinalysis.
4. Relate the symptoms and signs of acute glomerulonephritis.
5. Describe how immune mechanisms are suspected to be a causative factor in acute and chronic glomerulonephritis.
6. Distinguish between hemodialysis and peritoneal dialysis.
7. Identify the hallmark sign of nephrosis.
8. List some nephrotoxic agents.
9. Explain why acute renal failure or acute kidney injury is considered a clinical emergency.
10. Discuss treatment measures for prolonging the life of the patient with chronic renal failure.
11. Identify the etiology and diagnosis of pyelonephritis.
12. Describe hydronephrosis.
13. Describe the common symptoms of renal calculi and list the possible complications.
14. List the causes of infectious cystitis and urethritis.
15. Describe diabetic nephropathy.
16. Describe the polycystic kidney and discuss the treatment options.
17. Discuss urinary catheterization.
18. Contrast the neurogenic bladder with stress incontinence.
19. List and describe the symptoms of renal cell carcinoma (RCC) and bladder carcinoma.
20. Identify those most at risk for RCC and bladder tumors.

KEY TERMS

azotemia (ah-zoh-TEE-me-ah)
catheterization (kath-eh-ter-eye-ZAY-shun)

creatinine (kree-AT-in-in)
cystoscopy (sis-TOSS-ko-pee)

dialysate (dye-AHL-ih-sate)
glomeruli (gloh-MER-you-lye)
glomerulonephritis (gloh-mer-you-low-neh-FRY-tis)
glomerulosclerosis (gloh-mer-you-low-sklee-ROW-sis)
hemodialysis (he-moh-dye-AHL-ih-sis)
hydronephrosis (high-droh-neff-ROW-sis)
immunosuppressive (im-you-noh-sue-PRESS-ihv)

lithotripsy (LITH-oh-trip-see)
nephrectomy (neh-FRECK-toh-me)
nephropathy (neh-FROP-ah-thee)
nephrotoxic (neff-row-TOCKS-ick)
oliguria (ohl-ih-GOO-rhee-ah)
peritoneal dialysis (per-ih-toe-NEE-al dye-AHL-ih-sis)
pyelonephritis (pye-eh-low-neh-FRY-tis)

Orderly Function of the Urinary System

The urinary system is responsible for producing, storing, and excreting urine; these processes prevent the body from becoming toxic. The kidneys facilitate the reabsorption of necessary nutrients, water, and electrolytes, cleanse the blood of the waste products of metabolism, and regulate the water, salts, and acids in body fluids to ensure the body's homeostasis. Regulation of the volume of water in the body is also an essential function. The urinary system includes the kidneys, which manufacture urine and play a role in the regulation of systemic blood pressure and the accessory structures. The ureters transport urine, and the bladder stores urine until it is excreted voluntarily through the urethra. The organs and accessory structures of the urinary system consist of two kidneys, two ureters, the urinary bladder, and the urethra (Fig. 11.1).

Each kidney (Fig. 11.2) is composed of about 1 million microstructures called *nephrons* (Fig. 11.3). The nephrons are functional units of the kidneys and are responsible for the filtration, reabsorption, and secretion of urine. Fig. 11.4 depicts the formation of urine. Urine is transported from the nephron to the renal pelvis and then to the ureters. The kidney has many other functions, including the secretion of renin, a hormone that raises blood pressure, and erythropoietin, which acts as a stimulus for red blood cell (RBC) production. It also has a role in the activation of vitamin D.

Nephrons are composed of the glomerulus, Bowman capsule, proximal convoluted tubule, the loop of Henle, distal convoluted tubule, and collecting duct.

As a primary organ of the urinary system, each kidney filters blood to form urine, which contains waste products to be eliminated from the body (see Fig. 11.2). The bean-shaped organs, about the size of a fist, are located in the back retroperitoneally to the abdominal cavity and lateral to the spinal column. Each kidney is separated into three areas or regions: the cortex, the medulla, and the renal pelvis.

Blood enters the kidneys through the renal arteries. Refer to Figs. 11.1 and 11.2 for blood supply to and from the kidneys. The arteries divide again and again into smaller arteries that ultimately enter the nephrons. Blood leaves the kidneys through the renal veins.

Urine leaves the kidneys through two long, slender tubes, the ureters, which enter the urinary bladder. Peristalsis in the muscular walls of the ureters moves urine into the urinary bladder, where it is temporarily stored until it is passed from the body by way of the urethra. Urine is voluntarily excreted from the bladder in a process called *urination* or

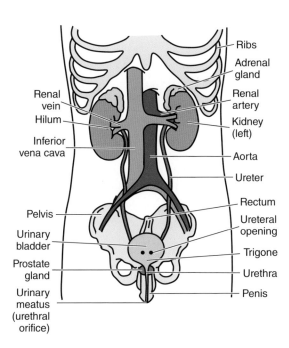

• **Fig. 11.1** Gross anatomy of the urinary system (male). (From Gould B: *Pathophysiology for the health professions*, ed 4, Philadelphia, 2011, Saunders/Elsevier.)

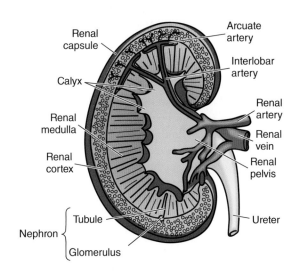

• **Fig. 11.2** Anatomy of the kidney. (From Gould B: *Pathophysiology for the health professions*, ed 4, Philadelphia, 2011, Saunders/Elsevier.)

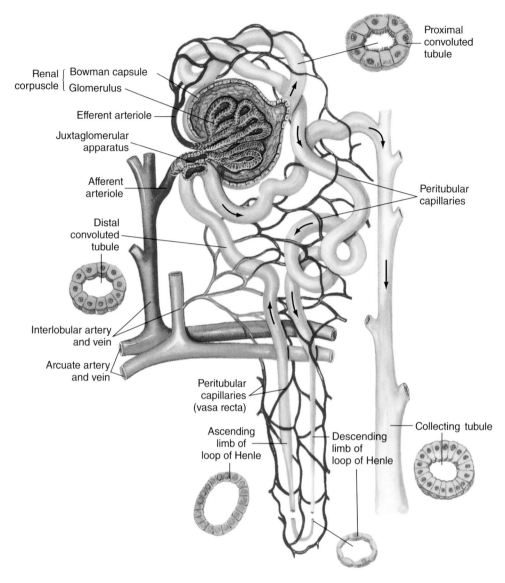

• **Fig. 11.3** The nephron. (From Patton KT, Thibodeau GA: *Mosby's handbook of anatomy and physiology,* ed 6, St. Louis, 2014, Mosby/Elsevier.)

micturition. The urethra is a tubular structure that extends from the base of the urinary bladder to the urinary meatus (urethral orifice) on the external surface of the body (see Fig. 11.1).

Infection, scarring, toxic necrosis, or trauma of the urinary tract can result in disturbances of renal function, and this allows urea (the nitrogenous waste of metabolism in urine) or extracellular fluid and electrolytes to accumulate in blood. Congenital or acquired structural defects and tumors cause obstructive diseases of the urinary system. Other important diseases of the urinary tract are immunologic disorders, circulatory disturbances, cystic disease, and metabolic disorders (e.g., diabetes mellitus).

The function of the urinary system often is evaluated by performing urinalysis (Table 11.1) and blood tests (Table 11.2). Normal results demonstrate proper filtration, absorption, elimination of metabolic waste, and precise fluid and electrolyte balance. Other tests for urinary tract disorders include culture and sensitivity tests to determine appropriate antibiotic therapy, radiologic tests that visualize structural and functional abnormalities, **cystoscopy** (see Enrichment box), and biopsy of lesions.

Usually symptoms of urinary diseases reflect an accumulation of waste products in blood and cause electrolyte imbalances in the body. Common symptoms include the following:

- Nausea
- Loss of appetite
- Fever
- Headache and body aches
- Flank or low back pain
- Bloody urine (hematuria)
- Edema
- Decreased urinary output
- Hypertension
- Pruritus

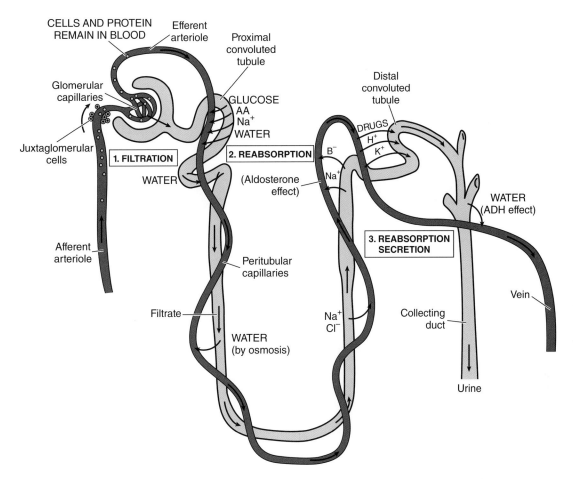

• **Fig. 11.4** Formation of urine. *AA,* Amino acids; *ADH,* antidiuretic hormone; *B⁻,* bicarbonate ions; *Cl⁻,* chloride ions; *H⁺,* hydrogen ions; *K⁺,* potassium ions; *Na⁺,* sodium ions. (From Gould B: *Pathophysiology for the health professions*, ed 4, Philadelphia, 2011, Saunders/Elsevier.)

Disorderly Function of the Urinary System

Acute Glomerulonephritis

Description

Acute **glomerulonephritis** is inflammation and swelling of the **glomeruli** (see Fig. 11.3) of the kidneys. It can be a primary disease of the kidney or may develop secondary to a systemic disease. This condition can follow a streptococcal bacterial infection of the throat or skin.

ICD-10-CM Code	N00.3 *(Acute nephritic syndrome with diffuse mesangial proliferative glomerulonephritis)* (N00.0–N00.5 = 6 codes of specificity)

Acute glomerulonephritis is coded according to sites and types of lesions. Refer to the physician's diagnosis for site and type of lesion and to the current edition of the ICD-10-CM coding manual.

Symptoms and Signs

Acute glomerulonephritis is marked by proteinuria (protein in urine), edema, and decreased urine volume. Hematuria can range from insignificant to a sudden onset of urine that is grossly bloody (gross hematuria). Urine may appear dark or may be described as coffee colored. Hypertension related to altered renal function and fluid retention is possible and is accompanied by headaches, visual disturbances, malaise, anorexia, and a low-grade fever. Flank or back pain develops as a result of swelling of the kidney tissue.

Patient Screening

Patients complaining of visible blood in urine accompanied by edema, headache, and flank or pelvic pain require prompt medical attention.

Etiology

This condition usually occurs after an infection caused by group A beta-hemolytic *Streptococcus*. It also can be idiopathic or may result from an immune reaction that causes circulating antigen-antibody complexes to become trapped within the network of capillaries of a glomerulus. In some cases, the antigen is endogenous (arising from within) as an accompaniment to tumors. The injury to the glomeruli results in a decrease in the rate of filtration of blood and, consequently, the retention of water and salts in the

TABLE 11.1	Routine Urinalysis[a]		
	Normal	**Abnormal**	**Pathology**
Characteristics			
Color and clarity	Pale to darker yellow and clear	Very pale Cloudy, milky, WBCs Hematuria, RBCs, reddish to reddish brown	Excessive water Leukocytes, UTI Bleeding in infection, calculi, or cancer
Odor	Aromatic	Foul Fruity Foul	Cystitis Diabetes mellitus UTI
Chemical nature	pH is generally slightly acidic, 6.5	Alkaline	Infections cause ammonia to form
Specific gravity	1.003–1.030—reflects amount of waste, minerals, and solids in urine	Higher—causes precipitation of solutes Lower—polyuria	Kidney stones, diabetes mellitus Diabetes insipidus
Constituent Compounds			
Protein	None or small amount	Albuminuria	Nephritis, renal failure, infection
Glucose	None	Glycosuria	Faulty carbohydrate metabolism, as in diabetes mellitus
Ketone bodies	None	Ketonuria	Diabetic acidosis
Bile and bilirubin	None	Bilirubinuria	Hepatic or gallbladder disease
Casts	None or small number of hyaline casts	Urinary casts composed of RBCs or WBCs, fat	Nephritis, renal diseases, inflammation, metal poisoning
Nitrogenous wastes	Ammonia, creatinine, urea, and uric acid	Azoturia, creatinine, and urea clearance tests disproportionate to normal BUN/creatinine ratio	Hepatic disease, renal disease
Crystals	None to trace	Acidic urine, alkaline urine, hypercalcemia, metabolism error	Not significant unless the crystals are large (stones); certain types interpreted by physician
Fat droplets	None	Lipiduria	Nephrosis

[a]Routine urinalysis is a physical, chemical, and microscopic examination of urine for abnormal elements that may help estimate renal function and provide clues of systemic disease. This table includes some important characteristics and elements screened for in basic urinalysis. Other normal constituents of urine that are studied routinely for diagnosis include calcium, urea, uric acid, creatinine, sodium chloride, hormones, potassium, magnesium, phosphates, and sulfates.
BUN, Blood urea nitrogen; *RBC*, red blood cell; *UTI*, urinary tract infection; *WBC*, white blood cell.

TABLE 11.2	Some Renal Diagnostic Tests
Test	**Designed to Evaluate**
Clearance test	Rate of glomerular filtration
Concentration and dilution tests	Functional capacity of renal tubular cells to adaptively retain and/or eliminate water
Serum creatinine and BUN	Capacity to eliminate end products of protein metabolism
Protein in urine	Permeability of glomerular membrane

BUN, Blood urea nitrogen.

body. Fig. 11.5 is a schematic representation of changes occurring in the nephron with acute poststreptococcal glomerulonephritis.

Diagnosis

Diagnosis is made on the basis of clinical findings, clinical history, and urinalysis results. Urine shows gross blood and the presence of RBCs, white blood cells (WBCs), renal tubular cells, and casts. Proteinuria may be present because of the increased permeability of the glomerular membrane. Blood tests show elevated blood urea nitrogen (BUN), hypoalbuminemia, and an elevated erythrocyte sedimentation rate. Kidney, ureters, and bladder (KUB) radiography and ultrasonography may reveal bilateral enlargement of the kidneys. Renal biopsy may help confirm the diagnosis (Fig. 11.6).

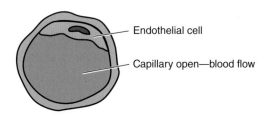

Endothelial cell

Capillary open—blood flow

Normal Glomerulus

Swollen endothelial cell and membrane

Narrow capillary lumen— GFR decreases

Immune complex deposits— inflammation

RBC and protein leaks into filtrate— hematuria and proteinuria

Mild Glomerulonephritis

Swollen cells

Immune complex deposits— severe inflammation

Cell proliferation

Little blood flow—oliguria

Severe Glomerulonephritis

• **Fig. 11.5** Schematic representation of changes occurring in the nephron with acute poststreptococcal glomerulonephritis. *GFR*, Glomerular filtration rate; *P*, protein, *RBC*, red blood cell. (From Gould B: *Pathophysiology for the health professions*, ed 4, Philadelphia, 2011, Saunders/Elsevier.)

Treatment

No specialized therapy is available for the poststreptococcal type of glomerulonephritis other than antibiotic therapy and rest. Diuretics help control edema and hypertension. Sodium intake is restricted to prevent circulatory overload and convulsions. Occasionally, corticosteroids are used if an immune reaction is the suspected cause. Patients should be instructed to consult their provider before taking any over-the-counter (OTC) medications, especially nonsteroidal antiinflammatory drugs (NSAIDs), because these agents can worsen renal function.

Prognosis

Most cases resolve within 2 weeks, and the patient experiences spontaneous recovery.

Prevention

Prevention depends on the cause of the condition. Streptococcal infections require medical intervention with antibiotics.

• **Fig. 11.6** Acute pyelonephritis. (From Stevens A, et al: *Core pathology*, ed 3, London, 2010, Mosby/Elsevier.)

Patient Teaching

Explain the underlying cause to patients and, if the patient is a child, the caregivers. Patients are instructed to complete the course of medications as prescribed. During the acute stage, bed rest should be instituted along with sodium intake restriction. Pregnant females with a history of acute glomerulonephritis require frequent medical evaluation.

Chronic Glomerulonephritis

Description

Chronic glomerulonephritis (CGN) is a slowly progressive, noninfectious disease that can lead to irreversible renal damage and renal failure. As an advanced stage of many kidney disorders, CGN results in inflammation, followed by progressive destruction of the glomeruli. This progressive destruction causes a reduction in the glomerular filtration rate (GFR), resulting in the retention of uremic poisons.

ICD-10-CM Code	N03.2 *(Chronic nephritic syndrome with diffuse membranous glomerulonephritis)* (N03.0–N03.5 = 6 codes of specificity)

Chronic glomerulonephritis is coded according to sites and types of lesions. Refer to the physician's diagnosis for site and type of lesion and to the current edition of the ICD-10-CM coding manual.

Symptoms and Signs

At first, CGN is *asymptomatic;* then subclinical progression of the disease leads to hypertension, hematuria, proteinuria, oliguria, and edema. In the later stages, with increasing renal failure, hypertension becomes severe, and azotemia develops. When the kidneys fail to remove urea from the blood (called *azotemia*), the body compensates by attempting to excrete urea through the sweat glands. Tiny crystals of urea appear on the skin; this condition is termed *uremic frost.* The patient experiences fatigue, malaise, nausea, vomiting, pruritus, and dyspnea.

Patient Screening

An appointment should be scheduled as soon as possible for any patient complaining of hematuria. Often hypertension symptoms, along with malaise and edema, are reported and indicate the need for prompt attention.

Etiology

Immune mechanisms are suspected to be a major cause of CGN; antigen-antibody complexes lodge in the glomerular capsular membrane, triggering an inflammatory response and glomerular injury. Primary renal disorders and multisystem diseases, such as systemic lupus erythematosus, are other possible causes. Toxins or medications can also cause this condition.

Diagnosis

The diagnostic studies used to detect CGN are the same as those used for acute glomerulonephritis: urinalysis, blood tests, radiographic studies, ultrasonography, and renal biopsy. The findings include signs of advanced renal insufficiency, rising BUN and serum creatinine levels, and grossly abnormal findings on urinalysis. A renal biopsy is valuable in determining the optimal treatment and the prognosis.

Treatment

The goals of treatment are to control edema, treat hypertension, and prevent congestive heart failure and uremia. The patient is given supportive measures for comfort. Medical treatment includes the administration of antihypertensives, diuretics, and antibiotics if a urinary tract infection (UTI) develops. Protein, salt (sodium [Na+] and phosphate), and fluid intake may be limited in the diet. Angiotensin-converting enzyme (ACE) inhibitors are often used to aid in the reduction of excess protein in urine. Guidance should be given to the patient to check with the health care provider before taking any OTC medications, especially NSAIDs because these medications can further worsen renal function. The patient may require dialysis (see Fig. 11.8) or may be a candidate for kidney transplantation.

Prognosis

Prognosis varies depending on the extent of destruction of the kidneys and the patient's response to therapy. Eventually, CGN will lead to end-stage renal disease (ESRD; Fig. 11.7). Dialysis may help the patient until kidney transplantation can be performed.

Prevention

Prompt treatment of acute glomerulonephritis, diabetes, and hypertension can help in the prevention of CGN.

Patient Teaching

Stress the importance of compliance with treatment regimens to reduce hypertension and the importance of seeking

• **Fig. 11.7** End-stage glomerulonephritis. (From Damjanov I: *Pathology for the health professions*, St. Louis, 2017, Elsevier.)

medical attention if needed. When dialysis is necessary, encourage the patient and the family to consider support groups. Advise patients to take diuretics in the morning to avoid disruption of sleep at night.

Nephrotic Syndrome (Nephrosis)

Description

Nephrotic syndrome, a disease of the basement membrane of the glomerulus, is secondary to a number of renal diseases and a variety of systemic disorders. Nephrotic syndrome encompasses a group of symptoms sometimes referred to as *protein-losing kidney.*

ICD-10-CM Code	N04.4 *(Nephrotic syndrome with diffuse endocapillary proliferative glomerulonephritis)* (N04.0–N04.5 = 6 codes of specificity)

Nephrotic syndrome is coded according to sites and types of lesions. Refer to the physician's diagnosis for site and type of lesion and to the current edition of the ICD-10-CM coding manual.

Symptoms and Signs

The patient with nephrotic syndrome loses excessive amounts of protein, mainly albumin, in urine (proteinuria). The excessive loss of protein in urine results in depressed plasma protein levels (hypoalbuminemia). Glomerular filtration becomes diminished, and water and sodium are retained, resulting in edema and hypertension. The syndrome includes microscopic or gross hematuria, hyperlipidemia, and a susceptibility to infections.

Nephrotic syndrome causes the patient to feel lethargic and depressed, with a loss of appetite. Abdominal pain may be present. There is also an increase in the chance of blood clots.

Dialysis and Kidney Transplantation

In the United States, ESRD affects thousands of people each year. In renal failure, the kidneys no longer can process blood and form urine. Therapy should begin before the development of ultimately fatal uremic symptoms. Dialysis or kidney transplantation, if successful, offers rehabilitation and extended life to patients with ESRD.

Dialysis

Dialysis filters out unwanted elements from blood by diffusion across a semipermeable membrane; the healthy kidneys usually remove these wastes. Thus the proper fluid, electrolyte, and acid-base balances are maintained in the body. Two methods used to perform blood dialysis are hemodialysis and peritoneal dialysis (Fig. 11.8).

• **Fig. 11.8** Dialysis. (A) Hemodialysis. (B) Peritoneal dialysis. (C) Principles of dialysis. *B*, Bicarbonate ion (buffer); *H+*, acids; *K+*, potassium ion; *N*, nitrogen wastes (urea); *Na+*, sodium ion; *P*, protein; *red dot*, blood cells. (A, From Ignatavicius D: *Medical-surgical nursing: patient-centered collaborative care*, ed 6, St. Louis, Saunders; B From Proctor D, et al: Kinn's the medical assistant, ed 13, St. Louis, 2017, Elsevier; C From Gould B: *Pathophysiology for the health professions*, ed 3, Philadelphia, 2005, Saunders/Elsevier.)

Beginning dialysis
(Blood enters)

No movement of cells and protein

Diffusion

Hi → Lo concentration

Osmosis and hydrostatic pressure

End of dialysis
(Blood leaves)

Time →

Semipermeable membrane

C

• **Fig. 11.8** (Cont'd)

Hemodialysis

Hemodialysis can take place in the patient's home or at a hospital. It removes impurities or wastes from the patient's blood by using an artificial kidney (hemodialyzer). Access to the bloodstream is created surgically in the arm, leg, or subclavian vein with an internal fistula, which allows blood to pass from the patient's body to the semipermeable membrane in the machine. The cleansed blood then returns to the patient in a procedure that takes 3 to 4 hours. The patient usually receives two or three sessions a week.

Peritoneal Dialysis

Peritoneal dialysis is carried out in the patient's own body with the use of a **dialysate** solution and the peritoneal membrane to filter out harmful toxins and excessive fluid. The clean dialyzing fluid passes into the peritoneal cavity through a permanent indwelling peritoneal catheter, and wastes diffuse across the peritoneal membrane into the fluid. The contaminated fluid then is drained and replaced with fresh fluid.

- Continuous ambulatory peritoneal dialysis takes place without a machine by allowing the solution to drain by gravity into a dialysis bag worn around the waist. This procedure takes about 15 minutes and is repeated three to four times a day and once at night.
- Continuous cycling peritoneal dialysis takes place while the patient sleeps, with the use of a cycling machine.
- Intermittent peritoneal dialysis takes several hours, is performed three to five times a week, and usually is done in a clinic.
- See Fig. 11.8C.

Continuous Renal Replacement Therapy

This type of dialysis, also called *hemofiltration*, is performed in a hospital setting. This typically takes place in the intensive care unit for patients with acute renal failure (ARF). Continuous renal replacement therapy dialysis takes place 24 hours each day, every day.

Kidney Transplantation

Kidney transplantation is the surgical placement of a donor kidney into a patient with irreversible renal failure. Used synergistically with clinical dialysis, kidney transplantation is one of medicine's success stories. Kidney transplantation leads the field of organ replacement, with many patients on waiting lists. **Immunosuppressive** agents are used to prevent or treat rejection syndrome. Sophisticated evaluation of the donor and the recipient to find a good match for human leukocyte antigen offers the best chances for a good prognosis.

Donor shortages continue and en bloc kidney transplants are performed when small recipients receive two kidneys, abdominal vena cava and aorta, ureters and bladder from the small donor. In some cases, en bloc kidney transplant only involves the kidneys, aorta and vena cava tissues. Current research is exploring the option of splitting the kidney prior to transplantation so that two patients can benefit from one kidney. This is, however, very rare in current practice.

Patient Screening

As previously mentioned, patients complaining of bloody urine that is accompanied by edema, headache, and flank or pelvic pain require prompt medical attention.

Etiology

Nephrotic syndrome is caused by increased permeability of the glomerulus, indicating renal damage. This condition may occur after an attack of glomerulonephritis, or it may be the result of exposure to certain toxins or drugs, pregnancy, or kidney transplantation (Box 11.1). Metabolic diseases, such as diabetes mellitus; certain infections; and allergic reactions are conditions that may lead to nephrotic syndrome.

Diagnosis

Diagnosis is based on the clinical findings and the presence of gross proteinuria and lipiduria (the presence of fatty casts) in a 24-hour urine specimen. Abnormal blood study serum values, including hypoalbuminemia and hyperlipidemia, support the diagnosis. If a renal tumor is suspected, renal biopsy with histologic study is indicated.

Treatment

Effective treatment begins by addressing the underlying cause. The dietary intake of protein is adjusted according to the GFR. Diuretics and decreased sodium intake help control edema. The use of ACE inhibitors is helpful in treating hypertension and usually reduces protein loss. A course of corticosteroids, such as prednisone, may have the positive effect of controlling proteinuria in some patients. Urine output must be monitored.

Prognosis

Prognosis varies depending on the extent of kidney destruction and the patient's response to therapy. There is no cure; however, some children who are diagnosed will "outgrow" the condition in late teens to early adulthood.

Prevention

Prompt treatment of glomerulonephritis is important to prevent this condition. Avoiding exposure to certain toxins or drugs helps prevent nephrotic syndrome, as does prompt treatment after exposure to these toxins (see Box 11.1). Monitoring kidney function in pregnant females and any patients with metabolic diseases (e.g., diabetes mellitus), certain infections, and allergic reactions may assist the physician in detecting malfunction early on, and thus treatment can be instituted early on.

Patient Teaching

Advise patients and their families to contact the physician immediately if any exacerbation of symptoms is noted. Encourage patients to remain active, to exercise, and to practice good skin care. Refer patients to a dietitian for instruction on planning a high-protein, low-sodium diet as prescribed.

Acute Renal Failure (Acute Kidney Injury)

Description

ARF also known as acute kidney injury (AKI) is a very sudden and severe reduction in renal function, which usually occurs quickly, in a matter of a few days. This is a common clinical emergency because nitrogenous waste products begin to accumulate in blood quickly.

ICD-10-CM Code	N17 *(Acute kidney failure)* (N17.0–N17.9 = 5 codes of specificity)

Acute renal failure is coded according to sites and types of lesions. Refer to the physician's diagnosis for site and type of lesion and to the current edition of the ICD-10-CM coding manual.

• BOX 11.1	Nephrotoxic Agents

Solvents	Neomycin
Carbon tetrachloride	Phenazopyridine
Methanol	Nonsteroidal antiinflammatory
Ethylene glycol	drugs
Heavy metals	Iodinated radiographic contrast
Lead	media
Arsenic	Antineoplastic agents
Mercury	Miscellaneous compounds
Pesticides	Acetaminophen
Antibiotics	Amphetamines
Kanamycin	Heroin
Gentamicin	Silicon
Polymyxin B	Cyclosporine
Amphotericin B	Poisonous mushrooms
Colistin	

Modified from Monahan F, et al: *Phipps' medical-surgical nursing, health and illness perspectives*, ed 8, St. Louis, 2007, Mosby.

Symptoms and Signs

The initial symptoms of AKI include oliguria, gastrointestinal disturbances, headache, drowsiness, confusion, and other alterations in the level of consciousness. A host of other symptoms can occur, depending on the underlying cause, the degree of impairment, and BUN levels.

Patient Screening

In many instances, patients with AKI are already under a physician's care or may even be receiving treatment as inpatients when initial symptoms occur. If not, anyone reporting sudden onset of these symptoms requires prompt attention.

Etiology

The causes of AKI are classified as those that result in diminished blood flow to the kidneys (e.g., circulatory shock or heart failure), those that involve intrarenal damage or disease (e.g., glomerulonephritis), and those that result from mechanical obstruction of urine flow. Of special concern is intrarenal damage, which can be prevented by control of exposure to substances known to be nephrotoxic, including drugs, insecticides, organic solvents, and cleaning agents (see Box 11.1). Whatever the cause, sudden renal dysfunction disrupts other body systems and, if left untreated, can lead to death. Certain antibiotics (i.e., aminoglycosides, vancomycin) can cause AKI in patients who have predisposing factors (i.e., existing kidney problems and old age) (Fig. 11.9).

Diagnosis

Blood tests and urinalysis reveal many abnormal findings associated with oliguria and the retention of nitrogenous wastes. BUN, serum creatinine, and potassium levels are elevated in the blood. Other diagnostic studies include renal ultrasonography, radiography (computed tomography [CT] or magnetic resonance imaging [MRI]) and intravenous pyelography (IVP). Monitoring of balanced

• **Fig. 11.9** Causes of acute renal failure. (A) Nephrotoxins. (B) Ischemia. (C) Pyelonephritis. *GFR,* Glomerular filtration rate. (From VanMeter: *Gould's pathophysiology for the health professions*, ed 5, St. Louis, 2015, Saunders.)

fluid intake and output is also important in determining kidney function.

Treatment

Determining the cause of AKI is crucial in the course of medical management to reduce the risk of permanent kidney damage. The ultimate goal is to reverse the decreased renal perfusion. All body systems are monitored and supported, as needed, through the uremic crisis. The patient may be evaluated for dialysis. Fluid intake and output are balanced to prevent overload. It is important to carefully manage nutritional support to ensure that protein is being replaced in the right proportions to prevent metabolic acidosis. Initiating a high-carbohydrate/low-protein diet will accomplish this. Sodium and potassium intake are controlled as well. Drug therapy may include antihypertensives, diuretics, intravenous (IV) fluids, and antiinfective agents because infection is a common complication of AKI.

Prognosis

In many cases, with prompt treatment AKI is reversible, and recovery is rapid and complete. Sudden renal dysfunction disrupts other body systems and, if left untreated, can lead to death.

Prevention

Prevention methods vary, depending on the causative factors. Promptly treating circulatory shock or heart failure and identifying conditions involving intrarenal damage or disease and those that result from mechanical obstruction of urine flow help prevent AKI. Additionally, controlling exposure to substances known to be nephrotoxic helps prevent acute renal injury.

Patient Teaching

Encourage patients who have recovered from AKI to be cognizant of the causative factors and aware of possible sources of toxins. Warn them of signs and symptoms of renal failure. Instruct them to immediately report such symptoms to the provider. Dietary guidelines should be discussed. Education materials should be shared with the patient.

Chronic Kidney Disease

Description

Chronic kidney disease (CKD) results from the gradual and progressive loss of nephrons, with irreversible loss of renal function and gradual onset of uremia. The systemic effects eventually can manifest in any and all body systems.

ICD-10-CM Code	N18 *(Chronic kidney disease)* (N18.1–18.9 = 7 codes of specificity)

Referral to the current edition of the ICD-10-CM coding manual is recommended to identify the manifestations of this disorder.

Symptoms and Signs

The patient with CKD may feel weak, tired, and lethargic. As the condition progresses, fluid retention in the body results in hypertension and edema. As uremic syndrome worsens, many other symptoms and signs are generated: arrhythmias, muscle weakness, dyspnea, metabolic acidosis, ulceration of the gastrointestinal mucosa, and hair and skin changes.

Patient Screening

Patients with chronic renal failure (CRF) probably have been diagnosed already, and routine follow-up visits may have been scheduled. Consulted specialist should schedule appointments as soon as possible.

Etiology

There are numerous causes of CRF CKD, including primary diseases or infections of the kidneys, such as glomerulonephritis, **pyelonephritis**, and polycystic kidneys. Often, CRF is the end stage of chronic renal diseases or chronic obstruction of the outflow of urine.

Diagnosis

Blood studies show elevated BUN, serum creatinine, and potassium levels, along with decreased hemoglobin and hematocrit levels. Urinalysis is grossly abnormal, with hematuria, excessive protein, glucose, leukocytes, and casts. The 24-hour urine volume has greatly decreased. Diagnostic studies include KUB radiography, renal ultrasonography, kidney scanning, IVP, and renal arteriography.

Treatment

The underlying cause, if known, must be treated. The patient is evaluated for dialysis or kidney transplantation to prolong life. Diet and nutritional modifications help control protein and sodium intakes to reduce the work of the diseased kidneys. Fluid intake and output are monitored and regulated. Drug therapy includes administration of diuretics, antihypertensives, antiinfectives, and antiemetics. Nausea, vomiting, and loss of appetite may be alleviated by a change in diet that includes more carbohydrate and fat calories and fewer protein calories. Severe anemia can occur with CKD, and often, the administration of erythropoietin, a protein that stimulates bone marrow, can help form new RBCs. Bone degeneration also can result from CKD, and calcitriol, a form of vitamin D, can be given to prevent bones from weakening.

Prognosis

The prognosis for CKD varies, depending on the etiology. No total cure for this condition is known. Preventing complications and providing supportive care are important.

Prevention

Promptly treating AKI and recognizing and treating the cause of intrarenal damage or diseases that result from mechanical obstruction of urine flow will help prevent further damage. Additionally, controlling exposure to substances known to be nephrotoxic can help prevent AKI and subsequent chronic failure.

Patient Teaching

Provide a list of support resources. Help them become aware of sources of possible toxic exposures that contribute to renal disease. Generate print-on-demand electronic materials, when possible, as teaching tools. Advise patients to consult their provider before taking any OTC medications, especially NSAIDs.

Pyelonephritis

Description

Pyelonephritis, the most common type of renal disease, is inflammation of the renal pelvis and connective tissues of one or both kidneys.

ICD-10-CM Code	N12 *(Tubulointerstitial nephritis, not specified as acute or chronic)* N10 *(Acute tubulointerstitial nephritis)* N11.0–N11.9 *(Chronic obstructive tubulointerstitial nephritis)*

Pyelonephritis is coded according to site and type of lesion. Refer to the physician's diagnosis for site and type of lesion and to the current edition of the ICD-10-CM coding manual.

Symptoms and Signs

Pyelonephritis occurs when pus collects in the renal pelvis, resulting in the formation of abscesses. The patient experiences rapid onset of fever, chills, nausea and vomiting, and flank (lumbar) pain. This usually is preceded by a UTI with urinary frequency or urgency and dysuria. The patient may report a foul odor with urination. Tenderness is noted in the suprapubic region, the abdomen becomes rigid, and palpation may reveal tender, enlarged kidneys. Urinalysis results show abnormal constituents, including urinary casts, nitrites, and leukocytes.

Patient Screening

Patients complaining of bloody or foul-smelling urine, accompanied by fever, chills, nausea, vomiting, and pelvic and flank pain, require prompt medical attention.

Etiology

Bacteria that ascend from the lower urinary tract to the kidneys usually cause pyelonephritis; it is less commonly caused by hematogenous or lymphatic spread of bacteria. Obstruction and stasis of urine by renal calculi (kidney stones), tumors, and benign prostatic hypertrophy predispose the kidneys to infection. Stasis of urine allows invading bacteria, usually *Escherichia coli*, to cause the infectious process. Pregnancy can also make one prone to pyelonephritis. Females are more at risk of bacterial contamination into the urinary tract. Catheterization or diagnostic procedures, such as endoscopic (cystoscopic) examination, can directly introduce organisms into the urinary bladder. The infection then moves upward in the urinary tract (ascending infection) to one or both kidneys (Fig. 11.10).

Diagnosis

The diagnosis is made by assessing the clinical findings and through urinalysis of a clean-catch urine specimen that shows increased WBCs and RBCs and the presence of bacteria, leukocytes, proteins, and casts. Blood culture and urine culture can identify the causative organism. Radiographic studies reveal kidneys that appear swollen or enlarged.

Treatment

The recommended antibiotic treatment for pyelonephritis is a 14-day treatment of trimethoprim and sulfamethoxazole, or a 7-day treatment of a fluoroquinolone such as ciprofloxacin. Increased fluid intake to dilute urine, along with bed rest, is urged. Unless patients are at high risk for UTIs, they respond well to treatment without recurrences. When pyelonephritis recurs, certain tests (e.g., IVP and/or renal ultrasonography) need to be performed to determine whether a renal abnormality (e.g., vesicoureteral reflux) is present. In more complicated cases, surgery may be indicated to relieve an obstruction or correct an anomaly.

Prognosis

Early detection and prompt treatment usually result in a good outcome. Untreated and recurrent pyelonephritis may be the cause of hypertension, bacteremia, and chronic pyelonephritis, leading to permanent kidney damage.

Prevention

Prevention includes drinking eight glasses of water a day. Those with a history of pyelonephritis are advised to void frequently. Proper use of toilet tissue after voiding (wiping from front to back for female patients) is important in the prevention of infection.

Patient Teaching

Patients who begin to experience symptoms should increase their fluid intake, especially of water. Females should be encouraged to wipe the perineum from the front to the back to avoid spreading fecal matter from the rectum to the urethral meatus.

Hydronephrosis

Description

Hydronephrosis is an abnormal dilation of the renal pelvis caused by pressure from urine that cannot flow past an obstruction in the urinary tract (Figs. 11.11 and 11.12).

ICD-10-CM Code	N13.3 (Other and unspecified hydronephrosis) (N13.30–N13.39 = 2 codes of specificity)

Symptoms and Signs

When the obstruction is severe and prolonged, fibrotic changes and loss of function of the involved nephrons occur. Hydronephrosis is usually a chronic condition characterized by the destruction of the kidneys that transpires without pain or symptoms. Its detection is often incidental, occurring during a radiographic examination or ultrasonography of the abdomen. A vague backache, diminished urine output, and difficulty urinating might be the only symptoms that the patient can identify. If an infection accompanies the condition, the patient may experience fever, chills, hematuria, and pyuria, and the kidney may be palpable.

Patient Screening

Many patients with hydronephrosis are asymptomatic for some time and request an appointment only when they begin to feel sick. A history of kidney stones may be noted by the patient.

As with many other kidney disorders, prompt medical attention is required for these patients.

Etiology

Dilation of the renal pelvis is caused by buildup of pressure in the kidneys due to an obstruction. The cause of the obstruction could be renal calculi, tumors, inflammation caused by infections, prostatic hyperplasia (enlargement), bladder tumors, blood clot, or congenital abnormalities. During pregnancy, the enlarged uterus can cause hydronephrosis.

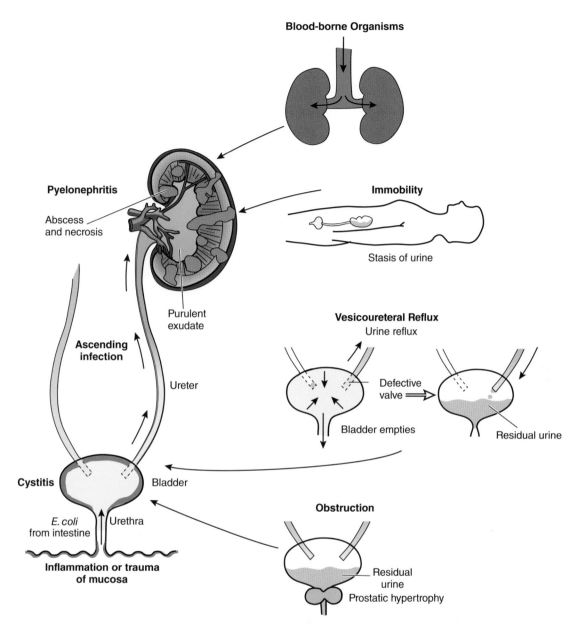

• **Fig. 11.10** Causes of infection in the urinary tract. (From Gould B: *Pathophysiology for the health professions*, ed 4, Philadelphia, 2011, Saunders/Elsevier.)

Diagnosis

The first indication of hydronephrosis is usually the result of investigating other abdominal structures. Follow-up contrast studies of the ureters and the kidneys need to be completed. Retrograde pyelography is necessary. Cystoscopy to rule out an obstruction by a tumor of the bladder or prostate is helpful (Fig. 11.13).

Treatment

The treatment of hydronephrosis depends on the underlying cause of the obstruction and the duration of the condition. When obstruction is discovered early, the source can be identified and removed by surgical intervention. A concurrent infection necessitates antibiotic therapy. When surgical intervention is not an option and/or the obstruction cannot be relieved, a nephrostomy tube may be inserted.

Prognosis

Once the obstruction causing the hydronephrosis has been resolved, the kidneys may return to normal function. If hydronephrosis has been present for an extended period, permanent damage may result.

Prevention

Preventing kidney stones and the subsequent obstruction of urine flow they can cause also helps prevent

• **Fig. 11.11** (A) Renal calculi and hydronephrosis. (B) Hydronephrosis with dilation of the renal pelvis and calyces and atrophy of renal tissue. (A, From Gould B: *Pathophysiology for the health professions*, ed 4, Philadelphia, 2011, Saunders/Elsevier; B From Cotran RS, Kumar V, Collins T: *Robbins pathologic basis of disease*, ed 6, Philadelphia, 1999, Saunders/Elsevier.)

• **Fig. 11.12** Renal calculi.

hydronephrosis. Urine and blood chemistry measurements and stone analysis provide clues that can help determine which preventive measures are likely to prevent recurring kidney stone formation. Additionally, modifications to the diet, increased exercise, and adequate fluid intake minimize the chance of stone formation. Prompt treatment of an enlarged prostate may prevent obstructions and the resulting hydronephrosis.

Patient Teaching

Encourage patients to follow the suggested diet and fluid regimen to prevent kidney stones. If a nephrostomy tube is in place, care instructions may be necessary.

Renal Calculi

Description

Renal calculi are stones in the kidney or elsewhere in the urinary tract formed by the concentration of various mineral salts (see Figs. 11.11–11.13).

ICD-10-CM Code	N20 (*Calculus of kidney and ureter*)
	(N20.0–N21.9 = 8 codes of specificity)

Renal calculi are coded according to location. Refer to the physician's diagnosis for location of the calculus and to the current edition of the ICD-10-CM coding manual.

Symptoms and Signs

Kidney stones can be solitary or multiple and vary in size. A larger stone formed in the shape of the renal pelvis is known as a *staghorn calculus* (Fig. 11.14). Small stones can be passed spontaneously, unnoticed. The patient's symptoms vary, depending on the degree of obstruction. If infection or blockage caused by the calculi is present, the patient experiences sudden severe pain in the flank area, known as *renal colic*, with urinary urgency and other urinary symptoms. Other symptoms include nausea and vomiting, hematuria, fever, chills, and abdominal distention. Blood in urine can be the result of trauma caused by the presence of small stones, which may be gravel-like in consistency, or larger stones, such as staghorn calculi. Hydronephrosis can develop if urine is prevented from flowing past the calculi.

Cystoscopy

Cystoscopy allows direct examination and treatment of the urinary bladder (see Fig. 11.13). A cystoscope is inserted through the urethra; this instrument has its own lighting system, a viewing scope, and a passage for catheters and surgical devices. Cystoscopy is used to obtain biopsy specimens for diagnosis and to remove stones or tumors.

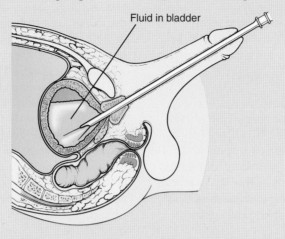

Fluid in bladder

• **Fig. 11.13** Cystoscopy. (From *Mosby's dictionary of medicine, nursing & health professions*, ed 8, St. Louis, 2013, Mosby.)

Staghorn calculus

A

B

• **Fig. 11.14** Staghorn calculi. (A) Drawing of a kidney with staghorn calculi. (B, From Stevens A, et al: *Core pathology*, ed 3, London, 2010, Mosby/Elsevier.)

Patient Screening

Pain caused by a kidney stone should be considered an emergency situation. If these patients cannot be seen in the office as soon as possible, they should be referred to an emergency care facility where they can receive analgesic intervention. The patient experiencing sudden onset of severe flank pain, pelvic pressure, accompanied by nausea and vomiting, requires immediate observation and treatment.

Etiology

Often, the cause of calculi is unknown, although a hereditary tendency for development of certain types of stones has been noted. Kidney stones are formed when there is an excessive amount of calcium or uric acid present in urine. Males are more prone to kidney stones compared with females. Calculi form when sources of crystals are found in urine, along with the absence of crystalline inhibitors, and urine is supersaturated with poorly soluble substances.

Risk factors include prolonged dehydration, prolonged immobilization, infection, urinary stasis from obstruction, long-term ingestion of certain medications, and metabolic factors, such as hyperparathyroidism and gout. (Gout is discussed in Chapter 7.)

Diagnosis

The diagnosis of renal calculi is made on the basis of family history, clinical findings, urinalysis, KUB radiographic studies, intravenous urography, renal ultrasonography, and CT. The patient is encouraged to strain the urine to capture any stones that are passed during urination so that the stones can be analyzed in a laboratory. The possible existence of metabolic disorders can be investigated by using blood and urine tests.

Treatment

The goals of medical care are to remove the calculi, treat pain and infection, and resolve the causative factors. These measures should prevent permanent kidney damage and the recurrence of calculi.

The treatment begins with analgesic therapy and hydration during the initial evaluation. Sometimes an alpha-blocker, such as Flomax, may be prescribed. These work by relaxing the muscles of the bladder, allowing the stone to pass. The location and size of the calculi indicate the course of treatment. Small calculi (<5 mm) may be treated with just observation and fluid hydration in the hope that the stones will pass spontaneously. Large calculi can be removed by any of several surgical procedures. Attempts are made to crush stones that are (1) too large to pass down the ureter, (2) lodged in the pelvis of the kidney, or (3) trapped in the proximal portion of the ureter. Extracorporeal shock wave lithotripsy is a procedure that breaks apart (crushes) the stones, thus allowing the small particles to be flushed out of the body naturally.

A surgical procedure using a ureteroscope to capture the stone in a basket and remove it is attempted for stones trapped in the distal aspect of a ureter. If the attempt to capture the stone is unsuccessful, electrohydraulic lithotripsy (EHL) or laser lithotripsy is used to attempt to break the stone apart into small particles that can be flushed out of the system. This procedure is usually done with the patient under general anesthesia and with the aid of fluoroscopy. After removal of the calculus, the ureter is visualized via the ureteroscope, and often the pelvis of the kidney is also inspected for any scarring, damage, or residual stone fragments. A stent that extends into the urinary bladder is placed in the pelvis of the kidney as a means of preventing edema and spasms of the ureter and subsequent occlusion of the ureter. The stent is removed in 2 to 5 days.

Stones in the urinary bladder often pass spontaneously. When this does not happen, an attempt to remove bladder stones is made during cystoscopy. When the previously mentioned procedures are unsuccessful in removing the calculi, surgical intervention in the form of percutaneous nephrolithotomy may be indicated to remove the stones before permanent damage is caused. A small incision is made into the kidney, and the stone is shattered by using ultrasound or EHL. Rarely, when the aforementioned procedures are unsuccessful, a surgical incision of the kidney is performed to remove the stones.

Depending on the chemical composition, some kidney stones can be dissolved or prevented from forming. Often the patient may pass small or microscopic stones naturally and without pain. The patient is encouraged to drink 8 to 12 glasses of water a day and may be given diuretics to prevent urinary stasis. Patients are encouraged to strain their urine to catch any stones or particles of stones that may be passed spontaneously. In that way, analysis of the calculi composition is made possible, which can help direct preventive measures.

Prognosis

The prognosis is good after the successful removal or spontaneous passage of the stones. However, additional stone formation is possible.

Prevention

Urine and blood chemistry measurements and stone analysis provide clues as to which preventive measures are likely to help. Prevention includes modification of diet, increased exercise, and adequate fluid intake to minimize the risk of stone formation in the future.

Patient Teaching

Instruct patients on the proper way to strain urine. Encourage intake of at least eight glasses of water a day. Explain the risk factors, such as UTI, stasis of urine, prolonged dehydration, prolonged immobilization, and long-term ingestion of certain medications. Patients should avoid food high in oxalates, purine, and phosphorus (Box 11.2). Referral to a dietitian for advice on dietary control is helpful. Some physicians prefer limiting the intake of calcium, whereas others place no restrictions on calcium intake.

Infectious Cystitis and Urethritis

Description

Cystitis, inflammation of the urinary bladder, and urethritis, inflammation of the urethra, are two common forms of lower UTI.

ICD-10-CM Code	N30.90 (Cystitis, unspecified without hematuria)
	N30.91 (Cystitis, unspecified with hematuria)

(N30.00–N30.91 = 14 codes of
specificity)
N34.1 *(Nonspecific urethritis)*
N34.2 *(Other urethritis)*
(N34.0–N34.3 = 4 codes of
specificity)

Cystitis and urethritis are coded according to type of infectious process. Refer to the physician's diagnosis for type of infectious process and to the current edition of the ICD-10-CM coding manual.

Symptoms and Signs

The inflammation and infection cause the patient to experience urinary urgency and frequency, dysuria, and possibly even incontinence. Patients often complain of pressure in the pelvis, pain in the pelvic region and low back, spasm of the bladder, fever and chills, and a burning sensation with urination. The color of the urine may be dark yellow, or pink or red if blood is present.

Patient Screening

Patients experiencing the classic symptoms of pain, frequency, and urgency require prompt attention. Advise them that they will need to provide a urine specimen on arrival at the office.

Etiology

The usual cause of cystitis and urethritis is an ascending bacterial invasion of the urinary tract. The most common causative microorganism is *Escherichia coli*, followed by *Klebsiella, Enterobacter, Proteus*, and *Pseudomonas* species. Some sexually transmitted diseases can cause cystitis and urethritis. Other causes of these conditions are viruses, fungi, parasites, and inflammation caused by chemotherapy

or radiation. Lesions can develop in the bladder secondary to inflammation, thereby intensifying the symptoms.

Diagnosis

The diagnosis is determined by evaluating the clinical findings, urinalysis of a clean-catch urine specimen, urine culture, and cystoscopy. Urinalysis shows dark yellow, pink, or red urine with abnormal urinary sediment and possibly blood and leukocytes. Microscopic examination of the urine specimen shows RBCs (occult blood), increased numbers of epithelial cells or leukocytes, bacteria, and nitrites. Urine may have a foul odor. The urine culture grows the causative agent for identification. Cystoscopy shows a reddened, inflamed bladder wall (Fig. 11.15). Tenderness in the suprapubic region and pain in the lower back may be elicited by palpation.

Treatment

Treatment consists of organism-specific antibiotic or urinary antiseptic therapy, such as trimethoprim-sulfamethoxazole, or nitrofurantoin. Penicillin derivatives are used to treat complicated cystitis, which tends to recur often. Treatment is a minimum of 3 to 5 days of medication for uncomplicated infections and 7 to 10 days for recurring infections. Antibiotics used to treat UTIs in females may affect the normal vaginal flora, causing yeast infections. Phenazopyridine (Pyridium), a urinary analgesic, also can be given to decrease dysuria or painful urination. Increased fluid intake and voiding frequently are encouraged.

Prognosis

Most lower UTIs respond well to antibiotic drug therapy.

Prevention

Prevention includes drinking eight glasses of water a day. Those who have a history of lower UTIs are advised to void frequently. Wiping from front to back after urinating is important in preventing infection. Females with frequent cystitis and urethritis are advised to use prophylactic antibiotic therapy (i.e., nitrofurantoin [Macrobid]) either

• **Fig. 11.15** Acute cystitis. The mucosa of the bladder is red and swollen. (From Damjanov I: *Pathology for the health professions*, St. Louis, 2017, Elsevier.)

consistently or directly after intercourse. Postmenopausal females are at higher risk for UTIs than other females.

Patient Teaching

Advise females to void (urinate) after engaging in sexual intercourse. Patients who begin to experience symptoms should increase their fluid intake, especially of water. Females should be encouraged to wipe the perineum from the front to the back to avoid spreading fecal matter from the rectum to the urinary meatus.

Diabetic Nephropathy

Description

Diabetic **nephropathy** refers to the renal changes resulting from diabetes mellitus, a systemic endocrine disease caused by the failure of the pancreas to release enough insulin into the body (see Diabetes Mellitus in Chapter 4). These changes, called **glomerulosclerosis**, can be expected to occur eventually in all patients with insulin-dependent (type 1) diabetes, which increases their morbidity and mortality. Additionally, many patients with noninsulin-dependent (type 2) diabetes also can develop this kidney disorder.

ICD-10-CM Code	E11.29 *(Type 2 diabetes mellitus with other diabetic kidney complication)* (E11.21–E11.29 = 3 codes of specificity) N08 *(Glomerular disorders in diseases classified elsewhere)*

It is important to code diabetes with renal manifestations first and then list the nephrotic syndrome.

Symptoms and Signs

Clinical manifestations, once they begin, include urinary retention, hypertension, nausea, and protein in the urine. UTI and pyelonephritis are common complications. Although nephropathy is more likely to develop in those afflicted by insulin-dependent diabetes mellitus, all patients with diabetes whose blood glucose levels and blood pressure are not controlled are at risk for this irreversible disorder.

Patient Screening

Those diagnosed with diabetes usually are scheduled for routine assessments by their health care provider. Patients with diabetes who report urinary tract symptoms require prompt assessment and should be scheduled as soon as possible.

Etiology

Diabetic glomerulosclerosis is a complication of diabetes mellitus; lesions of the glomeruli eventually cause the filtration rate to decrease. Insufficient control of blood glucose levels and high blood pressure in patients with diabetes may hasten the deterioration of renal function.

Diagnosis

Blood tests reveal an elevated BUN level and an increase in cholesterol levels. Urinalysis shows protein and leukocytes in urine. Urinary microalbumin signals the presence of urinary albumin, an indication of nephropathy. Hypertension is another factor to be noted. The diagnosis is confirmed by imaging, radiographic studies, and renal biopsy.

Treatment

In patients with diabetes, susceptibility to renal failure varies, so the treatment plan must be individualized. Medical control of diabetes, blood pressure, and infections is important. Drug intervention includes an ACE inhibitor for blood pressure control and prolongation of proper kidney function. Fluid intake and output should be balanced; diuretics may be prescribed if needed. Dialysis or evaluation for kidney transplantation may be part of the long-term plan.

Prognosis

Early detection and treatment lead to the best outcome. There is no cure, and when blood glucose and blood pressure are not kept under control, the outcome becomes bleaker. ESRD is the final outcome.

Prevention

Close monitoring of both blood glucose levels and blood pressure, with appropriate treatment intervention, is helpful for all patients with diabetes. Monitoring urine microalbumin is recommended yearly for all patients with diabetes.

Patient Teaching

Make patients with diabetes aware of the importance of maintaining blood glucose at appropriate levels. Also, advise them about the importance of monitoring blood pressure and keeping it at acceptable levels. Compliance with prescribed drug therapy is important.

Polycystic Kidney Disease

Description

Polycystic kidney disease is a slowly progressive and irreversible disorder in which normal renal tissue is replaced by multiple grapelike cysts (Fig. 11.16). The condition is bilateral, with cysts forming from dilated nephrons and collecting ducts. Eventually the kidneys become grossly enlarged, with compression of surrounding tissue leading to impaired renal function and renal failure.

ICD-10-CM Code	Q61.3 *(Polycystic kidney, unspecified)* (Q61.1–Q61.3 = 4 codes of specificity) Q61.2 *(Polycystic kidney, adult type)* Q61.19 *(Other polycystic kidney, infantile type)*

• **Fig. 11.16** Adult polycystic disease. (From Stevens A, et al: *Core pathology*, ed 3, London, 2010, Mosby/Elsevier.)

Symptoms and Signs

As the kidneys become dilated, they are palpable on physical examination. The patient experiences lumbar pain, abdominal pain and tenderness, hematuria, and systemic hypertension and is more prone to renal infections and renal calculi. These patients usually experience chronic high blood pressure and kidney infections.

Patient Screening

Patients complaining of blood in their urine accompanied by edema, headache, and flank or pelvic pain, require prompt medical attention.

Etiology

Polycystic kidney disease is inherited but may not manifest until adolescence or adulthood. It is not clearly understood why the cysts form. Acquired cystic kidney disease (noninherited) is a sequela of long-term kidney disease and/or long-term dialysis. Autosomal recessive polycystic kidney disease appears in infants and children and progresses rapidly to ESRD and death. Autosomal dominant polycystic kidney disease usually has its onset during the middle-age years.

Diagnosis

The diagnosis is made by evaluating the clinical findings and the results of renal function tests, such as urinalysis, which shows microscopic blood, proteinuria, and leukocytes. Radiography, abdominal CT, abdominal MRI, and IVP show enlarged kidneys with irregular outlines and a spidery appearance throughout.

Treatment

Treatment for this ESRD consists of managing symptoms. Dialysis and kidney transplantation are two options for the treatment. The kidneys may have to be surgically removed if the patient has intractable pain, renal stones, or persistent infections. Management of UTIs is necessary, as is the management of hypertension.

Prognosis

At the present time, no cure for polycystic disease is known.

Prevention

The majority of cases are inherited; therefore there is no prevention of inherited polycystic kidney disease. Acquired polycystic kidney disease, as a sequela to long-term kidney disease and/or dialysis, also has no means of prevention.

Patient Teaching

Suggest to patients and their families that they seek out community resources for those with kidney disease. Online or in-person support groups with other people dealing with a similar situation may provide emotional support. Be prepared to answer questions about the disease process and outcomes. Advise patients that emptying the bladder regularly is helpful in preventing UTIs. Monitoring urinary output, blood pressure, and weight may be recommended. The patient should also avoid becoming fatigued.

Neurogenic Bladder

Description

Neurogenic bladder is a dysfunction of the urinary bladder that causes difficulty with emptying the bladder or urinary incontinence.

ICD-10-CM Code	N31.9 *(Neuromuscular dysfunction of bladder, unspecified)*
	(N31.0–N31.9 = 5 codes of specificity)

Symptoms and Signs

Symptoms may include pain, persistent infections, diabetes, dribbling, and renal stones. Some patients with sensory-related problems experience hesitancy and decreased volume of the urinary stream. Others may experience urinary retention resulting from decreased or absent stimuli to void. If the condition is the result of motor paralysis, the patient has the sensation of a full bladder but is unable to initiate the stream to empty. The patient with an uninhibited neurogenic bladder is not able to control the voiding pattern and is persistently incontinent of small amounts of urine. In reflex neurogenic bladder, normal sensation is absent, with uncontrolled bladder contractions occurring, which results in spontaneous voiding of spurts of urine. With an autonomous neurogenic bladder, all sensations and contraction capabilities are absent, resulting in an inability to void without applying pressure to the suprapubic area (Valsalva and Credé maneuvers).

Patient Screening

In most circumstances, the inability to empty the bladder and urinary incontinence are stressful for the patient. Prompt assessment is indicated.

Etiology

An insult to the brain, the spinal cord, or the nerves supplying the lower urinary tract, whether by trauma or a disease process, may result in this condition. Damage may be caused by cerebrovascular accident, spinal cord trauma, tumors, neuropathies, herniated lumbar disks, poliomyelitis, spinal cord lesions, or myelomeningocele. Heavy metal poisoning and genetic nerve disorders can also play a role in this disorder.

Diagnosis

The diagnosis is based on a history of trauma or a disease process, clinical findings, and the results of urodynamic studies that assess bladder function. Urine flow rate may be evaluated by an uroflowmeter, a device for continuous recording of urine flow in milliliters per second.

Treatment

The treatment is directed toward preventing UTIs and attempts to restore some normalcy in function. Providing the means for storing urine and emptying the bladder are of primary importance. Catheterization, whether intermittent or indwelling, is necessary to help the patient maintain an acceptable quality of life (Fig. 11.17). Drug therapy with parasympathomimetic agents may be indicated in some cases. Surgery and the use of external collection devices are other alternatives. Possible complications include hydronephrosis and renal failure.

Prognosis

Usually, no cure for the neurologic defect that caused the bladder dysfunction is possible. Drug therapy may be helpful. Oxybutynin or tolterodine may be used in cases of urinary urge incontinence caused by muscle spasms of the bladder.

Prevention

Prevention varies, depending on the cause.

Patient Teaching

Patients may require instructions for self-catheterization or other techniques for emptying the bladder. Use customized, electronically generated educational materials, when available, to reinforce the treatment plan.

Stress Incontinence

Description

Stress incontinence is the uncontrollable leakage of urine from the urinary bladder during physical exertion or actions that stress the pelvic muscles, such as laughing, sneezing, coughing, lifting, stretching, or running.

ICD-10-CM Code	N39.3 (Stress incontinence [female] [male])
	N39.46 (Mixed incontinence)

Referral to the current edition of the ICD-10-CM coding manual is recommended to confirm the appropriate code.

Symptoms and Signs

Stress incontinence is a symptom, a sign, and a diagnosis. It occurs when increased abdominal pressure forces urine through the bladder sphincter. The patient (usually female) experiences leakage of urine when coughing, sneezing, laughing, lifting, or running, without feeling prior urgency. The patient is unable to control the leakage during physical exertion.

Patient Screening

Although not a urologic emergency, stress incontinence can seem like an emergency for the individual experiencing it. The patient should be scheduled for an appointment as soon as possible.

Etiology

Weakening of the pelvic floor muscles and the urethral structure causes this embarrassing disorder. Trauma to the area resulting from childbirth and pressure from an existing pregnancy can result in those changes. The hormonal changes of aging and menopause make the condition more common in older females. Certain medications and obesity can precipitate the disorder.

Diagnosis

The symptoms clearly point to the diagnosis. Endoscopy and urodynamic voiding cystourethrography reveal abnormal bladder position, with leakage provoked by coughing or straining.

Treatment

The treatment consists of exercises (Kegel exercises or pelvic floor muscle tightening), estrogen replacement (most effective when estrogen cream is inserted vaginally), drug therapy, surgical repair, or collagen injections. Drug therapy may include tolterodine, darifenacin, trospium, or solifenacin. Botox injections may also be used to tighten the neck of the bladder when other methods fail.

Prognosis

Prognosis varies depending on the etiology.

Prevention

Strengthening pelvic and perineal muscles is helpful. Medications can control the symptoms in some females; for others, there is no prevention.

Patient Teaching

Provide information on Kegel exercises and other exercises to strengthen pelvic and perineal muscles. Discuss diet and fluid intake modifications. Provide resources for support.

Renal Cell Carcinoma

Description

Renal cancer is a condition in which one or more malignant tumors develop in one or both kidneys. The most common

Urinary Catheterization

Urinary catheterization involves the insertion of a catheter into the urinary bladder through the urethra for the withdrawal of urine and for irrigation of the bladder with a therapeutic solution (see Fig. 11.17). A strict sterile technique is necessary to prevent cystitis. Urinary catheterization is indicated to empty the bladder before surgery, to obtain a sterile urine specimen, to relieve urinary retention, and to treat incontinence (an indwelling catheter is attached to a drainage bag).

Indwelling female catheterization

Male catheterization

• **Fig. 11.17** Urinary catheterization.

Urinary Incontinence

Normally, as the bladder distends with urine, a reflex is stimulated to initiate voluntary urination (micturition); the sphincters of the bladder and the pelvic diaphragm relax, the bladder muscles contract, and the bladder empties. Urinary incontinence is partial or total loss of voluntary control of the bladder with inability to retain urine. The causes vary, from muscle or sphincter impairment to nerve damage or structural abnormalities.

This condition is very prevalent in older adults, commonly because of overactivity of the bladder musculature, resulting in urgency and incontinence with an inappropriately small volume of urine. Incontinence sometimes is experienced temporarily after the stretching of muscles during childbirth. Children may experience a form termed *enuresis*, or bedwetting. Other types of overactive bladder, or frequency and urge incontinence, are the subject of much-noted current research. Neurologic damage, such as brain damage or spinal cord injury, may result in permanent incontinence.

Incontinence is treated or managed according to the degree, type, and cause. Antispasmodic agents, adult diapers, "bladder training," estrogen therapy for females, and pelvic muscle exercises are some of the therapeutic measures that may be tried. Chronic indwelling catheters are avoided in the management of incontinence because of the risk of infection.

primary tumor of the kidney occurs in the renal cortex and is termed *renal cell carcinoma* (RCC). Less common tumors include Wilms tumor, a congenital renal tumor of childhood, and cancer of the renal pelvis (Fig. 11.18).

ICD-10-CM Code	C64.9 *(Malignant neoplasm of unspecified kidney, except renal pelvis)* (C64.1–C65.9 = 6 codes of specificity)

Referral to the current edition of the ICD-10-CM coding manual is recommended to determine appropriate code according to the site and type of the carcinoma.

Symptoms and Signs
The classic triad of symptoms of RCC is hematuria, abdominal mass, and flank pain. Approximately 10% of patients have all three findings, and those that do are likely to have advanced disease. Other less common signs and symptoms are weight loss, anemia, fever, hepatic dysfunction, and hypercalcemia. Many patients with RCC experience no symptoms until the disease is advanced.

Patient Screening
Patients experiencing hematuria require prompt assessment, as do those reporting an abdominal mass and/or flank pain.

Overactive Bladder

Individuals with an overactive bladder experience urinary urgency or strong, sudden urges to urinate. This sudden, uncomfortable urge to urinate may occur during daytime hours or awaken the individual from sleep. The uncontrollable urge (urge incontinence) can result in urinary incontinence with the accidental loss or leakage of small amounts of urine. Frequency of urination may also be a symptom of overactive bladder.

Additionally, overactive bladder may present social, occupational, and psychosocial problems. The individual with overactive bladder symptoms may not be able to accommodate the urge to urinate. Some of these individuals are afraid to leave the safety of the nearness of their own lavatory or opt for bulky undergarment padding and absorbent protection when they go out in public.

Under normal circumstances, the bladder muscle transmits impulses to the brain, indicating that it is full and needs to be emptied. Overactive bladder muscles transmit false signals to the brain before the bladder is full, resulting in a strong urge to urinate, even to the point of urine leakage or incontinence.

The individual has options in treating this condition, including rehabilitation of pelvic muscles, learning behavior therapies to regain control of the bladder, and drug therapy. Rehabilitation of pelvic muscles and biofeedback trains the sphincter and may not produce the rapid effect that some individuals desire; therefore they decide to try to eliminate or at least lessen the problem with drug therapy.

Drug therapy involves treatment with three different medications. Estrogen may be helpful for postmenopausal females in combination with other drug therapy concepts; however, some may be reluctant to include estrogen in their therapy because estrogen replacement increases the risk of cancer in some females. Drugs available for therapy include tolterodine, oxybutynin, solifenacin, trospium, and darifenacin. These medications help alleviate the condition by relaxing the smooth muscle of the bladder and reducing the number of muscle spasms. Patients should be advised that anticholinergic side effects may occur with these medications (e.g., dry mouth and blurred vision). Discussions in regard to the benefits and side effects of each drug will be discussed.

• **Fig. 11.18** Wilms tumor. (From Damjanov I: *Pathology for the health professions*, St. Louis, 2017, Elsevier.)

• **Fig. 11.19** Renal cell carcinoma. Typical cross-section of yellowish, spherical neoplasm in one pole of the kidney. Note the tumor in the dilated, thrombosed renal vein. (From Kumar V, Cotran R, Robbins S: *Robbins basic pathology*, ed 8, Philadelphia, 2008, Saunders/Elsevier.)

Etiology

Around 95% of cases of RCC are sporadic, but some familial forms are known. The most common is a component of the von Hippel-Lindau (VHL) syndrome. Patients with this disorder are predisposed to the development of multiple bilateral renal cysts, carcinomas, and tumors in other locations (Fig. 11.19). Risk factors for sporadic RCC are smoking, obesity, hypertension, patients with acquired cystic kidney disease undergoing dialysis, and prolonged exposure to chemicals, such as asbestos and cadmium. RCC is more common in males, and the incidence varies geographically, with the highest rates found in the Czech Republic and North America.

Diagnosis

Increasing numbers of RCCs are being detected incidentally on radiologic examinations done for some other unrelated disease. Procedures used to diagnose suspected neoplasms are abdominal CT or abdominal ultrasonography. Once a diagnosis is made, the clinician must look for metastasis by using CT of the abdomen and chest; MRI, in some cases; and bone scanning. A biopsy or tumor resection is then done for histologic confirmation.

Treatment

The treatment of choice for RCC is surgical removal. Depending on the stage, the patient can be treated with partial **nephrectomy**, radical nephrectomy, energy ablative techniques, and targeted therapy using angiogenesis inhibitors to interfere with the growth process. Drug therapy may include the mTOR (mammalian target of rapamycin) inhibitors everolimus and temsirolimus, or protein kinase inhibitors such as sorafenib, sunitinib, or axitinib. Immunotherapy may also be used with interferon, interleukin-2, or molecularly targeted therapy, such as tyrosine kinase inhibitors.

Prognosis

The single most important determinant of prognosis is the pathologic stage at diagnosis. A pathologist usually determines this by histologic evaluation of the resected tumor. High levels of lactate dehydrogenase, serum calcium, and low hemoglobin are poor prognostic indicators.

Prevention

Individuals at high risk (those with VHL syndrome, history of kidney irradiation, ESRD, and 3 to 5 years on dialysis, or a strong family history of RCC) should undergo periodic screening with abdominal ultrasonography, CT, or MRI to detect early disease. Cessation of smoking and maintenance of a healthy weight are recommended.

Patient Teaching

Encourage regular checkups for other family members when a family history of cancer is known and provide resources for cancer support groups.

Bladder Tumors

Description

Bladder neoplasms usually involve the transitional epithelium (urothelium) that lines the surface of the bladder. The urothelium also lines the entire urinary tract from the renal pelvis to the prostatic urethra. Although the bladder is the most common site for a tumor to occur, it can develop at any site in the urothelium-lined urinary tract (Fig. 11.20).

ICD-10-CM Code	D49.4 *(Neoplasm of unspecified behavior of bladder)*
	C67.9 *(Malignant neoplasm of bladder, unspecified)*
	(C67.0–C67.9 = 10 codes of specificity)

As with other carcinomas, refer to the physician's diagnosis for specific type and site of carcinoma and to the current edition of the ICD-10-CM coding manual for appropriate code.

Symptoms and Signs

The most common symptom of a bladder tumor is gross, intermittent, painless hematuria. Pain in the flank or suprapubic area may occur as the carcinoma becomes locally advanced or metastatic. Voiding symptoms (e.g., dysuria, urgency, and increased frequency) are sometimes

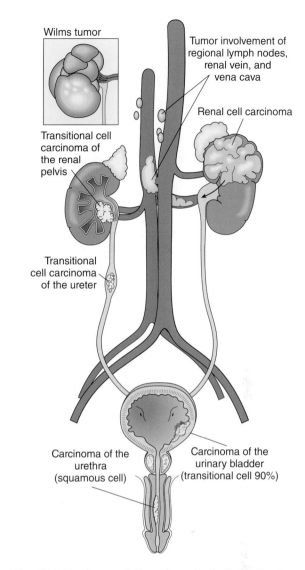

• **Fig. 11.20** Neoplasms of the urinary tract. (From Damjanov I: *Pathology for the health-related professions*, ed 4, St. Louis, 2012, Saunders/Elsevier.)

experienced. Symptoms of advanced disease include fatigue, weight loss, and anorexia.

Patient Screening

Patients reporting gross, intermittent, and painless hematuria, along with dysuria, urgency, and increased frequency should be assessed as quickly as possible.

Etiology

Environmental exposures are thought to account for most cases of bladder cancer because the surface epithelium is exposed to potential carcinogens excreted in urine (Fig. 11.21). Risk factors include: occupational exposure to aniline dyes or diesel exhaust, cigarette smoking, and a history of frequent bladder infections or prior bladder cancer. Human papillomavirus infection is associated with an increased risk of bladder cancer. According to the American Cancer Society, nine of 10 patients diagnosed with bladder cancer are older than 55 years old (2023 statistics).

• **Fig. 11.21** Bladder cancer. (A) Gross appearance of an intraluminal mass *(arrow)*. (B) Histologic examination reveals that the mass is a papillary transitional cell carcinoma. (From Damjanov I: *Pathology for the health-related professions*, ed 4, St. Louis, 2012, Saunders/Elsevier.)

Diagnosis

Unexplained hematuria should be investigated. Full urologic evaluation of the entire urinary tract is indicated. This consists of cystoscopy, urinary cytology (examination of transitional cells in the patient's voided urine), and IVP, renal ultrasonography, and/or CT. A biopsy sample can be taken of suspicious lesions during cystoscopy. Once the diagnosis is known, ultrasonography, CT, or MRI may be used to evaluate for extravesical extension and metastatic disease. Research continues to detect biomarkers in urine that can be used to diagnose bladder cancer. The most commonly used staging system is the TNM system proposed by the American Joint Committee on Cancer, in which T indicates the degree of invasion of the bladder wall. Accurate staging is necessary to direct treatment and predict prognosis.

Treatment

The treatment of bladder cancer has three main goals: (1) to eradicate the disease, (2) to prevent recurrence, and (3) to prevent the development of invasive disease. The standard initial treatment is tumor resection via transurethral resection of the bladder tumor (TURBT). This procedure involves a complete cystoscopic resection of any visible tumors and selected biopsies of the bladder mucosa. Recurrent tumors are removed by using TURBT. If the patient is at high risk for recurrence, bacillus Calmette-Guérin (BCG) is administered into the bladder. BCG, a mycobacterium modified to a less pathologic state, induces a local immune reaction that suppresses tumor growth. Cystectomy is indicated for patients with many recurrences and resistance to this intravesical therapy.

Invasive carcinoma confined to the bladder is treated with either radical cystectomy or partial cystectomy and adjuvant chemoradiotherapy. For patients with metastatic carcinoma, multidrug chemotherapy may result in tumor shrinkage and moderately increased survival, but not a cure.

Prognosis

Stage is the most important independent prognostic indicator for disease progression and overall survival. Once invasion outside the bladder or nodal disease is detected, outcomes without systemic therapy are poor. However, recurrence is a more common problem than progression. Lower-grade, well-differentiated tumors have a slower growth rate and a better prognosis.

Prevention

Screening for bladder cancer in asymptomatic individuals is not recommended. Efforts should be made to reduce occupational exposures and to cease cigarette smoking.

Patient Teaching

Encourage regular checkups for other family members when a family history of cancer is noted and provide information for cancer support groups.

Review Challenge

Answer the following questions:
1. How does the urinary system work specifically to maintain homeostasis?
2. What are some of the common symptoms of urinary system diseases?
3. Identify the unit of function of the kidney.
4. What are the etiologic factors of acute and CGN?
5. List some of the goals for the treatment of CGN?
6. What are some examples of abnormal findings in urinalysis?
7. Which individuals may require dialysis? Kidney transplantation?

8. What are possible treatment options for ESRD?
9. What are the classic clinical symptoms and signs of nephrosis? What causes nephrosis?
10. List some nephrotic agents.
11. Why is AKI considered a clinical emergency?
12. Discuss the difference between ARF or AKI and CRF.
13. When is renal failure irreversible?
14. How would a patient with pyelonephritis describe his or her symptoms?
15. How might organisms be introduced into the urinary tract and cause pyelonephritis?
16. Which condition is a complication of urinary tract obstruction? What are some causes of urinary tract obstruction?

17. What are the risk factors for renal calculi?
18. What are the etiologic sources of infectious cystitis and urethritis?
19. How does diabetes mellitus contribute to diabetic nephropathy?
20. How would you describe the polycystic kidney?
21. How would you compare the pathology of the neurogenic bladder with that of stress incontinence?
22. When may catheterization be indicated?
23. Describe overactive bladder.
24. What is the treatment and prognosis for RCC? For bladder tumors?
25. Why should children who are being toilet trained be taught to wipe from front to back?

Real-Life Challenge: Cystitis

A 35-year-old female reports pain in the pelvic region and lower back, frequency and urgency of urination, and burning on urination. The onset of symptoms was about four hours before the office visit.

Vital signs: temperature, 100.5°F; pulse, 96 beats/min; respirations, 18 breaths/min, blood pressure, 130/88 mm Hg. A clean-catch urine specimen is obtained, and it is pink in color and has a foul odor. The urine specimen is sent to the laboratory for urinalysis, culture, and sensitivity testing. Physical examination reveals tenderness over the bladder. Microscopic examination of the specimen reveals blood, leukocytes, and bacteria.

A diagnosis of cystitis is made, and trimethoprim-sulfamethoxazole (Bactrim DS) is prescribed. The patient is encouraged to force fluids and is instructed to call the office the next day to report her progress.

Questions

1. What is another term for cystitis?
2. What additional symptoms might a patient with cystitis exhibit?
3. What is the usual cause of cystitis?
4. Why is a urinalysis important in diagnosing cystitis?
5. Why would the patient's urine have a foul odor?
6. Why would culture and sensitivity testing be important in the treatment of cystitis?
7. What alternative drug therapy is available to treat cystitis?
8. Why would the patient be encouraged to force fluids?

Real-Life Challenge: Renal Calculus

The wife of a 42-year-old male called the office stating that within the last hour, her husband had a sudden onset of severe pain in his left side and back. He also has experienced nausea and vomiting. Questioning revealed the pain to be located in the left flank area and quite severe. The wife also reported that the pain radiated down toward her husband's scrotum and that he was experiencing pressure in the perineal area and a frequent urge to urinate. A renal calculus was suspected, and the patient's wife was advised to transport him to an emergency facility.

Vital signs were temperature, 99.6°F; pulse, 96 beats/min; respirations, 20 breaths/min; and blood pressure, 124/88 mm Hg. A urine specimen was obtained, and the dipstick indicated blood in urine. The abdomen was slightly distended, the left flank area exhibited tenderness on palpation, and tenderness was noted over the bladder. A renal calculus was suspected, and KUB radiography, IVP, and ultrasonography of the kidneys were ordered. An IV line was started, and the patient was given 2 mg of morphine sulfate IV push.

KUB radiography revealed a suspicious area 8 cm distal to the origin of the left ureter. IVP confirmed the presence of a 3.5-mm calculus distal to the ureteral origin. Renal ultrasonography indicated hydronephrosis of the left kidney. The patient was admitted for observation and for pain management.

Questions

1. What causes renal calculi to form?
2. What are the significant symptoms leading to suspicion of renal calculi?
3. What is renal colic?
4. Which conditions cause blood in the urine?
5. What is the cause of hydronephrosis?
6. Why would the patient be instructed to strain all the urine?
7. What are the treatment options for the patient with renal calculi?
8. Why is IV morphine administered?

Internet Assignments

1. Research the incidence and treatment of urinary incontinence at the websites of the National Kidney Foundation and the American Urological Association. Compare the information found on both sites.
2. Research the incidence, types of stones, and treatment of renal calculi at the websites of the National Kidney Foundation and the American Urological Association. Compare information found on both sites.
3. Research transplant donations, by both live and cadaver donors, at the websites of the National Kidney Foundation and the American Urological Association. Include the information about the expenses associated with transplantation.

Critical Thinking

1. Discuss the importance of drinking eight glasses of water daily.
2. List causes of obstructive diseases of the urinary system, and identify congenital or acquired structural defects and tumors, obstructive diseases of the urinary system, immunologic disorders, circulatory disturbances, cystic disease, and metabolic disorders (e.g., diabetes mellitus).
3. Discuss the importance of good perineal hygiene and emptying the bladder as a preventive measure with a female patient recently diagnosed with pyelonephritis.
4. The patient who has been diagnosed with CGN requires patient teaching about the progression and prognosis of the condition. Describe how you would approach the topic because the outcome of this condition is not a positive one. List some teaching aids that could be used to make the explanation more understandable to the patient.
5. Discuss with the patient the diagnosis of CGN.
6. The patient with ESRD may require special funding for treatment. Encourage the patient and the family to begin locating types of assistance that are available to patients with ESRD.
7. List the renal conditions that ultimately may cause ESRD, even if aggressively treated.
8. Identify some patients with diabetes, and discuss with them the renal complications caused by diabetes.
9. Explain the importance of straining urine to capture the kidney stone, "gravel," or sand that has been voided after a kidney stone attack.
10. Discuss with patients and their families the embarrassment issues and the products available to help deal with stress incontinence.

Prepare to discuss Critical Thinking case study exercises for this chapter that are posted on Evolve.

Credentialing Examination Questions

1. Which urinary structure is the functional unit of the kidney?
   A. Bladder
   B. Urethra
   C. Calyx
   D. Nephron
2. Which statement best describes nephrotic syndrome?
   A. Disease of the basement membrane of the glomeruli
   B. Caused by renal calculi
   C. Has symptoms of increased appetite
   D. Can be treated with antibiotics and will resolve
3. Which dipstick result is seen in various urinary tract disorders and infections?
   A. Hematuria
   B. High specific gravity
   C. Glucose
   D. Low specific gravity
4. Why is it important for female patients to use tissue wiping front to back after voiding?
   A. To feel cleaner
   B. Brings urine away from the front of the body
   C. Avoids transmitting fecal material toward the urethra
   D. Uses less tissue, which saves money
5. Which term is the accurate spelling for breaking up or crushing kidney stones using sound waves?
   A. Litotripsy
   B. Lithotripsy
   C. Lithography
   D. Litholysis
6. Lowering the chances of getting cystitis can be accomplished by drinking a minimum of which number of glasses of water per day?
   A. 3
   B. 5.
   C. 7
   D. 8
7. Which fruit does a polycystic kidney resemble?
   A. Strawberry
   B. Kiwi
   C. Grapes
   D. Blueberry
8. Which event may result in a neurogenic bladder?
   A. Spinal cord injury
   B. Injury to the brain
   C. Insult to the nerves supplying the lower urinary tract
   D. All of the above

9. Which triad of symptoms is seen in RCC?
   A. Proteinuria, glycosuria, flank pain.
   B. Hematuria, abdominal mass, and flank pain.
   C. Abdominal mass, hematuria and pyuria.
   D. Hematuria, pyuria, glycosuria.

10. Weakening of the pelvic muscle floor can cause which condition?
    A. Stress incontinence
    B. Pyelonephritis
    C. Diabetic nephropathy
    D. Urethritis

12

Diseases and Conditions of the Reproductive System

CHAPTER OUTLINE

LEARNING OBJECTIVES

After studying this chapter, you should be able to:

1. Identify risk factors for sexually transmitted infections (STIs).
2. Discuss male latex condoms and sexually transmitted diseases.
3. Explain what a silent STI is and give an example.
4. Name the complications of untreated gonorrhea.
5. Explain why females with genital herpes are advised to have regular Papanicolaou smears.
6. Explain why the human papillomavirus vaccine is recommended for girls and young females and, more recently, for males.
7. Describe the stages of untreated syphilis.
8. Explain why hepatitis B is classified as an STI.
9. List the possible causes of sexual dysfunction in males and females.
10. Name drugs that can contribute to impotence.
11. Discuss the possible causes of male and female infertility.
12. Explain how varicocele may contribute to male infertility.
13. Recall the best prevention of epididymitis.
14. Explain why torsion of the testicle is considered a medical emergency.
15. List some likely symptoms experienced by a male with benign prostatic hyperplasia.
16. Explain the value of prostate-specific antigen as a screening test.
17. Discuss the medical interventions for prostatic cancer.
18. Name the common first sign of testicular cancer.
19. Define mittelschmerz.
20. Explain what causes the dysmenorrhea associated with endometriosis.
21. Discuss the importance of early diagnosis and prompt treatment of pelvic inflammatory disease.
22. Explain the etiology of toxic shock syndrome.
23. Name the hormones that regulate the menstrual cycle.
24. Discuss the advantages and possible risks of hormone replacement therapy for the postmenopausal female.
25. Explain how uterine prolapse, cystocele, and rectocele may be corrected surgically.
26. List the risk factors for cervical cancer.
27. Name the leading cause of death attributed to gynecologic malignancies.
28. Name a condition considered a complication of pregnancy.
29. Discuss possible causes of spontaneous abortion (miscarriage).
30. List some possible causes of ectopic pregnancy.
31. Explain how a pregnant female is monitored for preeclampsia.
32. Describe abruptio placentae.
33. Name some problems associated with multiple pregnancies.
34. List the factors that place females at higher risk for breast cancer.

KEY TERMS

amenorrhea (ah-men-o-REE-ah)
autoinoculation (aw-toh-in-ock-u-LAY-shun)
chancre (SHANG-ker)
colporrhaphy (kol-POUR-ah-fee)
curettage (ku-reh-TAHZH)
dysmenorrhea (dis-men-oh-REE-ah)
dyspareunia (dis-pah-RUE-nee-ah)
dysuria (dis-YOU-ree-ah)
genitourinary (jen-ih-toe-YU-rih-nar-ee)
hysterosalpingography (hiss-ter-oh-sal-pin-GOG-rah-fee)
laparoscopy (lap-ar-OS-ko-pee)
leiomyoma (lye-o-my-OH-ma)
menorrhagia (men-oh-RAY-jee-ah)

metrorrhagia (met-roh-RAY-jee-ah)
orchitis (or-KYE-tis)
pessary (PESS-ah-ree)
prolapse (pro-LAPS)
prostatectomy (pros-tah-TECK-toh-me)
psychosexual (sigh-ko-SEKS-you-al)
salpingo-oophorectomy (sal-ping-go-oh-ouf-oh-RECK-toh-me)
septicemia (sep-tih-SEE-me-ah)
ultrasonography (uhl-tra-son-OGG-rah-fee)
urethritis (you-ree-THRYE-tis)
varicocele (VAR-ih-ko-seel)

The Normally Functioning Reproductive Systems

The reproductive process in humans is sexual and involves the union of two sex cells: one male and one female. As the fetus develops, male or female definition becomes evident. The organs of the reproductive system usually are classified into two groups: the gonads (testes and ovaries), which produce germ cells and hormones, and the series of ducts necessary for the transportation of the germ cells.

The male reproductive system functions to transfer the sperm cells to the female for fertilization of the ovum. The testes produce the sperm and the hormones necessary for the development and maintenance of the secondary sex characteristics. The sperm is transported through the series of ducts beginning with the epididymis, the ductus deferens, and the ejaculatory ducts. The seminal vesicles, the prostate gland, the bulbourethral glands, and the penis are accessory organs that help propel the sperm on its journey to meet the egg (Fig. 12.1).

The female reproductive system nourishes and enables the development of the fertilized ovum. The ovaries (which contain the female's lifetime supply of eggs) produce and release the egg and the hormones necessary for the development

• **Fig. 12.1** Normal male reproductive system.

of secondary sex characteristics and the maintenance of a pregnancy. The ductal system for transport, nourishment, and growth of the fertilized ovum includes the fallopian tubes and the uterus. Other principal parts of the female reproductive system include the cervix, the vagina, and the external genitalia (Fig. 12.2).

The breasts are accessory organs of reproduction and are the two milk-producing glands (Fig. 12.3). When a female is pregnant, the breast tissue is stimulated by both ovarian and placental hormones to prepare for lactation. After delivery, lactating hormones further stimulate the breast tissue to produce and release milk to nourish the infant.

The process of reproduction requires that the sperm fertilize the egg. After release from the ovary, the egg progresses down the fallopian tube. In a typical pregnancy, the egg is met in the fallopian tube by the sperm. After the sperm fertilizes the egg, the zygote continues to travel down the fallopian tube to the uterus, where it eventually attaches to the uterine lining (endometrium) to be nourished and to grow. The placenta forms within the uterine wall and provides a mechanism for the exchange of nourishment and waste products between the mother and the developing fetus. A normal gestational period is 38 weeks after conception, or 40 completed weeks after the start of the last menstrual period, at which time the birth process may begin with labor and subsequent delivery of the infant.

The anterior pituitary gland produces gonadotropic hormones that cause the ovaries to produce estrogen and progesterone, which regulate the menstrual cycle. During menstruation, the endometrium (the disintegrated endometrial cells along with secretions and blood cells) is shed via the vagina. This is followed by the next cycle of ovarian production of estrogen, produced from maturing ovarian follicles, which eventually release the mature ovum during ovulation. The corpus luteum then develops after the release

of the ovum, and progesterone is secreted into the bloodstream to stabilize the growth of the endometrium to prepare for implantation of the fertilized ovum. If pregnancy does not occur, the endometrium again is shed through menses.

Both the male and female reproductive systems are vulnerable to many diseases, including sexually transmitted diseases (STDs), malignancies, benign growths, and chemical imbalances. Abnormal function of the reproductive system sometimes results from functional, structural, dietary, or emotional causes. Complications often develop during pregnancy, some severe and some merely aggravating. This chapter explores the most common disease entities, conditions, and complications of both male and female reproductive systems.

> ⚠️ **ALERT!**
>
> **Risk Factors for Sexually Transmitted Diseases and Sexually Transmitted Infections (STIs)**
>
> - Sex with someone whose sexual history one does not know
> - Starting sexual activity at an early age
> - Drug use with sharing of needles
> - Sex with multiple partners
> - Sexual intimacy with someone who has been diagnosed with an STI or one who is being treated for an STI
> - Exposure to skin-to-skin contact in the presence of any open lesion, such as a chancre or a wart
> - Use of alcohol or other drugs that may cloud one's judgment about a sexual encounter
> - Hemophilia
> - Males having sex with males
> - Transfusion of blood or blood products
> - Babies being carried by a human immunodeficiency virus (HIV)–positive mother
> - Breast-fed infants of an HIV-positive mother
> - Lack of education or concern about risky sexual behavior

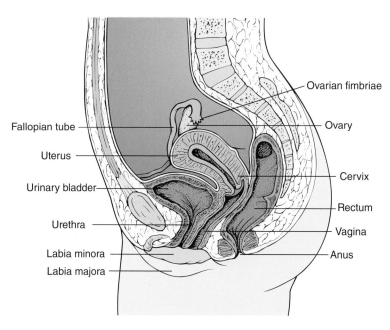

• **Fig. 12.2** Normal female reproductive system.

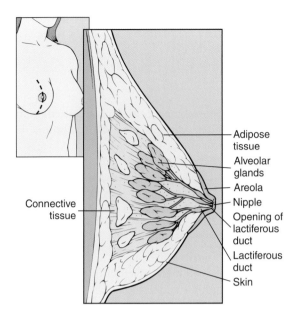

Connective tissue

Adipose tissue
Alveolar glands
Areola
Nipple
Opening of lactiferous duct
Lactiferous duct
Skin

• **Fig. 12.3** Normal female breast.

Abnormally Functioning Reproductive Systems

Sexually Transmitted Diseases

Many infectious diseases are spread by sexual contact, some of which are incurable and all of which can damage health or even threaten life. STDs, also referred to as STIs, are among the most common contagious diseases in the United States. In some cases, STIs are asymptomatic and are spread by individuals unaware that they are infected. These diseases represent a "silent epidemic." Untreated STIs can lead to serious long-term health consequences. The infections are transmitted from one person to another through body fluids, such as blood, semen, and vaginal secretions during vaginal, anal, or oral sex. Some are spread by direct contact with infected skin or for example, in the case of pubic lice, are transmitted by clothing, bedding, or infected hairs during coitus. Most STIs are treatable, but there is no cure for viral STIs, such as herpes and human immunodeficiency virus (HIV). Among the many concerns about STIs is the possible transmission by an infected mother to a fetus or a newborn, sometimes with dire consequences to the baby. All pregnant females should be screened for STIs.

STI rates in the United States are among the highest in the world and cases continue to rise. Attempts to control this rampant public health problem are focusing on research, education, and prevention campaigns. Requirements for reporting STIs vary from state to state. However, several STIs that, when diagnosed, must be reported to state health departments and the Centers for Disease Control and Prevention (CDC) for statistical purposes are chlamydia, gonorrhea, syphilis, chancroid, HIV infection, acquired immunodeficiency syndrome (AIDS), and hepatitis B. See Chapter 8 for a discussion of hepatitis B.

ⓘ ALERT!

Male Latex Condoms and Sexually Transmitted Diseases

The surest way to avoid transmission of sexually transmitted infections (STIs) is to abstain from sexual intercourse or to be in a long-term mutually monogamous relationship with a partner who has been tested and is known to be uninfected.

For people whose sexual behaviors place them at risk for STIs, correct and consistent use of the male latex condom can reduce the risk of STI transmission. Although no protective method is 100% effective, consistent condom use has proven to decrease risk. Incorrect condom use can lead to condom slippage or breakage, which reduces their protective effect. Inconsistent use (e.g., failure to use condoms with every act of intercourse) can lead to STI transmission, because transmission can occur with a single act of intercourse.

Condom use has been associated with a reduced risk of cervical cancer, but the use of condoms should not be a substitute for routine Papanicolaou (Pap) smears to detect and prevent cervical cancer.

Centers for Disease Control and Prevention (CDC). CDC Fact Sheet for Public Health Personnel: National Center for HIV, STI, and TB prevention. Available at: https://www.cdc.gov/condomeffectiveness/latex.html

Chlamydia

Description

Chlamydia, the most commonly reported notifiable STI in the United States, causes urethritis in males and urethritis and cervicitis in females.

ICD-10-CM Code	A74.9 *(Chlamydial infection, unspecified)* (A74.0–A74.9 = 4 codes of specificity)

Symptoms and Signs

Chlamydia sometimes is called the *silent STI* because it often has no symptoms, and thus it is sexually transmitted unknowingly. A high percentage of females have no symptoms before dangerous complications start, in contrast with males who typically do have symptoms. Chlamydia is a major cause of female sterility and a leading cause of pelvic inflammatory disease (PID). According to the CDC, chlamydia is the most commonly reported STI in the United States.

Early female symptoms include dysuria, an odorless, yellow vaginal discharge with a burning sensation, itching, abdominal pain, and dyspareunia. Infected males experience a thin, watery discharge from the penis, with a burning sensation and itching, and a burning sensation when urinating, the latter caused by urethritis. The scrotum may be swollen, and the patient may be feverish. The inguinal lymph nodes often are enlarged in both sexes. A small transient lesion and skin irritation may be noticed. Newborns can acquire chlamydia from the infected mother during birth, resulting in conjunctivitis, blindness, arthritis, or overwhelming infection.

Patient Screening

Symptoms usually start 1 or 2 weeks after exposure; they are likely to be mild, such as a burning sensation during urination and genital discharge in both males and females. An early appointment should be scheduled to confirm the diagnosis and begin treatment.

Etiology

Chlamydia trachomatis, an intracellular bacterium, is the cause of chlamydia and usually is transmitted through sexual contact. The site of primary infection is usually around the genitals, but it can be oral or anal, depending on sexual practice. The organism can be found in the cervix, throat, or rectum and can be transmitted unknowingly.

Diagnosis

Testing for chlamydia is most often done using a deoxyribonucleic acid (DNA) probe test, which is a test based on DNA detection. A Nucleic Acid Amplification Testing (NAAT) may also be performed.

Treatment

Antibiotic therapy is given to both partners, beginning with a single injection, and/or followed by a course of oral antibiotics, such as azithromycin, erythromycin, or a 7-day regimen of doxycycline. More severe cases may require hospitalization and treatment with intravenous (IV) antibiotics. Prompt treatment can cure the infection and prevent complications, such as PID and problematic pregnancy. Follow-up testing is recommended.

Prognosis

Chlamydial infection can be cured with a complete course of antibiotics when taken as directed, even after symptoms subside. Long-term consequences of untreated chlamydia are more serious for females who are prone to PID, which can result in infertility; they are also more likely to become infected by HIV, if exposed. Chlamydia left untreated in males can cause epididymitis, which may lead to infertility.

Prevention

Infected patients should inform their sexual contacts of the infection. See the risk factors for STIs. All states require reporting of cases of chlamydia to the public health department. The CDC recommends annual chlamydia screening for sexually active females under 25 years of age and for those over the age of 25 with multiple sex partners. Urine tests for chlamydia in males can help reduce the transmission of disease to females. In addition to compromising reproductive health in females, infection with chlamydia facilitates the transmission of HIV infection.

Patient Teaching

Emphasize the importance of taking the complete course of antibiotic therapy as prescribed. Recommend that patients abstain from intercourse until both partners are cured.

Inform patients that meticulous personal hygiene and frequent hand washing are necessary to prevent the spreading of the infection to the eyes.

Gonorrhea

Description

Gonorrhea, the second most commonly reported notifiable disease in the United States, is a sexually transmitted infection (STI) of the **genitourinary** tract.

ICD-10-CM Code	A54.00 *(Gonococcal infection of lower genitourinary tract, unspecified)* (A54.00–A54.29 = 11 codes of specificity)

Symptoms and Signs

Gonorrhea, also a common infection of the genitourinary tract, causes symptoms and complications similar to those of chlamydia in male and female patients. A purulent discharge from the male or female genitourinary tract and dysuria are often present but can vary in severity. Many patients are asymptomatic in the early stages of infection, so they may unknowingly continue to spread the infection. The disease also can infect the eyes and throat or become systemic.

Patient Screening

Males develop symptoms, if any, after an incubation period of 3 to 6 days. Symptoms in males vary but may include discharge from the penis, pain or burning with urination, and testicular pain or edema. Females may experience vaginal discharge, heavier menstrual periods, pain in the lower abdomen, dysuria, and urinary frequency.

Etiology

Infection with the common bacterium *Neisseria gonorrhoeae* usually results from sexual transmission. Gonorrhea can be transmitted via vaginal, anal, or oral intercourse with an infected individual. Because transmission is also possible during birth, newborns must be protected from eye infections that can lead to blindness (Fig. 12.4). Prophylactic erythromycin salve is administered routinely at birth.

• **Fig. 12.4** Gonorrhea ophthalmia. (From Grimes D: *Infectious diseases—Mosby's clinical nursing series*, St. Louis, 1994, Mosby.)

Diagnosis

Laboratory cultures from the infected site (cervix, rectum, or throat) of infectious body secretions and microscopic examination of exudate with a Gram stain are performed to identify the *N. gonorrhoeae* organism. Nucleic acid amplification testing (NAAT) can be used and is considered effective. A DNA-probe technique called *polymerase chain reaction (PCR)* identifies the genetic material of the bacterium.

Treatment

Curative treatment is recommended for the infected individual and any sexual partners as well. Throughout the years, gonorrhea has become more difficult to treat because of antibiotic-resistant strains. The CDC recommends an injection of ceftriaxone (500 mg) for uncomplicated cases of gonorrhea. After the antibiotic therapy, follow-up culture studies are ordered to ensure a complete cure, because some strains are becoming increasingly antibiotic resistant. Neglecting treatment of a gonococcal infection can lead to complications, including PID, septicemia, infertility, and septic arthritis. Salpingitis (inflammation or infection of the fallopian tube) is the most common complication of gonorrhea.

Prognosis

With early and complete treatment, the prognosis is excellent, even when there are complications.

Prevention

Safe sexual practices to prevent transmission to partners. Routine instillation of erythromycin 0.5% ophthalmic ointment into the eyes of newborns is practiced. Abstinence from sexual contact is maintained until treatment is complete and follow-up culture results are negative.

Patient Teaching

Emphasize the importance of complying with a complete treatment plan and follow-up testing to ensure a cure. Inform the patient of the risk factors (see the Alert box about Risk Factors for Sexually Transmitted Diseases) and that the organism can exist in the back of the throat (as a result of oral sex), in the genitals, and in the rectum.

Trichomoniasis

Description

Trichomoniasis is a protozoal infection of the lower genitourinary tract; the infection is usually vaginal in females and urethral in males.

ICD-10-CM Code	A59.9 *(Trichomoniasis, unspecified)*
	(A59.00–A59.9 = 7 codes of specificity)

The above code may be valid as a principal diagnosis. Refer to the physician's diagnosis and then to the current edition of the ICD-10-CM coding manual to ensure the greatest specificity of pathology.

Symptoms and Signs

Trichomoniasis is common among people who are sexually active. Most infected males and females, however, are asymptomatic. This contributes to the spread of the unrecognized infection and delays in treatment.

The initial symptoms for male and female patients may include urethritis with dysuria and itching. In addition, females may notice a profuse, frothy, greenish-yellow, odorous discharge from the vagina and vulvar irritation. In females, a characteristic "strawberry cervix" may be observable on colposcopy. A thin, whitish discharge from the penis may be noted by males. In either case, the discharge may subside without treatment, but the infection remains and can become chronic.

Patient Screening

Discomfort associated with the irritating discharge usually prompts a request for an appointment for an examination.

Etiology

Trichomoniasis is a protozoal infection caused by *Trichomonas vaginalis* and is usually transmitted through sexual contact. The incubation period is 5 to 28 days.

Diagnosis

A wet preparation of vaginal secretions from females or discharge from the urethra in males is studied for the microorganism *T. vaginalis*. Urinalysis also may reveal the organism if the urine is contaminated from vaginal discharge. The cervix is examined for the presence of small hemorrhages with a strawberry-like appearance.

Treatment

If the wet prep, urinalysis, or laboratory culture result is positive, antiprotozoal drugs are given. Metronidazole (Flagyl) or tinidazole (Tindamax) may be given as a single dose or as a multiday treatment. *Patients are cautioned never to consume products containing alcohol while taking these medications.*

Prognosis

The prognosis is good if both partners receive medical treatment, including a follow-up examination that ensures that the infection is cured completely. Failure to treat both partners causes reinfection, called "ping-pong" vaginitis. An increased risk for HIV transmission has been noted. Pregnant females with trichomoniasis can experience complications.

Prevention

Because this disease is transmitted primarily through sexual contact, prevention requires avoiding sex with someone whose sexual history one does not know. Latex condoms may help prevent the spread of trichomoniasis.

Patient Teaching

Advise the patient that consumption of alcohol is contraindicated while taking metronidazole or tinidazole. See the information in the Prevention and Prognosis sections.

Genital Herpes

Description

Genital herpes is an incurable, recurrent infection of the skin of the genital area, with ulcerations spread through direct skin-to-skin contact, causing painful genital sores similar to cold sores (Fig. 12.5).

ICD-10-CM Code	A60.9 *(Anogenital herpesviral infection, unspecified)*

(A60.00–A60.9 = 8 codes of specificity)

Genital herpes is coded according to the site of the lesion(s). Refer to the physician's diagnosis and then to the current edition of the ICD-10-CM coding manual to ensure the greatest specificity of pathology.

Symptoms and Signs

Genital herpes is caused by herpes simplex virus type 2 (HSV-2), and less frequently by HSV-1, and is a recurrent, incurable viral disease. A large percentage of infections is subclinical, so the initial episode may go unnoticed. More often, one or more blisterlike lesions are noted somewhere on the genitals or around the anus. The painful ulcers and blisters usually occur 2 to 30 days after sexual contact with an infected person. Often the first episode is accompanied by systemic influenza symptoms, swollen glands, fever, headache, and painful urination. The condition is infectious when sores are present, but some people without symptoms, called *shedders*, can transmit the virus. Herpetic lesions occur more often in females than in males, and the infection tends to be more severe in females. Subsequent outbreaks can occur for months or years because the virus hides in the nervous system and lies dormant between flare-ups.

• **Fig. 12.5** Genital herpes in the female *(left)* and the male *(right)*. (From Behrman RE, Kliegman RM, Arvin AM: *Slide set, Nelson textbook of pediatrics*, ed 15, Philadelphia, 1996, Saunders.)

Patient Screening

Systemic symptoms may be present during the acute stage. When fever, headache, muscle aches, and swollen glands are present, an appointment for the individual is scheduled promptly for investigative medical evaluation.

Etiology

HSV-2 usually is transmitted sexually via virus-infected body fluids during skin-to-skin contact. Cross-infection may result from oral-genital or anal sex, and the infection is permanent. Genital herpes can also be caused by HSV-1, especially in the younger population.

The presence of open lesions increases the risk of contracting AIDS during sexual acts between persons infected with HSV-2 and those who are positive for HIV infection.

Diagnosis

Physical examination notes the presence of characteristic lesions on the male or female genitalia. An antigen test or tissue culture laboratory techniques can identify HSV-2. PCR and a rapid fluorescent test are also used to identify HSV-2.

Treatment

There is no cure, but prescription drugs that reduce the duration and frequency of outbreaks are currently available. These drugs include acyclovir (Zovirax), famciclovir (Famvir), and valacyclovir (Valtrex). Females with genital herpes must be monitored more carefully for cervical cancer. A Papanicolaou (Pap) smear every 6 months is recommended. Finally, a cesarean section may be indicated, because the virus is dangerous to the newborn.

Prognosis

Recurrent herpes usually has prodromal symptoms, such as tingling, itching, or burning 1 to 5 days before the lesion(s) appear. Recurrent episodes are common but tend to be milder and often are triggered by fatigue and stress. Generally, the infection poses no serious problems for healthy adults.

Prevention

The only absolute prevention is by practicing sexual abstinence and mutual monogamy. Condoms do not necessarily provide a complete barrier against skin-to-skin contact. After years of research, attempts to develop a vaccine have been disappointing. There is no effective vaccine for prevention of herpes, however research continues.

> **NOTE**
>
> Unprotected exposure of healthcare workers to oral and genital secretions when providing care to patients with HSV infection can result in an intensely painful infection of fingers called *herpetic whitlow*. This is usually caused by **autoinoculation** or other direct contact between HSV and a break in the skin, such as a torn cuticle.

Patient Teaching
Counsel the patient about the preventive measures and the prognosis. Recommend frequent and thorough hand washing; the infection could spread to the eyes and other areas of the skin. Provide the patient with educational material on how to cope with the disease. Address any concerns about how the disease affects personal relationships and the need to inform anyone they have sex with about their genital herpes. Inform the patient the virus can be shed even while he or she is asymptomatic.

Genital Warts (Condylomata Acuminata)
Description
Condyloma acuminatum is a genital infection that causes raised cauliflower-like growths in or near the vagina or rectum or along the penis (Fig. 12.6). It has become one of the most common STIs in the world.

ICD-10-CM Code   A63.0 *(Anogenital [venereal] warts)*
(A63.0–A64 = 3 codes of specificity)

Symptoms and Signs
These genital warts are usually painless, and many females have no obvious symptoms. Sometimes the lesions may cause itching or burning. These contagious lesions appear several weeks to several months after direct skin-to-skin contact during sexual intercourse with an infected person. The discomfort experienced varies, depending on the size, number, and location of the warts (see Fig. 12.6).

Patient Screening
Schedule the male or female patient for an examination.

Etiology
Human papillomavirus (HPV) is the cause of genital warts and usually is transmitted sexually. It has a prolonged incubation period of 1 to 6 months. HPV infects epithelial cells. Risk factors for acquiring persistent infection with HPV are early age at initiation of sexual activity and having multiple sexual partners. Coinfection with HIV causes a further increase in the risk for HPV-related cancer.

Many types of HPV have been identified by scientists. The same types of HPV that infect the genital areas can infect the mouth and the throat. Some are low-risk types, whereas the high-risk types can cause cancer.

Diagnosis
Genital warts can be identified by their appearance, but biopsy sometimes is suggested to rule out carcinoma. The wart must be differentiated from a syphilitic lesion. Identification of the genetic material (DNA) of the virus confirms HPV infection.

Treatment
Some genital warts go away without treatment, but the underlying virus is never completely eliminated. The treatment is chemical or surgical removal of the warts, but recurrence is common. Topical drug therapy to remove the warts includes a keratolytic agent, such as podofilox and trichloroacetic acid. Imiquimod is indicated for the treatment of external genital and perianal warts or condyloma acuminata in patients aged 12 years. This is widely used to stop new genital warts from forming. Surgical procedures for wart removal include cryosurgery, which involves the freezing and removal of affected tissue. Electrodesiccation is a process that uses a laser to remove larger warts and is also very effective. Some genital warts go away without treatment.

Studies have shown that females with genital HPV infection are at greater risk for cervical cancer. Because the warts spread more rapidly during pregnancy, a cesarean section may be necessary if the warts occlude the birth canal.

Prognosis
Genital warts have no complications, but the disease tends to recur. Even after treatment, recurrence of symptoms is possible. Pregnancy promotes the growth and spread of the lesions.

Prevention
Sexual contact with an infected individual and with someone whose sexual history is unknown should be avoided. The long incubation period introduces an added risk of infecting others or contracting the disease.

A vaccine to help prevent HPV infection is recommended. (see the Enrichment box about Human Papillomavirus Vaccine and Cervical Cancer).

Patient Teaching
Counseling about all aspects of the prevention and transmission of genital warts is important.

• **Fig. 12.6** Genital warts. (From Behrman RE, Kliegman RM, Arvin AM: *Slide set, Nelson textbook of pediatrics*, ed 15, Philadelphia, 1996, Saunders.)

Human Papillomavirus Vaccine and Cervical Cancer

There are many types of human papillomavirus (HPV), some of which are known to cause cancers of the cervix, anus, vagina, vulva, and penis. HPV infection is most often associated with cervical cancer. Although an invasive neoplasm will not develop in most people infected with HPV, it is important to reduce the risk of infection. The virus may be spread not only via unprotected intercourse but also through close physical contact with an infected area of the body and probably through digital/anal, oral/anal, and digital/vaginal contact as well. Using barrier contraception and limiting the number of sexual partners are recommended to reduce the risk of infection. No antiviral drugs currently are available to treat HPV infection. Those who are infected should know the risk of cancer and should follow up periodically with their physician to monitor for premalignant neoplastic changes.

Although the use of annual Pap smear tests to screen for cervical cancer has drastically reduced the number of deaths from cervical cancer in developed countries, cervical cancer remains a leading cause of cancer-related death in countries without these programs. The HPV vaccine is given to prevent the most common types of HPV that can lead to these cancers. This vaccine was approved by the US Food and Drug Administration (FDA) and is recommended by the Centers for Disease Control and Prevention for both female and male patients. The vaccine is usually administered at age 11 to 12 years but may be administered as early as age 9 years. Those receiving the injection at age 11 to 12 years, should receive two doses of the vaccine, with the second vaccine 6 to 12 months after the initial dose.

Patients who start the vaccination at age 15 years or later should receive a three-dose series within 6 months. The second dose is administered 1 to 2 months after the initial vaccination, and the third dose is administered 6 months after the first vaccination. Although the HPV vaccine is a major advance in the prevention of cervical cancer, it will not replace the need for other preventive strategies, such as annual screening with Pap smear tests for early detection of abnormal cells.

• **Fig. 12.7** A chancre of primary syphilis. (From Kumar V, et al: *Robbins basic pathology*, ed 10, St. Louis, 2018, Elsevier.)

• **Fig. 12.8** Secondary syphilis. (From Grimes D: *Infectious diseases—Mosby's clinical nursing series*, St. Louis, 1994, Mosby.)

Syphilis

Description

Syphilis is a chronic, systemic STI that has four stages.

ICD-10-CM Code A51.0 *(Primary genital syphilis)*
(A51.0–A52.09 = 24 codes of specificity)
A51.49 *(Other secondary syphilitic conditions)*
A53.0 *(Latent syphilis, unspecified as early or late)*
(A53.0–A53.9 = 2 codes of specificity)
Refer to the physician's diagnosis and then to the current edition of the ICD-10-CM coding manual to ensure the greatest specificity of pathology.

Symptoms and Signs

Syphilis begins with the presence of a painless but highly contagious local lesion called a chancre on the male or female genitalia (Fig. 12.7). Without early treatment during the primary stage, it becomes a systemic, chronic disease that can involve any organ or tissue. In 1 to 2 months, when the primary lesion heals, the causative organism (the spirochete *Treponema pallidum*) has disseminated throughout the body and multiplied, producing lesions wherever the organisms are most prevalent, including the skin, lymph nodes, cardiovascular system, brain, and spinal cord.

The disease continues to be contagious during the second stage, when there is systemic manifestation. This stage can present many symptoms, including fever, headaches, aching of joints, mouth sores, and rashes on the palms of the hands and soles of the feet (Fig. 12.8). The third stage is a latent period, which can last years, during which the infection is generally subclinical or asymptomatic. In the last stage, the lesions, called *gummas*, have invaded body organs and systems, causing widespread damage to the point of being debilitating and life threatening.

When a fetus is infected, the child may die in utero or be born with congenital syphilis and multiple abnormalities.

Patient Screening

It is important to treat syphilis in the early stages. Syphilis cases continue to be reported in the United States, especially among males.

Etiology

Syphilis is caused by infection with the spirochete *T. pallidum* through sexual contact or other direct contact with infected lesions or infected body fluids. It is highly contagious when a chancre is present (see Fig. 12.7). Congenital transmission can occur during pregnancy.

Diagnosis

Standard screening tests are the Venereal Disease Research Laboratory (VDRL) test and the rapid plasminogen reagent test. A smear taken from the primary lesion is examined microscopically for *T. pallidum*. Antibodies can be detected in the patient's serum. Further testing confirms the diagnosis and provides a titer to monitor response to treatment. Worldwide, the diagnosis of syphilis requires concurrent HIV testing as well.

Treatment

Syphilis can be easily cured in its early stages with a course of antibiotic therapy by using penicillin G. If the patient is allergic to penicillin, other antibiotics are used, such as doxycycline, azithromycin, and ceftriaxone. The disease is best treated in the primary and secondary stages, before it causes irreversible damage to the body. Patients are monitored with follow-up blood tests for the presence of *T. pallidum* for up to a year.

Prognosis

Treatment can cure syphilis. Untreated syphilis progresses to long-term severe systemic complications. Syphilis facilitates the spread of HIV infection.

Prevention

Sexual contact with an infected individual and contact with body fluids should be avoided. Syphilis can be transmitted in the first few years of the latent stage and in the first two stages. When in doubt, a VDRL test should be performed to detect infection. See the list of risk factors for STIs. Syphilis cases are reportable to the local Department of Health.

Patient Teaching

Emphasize the importance of finishing the course of medication, even if symptoms are alleviated. Urge the patient to inform his or her sexual partners about the infection so that they can seek treatment, if needed. Instruct the patient to avoid all risk factors for STIs.

Chancroid

Description

Chancroid, also called *soft chancre*, is a bacterial infection of the genitalia that causes necrotizing ulceration and lymphadenopathy.

ICD-10-CM Code   A57 *(Chancroid)*

Symptoms and Signs

The shallow and painless lesion appears on the skin or mucous membrane at the site of entry, 7 to 10 days after sexual contact with an infected person (Fig. 12.9). Tender, superlative inguinal adenopathy is noted on physical examination. The ulcer usually deepens and becomes purulent and can be spread to other areas of the body via autoinoculation.

Patient Screening

The presence of a lesion on or near the genitalia usually prompts a request for an appointment for an examination.

Etiology

The causative agent of chancroid is the bacterium *Haemophilus ducreyi*.

Diagnosis

The diagnosis is based on the clinical appearance of the lesions. In the laboratory, Gram staining of smears of the exudate is performed to confirm the cause of infection. The presence of syphilis or HSV infection is ruled out.

Treatment

The patient usually responds well to antibiotic therapy (i.e., azithromycin, clarithromycin, or ceftriaxone). The lesions sometimes must be drained surgically. Good personal

• **Fig. 12.9** Chancroid: male. (From Grimes D: *Infectious diseases—Mosby's clinical nursing series*, St. Louis, 1994, Mosby.)

hygiene is advised. The patient is told to keep the infected areas clean and dry and to refrain from sexual contact during the entire time of treatment.

Prognosis

Antibiotic therapy is usually curative. Severe infection may cause scarring.

Prevention

No vaccine is available. The use of a condom helps prevent the spread of infection. Chancroid is a reportable STI.

Patient Teaching

All regular sexual partners should be examined and treated, if needed. Serologic testing for HIV is recommended for patients treated for chancroid.

Hepatitis B

See Chapter 8 for a discussion about hepatitis B.

Sexual Dysfunction

The most common male and female sexual dysfunctions are discussed briefly. Sexual health and proper sexual functioning are important to human beings for the pleasure they provide, for the intimacy they nurture in a relationship, and for reproduction. To fulfill these purposes, individuals must be free from organic disease and **psychosexual** disorders.

Ideally, the human sexual response cycle progresses from a state of desire or arousal, through orgasm, to resolution or a feeling of well-being and relaxation. This cycle depends on a balance and interplay among physical, mental, and emotional factors.

Erectile Dysfunction/Impotence

Description

Erectile dysfunction (ED)/impotence is a consistent or recurrent inability to achieve or maintain penile erection.

ICD-10-CM Code	N52 *(Male erectile dysfunction)*
	N52.0 *(Vasculogenic erectile dysfunction)*
	N52.01 *(Erectile dysfunction due to arterial insufficiency)*
	N52.02 *(Corporo-venous occlusive erectile dysfunction)*
	N52.03 *(Combined arterial insufficiency and corporo-venous occlusive erectile dysfunction)*
	N52.1 *(Erectile dysfunction due to diseases classified elsewhere)*
	N52.2 *(Drug-induced erectile dysfunction)*
	N52.3 *(Postsurgical erectile dysfunction)*
	N52.31 *(Erectile dysfunction following radical prostatectomy)*
	N52.32 *(Erectile dysfunction following radical cystectomy)*
	N52.33 *(Erectile dysfunction following urethral surgery)*
	N52.34 *(Erectile dysfunction following simple prostatectomy)*
	N52.39 *(Other postsurgical erectile dysfunction)*
	N52.8 *(Other male erectile dysfunction)*
	N52.9 *(Male erectile dysfunction, unspecified)*

Impotence is coded by specific disorders. Refer to the physician's diagnosis and then to the current edition of the ICD-10-CM coding manual to ensure the greatest specificity of pathology.

Symptoms and Signs

ED/impotence is the inability of a male to perform in sexual intercourse, usually because he is unable to attain or maintain an erection of the penis sufficient for satisfactory sexual activity. It is the most common male sexual disorder, affecting most males at some time during their lives. The condition can be temporary or may become chronic.

Patient Screening

A complete physical examination or a private consultation may be scheduled.

Etiology

Sexual arousal causes the arteries in the penis to relax and dilate, thus allowing an increased blood flow to the penis. The expansion and hardening of the penis causes a compression of the veins carrying blood away from the penis, resulting in an erection. Anything that impedes the nerve response or that alters the necessary pattern of blood flow results in failure to achieve an erection.

Medical conditions affecting the blood vessels and restricting blood flow to the penis include diabetes mellitus, hypertension, heart disease, obesity, smoking, and hypercholesterolemia. Neurologic elements (e.g., nerve insult resulting from prostate surgery and spinal cord, pelvic, or perineal trauma) may interrupt the impulse transmission between the central nervous system and the penis. Side effects of medications prescribed to treat hypertension and depression can also lead to ED. Other common causes are alcohol, recreational drugs, antihistamines, and diuretics.

ED/impotence may also have a psychosocial basis that is not directly related to the mechanical functioning of the penis. The most common contributing factors include depression and stress.

Diagnosis

A medical history and physical examination to reveal any underlying medical causative factors are necessary. The history should include patient and family history of diabetes mellitus or other endocrine disorders, hypertension, heart disease, cerebral vascular accidents, spinal cord injuries, and vascular or renal disease; any surgery or trauma to the pelvic area; medications that the patient currently is taking or previously has taken; lifestyle, including smoking habits and alcohol consumption; stress levels; and relationship with the sexual partner. Laboratory tests to rule out organic disease help the physician make the diagnosis. Measurement of the testosterone level in blood is helpful, especially if the patient indicates low sexual desire.

Treatment

The treatment may first require management of underlying medical disorders or changing/ discontinuing current medications. Testosterone therapy is used for males with androgen deficiency. Other courses of remedies, such as programs for substance abuse or psychological counseling, are more complex and time consuming. Interventions, such as psychoanalysis, discussion, behavioral modification, and sensate exercises, are aimed at restoring the patient's ability to complete the entire sexual response cycle. Other approaches include penile implants, external vacuum devices, and penile injection therapy.

A more recent approach is oral drug therapy with medication, such as sildenafil citrate (Viagra), vardenafil (Levitra), and tadalafil (Cialis). During sexual stimulation, nitric oxide is released in the corpus cavernosum, initiating an enzymatic cascade, ultimately resulting in the relaxation of the smooth muscle of the corpus cavernosum and an inflow of blood. This class of medication (phosphodiesterase-5 [PDE5] inhibitors) increases the effect of nitrous oxide, consequently helping the male to have an erection satisfactory for desired sexual activity. Sexual stimulation is needed for these drugs, taken at the recommended dosage, to assist with achieving an erection; they have no effect in the absence of sexual stimulation. See the Alert box about Precautions Concerning Sildenafil Citrate (Viagra), Vardenafil, and Tadalafil (Cialis).

Prognosis

The prognosis varies greatly, depending on the cause. Effective therapy is available in many cases. The prevalence increases with advancing age.

> **NOTE**
>
> There is growing evidence linking erectile dysfunction (ED) to the eventual onset of the clinical manifestation of coronary artery disease.

Prevention

Impotence is usually secondary to one of many diseases and conditions.

Patient Teaching

If the cause is psychogenic, refer the patient to counseling. Direct other patient teaching toward treating the organic cause.

Male and Female Infertility

Description

Infertility may be defined as the involuntary inability to conceive.

ICD-10-CM Code	N46.9 *(Male infertility, unspecified)* (N46.8–N46.9 = 2 codes of specificity) N97.9 *(Female infertility, unspecified)* (N97.0–N97.9 = 5 codes of specificity)

Symptoms and Signs

With regular, unprotected intercourse, about 90% of couples conceive within 1 year. The inability of a couple to conceive can originate from female factors, male factors, or both.

Patient Screening

A complete medical evaluation should be scheduled for both partners.

---

❶ ALERT!

Precautions Concerning Sildenafil Citrate (Viagra), Vardenafil, and Tadalafil (Cialis)

Males who have underlying cardiovascular disease and are advised against sexual activity should not take sildenafil, vardenafil, or tadalafil. In addition, males who have had a heart attack, stroke, or life-threatening arrhythmia in the past 6 months also are warned not to take these drugs, which are classified as phosphodiesterase-5 (PDE5) inhibitors. This class of medication is also contraindicated in patients taking nitrites, both regularly and intermittently, because the combination of the two drugs may lead to severe hypotension.

Other preexisting conditions that may preclude the use of these medications are hypotension, hypertension, unstable angina, liver or kidney impairment, retinitis pigmentosa, or any anatomic deformity of the penis.

Side effects, in order of likelihood of occurrence, may include headache, stomach pain, flushing, nosebleeds, or mild temporary vision changes, including color perception changes and blurred vision. Males are advised to take the smallest possible dose to achieve an erection. In addition, a prolonged erection (lasting longer than 4 hours) is an indication to notify the physician.

Any male experiencing chest pain or other serious side effects after taking these medications should seek immediate emergency medical assistance and should advise emergency personnel of the use of these drugs (sildenafil, vardenafil, or tadalafil). Concurrent use of any form of nitrate drug therapy or short-acting nitrate drug to treat chest pain may cause life-threatening hypotension.

Etiology

The causes of infertility in males may be subdivided into different categories. The most common cause for infertile males is idiopathic, meaning that there is no identifiable disorder of sperm number, function, or morphology. Testicular dysfunction, including congenital disorders of the testes, certain developmental disorders, chromosomal abnormalities, and varicoceles, is the next most prevalent cause. The two final categories are disorders of sperm transport and diseases of the hypothalamus or the pituitary gland. Environmental factors, such as certain drugs, radiation, smoking, or pollutants, can also be implicating factors in infertility.

In a female, common causes include fallopian tube dysfunction, ovulation disorders, and uterine abnormalities.

Diagnosis

After a physical examination and an interview of both partners, specific testing procedures are chosen. In males, a complete history, with special attention to childhood diseases, is followed by a thorough physical examination for any structural abnormalities. It is pertinent to inquire about any personal or familial genetic or endocrine disorders. A full semen analysis is essential and, if relevant, possibly chromosome and testosterone testing.

In females, ovulatory function is established by charting of the menstrual cycle. Hormone levels are studied through blood tests. The fallopian tubes and uterine cavity are visualized through **hysterosalpingography** to determine tubal patency. In some cases, **laparoscopy** may be necessary to rule out endometriosis or chronic infection.

Treatment

Each treatment plan is unique, depending on the problems that are identified in the medical and psychological evaluations. The course of action to achieve pregnancy may include treatment of infection, surgery to remove the blockage, the use of fertility drugs (e.g., follicle-stimulating hormone [Follistim]); intrauterine insemination (IUI); or in vitro fertilization (IVF). Many other new assisted reproductive technologies are offered by clinicians specializing in infertility treatment.

Prognosis

Many couples who seek treatment for infertility do achieve pregnancy. Some have untreatable causes, or in some, it may take as long as 3 years to achieve pregnancy.

Prevention

When possible, preventing the causative factors that lead to sterility is preferable. Methods of preventing male infertility include maintaining good overall health to reduce obesity and cardiovascular disease, regular physical examinations, and protection of the testicles during sports. Early and complete treatment of any STI is important for males and females.

Patient Teaching

Much of the patient teaching involves answering questions about the complexity of the medical evaluation and the selected therapeutic approach.

Contraception/Birth Control

Many visits to the medical office are to inquire about contraception methods, also known as *birth control*. There are multiple options available, with each being chosen over another based on the personal preference of the patient, effectiveness, and benefits or risks. Birth control can be considered temporary or permanent. Some permanent methods are reversible, whereas others are not. The patient should be educated on the various methods available and on the benefits and risks of use. Barrier methods of contraception are effective against STIs, such as HIV infection. Nonbarrier methods are used to prevent pregnancy, but they do not protect against STIs.

Sterilization is a permanent option of birth control for either partner. Female sterilization consists of tubal ligation, commonly referred to as *tying the tubes*. This procedure is accomplished when the physician cuts and closes the fallopian tubes. Sperm are unable to reach the egg for fertilization and immediate sterilization results. Hysterectomy, the removal of the uterus, is another method of permanent sterilization.

Vasectomy is the method for permanent sterilization of a male patient. Vasectomy involves cutting the vas deferens so that sperm cannot travel to the female during intercourse. Both vas deferens are cauterized or sutured shut. After a vasectomy, the patient should have a postvasectomy sperm count to ensure that the procedure was successful and that no sperm are present in the semen.

Other methods of contraception are reversible. Intrauterine devices (IUDs); barriers; and fertility awareness–based, hormonal, and lactation amenorrhea are all methods of reversible birth control. Emergency postcoital contraception is also an option if intercourse has taken place without the use of contraception.

An IUD is placed into the uterus to prevent pregnancy. Currently, two categories of IUDs are acceptable and approved by the FDA: copper and hormonal.

The copper T IUDs are small, shaped like the letter T, and inserted through the cervix. This system works by triggering the immune system to prevent pregnancy. This IUD has to be removed after a certain number of years (e.g., it can be left in place for up to 10 years) or if pregnancy should occur while the IUD is in the uterus. (2) There are four other FDA-approved IUD systems that release progestin daily, thus preventing pregnancy. They make the mucous thicker, and also prevent ovulation from taking place. These IUDs should only be left in for a certain number of years, each according to the schedule from the manufacturer, and should be removed as instructed.

Barrier methods of contraception prevent sperm from entering the cervix by blocking the cervix. The diaphragm (cervical cap) and contraceptive sponge are placed next to the cervix in the vagina before sexual intercourse. Condoms that are now available for male and female partners also provide barrier protection. Spermicide is used with any of these methods, and all instructions for use should be followed with each method.

Fertility awareness–based contraception methods can be used by females who are cognizant of their menstrual cycles. The fertility pattern includes which days of the month a female cannot get pregnant, or days she is not likely to get pregnant, and which days are considered fertile days, or days when conception can take place.

Hormonal Methods

Hormonal methods of birth control are also popular among females. Implants, progesterone injections, progesterone pills, combined oral contraceptives (containing both progesterone and estrogen), patches, and vaginal rings are all methods indicated for prevention of pregnancy.

Implants are placed under the skin. The progesterone in the small, thin rod is released over 3 years and then can be replaced. Progesterone injections are administered every 3 months. Birth control pills are dispensed in 21- or 28-day packages. The combined form contains both estrogen and progesterone. The pill containing only progesterone is prescribed for females who cannot take estrogen. Patches containing estrogen are placed on the buttocks or on the upper body. The patches have an adhesive material and are changed every week for 3 weeks. The fourth week is patch-free. Patches cannot be placed on the breast area. Patients who weigh more than 198 lb (90 kg) should be aware that patches may be less effective in preventing pregnancy.

The contraceptive vaginal ring is inserted, releases estrogen and progesterone very slowly for 3 weeks, and is removed during the menstrual cycle.

New mothers who are nursing full-time can use the lactational amenorrhea method of birth control. This option is best for mothers within a 6-month postpartum period and not experiencing menstruation.

Emergency Contraception

Emergency contraception may be used when no contraceptive method was used during sexual intercourse. A copper T IUD can be inserted within 5 days after unprotected intercourse. A second option is the "morning after" pill. The pill can be taken within 3 days after unprotected sex. The pill should be taken as a single dose within 72 hours after unprotected sexual intercourse. The sooner it is taken, the less likely a person is to become pregnant. Also, some emergency contraception pills may not work for individuals who weigh over 155 pounds.

Male Reproductive Diseases

The most common diseases of the male reproductive system are those affecting the prostate gland. The gland can become inflamed or enlarged as a result of bacteria and can cause urinary problems. Common symptoms are as follows:
- Any urinary symptoms, such as frequency, urgency, incontinence, and dysuria
- Pain, swelling, or enlargement of any of the reproductive organs
- Any sexual dysfunction, such as ED/impotence

Epididymitis
Description
Epididymitis is inflammation of the epididymis, the excretory duct of the testicles.

ICD-10-CM Code	N45.1 *(Epididymitis)*
	N45.2 *(Orchitis)*
	N45.3 *(Epididymo-orchitis)*

The above code may be valid as a principal diagnosis. Use an additional code to identify the causative organism. Refer to the physician's diagnosis and then to the current edition of the ICD-10-CM coding manual to ensure the greatest specificity of pathology.

Symptoms and Signs
Symptoms of epididymis inflammation can include scrotal pain and discomfort that radiates into the groin and pain with ejaculation. It is the most common cause of scrotal pain in males seen in the outpatient setting. The epididymis may become enlarged, tender, and firm to palpation. The patient may have groin and scrotal tenderness with severe pain in the testes. Walking may be difficult for the patient as he tries to protect a painful scrotum.

Patient Screening
The patient often experiences great discomfort during the acute phase, requiring a same-day appointment, if possible.

Etiology
The most common cause of epididymitis is an infection; however, it can also be a result of noninfectious etiologies, including trauma or autoimmune disease. STIs by *N. gonorrhoeae* and *C. trachomatis* are the most common bacterial causes of epididymitis. *Escherichia coli* and *Pseudomonas* are other bacterial causes of this condition in older males. Urinary tract infections, tuberculosis, mumps, removal of the prostate gland (**prostatectomy**), trauma, and the prolonged use of an indwelling catheter also may predispose the patient to epididymitis. A viral infection associated with HIV infection can also cause epididymitis.

Diagnosis
Physical examination, urinalysis, urine culture, and urethral swabs for chlamydia and gonorrhea are used to make the diagnosis of epididymitis. The patient also may have an elevated white blood cell (WBC) count.

Treatment

Antibiotic treatment for infectious causes, combined with the administration of antiinflammatory drugs and rest, is beneficial. The use of scrotal support or elevation also may help to lessen tension on the spermatic cord. Scarring may occur, which can lead to sterility if treatment is delayed. This is especially true if the disease is bilateral.

Prognosis

The prognosis is usually good with early treatment. Possible complications include sterility.

Prevention

The best prevention for epididymitis is the early treatment of urinary and STIs. Condom use during sexual intercourse also is recommended.

Patient Teaching

Advise using comfort measures, including ice packs, scrotal support, lightweight clothing, and elevation of the scrotum while at rest. List the warning signs of complications: increased pain, swelling, or discharge.

Orchitis

Description

Orchitis is infection of the testis.

> ICD-10-CM Code   N45.1 *(Epididymitis)*
>   N45.2 *(Orchitis)*
>   N45.3 *(Epididymo-orchitis)*
> *The above code may be valid as a principal diagnosis. Use an additional code to identify the causative organism. Refer to the physician's diagnosis and then to the current edition of the ICD-10-CM coding manual to ensure the greatest specificity of pathology.*

Symptoms and Signs

Inflammation of the testes is caused by viral or bacterial infection and injury. It may affect one or both testes, causing swelling, tenderness, and acute pain. The patient also may experience chills, fever, nausea, vomiting, and general malaise.

Patient Screening

Prompt treatment to alleviate pain and appropriate antibiotic therapy are indicated.

Etiology

Viruses and bacteria can cause this condition, and it may follow epididymitis in sexually active males. Sexual behavior that puts one at risk for STIs may also result in orchitis. Isolated orchitis may be a consequence of infection by the mumps virus. Scrotal atrophy, scrotal abscess, and infertility are complications if left untreated.

Diagnosis

A clinical history to determine the patient's exposure to STIs and mumps or other related diseases, and a physical examination, usually indicate the diagnosis. Further testing in sexually active males should include urethral swabs for chlamydia and gonorrhea. Urinalysis, serologic study, throat culture, or serum antibody testing may be used to isolate or identify causative agents, such as the mumps virus, but is rarely necessary. Immediate differentiation of orchitis from testicular torsion can be accomplished with Doppler ultrasonography.

Treatment

If the cause of orchitis is bacterial, appropriate antibiotic treatment with cephalexin or ciprofloxacin should be started immediately. Orchitis caused by the mumps virus has no specific treatment other than supportive care. Bed rest is usually prescribed, along with certain antiinflammatory drugs to reduce fever and swelling in severe cases. The use of scrotal support also may help.

Prognosis

Healing follows successful treatment with antibiotics, but scarring may compromise fertility.

Prevention

Risk factors for STIs should be avoided. To prevent orchitis related to the mumps virus, all adult males who have not had mumps should be vaccinated.

Patient Teaching

Emphasize the importance of finishing the entire course of antibiotics as prescribed. Suggest comfort measures, such as scrotal support and the use of ice packs. Explain the importance of follow-up appointments for urologic care.

Torsion of the Testicle

Description

Torsion of the testicle is a condition in which one testicle is twisted out of its normal position (Fig. 12.10A).

> ICD-10-CM Code   N44.00 *(Torsion of testis, unspecified)*
>   (N44.00–N44.04 = 5 codes of specificity)

Symptoms and Signs

The primary symptom is a sudden, severe pain in one testicle. The pain can be so severe that it causes nausea and vomiting, and it is usually constant. When the torsion occurs, the scrotum becomes swollen, red, and tender. Torsion can cause the blood vessels supplying the testicle to become kinked, which, in turn, prevents the blood flow to and from the affected testicle.

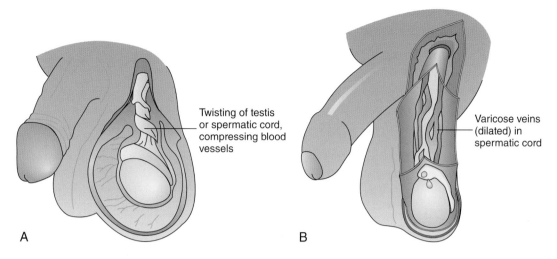

Twisting of testis
or spermatic cord,
compressing blood
vessels

Varicose veins
(dilated) in
spermatic cord

A   B

• **Fig. 12.10** (A) Torsion of testis. (B) Varicocele. (From Gould BE, Dyer RM: *Pathophysiology for the health professions*, ed 4, St. Louis, 2012, Saunders.)

Patient Screening
Emergency treatment is required.

Etiology
This condition occurs when the testis rotates on the spermatic cord, causing a sudden, extreme twist or torsion. It can happen spontaneously or as a result of trauma. The arteries and veins are compressed, ischemia develops, and the scrotum swells.

Diagnosis
Diagnosis is based on the patient's history and a gentle physical examination by the physician. The testicle usually has an abnormal appearance in the scrotum. Because the symptoms of testicular torsion and epididymitis are similar, Doppler ultrasonography may be performed to determine whether testicular torsion is the cause of the pain and swelling. In torsion of the testicle, ultrasonography shows little or no blood flow to the testicle.

Treatment
Immediate consultation with urology is required, followed by surgical intervention for both testes. Surgery should never be delayed, because the delay may result in permanent damage to the testicle. The patient will require bilateral orchiopexy (untwisting and stitching the testes into the proper position) for fixation to reduce the risk of torsion in the future.

Prognosis
The prognosis is good if surgical interventions are performed after a confirmed diagnosis.

Prevention
No prevention is known.

Patient Teaching
Give as much preoperative information as possible by answering questions and giving directions to the patient or the family. The patient also will need information about postoperative care.

Varicocele
Description
In **varicocele**, the veins of one of the testicles become abnormally distended, causing swelling around the testicle that expands within the scrotal sac (see Fig. 12.10B).

ICD-10-CM Code	I86.1 *(Scrotal varices)*

Symptoms and Signs
This is a disorder that is more uncomfortable than painful. A varicocele may be especially uncomfortable in hot weather or after exercise and may be temporarily relieved by lying down. Because the increased presence of venous blood raises the temperature within the scrotum, varicocele may contribute to a lower sperm count or infertility. Decreased testosterone is another symptom. It is more common on the left side because of the anatomy of the vascular supply.

Patient Screening
The condition often is asymptomatic. If a vein ruptures as a result of local injury, pain and swelling in the scrotum cause the patient to seek prompt medical intervention.

Etiology
Incompetent venous valves can cause dilation of the large scrotal veins and venous stasis. Varicoceles can also be congenital.

Diagnosis
Patient history, physical symptoms, and examination by the physician confirm the diagnosis.

Treatment
Treatment consists of measures to relieve the symptoms. These can include the wearing of tight-fitting underwear

or the use of an athletic supporter. If the varicocele affects fertility, surgery can remove the distended veins, but the results may not justify the risks of the surgery. Results vary, depending on the severity of the distention.

Prognosis
In some cases, surgical repair has been reported to improve fertility and decrease pain. In some cases, the patient will not need any intervention.

Prevention
No prevention is known.

Patient Teaching
Encourage the patient to use comfort measures to relieve the symptoms. If the patient undergoes surgical repair, review the postoperative care.

Prostatitis

Description
Prostatitis is an acute or chronic inflammation of the prostate gland.

ICD-10-CM Code	N41.0 *(Acute prostatitis)*
	N41.1 *(Chronic prostatitis)*

Refer to the physician's diagnosis and then to the current edition of the ICD-10-CM coding manual to ensure the greatest specificity of pathology.

Symptoms and Signs
Inflammation of the prostate gland is more common in males older than 50 years of age but can occur in males of any age. The prostate may be enlarged and tender, and in some instances, discharge may be seen at the tip of the penis. The patient may be asymptomatic or may experience acute symptoms in mild or sporadic forms and has pain and a burning sensation during urination. Other common symptoms include low back pain, perineal pain, fever, muscular pain or tenderness, and urinary frequency with urgency. There may be blood in the urine.

Patient Screening
When a patient has acute symptoms of pain and other urinary symptoms, prompt medical evaluation is indicated.

Etiology
The cause of inflammation of the prostate is not always known but is usually infection. Infection may be either bacterial or nonbacterial. Bacterial causes may include, most commonly, *E. coli* that has caused a urinary tract infection, gonococci from a patient with gonorrhea, *Staphylococcus, Streptococcus,* or *Pseudomonas.*

Diagnosis
The prostate gland is gently palpated on physical examination. Urinalysis, blood culture, and a WBC count are ordered. Ultrasonography to measure postvoid residual urine may be ordered.

Treatment
The usual treatment of acute prostatitis is a fluoroquinolone antibiotic such as levofloxacin (Levaquin), or trimethoprim-sulfamethoxazole therapy. The physician also may order sitz baths, rest, an increase in fluid intake, and the administration of analgesics and antiinflammatory drugs. Patients acutely ill on presentation are hospitalized for IV fluids and antibiotics.

Chronic prostatitis can potentially develop from recurrent urinary tract infections, urethral obstruction, and acute urinary retention.

Prognosis
The prognosis for acute prostatitis is good because it responds well to treatment. The outlook for the less common chronic prostatitis is not as favorable. Complications, such as epididymitis, bacteremia, or prostatic abscesses, can occur.

Prevention
The best prevention for prostatitis is the early treatment of urinary tract infections with the prescribed antibiotics.

Patient Teaching
Emphasize the need for strict adherence to the prescribed medications.

Benign Prostatic Hyperplasia

Description
Benign prostatic hyperplasia (BPH) is nonmalignant, noninflammatory hypertrophy of the prostate gland.

ICD-10-CM Code	N40.0 *(Enlarged prostate without lower urinary tract symptoms [LUTS])*
	N40.1 *(Enlarged prostate with lower urinary tract symptoms [LUTS])*

Symptoms and Signs
Enlargement of the prostate gland is a common condition in males older than 50 years of age, and the frequency increases with age. BPH usually progresses to the point of causing compression of the urethra with urinary obstruction and resulting urinary retention (Fig. 12.11). Common signs and symptoms may include difficulty starting urination, a weak stream of urine, or an inability to empty the bladder completely. Urinary frequency, including nocturia, and in severe cases, inflammation and symptoms of renal disease have been observed.

Patient Screening
A routine physical examination is appropriate to evaluate BPH.

• **Fig. 12.11** Benign prostatic hyperplasia. (From Kumar V, Cotran RS, et al: *Robbins basic pathology*, ed 7, Philadelphia, 2003, Saunders.)

• **Fig. 12.12** Cancer of the prostate. (From Kumar V, Cotran RS, et al: *Robbins basic pathology*, ed 7, Philadelphia, 2003, Saunders.)

Etiology

The cause of BPH is not completely understood, but the condition seems to be associated with the aging process and hormonal and metabolic changes. As the prostate gland enlarges, it compresses either the neck of the bladder or the urethra, causing obstruction of the urinary flow.

Diagnosis

The usual diagnosis is based on patient history and a rectal examination for prostatic abnormalities. Routine tests include urinalysis, urine culture, renal function studies, and prostate-specific antigen (PSA) serum levels to screen for prostatic cancer. Urinary flow test, postvoid residual volume test, 24-hour voiding diary completion, transrectal ultrasound, prostate biopsy, and cystoscopy are other tests that will provide more information for the provider.

In many cases, the International Prostate Symptom Score is used to determine the subjective degree of symptoms and their impact on the patient's quality of life.

Treatment

Treatment of BPH may be watchful waiting when symptoms are not bothersome. Lifestyle changes that are recommended include control of fluid intake before bedtime and avoiding medication that may cause urinary retention, such as decongestants. Drug therapy with alpha-adrenergic blockers, including tamsulosin hydrochloride (Flomax), doxazosin mesylate (Cardura), and terazosin hydrochloride, may be prescribed to relax the tightened muscles inside the prostate and relieve symptoms. Another class of drugs is the 5-alpha-reductase inhibitors, which are dutasteride (Avodart) or finasteride (Proscar) that work by reducing the size of the prostate. When symptoms are moderate to severe, a highly effective surgical treatment, transurethral resection

of the prostate (TURP), may be performed to remove the obstructive part of the prostate.

Prognosis

The prognosis for BPH is good with intervention. Severe symptoms, if left untreated, can progress to urinary retention and infection, which may reach the kidneys. Complications of this condition may include cystitis, dilation of the ureters, pyelonephritis, hydronephrosis, and uremia.

Prevention

The possibility of prevention of BPH is unknown. Physicians strongly recommend that older males have regular prostate examinations to detect any enlargement.

Patient Teaching

Inform the patient that ingestion of decongestants, antidepressants, tranquilizers, alcohol, and anticholinergics tends to increase urinary obstruction.

If a prostatectomy is scheduled, review with the patient the physician's explanation of the procedure, and give appropriate information about presurgical and postsurgical care, including possible complications that should be reported to the physician.

Prostate Cancer

Description

Prostate cancer is a malignancy of the small gland located below the bladder and anterior to the rectum in males, known as the *prostate gland*. Although this is a very common cancer, it grows so slowly that only 1 in 41 males diagnosed with prostate cancer will die as a result of it. Nonetheless, after lung cancer, prostate cancer is the second leading cause of cancer-related death in males (Fig. 12.12).

ICD-10-CM Code	C61 *(Malignant neoplasm of prostate)*

TABLE 12.1	Age-Specific Reference Ranges for Serum Prostate-Specific Antigen (PSA)		
Age Range (years)	Reference Range (ng/mL)[a]		
	Blacks	Whites	Japanese
40–49	0.0–2.0	0.0–2.5	0.0–2.0
50–59	0.0–4.0	0.0–3.5	0.0–3.0
60–69	0.0–4.5	0.0–4.5	0.0–4.0
70–79	0.0–5.5	0.0–6.5	0.0–5.0

[a]PSA blood tests are reported as nanograms per milliliter.

Symptoms and Signs

Prostate cancer is often asymptomatic at diagnosis because it is usually detected clinically by abnormalities on routine digital rectal examination (DRE) or by detecting a high concentration of PSA in serum. Asymmetric areas of induration and nodules felt on DRE suggest prostate cancer, and malignant prostate tissue generates more PSA than normal or hyperplastic tissue does (refer to Table 12.1 for PSA values). The usual symptoms, when present, are those associated with urinary obstruction. These include weak or interrupted urine flow, urinary frequency, urinary retention, dysuria, nocturnal enuresis, and hematuria. However, these symptoms also often are common to BPH or an infection or inflammation of the prostate gland.

Patient Screening

Schedule a physical examination with screening for prostate cancer annually for patients 50 years of age or older considered at average risk. Those considered at higher risk for prostate cancer should be screened at age 40 if they have more than one first-degree family (brother or father) member with prostate cancer and age 45 if they are African American or have one first-degree family member with prostate cancer.

Etiology

Risk factors for prostate cancer include race, ethnicity, age, gene changes or heredity, geographic location, and lifestyle. Prostate cancer is more common in older males and rarely occurs before age 40 years. Ethnicity is also important because prostate tumors are much more common in African American males than in white or Hispanic males. Risk is also higher in males who have particular mutations in the *BRCA1* or *BRCA2* genes (breast cancer susceptibility genes). Although many dietary risk factors have been studied, a diet high in animal fat is the most consistent link. Many studies are being done to evaluate other genetic factors, exposures, and infections as possible risk factors.

Diagnosis

Although abnormally high PSA levels and abnormal DRE are highly suggestive findings, prostate biopsy is necessary to diagnose cancer. A biopsy is advised if the PSA level is greater than 4 ng/mL and should be performed at lower values if clinical suspicion is high. A transrectal ultrasound-guided biopsy is usually performed. If the biopsy result is negative but the PSA level remains high, a repeat biopsy is often performed several weeks to months later, because prostate cancer can be missed on the initial biopsy. If a biopsy specimen is found to contain carcinoma, further evaluation and clinical staging are needed to select the appropriate treatment strategy. The TNM (tumor-node-metastasis) staging system proposed by the American Joint Committee on Cancer (AJCC) is the most popular method used for staging. Clinical staging uses DRE, PSA measurement, and imaging studies. Analysis of the tumor histology (the Gleason score) leads to a scoring system based on the degree of glandular differentiation and structural architecture. The Gleason score and the PSA level are incorporated into the TNM stage determination as well.

Treatment

Treatment of prostate cancer depends on the stage of the disease, the Gleason score, the PSA level, the age and physical condition of the patient, and the risks and benefits of each treatment option. Options for early-stage prostate cancer include radical prostatectomy, radiation therapy, brachytherapy (the direct implantation of a radiation source into the prostate), or active surveillance. Radical prostatectomy and radiation have potential complications of ED/impotence and urinary symptoms. Active surveillance with initiation of treatment at any sign of disease progression may be preferred for those with low-risk disease or significant comorbidities.

For patients with metastatic prostate cancer, first-line treatment involves androgen deprivation therapy (ADT) by either surgical orchiectomy (removal of a testicle) or medical orchiectomy (use of hormones to suppress the release of testosterone). The purpose of ADT is to reduce the amount of androgen hormones in the body or prevent the body from responding to them as a method to inhibit the growth of cancer cells. If the cancer becomes resistant to ADT, there are a number of other recently approved medicines that can be tried, with or without chemotherapy, including the Sipuleucel-T cancer vaccine. Patients should be followed up with PSA measurements every 3 to 12 months to monitor the efficacy of treatment and to detect recurrences.

Prognosis

The most important predictors of disease progression are TNM stage, Gleason score of the biopsy specimen, and serum PSA level. For early-stage tumors, radiation therapy and prostatectomy offer similar 10-year survival rates. The overall 5-year survival rate is nearly 100%, because many prostate cancers are diagnosed in early stages as a result of the current screening procedures. The survival rate declines, however, with longer follow-up.

Prevention

There is no 100% proven prevention. Risk studies give varying information; however, some studies indicate eating a healthy diet high in fruits and vegetables and low in fat may lower one's risk when combined with a healthy exercise program.

Patient Teaching

Emphasize the risks and benefits of annual screening for prostate cancer after the age of 50 years. Describe and explain diagnostic procedures. Review the information given by the physician about the mode of treatment and the likely side effects. Explain the warning signs of complications that should be reported to the physician and encourage open communication.

Testicular Cancer

Description

The testicles are the male gonads that produce sperm and are the primary source of male hormones. Cancer of the testicle is one of the most curable solid neoplasms, but it still has a significant effect on the physical and emotional status of the young population it usually affects. Nearly all testicular tumors are germ cell tumors, equally distributed between two main types: seminomas and all others, termed *nonseminomatous germ cell tumors (NSGCTs)*.

ICD-10-CM Code	C62.10 *(Malignant neoplasm of unspecified descended testis)* (C62.10–C62.12 = 3 codes of specificity) C62.90 *(Malignant neoplasm of unspecified testis, unspecified whether descended or undescended)* (C62.90–C62.92 = 3 codes of specificity)

Symptoms and Signs

The most common presentation is a nodule or painless swelling of one testicle. Some patients complain of a dull ache or a heavy sensation in the abdomen, perianal area, or scrotum. Fewer patients have acute pain or gynecomastia. Symptoms of advanced disease include enlarged lymph nodes in the neck, dyspnea or cough, anorexia, bone pain, and lower extremity swelling.

Patient Screening

When a patient reports a nodule or the swelling of a testicle, the next available appointment should be scheduled for a medical evaluation.

Etiology

Testicular neoplasms are most common in males between ages 15 and 45 years (Fig. 12.13). Risk factors include

Spermatic cord   Malignant tumor

• **Fig. 12.13** Cancer of the testes. (From Gould BE, Dyer RM: *Pathophysiology for the health professions*, ed 4, St. Louis, 2012, Saunders.)

cryptorchidism (undescended testicle), personal and family histories of testicular cancer, previous GCT(s), infertility, and HIV infection. Down syndrome and Klinefelter syndrome may predispose affected males to the development of testicular cancer. Children with cryptorchidism are at a higher risk for the disease, even if the testicle is brought to its anatomic position in the scrotum.

Diagnosis

Diagnosis begins with a physical examination of the testes and palpation for nodal involvement. Any firm, hard area in the affected testis is cause for concern. The diagnostic evaluation of suspected testicular cancer continues with scrotal ultrasonography, computed tomography (CT) of the abdomen and pelvis, chest radiography, and measurement of serum tumor markers. Radical orchiectomy also is performed to provide histologic evaluation of the tumor, and retroperitoneal lymph node dissection identifies nodal metastasis. Biopsy is not attempted because of the risk of causing tumor spread. In young males for whom future fertility is important, efforts should be made to perform a baseline sperm count and sperm banking before radiographic procedures so that radiation does not damage sperm. Serum tumor markers that are elevated in many testicular cancers are alpha-fetoprotein (AFP), the beta-subunit of human chorionic gonadotropin (beta-hCG), and lactate dehydrogenase (LDH). These markers help in initial diagnosis, but they are more useful for subsequent disease follow-up.

The TNM staging system for testicular cancer developed by the AJCC considers the primary tumor, nodal involvement, distant metastases, and the serum tumor marker values for AFP, beta-hCG, and LDH. These parameters define stages I to III, which define good, intermediate, and poor prognoses, respectively. Metastatic tumors are staged under a separate system.

Treatment

Testicular NSGCTs are highly chemosensitive. Cisplatin-based combination chemotherapy can cure up to 80% of patients, even those with distant metastases. For those with advanced disease, residual masses may remain after chemotherapy. Surgical resection may be performed to excise the masses, remove any histologically malignant elements, and prevent compression of adjacent structures. Seminomas are radiosensitive, so the patient may be treated with radiation, with or without chemotherapy. For males with elevated levels of a serum tumor marker, monitoring the level throughout treatment often produces the best indication of treatment effectiveness.

As a result of the high cure rate for testicular cancer, posttreatment follow-up is an important part of the care for these patients. Periodic follow-up includes history and physical examination, serum tumor marker measurement, and radiographic studies for a minimum of 5 years after orchiectomy. The optimal surveillance schedule is determined by tumor type and pretreatment disease stage.

Prognosis

The 5-year relative survival rate is greater than 95% in the United States. Factors that affect the prognosis include initial serum concentration of tumor markers, time between diagnosis and treatment, age of the patient, extent of visceral organ involvement, and number of distant metastases.

Prevention

There is no known prevention or screening for testicular cancers. Patients are recommended to check for lumps or changes in a warm shower once a month and report any changes to the physician promptly.

Patient Teaching

Explain all diagnostic and treatment procedures. Review the physician's explanations, and encourage questions. Give the patient information about fertility and sexual potency. Emphasize the importance of the long-term surveillance schedule.

Female Reproductive Diseases

The female reproductive organs are affected by disease in several ways: (1) microorganisms can invade the pelvis or vagina, causing infection and (2) tumors, either benign or malignant, may occur anywhere in the reproductive tract. Symptoms that may require further evaluation are:
- Symptomatic vaginal discharge, with or without odor
- Lower pelvic or abdominal pain
- Pelvic symptoms, such as menstrual pain (**dysmenorrhea**), absence of menstruation (**amenorrhea**), scanty menstruation (**oligomenorrhea**), bleeding between

menses (**metrorrhagia**), and heavy or prolonged menstrual flow (**menorrhagia**)
- Fever
- Pain during sexual intercourse (dyspareunia) or other sexual dysfunction

Premenstrual Syndrome

Description

Premenstrual syndrome (PMS) is a constellation of physical and emotional symptoms that may appear shortly after ovulation and subside with the onset of menstruation or shortly thereafter.

ICD-10-CM Code	N94.3 *(Premenstrual tension syndrome)*

Symptoms and Signs

During the menstrual cycle, fluctuating hormone levels alter mood, sexual desire, and energy levels and may affect physical functioning. Troublesome symptoms related to these hormone shifts include anxiety, anger, sadness, bloating, food cravings, breast pain, irritability, and fatigue. Some females experience edema (swelling related to fluid retention), bloating, and abdominal pain as well. When these cyclic symptoms become severe and fit certain psychological criteria, the diagnosis shifts from PMS to premenstrual dysphoric disorder (PMDD).

Patient Screening

Consultation with a physician and a pelvic examination are scheduled.

Etiology

PMS is related to fluctuations in the levels of estrogen and progesterone and their subsequent impact on levels of neurotransmitters, such as dopamine, serotonin, and norepinephrine in the brain and other parts of the body. There are also alterations in other compounds in the body that lead to sodium and fluid retention. PMS occurs only in ovulating females.

Diagnosis

One of the best ways to make the diagnosis is to have the patient keep a record of her symptoms as they relate to her menstrual cycle. There are no specific medical tests to diagnose PMS, but blood tests, careful history, and physical examination may help rule out other medical conditions.

Treatment

The treatment of PMS is directed toward the relief of symptoms. Reduced dietary intake of sodium, increased calcium consumption, moderate exercise, use of mild analgesics and diuretics, and emotional support all help. In addition, some females notice less breast tenderness when they eliminate caffeine from their diet. In some cases, treatment with antidepressants, such as fluoxetine or sertraline, may be indicated, especially if the patient meets the criteria for PMDD.

Medical treatment may include a prescription for birth control pills. Other therapies include using extended-cycle birth control pills. These contraceptives are packaged so that the female will have only four periods per year compared with the normal 12 per year.

Prognosis

Most PMS can be managed with dietary modification. In some females, PMS worsens with age, and for others, it does not appear until they are older. PMS resolves when a female reaches menopause.

Prevention

There is no prevention available.

Patient Teaching

Some females benefit from a stress-reduction program or counseling to better cope with symptoms. Assure the patient a large percentage of menstruating females experience PMS in some form.

Amenorrhea

Description

The absence of menstrual periods, whether temporary or permanent, is known as *amenorrhea*.

ICD-10-CM Code   N91.2 *(Amenorrhea, unspecified)*
(N91.0–N91.2 = 3 codes of
specificity)

Symptoms and Signs

Primary amenorrhea is no menses by age 15 years. Secondary amenorrhea is no menses for 3 months, after a female has been having monthly menstrual cycles. Short periods of amenorrhea may be normal between menarche (the onset of menstruation) and regular menstrual cycling, which is established usually by age 18 years or later. Amenorrhea has no symptoms, and the only sign is a lack of cyclic bleeding.

The term *postpill amenorrhea* refers to failure to resume menses within 3 months of discontinuation of oral contraception.

Patient Screening

A medical consultation and physical examination are indicated for a female having amenorrhea.

Etiology

In primary amenorrhea, the cause is generally late onset of puberty. It also can be caused by an abnormality in the reproductive system or hormonal imbalances. These conditions usually are not suspected unless the girl has reached the age of 15 years and is still not having her periods. Obstruction of the uterus or vagina or chromosomal/developmental/endocrine abnormalities are ruled out as a cause of primary amenorrhea. Cases of secondary amenorrhea are mainly hormone related. After pregnancy is ruled out, other conditions (e.g., thyroid disease, excess weight loss, poor nutrition, excessive athletic training, psychological stress, or pituitary tumors) should be ruled out.

Diagnosis

Pregnancy should be ruled out in all sexually active females in their reproductive years. Premature ovarian failure, also referred to as primary ovarian insufficiency, should be ruled out in females younger than 40 years of age. The diagnosis of amenorrhea is based on the patient history, whereas the etiology requires blood tests, physical examination, and occasionally radiographic evaluation.

Treatment

The treatment of primary or secondary amenorrhea is to correct the underlying condition that caused it, if possible. When this is not possible, then contraceptive hormones or cyclic progesterone may be used to induce menstruation.

Prognosis

The prognosis of amenorrhea is excellent when the underlying cause is corrected or if cyclic hormones are used to induce menses.

Prevention

Management of weight, proper nutrition, and reducing stress can help prevent amenorrhea.

Patient Teaching

Reinforce any medical regimen as prescribed, and review any adverse effects of hormonal therapy that should be reported to the physician.

Dysmenorrhea

Description

Dysmenorrhea, a common gynecologic disorder, is pain and cramping associated with menstruation and affects about 60% of postpubertal females.

ICD-10-CM Code   N94.6 *(Dysmenorrhea,*
unspecified)
(N94.4–N94.6 = 3 codes of
specificity)

Symptoms and Signs

Dysmenorrhea is pain or cramping that begins either shortly before or shortly after the onset of the menstrual flow. Primary dysmenorrhea describes the onset with the initiation of menses, and secondary dysmenorrhea occurs later, after years of normal nonpainful menses. The discomfort can be located just in the uterine area or diffusely throughout the lower pelvis and back, and with occasional radiation to the thighs or buttocks. Some patients may experience headache, nausea, or dizziness. The symptoms normally lessen and abate by the end of menstruation.

Patient Screening

Severe pain associated with menstruation can result in loss of time at work or inability to perform usual daily activities in a small percentage of people. An appointment should be scheduled for an initial evaluation to diagnose the cause and select the proper management.

Etiology

In primary dysmenorrhea, the cause is thought to be the underlying muscular structure of the uterus and how it reacts to the various chemicals, such as prostaglandins, produced during the cycle. Secondary dysmenorrhea is more likely to be caused by an underlying disorder or disease condition, including pelvic infections, fibroids, and cervical stenosis, but most commonly by endometriosis.

Diagnosis

The diagnosis is made from patient history. Medical causes of dysmenorrhea should be eliminated first. The etiology may be determined from careful history and physical examination, pelvic ultrasonography, and even diagnostic laparoscopy. In some cases, psychiatric evaluation may be indicated to evaluate the patient for anxiety and depression.

Treatment

Nonsteroidal antiinflammatory drugs (NSAIDs), whether prescription or over the counter, and hormonal birth control are generally beneficial for pain relief. Using a heating pad on the abdomen also may help. If an underlying organic reason that is causing the pain is found, then that disease process is treated. For endometriosis, birth control pills, progestins, gonadotropin-releasing hormone (GnRH) analogs, and surgery may all be used to alleviate pain. Fibroids may be removed surgically or reduced in size with high-frequency ultrasound ablation or embolization. Newer techniques, such as laparoscope-guided fibroid diathermy are only available for the right patient. Progesterone receptor antagonists have also shown promise in clinical studies and may soon be available to manage fibroids.

Prognosis

The prognosis for dysmenorrhea is good when the underlying causes are corrected. Even when a cause is not found, the response to NSAIDs and birth control pills is excellent. Primary dysmenorrhea often improves after childbirth.

Prevention

The initial occurrence of dysmenorrhea cannot be prevented; however, if menses are eliminated, then recurring dysmenorrhea can be eliminated.

Patient Teaching

In mild cases, comfort measures are individualized. Help the patient understand the use of analgesics or hormonal contraceptives. When surgery is required, provide preoperative and postoperative counseling.

Ovarian Cysts

Description

Ovarian cysts are fluid-filled, semisolid, or solid masses that originate on or within the ovary. Follicles that occur during a normal menstrual cycle are often called *cysts* during radiologic evaluation, but it is best to think of them as follicles unless they are outside the physiologic norm in size or appearance (Fig. 12.14).

ICD-10-CM Code	N83.20 *(Unspecified ovarian cysts)*
	N83.29 *(Other ovarian cysts)*

Refer to the physician's diagnosis and then to the current edition of the ICD-10-CM coding manual to ensure the greatest specificity of pathology.

Symptoms and Signs

Most small cysts will go unnoticed by the patient. The size at which a cyst becomes symptomatic depends on many factors, including how quickly it develops, the underlying cause, and its association with adjacent structures or other intrapelvic pathology. Rarely, urinary retention can result when a large cyst presses on the area near the bladder. If the cyst produces hormones, then it can affect the body functions associated with those hormones. Larger cysts can undergo a process known as *torsion* or *twisting*, which can cause pain, nausea, and vomiting. Torsion is resolved with surgery and occasionally removal of the ovary. Torsion of the ovary can be as serious as torsion of the testicle.

Patient Screening

The pain and other symptoms associated with an ovarian cyst, or possible complications, prompt the call for medical intervention.

Etiology

There are two basic types of ovarian cysts: physiologic cysts (those caused by normal functioning of the ovary) and neoplastic cysts. Neoplastic cysts are either benign or malignant. Occasionally cancer from other parts of the body metastasizes to the ovary. Most ovarian cysts are physiologic, resulting from ovarian follicle growth or a corpus luteum that persists too long. Cysts that occur in a postmenopausal female and those greater than 10 cm in size are more concerning with regard to possible malignancy. The cause of malignant or benign ovarian tumors is not certain.

Diagnosis

A pelvic mass may be noted during a pelvic or rectal examination. Ultrasonography is the best way to assess the presence and nature of ovarian cysts. Magnetic resonance imaging (MRI) or CT can also help detect cysts. Laparoscopy with direct vision of the ovaries may be appropriate if a cyst must be removed.

• **Fig. 12.14** (A and B) Ovarian serous tumors. (C) Dermoid cyst of the ovary. (Courtesy Dr. Christopher Crum, Brigham and Women's Hospital, Boston, Massachusetts.)

Treatment

Benign physiologic cysts are common, and small cysts seldom require any treatment. Large cysts sometimes can be drained during laparoscopy or even removed. This often can be performed without affecting the ovary. Cysts that are drained are more likely to recur than those that are removed. Small physiologic cysts usually disappear spontaneously. Birth control pills can control ovulation which may lower risk, but they cannot treat existing cysts. Cysts that are cancerous require surgery, often with removal of the uterus, omentum, appendix, and lymph nodes.

Prognosis

For nonmalignant cysts, the outcomes are generally excellent. For cysts related to endometriosis, the outcome depends on the success of treating the endometriosis, and these cysts have a high percentage of recurrence. In the case of cancerous cysts, the prognosis depends on the stage of the disease, the origin of the tumor's cell line, and the degree of cellular abnormality.

Prevention

No prevention is known, although taking birth control pills may reduce the occurrence of physiologic cysts.

Patient Teaching

Encourage the patient to use the analgesic medication, as prescribed, for comfort. Offer appropriate assurance about the prognosis. Give preoperative and postoperative instructions when surgery is scheduled.

❖ ENRICHMENT

Mittelschmerz

Mittelschmerz is the term for unilateral pain that occurs in the region of an ovary during ovulation, usually midway through the menstrual cycle. This dull pain has a duration of a few minutes to a few hours and can indicate the time of ovulation for couples attempting to conceive.

Although the etiology is unknown, leakage of follicular fluid into the abdomen during ovulation or stretching and rupturing of the ovarian cortex may be the cause. The pain occasionally is severe enough for the female to seek medical care. A history of occurrence at the midpoint of the menstrual cycle and the elimination of other pelvic or abdominal causes lead to the diagnosis of mittelschmerz. Mild analgesics provide pain relief.

Endometriosis

Description

Endometriosis is a chronic condition characterized by extrauterine endometrial tissue. The implants of the endometrium are found most commonly in the pelvis but may occur in distant sites (Fig. 12.15).

ICD-10-CM Code   N80.9 *(Endometriosis, unspecified)*
 (N80.0–N80.9 = 9 codes of specified)

• **Fig. 12.15** Endometriosis (ectopic sites). (From Gould BE, Dyer RM: *Pathophysiology for the health professions*, ed 4, St. Louis, 2012, Saunders.)

Endometriosis may be coded by site and the pathology. Refer to the physician's diagnosis and then to the current edition of the ICD-10-CM coding manual to ensure the greatest specificity of pathology.

Symptoms and Signs

Although endometriosis is considered a benign condition, it can be acute or chronic. Secondary dysmenorrhea is a classic symptom. Painful intercourse, painful defecation due to adherence near the rectum, and even infertility can be related to this disease. The cyclical inflammation and scarring eventually can lead to symptoms even when a female is not menstruating. Complications include infertility, ectopic pregnancy, pelvic scarring, and adhesion formation.

Patient Screening

When a patient has progressively painful menstruation, a pelvic examination should be scheduled. Infertility may be the only complaint in some patients.

Etiology

There are differing theories regarding the cause of endometriosis. Retrograde menstruation is believed to be the most likely cause for most cases of this condition. When functioning endometrial tissue grows outside the uterine cavity, it responds to the ovarian hormones as the endometrium (lining of the uterus) does during the normal menstrual cycle. The cyclic swelling, inflammation, bleeding, and subsequent scarring are the reasons for the pain. Risk factors include a family history of the disease, menstrual cycles being shorter than 28 days or lasting longer than 7 days, and uterine structural abnormalities that interfere with the normal flow of menstrual blood out of the uterus. Fibroids and diseases of the immune system, such as systemic lupus erythematosus (SLE), have also been associated with an increased incidence of endometriosis.

Diagnosis

During the pelvic examination, the physician may be able to detect tender areas, nodules, or even thickened scar tissue. Enlarged ovaries may represent endometriomas, and a retroflexed uterus may be scarred and immobile. Good history and physical examination, combined with ultrasonography, can help accurately diagnose advanced endometriosis in the majority of patients. Laparoscopy may be used to confirm the diagnosis and help stage the extent of the disease (Fig. 12.16). Treatment can then be tailored to the female's needs depending on her age, general health, and severity of symptoms.

Treatment

Conservative treatment with various hormones is indicated for younger patients who wish to have children. NSAIDS and analgesics may help with pain. Hormonal contraception, GnRH analogs, and progestin-releasing intrauterine devices (IUDs; Fig. 12.17) or subdermal progestin-releasing

• **Fig. 12.16** Laparoscopy.

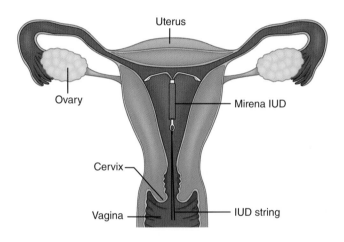

• **Fig. 12.17** Mirena intrauterine device (IUD). (From Proctor D, et al: *Kinn's the medical assistant*, ed 13, St. Louis, 2017, Elsevier.)

implants can all be used to manage the symptoms associated with this disease. Danazol (a testosterone derivative) may also be used be used to manage symptoms. However, it is not considered a first-line treatment due to the high incidence of side effects. Another alternative is the use of aromatase inhibitors. Although these agents are normally used for the treatment of breast cancer, they can decrease the conversion of other hormones to estrogen. Blocking estrogen may prevent the endometriosis from growing. Surgery can remove endometrial implants, deep nodules, and adhesions. Although there is no cure, pregnancy, breast-feeding, or menopause may bring remission of symptoms because the aberrant tissue tends to shrink under these conditions. Surgery can be used to remove or destroy endometrial growths. In severe cases, a total hysterectomy with bilateral **salpingo-oophorectomy** may be indicated.

Prognosis

Although no cure for endometriosis is known, a variety of treatment options are available. Generally the prognosis is good.

• **Fig. 12.18** Pelvic inflammatory disease. (From Kumar V, et al: *Robbins basic pathology*, ed 10, St. Louis, 2018, Elsevier.)

Prevention

No effective prevention is known. Eliminating menstruation may help reduce disease recurrence.

Patient Teaching

Review with the patient the issues surrounding the disease and inform her that it can progress or even regress over time. Provider instructions need to be followed.

Pelvic Inflammatory Disease

Description

PID is an infection of a female's pelvis. The tubes, ovaries, and surrounding tissue are involved in the infection, which can be self-limiting or, in cases of abscess formation, life threatening (Fig. 12.18).

ICD-10-CM Code	N73.9 *(Female pelvic inflammatory disease, unspecified)*
	(N73.8–N74 = 3 codes of specificity)

Symptoms and Signs

The infection is most common in young sexually active females, especially those with more than one sexual partner. Initially, the patient may experience low abdominal pain. Other symptoms are those of an active infection: fever, chills, malaise, a foul-smelling vaginal discharge, backache, and a painful, tender abdomen. Often even walking is painful, and the patient may walk with a shuffling gait. If an abscess has developed, a soft, tender pelvic mass may be palpated. The WBC count and the erythrocyte sediment rate (ESR) are usually elevated.

Patient Screening

The patient with PID reports constitutional symptoms and pain. When symptoms are severe, arrange for immediate medical intervention.

Etiology

The initial infection is usually an STI (e.g., gonorrhea, chlamydia), but then the etiology becomes multibacterial, with the involvement of both aerobic and anaerobic organisms.

Diagnosis

The pelvic examination demonstrates tenderness, usually bilaterally. Most commonly, the cervix is tender to manipulation or movement. Cervical cultures may or may not be positive for an STI. Ultrasonography can help rule out abscess formation. Fever, elevated WBC count, and physical examination are usually sufficient to make the diagnosis and begin treatment. Sometimes the symptoms or signs are not clear; in that case, laparoscopy can be helpful in confirming the diagnosis.

Treatment

Early diagnosis and prompt treatment lessen the damage to the reproductive system. Treatment consists of antibiotics given either intravenously or orally, depending on the severity of the infection.

Prognosis

Without effective treatment, serious complications may develop. The inflammation of the female reproductive organs can cause scar tissue (adhesions) to form. If adhesions form in or around the fallopian tubes, they can cause infertility or increase the risk of ectopic pregnancy. Peritonitis, septicemia, and even death may result. Early and aggressive therapy can improve the prognosis.

Prevention

The best prevention of PID is to not acquire an STI.

Patient Teaching

Inform the patient that infection typically begins intravaginally and ascends through the entire genital tract. Review all risk factors. Sexually active females with multiple partners should be told that PID is frequently associated with STIs. There is a small risk of developing PID after IUD insertion but this risk only lasts a few weeks after insertion.

Description

Leiomyomas (fibroids) are noncancerous (benign) tumors of the smooth muscle within the uterus. They may vary in number, size, and location within the uterus. They are the most common tumors of the female reproductive tract and can occur in a large percentage of females before the age of 50. (Fig. 12.19).

ICD-10-CM Code	D25.9 *(Leiomyoma of uterus, unspecified)* (D25.0–D25.9 = 4 codes of specificity)

Leiomyomas are coded according to site. Refer to the physician's diagnosis and then to the current edition of the ICD-10-CM coding manual to ensure the greatest specificity of pathology.

• **Fig. 12.19** Leiomyomas. (From Cotran RS, Kumar V, Collins T: *Robbins pathologic basis of disease,* ed 6, Philadelphia, 1999, Saunders.)

Symptoms and Signs START

Most fibroids are asymptomatic. If symptoms do occur, they may include pelvic pain, pressure, constipation, urinary frequency, abnormal bleeding, and heavy or prolonged periods. The latter symptom is the most common. The severity of symptoms is related to the number, size, and location of the tumors.

Patient Screening

Schedule a gynecologic examination and medical consultation for a female experiencing the symptoms mentioned previously. Ask the female if she is pregnant or could be pregnant.

Etiology

The cause of leiomyomas and fibroids is unknown. Their development is stimulated by estrogen, and they typically regress after menopause. Birth control pills and hormone replacement therapy do not appear to have much of an impact on the growth or size of fibroids.

Diagnosis

The diagnosis is based on pelvic examination and patient history. A definitive diagnosis is based on ultrasonography and tissue biopsy.

Treatment

Treatment generally depends on the severity of the symptoms, the patient's age, and her desire to have children. In females of childbearing age, surgery can be performed to remove the tumors. In a female who does not want to have children, MRI-guided high-frequency ultrasound ablation may be useful. Uterine artery embolization, once considered useful only in females who are through with childbearing, may be finding a niche in females who want to have children. Hysterectomy is the only definitive treatment because fibroids can recur after other procedures. The route of hysterectomy depends on many factors; however, modern techniques allow many females to undergo surgery as an outpatient.

Prognosis

In general, fibroids do not need to be removed. The rate of malignancy within a fibroid is very rare. In cases where they are removed, there is a chance of recurrence. The risk of recurrence is greater when multiple fibroids are present. With the removal of the uterus, there is essentially no risk of recurrence.

Prevention

No method for the prevention of leiomyomas is known.

Patient Teaching

Teach the patient about the signs of complications, such as hemorrhage or sudden onset of pain and fever.

Vaginitis
Description

Vaginitis is inflammation and/or infection of the vaginal tissues.

ICD-10-CM Code	N76.0 *(Acute vaginitis)*
	N76.1 *(Subacute and chronic vaginitis)*
	N76.2 *(Acute vulvitis)*
	N76.3 *(Subacute and chronic vulvitis)*

Refer to the physician's diagnosis and then to the current edition of the ICD-10-CM coding manual for an additional code to identify the causative organism.

Symptoms and Signs

Inflammation of the vagina is common, and all age groups are at risk. It is generally not perilous, but it can be irritating and painful. Vaginal discharge, with local itching, burning, and odor, is the principal symptom. Depending on the causative agent, the discharge may be white, gray, or green; almost absent to copious; and odorless or malodorous. The discharge may cause irritation and soreness of the vulva. Fever may be present.

Patient Screening

The discomfort and irritation secondary to vaginal infection prompt the earliest possible appointment for a pelvic examination, diagnosis, and treatment.

Etiology

Fungal infections, such as candidiasis, are one of the most common causes of vaginitis. Another common cause is bacterial vaginosis, which occurs when there is bacterial overgrowth and the balance of "good" and "bad" bacteria normally found in the vagina is affected. Another infection

is caused by a protozoan called *Trichomonas*. Cervical infections in chlamydia or gonorrhea can produce a discharge that is irritating and may be mistaken for vaginitis. In postmenopausal females, the absence of estrogen can cause thinning of the vaginal lining and alterations in the normal flora, leading to increased susceptibility to infections. This condition is referred to as *atrophic vaginitis.*

Diagnosis

After taking the medical history, the physician performs a pelvic examination and swabs the vagina. Specimens from the vagina and cervix are analyzed for the presence of bacteria and fungus, and the pH of the discharge is assessed. The discharge can also be assessed for odor and a slide may be prepared to look at in the office. Specifically, *Gardnerella* infection causes a strong "fishy" odor. If the diagnosis is in doubt, a specimen can be sent to the laboratory for culture.

Treatment

Depending on the results of the culture and wet preparation examination, treatment may consist of an antifungal, antibacterial, or hormone therapy (in the case of atrophic vaginitis). More specifically, appropriate treatment for bacterial vaginosis would be metronidazole or clindamycin (oral or vaginal). Yeast infections may be treated with miconazole, clotrimazole (vaginally), or fluconazole (orally). Trichomoniasis may be treated with metronidazole or tinidazole. Patients taking metronidazole or tinidazole are cautioned not to consume any alcohol-based products in any form.

Prognosis

With proper treatment, the inflammation usually clears up in about a week. However, vaginitis may be a recurring problem in some females.

Prevention

Preventive measures are directed toward known causes, avoidance of STIs, maintenance of good hygiene, avoidance of known chemical irritants, and recognition of risk factors for postmenopausal females. Douching interrupts the normal pH of the vagina and may contribute to *Gardnerella* infection.

Patient Teaching

Give information to the patient according to the determined etiology. Emphasize the importance of complying with the prescribed medication therapy exactly as directed after the infection has been identified. Review the risk factors for STIs, if appropriate. Advise the patient to avoid mechanical or chemical irritants, which may be found in douches, deodorant sprays, spermicides, latex condoms, detergents, or bubble bath products. Tight, nonporous underclothing and poor personal hygiene can promote bacterial growth. The use of a nonirritating vaginal lubricant during intercourse may help the postmenopausal female.

Toxic Shock Syndrome

Description

Toxic shock syndrome (TSS) is an acute, systemic infection with *Staphylococcus aureus* or streptococcal toxic-like syndrome. The condition occurs in young, healthy persons aged 20 to 50 years.

> ICD-10-CM Code   A48.3 *(Toxic shock syndrome)*
> *Refer to the physician's diagnosis and then to the current edition of the ICD-10-CM coding manual for an additional code to identify the bacterial agent.*

Symptoms and Signs

Symptoms may vary from one person to another. The sudden onset is characterized by high fever, headache, muscle aches, confusion, redness of throat, mouth, and eyes, and a rash. The syndrome progresses rapidly to hypotension and shock. Other symptoms and signs that the patient might experience are gastrointestinal (GI) symptoms, diarrhea, neuromuscular disturbances, abnormal kidney function, and an elevation of the liver enzyme levels. Without treatment, the disease may become life threatening.

Patient Screening

Immediate medical treatment is indicated.

Etiology

Toxic shock syndrome can result from an increase in *S. aureus* colonization, *S. pyogenes*, and *C. sordellii*. The toxins produced by the bacteria create the illness. Historically initial infections were primarily associated with the use of superabsorbent tampons, but those incidences have decreased since tampons are now made with different types of materials. Other things that put a person at risk include recent surgery, use of diaphragms or contraceptive sponges, and viral infections.

Diagnosis

A diagnosis of TSS is based on clinical evaluation and laboratory tests.

Treatment

Therapy for TSS is supportive and includes the replacement of fluids to counteract shock and the use of antibiotics to treat the infection. Currently, physicians are treating staphylococcal toxic shock with IV vancomycin to cover methicillin-resistant *Staphylococcus aureus* (MRSA).

Prognosis

Prompt diagnosis followed by antibiotic treatment offers the best prognosis. However, TSS can result in neurologic, renal, and respiratory complications, and if treatment is delayed, death from shock.

Prevention

Physicians advise females to use tampons that are just absorbent enough to handle their menstrual flow and to avoid the superabsorbent type. Tampons are best used during the daytime and should be changed frequently. Keep surgical wounds clean and follow directions for using contraceptive diaphragms or sponges.

Patient Teaching

Explain the importance of taking the entire course of antibiotics as prescribed and following the provider's instructions.

Menopause START

Description

Menopause (change of life, or *climacteric*) is the cessation of menstrual periods for 1 year, with evidence of ovarian failure. The average age of menopause is 51 years in the United States and it is not considered premature unless it occurs before age 40 years.

> ICD-10-CM   N95.1 *(Menopausal and female*
> Code   *climacteric states)*
> (N95.0–N95.9 = 5 codes of
> specificity)

Symptoms and Signs

Many females experience the onset of menopause between the ages of 45 and 55 years. Fluctuation in the menstrual cycle and flow is noted, with periods often becoming lighter and less frequent. Hot flashes and night sweats often are reported as a mild to intolerable nuisance in about 75% of females going into menopause. Vaginal dryness and skin changes may appear. Many females experience transient to troublesome psychological symptoms, including depression, poor memory, anxiety, sleep disorders, and loss of interest in sex. By definition, females who are still menstruating but have symptoms of menopause are not menopausal. They are more properly classified as perimenopausal. Once they have stopped menstruating, then they are considered menopausal.

Patient Screening

Schedule a medical examination and consultation with the physician. Inform the patient that a pelvic examination may be required.

Etiology

Starting as early as age 30 years, changes occur in the ovarian production of certain hormones. This creates alterations in the pituitary levels of follicle-stimulating hormone (FSH), driving the failing ovary to produce more follicles. This altered balance between ovarian estrogen, follicle generation, and pituitary level of FSH leads to fluctuations in the menstrual cycle hormones. These changes create the symptoms that females experience as they approach menopause. Once the ovarian reserve has been exhausted and the ovary can no longer produce viable eggs, then ovulation halts and menstruation ceases. Chemotherapy or radiation treatment for certain cancers can also bring on menopause. Surgical menopause (i.e., a total hysterectomy) is a sudden event and may be associated with an increase in hot flashes and nuisance symptoms compared with natural menopause, if not treated with hormones.

Diagnosis
Patient history suggests menopause. The blood serum levels of FSH are elevated, and the estrogen levels are low.

Treatment
The treatment of menopause is really the management of the symptoms related to the condition. Hot flashes and other symptoms related to estrogen withdrawal may be managed with estrogen products or a low-dose selective serotonin reuptake inhibitor (SSRI) such as paroxetine mesylate (Brisdelle). Because there is ongoing debate regarding the potential for cancer with hormone treatment, the patient should be involved in the final decision regarding whether or not to use hormones. Estrogen may not be recommended for long-term use in all patients. Vaginal changes can be managed with local estrogen products and lubricants or the newer selective estrogen receptor modulator (SERM) ospemifene (Osphena). Bone loss can be effectively treated with bisphosphonates: alendronate (Fosamax), risedronate (Actonel), ibandronate (Boniva), SERMs such as raloxifene (Evista), or salmon calcitonin. With very low bone density, other agents, such as denosumab (Prolia, a rank ligand inhibitor) or teriparatide (Forteo, a synthetic parathyroid hormone), may be required. Weight-bearing exercise and dietary calcium or calcium supplementation with adequate vitamin D_3 can also help reduce the rate of bone loss in sedentary patients or those with poor calcium intake and low vitamin D levels.

Prognosis
Menopause is a normal condition with a variable course. Cigarette smokers experience menopause about 2 years earlier compared with nonsmokers.

Prevention
Menopause cannot be prevented. Patients who have a total hysterectomy experience menopause after surgery as a result of the removal of the ovaries.

Patient Teaching
Pros and cons of hormone replacement therapy and alternatives to hormone replacement therapy should be shared. Encourage questions about symptoms experienced. Recommend a healthy lifestyle as the first line of defense against changes related to aging.

Uterine Prolapse
Description
Prolapse of the uterus is the downward displacement of the uterus from its normal location in the pelvis.

ICD-10-CM Code	N81.2 (Incomplete uterovaginal prolapse) (N81.2–N81.4 = 3 codes of specificity)

Symptoms and Signs
Most patients with mild degrees of prolapse have no symptoms. On occasion, the patient may feel increased vaginal or pelvic pressure as the uterus descends into the vagina. When the prolapse is at the point where the cervix is exiting the vagina, the female may feel it while wiping herself after urination. Sometimes the prolapsed uterus can cause pain during intercourse or generalized pelvic discomfort.

Patient Screening
Schedule a routine appointment and a pelvic examination for the patient.

Etiology
Uterine prolapse occurs when the normal support of the uterus weakens as a result of trauma (childbirth), aging, or genetic factors. The weakening of these supports allows the uterus to move down the vaginal canal, pulling the vagina where the cervix is attached along with it. When the uterus is completely outside the vagina, it is termed *complete procidentia* (Fig. 12.20). If it is less than complete, then it is graded on the basis of the distance that it has traveled down the vagina in comparison with the normal anatomic position in relation to the introitus (opening of the vagina).

Diagnosis
The prolapse is visible on pelvic examination.

Treatment
There is no way to have the prolapse reverse itself once it has occurred. Losing weight, reducing coughing, correcting constipation by using the Valsalva maneuver, or targeted physical therapy can help slow down the progression of the process. The use of a pessary may help alleviate some of the symptoms of prolapse, but it does not correct the problem. This device is inserted into the vagina to support the uterus and prevents it from prolapsing. Surgery is the only way to correct prolapse. In females who no longer need the uterus, a hysterectomy is commonly performed, with or without reattaching the vaginal apex to the sacrum or to the sacrospinous ligaments.

Prognosis
The prognosis is good even if surgery is required.

Prevention
Exercises that strengthen the muscles of the pelvic floor after childbirth are recommended. Smoking cessation to reduce coughing and high-fiber diets with adequate fluid intake to reduce constipation can help.

A   B   C

• **Fig. 12.20** Uterine prolapse. (A) First degree. (B) Second degree. (C) Complete prolapse. (From Seidel HM, et al: *Mosby's guide to physical examination*, ed 8, St. Louis, 2014, Mosby.)

Patient Teaching

Review the anatomy and nature of the condition, and make sure the patient understands how to perform Kegel exercises. Surgical options should be shared if this is recommended.

Cystocele

Description

Cystocele is the downward displacement and protrusion of the urinary bladder into the anterior wall of the vagina (Fig. 12.21).

Bladder pushing into vagina

Cystocele

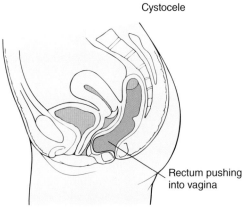

Rectum pushing into vagina

Rectocele

• **Fig. 12.21** Cystocele and rectocele.

ICD-10-CM Code	N81.9 *(Female genital prolapse, unspecified)* (N81.10–N81.12 = 3 codes of specificity)

Symptoms and Signs

This disorder causes the female patient to experience pelvic pressure. It may cause bladder symptoms, such as urinary leakage, urgency, or discomfort during intercourse. In severe cases with urethral or bladder neck kinking, the bladder cannot be emptied completely. This can cause overdistension of the bladder with resultant nerve and/or muscle damage or increased incidence of bladder infections.

Patient Screening

Schedule a routine appointment and a pelvic examination for the patient. Symptoms of cystitis, such as painful and frequent urination, may require an earlier appointment.

Etiology

This condition results from trauma to the fascia, muscle, and pelvic support structures during pregnancy and delivery or from atrophy of these structures as a result of aging and genetic predisposition.

Diagnosis

Diagnosis is based on the clinical picture and findings of the physical examination.

Treatment

The treatment options for cystocele are the same as those for uterine prolapse. Symptoms of incontinence may be improved by performing Kegel exercises; however, surgery or pessary insertion are methods of treatment. Surgery to return the bladder to its normal position may be done with or without applying surgical mesh. Each type of mesh carries its own benefits and risks. A candid discussion of these risks and benefits is necessary before surgical intervention.

Prognosis

The prognosis is good.

Prevention

Exercises that strengthen the pelvic floor muscles after childbirth may help. The tissue changes associated with aging cannot be prevented. Avoiding traumatic vaginal delivery may also help reduce the incidence of this condition.

Patient Teaching

Review the prescribed exercises. Give preoperative and postoperative instructions to candidates for **colporrhaphy**, a surgical procedure that involves suturing of the vagina to narrow it.

Rectocele

Description

A rectocele is the protrusion of the rectum into the posterior wall of the vagina.

ICD-10-CM Code	N81.6 *(Rectocele)*

Symptoms and Signs

The rectocele causes the female patient to experience a bearing-down feeling, fullness in the vagina, back pain, pelvic pressure, and difficulty evacuating the rectum (see Fig. 12.21).

Patient Screening

Schedule a routine appointment and a pelvic examination as soon as possible.

Etiology

Similar to a cystocele, a rectocele occurs when the posterior wall of the vagina is weakened, allowing protrusion of the rectum into the vagina. This most commonly occurs as a result of childbirth, aging, or genetic predisposition.

Diagnosis

Diagnosis is based on the clinical picture and the findings of the physical examination.

Treatment

Treatment consists of surgical repair of the posterior wall of the vagina (posterior colporrhaphy). A pessary can also be used if surgery is not desired.

Prognosis

The prognosis is good with surgical repair.

Prevention

No prevention is known. Reduction in coughing and in constipation may help decrease the severity or delay onset in predisposed patients.

Patient Teaching

Give the patient appropriate preoperative and postoperative instructions. Anticipate questions, and reassure the patient concerned about how the procedure may affect sexual intercourse.

Cervical Cancer

Description

The cervix is the lower part of the uterus, extending from the uterine isthmus into the vagina. It functions to allow sperm into the uterine cavity and the infant to pass into the birth canal. Most cervical cancers are either squamous cell carcinomas that arise in the transitional zone between the different epithelial types of the uterus corpus and the vagina or adenocarcinoma (Fig. 12.22).

ICD-10-CM Code	C53.9 *(Malignant neoplasm of cervix uteri, unspecified)* (C53.0–C53.9 = 4 codes of specificity)

• **Fig. 12.22** Cancer of the cervix. (From Cotran RS, Kumar V, Collins T: *Robbins pathologic basis of disease*, ed 6, Philadelphia, 1999, Saunders.)

Symptoms and Signs

The two main symptoms of cervical cancer are (1) a watery, bloody, or purulent vaginal discharge that may be heavy and foul smelling and (2) bleeding between menstrual periods, after intercourse, or after menopause. The most common sign is an abnormal Pap smear test result. The appearance of the cervical lesion varies, but it is often a mass or an ulcer on the surface of the cervix. Signs and symptoms of advanced disease include pelvic or lower back pain, hematuria, dysuria, or rectal bleeding.

Patient Screening

Encourage females to have regular screening with cervical Pap smear tests. Schedule a prompt gynecologic examination for the female experiencing abnormal vaginal bleeding such as prolonged or intermittent periods, bleeding after intercourse, or a period after menopause.

Etiology

Invasive cervical cancer is often considered a preventable disease because it has a long premalignant stage (often 10 years or longer) and an effective screening program and effective therapies. Therefore the biggest risk factor for invasive cervical carcinoma is the lack of regular screening with cervical Pap smear tests. The other major risk factor is exposure to oncogenic types of HPV, such as HPV-16, -18, -31, and -45. Infections by these HPV types are more common in individuals who have had early and frequent unprotected sexual activity with multiple partners. HPV DNA is detected in nearly all invasive cervical cancers. HPV infection is often found with other risk factors, such as smoking, immunosuppression, low socioeconomic status, early and multiple parity, prolonged use of oral contraceptives, and/or other STIs. The most common age at diagnosis is 45 to 55 years, but it is also a significant problem in females older than 65 years of age, who are less likely to undergo Pap smear tests. The premalignant lesion for cervical cancer is called *cervical intraepithelial neoplasia* (CIN), and it involves dysplasia or atypical changes in the cervical epithelium.

Diagnosis

The Pap smear test was developed specifically to detect cervical cancer. The diagnosis of cancer is then confirmed through colposcopy and directed biopsy of the cervical lesion. The stage is determined clinically through physical examination of the patient, chest x-ray, intravenous pyelography (IVP), cystoscopy, and proctoscopy. Lymph node sampling also may be performed. The International Federation of Gynecologists and Obstetricians developed the staging system that is currently used. It differs from the commonly used TNM system in that it relies on clinical evaluation rather than the pathologic features of the tumor. This is because cervical cancer is most common in developing countries where more modern techniques are not available for staging the tumor.

Treatment

Treatment is determined by stage. Low-grade CIN is followed with repeat cytology at 6 and 12 months. For high-grade CIN, loop electrosurgical excision procedure is preferred, and other treatments include laser therapy and cryoablation. Radical hysterectomy (removal of the uterus, cervix, and upper vagina) is usually performed to treat CIN in the early invasive stages. For carcinomas that have invaded the pelvic wall or have distant metastases, radiation therapy is included in the treatment. Cisplatin-based chemotherapy often is used in conjunction with radiotherapy. Patients should be followed up with periodic physical examinations and Pap smear tests to detect recurrences.

Prognosis

Stage is the most important determinant of prognosis, followed by lymph node status, tumor volume, and depth of tumor invasion. HPV subtype also may affect the prognosis, with HPV-18 having a poorer prognosis compared with the other subtypes. The 5-year survival rate is 91% if diagnosed early. The 5-year survival rate if diagnosed after the cancer has spread to nearby tissues and lymph nodes is 60%. The 5-year survival rate is 19% the cancer has spread to distant tissues. Recurrence is usually local (e.g., cervix, uterus, and/or vagina) and carries a very poor prognosis.

Prevention

Primary prevention of cervical cancer can be achieved through vaccination with one of the two FDA-approved vaccines against HPV (see the Enrichment box about Human Papillomavirus Vaccine and Cervical Cancer). All sexually active females should undergo an annual Pap smear test and pelvic examination at 21 years or earlier if recommended by their physician. After three or more consecutive normal Pap smear test results or after age 30 years, screening can be performed less often, at the discretion of the physician, but should be done at least every 3 years. HPV testing can be performed at the same time as the Pap smear test to detect infection by high-risk subtypes of HPV. Females with a Pap smear test result suggesting CIN should be evaluated with colposcopy and biopsy of any lesion detected. For females with no risk factors and at least three normal smear test results, screening can cease around age 65 or 70 years. Unfortunately, screening programs are often lacking in developing countries.

Patient Teaching

Emphasize that with early diagnosis, the survival rate for cervical cancer is excellent. Females diagnosed with invasive stages of cervical cancer require information about treatment and possible complications. Explain preoperative and postoperative instructions for hysterectomy, radiation therapy, and/or chemotherapy.

Vaginal Cancer

Description

Primary cancer of the vagina is rare, and malignancy usually results from metastasis from neoplasms of adjacent structures. Most primary tumors are squamous cell carcinomas, but other types, such as melanoma or adenocarcinoma, may be seen.

ICD-10-CM Code   C52 *(Malignant neoplasm of vagina)*

Symptoms and Signs

Most patients have vaginal bleeding, usually postcoital or postmenopausal bleeding. Other symptoms include a malodorous or watery vaginal discharge; urinary symptoms, such as dysuria or frequency; constipation; melena; or a vaginal mass. The tumor itself presents as a mass, plaque, or ulcer on the vaginal wall. The posterior wall of the upper one-third of the vagina is the most common site.

Patient Screening

Unusual vaginal bleeding, pelvic pain, or the symptoms mentioned earlier require diagnostic evaluation which includes a pelvic examination.

Etiology

Risk factors for primary vaginal cancer include HPV infection (particularly subtypes 16 and 18), prior history of gynecologic malignancy, advanced age, multiple lifetime sexual partners, early age at first intercourse, and cigarette smoking. Vaginal intraepithelial neoplasia (VAIN), which comprises atypical squamous cells without invasion, may be a premalignant lesion for vaginal cancer. It is usually asymptomatic but can be associated with postcoital spotting or vaginal discharge.

Diagnosis

Diagnosis is difficult because the malignant lesion may be small and missed on gynecologic examination. Pap smear tests may reveal malignant cells of the vagina incidentally when screening for cervical cancer. Definitive diagnosis is accomplished through colposcopic examination and direct biopsy of the lesion. A cervical biopsy also must be performed to rule out primary cervical cancer. Carcinomas are staged by means of physical and pelvic examinations, cystoscopy, proctoscopy, chest radiography, and bone scanning. The TNM staging system is used, where T reflects the extent of tumor penetration through the vaginal wall.

Treatment

Treatment is based on the location, size, and clinical stage of the tumor. Surgery usually includes hysterectomy, upper vaginectomy, and bilateral pelvic lymphadenectomy and may be performed with adjuvant radiation therapy. Radiotherapy alone may be sufficient to treat early-stage vaginal cancers.

Prognosis

The major indicator of prognosis is the stage at the time of diagnosis, although lymph node status, age, and lesion location are also important. Because many vaginal cancers are diagnosed at an advanced stage and because a high percentage of locally advanced cancers recur within 6 months of initial treatment, the overall relative 5-year survival rate for squamous cell vaginal cancer is around 57%.

Prevention

Undergoing regular screening with Pap smear tests, using barrier contraceptives, and limiting the number of sexual partners may reduce the risk of vaginal cancer. Diagnosis and treatment of VAIN with surgical excision, laser ablation, or topical 5-fluorouracil may prevent progression to invasive disease. Periodic follow-up should be performed to look for recurrent VAIN or invasive disease.

Patient Teaching

Enforce the physician's recommendation for a screening schedule based on the patient's history of risk factors, and referrals if indicated. Review with the patient the physician's explanation of procedures and possible complications of therapy.

Labial or Vulvar Cancer

Description

The vulva is the area of the female external genitalia. Any condition that can affect the skin on other parts of the body can affect the vulva. Greater than 90% of vulvar malignancies are squamous cell carcinomas.

ICD-10-CM Code   C51.0 *(Malignant neoplasm of labium majus)*
C51.1 *(Malignant neoplasm of labium minus)*
C51.9 *(Malignant neoplasm of vulva, unspecified)*

Symptoms and Signs

Most patients have a nodule or ulcer, usually on the labia majora. The lesion may be associated with pruritus. Less common symptoms and signs include vulvar bleeding, discharge, dysuria, and enlarged lymph nodes in the groin.

Patient Screening

The patient may complain of a sore or nodule on the labia causing discomfort; schedule a gynecologic examination.

Etiology

Vulvar neoplasms are encountered most often in postmenopausal females. The average age at diagnosis is 65 years. Risk factors include cigarette smoking; HPV (usually subtypes 16 and 33) or HIV infection; multiple sexual partners; prior history of cervical cancer; and northern European ancestry. Vulvar intraepithelial neoplasia (VIN), which is noninvasive epithelial dysplasia of the vulva, is thought to be a premalignant lesion for invasive carcinoma.

Diagnosis

Diagnosis requires a biopsy of the lesion. Colposcopy may be used to define areas for biopsy. After the diagnosis of cancer is confirmed, a physical examination for the involvement of regional lymph nodes is mandatory. Evaluation also includes colposcopy to assess for multifocal lesions and MRI or positron emission tomography with CT. A Pap smear test is performed to check for cervical cancer. The tumor is staged surgically, because lymph node involvement is the most important prognostic indicator.

Treatment

The usual treatment of vulvar carcinoma is either surgical removal of the growth and surrounding skin or removal of all or part of the vulva itself. Inguinofemoral lymphadenectomy is usually performed. Depending on the stage of the disease, radiation therapy, with or without chemotherapy, is added. Patients with distant metastases or recurrences typically have a poor rate of response.

Prognosis

Inguinofemoral lymph node status is the most important indicator of prognosis, regardless of stage. Tumor size and depth of invasion are also important.

Prevention

The risk for vulvar carcinoma is reduced by the use of barrier contraceptives, regular gynecologic examinations, and treatment of VIN with excision, laser therapy, or topical 5-fluorouracil.

Patient Teaching

Explain the medical treatment which may include preoperative and postoperative instructions, the use of analgesics, and the side effects to expect from radiation therapy or chemotherapy. Emphasize the importance of follow-up care.

Ovarian Cancer

Description

Ovarian cancer accounts for more deaths than any other gynecologic malignancy. Because of the location of the ovaries deep within the pelvis, the cancer is often asymptomatic until the more advanced stages.

ICD-10-CM Code	C56.9 (Malignant neoplasm of unspecified ovary) (C56.1–C56.9 = 3 codes of specificity)

Symptoms and Signs

Ovarian neoplasms may cause nonspecific symptoms, such as lower abdominal discomfort, bloating, constipation, lower back pain, irregular menstrual cycles, urinary frequency, or dyspareunia. The most common sign is an enlargement of the abdomen caused by the accumulation of fluid (ascites), but this usually indicates advanced disease. Persistent, vague digestive disturbances (e.g., discomfort, gas, or distention that cannot be explained by any other cause) should be evaluated for ovarian cancer.

Patient Screening

For a female experiencing the nonspecific symptoms listed previously, schedule a physical examination, including a pelvic examination.

Etiology

Most ovarian cancers occur in females older than 55 years of age. The etiology is largely unknown, but multiple risk factors have been identified. Females who have had breast cancer or who have a family history of breast or ovarian cancer have an increased risk. They may have mutations in *BRCA1* or *BRCA2*, the breast cancer susceptibility genes. People with hereditary nonpolyposis colon cancer also have an increased risk for ovarian cancer. Pregnancy, breast-feeding, prolonged use of oral contraceptives, and tubal ligation may reduce the risk of development of ovarian cancer.

Diagnosis

Early-stage ovarian cancer is sometimes diagnosed on palpation of an abnormal adnexal mass during a routine pelvic examination. Because of the deep anatomic location of the ovary, however, early-stage tumors often are not discovered. The finding of a pelvic mass usually leads to pelvic ultrasonography and the use of serum tumor markers to help distinguish malignant masses from benign masses. Serum CA-125, a glycoprotein tumor marker that is elevated (> 65 units/mL) in greater than 80% of ovarian cancers, should be measured. The TNM stage is based on surgical evaluation during a surgical diagnostic procedure (usually laparotomy). Therapeutic cytoreduction (surgical reduction of tumor volume) also is performed at this time.

Treatment

Optimal therapy for ovarian cancer is determined by the extent of the disease at the time of diagnosis and by the size and location of any residual tumor after the surgical staging procedure. Early-stage disease (stages I and II) is treated with surgical removal of the ovaries and fallopian tubes (bilateral salpingo-oophorectomy) and the uterus (hysterectomy), although only one ovary may be removed if the cancer is diagnosed in a very early stage and the female still wishes to have children. The risk of relapse is reduced by adjuvant chemotherapy with platinum-based compounds. Treatment for advanced disease may also include intraperitoneal chemotherapy. The efficacy of treatment is evaluated through radiography and is indicated by a decline in the serum CA-125 level. Patients should be followed up regularly with physical examinations and CA-125 level measurements to detect recurrent disease.

Prognosis

The survival rate depends on the stage diagnosed and whether the cancer is localized or spread.

Other important factors for a better prognosis include young age, absence of ascites, and low volume of residual disease after surgery. Females with ovarian cancer and *BRCA1* or *BRCA2* mutations often have a more favorable prognosis because of better response to chemotherapy.

Prevention

There is no prevention for ovarian cancer, but avoiding certain risk factors, if possible, may make a difference in the likelihood of occurrence. Oral contraception, breast-feeding, tubal ligation (if performed for medical reasons), and having a healthy weight or body mass index can reduce risks, as cannot taking hormone replacement therapy after menopause. Screening is recommended only for females with known *BRCA1* or *BRCA2* gene mutations after discussions with their physicians about the benefits and risks of screening. Screening is done with transvaginal ultrasonography and serum CA-125 measurements every 6 to 12 months, beginning at age 30 to 35 years, or 5 to 10 years before the earliest age at the first ovarian cancer diagnosis in the family. Alternatively, females at high risk for ovarian cancer may choose to have prophylactic oophorectomy by age 35 years, although it does not completely eliminate the risk of cancer.

Patient Teaching

Emphasize the importance of regular gynecologic examinations. If a pelvic mass is found, provide a complete explanation of the diagnostic procedures. Explain the presurgical and postsurgical instructions.

Endometrial Cancer

Description

Endometrial cancer (also known as *uterine cancer*) involves the lining of the uterus, which undergoes cyclic changes as a result of hormonal stimulation. It is the most common gynecologic malignancy (Fig. 12.23). Endometrial cancer is typically grouped into 1 of 4 categories: p53 mutation, copy number low, copy number high, and POLE mutation.

ICD-10-CM Code	C54.1 *(Malignant neoplasm of endometrium)*
	C54.2 *(Malignant neoplasm of myometrium)*
	C54.3 *(Malignant neoplasm of fundus uteri)*
	C54.9 *(Malignant neoplasm of corpus uteri, unspecified)*

Symptoms and Signs

Endometrial cancer causes ulcerations in the uterus. As blood vessels erode, vaginal spotting or bleeding occurs. The most common presenting symptom is abnormal

• **Fig. 12.23** Endometrial cancer. (From Cotran RS, Kumar V, Collins T: *Robbins pathologic basis of disease*, ed 6, Philadelphia, 1999, Saunders.)

perimenopausal or postmenopausal uterine bleeding. Late manifestations of this cancer include pain and systemic symptoms. The disease may be revealed by the presence of atypical endometrial cells observed on routine Pap smear testing.

Patient Screening

Schedule a gynecologic examination and a Pap smear test for the female having abnormal uterine bleeding, especially after menopause has occurred.

Etiology

There are several possible causes that have been identified to increase the risk of endometrial cancer. These include a personal history of breast or ovarian cancer, history of radiation therapy for pelvic cancer, tamoxifen use for breast cancer, hormone imbalance, never having been pregnant, infertility, estrogen replacement therapy, starting period before age 12, late menopause, diabetes, and a diet which includes large amounts of animal fat. A family history of endometrial, ovarian, and/or colon cancers also puts one at higher risk. A personal history of polycystic ovary syndrome or atypical endometrial hyperplasia can result from several possible causes. Excessive

Endometrial cancer is primarily a disease of postmenopausal females. The median age at diagnosis is 61 years. A person with a family history of Lynch syndrome is at higher risk for endometrial cancer. Type 2 diabetes, obesity, and hypertension also lead to an increased risk. Pregnancy and the use of oral contraceptives for at least 12 months appear to offer a protective effect.

Diagnosis

After a pelvic examination to assess for pelvic masses or other causes of uterine bleeding, endometrial biopsy is usually performed on all females with abnormal uterine bleeding or abnormal endometrial cells observed on the Pap smear test. Transvaginal ultrasonography may be helpful as an initial study in postmenopausal females. Dilation and curettage (D&C) remains the gold standard and is usually performed when endometrial biopsy is nondiagnostic. TNM staging requires total hysterectomy with bilateral salpingo-oophorectomy, along with lymph node dissection, to fully evaluate the extent of the disease. The serum tumor marker CA-125 also may be measured to predict the spread of disease beyond the uterus.

Treatment

Very early-stage endometrial cancer is treated with surgery alone, whereas adjuvant radiation therapy with or without chemotherapy is recommended for those with more advanced disease. A radioactive implant can be inserted into the vagina and left in place for the duration of treatment while the patient is in the hospital (vaginal brachytherapy). Hormone therapy is another alternative. The risk of recurrent disease is greatest within the first 3 years of diagnosis. A follow-up physical examination, including pelvic examination, should be performed initially every 3 to 6 months to detect recurrence.

Prognosis

The prognosis is determined by the stage of the disease and the tumor grade.

Prevention

Routine screening is not recommended for most females because no good noninvasive test is available. For those with Lynch Syndrome annual endometrial biopsy is recommended, starting at age 35 years. These females should also be counseled about prophylactic hysterectomy with salpingo-oophorectomy after completion of childbearing.

Patient Teaching

Counsel patients about the symptoms of endometrial cancer, and instruct them to report any abnormal bleeding or spotting to the healthcare provider. After endometrial cancer is diagnosed, give preoperative and postoperative instructions. Explain the benefits of radiation therapy if indicated by the provider. Explain the purpose, duration, and possible side effects of any therapeutic regimen. Support groups for cancer may be helpful.

Conditions and Complications of Pregnancy

Most pregnancies progress to term uneventfully (Fig. 12.24). Complications ranging from worrisome or annoying conditions to life-threatening conditions affecting the mother or the fetus occasionally occur. Complications can develop at any point during pregnancy, which underscores

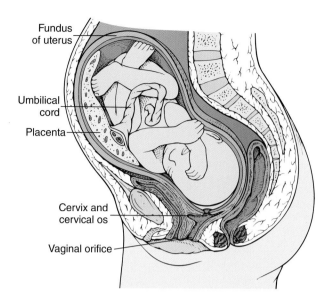

• **Fig. 12.24** Normal uterine pregnancy.

• **Fig. 12.25** Amniocentesis. In amniocentesis, a syringe is used to collect amniotic fluid. Ultrasound imaging is used to guide the tip of the syringe needle to prevent damage to the placenta and fetus. Fetal cells in the collected amniotic fluid can then be chemically tested or used to produce a karyotype of the developing baby. (From Patton KT, Thibodeau GA: *The human body in health and disease*, ed 6, Maryland Heights, Missouri, 2014, Elsevier.)

the importance of early and continual prenatal care and patient education.

Prenatal diagnostic tests can help identify fetal genetic or chromosomal abnormalities and detect complications:

* Amniocentesis: A small amount of amniotic fluid is extracted for laboratory analysis (Fig. 12.25).

Ultrasonography

Ultrasonography is a technique in which high-frequency intermittent sound waves are reflected off tissues and are read by scanners. The various densities of the tissue then are displayed on a screen, and still pictures can be taken to record the real-time image.

Pelvic ultrasonography is specific for the lower abdominal tissues, including the uterus, adnexa, and fetus. This safe technique helps diagnose fetal anomalies; determine fetal age, size, and position; evaluate the condition and placement of the placenta; and identify many other conditions of the female reproductive system. 3D prenatal ultrasonography produces images of the fetus as photographs (see Fig. 12.26). Four-dimensional ultrasonography adds the dimension of time to the process. Parents can now see live-action images of their unborn child or of any internal anatomy.

• **Fig. 12.26** 28-Week three-dimensional ultrasonography. Note distortion of the right forehead, which is caused by the uterine wall. (Courtesy Carli Reed.)

- Chorionic villus sampling (CVS): a biopsy procedure to excise placental tissue for laboratory analysis
- Maternal serum fetal-free DNA analysis
- Doppler ultrasonography: noninvasive real-time, three-dimensional (3D) fetal imaging (see Fig. 12.25)

The first two procedures carry a low risk for miscarriage and infection; the maternal serum test has no risk of fetal loss. Recent recommendations regarding ultrasonography are that it should be performed only for medical reasons, with time and power output kept to a minimum.

Morning Sickness

Description

Morning sickness is the nausea and vomiting associated with pregnancy. It is quite common, affecting up to 70% of pregnant females. The symptoms may begin before the first missed menses but normally resolve by the end of the first trimester or 13th week. If the nausea and vomiting are

severe enough to cause excessive weight loss or metabolic imbalance, then it is called *hyperemesis gravidarum (HG)*.

ICD-10-CM Code	O21.0 *(Mild hyperemesis gravidarum)* (O21.0-O21.9 = 5 codes of specificity)

Symptoms and Signs

The symptoms of nausea and vomiting can occur anytime during the day. Sometimes the nausea is short lived and occurs in waves; at other times, the patient may feel nauseated for hours at a time. If she is dehydrated, urine can look dark; ketones may be present on urine testing; and if the vomiting is severe enough, blood tests may show evidence of metabolic and electrolyte abnormalities. Signs to watch for are rapid pulse, poor skin turgor, decreased urine output, and constipation. These are all signs of dehydration.

Patient Screening

If the patient is experiencing excessive nausea and vomiting, make a prompt appointment for a regular pregnancy checkup. If a female experiences weight loss greater than 10% of her prepregnancy weight, she may need to have a more complete evaluation and management in a hospital setting.

Etiology

The etiology of morning sickness has yet to be clearly defined; however, it is believed that hCG or one of its forms and estrogen (estradiol) are the main culprits responsible for this condition. Psychological problems can also cause nausea and vomiting in pregnancy or make it worse. Patients with underlying GI conditions may also experience more nausea and GI symptoms.

Diagnosis

The diagnosis is based on symptoms and a positive pregnancy test result.

Treatment

In most cases of simple morning sickness, hydration, rest, and eating small amounts of food are sufficient to help the female cope with the process. Avoiding certain foods, smells, and other environmental triggers can also be of benefit. The use of ginger, hypnosis, wristbands, and vitamins B_6 and B_{12} can all help reduce the severity of this condition. If symptoms are severe the provider may use other drugs to help alleviate symptoms. Most of these drugs are considered safe in pregnancy, although none has undergone specific testing for this indication.

Prognosis

The condition usually is self-limiting and resolves gradually. If the condition becomes severe, it can lead to esophageal tears, peripheral neuropathies, encephalopathy, and even death.

Prevention

No prevention is known.

Patient Teaching

Instruct the pregnant female to keep her scheduled appointments, notify the provider of any worsening of nausea and vomiting, and monitor her weight.

Hyperemesis Gravidarum

Description

HG is the more severe stage of morning sickness; it usually does not respond to over-the-counter remedies and requires prescription medications and even hospitalization.

ICD-10-CM Code	P05.2 *(Newborn affected by fetal [intrauterine] malnutrition not light or small for gestational age)* *(P05.00-P05.9 = 20 codes of specificity)* O21.1 *(Hyperemesis gravidarum with metabolic disturbance)*

Symptoms and Signs

HG occurs when the pregnant patient experiences frequent, severe episodes of nausea and vomiting, weight loss, and dehydration and is unable to keep either food or liquid in the stomach. If left untreated, fluid and electrolyte imbalances can cause acid-base disturbances in the fetus and the mother. Abnormal urine osmolality, the excretion of moderate or high levels of ketones into urine, is usually noted during the evaluation of these patients. Laboratory tests may indicate an increase in the number of red blood cells (hemoconcentration), mild elevations in the WBC count, and abnormalities in other blood chemistries as a result of excessive vomiting and dehydration. Abnormal liver enzymes and thyroid laboratory values may also be present.

Patient Screening

Severe nausea and vomiting during pregnancy require prompt medical evaluation.

Etiology

The etiology is unknown. As with morning sickness, elevated estrogen and hCG levels are believed to be responsible for this condition. Patients with underlying emotional disturbances or those in abusive relationships have a higher incidence of this condition.

Diagnosis

Diagnosis is based on symptoms, weight loss, and signs of dehydration, which disturb the serum electrolyte balance. Any pregnant patient with severe nausea and vomiting not responding to standard measures and who continues to lose weight can be classified as having HG.

Treatment

In severe cases, the patient is hospitalized for reversal of dehydration with IV fluids. Any electrolyte imbalance can also be corrected with proper infusion of necessary salts. Other metabolic disturbances, such as hyperthyroidism, can be ruled out at this time. Antiemetics can be given intravenously until the female feels able to take oral liquids. Once the patient is able to tolerate oral agents without vomiting and when her weight stabilizes, she may be sent home. Home nursing then can be used to continue any IV treatments. Most patients are managed outside of the hospital for this condition.

Prognosis

The prognosis is excellent because the condition resolves spontaneously as the pregnancy progresses. As long as the patient is treated in an expedient fashion, complications from dehydration and excessive electrolyte disturbances should be avoidable. If treated nonaggressively or unsuccessfully, profound maternal and fetal complications can result. Research studies indicate females who experience this type of problem during pregnancy are at an increased risk for depression during pregnancy and postpartum.

Prevention

Timely medical intervention can prevent complications from affecting the mother and her fetus.

Patient Teaching

After the patient's condition becomes stable, instruct the patient to eat small, frequent meals of bland food. Suggest that portions be increased as tolerated. Warn the mother to report signs of dehydration or recurrence of symptoms.

Spontaneous Abortion (Miscarriage)

Description

Spontaneous abortion is a naturally occurring loss of a fetus before the 20th week of pregnancy. Spontaneous abortions are classified as missed (no tissue has passed), incomplete (some tissue has passed), or complete (all tissue has passed).

ICD-10-CM Code	O03.9 *(Complete or unspecified spontaneous abortion without complication)* *(O03.0-O03.9 = 28 codes of specificity)*

Coding spontaneous abortion requires modifiers to identify stage. Refer to the physician's diagnosis and then to the current edition of the ICD-10-CM coding manual to ensure the greatest specificity of pathology.

Symptoms and Signs

In cases of incomplete or complete abortion, the patient has vaginal bleeding and pelvic cramping.

Excessive bleeding may lead to hypovolemia, which causes a rapid pulse and low blood pressure. In the hospital, a complete blood count (CBC) will verify the extent of blood loss. In severe cases with extensive hemorrhage, shock is a concern. A positive pregnancy result on urine or blood tests is important to verify that the patient is/ was pregnant. Examination of the cervix may reveal blood in the vagina, with or without any visible products of conception. It is always important to realize that a patient with an ectopic pregnancy may have very similar symptoms.

Patient Screening

Vaginal bleeding and cramping during pregnancy should be reported to the attending physician immediately, and the patient should be directed to prompt medical care.

Etiology

The etiology is usually unknown, with about 10% to 20% of all known pregnancies ending in spontaneous abortion. The majority of spontaneous miscarriages result from abnormal chromosomes. Infection, metabolic disturbances, and maternal antibody production (e.g., in SLE or clotting disorders) have been associated with an increased risk of abortion. Drugs and most prescribed medications do not normally cause abortions. Travel, exercise, and intercourse are also not associated with miscarriage.

Diagnosis

The diagnosis is based on the clinical picture and pelvic ultrasonography. Ultrasonography can help determine fetal viability or the amount of remaining tissue within the uterus. Depending on the level of serum hCG, it may also be helpful in ruling out ectopic pregnancy.

Treatment

If bleeding is not severe, the mother is treated conservatively by allowing the products of conception to pass on their own. The female may also be given medications to help expedite the passage of fetal and placental tissues. In cases of complete abortion, there usually is no need for medications. If bleeding is severe or the expulsion of the contents of the uterus is incomplete, surgical intervention (D&C) may be indicated. In many instances of missed abortion, the female may elect to have surgical removal of the products of conception to avoid the uncertainty and discomfort associated with the spontaneous passage of the pregnancy. It is important to know the female's blood type, because Rho(D) immune globulin (RhoGAM) may be indicated if she is Rh negative.

Prognosis

The prognosis in all three types of spontaneous abortion is excellent. Even when a D&C is required or requested, the impact on future pregnancies is minimal.

Prevention

The cause often is not certain, but good prenatal care is recommended. Alcohol, tobacco, abuse of inhalants, and drugs, are contraindicated during pregnancy. Herbs and prescription drugs should be taken with caution and only with physician approval.

Patient Teaching

Instruct the patient to report any increased vaginal discharge, bleeding, or progressive cramping to the provider. After spontaneous abortion, alert the patient to the signs of infection, which should be reported immediately. Provide referral for grief counseling.

Ectopic Pregnancy

Description

An ectopic pregnancy occurs when the fertilized ovum implants and grows outside the endometrial canal, most often the fallopian tube (Fig. 12.27).

ICD-10-CM Code	P01.4 *(Newborn [suspected to be] affected by ectopic pregnancy)* O00.9 *(Ectopic pregnancy, unspecified)* (O00.0-O00.9 = 5 codes of specificity)

Symptoms and Signs

The female with a positive pregnancy test result and pelvic pain is the most common presentation for an ectopic pregnancy. When pain is present, it is usually on one side.

• **Fig. 12.27** Sites of ectopic (tubal) pregnancy.

Cramping of the uterus, with or without bleeding, can also occur. If there is bleeding into the abdomen, then the patient may experience diffuse pelvic pain. A level of the serum beta-hCG greater than 1500 to 2500 units, with an empty uterus seen on transvaginal ultrasonography, is suspicious for ectopic pregnancy. It should also be noted that in rare cases, the ectopic pregnancy will occur in a C-section scar. An abnormal rise in the level of beta-hCG over 48 hours can also be an early sign of an ectopic pregnancy.

Patient Screening

The sudden onset of severe lower abdominal pain accompanied by vaginal bleeding signals the need for prompt medical evaluation. Most patients will be referred to an emergency department.

Etiology

The cause is unknown; however, any fertilized egg that cannot make it into the uterus but is able to implant itself and grow will become ectopic. Pelvic adhesions, the presence of damaged fallopian tubes, progesterone contraception, previous tubal ligation, previous pelvic infection, prior pelvic surgery, and IUDs are all associated with an increased incidence of ectopic pregnancy.

Diagnosis

The diagnosis of ectopic pregnancy can be very difficult. If it is not ruptured and not causing pain, then serial ultrasound examinations with serial blood pregnancy tests may help make the diagnosis. In cases of ruptured ectopic pregnancies or those associated with pain, the diagnosis may be less difficult. Transvaginal ultrasonography is the mainstay in diagnostic imaging. In areas where the diagnosis remains unclear or ultrasonography is not available, then a frozen D&C may be performed to look for evidence of intrauterine gestational tissue. Culdocentesis (placing a needle into the space behind the uterus) can likewise be used in some cases where the diagnosis is uncertain. If the diagnosis still remains in question, then laparoscopy may be performed to directly visualize the pelvis and the fallopian tubes.

Treatment

The treatment of ectopic pregnancy depends on many factors. In early unruptured ectopic pregnancies, a medication (methotrexate) may be administered. This drug causes the placenta to die and the products to be reabsorbed by the body. Laparoscopic surgery is one of the most common ways of treating ectopic pregnancy. If the tube is unruptured, then tubal conservation may be possible. In many cases, the tube is sacrificed, but rarely is it necessary to remove the ovary. Even when there has been internal bleeding, surgery can still be accomplished through the laparoscope. Blood transfusion is rarely needed unless the blood loss has been excessive. If the fallopian tube is preserved, then the female is at increased risk for another ectopic pregnancy in that tube. In some instances of known ectopic pregnancy with falling beta-hCG levels,

close observation may be warranted without the use of methotrexate or surgery. This is, however, clearly reserved for special circumstances.

Prognosis

The prognosis is good with prompt medical intervention. The chances of conception and a normal intrauterine pregnancy are generally excellent in most cases. There is not a lot of concrete research in regard to pregnancy after C-section scar ectopic pregnancies because they are so rare. If there is underlying tubal disease or extensive pelvic adhesions, then the chances of pregnancy are reduced. A prior ectopic pregnancy increases the risk of subsequent ectopic pregnancies. Clearly, massive internal bleeding from ruptured ectopic pregnancy can be life threatening.

Prevention

One of the major risk factors for ectopic pregnancy is a history of PID. Preventing this infection can reduce the risk of ectopic pregnancy. Most causes of ectopic pregnancy cannot be altered.

Patient Teaching

During emergency medical care, provide reassurance to the patient in pain and distress through frequent updates and explanations of the procedures being performed and the reasons. Give analgesics as prescribed. Anticipate the normal emotional response to a terminated problem pregnancy.

Premature Labor

Description

Premature labor is contractions leading to cervical change occurring before 37 completed weeks of pregnancy.

ICD-10-CM Code	O60.00 (Preterm labor without delivery, unspecified trimester) (O60.00-O60.23 = 10 codes of specificity)

Symptoms and Signs

Premature labor occurs when the pregnant female begins experiencing contractions that are generally regular and painful and that lead to changes in the size of the cervical opening or length of the cervix. Sometimes the female has contractions that she cannot feel and are only evident on a fetal monitor. She may have an increase in vaginal discharge or spotting. Vaginal examination may reveal cervical changes, as mentioned previously. Ultrasonography can also be used to assess cervical length and can reveal dynamic changes in this length with abdominal pressure or contractions.

Patient Screening

A patient with premature contractions must be brought to the attention of the physician or the nurse for immediate instructions for medical intervention.

Etiology

Most cases of premature labor are of unknown etiology. Predisposing conditions include maternal infection, uterine abnormalities, uterine fibroids, uterine bleeding, prior history of preterm birth, multifetal pregnancy, advanced maternal age, gum disease, vaginal colonization with certain bacteria, lack of prenatal care, and preterm cervical dilation or effacement. Other possible contributing factors include smoking, stress, and domestic violence.

Diagnosis

The diagnosis is made by demonstrating cervical change in the presence of uterine contractions. Many physicians treat painful regular contractions even when there is no cervical change if risk factors are present. A substance produced by the fetal membranes called *fetal fibronectin* can help predict the risk of preterm delivery and may be used to manage a patient who is experiencing contractions without cervical change, depending on the risk profile. A cervical length change on ultrasonography is as useful as a pelvic examination to make the diagnosis.

Treatment

There is no effective treatment for preterm labor once the cervix is thinned and dilated. However, measures can be taken to slow preterm labor. Preterm contractions may be managed with terbutaline (while the patient is in the hospital), indomethacin (Indocin), calcium channel blockers, and magnesium sulfate. Current data have called into question the use of magnesium sulfate, although it may be neuroprotective in premature infants. Intramuscular injections of steroids are given to the mother to reduce the complications of prematurity to the fetus if labor cannot be stopped and the patient is about to deliver a very premature fetus (≤34 weeks). In April of 2023 the FDA released a statement after many years of practice that progesterone injections should no longer be used to treat preterm labor. These shots were known by the generic name 17-OHPC (17-alpha hydroxyprogesterone caproate) and the brand name Makena.

◆ ENRICHMENT

Fetal Movement

Studies have shown fetal movement is an indicator of the oxygenation and well-being of the fetus. Some physicians have the expectant mother chart fetal movement or kicks beginning at 28 weeks of gestation and continuing until the day of delivery. Kick counting methods vary and an individual provider will explain how they prefer the mother count movements. The number of perceptible fetal movements varies from patient to patient. The mother is instructed to contact her physician if she notices fewer kicks or the absence of fetal movements. It should also be noted that more movement may take place after a meal.

Prognosis

The outcome for the fetus depends on the age at delivery, underlying presence of infection, birth defects, and cause of the labor. The earlier the gestational age, the more guarded the prognosis. The addition of steroids before birth can improve neonatal outcomes.

Prevention

The causes of premature labor are not clearly understood. Treatment of underlying infections; bed rest; judicial use of tocolytics (to inhibit uterine contractions); use of steroids, when appropriate; and enhanced fetal surveillance may all help prevent some cases of preterm labor and preterm birth.

Patient Teaching

Help the patient set goals for a healthy outcome for mother and infant. Give written instructions regarding when to call the physician, or seek emergency care.

Preeclampsia and Eclampsia

Description

The term *preeclampsia* refers to a serious disease of pregnancy characterized by hypertension and proteinuria. This condition occurs most commonly in the third trimester but can occur any time after 20 completed weeks of pregnancy.

Eclampsia is the occurrence of a seizure or coma in a patient with preeclampsia.

ICD-10-CM Code	O14.00 (*Mild to moderate preeclampsia, unspecified trimester*)
	O14.90 (*Unspecified preeclampsia, unspecified trimester*)
	(O14.00–O14.93 = 12 codes of specificity)
	O15.9 (*Eclampsia, unspecified as to time period*)
	(O15.00–O15.9 = 6 codes of specificity)

Symptoms and Signs

Preeclampsia can be preceded by increased weight gain, usually noted as peripheral swelling or edema. Not all patients with preeclampsia will have edema. Elevation of blood pressure to a level greater than 140/90 mm Hg is a sign that also indicates this condition. When there is greater than 300 mg of protein in urine over a 24-hour period, then the conditions for the diagnosis of preeclampsia are present. The presence of other symptoms, such as persistent headache, visual disturbances, or epigastric pain, can also be present. When blood pressure and urinary protein levels become markedly elevated, the disease may have a more severe course and a potentially worse prognosis. The deep tendon reflexes may also be more exaggerated; and in patients who are severely affected, clonus may be present. If the patient has a seizure, it is usually of the grand mal type and can demonstrate the usual postictal manifestation of confusion and disorientation. These patients are also at increased risk for stroke, and thus any symptom of a central neurologic nature needs to be evaluated for the presence of stroke. In addition, some patients may have symptoms that include HELLP syndrome. Hemolysis of red blood cells, elevated liver enzymes, and low platelet count are present. This is thought to have a relationship to preeclampsia, but research continues to identify all aspects of this condition.

Patient Screening

The female who is pregnant or suspects pregnancy and reports the onset of edema, sudden weight gain, headaches, or sudden elevation of blood pressure should be evaluated by the physician promptly. The onset of seizures requires emergency intervention.

Etiology

The etiology of preeclampsia remains unknown. It is believed to be related to the blood vessels in the placenta not working properly. The presence of a placenta is necessary for this condition to occur. Once the placenta is delivered, the condition typically begins to resolve after 24 to 48 hours, although there are cases of persistent preeclampsia that last for 7 days or even up to 6 weeks after delivery.

Diagnosis

The diagnosis is based on the clinical picture, history, elevated urinary protein level, elevated blood pressure, neurologic symptoms, and/or abnormal laboratory results.

Treatment

The treatment for preeclampsia is delivery of the infant and the placenta. If the disease is mild and the female is far from her due date, then bed rest, frequent monitoring of the fetus and the mother, monitoring of blood tests, and delay of delivery until fetal lung maturity may be necessary. In cases of more severe disease, immediate delivery may be warranted. Laboring females with preeclampsia may require medications, such as magnesium sulfate, which dramatically reduce the risk of a seizure. After delivery, the disease usually remits; however, it may worsen over the immediate 24 to 48 hours before improving. There can even be new-onset disease up to 6 weeks after delivery.

Prognosis

Early diagnosis and treatment of preeclampsia offer the best prognosis for mother and baby. The prognosis is poorer with severe disease, which may result in maternal and/or fetal death.

Prevention

If at risk, possible preventive steps include low-dose aspirin (81 mg) therapy. Good nutrition may also be of some value.

Patient Teaching

Emphasize the advantages of early and regular prenatal care to monitor weight, blood pressure, and urinary protein levels. If a pregnant female is considered to be at risk for eclampsia, educate the female about the warning signs to report: sudden weight gain, edema, headache, and increased blood pressure.

Abruptio Placentae

Description

Abruptio placentae is premature detachment of a normally positioned placenta during pregnancy.

ICD-10-CM Code	P02.1 *(Newborn [suspected to be] affected by other forms of placental separation and hemorrhage)*
	O45.8X9 *(Other premature separation of placenta, unspecified trimester)*
	(O45.001–O45.93 = 24 codes of specificity)

Symptoms and Signs

When the placenta separates prematurely from the uterine wall, it can cause hemorrhage, abdominal pain, fetal distress, and even fetal death. The degree of bleeding can vary quite considerably, with most cases being mild to moderate. The uterus usually contracts when there is an abruption, and these painful contractions are often very closely spaced and come on rather suddenly. Monitoring of the fetal heart rate may show some abnormalities; however, early on, there may be a normal heart rate and pattern. If the abruption is extensive, then fetal death may ensue, and the large clot that forms under the placenta may lead to excessive blood loss in the mother and consumption of clotting factors, leading to coagulopathy. In more severe cases, the mother's blood is unable to clot. Some abruptions do not have any associated external bleeding, and the only signs are fetal heart rate abnormalities or even fetal death. Occasionally, a large abruption may be detected with ultrasonography.

Patient Screening

The signs of abruptio placentae represent a medical emergency for the mother and fetus. Emergency care is needed as soon as possible.

Etiology

Abruptio placentae is a complete or partial separation of the placenta from the uterine wall (Fig. 12.28). In many cases, the cause is unknown; however, hypertension, preeclampsia, trauma, maternal vascular disease, infection, drug use (cocaine), and multiple gestation all predispose a female to placental abruption.

Diagnosis

The diagnosis is usually made by the constellation of risk factors, fetal heart rate pattern, the mother's symptoms, contraction pattern, and presence of bleeding. In many

• **Fig. 12.28** Abruptio placentae.

instances, the diagnosis is only suspected and is confirmed or refuted at the time of delivery. Ultrasonography rarely helps in the diagnosis of small or moderate abruptions, but it can identify large subplacental bleeds.

Treatment
The care of the patient with suspected abruption depends on the degree of placental separation, proximity to the due date of delivery, and maternal and fetal stability. In mild cases, labor may continue with anticipated vaginal delivery. An operating room must be readily available in these cases, because the clinical picture may deteriorate rapidly in these patients. In significantly preterm patients not in labor, hospitalization with careful monitoring may be appropriate. Most cases are treated by immediate surgical delivery. Massive blood loss and coagulopathy are treated with the replacement of blood and clotting factors.

Prognosis
The prognosis depends on the degree of abruption and the gestational age of the fetus. As long as the abruption is small, and the fetus is beyond 34 weeks gestation, then the outlook is excellent. In very premature infants and those in whom the abruption compromises oxygenation, the prognosis may be more guarded.

Prevention
Good prenatal care with individualized attention to risk factors may help prevent abruptions in some cases.

Patient Teaching
Reinforce the principles of prenatal care, and instruct the patient to report unexpected symptoms, such as sudden bleeding or abdominal pain, immediately.

Placenta Previa
Description
Placenta previa is the placenta covering the opening to the cervix. In a partial previa, the majority of the placenta is away

from the opening (os), and in a complete or central previa, the more central portion of the placenta covers the os.

ICD-10-CM Code	O44.00 *(Placenta previa specified as without hemorrhage, unspecified trimester)* (O44.00–O44.13 = 8 codes of specificity)

Symptoms and Signs
The patient experiences painless, bright vaginal bleeding, usually in the first or second trimester of pregnancy. Occasionally the patient experiences painless vaginal bleeding in the third trimester as the first sign. The abdomen is soft and nontender. In cases of excessive bleeding, vital signs may indicate shock, with a rapid and thready pulse and falling blood pressure. The fetal heart rate may indicate that the blood supply to the fetus is compromised.

Patient Screening
The onset of bright-red vaginal bleeding during pregnancy requires immediate attention, close observation, and diagnostic evaluation. The attending physician is notified.

Etiology
This condition is caused by low implantation of the blastocyst in the uterine cavity. A prior cesarean delivery increases the risk of previa, as does previous childbirth or multiple gestation.

Diagnosis
The diagnosis is based on a pelvic ultrasonogram showing the placenta being implanted over the cervical os. In a complete placenta previa, the placenta totally overlies the os (Fig. 12.29). In a partial placenta previa, the placenta is implanted low in the uterus but does not entirely overlap the os. As the cervix begins to dilate, the vessels tear loose, and the placenta bleeds. It is critical that a cervical examination not be performed until the location of the placenta has been verified on ultrasonography.

Internal cervical os   Placenta

• **Fig. 12.29** Placenta previa.

Treatment

In many pregnancies with a known history of placenta previa, the female may go about her daily activities as long as she is not bleeding. Exercise and intercourse are avoided; and if bleeding occurs, then prompt evaluation in the hospital is usually warranted. If the bleeding stops and the fetus is stable, then the patient may be monitored as an outpatient, with activity restriction and regular visits. If the bleeding is more significant, then hospitalization may be required until the fetus is deemed mature. Often, in stable previa, delivery is accomplished around the 36th week to avoid the potential for catastrophic bleeding that may occur if labor ensues. For any massive hemorrhage with fetal or maternal compromise, immediate delivery by cesarean section is warranted. At no time is vaginal delivery of a viable fetus allowed when there is placenta previa present.

Prognosis

In most cases of previa, the outcomes are excellent. Clearly, the prognosis becomes more guarded if there is excessive blood loss and fetal compromise requiring immediate delivery, especially if the infant is premature.

Prevention

No prevention is known.

Patient Teaching

Explain all procedures, and offer reassurance throughout. Conservative treatment may require bed rest and lifestyle modification for an extended period during pregnancy; reinforce the purpose of the treatment, and address the need for home care referrals. Vaginal intercourse may be contraindicated.

❖ ENRICHMENT

Usual and Unusual Presentations

Most fetuses present in the cephalic, or vertex (head first), position; however, some present in other positions, such as footling breech (feet first), frank breech (buttocks), or transverse lie (across the uterus). Even some of the cephalic presentations (brow or chin) cause complications that may preclude normal vaginal delivery (Fig. 12.30). In cases of abnormal presentations, delivery is accomplished with a cesarean section.

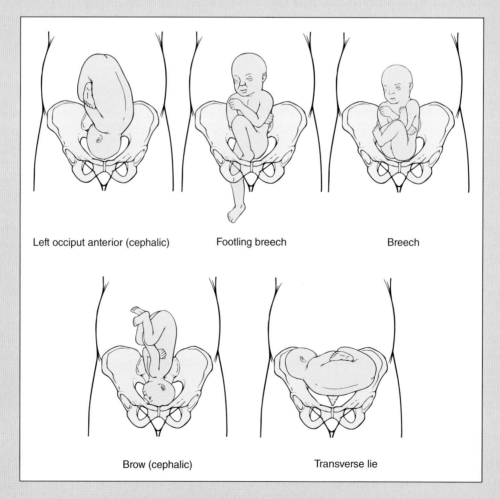

| Left occiput anterior (cephalic) | Footling breech | Breech |

| Brow (cephalic) | Transverse lie |

• **Fig. 12.30** Fetal presentations.

❖ ENRICHMENT

Problems Associated with Multiple Pregnancies

The incidence rate of multiple (gestation) pregnancies is increasing. Infertility treatment contributes to this increase because fertility drugs, such as follicle-stimulating hormone (FSH; Follistim), are given to stimulate ovulation. These drugs often cause several ova to be released at ovulation, thus giving sperm multiple opportunities for fertilization. During the process of in vitro fertilization (IVF), several fertilized ova are implanted in the hope that at least one successful pregnancy will result. The ovaries sometimes release more than one ovum in the natural course of events. Finally, a fertilized zygote sometimes divides to produce identical twins (Fig. 12.31).

Many problems are associated with multiple (gestation) pregnancies. The mother is at greater risk for toxemia (preeclampsia) and for complications such as dyspnea, urinary frequency, constipation, edema of the feet and legs, and heartburn earlier in the pregnancy compared with the mother with a single fetus. The expectant mother of triplets, quadruplets, quintuplets, or sextuplets often is hospitalized by the beginning of the third trimester and restricted to bed rest. The fetuses are monitored frequently and usually must be delivered by cesarean section. The size of the multiple pregnancies generally prevents the pregnancy from continuing to term. This may result in very small, immature infants who need intensive nursing care and monitoring.

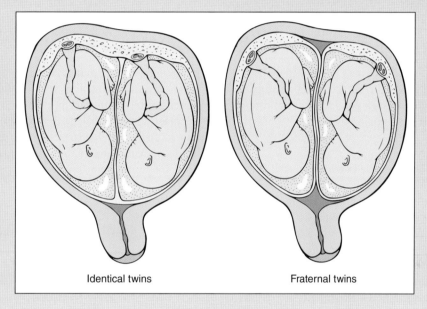

Identical twins   Fraternal twins

• **Fig. 12.31** Twin pregnancies.

Hydatidiform Mole

Description
A hydatidiform mole is an abnormal proliferation of the placental tissue that can take on the characteristics of a malignancy. The placenta has a "cluster of grapes" type of appearance on ultrasonography, or the diagnosis may be based on pathologic evaluation after a miscarriage or pregnancy termination.

ICD-10-CM Code	O01.9 *(Hydatidiform mole, unspecified)*
	(O01.0–O01.9 = 3 codes of specificity)
	D39.2 *(Neoplasm of uncertain behavior of placenta)*

Symptoms and Signs
The patient with a hydatidiform mole experiences symptoms just like any other pregnant female. Occasionally there may be more nausea and vomiting and more vaginal bleeding than usually seen. On physical examination, the uterus may

feel larger than expected, based on the last menstrual period. In cases of complete molar pregnancy, no fetus develops, and ultrasonography shows an empty or absent sac and an abnormal-appearing placenta. An incomplete mole is one that occurs with a living fetus, so it may be more difficult to detect. If the blood hCG level is measured, it may be greatly elevated, out of proportion to what would be expected on the basis of the stage of pregnancy.

Patient Screening
If a pregnant female reports vaginal bleeding, an appointment for ultrasonography is scheduled to evaluate the uterus.

Etiology
The cause of a molar pregnancy is a genetic anomaly in fertilization. The placenta develops abnormally as a mass of clear grapelike vesicles (Fig. 12.32). Usually no fetus is present.

A   B

• **Fig. 12.32** Hydatidiform mole. (A) Abnormal proliferation of placental tissue in a hydatidiform mole. (B) "Cluster of grapes" type appearance of hydatidiform mole. ((B) From Damjanov I, Linder J: *Pathology: a color atlas*, St. Louis, 1999, Mosby.)

Diagnosis

The diagnosis is based on the clinical picture; the absence of fetal heart tones (FHTs) in a complete mole; abnormally elevated hCG levels; and, most importantly, the appearance of the placenta on the ultrasonogram.

Treatment

The mole normally is not expelled spontaneously, so surgical intervention is indicated, the usual treatment being evacuation of the uterus by D&C. Observation for hemorrhage is important. If the molar tissue persists after evacuation, then chemotherapy may be indicated to prevent further growth and spread of the tissue. On occasion, persistent trophoblastic tissue that does not respond to chemotherapy may necessitate hysterectomy. In cases of uterine evacuation, then serial beta-hCG assessments are required until the values fall below detectable amounts. Pregnancy should be avoided for at least 6 months after removal of a hydatidiform mole.

Prognosis

Most hydatidiform moles do not persist, and the prognosis is good with early treatment. Complications, such as infection and bleeding, can occur. When a fetus is present, preeclampsia may occur before 20 weeks gestation, raising concerns about an incomplete mole. This condition can be a precursor to choriocarcinoma, and the patient must be instructed to have frequent follow-up examinations.

Prevention

No prevention is known. Hydatidiform moles occur in about 1 in 1000 pregnancies in the United States.

Patient Teaching

Explain the surgical procedure. Anticipate emotional responses to the diagnosis of a "false pregnancy." Emphasize the importance of follow-up care.

Diseases of the Breast

Ranging from mild to fatal, diseases of the breast necessitate age-appropriate screening, with routine mammography, as prescribed by the physician. Although diseases of the breast are most common in females, diseases of the breast occur also in males. Any changes in the breast tissue, such as lumps, indentations, nipple crusting, or leaking, should be cause for concern and investigation.

Fibrocystic Breast Condition

Description

Fibrocystic breast condition is a common, benign breast disorder.

ICD-10-CM Code	N60.19 *(Diffuse cystic mastopathy of unspecified breast)* (N60.11–N60.19 = 3 codes of specificity)

Symptoms and Signs

The female patient with mammary fibroplasia experiences an uncomfortable feeling in the breasts. Lumps and cysts, single or multiple, smooth and rounded, can be palpated in one or both breasts. The breasts are tender on palpation, and the patient may experience shooting pains in the breast tissue. Tenderness is usually more intense during the premenstrual period. After menopause, the condition becomes less of a problem.

Patient Screening

A female who discovers one or more breast lumps is scheduled for a breast examination.

Etiology

The etiology of this condition is unknown. An increase in the formation of fibrous tissue and hyperplasia of the epithelial cells of the ducts and glands result in dilation of the ducts. Cystic disease is the most common disease of the

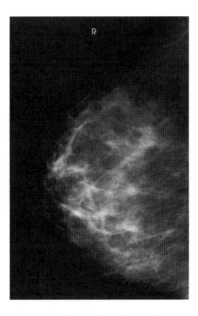

• **Fig. 12.33** Mammogram. (From *Mosby's medical, nursing, and allied health dictionary*, ed 8, St. Louis, 2010, Mosby.)

	American Cancer Society	U.S. Preventive Services Task Force
Test		
Mammography		
40–49 years	Annual	Insufficient evidence to support
>49 years	Annual, if healthy	Every 2 years; 50–75 years
Clinical breast examination	Every 3 years; 20–39 years Annually, ≥40 years	Insufficient evidence to support
Breast self-examination	Optional	Not recommended

TABLE 12.2   Breast Cancer Screening

From Goldman L, Schafer AI: *Goldman's Cecil medicine*, ed 24, Philadelphia, 2012, Elsevier/Saunders.

female breast, usually occurring between ages 30 and 50 years and is related to normal hormonal variations.

Diagnosis
Prompt diagnosis is based on palpation and mammography (Fig. 12.33 and Table 12.2) to differentiate cystic disease from a malignant neoplasm. Ultrasonography may be performed to determine whether the lump is solid or hollow. This can help distinguish between cysts and tumors of the breasts.

Treatment
No specific treatment for this condition is known. The goal of treatment is to relieve breast pain and correct menstrual irregularity. Antiinflammatory medication or oral contraceptives may be ordered. In some cases, physicians aspirate the cysts with a needle. The patient is advised to wear a firm, supporting bra and restrict caffeine intake.

Prognosis
The condition is benign, and most fibrocystic breast conditions never result in malignancy; however, microscopic findings that show atypical cells or hyperplasia are associated with an increased risk for breast cancer.

Prevention
No universal means of prevention is known. Some females notice an improvement with caffeine restriction.

Patient Teaching
Teach the patient about the importance of breast self-examination and of annual mammography. Emphasize the need for careful surveillance, because the lumps and cysts of the disease can mask malignancy.

Mastitis
Description
Mastitis is inflammation of one or more mammary glands of the breast.

ICD-10-CM Code   N61 *(Inflammatory disorders of breast)*

Symptoms and Signs
Acute puerperal (postdelivery) mastitis is inflammation of breast tissue during postpartum lactation. The nursing mother experiences sudden pain, redness, and heat in the breasts at either the beginning or the end of lactation. The breasts are hot and feel doughy and tough, and the axillary lymph nodes may be enlarged. There is a discharge from the nipple. Other symptoms are fever and malaise.

Patient Screening
Schedule a same-day appointment for a female experiencing symptoms of mastitis.

Etiology
Mastitis often is caused by a streptococcal or staphylococcal infection. However, other pathogens can also cause mastitis. Bacteria invade the milk ducts and cause inflammation and occlusion. Milk stagnates in the lobules, producing a dull pain.

Diagnosis
The diagnosis is based on the clinical picture.

Treatment
A firm, supportive bra should be worn, heat may be applied to the area, progesterone may be prescribed, and drug therapy in the form of antibiotics is implemented in

some cases. Palliative care includes rest, analgesia, and warm soaks. Breast-feeding need not be discontinued if there is improvement.

Prognosis
The prognosis for this benign condition is good with treatment. Abscesses may form with inadequate treatment.

Prevention
Anyone in contact with a nursing mother should practice infection prevention techniques.

Patient Teaching
Instruct the mother in good personal hygiene, especially in hand-washing techniques. Emphasize the importance of taking the complete course of antibiotics as prescribed.

Fibroadenoma of the Breast

Description
Fibroadenoma is a nontender benign tumor of the breast (Fig. 12.34).

ICD-10-CM Code	D24.9 *(Benign neoplasm of unspecified breast)* (D24.1–D24.9 = 3 codes of specificity)

Symptoms and Signs
Fibroadenoma of the breast is the most frequent breast tumor in adolescents and young females. The female patient feels a firm, round, encapsulated, movable mass in the breast. She experiences no pain or only slight tenderness.

Patient Screening
Schedule an appointment for a breast examination to evaluate the breast mass.

Etiology
The etiology is unknown, but fibroadenomas are hormonally responsive, growing in size during the late phases of the menstrual cycle or during pregnancy.

• **Fig. 12.34** Fibroadenoma of the breast. (From Damjanov I, Linder J: *Pathology: a color atlas*, ed 6, St. Louis, 2006, Mosby.)

Diagnosis
The diagnosis is based on palpation, the clinical picture, and mammography. Core biopsy is highly specific to distinguish breast masses, such as fibroadenoma, from malignancy.

Treatment
Treatment of this benign tumor of the breast is surgical removal of the tumor with the patient under local anesthesia. The pathology report confirms the diagnosis.

Prognosis
The prognosis is usually good, and there are no complications.

Prevention
No prevention is known.

Patient Teaching
Discuss the surgical course of action with the patient. Assure the patient that the physician or the nurse will tell her the results of the pathology report as soon as possible.

Cancer of the Breast

Description
Breast cancer usually arises from the terminal ductal lobular unit (TDLU) of the breast, the functional unit of the breast tissue, which is very hormonally responsive.

ICD-10-CM Code	C50.919 *(Malignant neoplasm of unspecified site of unspecified female breast)* (C50.011–C50.919 = 27 codes of specificity) C50.929 *(Malignant neoplasm of unspecified site of unspecified male breast)* (C50.021–C50.929 = 27 codes of specificity)

Symptoms and Signs
Physical symptoms and signs of breast cancer include a lump, swelling, or tenderness of the breast; irritation or dimpling of the breast skin *(peau d'orange);* and pain, ulceration, or retraction of the nipple. Visual examination may reveal that the breasts are asymmetric. The earliest sign, however, is an abnormality seen on a mammogram, which usually appears before the female or her physician can feel a lump. In advanced stages of untreated lesions, the nodule becomes fixed to the chest wall, and axillary masses and ulceration develop (Fig. 12.35). Breast pain is not a common factor in early breast cancer.

Patient Screening
A female (or male) presenting with any lump, nodule, dimpling, abnormal nipple discharge, or change in breast shape, with or without pain, should be given the first available appointment for diagnostic evaluation. The same applies to a patient with abnormal findings on screening mammography.

• **Fig. 12.35** (A) Patient with lump and nipple retraction in the left breast. (B) Patient with altered nipple height resulting from breast cancer in left breast. (From Seidel HM, et al: *Mosby's guide to physical examination*, ed 7, St. Louis, 2011, Mosby.)

Etiology

Breast cancer is the most common cancer and the second leading cause of cancer-related death among females in the United States. The two greatest risk factors for breast cancer are increased age and female sex. Breast cancer is 100 times more common in females than in males.

Other risk factors have to do with hormonal, reproductive, and genetic factors. Prolonged exposure to and higher concentrations of endogenous estrogen increases the risk of breast cancer. Therefore younger age at menarche, older age at first full-term pregnancy, and older age at menopause are risk factors. Long-term (>5-year) use of combined estrogen/ progesterone hormone replacement therapy causes a modest increase in the risk of breast cancer. Those with a history of breast cancer have an increased risk of breast cancer in the other breast. The use of alcohol increases the risk. Family history is important in determining risk, although only about 15% of females diagnosed with breast cancer have a positive family history. About 3% of breast cancers are associated with mutation of *BRCA1* or *BRCA2*, the inherited breast cancer susceptibility genes.

Ductal carcinoma in situ (DCIS), defined as a malignant population of cells that lack the capacity to invade through the basement membrane, is a precursor lesion for breast cancer. These cells can spread through the duct system to involve an entire sector of the breast, or they can even migrate up to involve the nipple skin, possibly leading to Paget's disease of the breast.

The risk of breast cancer is lower in males because the male breast is much less sensitive to hormonal influences. In addition, the normal male breast does not have lobules; thus it has no TDLU. Risk factors for male breast cancer are Klinefelter syndrome, gynecomastia, testicular dysfunction, radiation exposure at a young age, and *BRCA2* gene mutation.

Diagnosis

Approximately 87% of breast cancers are diagnosed on the basis of abnormal findings on mammography, with the remainder being detected on physical examination. Because not all mammographic findings indicate cancer,

further evaluation (e.g., diagnostic mammography and ultrasonography) is used to determine the need for biopsy. Ultrasonography is used to differentiate solid masses from cystic masses and to determine whether malignant features are present, although contrast-enhanced MRI may need to be performed in females with dense breasts. Biopsy of all suspicious lumps should be performed for a definitive diagnosis. Breast cancer is staged according to the TNM system. Staging mammography for both breasts is important in patients considering breast-conserving therapy (BCT).

If the disease is suspected to be at an advanced stage, CT of the chest and/or abdomen and pelvis, and bone scanning should be performed, depending on the patient's symptoms. The tumor's estrogen receptor and progesterone receptor status and expression of the oncogene *c-erbB-2* and its protein product HER2/neu should be measured because they have both predictive value and prognostic value.

Treatment

DCIS should be treated with either mastectomy or BCT (wide excision followed by radiation therapy) and, in many cases, tamoxifen to prevent progression to invasive cancer. Treatment of invasive breast cancer takes into account stage and patient preferences. Surgical resection of the tumor via mastectomy or BCT with removal of any affected axillary lymph nodes is almost always part of the treatment plan. Surgery is usually combined with radiation therapy, hormone therapy (depending on the estrogen/progesterone receptor status of the tumor), and/or chemotherapy. Trastuzumab (Herceptin) is a humanized monoclonal antibody directed against *c-erbB-2* and may be effective against tumors that overexpress this oncogene. Patients with hormone receptor-positive tumors may benefit from treatment with an aromatase inhibitor. Close follow-up after completion of treatment is necessary to assess for disease recurrence.

Prognosis

Axillary lymph node positivity is the most important prognostic indicator. The presence of estrogen and progesterone receptors is associated with a better prognosis and tumor responsiveness to hormone therapy, although this difference is becoming smaller as a result of advances in chemotherapy. Other factors associated with prognosis are tumor size and grade. Many new prognostic factors are in use or being studied. One such test, the 21-gene recurrence score assay, is performed on breast tissue in patients with newly diagnosed, lymph node-negative, estrogen receptor-positive breast cancer to predict recurrence risk. It can also be used to predict response to chemotherapy and identify those who may benefit from prolonged endocrine therapy.

Localized breast cancer has a 5-year survival rate of 99%. Regional spread reduces the rate to 86%, and distant metastasis results in a 5-year survival rate of around 30%. Some females may report a condition called *postbreast therapy pain syndrome* after surgery for breast cancer. The pain can develop weeks or years after surgery, and nerve damage is suspected to be the cause.

Prevention

Some lifestyle changes may reduce the risk of breast cancer, such as having a child before age 25 years, breast-feeding for at least 6 months, avoiding weight gain, and limiting alcohol consumption. Females at very high risk can reduce their risk by 50% by taking tamoxifen or approximately 38% by taking raloxifene for 5 years. Both drugs are approved by the FDA for the prevention of breast cancer. General screening of the population for *BRCA1* or *BRCA2* mutations is not recommended.

Regular screening with mammography can reduce the risk of death from breast cancer. Mammography can identify breast cancer at an early stage, before physical symptoms develop. Tomosynthesis, also referred to as *3D mammography* provides a clearer, more accurate, and detailed view of the breast. The screening recommendation from the American Cancer Society is that females aged 40 to 44 years should have the option to begin mammogram screenings. Those 45 to 55 years of age should undergo mammography every year. Those older than 55 should continue every 2 years, or yearly. Screening should continue as long as females are healthy and expected to live 10 more years or longer. Females should report any changes in their breasts to their healthcare provider whether they do regular self-examinations or not. In addition to breast mammography, annual MRI should be offered to patients at high risk of breast cancer. For patients with *BRCA1* or *BRCA2* mutations, prophylactic double mastectomy can reduce breast cancer risk by 90%. The risks and benefits of this procedure need to be discussed in detail with an experienced healthcare provider.

Patient Teaching

Review and reinforce the preventive measures mentioned earlier. Provide information to females diagnosed with localized tumors about the local resection procedure and the importance of follow-up care, including regular mammography and/or ultrasonography, and clinical breast examinations by a healthcare professional.

More aggressive therapy for invasive or metastatic disease requires a great deal of teaching. Explain the purpose of the procedures and any discomfort that normally may be experienced as a result of surgery, radiation, chemotherapy, or hormone therapy. Most patients express great concern about their prognosis; this issue is always referred to the attending physician, as are questions about breast reconstruction.

Paget Disease of the Breast

Description

Paget disease of the breast is a characteristic breast lesion that signifies the presence of malignant adenocarcinoma cells. Underlying carcinoma of the breast is present in 93% to 100% of cases.

ICD-10-CM Code	C50.019 *(Malignant neoplasm of nipple and areola, unspecified female breast)*

Symptoms and Signs

The skin of the nipple develops an erythematous, eczematous, scaly, or ulcerated lesion (Fig. 12.36). The lesion, often unilateral, may heal spontaneously, or topical treatments may mask the inflammation, but this does not mean that Paget disease is not present. Signs of more advanced disease include bloody discharge from the nipple and nipple retraction. Some patients may have only persistent pain or pruritus of the nipple. The patient also may have a palpable breast mass or abnormality on mammography.

Patient Screening

Schedule a breast examination for any patient reporting redness, scaling, or lesions of the nipple, discharge from the nipple, or changes in the shape of the nipple; this is important even when the patient reports an eventual improvement in the condition.

• **Fig. 12.36** Paget's disease of the breast. (From Habif T: *Clinical dermatology*, ed 4, Philadelphia, 2004, Mosby.)

Etiology

It is not known whether Paget cells arise from underlying mammary adenocarcinoma (the most widely accepted theory) or whether they represent a carcinoma in situ that is independent of any underlying carcinoma. The peak age of disease onset is 50 to 60 years.

Diagnosis

The diagnosis can be established by biopsy or nipple scrape cytology. Mammography or MRI can detect an associated breast mass. Paget cells are often tested for estrogen and progesterone receptor positivity and for overexpression of HER2.

Treatment

Historically, treatment has consisted of simple mastectomy, but breast-conserving surgery used to treat breast cancer is now being used to treat Paget disease as well. Axillary lymph node dissection should also be performed if carcinoma is suspected. Whole-breast irradiation may be performed in addition to surgery. The underlying breast carcinoma must also be treated.

Prognosis

The prognosis is affected by the presence of invasive ductal carcinoma and by metastasis to the axillary nodes.

Prevention

Females should be educated to report nipple changes to aid in the detection of lesions in the early stages of the disease.

Patient Teaching

Review the value of reporting nipple and breast changes, especially for females between ages 50 and 60 years. Clarify the purpose and procedure of the biopsy of the nipple lesion. Additional teaching should be provided to explain the treatment decision; this could include patient preparation for breast surgery and radiation therapy.

Review Challenge

Answer the following questions:

1. What are the risk factors for sexually transmitted infections (STIs)?
2. Why is chlamydia called the *silent STI*?
3. What are the possible complications of untreated gonorrhea?
4. What is meant by the term *ping-pong vaginitis?*
5. What is the pathologic course of genital herpes? How is it treated? Can it be cured?
6. How is genital herpes contracted?
7. Why is early diagnosis and treatment of syphilis important?
8. List the causes of dyspareunia in males and females.
9. Which drugs may contribute to male impotence?
10. What are the possible causes of male and female infertility? Are any preventable?
11. How is benign prostatic hyperplasia treated? What are the possible complications?
12. What are the possible causes of epididymitis? Of orchitis?
13. What are the symptoms and signs of torsion of the testicle?
14. What is a varicocele? How may it be a factor in male infertility?
15. Why is prostate-specific antigen screening valuable? Why is early detection of prostatic cancer vital? Name the diagnostic criteria.
16. What is often the first sign of testicular cancer?
17. List the common symptoms of female reproductive diseases.
18. Explain the difference between primary and secondary dysmenorrhea.
19. How is mittelschmerz related to ovulation?
20. What is the pathology associated with endometriosis?
21. Why is pelvic inflammatory disease a serious condition? What is the etiology?
22. What are the most common tumors of the female reproductive system?
23. What organism is commonly the cause of vaginitis?
24. What is toxic shock syndrome?
25. How has medical opinion changed recently regarding the use of hormone replacement therapy during menopause?
26. Which etiologic factors do uterine prolapse, cystocele, and rectocele have in common?
27. What are the risk factors for cervical cancer? How is cervical cancer detected by the Papanicolaou smear?
28. What is the leading cause of death attributed to female reproductive system disorders? Why is it called a *silent* cancer?
29. What are the possible causes of ectopic pregnancy?
30. What are the clinical indications of toxemia?
31. What is the life-threatening complication that may occur in abruptio placentae? In placenta previa?
32. What are the factors that place females at a higher risk for cancer of the breast?

Real-Life Challenge: Benign Prostatic Hyperplasia

A 60-year-old male reports urinary frequency and nocturia three to four times a night. On questioning, he reveals having difficulty starting urination and a weak stream of urine. He also reports that he thinks he is not completely emptying his bladder. The symptoms have had an insidious onset.

The examination reveals a well-nourished, 60-year-old male with vital signs as follows: temperature, 98.6°F; pulse, 72 beats per minute; respirations, 14 breaths per minute; and blood pressure, 116/78 mm Hg. His skin is warm, dry, and pink. The prostate-specific antigen (PSA) test is ordered, and results return at 5 ng/mL. The subsequent digital rectal examination (DRE) reveals an enlarged prostate gland with no nodules or depressions. The urinalysis results are normal, and the urine culture results are negative.

Drug therapy with tamsulosin hydrochloride (Flomax) is ordered. The patient is instructed to have a repeat PSA test in 6 weeks and to return for follow-up DRE. The diagnosis is possible benign prostatic hyperplasia (BPH).

Questions

1. What is the underlying reason for the urinary symptoms?
2. What are the normal results for PSA?
3. What causes the prostate to enlarge?
4. Why is the PSA drawn before the DRE?
5. What are treatment options other than drug therapy?
6. What are the possible side effects of drug therapy?
7. What might be the side effects of surgical treatment of BPH?
8. What symptoms of BPH are similar to symptoms of prostate cancer?

Real-Life Challenge: Endometriosis

A 35-year-old female has dysmenorrhea, often having onset of pain the day before the onset of menses. The pain occasionally continues a few days after the end of menses. She describes the pain as a constant cramping type of pain in the lower abdomen, vagina, and back. The patient describes her menstrual flow to be unusually heavy and also states that she has pain during defecation.

The patient is a gravida III, para II, with a history of a miscarriage 5 years ago. Her living children are 7 and 11 years of age. The patient also states that she has been unable to conceive after 3 years of unprotected intercourse. She also reveals a history of tampon use during the past 10 years.

The pelvic examination reveals generalized tenderness throughout the pelvis. Vital signs are temperature, 98.8°F; pulse, 88 beats per minute; respirations, 16 breaths per minute; and blood pressure, 106/74 mm Hg. Endometriosis is suspected, and the patient is given the choice of conservative treatment with hormones or laparoscopy to visualize the condition of the reproductive organs. The Pap smear result is negative.

Questions

1. What is the cause of endometriosis?
2. What is the significance of the obstetric history?
3. Why would the patient experience pain before menses?
4. What other pelvic organs might be involved?
5. Why would hormone therapy be prescribed?
6. What other types of treatment may be used?
7. What is the significance of the patient being unable to conceive?

Internet Assignments

1. Explore a medical website, such as Medicinenet.com, to research the latest findings on hormone replacement therapy for females experiencing menopause or perimenopause.
2. Visit the Women's National Health Resource Center website, select a health topic of interest to you, and research it. Report a summary of your findings to the class.
3. Visit the National CDC website, and research the latest campaign to stop the spread of genital herpes through a STI awareness outreach.
4. Visit the American Society for Reproductive Medicine website, and go to *Headlines in Reproductive Medicine* to research a topic of current interest, such as the risks of midlife motherhood.

Critical Thinking

1. Breast cancer is the most common cancer, except for skin cancer, and the second leading cause of cancer-related death among females in the United States. Explain the facts you know about what factors, such as age, affect the mortality rate. Discuss the risk factors for breast cancer. What percentage of breast cancers are diagnosed through abnormal mammography findings?

2. Name some specific symptoms and signs that may signal the onset of certain complications of pregnancy.

3. There are many causes of infertility. Are the causes more easily identified in males or in females? Which causes are preventable? In many cases, can a couple seeking help to achieve pregnancy be offered reasonable hope?

4. In a patient teaching session with a female with a trichomoniasis infection, why is it necessary to explain how to avoid "ping-pong" vaginitis?

5. For patients with metastatic prostate cancer, how would you explain how first-line treatment with androgen deprivation therapy (ADT) works against the cancer?

Prepare to discuss Critical Thinking case study exercises for this chapter posted on Evolve.

Credentialing Examination Questions

1. A patient is using emergency contraception. Which time frame after intercourse takes place, is best to take the contraceptive pill for the best outcome?
   A. Within 24 hours
   B. 24 to 48 hours
   C. 48 to 72 hours
   D. 72 to 96 hours

2. Which sexually transmitted infection is called "silent" because it often has no symptoms?
   A. Syphillis
   B. Gonorrhea
   C. Chlamydia
   D. HIV

3. Which method of birth control is best for the prevention of sexually transmitted infections?
   A. Birth control pills
   B. Diaphragm
   C. IUD
   D. Male latex condoms

4. Which STD is not curable?
   A. Gonorrhea
   B. Syphilis
   C. Herpes
   D. Chlamydia

5. Which type of cancer is associated with HPV infection?
   A. Prostate
   B. Cervical
   C. Ovarian
   D. Testicular

6. Which class of medication is used to treat some types of ED?
   A. Antibiotic
   B. Antifungal
   C. Antihypertensive
   D. Phosphodiesterase-5 inhibitor

7. Which problems have been linked to female infertility?
   A. Fallopian tube dysfunction
   B. Ovulation disorders
   C. Uterine abnormalities
   D. All of the above

8. Which type of gynecological cancer is the most common?
   A. Uterine
   B. Ovarian
   C. Cervical
   D. Vulvar

9. A pregant female is told her baby is in the breech position at her checkup. Which part of the baby is toward the cervix?
   A. Head
   B. Arm
   C. Chin
   D. Feet

10. Which diagnostic screening test successfully identifies the majority of cases of breast cancer?
    A. MRI
    B. Mammography
    C. Breast ultrasound
    D. Breast self-examination

13

Neurologic Diseases and Conditions

CHAPTER OUTLINE

LEARNING OBJECTIVES

After studying this chapter, you should be able to:

1. Name the main components of the nervous system.
2. Describe how data are collected during a neurologic assessment.
3. Name the common symptoms and signs of a cerebrovascular accident (CVA).
4. Name the three vascular disorders that may cause a CVA.
5. Define a transient ischemic attack.
6. List some of the problems to which the nervous system is susceptible.
7. Distinguish between (1) epidural and subdural hematomas and (2) cerebral concussion and cerebral contusion.
8. Describe three mechanisms of spinal injuries.
9. Name the goals of treatment of spinal cord injuries.
10. Explain the neurologic consequences of the deterioration or rupture of an intervertebral disk.
11. Explain why cephalalgia is sometimes considered a symptom of an underlying disease.
12. Describe the symptoms of a migraine.
13. Describe first aid for seizures.
14. Explain how the symptoms of Parkinson disease are controlled.
15. Describe the progression of amyotrophic lateral sclerosis.
16. Discuss restless legs syndrome.
17. Discuss transient global amnesia.
18. Distinguish between trigeminal neuralgia and Bell palsy.
19. List the diagnostic tests used for meningitis and explain how the causative organism is identified.
20. Name the common causes of encephalitis.
21. Explain the pathologic course of Guillain-Barré syndrome.
22. Explain what is meant by postpolio syndrome.

KEY TERMS

aphasia (ah-FAY-zee-ah)
aura (AW-rah)
autonomic (aw-toe-NOM-ic)
cephalalgia (sef-ah-LAL-jee-ah)
chorea (ko-REE-ah)

concussion (kon-KUSH-un)
contusion (kon-TOO-zhun)
contrecoup (KON-trah-koo)
craniotomy (kray-nee-OTT-toe-me)
demyelination (dee-my-eh-lih-NAY-shun)

diplopia (dip-LOW-pee-ah)
epidural (ep-ih-DUR-al)
fasciculation (fa-sik-you-LAY-shun)
hematoma (hem-ah-TOE-mah)
hemiparesis (hem-ee-PAR-ee-sis)
hemiplegia (hem-ee-PLEE-jee-ah)

neurotransmitter (new-roh-TRANS-mit-er)
paraplegia (par-ah-PLEE-jee-ah)
parasympathetic (par-ah-sim-pa-THET-ik)
paresis (pah-REE-sis)
quadriplegia (kwod-rih-PLEE-jee-ah)
tetraplegia (tet-ra-PLEE-jee-ah)

Orderly Function of the Nervous System

The nervous system is a complex, sophisticated, and elaborate network of many interlaced nerve cells (neurons) that make up the brain (Fig. 13.1A), the spinal cord (see Fig. 13.1B), and the nerves. Electrical impulses are carried throughout the body by the neurons (see Fig. 13.1C; Fig. 13.2). This entire system regulates and coordinates the body's activities and produces responses to stimuli, which help the body adjust to changes in its environment, both internal and external.

The nervous system is composed of two divisions: the central nervous system (CNS) and the peripheral nervous system (PNS). The CNS includes the brain and spinal cord. Its function is to process and store sensory and motor information and to govern the state of consciousness. The frontal lobe of the cerebrum controls intellectual functions, such as thinking, willing, remembering, and deciding, and those that control personality. Coordination, equilibrium, and posture are coordinated in the cerebellum area of the brain. The hypothalamus regulates the secretion of hormones from the pituitary gland and regulates many visceral activities.

The medulla oblongata contains vital centers that help regulate heart rate, blood pressure, and respiration. Five pairs of the 12 cranial nerves originate in the medulla oblongata. It is considered an extension of the spinal cord. All the sensory and motor nerve fibers pass through the medulla oblongata, connecting the brain and the spinal cord. The spinal cord, a continuation of the medulla oblongata, extends to the first lumbar vertebra. It is divided into 31 segments, each giving rise to a pair of spinal nerves or reflex centers, carrying impulses to and from the brain (see Fig. 13.1D).

The vast network of nerves throughout the rest of the body is part of the PNS (Fig. 13.3A). Peripheral nerves connect with the spinal cord at many levels and the information (impulses) they carry travels to and from the brain and spinal cord. Sensory (afferent) nerves transmit impulses from parts of the body (e.g., skin, eye, ear, and nose) to the spinal cord and brain. Motor (efferent) nerves transmit impulses away from the CNS and produce responses in muscles and glands. The PNS contains 12 pairs of cranial nerves (see Fig. 13.3B), and 31 pairs of spinal nerves (see Fig. 13.3C). Refer to Fig. 6.14 to compare innervations of spinal nerves and the sympathetic and parasympathetic nerves.

The sympathetic and parasympathetic nerves make up the autonomic nervous system (ANS), which regulates the involuntary muscle movements and glandular actions of the body. The PNS also controls all conscious activities, which greatly affect unconscious processes, such as heart rate, breathing, and bowel functions (see Fig. 13.3D).

Four major blood vessels on each side of the head supply the brain with essential oxygen and nutrients. The carotid arteries (two internal and two external) originate from the two common carotid arteries and are located in the anterior portion of the neck; the two vertebral arteries (Fig. 13.4), join with the two anterior and posterior cerebral arteries, and the two anterior and posterior communicating arteries to form the brain's vascular system in a roughly circular configuration of arteries known as the *circle of Willis*. Branches from the circle of Willis supply blood to all portions of the brain (Fig. 13.5). Areas of the brain that depend on a single branch for survival are especially susceptible to disruption in the blood flow (e.g., thrombus or embolus).

The nervous system is susceptible to a variety of problems. Defects in the circulatory system of the brain can lead to vascular disorders and damaged brain cells. The brain also can be damaged by injuries, infections, metabolic derangement, inherited defects, congenital defects, degeneration, and tumors. Because of the complex nature of the CNS and the PNS, damage to either of the systems can cause extremely diverse symptoms.

Common problems within the nervous system that necessitate attention from health care providers include the following:
- Headaches
- Dizziness
- Muscle weakness
- Tremors
- Motor disturbances, other disturbances of movement, or paralysis
- Radiating pain
- Memory impairment
- Altered levels of consciousness
- Drowsiness
- Sensory disturbances or numbness
- Speech disturbances
- Visual disturbances

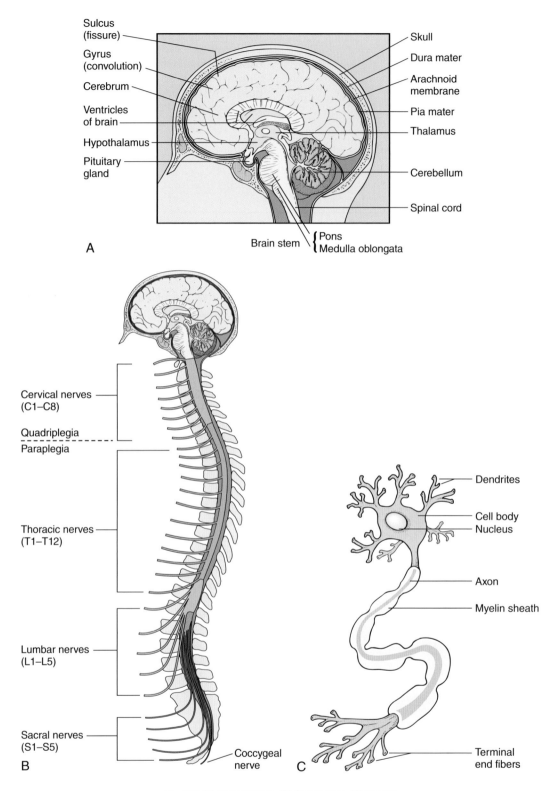

• **Fig. 13.1** (A) Normal brain. (B) Spinal cord. (C) Neuron.

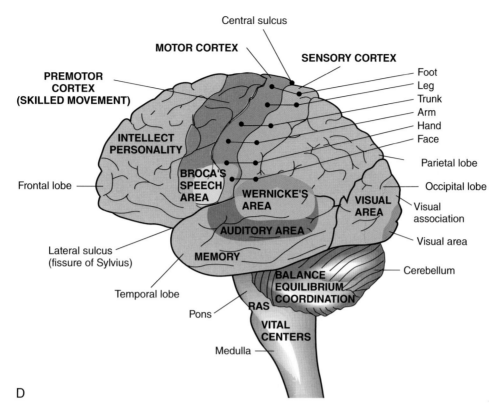

• **Fig. 13.1, cont'd** (D) Functional areas of the brain. *RAS*, Reticular activating system. (D, From Gould BE, Dyer RM: *Pathophysiology for the health professions*, ed 4, St. Louis, 2012, Saunders.)

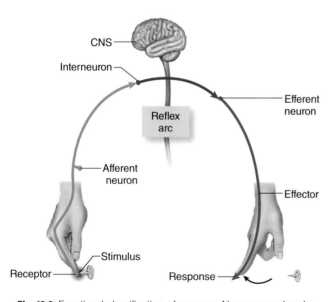

• **Fig. 13.2** Functional classification of neurons. Neurons can be classified according to the direction in which they conduct impulses. The most basic route of signal conduction follows a pattern, called *reflex arc. CNS*, Central nervous system. (From Patton K, Thibodeau G: *Anatomy & physiology*, ed 9, St. Louis, 2016, Mosby.)

Disorderly Function of the Nervous System

Vascular Disorders

Cerebrovascular Accident (Stroke)

Description

A cerebrovascular accident (CVA), or stroke, is a neurologic emergency, which occurs when the brain is damaged by a sudden disruption in the flow of blood to a part of the brain (embolic) or by bleeding inside the head (hemorrhagic). Sometimes a stroke may be referred to as a cerebrovascular insult or *brain attack*.

ICD-10-CM Code	I63.50 *(Cerebral infarction due to unspecified occlusion or stenosis of unspecified cerebral artery)*
	(I63.00–I63.9 = 72 codes of specificity)

Symptoms and Signs

CVAs are the number one cause of adult disability. Because of the inadequate blood supply, the physical and mental functions controlled by the affected area of the brain fail to operate properly (Fig. 13.6A).

The symptoms and signs of a stroke reflect the portion of the brain affected (see Fig. 13.6B). Common stroke symptoms include the following:
- Sudden severe headache
- Sudden aphasia, *dysphasia*, or difficulty understanding language

- Sudden weakness, numbness, or paralysis of the face, including one-sided drooping mouth and eyelid (hemiparesis)
- Sudden confusion or impaired consciousness
- Sudden loss of vision, blurred vision, unequal pupils, or diplopia

Neurologic Assessment

Neurologic assessment relies on a step-by-step collection of data to evaluate the neurologic status and cognitive function of a person. The examination is appropriate after head trauma occurs, cranial surgery is performed, or when a neurologic disorder, such as a brain tumor or stroke, is suspected. Observations and findings are graded on a scale and documented.

Neurologic assessment begins with a thorough medical history, noting past and current problems and recording

medications, vitamins, and supplements being taken. The patient's comprehension and judgment are noted during the examination.

The patient's mental status may be graded with the Glasgow coma scale, which is a standardized system for assessing responses to stimuli.

Next, the more sophisticated mental functions, including speech, language, and writing skills, are tested. Is the patient having difficulty putting words together, or is speech

Major Components of Cranial Nerves

NUMBER	NAME	TYPE OF FIBERS	FUNCTION
I	Olfactory	Sensory	Special sensory—smell
II	Optic	Sensory	Special sensory—vision
III	Oculomotor	Motor	Eye movements
			Four extrinsic eye muscles
			Upper eyelid—levator palpebrae muscle
		PNS	Iris—pupillary constrictor muscle
			Ciliary muscle—accommodation
IV	Trochlear	Motor	Eye movements—superior oblique eye muscle
V	Trigeminal	Sensory	General sensory—eye, nose, face and oral cavity, teeth
		Motor	Muscles of mastication with sensory proprioceptive fibers; speech
VI	Abducens	Motor	Eye movements—lateral rectus eye muscle
VII	Facial	Sensory	Special sensory—taste, anterior two-thirds of tongue
		Motor	Muscles of facial expression
			Scalp muscles
		PNS	Lacrimal gland, nasal mucosa, salivary glands (sublingual and submandibular)
VIII	Vestibulocochlear	Sensory	Special sensory—hearing and balance (inner ear)
IX	Glossopharyngeal	Sensory	Special sensory—taste, posterior one-third of tongue
			General sensory—pharynx and soft palate (gag reflex)
			Sensory—carotid sinus for baroreceptors and chemoreceptors
		Motor	Pharyngeal muscles—swallowing
		PNS	Salivary gland (parotid)
X	Vagus	Sensory	Special sensory—taste, pharynx, posterior tongue
			General sensory—external ear and diaphragm
			Visceral sensory—viscera in thoracic and abdominal cavities
		Motor	Pharynx and soft palate—swallowing and speech
		PNS	Heart and lungs, smooth muscle, and glands of digestive system
XI	Spinal accessory	Motor	Voluntary muscles of palate, pharynx, and larynx
			Head movements—sternocleidomastoid and trapezius muscles
XII	Hypoglossal	Motor	Muscles of tongue

PNS, parasympathetic nervous system.
From Gould: *Pathophysiology for the Health Professions*, ed 4, St. Louis, 2011, Saunders.

slurred? Do the patient's ideas and thoughts make sense? Behavior, emotional state, long-term and recent memory, and attention span are observed.

The cranial nerves are assessed by testing the patient's sense of smell, visual acuity, eye movements, muscles of mastication, taste perception, facial muscles, hearing, tongue movements, and swallowing.

Motor function is evaluated by testing muscle tone and strength. Significant asymmetry in the size, shape, or strength of corresponding muscles may be noted. Changes in muscle extension and flexion and spasticity or flaccidity are also noted.

Coordination and balance are assessed by watching for unsteadiness, a shuffling gait, or the dragging of a foot. The patient is asked to perform rapid alternating movements and tasks to demonstrate fine motor coordination. A reflex hammer is used to test deep tendon reflexes in the arms and legs.

Sensory examination determines diminished or abnormal sensation. A cotton ball may be brushed against the skin at different points. A slight pin stick tests for superficial pain. Temperature and vibration tests also are done.

Findings lead the clinician to begin focusing on any problem area. As abnormal assessment findings emerge, the need for further testing is also indicated.

- Sudden onset of dizziness, loss of balance, or loss of coordination

A severe stroke can result in coma and death. Early recognition of symptoms and prompt medical intervention can help reduce the risks of disability and death.

Patient Screening

Any individual experiencing a sudden onset of weakness, numbness or paralysis, difficulty speaking or understanding language, confusion or loss of consciousness, loss of vision or double vision, loss of balance or coordination, or dizziness requires immediate assessment and aggressive intervention. These individuals should be immediately entered into the emergency medical system (EMS) by the medical office or a family member for treatment. Occasionally the onset of symptoms may be insidious over a period of a few hours or even a day.

❗ ALERT!

FAST Method for Recognizing and Responding to Stroke Symptoms

Use the letters in F.A.S.T. to spot a Stroke

F = Face Drooping—Does one side of the face droop or is it numb? Ask the person to smile. Is the person's smile uneven?

A = Arm Weakness—Is one arm weak or numb? Ask the person to raise both arms. Does one arm drift downward?

S = Speech Difficulty—Is speech slurred?

T = Time to call 911—Stroke is an emergency. Every minute counts. Call 911 immediately. Note the time when any of the symptoms first appear.

Stroke symptoms, act FAST. National Stroke Association website: https://www.stroke.org/en/about-stroke/stroke-symptoms. Accessed November 9, 2023.

Etiology

A CVA is usually the result of one of three types of vascular disorders: (1) occlusion of an artery caused by an atheroma;

(2) sudden obstruction by an embolus, including a cerebral thrombosis (clot), embolism (moving clot), or other moving emboli; or (3) cerebral bleeding. These vascular disorders most often are caused by atherosclerosis (see the Atherosclerosis section in Chapter 10) and hypertension (high blood pressure). Strokes also can result from blood disorders, arrhythmias such as atrial fibrillation, systemic diseases (e.g., diabetes mellitus and neurosyphilis), hyperlipidemia, rheumatic heart disease, or head trauma. A high-fat diet, lack of exercise, cigarette smoking, obesity, and a family history of atherosclerotic disease are contributing factors.

CVAs caused by an embolus or hemorrhage often have a sudden onset, whereas strokes caused by a thrombus may appear more gradually. Cerebral thrombosis occurs if one of the cerebral arteries becomes narrowed because of plaque buildup from atherosclerotic disease. This thrombus, or clot, can enlarge until it partially or completely blocks blood flow to the artery, thereby starving the tissue it feeds of oxygen.

Cerebral embolism is also a blockage, but it is caused by a foreign object or embolus. This embolus can be a piece of the arterial wall, a small blood clot from a diseased heart, or a bacterial clot; usually, platelet fibrin from an ulcerated arterial wall of the heart or valve of the heart is the causative factor. Atrial fibrillation may be a cause of the release of the embolus from the inner chambers of the left side of the heart. It is carried in the bloodstream until it becomes wedged in a blood vessel and obstructs the flow of blood to an area of the brain.

With cerebral hemorrhage, the cerebral artery is not blocked but instead ruptures, flooding the surrounding brain tissue with blood (see Fig. 13.6C). The initial effects of a hemorrhage may be more severe than those of a thrombosis or embolism, and the long-term effects are much more serious (see Fig. 13.6D). (Refer to the Enrichment box about Arteriovenous Malformations.)

Diagnosis

Physical examination of the patient leads the physician to suspect a CVA and to gauge the impairments on a functional scale. It can be confirmed with magnetic resonance imaging

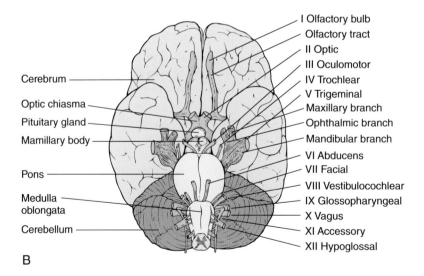

Brachial plexus
(C5–C8 and T1)

Phrenic

Axillary

MAJOR NERVES OF SHOULDER

Musculocutaneous

Axillary

Radial
Median
Ulnar

Radial

Median

Ulnar

Lumbar plexus
(T12 and L1–L5)

Sacral plexus
(S1–S4)

Femoral
Sciatic

Common peroneal

Superficial
peroneal

Tibial

Deep
peroneal

Saphenous

A

Cervical
plexus
(C1–C4)

Brachial
plexus
(C5–T1)

Lumbar
plexus
(L1–L4)

Sacral
plexus
(L5–S3)

Cervical nerves
(8 pairs)

Thoracic nerves
(12 pairs)

Lumbar nerves
(5 pairs)

Sacral nerves
(5 pairs)

Coccygeal
nerves
(1 pair)

C

Cerebrum

Optic chiasma

Pituitary gland

Mamillary body

Pons

Medulla
oblongata

Cerebellum

I Olfactory bulb
Olfactory tract
II Optic
III Oculomotor
IV Trochlear
V Trigeminal
Maxillary branch
Ophthalmic branch
Mandibular branch
VI Abducens
VII Facial
VIII Vestibulocochlear
IX Glossopharyngeal
X Vagus
XI Accessory
XII Hypoglossal

B

• **Fig. 13.3** (A) Peripheral nervous system. (B) Cranial nerves. (C) Spinal nerves.

Sympathetic division

Parasympathetic division

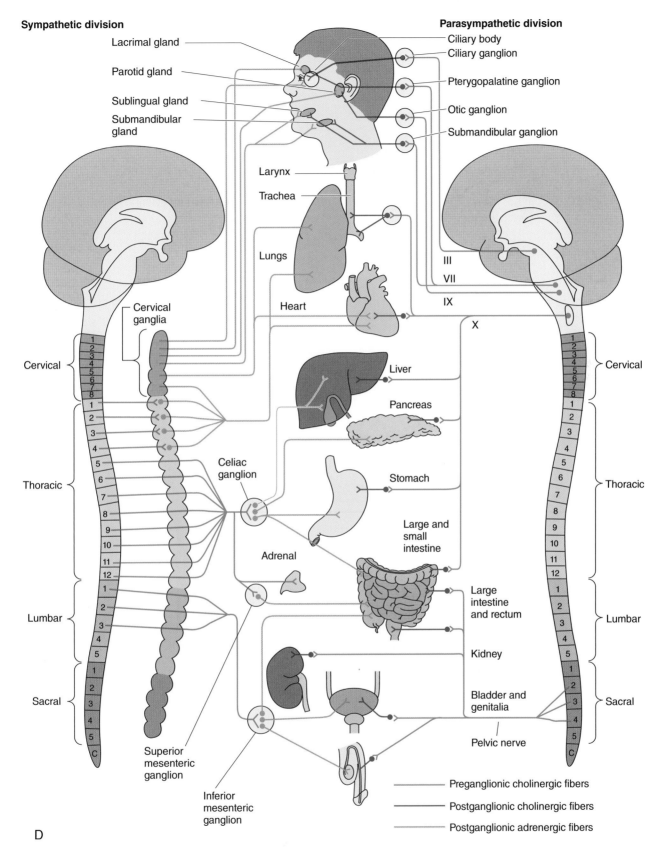

• **Fig. 13.3, cont'd** (D) Autonomic nervous system.

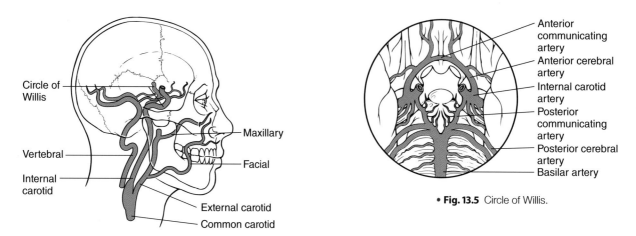

Circle of
Willis

Maxillary

Vertebral

Facial

Internal
carotid

External carotid

Common carotid

• **Fig. 13.4** Cerebral circulation. Major arteries of the head and neck.

Anterior
communicating
artery

Anterior cerebral
artery

Internal carotid
artery

Posterior
communicating
artery

Posterior cerebral
artery

Basilar artery

• **Fig. 13.5** Circle of Willis.

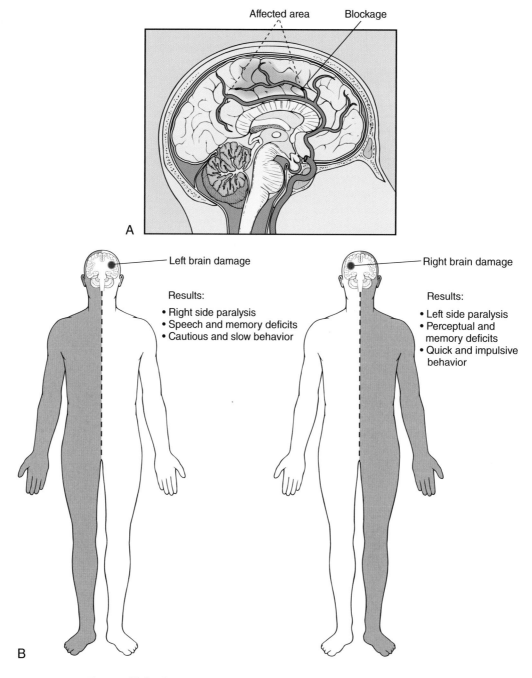

Affected area   Blockage

A

Left brain damage

Results:
• Right side paralysis
• Speech and memory deficits
• Cautious and slow behavior

Right brain damage

Results:
• Left side paralysis
• Perceptual and
  memory deficits
• Quick and impulsive
  behavior

B

• **Fig. 13.6** (A) Cerebrovascular accident (CVA). (B) Areas of the body affected by CVA

• **Fig. 13.6, cont'd** (C) Cerebral hemorrhage. Massive hypertensive hemorrhage rupturing into a lateral ventricle. (D) Arteriovenous malformation. (C and D, From Kumar V, et al: *Robbins basic pathology*, ed 8, Philadelphia, 2009, Saunders.)

(MRI), computed tomography (CT), cerebral angiography, or electroencephalography (EEG). Blood tests for bleeding and clotting disorders may be performed. Cardiac monitoring may show atrial fibrillation or other arrhythmias. Providers may order an agitated saline contrast echocardiogram. This is referred to as a *"bubble study or bubble test"*. This test allows the physician to see if there is a problem with the way the blood is traveling through the heart. Some individuals have a small hole which usually closes a few weeks after birth. In many patients, it never poses any problem. When a patient has no explained reason or strong risk factors for stroke, the bubble test can help identify if the hole is still present, potentially allowing blood to travel the wrong way, resulting in stroke. This is referred to as a *patent foramen ovale* when the hole or tunnel is present between the right and left atria.

Treatment

Treatment for a hemorrhagic stroke is different than treatment for an ischemic stroke. When the patient is diagnosed with an ischemic stroke, blood thinning drugs are administered. The patient may be given a drug called recombinant tissue plasminogen activator. This may also be referred to as alteplase (Activase). This medication must be administered within 3 hours of the stroke symptoms. In some cases may be administered up to 4.5 hours after the symptoms begin. This is why it should be noted what time the first stroke symptom occurred. This medication also poses a risk of bleeding into the brain and is used cautiously with benefits and risks weighed carefully by the provider prior to administration.

Surgery to improve circulation within the cerebral arteries or to remove clots is considered. If the patient has a positive bubble test, the patent foramen ovale can be closed between the atria.

Other therapeutic measures include surgery to repair broken or bleeding blood vessels and drugs to prevent or reverse brain swelling. Antiarrhythmic drugs are administered for arrhythmias. Long-term treatment for CVA depends on the size and location of the stroke and the presence and severity of impairments. The goal of medical treatment is to restore lost functions and treat underlying disorders. A team approach to rehabilitation includes help from family members' therapists. Inpatient rehabilitation is needed for patients who need daily therapy to become stronger and more independent after a stroke.

Prognosis

Recovery varies in rate of improvement and degree of rehabilitation. Some permanent disability may remain even after rehabilitation efforts. Strokes do cause brain damage. Brain cells that are destroyed do not recover and are not replaced; patients can learn new ways of functioning by using other undamaged brain cells.

Prevention

Prevention of stroke includes positive lifestyle changes to reduce controllable risk factors, such as hypertension, smoking, excesses in diet and alcohol consumption, and uncontrolled diabetes. Other risk factors over which the individual has no control include age and family history of stroke. Medication regimens are helpful in some cases caused by hypertension and atrial fibrillation. According to the Centers for Disease Control and Prevention, approximately 80% of CVAs are preventable with patient education and control or modification of risk factors.

Patient Teaching

Review the warning signs of a stroke with the patient and the family. Instruct them about the importance of quickly seeking medical intervention for any signs of impending stroke and to note the time the symptoms began.

Assist the family in finding resources for therapy and appropriate medical equipment for home use that will facilitate the home care and safety of the patient. Occupational, physical, and speech therapy referrals may be facilitated.

ENRICHMENT

Arteriovenous Malformations

Formed during fetal development, arteriovenous malformations (AVMs) are abnormal structures of the blood vessels. The etiology of this congenital condition, which is usually discovered between ages 10 and 40 years of age, is unknown, but research is ongoing to learn as much as possible about the cause. Although usually found in the brain, AVMs may be located in any vascular structure. Blood normally flows from the artery through the capillaries to the veins. In AVMs, there is an abnormal connection in which the capillaries are lacking. As a result, arterial blood moves directly into the veins, giving the blood vessels the appearance of a tangled mass of arteries and veins. These fragile vascular structures have a tendency to bleed, and this often results in hemorrhage. When AVMs are located in the brain, the symptoms of bleeding are similar to those of a stroke. The patient complains of generalized or region-specific headache or the worst headache of their life. Nausea and/or vomiting, stiff neck, confusion, lethargy, generalized weakness, visual problems, and irritability may be noted. As the bleeding progresses, speech may become impaired, muscle weakness and paralysis may be noted in the face, ringing in the ears may be reported, and dizziness and syncope may follow. Some patients may lose consciousness.

Diagnosis is made through assessment of the clinical signs and imaging studies, including CT and MRI of the brain. Prompt treatment is required and includes surgical intervention, radiation therapy, or embolization of the involved vessel. Cerebral AVMs have a mortality rate of approximately 10% if ruptured. Additionally, residual conditions caused by the insult of oxygen and nutrition deprivation of the brain tissue are possible. Seizure activity and other neurologic problems may follow. No method of prevention is known for this condition. AVM may also be misrecognized in infancy as a capillary malformation, which are commonly called "port wine stains."

 ENRICHMENT

Cerebral Aneurysms

A cerebral aneurysm, a cerebrovascular condition, is an abnormal localized weakening, thinning, or dilation of the wall of a cerebral artery or vein, resulting in ballooning of the blood vessel. Leakage or spilling of blood results in hemorrhage in the brain.

Pressure caused by the bulging vessel is placed on a nerve or brain tissue. Cerebral aneurysms often cause no symptoms and go unnoticed until rupture or leakage occurs, with blood being released into the brain, causing a stroke and resulting brain damage. Cerebral aneurysms can occur in any part of the brain; however, many commonly occur near the base of the brain in the circle of Willis (see Fig. 13.5).

The etiology may be a congenital defect, atherosclerosis, hypertension, infection, cancer, drugs, or trauma to the head. Although most often occurring in adults, children also may experience cerebral aneurysms.

Diagnosis of a cerebral aneurysm usually occurs with the onset of symptoms of cerebral bleeding. Occasionally diagnosis is made incidentally on imaging examination for other causes. The treatment is surgical repair of the vessel. Frequently the rupture is so acute with rapid onset that surgical intervention is unsuccessful, and brain damage occurs.

Transient Ischemic Attack

Description

Transient ischemic attacks (TIAs) are temporary episodes with a duration of a few minutes of impaired neurologic functioning caused by inadequate flow of blood to a portion of the brain.

ICD-10-CM Code	G45.0 *(Vertebrobasilar artery syndrome)* *(G45.0–G45.9 = 7 codes of specificity)*

Symptoms and Signs

Transient cerebral ischemia can occur in various sites, and therefore various diagnostic codes are used. After the physician has diagnosed the site of the ischemia, refer to the current edition of the *International Classification of Diseases, 10th Revision, Clinical Modification* (ICD-10-CM) coding manual to confirm the appropriate code for transient cerebral ischemia. TIAs often are referred to as *little strokes* or *mini-strokes* because they resemble a stroke caused by an embolism but they are not to be disregarded as unimportant. They can serve as an indicator of future ischemic stroke. The individual may report sudden weakness and numbness down one side of the body, dizziness, dysphagia, confusion, difficulty seeing with one eye, and/or loss of balance. The individual may complain of a sudden-onset headache. Usually, TIAs do not cause unconsciousness. These TIAs often manifest as recurring episodes, lasting from just seconds to a few minutes, with symptoms gradually subsiding. The symptoms, like those of a stroke, depend on which part of the brain is affected. Differentiation between a stroke and a TIA is the duration of symptoms and the absence of permanent brain damage.

Patient Screening

As with individuals complaining of CVA type of symptoms, individuals experiencing TIAs require immediate assessment and intervention to reduce residual effects. Instruct them or their families to contact the EMS or to be transported immediately to an emergency facility.

Etiology

The most common cause of a TIA is a piece of plaque, formed by atherosclerosis, which breaks away from the wall of an artery or heart valve and travels to the brain (Fig. 13.7). This is known as an *embolus*, or a moving clot. Platelet fibrin emboli from an arterial ulcer are often the causative factor. Arterial vascular spasms and minute blood clots also may be etiologic factors. Unlike strokes, TIAs do not normally cause permanent damage to the brain tissue.

Diagnosis

Physical examination and history are the first steps in diagnosing the problem. Next is determining the source of a possible embolus. The carotid arteries are a likely source of emboli. Cranial MRI, CT, carotid ultrasonography, and EEG are all helpful in confirming the diagnosis; however, all results can appear normal.

Treatment

Treatment depends on the location of the TIA and the underlying cause. Anticoagulants and antiplatelets are commonly used during an episode to lessen the frequency or risk of recurrences. Therapy may include heparin, enoxaparin, warfarin, aspirin, dipyridamole, apixaban, and clopidogrel.

Prognosis

The prognosis varies, depending on the extent and duration of the ischemia. Most attacks resolve with minimal residual effects. TIAs should be considered warning signals for future CVAs.

Prevention

As with CVAs, prevention includes positive lifestyle changes to reduce controllable risk factors, such as smoking, excesses in diet and alcohol consumption, untreated high blood pressure, and uncontrolled diabetes. Management of heart arrhythmias can also prevent stroke. Oral contraceptives may increase the risk of strokes.

Patient Teaching

Instructions should be given concerning possible symptoms of an impending stroke. Family members should be instructed to seek immediate medical intervention for the patient at the first sign of a stroke. Give instructions for monitoring blood pressure, and emphasize the importance of complying with the prescribed drug therapy. Go over stroke FAST information with the patient and family.

Head Trauma

Head trauma may result in brain injury, also known as a traumatic brain injury (TBI). Ranging from mild to life threatening or fatal, TBIs may be the result of several types of insults to the head. Included in the forms of TBI are concussions, contusions, closed-head injuries, open-head injuries, linear fractures, comminuted fractures, compound fractures, and contrecoup injuries. Concussions, contusions, and injuries in which the cranial vault is not violated are types of closed-head injuries; fractures to the cranial vault are open-head injuries and include linear, depressed, comminuted, compound, and basilar skull fractures (see Fig. 13.11).

Professional sports organizations are now actively exploring the results of TBIs and concussions that have occurred and are occurring in various sports activities. Recommendations are forthcoming on how long an individual should be kept inactive after a TBI. Research continues to determine all the cumulative effects of TBI.

Epidural and Subdural Hematomas

Description

An epidural hematoma is a collection or mass of blood that forms between the skull and the dura mater, the outermost of the three meningeal layers covering the brain. With a subdural hematoma, the blood collects or pools between the dura mater and the arachnoid membrane, the second meningeal membrane (Fig. 13.8).

ICD-10-CM Code	S06.6X0A (Traumatic subarachnoid hemorrhage without loss of consciousness, initial encounter) (S06.6X0 [7th digit]–S06.6X9 [7th digit] = 10 codes of specificity) S06.4X0A (Epidural hemorrhage without loss of consciousness, initial encounter) (S06.4X0 [7th digit]–S06.4X9 [7th digit] = 10 codes of specificity) S06.5X0A (Traumatic subdural hemorrhage without loss of consciousness, initial encounter) (S06.5X0 [7th digit]–S06.5X9 [7th digit] = 10 codes of specificity)

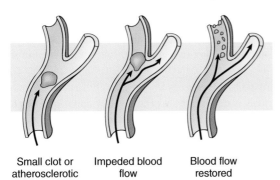

Small clot or atherosclerotic plaque embolus | Impeded blood flow | Blood flow restored

• **Fig. 13.7** Embolus causing transient ischemic attack.

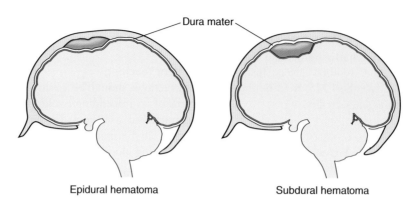

Dura mater

Epidural hematoma   Subdural hematoma

• **Fig. 13.8** Hematomas (two types).

Intracranial injuries are coded according to site, type of wound, state of consciousness, or length of unconsciousness. Refer to the current edition of the ICD-10-CM coding manual for verification of the appropriate code once the diagnosis has been confirmed.

Symptoms and Signs

Pressure on the brain resulting from either of these hematomas can result in impaired functioning of the brain or possibly death.

Symptoms of an epidural hematoma typically appear within a few hours of head trauma. They include sudden headache, dilated pupils, nausea and often vomiting, increased drowsiness, and perhaps hemiparesis. If the hematoma is not treated promptly, unconsciousness, coma, and death occur. Deterioration of the patient's condition can be rapid. This is a neurologic emergency.

Subdural hematomas often exhibit symptoms similar to those of an epidural hematoma, except the onset is delayed because of slower accumulation of blood. This delayed onset may mimic the symptoms of a TIA, stroke, or dementia. Diplopia is a common occurrence in patients with a subdural hematoma.

Patient Screening

Most trauma victims with closed and open-head injuries are transported to an emergency facility for treatment. When a head injury is not obvious, the onset of symptoms may be insidious. When a family member, or possibly the injured individual himself or herself, calls in complaining of pain in the head and onset of other neurologic symptoms after head trauma, instruct the family member to have the trauma victim transported to an emergency facility for immediate assessment. Emphasize that the victim should not drive. The victim of any acceleration-deceleration type injury, such as motor vehicle accidents (MVAs) or falls, requires prompt assessment and intervention.

Etiology

Both types of hematomas can result when blood from ruptured vessels seeps into and around the meningeal layers. Head trauma is the usual cause; a blow to the head can cause an epidural hematoma, or the head striking an immovable object (sudden acceleration or deceleration injury) can cause a subdural hematoma. Sudden acceleration or deceleration injury results in the brain striking the skull or tearing of the vessels within the brain or meninges. Subdural hematomas often occur among older adults or alcoholics as a result of falls. Cerebral hematoma often follows a skull fracture.

Diagnosis

The clinical findings noted on examination of the patient, along with a history of recent head trauma, suggest to the physician the possibility of either an epidural hematoma or a subdural hematoma. Cranial radiography, CT, MRI, and cerebral arteriography help locate the hematoma and rule out other causes of the symptoms. Prompt investigation of the condition is vital. Obtaining the history of the mechanism of injury and time of the initial insult is an additional aid in determining the diagnosis.

Treatment

If the person loses consciousness because of head trauma, rapid medical attention is needed. A craniotomy and/or cranial *trephination* (i.e., making a burr hole in the skull with a drill to relieve pressure by draining off the blood that has accumulated), may be necessary. This procedure is performed to remove the accumulated blood and to cauterize the bleeding vessels if increasing intracranial pressure indicates a life-threatening situation. When this procedure is performed promptly, complete recovery is possible. A patient not losing consciousness but displaying symptoms, either immediate or delayed, should be seen by a physician as soon as possible for evaluation.

Prognosis

Prognosis is dependent on the level of consciousness of the patient, age, size of the hematoma, whether or not brain damage occurred, and how quickly treatment is initiated.

Patient Teaching

Provide postsurgical instructions for care of the incision. Instruct caregivers to assess for indications of neurologic changes and other signs of increased intracranial pressure. Encourage the use of seat belts, child restraint seats, and helmets in contact sports and cycling, skiing, boarding, or any such activity.

Cerebral concussion

Description

Cerebral concussion is bruising of the cerebral tissue caused by back-and-forth movements of the head, as in an acceleration-deceleration insult. Blunt force trauma and falls also may result in cerebral concussion.

ICD-10-CM Code	S06.0X9A (Concussion with loss of consciousness of unspecified duration, initial encounter) (S06.0X0 [7th digit]-S06.0X9 [7th digit] = 10 codes of specificity)

Cerebral concussions have various codes according to the level of consciousness and duration of any periods of unconsciousness and are designated by the addition of the fourth digit. Refer to the current edition of the ICD-10-CM coding manual to determine the appropriate code.

Symptoms and Signs

With cerebral concussion, patients may experience loss of consciousness. It often is referred to as *being knocked out*. This state may last from a few seconds to several minutes and may be followed by periods of amnesia. Respirations become shallow, the pulse rate drops, and muscle tone is flaccid. Symptoms appearing after the person has regained consciousness may include headache, nausea, vomiting, ringing in ears, diplopia or blurred vision, and photophobia (sensitivity to light). Persons with this injury may exhibit irritability, decreased levels of concentration, and amnesia. Children may have vomiting, episodes of crying, a blank look on their face, disinterest in toys, seizures, or other atypical behavior.

Patient Screening

Individuals who have suffered a head injury and experienced loss of consciousness need immediate assessment and intervention. In most cases, treatment at an emergency care facility is the optimal choice.

Etiology

Cerebral concussion is an injury resulting from impact with a blunt object, either by receiving a blow to the head or by falling. This results in disruption of the normal electrical activity in the brain, but the brain itself usually is not permanently injured (Fig. 13.9). *Mild traumatic brain injury (MTBI)* is a term that can be applied to this injury.

Diagnosis

A complete neurologic examination, along with a history of the injury, is required. CT and MRI indicate no evidence of damage to the brain tissue. MRI called functional neurocognitive imaging can detect postconcussion syndrome. History from others (e.g., relatives, friends, observers, and ambulance staff) is vital.

Concussion

Contusion

• **Fig. 13.9** Head injuries.

Treatment

The usual treatment for concussion is quiet bed rest, with observation of the patient for signs of behavioral changes. Current recommendations suggest that it is acceptable to allow the patient to sleep, but it is important to make sure that the patient awakens fully when roused. Avoiding sports and other physical activities is recommended. Any changes noted, including changes in the level of consciousness, could indicate a progressive brain injury.

Prognosis

The prognosis is unpredictable and depends on the extent of the insult and any additional trauma. Cumulative effects may occur with successive MTBIs, resulting in more severe symptoms. Although most symptoms disappear after a few days or weeks, some individuals may experience postconcussion syndrome for weeks or months. Many people recover with no residual damage.

Prevention

Cerebral concussions are difficult to prevent. Consistent use of seat belts, child restraint seats, and helmets may help reduce the severity of the injury. Never drive under the influence of alcohol. Elderly patients can reduce the risk of falls to prevent concussions. Individuals who have experienced concussions are encouraged to avoid situations where another blow to the head could occur.

Patient Teaching

Encourage all patients to consistently use seat belts, secure children in child restraint seats, and wear helmets while playing contact sports or cycling. Avoid situations where another head injury is likely. Provide family members or other caregivers with written information about the care of the individual with a closed-head injury. Notify the patient and caregiver of things to look for and complications that should be reported to the medical office.

Cerebral Contusion

Description

Cerebral contusion is more serious than concussion. This injury to the brain involves bruising of tissue along or just beneath the surface of the brain. It may also be termed a *contrecoup (counterblow) insult.*

ICD-10-CM Code	S06.330 A *(Contusion and laceration of cerebrum, unspecified, without loss of consciousness, initial encounter)* (S06.300 [7th digit]–S06.389 [7th digit] = 90 codes of specificity)

Cerebral lacerations and contusions are coded according to site, type of wound, state of consciousness, or length of unconsciousness. Once the diagnosis has been confirmed, refer to the current edition of the ICD-10-CM coding manual for assistance in verifying the appropriate code.

Symptoms and Signs

The symptoms and signs of contusion vary, depending on the site and extent of the injury, and persist for longer than 24 hours. They may range from temporary loss of consciousness to coma. When conscious, the person may report a severe headache and hemiparesis. The symptoms may be progressive in nature. The person may appear drowsy and lethargic or hostile and combative.

Permanent damage to the brain may result from cerebral contusions caused by subdural and epidural hematomas (see the Epidural and Subdural Hematomas section), causing impaired intellect, dysphasia, paralysis, epilepsy, impaired gait, and continuing stupor.

Patient Screening

Individuals who have suffered a head injury and complain of severe headaches experience one-sided paralysis and a period of unconsciousness and are in need of immediate assessment and intervention. In most cases, treatment at an emergency care facility is the optimal choice. The unconscious individual should be taken to an emergency facility.

Etiology

Contusion of the brain is caused by a blow to the head or by impact against a hard surface, as occurs in an automobile

• **Fig. 13.10** Cerebral contusions associated with smear subdural hemorrhage and subarachnoid hemorrhage. (From Houck M: *Encyclopedia of forensic sciences*, ed 3, 2023, Elsevier.)

accident. The twisting or shearing force against the two hemispheres of the brain that occurs when it collides with the cranial bones may damage the structures deep within the brain (see Fig. 13.9). Cerebral contusion often is associated with a skull fracture (Fig. 13.10). This TBI may be observed in child, spouse, partner, or elder abuse.

Diagnosis

A thorough neurologic examination is necessary, along with obtaining the history of the mechanism of the injury. CT reveals the location and extent of brain damage and cranial radiography helps rule out a possible skull fracture.

Treatment

Patients with cerebral contusion need to be hospitalized so that their vital signs can be monitored and rapid medical intervention can be provided if required. Specific treatment depends on the site and severity of the contusion.

Prognosis

The prognosis is unpredictable and depends on additional trauma and the health of the individual. Underlying pathology may compromise the possibility of a favorable outcome. Increased intracranial pressure and possible herniations are complications that may follow the injury.

Prevention

As with cerebral concussions, cerebral contusions are difficult to prevent. The consistent use of seat belts, child restraint seats, and helmets may help reduce the severity of the injury.

Patient Teaching

As with cerebral concussions, all individuals should be encouraged to consistently use seat belts, secure children in child restraint seats when traveling by car, and wear helmets when engaging in contact sports or cycle riding. Provide family members or caregivers with written information about the care of a victim with a closed-head injury. Instruct family members or caregivers to seek immediate medical attention for the victim if the symptoms worsen.

Depressed Skull Fracture

Description

A fractured skull occurs with a break or fracture in one of the bones of the cranium (Fig. 13.11). When the skull bones are depressed or torn loose, they are pushed below the normal surface of the skull.

ICD-10-CM Code	S02.91XA (Unspecified fracture of skull, initial encounter for closed fracture) (S02.0 [7th digit]–S02.92 [7th digit] = 32 codes of specificity)

Once a diagnosis has been made specifying site and type of skull fracture, refer to the current edition of the ICD-10-CM coding manual to determine the highest specificity.

Symptoms and Signs

When a portion of the skull is broken and is pushed in on the brain, causing injury, it is said to be a *depressed skull fracture* (see Fig. 13.11). The symptoms depend on the site of the fracture. For example, a bone fragment pressing on the motor area of the brain may cause hemiplegia (Fig. 13.12). Characteristically, symptoms from a depressed fracture are not progressive. They tend to remain static until the depressed bone is elevated and the pressure is relieved. Seizures are a common complication of depressed skull fractures.

Signs include bleeding from the wound, ears, nose, or around the eyes; changes in pupils (either nonreactive or unequal); bruising behind the ears *(Battle sign)* or around and under the eyes *(raccoon eyes)*; and clear or bloody drainage from the ears or the nose. Other signs include headache, stiff neck, nuchal rigidity (neck stiffness), nausea, vomiting, visual disturbances, slurred speech, confusion, restlessness, irritability, difficulty balancing, drowsiness, seizures, and/or loss of consciousness.

Patient Screening

Patients with head injuries are in need of prompt intervention. Immediate transfer to an emergency facility is recommended. Head injuries should always be considered life threatening until ruled otherwise.

Etiology

Direct impact on the skull by a blunt object is the most common cause of depressed fractures. Industrial and automobile accidents are two of the many possible causes. Child, domestic, intimate partner, or elder abuse may also be a causative factor. The fractured bone may cut an artery or vein, causing hemorrhage in the brain.

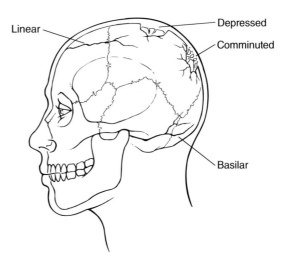

• **Fig. 13.11** Skull fractures.

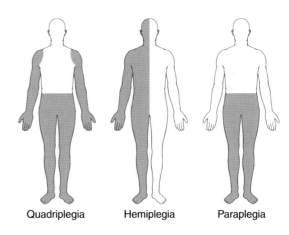

• **Fig. 13.12** Types of paralysis.

Diagnosis

Physical examination of the patient most likely reveals a defect in the skull. Cranial radiography indicates whether and where the brain is being crushed. CT shows the presence of life-threatening cerebral edema.

Treatment

Treatment is aimed at relieving intracranial pressure. A craniotomy is performed, and the depressed bone is elevated back into place. Head protection is worn until the fracture has healed at least partially.

Prognosis

The prognosis is unpredictable; it depends on the extent of the insult, timely intervention, possible complications, additional trauma, and any underlying medical conditions. Successful surgical intervention to relieve intracranial pressure and arrest bleeding usually has a positive outcome.

Prevention

Prevention is difficult because of the accidental nature of the fracture. Consistent use of seat belts and child restraint seats when in motor vehicles; wearing helmets during cycling,

Basilar Skull Fracture

A basilar skull fracture is a fracture of the bones of the floor of the cranial vault (see Fig. 13.11). This injury usually results from a massive insult to the cranium during a motor vehicle accident or other violent trauma in which the head is struck anteriorly or laterally in the midportion. As with other head injuries, symptoms, signs, and treatment depend on the area involved and the extent of the fracture. "Raccoon eyes" and "battle sign" are manifestations of basilar skull fracture and alert the physician to order imaging of the cranial vault for further investigation. Cerebrospinal fluid flowing from the ears or nares may be associated with a skull fracture. The level of consciousness is assessed, as are other neurologic signs. Treatment is like that of head injuries, including surgical intervention to relieve intracranial pressure. Occasionally the severity of the fracture causes severing of the pituitary stalk, resulting in panhypopituitarism.

skiing, skateboarding, or similar activities; and wearing full protective gear when playing contact sports will all help reduce the extent of damage in a head injury.

Patient Teaching

Reinforce to parents the potential dangers of head injuries in children, and remind them of the importance of children wearing helmets while cycling, skiing, skateboarding, or similar activities and while playing contact sports. Advise parents and others to seek professional emergency intervention in the event of a head injury in their children. Provide the patient and the family with visual aids depicting the neurologic system and its functions.

Spinal Cord Injuries

Paraplegia and Quadriplegia (Tetraplegia)

Description

Injuries to the spinal cord affect the innervation of any spinal nerves distal to the point of insult. The extent of the injury and consequential edema often result in the failure of spinal nerve functioning, with resulting loss of motor and sensory function. Paraplegia is loss of nerve function in areas below the waist and paralysis of the lower trunk and legs. Quadriplegia/Tetraplegia is a loss of nerve function at the cervical region resulting in paralysis of the arms, hands, trunk, and legs.

ICD-10-CM Code	G82.20 *(Paraplegia, unspecified)* (G82.20–G82.22 = 3 codes of specificity) G82.50 *(Quadriplegia, unspecified)* (G82.50–G82.54 = 5 codes of specificity)

Quadriplegia/Tetraplegia is coded by site and type. Once diagnosis confirms site and type, refer to the current edition of the ICD-10-CM coding manual for the appropriate code.

Symptoms and Signs

When the spinal cord is injured, one or more parts of the body inferior to the point of injury may be affected. The damage to the cord may be only temporary, but it usually leads to some degree of permanent disability, because nerve pathways control many body functions and actions. Paraplegia results in the loss of motor and sensory control of the trunk of the body and lower extremities. Loss of bowel, bladder, and sexual function is also common. Quadriplegia/tetraplegia results in paralysis of the lower extremities and usually the trunk, with either partial or total paralysis of the upper limbs. Hypotension, hypothermia, bradycardia, and respiratory problems also may be present. In some patients, respiration is maintained or assisted by mechanical ventilation.

Patient Screening

Individuals who sustain the acceleration-deceleration type of injury require stabilization for transport to an emergency care facility. Appointments for recovering patients will be scheduled for follow-up as necessary.

Etiology

Generally spinal cord injuries that cause paraplegia and quadriplegia/tetraplegia are the result of vertebral fractures or vertebral dislocation. The site of the injury, the type of trauma to the cord, and the severity of the trauma determine whether paraplegia or quadriplegia/tetraplegia will occur (see Fig. 13.12).

Trauma to the thoracic and lumbar regions of the spine (T1 and below) usually results in paraplegia (see Fig. 13.1B). Vertical compression and hyperflexion of the spine usually produce this injury. Trauma to the cervical vertebrae (C5 or above) may result in quadriplegia/tetraplegia. Injuries between C5 and C7 in the cervical vertebrae may produce varying degrees of paresis to the shoulders and arms. Damage occurring above C3 is usually fatal. The usual cause of this fatal injury is hyperextension or flexion of that portion of the spine. Mechanisms of spinal cord injury are presented in Fig. 13.13.

Diagnosis

A complete assessment of neurologic functioning is needed. Spinal radiography, MRI, and CT are ordered to determine the type and extent of injury. Fig. 13.14A and B show the effects of spinal cord damage.

Treatment

The goals of treatment for all spinal cord injuries include restoring the spine's normal alignment and stability, decompressing the spinal cord, nerves, and vertebrae, and early rehabilitation of the patient. These goals may involve surgery or using specialized medications and procedures.

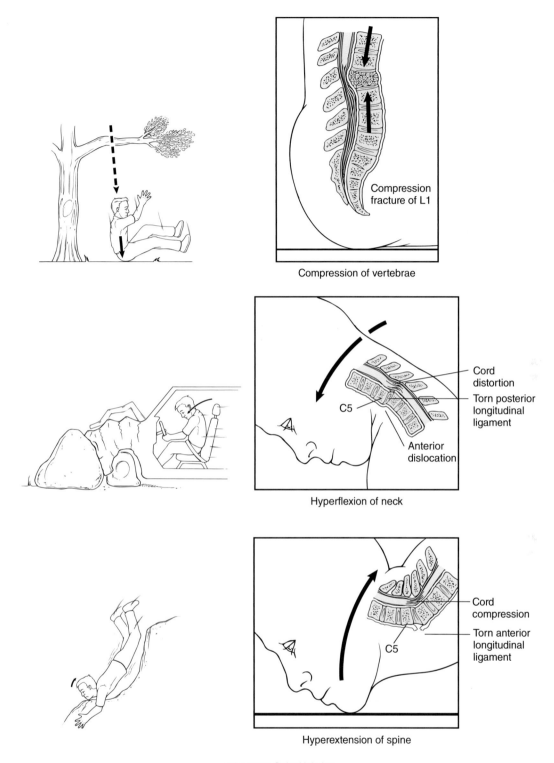

Compression of vertebrae

Hyperflexion of neck

Hyperextension of spine

• **Fig. 13.13** Spinal injuries.

Immediate spinal cord trauma intervention includes stabilization of the neck and spine before any movement to prevent secondary damage. Another intervention may include inducing a hypothermic state to the injured area in hopes of preventing edema of the spinal cord area. The location of the injury will also bear an impact on treatment.

When the patient is discharged they will need physical and occupational therapy to become stronger. Mental health counseling may also be necessary to help the patient deal with the frustrations of losing the capability of walking and caring for theirself.

Prognosis

The prognosis for a person with a spinal cord injury always is guarded. However, the earlier treatment is begun, the better the prognosis. Research focused on improving outcomes for spinal cord injuries is ongoing. The partial or total severing of the spinal cord results in

• **Fig. 13.14** The effects of spinal cord damage. (A) During spinal shock (period immediately after injury). (B) Overview of permanent effects (after spinal shock). *SNS,* Sympathetic nervous system. (From Gould BE, Dyer RM: *Pathophysiology for the health professions,* ed 4, St. Louis, 2012, Saunders/Elsevier.)

permanent, irreversible damage and paralysis of areas below the insult.

Prevention

Absolute prevention of spinal cord injury is not possible. Preventing injury beyond the initial insult is avoided by immediate stabilization of the injured person before any form of movement or transport to an emergency facility is attempted.

Patient Teaching

Patient teaching will be adapted to each individual situation in regard to where the injury or insult occurred and whether or not the patient has hemiplegia, paraplegia, or quadriplegia. Becoming as independent as possible will be important to both the patient and caregiver. The safety of the patient is important to prevent further injury or complications. Physical and occupational therapy should be included. Teaching the patient and caregiver how to prevent pressure sores is important for spinal cord injuries. Equipment for

◆ **ENRICHMENT**

Wounded Warrior Project

The Wounded Warrior Project provides opportunities to veterans with quadriplegia or other physical or emotional injury to stay in an underwater cage and interact with some species of sharks and swim with whale sharks, manta rays, and other species of fish, in conjunction with rehabilitative therapy after injury. In cases of paralysis, water therapy allows these individuals, who are no longer able to move on land, to move in the water. There are some programs that involve dives while in underwater cages, and other programs, such as the one at the Georgia Aquarium, which allows swimming in the water with marine life species, but without the use of cages.

home use should be ordered which can make day-to-day living easier. Teaching can assist the patient in learning to navigate their new "normal." This will take much time and the medical staff should assist the patient and caregiver with resources. Information should be given in regard to when the provider should be notified if there are concerns.

Intervertebral Disk Disorders

Degenerative Disk Disease

Description
The degeneration or deterioration of an intervertebral disk may result in pain in the areas served by the spinal nerves exiting at or below that disk space. Degenerative disk disease is a natural part of aging, occurring in almost everyone over time.

ICD-10-CM Code	M51.34 (Other intervertebral disk degeneration, thoracic region)
	M51.35 (Other intervertebral disk degeneration, thoracolumbar region)
	M51.36 (Other intervertebral disk degeneration, lumbar region)
	M51.37 (Other intervertebral disk degeneration, lumbosacral region)

Degenerative disk disease is coded by site. Once the site is confirmed by diagnosis, refer to the current edition of the ICD-10-CM coding manual for the appropriate code.

Symptoms and Signs
When pain occurs, it radiates down the nerve path (dermatome); may be described as burning; and can become intractable. The constant back pain and severe pain that radiates down one or both legs may be accompanied by loss of some motor functions in the legs. Additionally, the individual may also experience some numbness and tingling associated with weakness. There can also be bowel or bladder issues. Ask about any incontinence (urinary or fecal) or constipation.

Patient Screening
Patients complaining of severe back pain require prompt assessment. An appointment should be scheduled as soon as possible or according to office policy. A report of loss of motor function in the legs requires prompt assessment. That patient should be referred to an emergency treatment facility.

Etiology
As a person ages, the fluid in the disk decreases, causing degenerative disk disease. The degeneration may be mechanical and the result of constant wearing on the disk. Misalignment of vertebrae causes continual rubbing on the disk involved, resulting in inflammation and gradual destruction of the disk. The resulting inflammation eventually involves the spinal nerve roots and may cause scarring. A sequela is a spinal stenosis, in which there is a narrowing of the vertebral canal, the nerve root canals (foramen), or intravertebral foramina, causing the nerve roots to become trapped in the foramen as they leave the spinal canal.

Diagnosis
The clinical findings and a history of previous back injury lead to investigation with various types of imaging. This may include radiography, most often MRI, myelography with contrast to show the disk status, and rarely, CT. The narrowing of the intervertebral spaces is consistent with the condition. Electromyography (EMG) and neurologic examinations demonstrate the involvement of the dependent nerves and also measure nerve conduction. The observation of neurologic deficits, including foot drop and the dragging of a leg when walking, adds to the suspicion of nerve damage.

Treatment
Current treatment includes advising patients to be as active as possible. Narcotic analgesics and nonsteroidal antiinflammatory drugs (NSAIDs) are prescribed for pain relief. Oral steroids also may be prescribed. Epidurals or selective nerve root blocks for disk pain or spinal stenosis may be recommended. Physical therapy is also very helpful. Transcutaneous electrical nerve stimulation (TENS) is used with positive results. (Refer to Enrichment box about Transcutaneous Electrical Nerve Stimulation; and see the Enrichment box about Physical Therapy later in the chapter.) Bracing the back may be helpful. Surgical intervention includes spinal fusion and freeing of the spinal nerve roots from entrapment. When surgical intervention is not an option, lidocaine topical (Lidoderm) patches may be prescribed for placement over the affected area of the back for some relief. TENS units are offering a measure of relief to some individuals. Ablation is performed for the medial branch to treat facet pain, not nerve impingement. Pain pumps are the last resort. A continuous infusion of morphine via a pump into the epidural space may be employed as the last resort to treat intractable pain. Implantation of a spinal cord stimulator, a device that masks pain, is used to control chronic pain that cannot be relieved surgically or medically.

Prognosis
The prognosis varies depending on the extent of the degenerative process and the patient's response to treatment.

Prevention
Prevention is difficult because this is a degenerative process and is common in aging. Encouraging proper body mechanics may be helpful.

Patient Teaching
Encourage patients to be compliant with the physical therapy prescribed and to take medications as prescribed. Provide them with information about pain control measures. When a surgical procedure is involved, discuss wound care.

Herniated and Bulging Disk

Description
A herniated disk, also known as a *ruptured* or *slipped disk*, is the rupture of the nucleus pulposus through the annular wall of the disk and into the spinal canal (Fig. 13.15A and C).

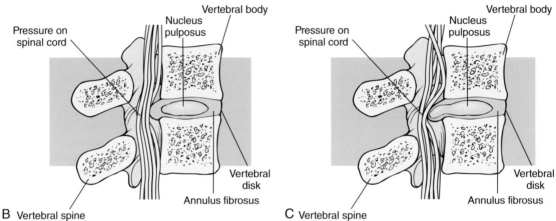

• **Fig. 13.15** (A) Herniated disk. The nucleus pulposus protrudes through the annulus fibrosus, putting pressure on the spinal cord and the spinal nerve. (B) Bulging disk (lateral view). Nucleus pulposus is contained in the annulus fibrosus. (C) Herniated disk (lateral view). Nucleus pulposus through the annular wall (annulus fibrosus) and pressure on the spinal cord.

❖ ENRICHMENT

Transcutaneous Electrical Nerve Stimulation

Transcutaneous electrical nerve stimulation (TENS) is prescribed as a nondrug alternative pain relief intervention. This involves use of small electronic units that operate with 9-V power to produce high-frequency electrical impulses, which are transmitted to the surface of the skin through electrodes placed on the skin into underlying nerve fibers. This concept of electrotherapy allows for placement of a unit where the pain occurs.

Two concepts are thought to be involved in pain relief. First the impulse or stimulation that is transmitted to the nerve fibers blocks the pain signal from being sent to the brain. When the signal is blocked, pain is not perceived. Second, the body has its own method of suppressing pain by releasing endorphins, natural chemicals that have analgesic activity. The impulses transmitted by the TENS unit stimulate the release of endorphins.

The use of TENS, a nondrug therapy option, permits many with chronic pain to return to a fairly normal life and

activities. The unit is small, measuring 2 to 2½ inches wide, 4 to 4½ inches long, and less than 1 inch thick. The units are programmable for strength and frequency of impulse to be delivered. Dual-chamber units have two lead wires that can be attached to the unit, and each has the capacity to be attached to two electrode leads. The electrodes are attached to the lead wires by small connecting wires. The unit can be hung from the waistband or from a belt. The electrodes are patches of various sizes, with adhesive on the back for attachment to the skin.

TENS units may be ordered for relief of chronic back pain, spinal stenosis, sciatica, arthritis, and postherpetic neuralgia. TENS units should *not* be used on patients with pacemakers or implantable cardioverter-defibrillators. Caution is recommended regarding their use in a pregnant female, especially around the developing fetus. The physician or physical therapist will provide instructions regarding use, settings, and safety measures.

ICD-10-   M51.9 *(Unspecified thoracic,*
  CM   *thoracolumbar, and lumbosacral*
  Code   *intervertebral disk disorder)*
              (M51.84–M51.9 = 5 codes of specificity)

Herniated intervertebral disk disorders are coded according to sites and involvement of myelopathy. Once diagnosis has been confirmed, refer to the current edition of the ICD-10-CM coding manual for the appropriate code.

Symptoms and Signs

Intervertebral disks are soft pads of cartilage and gelatinous material located between each of the vertebrae that make up the spine. Each disk acts as a shock-absorbing cushion for the vertebrae and gives the back its flexibility for movement. Within each of these disks is a gelatinous center called the *nucleus pulposus*, which is surrounded by an annulus, a circular wall-like structure. The nucleus pulposus is contained within the annular wall in a bulging disk (see Fig. 13.15B); thus the protrusion into the spinal canal is not as severe. The rupture can cause severe back pain and even disability if it presses against or pinches the spinal nerves. Sudden, sharp pain that worsens with movement or in certain positions may radiate from the back to the buttocks, thighs, and legs following the course of the impinged nerve, causing pain, paresthesia, and muscle weakness in the leg, in a dermatomal pattern. When this pain results from pinching of the nerve roots that form the sciatic nerve, it is known as *sciatica* (Fig. 13.16). In most cases, herniation of disks occurs in the lower back, between the fourth and fifth lumbar vertebrae, or between the fifth lumbar and first sacral vertebrae (lumbosacral area). Ruptured disks in the cervical region of the spine often produce pain and weakness in the arms and the neck. Pain from injury to a disk can be either unilateral or bilateral.

Patient Screening

A herniated disk is a painful and serious condition that necessitates immediate medical attention. The patient complaining of back pain should be given the next available appointment. If the patient is unable to walk or is in severe pain, a referral to the emergency services may be needed if a quick appointment is not available.

Etiology

Herniated and bulging intervertebral disks usually result from accumulated trauma (e.g., improper body mechanics when lifting) or sudden impact. Poor posture and the aging process can cause the disks to degenerate. The rupture may occur at the time of the trauma or shortly thereafter.

Diagnosis

A thorough history of the back pain is important. Physical examination of the back is performed to rule out other possible causes of the patient's symptoms. A diagnosis of lumbar disk herniation can be considered if the patient has sciatic pain when the

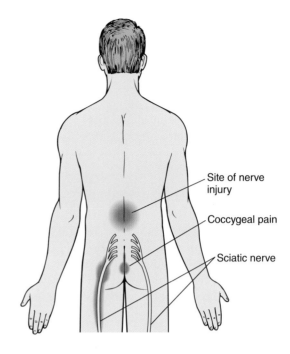

• **Fig. 13.16** Radiation of sciatic nerve pain.

physician performs the straight leg raise test. The physician may order MRI, CT, or myelography to help confirm the diagnosis.

In a bulging disk, the disk material is herniated through the inner annulus but not the outer annulus, so the contained material can still distort the path of the nerve with resulting pain. In more severe herniation, which is considered noncontained, the nucleus pulposus penetrates both the inner and outer layers of the annulus.

Treatment

Conservative treatment consists of the use of hot or cold packs and the administration of muscle relaxants and analgesics, such as aspirin, ibuprofen, or oral prednisone. Additional conservative treatment includes epidural injections and physical therapy.

When conservative treatment is not successful, surgical excision of the herniated disk may be needed. Procedures include percutaneous diskectomy, in which a needle is introduced into the intravertebral space and the encroaching portion of the nucleus pulposus is aspirated (for uncomplicated disk herniation); microdiscectomy, involving a small surgical incision, allowing the offending material to be aspirated; diskectomy as a surgical procedure combined with laser ablation and evaporation of the disk; or removal of the disk along with a laminectomy, with fusion of the vertebrae.

Often the pain from bulging disks resolves with rest and drug therapy.

Prognosis

The prognosis varies depending on the extent and duration of herniation. In many cases, the herniation resolves with conservative care. When surgical intervention is necessary, the outcome is usually favorable.

Prevention

The use of good and proper body mechanics is helpful in prevention; however, accidental slips and falls cannot always be avoided.

Patient Teaching

Provide these patients with information about good and proper body mechanics. Encourage those for whom rest and physical therapy are prescribed to be compliant. Share electronic or printed resources.

Sciatic Nerve Injury—Spinal Stenosis

Description

Sciatic nerve injury is a pathologic condition caused by trauma, degeneration, or rupture of the nucleus pulposus within the intervertebral disks. Spinal stenosis, a narrowing of the spinal canal or the nerve root foramen, is often termed *sciatica* because of the compression on the spinal cord and spinal nerve roots.

ICD-10-CM Code	S74.00XA *(Injury of sciatic nerve at hip and thigh level, unspecified leg, initial encounter)* (S74.00 [7th digit]–S74.92 [7th digit] = 15 codes of specificity)

Spinal stenosis is coded by region. Once the diagnosis has confirmed the affected region, refer to the current edition of the ICD-10-CM coding manual for the appropriate code.

Symptoms and Signs

Rupture or degeneration of the nucleus pulposus produces severe, sharp pain radiating from the sciatic nerve down the leg and to the foot (see Fig. 13.16). The pain may be continuous or intermittent, and areas of the skin supplied by the affected nerves may feel numb. A rupture of the nucleus pulposus posteriorly toward the neural canal results in pressure on the nerve root, causing sciatica symptoms or affecting the sciatic nerve, causing low back pain and leg pain. Anterior or lateral ruptures may or may not produce symptoms. The resulting symptoms depend on the extent of the rupture and the proximity of the nerves to the site. Nerve injury can produce severe disability, which may be temporary or permanent. Persons with sciatic nerve involvement may be so uncomfortable that they are unable to sit or stand without pain.

Patients with spinal stenosis also report pain in the back, radiating down the legs, and pain in the buttocks, thighs, or calves; the pain increases with standing, walking, or exercise. Additionally, they may experience numbness in these areas that becomes worse when standing, walking, or exercising. A weakness in the legs may be noted. Reflexes in the lower extremities often are asymmetric, and sensation may be decreased.

Patient Screening

Patients reporting lower back pain that radiates down the leg require prompt assessment for pain relief and to prevent further exacerbation of the condition. If an appointment is not available on the day of request, the patient should be referred to an emergency facility for evaluation and treatment.

Etiology

Trauma to the sciatic nerve may result from a fall, poor body mechanics, or gunshot or stab wounds. The aging process can lead to degeneration of disks or the nucleus pulposus. An inflammatory autoimmune response may prompt more rapid degeneration within a disk. The aging process, along with arthritic changes, may cause a narrowing of the spinal canal and the foramen where the spinal nerves exit the vertebrae. Formation of osteophytes on the foramen where the spinal nerves exit also can cause pain that radiates down the leg. Congenital narrowing of the spinal canal may be involved as well.

Diagnosis

After obtaining the medical history and performing a physical examination, the physician may order several diagnostic tests. These tests may include spinal radiography, MRI, CT, myelography, and blood serum studies. Vascular integrity is assessed, and insufficiency is ruled out. Often radiography of the spine shows degenerative changes along with a narrowed spinal canal. EMG studies may show neurologic changes.

Treatment

Conservative treatment may include oral corticosteroids (prednisone, methylprednisolone) and physical therapy, including ultrasound diathermy with massage or acupuncture. After the acute pain and inflammation have subsided, an exercise program to strengthen the back and abdominal muscles may be ordered. Drug therapy may also consist of analgesics such as acetaminophen, muscle relaxants (e.g., diazepam, cyclobenzaprine, and methocarbamol), and NSAIDs (e.g., ibuprofen, naproxen, indomethacin, celecoxib, or meloxicam). For severe pain not controlled by the aforementioned medications, a referral to a pain management specialist may be made. In some cases, stronger medications such as tramadol, hydrocodone-acetaminophen, or oxycodone-acetaminophen may be prescribed.

Physical therapy, including applications of heat and cold or gentle massage (myofascial release), may help relieve acute pain. Corticosteroid epidural injections may relieve pain and reduce inflammation of the spinal nerve. This option, many times, does not cure spinal stenosis or sciatica. Leaning forward or sitting often helps relieve the back pain.

Disabling pain or increasing weakness may necessitate surgical intervention. If a disk is causing the pain, then the removal of part or all of the disk or nucleus pulposus (diskectomy or microdiscectomy) spinal fusion may be helpful. Decompression of the spinal nerve foramen can be used to free the trapped spinal nerves. Surgery may not relieve low back pain caused by underlying conditions, such as osteoarthritis.

See the Enrichment box about Physical Therapy.

Physical Therapy

Normal physical activity and function can be compromised by the aging process and by disease or injury. Physical therapy is a branch of rehabilitative health used to help patients maintain or restore their physical abilities. Physical therapists are trained and certified to help plan programs and set goals for improvement in the individual's body strength and ability to function in daily activities. This process of rehabilitation can be challenging, but many experience positive physical and psychological rewards with good compliance.

Physical therapy is prescribed to help with recovery from insult to the musculoskeletal and/or the nervous system. Trauma to the musculoskeletal system often involves injury to the nerves in proximity. These insults may be traumatic in nature, resulting from a motor vehicle accident, a fall, a strain or sprain, or any other type of trauma. After surgical procedures with joint replacement or stabilization of fractures, physical mobility, and healing often are improved with regular therapy. Sports and work-related injuries are common reasons for the use of the intervention techniques of physical therapy. The aging process brings about mechanical changes to the body and causes interference in the individual's normal daily activities. The condition of individuals who are in the poststroke phase or who have other neurologic conditions often improves with physical therapy.

After assessment of the individual's gait, posture, range of motion, reflexes, strength, and the physical insult to the tissue, the therapist develops a plan of action to discuss this with the individual. Realistic goals are identified, along with time that can be committed to the therapy. The goal of the therapy is to improve the use of bones, joints, muscles, and nerves and to reduce the level of pain experienced by the individual. Restoration of function, improving the ability to move, and prevention of disability are also part of the goal. The therapist incorporates treatment modalities, including specially designed exercises; heat, light, massage, or ultrasound therapy; electrical stimulation; and/or aquatic therapy. Instruction and advice on proper body mechanics, posture, and motion may be included in the therapy. Individuals are provided with instructions for home exercise and exercise techniques for continuing therapy at home. Following all instructions is recommended for the best outcome.

Physical therapists also provide assistive devices for ambulation and instruction in their use. Individuals requiring ambulation devices are measured for them, and the device is then assembled to fit the patient. Crutch, walker, and cane walking will be taught for safe ambulation by the individual.

Prognosis

The prognosis varies, depending on the extent of the degeneration and traumatic insult. Surgical intervention may provide relief from pain.

Prevention

Preventing injury associated with traumatic insults is difficult. Degeneration of disks in aging is unavoidable.

Patient Teaching

Provide instructions for good and proper body mechanics. Encourage compliance with prescribed physical and drug therapy. Share links for electronic materials or printed material as teaching tools.

Functional Disorders

Headache

Description

Headache (cephalalgia) is a pain in the head that is not confined to any one specific nerve distribution area.

ICD-10-CM Code	G44.1 *(Vascular headache, not elsewhere classified)*
	(G44.1–G44.89 = 26 codes of specificity)
	R51 *(Headache)*

Symptoms and Signs

Headaches may be acute or chronic and located in the frontal, temporal, or occipital regions of the head or a combination of these. Cephalalgia also may be confined to only one side of the head or may be located above one or both eyes. The type of pain may vary from dull and aching to almost unbearable. It can be an intense intermittent pain, throbbing pain, pressure pain, or penetrating pain driving through the head. Brain tissues themselves never ache because they do not contain sensory nerves; however, the meninges do have pain receptors. Sensitivity in this area exists in only the meninges, the skin and muscles covering the skull, and the numerous nerves that travel from the brain to the head and the face.

Headaches are commonly experienced and usually are self-limiting. Cephalalgia, or secondary headache, is sometimes a symptom of an underlying disorder or disease (e.g., sinus infection or congestion, temporomandibular joint syndrome, hypertension, stroke, brain tumor, meningitis, and encephalitis). In most cases, however, headaches are caused by nothing more serious than fatigue or tension.

Some types of headaches are not symptoms of underlying disorders but are considered specific diseases. One of these is a cluster headache. In a cluster headache, the pain is generally severe, developing around or behind one eye, and having abrupt onset and cessation. The affected eye may tear. Cluster headaches usually occur at night, continue occurring for several weeks or months, and then disappear for some time. They may also be more common in a specific season or time of the year. Another example of a severe type of headache is migraine (see the Migraine section).

Patient Screening

Patients complaining of intractable head pain require prompt assessment. An appointment should be scheduled as soon as possible. If a same-day appointment is not possible and the patient needs to be seen sooner, the patient should be referred to an emergency treatment facility.

Etiology

Many factors, either alone or in combination, can irritate the pain-sensitive tissues or structures in the head and produce headaches. Examples are stress; too little or too much sleep; overeating or overdrinking; a stuffy or noisy environment; and heavy physical labor, either indoors or outdoors. Some affected individuals may also be suffering from caffeine withdrawal or sensitivity to scents. From a physiologic standpoint, however, there are only two causes of headaches. The first cause is a strain on the facial, neck, and scalp muscles resulting from tension. The headache that results is called a *tension headache*. The second cause is edema within the blood vessels of the head, which results in a change in arterial size. The headache that results is called a *vascular headache*.

Diagnosis

The medical history is vitally important in identifying a pattern of headaches and is helpful in detecting any underlying causes. Physical examination and neurologic testing are necessary if a recurring pattern of headaches is revealed. Cranial and spinal radiography, EEG, CT, and MRI may be ordered to rule out organic causes.

Treatment

The cause of the headache determines the type of treatment chosen. If the physician does not find an underlying cause of the headache, analgesics (e.g., aspirin, acetaminophen, and NSAIDs), muscle relaxants, minor tranquilizers, muscle massages, and relaxation with a warm bath are effective in providing temporary relief from headache. Lying in a dark room may help with headaches if the light seems to make the headache worse.

Prognosis

The prognosis for the typical headache is good. The prognosis for intractable head pain varies, depending on the cause. Drug therapy often helps relieve the pain. Stress reduction and relaxation techniques may lead to a positive outcome.

Prevention

Prevention involves avoiding known or suspected trigger factors. A diary kept by the patient may uncover triggers that should be avoided if a pattern is identified.

Patient Teaching

Provide patients with information on relaxation techniques and stress reduction. Use customized electronically generated educational materials or digital tools to reinforce the treatment plan.

Migraine

Description

Periodic severe headaches that may be completely incapacitating and almost always are accompanied by other symptoms, such as nausea and vomiting, sensitivity to light and sound, anorexia, intense hemicranial or bilateral throbbing pain, and visual signs and symptoms (or auras), are known as *migraine headaches*.

> ICD-10-CM Code — G43.909 (Migraine, unspecified, not intractable, without status migrainous) (G43.001–G43.919 = 40 codes of specificity)
>
> *Refer to the current edition of the ICD-10-CM coding manual for the most specific code.*

Symptoms and Signs

Patients who experience migraine headaches complain of intense throbbing pain. The pain may be on one or both sides of the head and nausea and vomiting may occur. Light and noise may make the headache worse. Before the onset of headaches, many persons who experience migraine headaches have visual **auras**: flashing lights, zigzagging lines, or areas of total darkness. Photophobia is another warning sign. The nature of each attack varies from person to person, but usually, there is a warning period during which the person feels abnormally fatigued and notices a mood change, fluid retention, neck stiffness, constipation, increased urination, and food cravings. Other less common symptoms that occur occasionally are numbness or tingling in one arm or on one side of the body, dizziness, and temporary mental confusion.

These headaches may begin in adolescence or early adulthood and cause pain so severe the individual cannot go to school or work.

Patient Screening

Patients known to experience migraine headaches and those reporting typical migraine headache symptoms require prompt treatment. If a patient who has never been diagnosed with migraine complains of the onset of severe headache, the patient should be referred to an emergency treatment facility to rule out other causes of extreme head pain.

Etiology

Recent research studies have confirmed that migraine headaches do occur in families and there is a genetic link. There are also times when a person suffers from migraine headaches, and no one else in the family is known to have migraines. A combination of factors appears to be involved in many cases. In some cases, certain foods (e.g., aged cheese, chocolate, and red wine) have been found to induce an attack.

The biological cause of migraines may be changes in cerebral blood flow, which is presumably attributable to vasoconstriction followed by vasodilation of the cerebral and cranial arteries.

Research continues to learn more about a rarer form of migraine and familial tendency. Familial hemiplegic migraines cause the symptom of weakness or hemiplegia on one side before the onset or during the headache. It has been discovered that there are three genes definitely involved in this familial occurrence.

Diagnosis

A medical history of recurring, severe headaches, preceded by any combination of the aforementioned symptoms or signs, suggests the diagnosis. EEG, CT, and MRI may be ordered to rule out any organic conditions.

Treatment

In some cases, the treatment is simply bed rest in a quiet, darkened room and the use of analgesics at the first sign of attack. Migraine treatment is multifaceted and may include many different drug classes. Triptans (sumatriptan, zolmitriptan, eletriptan, naratriptan, and frovatriptan) are often utilized in the initial therapy regimen. For other patients, drug therapy in the form of vasoconstrictors to constrict dilated blood vessels is effective in relieving pain. Antiemetics to control vomiting may be needed. Relaxation therapy or biofeedback has been used successfully to lessen the frequency of migraines in some patients. Calcitonin gene–related peptide inhibitors are the newest class of migraine medications to be approved by the US Food and Drug Administration (FDA). These medications are used to reduce migraine frequency and are indicated for patients who experience four or more migraine days per month. Currently, three of these drugs are available: erenumab (Aimovig), galcanezumab (Emgality), and fremanezumab (Ajovy).

Prevention

Patients should be advised to avoid the "trigger" factors, if possible. The value of implementing drug therapy and relaxation techniques at the first sign of a headache should be stressed. If additional drug therapy is required for pain relief, it should be employed as soon as possible. The prognosis is usually favorable when the patient complies with drug therapy and the instruction to rest.

Patient Teaching

Provide patients with information on stress reduction. Advise them on the importance of taking preventive medications on a regular basis if indicated. Tracking headache onset and duration, as well as other information regarding headaches, can help the provider narrowing down triggers.

Epilepsy

Description

Epilepsy, a seizure disorder, is a chronic brain disorder characterized by sudden episodes of abnormal, intense electrical activity in the brain, which results in seizure activity.

| ICD-10-CM Code | G40.901 (*Epilepsy, unspecified, not intractable, with status epilepticus*) G40.909 (*Epilepsy, unspecified, not intractable, without status epilepticus*) (G40.301–G40.919 = 21 codes of specificity) |

Epilepsy is coded according to type. Both fourth and fifth digits are required. Once the diagnosis has been confirmed, refer to the current edition of the ICD-10-CM coding manual for the appropriate code.

Symptoms and Signs

Epilepsy has many forms and a variety of manifestations; greater than 30 types of seizures are known, and it is possible for a person to have more than one type. Seizures are now classified into three types: generalized onset, focal onset, and unknown onset. The classification is determined by the onset or beginning of a seizure, a person's level of consciousness or awareness during the seizure, and whether there is movement or no movement during the seizure.

Generalized onset seizures can affect both sides of the brain at one time and are further identified as absence, tonic, atonic, clonic, myoclonic, and tonic-clonic.

Absence seizures, previously called petit mal epilepsy or petit mal seizures, consist of a brief change in the level of consciousness indicated by staring, blinking, or blankly staring with a loss of awareness of surroundings. The episodes last only a few seconds and can occur many times a day (hundreds), if not treated. Absence seizures occur most often in children and young adults.

Tonic seizures cause a person's muscles to become stiff. The patient may become unconscious and fall to the ground during this type of seizure. In contrast, atonic seizures, which may be referred to as *drop seizures*, cause the muscles to become lax, weak, or the individual will have no muscle control.

Clonic seizures are identified by jerking of the muscles which occur in repetition. The arms, face and neck are typically affected and the movements are on each side of the body. Myoclonic seizures may not cause an individual to become unconscious, however twitching or jerks in the legs and arms can be observed.

Tonic-clonic seizures, historically referred to as *grand mal seizures* may begin with a loud cry, followed by falling to the ground and loss of consciousness. Prolonged contraction of the respiratory muscles causes the patient to become cyanotic. Generalized rhythmic muscle spasms occur, followed by relaxation. The patient may be incontinent of urine and/or feces. The seizure subsides in 1 to 2 minutes, but consciousness may be regained slowly. The person may be drowsy, confused, and weak; report a headache; and have no memory of the event afterward.

Focal onset seizures are those which are described as not involving the entire brain but arising from a localized area in the brain. They can be divided further into focal onset "aware" seizure or focal onset "impaired awareness" depending on whether or not the person who has the seizure is aware of what is taking place, or awake versus not having awareness or being confused about what happened or is going on during the seizure. Muscle twitching or other symptoms may be observed with focal onset seizures.

The other classification is u*nknown* onset seizures. This classification is used when there is limited information about the seizure, or the symptoms experienced because no one actually witnesses what took place. This occurs when someone lives independently or a seizure occurs during the night. Once more is known about the seizure activity, it may be then classified as generalized onset or focal onset. In all three classifications, generalized, focal, and unknown onset, the seizures can be either motor or nonmotor.

While most people will come out of a seizure quickly, status epilepticus can occur with a seizure. This happens when one seizure follows another with no recovery of consciousness between attacks. This is considered a medical emergency that requires immediate anticonvulsant therapy to prevent cerebral anoxia, hyperpyrexia, vascular collapse, and even death.

Patient Screening

Patients experiencing any form of seizure activity need immediate assessment and intervention.

Etiology

In some patients, no apparent cause for the abnormal electrical discharge in the brain is found. It has been identified though, that there is a greater incidence in some families with genetic changes in some individuals with epilepsy.

Epilepsy or seizures can also result from an abnormality in the brain resulting from a pathologic process, genetic or acquired, that seems to trigger seizures. Pathologic conditions associated with seizure disorder include scar tissue on the cerebral cortex from infection or head trauma, cortical neoplasms, cerebral edema, TIAs, and CVAs (strokes). Other possible causes are birth trauma (cerebral palsy), drug toxicity (e.g., alcohol), diabetes, hypoglycemia, and other conditions that deprive the brain of oxygen.

Diagnosis

Not all seizures imply epilepsy; thus a medical history is essential for determining the diagnosis. EEG shows semi-specific brain activity, suggesting epilepsy; MRI also may be helpful. Classification of epilepsy is based on the location of the abnormal activity and its duration. CT shows structural changes in the brain, such as tumors, scars, and malformations. Cerebral angiography may identify vascular changes in the brain. Skull radiography may reveal evidence of fracture, separation of cranial sutures, or movement of

the pineal gland. Blood serum chemistry changes may indicate metabolic disease, drug toxicity, or hypoglycemia.

Treatment

Anticonvulsant medications are the treatment of choice for epilepsy. Commonly used medications include phenytoin, carbamazepine, valproic acid, divalproex, levetiracetam, gabapentin, topiramate, and oxcarbazepine. Close monitoring and adjustments of dosage to attain effective therapeutic control are essential. Patients are instructed to adhere to their medication schedules and take their medications as directed.

Side effects from anticonvulsants can vary, and patients should be instructed to review concerns with their prescribers. Other procedures include vagus nerve stimulation, DBS, responsive neurostimulation.

In rare cases, surgical intervention may be necessary to excise an identified lesion in the brain. MRI-guided stereotactic laser ablation may be used to help symptoms when surgery cannot be performed due to risk. Some children with epilepsy follow a ketogenic diet. Researchers believe the change in diet results in chemical changes in the brain that reduce seizures. The diet should be fully discussed with the physician.

Prognosis

The prognosis varies. Drug therapy often can control seizure activity. Status epilepticus is a life-threatening event. Immediate intervention may afford a positive outcome.

Prevention

Prevention of the initial onset of seizure activity is impossible. Compliance with drug therapy has a positive effect in preventing seizures once they are diagnosed.

Patient Teaching

Because this disease often is feared and misunderstood, education is necessary to dispel myths. Talk about first aid instructions that are available and can teach family members how to care for the patient in the event of grand mal seizures (Fig. 13.17). Emphasize abiding by state law restrictions regarding driving a motor vehicle if seizure activity is not in control. For example, in Alabama, one must be seizure-free for 6 months to drive a motor vehicle. Additionally, stress the importance of drug therapy compliance, and having laboratory levels drawn as instructed by the physician to ensure medication levels are in therapeutic range if indicated.

Parkinson Disease
Description

Parkinson disease is a common, slowly progressive neurologic disorder characterized by the onset of recognizable disturbances: "pill-rolling" tremor of the thumb and forefinger, muscular rigidity, slowness of movement, and postural instability.

| ICD-10-CM Code | G20 (Parkinson disease) |

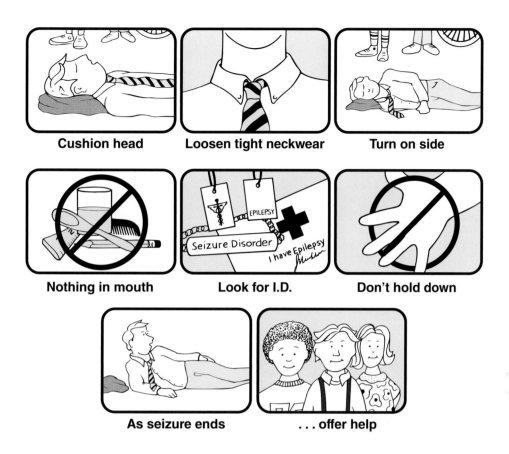

Cushion head **Loosen tight neckwear** **Turn on side**

Nothing in mouth **Look for I.D.** **Don't hold down**

As seizure ends **. . . offer help**

Most seizures in people with epilepsy are not medical emergencies. They end after a minute or two without harm and usually do not require a trip to the emergency room.

But sometimes there are good reasons to call for emergency help. A seizure in someone who does not have epilepsy could be a sign of serious illness.

Other reasons to call an ambulance include:
- A seizure that lasts more than 5 minutes
- No "epilepsy" or "seizure disorder" I.D.
- Slow recovery, a second seizure, or difficulty breathing afterward
- Pregnancy or other medical I.D.
- Any signs of injury or sickness

• **Fig. 13.17** First aid for seizures. *I.D.*, Identification. (Courtesy Epilepsy Foundation, www.epilepsy.com.)

Symptoms and Signs

Usually insidious in onset, Parkinson disease symptoms, which vary from person to person, may be associated with aging until the recognizable paradigm of Parkinson disease emerges. A primary symptom is tremors or trembling in hands, arms, jaws, face, and legs. Additionally there is rigidity or stiffness of limbs and trunk, causing a stooped posture. The patient moves slowly, with a peculiar shuffling gait: the head is bowed, the body is flexed forward, the knees are slightly bent, and the patient tends to fall as a result of impaired balance and coordination (Fig. 13.18). The face takes on a masklike or expressionless appearance, speech is muffled, and swallowing is difficult. Gradual changes in behavior and mental activity are noted in some patients as

the disease progresses. The mean age at onset is 60 years, but approximately 5% to 10% of cases appear in people who are less than 50 years old. Parkinson disease afflicts males twice as much as it affects females but sometimes females are not diagnosed as quickly as male patients.

Patient Screening

Because of the insidious onset of Parkinson disease, patients and family members may contact the office for an appointment because of the vague neurologic symptoms. The next available appointment should be scheduled for these individuals. Those already identified as having the disease will have appointments scheduled for routine follow-up care.

• **Fig. 13.18** Typical shuffling gait and posture of patients with Parkinson disease.

• **Fig. 13.19** Degenerative diseases of the brain involve preferentially various parts of the brain. Alzheimer disease causes atrophy of the frontal and occipital cortical gyri. Huntington disease affects the frontal cortex and basil ganglia. Parkinson disease is marked by changes in the substantia nigra. Amyotrophic lateral sclerosis affects the motor neurons in the anterior horn of the spinal cord, the brainstem, and the frontal cortex of the brain. (From Damjanov I: *Pathology for the health-related professions*, ed 4, St. Louis, 2011, Saunders/Elsevier.)

Etiology

What causes the degeneration of nerves in the motor system of the brainstem is not known. A combination of exposure to toxins, genetics, and environmental influences may all be factors contributing to Parkinson disease. The substantia nigra is the area of the brain where dopamine, a neurotransmitter is produced. A deficiency of dopamine has been clinically demonstrated in patients with Parkinson disease. Parkinsonism (as a syndrome) also can occur after ingestion of poison, after encephalitis, and after taking certain major tranquilizers and certain antihypertensive drugs. Degenerative diseases of the brain involve preferentially various parts of the brain (Fig. 13.19). Although Parkinson disease is a neurodegenerative brain disorder that progresses slowly in most people, the term *parkinsonism* refers to a group of neurologic disorders that cause movement problems, such as tremors, slow movement, and stiffness, similar to those seen in Parkinson disease.

Diagnosis

The diagnosis is based on the characteristic history and a careful neurologic examination. Decreased dopamine levels may be noted.

Treatment

Because Parkinson disease has such a wide variety of symptoms, treatment is individualized for each patient. Parkinson disease cannot be cured; therefore medical management consists of supportive measures and control of symptoms with the use of drugs. Carbidopa-levodopa, dopamine agonists such as pramipexole and ropinirole, and MAO B inhibitors such as selegiline and rasagiline are among the most prescribed medications. Physical therapy helps the patient maximize mobility within the limitations of the disease. The patient is given every possible supportive measure to encourage independence and self-care.

A treatment called *deep brain stimulation (DBS)* has been approved by the FDA. Electrodes are implanted into the brain and connected to a small pulse generator, which can reduce the need for levodopa and decrease involuntary movements (dyskinesias). The pulse generator is carefully programmed externally to lessen the symptoms.

Prognosis and Prevention

At the present time, no cure for Parkinson disease is known. There is ongoing research to find a cure. No method of preventing Parkinson disease is known.

Patient Teaching

Assist the patient and family in locating and contacting available community resources and medical resources. Encourage family members to be supportive of the therapy prescribed to help the patient remain independent as long as possible.

Huntington Chorea

Description

Huntington chorea (Huntington disease) is a hereditary degenerative disease of the cerebral cortex and basal ganglia, resulting in progressive atrophy of the brain.

ICD-10-CM Code   G10 *(Huntington disease)*

Symptoms and Signs

The chronic, progressive chorea (ceaseless, uncontrolled, involuntary movements) has an insidious onset, with loss of musculoskeletal control exhibited by subtle, semipurposeful movements that may be described as "dance-like" movements. Typically, the arms and the face are the first areas to be involved, with movements ranging from mild fidgeting to tongue-smacking. An individual may also have a fixed posture caused by involuntary muscle contraction called dystonia instead of chorea. Difficulty swallowing may occur. Speech difficulties are experienced, and the emotional state deteriorates, and dementia occurs eventually. Disruption of personality is displayed by the untidy and careless appearance of the individual. Personality changes noted are described as apathetic, moody behavior; loss of memory; and onset of paranoia. The onset of symptoms typically begins in early middle age.

Patient Screening

The insidious onset of Huntington chorea results in vague symptoms; therefore the condition may be found by chance during a routine visit. Because it is a familial-type disease, patients with a family history of the disease may be aware of the progression of symptoms and request an appointment. Although not considered an emergency, the occurrence of symptoms can create high levels of anxiety in patients, so the next available appointment should be scheduled for this patient.

Etiology

Although the exact etiology of this condition is uncertain, it is transmitted by an autosomal dominant trait that can be inherited by either sex. The HTT gene provides instructions for making a protein called huntingtin. There is a DNA sequence identified as the CAG (cytosine, adenine, guanine) trinucleotide repeat. People with Huntington disease have 36 to over 120 more repeats of CAG on the HTT gene. This is significant when compared to those individuals without Huntington disease which have the normal 10 to 36 repeats of CAG on the HTT gene.

Diagnosis

No definitive method of diagnosis is known, except by careful neurologic appraisal and by detection of the defective gene through deoxyribonucleic acid (DNA) analysis. A history of progressive chorea and dementia, along with a familial trait for the disease, leads to further investigation. MRI and CT demonstrate brain atrophy.

Treatment

No cure for this progressively deteriorating condition is known; therefore treatment is supportive, symptomatic, and protective. Haloperidol (Haldol) may be prescribed in an attempt to control choreic movements and to reduce agitation. Tetrabenazine may also used to treat the symptoms of chorea. Selective serotonin reuptake inhibitor antidepressants, benzodiazepines, and atypical antipsychotic medications are used to treat the psychiatric symptoms of the disease. Some authors have advocated using physical therapy, occupational therapy, speech therapy, and psychosocial support.

Prognosis

At the present time, no cure for Huntington chorea is known. Drug therapy may help control agitated behavior. Individuals are known to live 10 to 30 years after diagnosis. Those diagnosed with juvenile Huntington disease live on average, 10 years after diagnosis.

Prevention

Because this is an inherited familial-type disorder, there are limited options to prevent this condition. Couples can choose to have genetic counseling prior to becoming pregnant. Some couples may choose in vitro fertilization and preimplantation genetic diagnosis. This will determine if an embryo has the gene for Huntington disease prior to implantation.

Patient Teaching

Provide the patient and the family with accurate information about the disease, its symptoms and progression in order for them to plan for the future.

Amyotrophic Lateral Sclerosis

Description

Amyotrophic lateral sclerosis (ALS), also known as *Lou Gehrig disease*, is a progressive, destructive motor neuron disease that results in muscular atrophy.

ICD-10-CM Code	G12.21 *(Amyotrophic lateral sclerosis)* (G12.20–G12.29 = 4 codes of specificity)

Symptoms and Signs

Fasciculations (small local involuntary muscular contractions) and accompanying atrophy and weakness are noted in the forearms and hands. This condition progresses to cause difficulties in speech, chewing, swallowing, and breathing; eventually, a ventilator is required. No sensory neuron involvement is noted, and functioning of the mind is not affected. The average age range for diagnosis of ALS is between the ages of 40 and 70; however, there are cases where diagnosis may be confirmed after age 20.

Patient Screening

Patients complaining of weakness and involuntary muscular contractions of the hands and arms should be assessed promptly. Anyone complaining of difficulty breathing and swallowing requires immediate assessment and should be transferred to the EMS for immediate treatment and transport to an emergency facility.

Etiology

Research indicates approximately 10% of people have a gene known to be linked to ALS. The other 90% of cases are not linked to family history or genetic mutation.

Diagnosis

Clinical findings, including upper and lower motor neuron involvement without any sensory neuron involvement, will lead to further investigation. EMG, nerve conduction study (NCS), MRI, blood and urine tests, spinal tap, nerve and muscle biopsy are methods used to confirm nerve, not muscle, involvement. The tests performed can rule out other causes for similar symptoms before a final diagnosis is determined which may take several months.

Treatment

There is no cure for ALS. Supportive measures and physical, occupational, and speech therapy directed at controlling symptoms and increasing quality of life are used in conjunction with approved medications. Recent drug therapies such as riluzole (Rilutek), edaravone (Radicava) and sodium phenylbutyrate/taurursodiol (Relyvrio) have shown promise in slowing the progression of the disease and extending life. Other drug therapy includes tizanidine and baclofen, which are muscle relaxants that help relieve muscle spasticity. Other medications are used to reduce fatigue, spasticity, pain, sleep difficulties, and excess salivation. Pulmonary management is vital. As breathing becomes more difficult the patient may use mechanical ventilation to assist as muscles become weaker.

Prognosis

No cure for ALS is known, and death usually occurs within 6 to 10 years after diagnosis.

Prevention

No method of prevention is known, however there is a 50% chance that children born to someone with the genetic form of ALS will inherit the gene. Risk factors are smoking, environmental toxins, and having served as a veteran. The reason those who have served in the military are at higher risk is not fully understood but is believed to be from some type of exposure to chemicals, toxins, viral infections, or trauma that took place during their service years.

Patient Teaching

Provide the patient and the family with information about the disease. Assist them in locating and contacting community resources.

Restless Legs Syndrome

Description

Restless legs syndrome (RLS) is a neurologic condition characterized by an overwhelming urge to move the legs. This irresistible urge to move the legs or body part is to stop an uncomfortable or odd sensation.

| ICD-10-CM Code | G25.81 *(Restless legs syndrome)* |

Symptoms and Signs

RLS is characterized by a group of symptoms that cause the individual to move the legs. There are feelings that often are described as itching, burning, jittery, creepy-crawly, pulling, tugging, and/or painful sensations in the legs. Occasionally the sensations may be felt in the arms, hips, or face. The awareness of the sensations may be intermittent, or it may occur on a daily basis. The inability to sit for extended periods often interferes with normal activities of life. These symptoms usually occur at night; during the day, they usually occur after long periods of sitting. Walking or moving the legs often relieves the symptoms. Many patients with RLS also experience periodic limb movement disorder during sleep.

Patient Screening

Patients requesting an appointment for difficulty and pain in the legs while sitting still may be experiencing RLS. They may also complain of unusual feelings in the legs that are relieved by standing and moving. Schedule an appointment as soon as convenient for both the patient and the physician. Request that the patient keep a daily record of symptoms, noting when they occur and what helps provide relief.

Etiology

The exact cause of RLS is unknown. The incidence of RLS appears to increase after middle age. Nerve damage from diabetes, underlying conditions of the kidney and sleep disorders, alcoholism, medications and pregnancy may play a part in the disorder. Stressful events may precipitate the onset of symptoms.

Diagnosis

Medical history and physical examination are useful in making the diagnosis. Symptoms occur most frequently in the evening or at night while the individual is relaxed or sleeping. Movement of the legs provides only temporary relief. A daily diary of symptoms noting when they occur and what helps provide relief is helpful in diagnosis.

Blood tests may show low blood iron levels. Secondary causes, including iron deficiency, varicose veins, folate and magnesium deficiencies, sleep apnea, uremia, diabetes, peripheral neuropathy, Parkinson disease, thyroid disease, and certain autoimmune disorders, need to be identified. Some drugs also may cause the symptoms.

Treatment

There is no cure for this condition. Treatment involves identifying and managing the underlying cause of the disorder. Drug therapy, including levodopa, dopamine agonists, and ropinirole may help alleviate or lessen some symptoms. Regular exercise, including leg stretching and massage along with application of heat, may provide relief. Cold application may be an alternative for some individuals.

Prognosis

Although there is no cure for this lifelong disorder, it is possible that symptoms may worsen as the individual ages. Therapies currently available may provide control and minimize symptoms. Some patients may experience periodic remissions of symptoms.

Patient Teaching

Encourage patients to be compliant with recommended medications and exercises. Provide information concerning possible side effects of medications, and instruct patients to report any side effects as soon as possible.

Transient Global Amnesia

Description

Transient global amnesia, although frightening and anxiety-provoking, usually is a benign event. As the name implies, the event is transient or temporary, with a duration of 1 to 6 (maybe even up to 12) hours. It is global in nature because it encompasses the entire memory of current events. The amnesia manifests as a total loss of recent memory; the learning process is completely blocked. Memory disturbances are involved.

| ICD-10-CM Code | G45.4 (Transient global amnesia) |

Symptoms and Signs

The individual experiencing the onset of transient global amnesia has a sudden onset of memory loss, primarily of both current and recent events. Repetitive asking of such questions as "Where are we going?" "Why are we going there?" "Where am I?" and "Why did we do that?" is typical. Confusion is apparent; nevertheless, the individual has recall of personal identity and orientation to place if the place is a normal environment. Memory loss may encompass the preceding 3 to 5 years and specific events. Usual tasks, including those requiring mechanical abilities, often are performed without difficulty. Neurologic signs are normal; no numbness, tingling, or weakness (unilateral or total) is noted; PERLA (pupils are equal and react to light and accommodation) and vocalization are normal. Communication skills concerning current events and status are affected by the amnesic event, which begins and ends abruptly. Memory usually returns within less than 24 hours. This also may be true of events that occurred a few hours to a few days before the amnesic event. Some patients complain of headaches.

Patient Screening

If the office schedule allows, the patient should be seen as soon as possible. This permits observation of the symptoms and helps reduce anxiety in both the patient and the family. Neurologic signs need to be observed, evaluated, and recorded. If an immediate appointment is not possible, the patient should be referred to an emergency facility for prompt observation and to rule out TIA and CVA.

Etiology

The etiology is unknown; however, evidence points to the precursors, such as experiencing stress or emotional events, swimming or immersion in cold or hot water, driving a motor vehicle, or having sexual intercourse. The individual may have experienced migraine headaches on previous occasions, usually without nausea, vomiting, or photosensitivity.

◆ ENRICHMENT

Chiari Malformation

Chiari malformation is diagnosed when the brain tissue is pressed down into the spinal cord. This is caused by an abnormally shaped or smaller-than-normal skull. The skull puts pressure on the brain and displaces it into the spinal cord. Chiari malformation is classified as type I, II, or III, depending on the severity of displacement of the brain. Type I involves the smallest amount of brain tissue in the spinal cord. Type II involves more brain tissue displacement than type I. Type III is congenital and is the rarest of the three types. A portion of the brainstem or cerebellum extends out from the skull through an abnormal opening. Type III has the worst outcome, with a high rate of death. It should also be noted that type II is also seen in the myelomeningocele form of spina bifida. Typically severe headache, which occurs after a person sneezes, coughs, or strains, is one main symptom. Lack of fine skill coordination, difficulty balancing, neck pain, tingling of feet and hands, numbness, dizziness, difficulty swallowing, and other neurologic symptoms may be experienced.

Diagnosis

Diagnosis is made by observing the symptoms and signs and obtaining a negative result on a neurologic examination. TIA, CVA, and seizure activity are to be ruled out first.

Prognosis

The prognosis is good; recurrence is very unlikely. The individual probably will never regain memory of the events that occurred during the episode or during the hours or days immediately preceding the episode.

Treatment

Treatment is supportive; the patient is given reassurance during and after the episode.

Prevention

No method of prevention is known. All patients are encouraged to reduce stress factors in their lives. Those with a history of migraine headaches and individuals over the age of 50 are at higher risk.

Patient Teaching

Reassurance should be given to the patient and family that this event is transient in nature and likely will not occur again. Instructions should be given to the family or caregiver to return if symptoms do recur.

Peripheral Nerve Disorders

Peripheral Neuritis/Neuropathy

Description

Peripheral neuritis/neuropathy is the degeneration of the peripheral nerves. Based on symptoms and prognosis, it is divided into four categories: motor, sensory, autonomic, and combination. The term encompasses many different disorders resulting from peripheral nerve damage.

> ICD-10-CM Code G60.9 *(Hereditary and idiopathic neuropathy, unspecified)*
> (G60.0–G60.9 = 6 codes of specificity)

Symptoms and Signs

Peripheral neuritis/neuropathy is the degeneration of peripheral nerves and affects the distal muscles of the extremities. Numbness, tingling, weakness, burning, pins and needles sensation, and loss of sensation in the hands and feet can be experienced. These symptoms can also be followed by flaccid paralysis and wasting of muscles in these areas. Deep tendon reflexes become diminished, and tenderness is noted in the atrophied muscles. The skin may take on a glossy, red appearance, and sweating is decreased. With leg and foot involvement, foot drop may be experienced. Some patients have pain in the affected regions. Diabetic neuropathy is one of the most common types of neuropathy.

Patient Screening

Patients reporting symptoms should be promptly assessed. Schedule an immediate appointment, according to office policy.

Etiology

Chronic alcohol intoxication; toxicity from arsenic, lead, carbon disulfide, benzene, or phosphorus; infectious diseases, including mumps, pneumonia, and diphtheria; metabolic or inflammatory disorders, including diabetes, rheumatoid arthritis, gout, and systemic lupus erythematosus; and certain nutritional deficiency diseases are all causative factors. The nerve degeneration leads to muscle weakness and sensory loss.

Diagnosis

The history, combined with the clinical findings characteristic of motor and sensory involvement, leads to additional investigation. Neurological testing to check for skin sensation, muscle strength, deep vibratory sensation and deep tendon reflex may be performed. Motor and sensory nerve impairment is usually detected by EMG and a NCS.

Treatment

The first step in effective treatment is to ascertain the cause and, if possible, to correct or eliminate the condition. Toxic substances need to be removed, if possible, and vitamin and nutritional deficits corrected. Underlying disease processes, especially diabetes, are treated or controlled. When chronic alcoholism is the cause, the patient must avoid all alcohol in any form. Supportive measures, such as administration of anticonvulsants and tricyclic antidepressants and getting rest and physical therapy, are employed to relieve pain.

Prognosis

Control of underlying causes may provide relief of symptoms. Proper nutrition is helpful and supports nerve health.

Prevention

Prevention is difficult when the etiology is a preceding disease process or exposure to toxic substances. Avoidance of alcohol may help prevent the recurrence of neuritis.

Patient Teaching

Encourage patients to be compliant with drug and physical therapy as prescribed.

Trigeminal Neuralgia (Tic Douloureux)

Description

Trigeminal neuralgia, or tic douloureux, is pain in the area innervated by the cranial nerve V (CN V), the trigeminal nerve.

> ICD-10-CM Code G50.0 *(Trigeminal neuralgia)*
> (G50.0–G50.9 = 4 codes of specificity)

Symptoms and Signs

The transient, excruciating pain of trigeminal neuralgia radiates along the distribution of the CN V and can affect any of the three CN V branches, although it usually affects the second and third branches (Fig. 13.20). When the ophthalmic branch is affected, pain is experienced in the eye and the forehead. The maxillary branch involves the nose, upper lip, and cheek. The mandibular branch involves the lower lip, the outer portion of the tongue, and the area of the cheek close to the ear. Additionally, more than one branch may be involved. The pain is always unilateral and does not cross the midline because only one side of the face is involved. The sudden onset of pain is triggered by mechanical or thermal stimulation. An affected person sleeps poorly and may

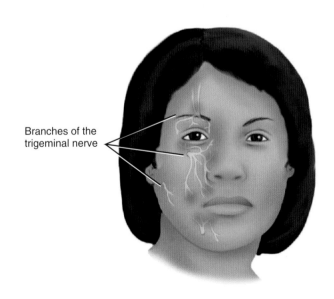

Branches of the trigeminal nerve

• **Fig. 13.20** Trigeminal nerve (cranial nerve V) and branches. (From Shiland B: *Mastering healthcare terminology*, ed 5, St. Louis, 2015, Elsevier.)

be undernourished and dehydrated because chewing, swallowing, or any touching of the area may set off the pain.

Patient Screening

The pain of trigeminal neuralgia is so severe that affected individuals require immediate pain relief. When an immediate appointment is not available, the patient should be referred to an emergency facility for assessment and treatment with medications for pain relief.

Etiology

There are various causes of trigeminal neuralgia, one of which is a compressed blood vessel. Trigeminal neuralgia may result from multiple sclerosis or another condition where the myelin sheath is impaired. A tumor or brain lesion can also press on the nerve and cause this pain. Stroke, injuries, or facial trauma can also cause trigeminal neuralgia. Some people may experience trigeminal neuralgia due to a brain lesion or other abnormalities. In other cases, surgical injuries, stroke, or facial trauma may be responsible for trigeminal neuralgia.

Diagnosis

The reports of excruciating pain that has an abrupt onset and duration of seconds to minutes on one side of the face suggest trigeminal neuralgia. Observation of the patient, both during an attack and at normal times, demonstrates the presence of pain. The patient avoids touching the face to prevent triggering an attack. MRI is useful in diagnosis determination.

The face should be protected and temperature extremes avoided. The episodes may last from months to years and then subside. Infection of a sinus or a tooth and tumors must be ruled out.

Treatment

Analgesics are prescribed for pain. Some authors have reported that many patients respond well to carbamazepine. Current drug therapy includes the use of anticonvulsant drugs to control the pain. Side effects may include dizziness, nausea, double vision, and sleepiness. The addition of muscle relaxants may be more effective; however, side effects include depression, confusion, and severe drowsiness. Botox injections have been administered to small numbers of patients who had little relief from traditional medications.

When relief cannot be obtained, surgical intervention to dissect the nerve roots is performed. Patients who smoke are advised to cease smoking.

Prognosis

The prognosis varies, depending on the underlying causative factors. Some cases resolve spontaneously, and some others may respond to drug therapy. Surgical intervention such as microvascular decompression, brain stereotactic radiosurgery and rhizotomy are also treatments which may afford pain relief, however there are side effects which may result in facial numbness in some cases where the affected nerve is compromised as a result. Pain may also return after some

procedures. Acupuncture and other alternative treatments have been successful in helping some patients but there is limited research on these treatments and how well they work.

Prevention

No method of prevention is known. Individuals are encouraged to avoid activities that trigger their pain.

Patient Teaching

Provide information about the condition and methods of treatment available as applicable.

Bell Palsy

Description

Bell palsy is a disorder of the facial nerve (CN VII) that causes a sudden onset of weakness or paralysis of facial muscles.

ICD-10-CM Code	G51.0 *(Bell palsy)*

Symptoms and Signs

The severity of paralysis in Bell palsy varies widely. The patient may be aware of pain or a drawing sensation behind the ear, followed by an inability to open or close the eye, drooping of the mouth, and drooling of saliva. Often the disorder is first noticed in the morning, having developed overnight. Initially the patient is unable to smile, whistle, or grimace, and the facial expression is distorted (Fig. 13.21).

Taste perception may be diminished, contributing to loss of appetite. The condition is usually unilateral. It may be transient or permanent and usually occurs between ages 15 and 60 years, in all sexes.

Patient Screening

The individual reporting sudden onset of one-sided facial paralysis requires prompt assessment to rule out a CVA. Referral is usually to an emergency facility for diagnosis.

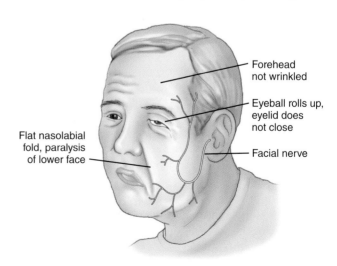

• **Fig. 13.21** Bell palsy. (From Shiland B: *Mastering healthcare terminology*, ed 5, St. Louis, 2015, Elsevier.)

The next available appointment should be scheduled to discuss the condition after a confirmed diagnosis.

Etiology

The cause of Bell palsy is not always certain. The symptoms result from blockage of impulses from the facial nerve (CN VII) caused by compression of the nerve in the bony canal. Bilateral facial paralysis has been noted in a small percentage of people with Lyme disease. EMG to determine the extent of the nerve involvement

Blood tests to determine if another condition such as diabetes or Lyme disease is present.

MRI or CT to determine if there is a structural cause for your symptoms.

Diagnosis

Bell palsy is diagnosed from symptoms, signs, and characteristic history. Laboratory blood testing, EMG to determine nerve involvement and MRI may be performed to rule out other conditions such as CVA and tumor.

Treatment

Early treatment is critical. The application of warm moist heat, gentle massage, and facial exercises to stimulate muscle tone is recommended. Prednisone may be prescribed to reduce inflammation of the facial nerve. Antiviral medications may be prescribed. Analgesics also may be required. The inability to close the eye may result in dry, sore eyes; artificial tears and an eye patch for protection from outside elements may be needed unless symptoms are mild. Electrotherapy stimulates the nerve and prevents atrophy of muscles.

Prognosis

Complete recovery is possible if the disease is treated early, and recovery often occurs spontaneously, especially in younger individuals. Nevertheless, residual effects may remain for an undetermined period.

Prevention

No method of prevention is known.

Patient Teaching

Provide information about the condition to the patient and the family. Patients should follow the recommended treatment plan.

Infectious Disorders

Meningitis

Description

Meningitis is inflammation of the meninges, the membranous coverings of the brain and spinal cord.

ICD-10-CM Code	G03.9 *(Meningitis, unspecified)* (G03.0–G03.9 = 5 codes of specificity)

Meningitis is coded according to cause or type. Once the diagnosis has confirmed the cause and type, refer to the current edition of the ICD-10-CM coding manual for the appropriate code.

Symptoms and Signs

Early symptoms of meningitis include vomiting and a headache that increases in intensity with movement or shaking of the head. Attempts of the examiner to move the head reveal nuchal rigidity, which is stiffness of the neck with resistance to any sideways or flexion-extension movements of the head; this is a classic sign. Positive *Kernig sign* (resistance to leg extension after flexing the thigh on the body) and *Brudzinski sign* (neck flexion causing flexion of the hips from the supine position) indicate meningeal irritation. Deep tendon reflexes increase, and the patient exhibits irritability, photophobia, and hypersensitivity of the skin. Seizures caused by cortical irritation can be late manifestations of the process. Drowsiness may progress to stupor and coma. Infants may have a bulge in the soft spot, be irritable, continually cry, have a high temperature, be inactive and their body and neck may be stiff.

Patient Screening

Early symptoms of meningitis are easily overlooked and may not appear severe enough to demand immediate assessment at first. As the symptoms and signs increase in nature, prompt assessment and intervention are necessary. The patient should be referred to an emergency facility without delay.

Etiology

Meningitis can be either bacterial or viral. The infection can originate directly from the brain, spinal cord, or sinuses. Some cases result after ear infections, skull fractures, or, rarely, after surgery. Open-head injuries are additional portals of entry for the offending bacteria. *Haemophilus influenzae, Neisseria meningitidis, Streptococcus pneumonia,* and *Listeria monocytogenes* are the bacteria responsible for most meningeal infections; however, the causative microorganism can be either bacterial or viral (Fig. 13.22). Fungi or parasites can also cause meningitis but these are not common causes. Drug allergies, inflammatory diseases, some cancers, and chemical reactions have also been identified as causing meningitis.

Diagnosis

The clinical findings alert the physician to the possibility of meningitis. Diagnostic lumbar puncture reveals increased CSF pressure and the presence of white blood cells (WBCs), protein, and low glucose in CSF. A culture of CSF showing the growth of microbes confirms the diagnosis. CSF may appear cloudy because of the presence of WBCs. Blood tests and CT scan of brain also help in determining diagnosis.

Treatment

Bacterial meningitis is treated aggressively with intravenous (IV) antibiotic therapy. Anticonvulsive drugs are

• **Fig. 13.22** Bacterial meningitis. The surface of the brain is covered with pus. (From Kumar V, Cotran RS, Robbins SL: *Robbins basic pathology*, ed 7, Philadelphia, 2003, Saunders.)

administered to control seizure activity. Glucocorticoids (dexamethasone, prednisone, and methylprednisolone) may be administered to reduce cerebral inflammation and edema. Aspirin, an NSAID, or acetaminophen is given for the headache. External stimuli are kept to a minimum and the room dark and quiet. Severe viral meningitis may also be treated with hydration IVs, oxygen, and steroids.

Prognosis

The prognosis is unpredictable and depends on the source of the infection and the patient's response to drug therapy. Bacterial meningitis, if untreated, has a high mortality rate.

Prevention

Vaccinations are recommended for Preteens and Teenagers to prevent meningitis. Certain populations at high risk for meningitis are also included in the category of those who can benefit from the protection of vaccination. Vaccinations approved and available in the United States are meningococcal conjugate (MenACWY) and serogroup B meningococcal (MenB). Individuals who have had contact with people known to have meningitis of often prescribed prophylactic antibiotics. Good handwashing techniques are always helpful in preventing the spread of any bacterial or viral infection.

Patient Teaching

Stress the importance of completing a prescribed regimen of antibiotics. Discuss isolation guidelines, if recommended to prevent transmission to other individuals.

Encephalitis

Description

Encephalitis is inflammation of the brain tissue.

ICD-10-CM Code   G04.90 *(Encephalitis and encephalomyelitis, unspecified)*
G04.91 *(Myelitis, unspecified)*
(G04.00–G04.01; G04.81–G04.91 = 6 codes of specificity)

Once the diagnosis has confirmed the cause and type, refer to the current edition of the ICD-10-CM coding manual for the appropriate code.

Symptoms and Signs

Encephalitis, an inflammation of the brain tissue, may have an insidious or sudden onset. Primary symptoms include headache and an elevated temperature. The patient experiences stiffness of the neck and back, muscular weakness, restlessness, visual disturbances, confusion, disorientation, and, in some cases, coma.

Patient Screening

Symptoms of stiffness in the neck and back, muscle weakness, accompanied by headache, fever, restlessness, visual disturbances, and lethargy indicate referral to an emergency facility is needed.

Etiology

Inflammation leads to cerebral edema and subsequent cell destruction. It is caused by viruses or toxins from chickenpox, measles, or mumps. Most cases are the result of a bite from an infected mosquito or tick. In rare cases, encephalitis is caused by a parasite, fungus, or bacteria.

Diagnosis

The clinical findings lead the physician to further investigation, including a lumbar puncture; blood and CSF studies reveal the presence of the virus. EEG and MRI are performed to evaluate the brain and rule out other pathology. Body scans using MRI, ultrasound, CT, and CT-PET (positron emission tomography) can rule out tumors that lead to autoimmune encephalitis. Brain biopsy may also be used in rare cases where the patient is declining and not responding to treatment.

Treatment

Antiviral agents such as ganciclovir, acyclovir, and foscarnet are used in treating encephalitis but these medications are not effective in all viral encephalitis cases. Autoimmune encephalitis is treated with IV or oral corticosteroids, plasma exchange, and IV immunoglobulin. Otherwise, treatment is symptomatic, with mild analgesics for pain, bed rest, antipyretic drugs for elevated temperature, anticonvulsants for seizure activity, and antibiotics for any intercurrent infection.

Prognosis

The prognosis is unpredictable and depends on the type of infection and response to drug therapy. Most viral forms run their course. Residual damage to the brain tissue may result.

Prevention

Prevention is difficult. Avoiding environments heavily populated by mosquitoes may prevent the bites. Use of mosquito spray and wearing long-sleeved shirts and long pants may prevent bites. Vaccination when traveling to areas known to have cases of encephalitis and good handwashing are recommended. Preventing mosquito breeding sites by eliminating standing water helps control the mosquito population. Community boards of health monitor the mosquito population and those of other vectors, such as birds that carry the West Nile virus.

Patient Teaching

Prevention is important. Stress the use of mosquito repellant when in an outdoor environment. Encourage patients and their families to be aware of encephalitis outbreaks in the community. Generate print-on-demand electronic materials, when possible, as teaching tools.

Guillain-Barré Syndrome

Description

Guillain-Barré syndrome is an acute, rapidly progressive disease of the PNS.

ICD-10-CM Code   G61.0 *(Guillain-Barré syndrome)*

Symptoms and Signs

The individual with Guillain-Barré syndrome experiences numbness and tingling of the feet and hands at the onset of the disease, followed by increasing muscle pain and tenderness. Progressive muscle weakness and paralysis usually start in the lower extremities and move up the body in 24 to 72 hours. Although most patients experience ascending paralysis, occasionally some patients experience descending weakness and paralysis. Respiratory insufficiency is possible, as is difficulty swallowing.

Patient Screening

Individuals reporting numbness and tingling of the feet and hands, followed by increasing muscle pain and tenderness and subsequent progressive muscle weakness and paralysis, need immediate assessment and intervention. The patient should be referred to an emergency facility for prompt care.

Etiology

Knowledge of the etiology is limited, but the syndrome is thought to have an autoimmune basis. The condition has been known to follow an infection with a virus or bacteria. Demyelination of nerves occurs with the syndrome.

Diagnosis

Confirmation is made by the finding of an elevated protein level in CSF, however the leukocyte count is normal.

Treatment

Hospitalization usually is required for observation. Treatment is supportive. Plasmapheresis washes plasma to remove antibodies, thereby shortening the time required for recovery. IV human immune globulin (IVIG) may be beneficial.

Prognosis

The prognosis varies, but recovery is usually complete.

Prevention

No method of prevention is known.

Patient Teaching

Encourage patients to keep follow-up appointments as scheduled. Explain the progression of the syndrome and the treatments available.

Brain Abscess

Description

A brain abscess, a collection of pus, can occur anywhere in the brain tissue (Fig. 13.23).

ICD-10-CM   G06.0 *(Intracranial abscess and*
Code   *granuloma)*

Symptoms and Signs

The primary symptom of a brain abscess is headache. Other symptoms and signs depend on the location and extent of the abscess. Generally, the patient exhibits symptoms and signs of increased intracranial pressure, including nausea and vomiting, visual disturbances, unequal pupil size, confusion, weakness on one side, changes in personality, and seizures. Many times, the eyes look toward the area of insult, that is, toward the side of the head where the abscess is located. *Nuchal rigidity* (stiffness of neck with resistance to moving head side to side or up and down) may be noted.

Patient Screening

Individuals who complain of an unusual headache and other symptoms listed above should be given an appointment as

• **Fig. 13.23** Brain abscess.

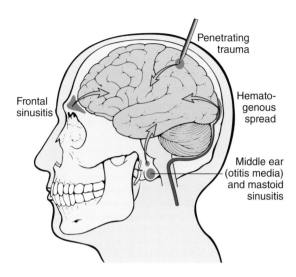

• **Fig. 13.24** Bacterial infections of the central nervous system. Infectious organisms may reach the brain through several routes: hematogenously; by direct entry because of penetrating trauma; or by direct spread from adjacent structures, such as the inner ear or the nasal sinuses. (From Damjanov I: *Pathology for the health-related professions*, ed 4, St. Louis, 2011, Saunders/Elsevier.)

soon as possible. When reports of one-sided weakness, nausea, vomiting, visual disturbances, stiff neck, unequal pupil size, and seizures are relayed, the disease has progressed to a stage that requires prompt assessment and intervention. The patient should be referred to an emergency facility or advise the individual or the family to call 911 and enter the individual into the EMS system.

Etiology
CNS abscesses may be the result of a local infection or may be secondary to infections elsewhere in the body. Any occurrence that breaches the integrity of the CNS, including head trauma and a craniotomy wound, may be the portal of entry for the microorganisms. The abscess may be secondary to another infectious process, such as sinusitis, otitis, dental abscess, subdural empyema, and bacterial endocarditis (Fig. 13.24).

Diagnosis
A history of infection, especially of the sinuses or the ear, or an insult to the CNS, coupled with the characteristic clinical features of increased intracranial pressure, suggests an abscess. EEG and CT are used to verify the diagnosis. Lumbar puncture is contraindicated because the resulting increase in intracranial pressure may cause the brainstem to herniate, resulting in death. Blood cultures may also be ordered.

Treatment
IV antibiotics are administered to resolve the infection. Mannitol or steroids are prescribed to reduce cerebral edema. Surgical drainage of the abscess may be necessary to relieve intracranial pressure and to culture the offending organism. Additional treatment is supportive.

Prognosis
The prognosis varies, depending on the location, size, and causative agent of the abscess. Underlying pathology and the health status of the patient also affect the recovery process. Earlier treatment provides the best outcome.

Prevention
Prompt treatment of infections helps in prevention.

Patient Teaching
Encourage prompt reporting of infectious processes involving the head so that treatment can resolve these potential sources of the abscess in a timely manner.

Enrichment

Poliomyelitis and Postpolio Syndrome
Poliomyelitis, a viral infection of the anterior horn cells of the gray matter of the spinal cord, causes selective destruction of the motor neurons. This highly contagious disease is no longer the threat to humankind that it was before the 1960s. The Salk and Sabin vaccines have virtually eliminated poliomyelitis in the Western world, making its occurrence rare.

Administration of the polio vaccines has helped to significantly reduce the incidence of polio. The World Health Organization's goal is to eradicate polio throughout the world with immunization. Three distinct serotypes of poliovirus exist: types 1, 2, and 3. Types 2 and 3 have been eradicated with type 1 still existent in two countries. Persons with immunosuppressive conditions should not be given the trivalent vaccine because they are at risk of contracting poliomyelitis. Additionally, any immunosuppressed person should not come in contact with the feces or nasal secretions of a recently vaccinated person. Two poliovirus vaccines currently are licensed in the United States: inactivated poliovirus vaccine and oral poliovirus vaccine.

Intracranial Tumors (Brain Tumors)

Description
Brain tumors can be primary tumors, neoplasms that originate in the brain itself, or secondary tumors, cancers that have metastasized from another area of the body, such as the lung, liver, kidney, or skin. Primary tumors can arise from any cell within the CNS (Fig. 13.25). They are named according to the tissues from which they originate.

ICD-10-CM Code	D49.6 (*Neoplasm of unspecified behavior of brain*)

Symptoms and Signs
Regardless of the tumor cell type, symptoms and signs result from displacement and compression of normal brain tissue by the tumor, causing progressive neurologic deficits, expansion of the brain (cerebral edema), and increased

• **Fig. 13.25** Brain tumor.

• **Fig. 13.26** Increased intracranial pressure and possible herniations. (From Gould BE, Dyer RM: *Pathophysiology for the health professions*, ed 4, St. Louis, 2012, Saunders/Elsevier.)

intracranial pressure, leading to possible herniation (Fig. 13.26). Common symptoms include headache (usually dull, constant, and worse at night); focal or generalized seizures (common in gliomas and secondary tumors); nausea and vomiting; syncope; cognitive dysfunction (including memory problems and personality changes); muscle weakness; sensory loss; aphasia; and visual dysfunction. The classic symptoms of cerebellar tumors (e.g., medulloblastoma) often are gait disturbance, nystagmus, lethargy, dysarthric speech pattern, and balance difficulty. Glioblastoma causes such symptoms as seizures, nausea, vomiting, and headache. This type of tumor is very aggressive and difficult to treat.

Patient Screening

Symptoms of early brain tumors are somewhat vague. Individuals complaining of constant headaches with increasing severity and worsening at night require prompt assessment. Reports of seizures, loss of consciousness, and reduced cognitive functioning also require prompt assessment, and the patient should be referred to an emergency facility.

Etiology

Primary brain tumors are classified histologically according to the predominant cell type: Gliomas, tumors derived from glial cells; meningiomas, tumors arising from the arachnoid membrane; and embryonal tumors, neoplasms that arise in children. Together they account for the majority of all cancerous primary brain tumors in the population. The most common type of malignant brain tumor is glioblastoma.

Diagnosis

The evaluation of a patient with a suspected brain tumor includes a detailed history, a neurologic examination, and diagnostic neuroimaging studies. Neurologic examination findings are associated with particular regions affected by the destruction of neural tissue. Cranial MRI is the diagnostic imaging modality of choice. Functional MRI, which measures blood flow through regions of the brain during various activities, or PET can be helpful in preoperative planning. Tissue obtained during surgery or through stereotactic biopsy is necessary for correct histologic diagnosis of the tumor type. Only tumor grade and histologic classification are considered definitive factors to determine the malignant potential of the tumor.

Although brain tumors can be malignant or benign, the distinction is blurred. Unlike benign neoplasms in other locations of the body, benign brain tumors may cause the same symptoms as malignant tumors, such that distinguishing between the benign and malignant types on clinical grounds can be very difficult. Even a benign tumor with little to no metastatic potential can be lethal if it occurs in a region of the brain that precludes full surgical resection.

Treatment

Benign and malignant neoplasms are often treated similarly. Patients with primary brain tumors must be treated for their symptoms and for the neoplasm. Symptomatic treatment includes the use of anticonvulsants to treat seizures and corticosteroids to decrease intracranial pressure. Surgery is the initial treatment for most tumors, providing tissue samples for definitive diagnosis and relieving symptoms by reducing tumor size. Surgery is usually followed by radiotherapy and/or chemotherapy, depending on the tumor type and stage. Staging of most brain tumors uses the modified TNM (tumor-node-metastasis) system. Immunotherapy has been successful in treating some cancers but has not been proven effective for glioblastoma.

Treatment of secondary brain tumors focuses on relief of neurologic symptoms and long-term tumor control.

Treatment choice is based on the location, size, and number of metastases; the patient's age; the patient's neurologic status; and the extent of systemic cancer. In general, patients with solitary brain lesions and no metastases at other sites are candidates for treatment with surgery and whole-brain radiation therapy. Although the patient may still be affected by extracranial disease, this treatment improves quality of life and reduces the likelihood of death resulting from neurologic causes. Patients with multiple or recurrent metastases are often treated with surgery or radiation with palliative intent.

Prognosis

The overall 5-year survival rate for all types of brain tumors combined varies, depending on the type of tumor and the age and sex of the patient. Poor prognostic indicators include a high tumor grade, the presence of mental changes at the time of diagnosis, large tumor size, and the inability to fully resect the tumor during surgery. Despite continued research to successfully treat glioblastoma, the 5-year survival rate is only 6.9%.

Prevention

No methods are known to prevent intracranial neoplasms.

Patient Teaching

Assist the patient and the family members in locating and contacting available community resources. Discuss the neurocognitive functional deficits resulting from insults to the brain and the delayed growth and learning disabilities that may occur in children. Encourage compliance with any prescribed drug or physical therapy. Use customized electronically generated educational materials, when available, to reinforce the treatment plan.

Review Challenge

Answer the following questions:

1. What is the central nervous system composed of? The peripheral nervous system?
2. What are some possible causes of diseases of the nervous system?
3. How is the nervous system evaluated during a diagnostic examination?
4. What are the three vascular disorders that may result in a cerebrovascular accident (CVA)?
5. How does a transient ischemic attack differ from a CVA?
6. What are some of the likely causes of epidural and subdural hematomas? Which condition is more likely to have a delayed onset of symptoms?
7. Which condition is more serious, cerebral concussion or cerebral contusion? Why?
8. What is the relationship between the location of a spinal cord injury and the signs and symptoms?
9. Which diagnostic findings may indicate degeneration or rupture of an intervertebral disk?
10. How does spinal stenosis contribute to sciatic pain?
11. Are headaches always a symptom of an underlying disease? What are some causative factors of cephalalgia?
12. What are the classic signs and symptoms of migraine?
13. What are the different types of epileptic seizures? What are the first aid guidelines?
14. What are the characteristic signs and symptoms of (1) Parkinson disease, (2) Huntington chorea, and (3) amyotrophic lateral sclerosis?
15. What are the suggested causes of and treatment interventions for transient global amnesia?
16. What are some causative factors of peripheral neuritis?
17. How does a patient with trigeminal neuralgia typically describe the pain?
18. What is the clinical appearance of a person with Bell palsy?
19. What is the diagnostic significance of nuchal rigidity in the presence of headache and photophobia?
20. What are the possible etiologic agents of encephalitis?
21. What is the pathologic progression of Guillain-Barré syndrome?
22. How do infectious organisms reach the brain? How is a brain abscess treated?
23. How are intracranial tumors classified, and what determines the symptomatology?
24. What is the 5-year survival rate for brain tumors identified as gliomas?

Real-Life Challenge: Epilepsy

A 26-year-old male had been (2 weeks earlier) in an MVA and had suffered a closed-head injury. Recovery was uneventful, and the patient was discharged from the hospital. The patient returned to work 2 days ago. The patient's wife called the office to state that she had awakened this morning to find her husband having a seizure. The patient was responsive but appeared confused.

The patient was transported to a hospital. Vital signs were temperature, 98.4°F; pulse, 72 beats per minute; respirations, 18 breaths per minute; and blood pressure, 116/78 mm Hg. The patient was responsive but not oriented to time, place, or person and appeared postictal. EEG was ordered, as was cerebral CT. The patient was diagnosed with seizure activity (epilepsy) secondary to the cerebral trauma suffered in the MVA. The patient was placed on antiseizure medication and admitted for observation.

Questions

1. What patient or family teaching regarding patient activity is indicated?
2. What is the significance of cerebral trauma to the onset of seizure activity?
3. What type of epilepsy is this seizure activity classified as?
4. Compare the three types of epilepsy with regard to seizure activity, treatment, and predisposing factors.
5. Which other diagnostic tests might be ordered?
6. Describe appropriate first aid intervention for a patient with grand mal seizure.
7. Explain status epilepticus.

Real-Life Challenge: Transient Ischemic Attack

The wife of a 67-year-old male called the office and reported that her husband awoke this morning with weakness and numbness on the right side. He had difficulty getting out of bed and complained of intermittent episodes of dizziness. He also was experiencing difficulty speaking. The patient had a history of hypertension and was taking enalapril (Vasotec) and propranolol (Inderal). The wife was advised that her husband should be seen in an emergency care facility, and an ambulance was called for transport.

On examination in the emergency facility, the patient was found to have diminished strength in the right hand and foot, diminished movement in the right arm and leg, and slurred speech. Vital signs were temperature, 98.6°F; pulse, 106 beats per minute and irregular; respirations, 22 breaths per minute; and blood pressure, 172/96 mm Hg. Oxygen therapy was started. Reflexes were diminished, as was pain response on the right side, including the extremities.

Cerebral MRI, CT, EEG, skull radiography, and ECG were ordered. ECG showed atrial fibrillation. Approximately 6 hours after onset, the symptoms began to resolve, with improvement seen in feeling and movement of the right extremities. Speech slowly became less slurred. The patient was diagnosed as having a transient ischemic attack (TIA), and an appointment was scheduled for follow-up evaluation. He was started on anticoagulant therapy.

Questions

1. What is the importance of the right-side involvement and slurring of speech?
2. Why would ambulance transportation to an emergency facility be recommended?
3. What is the significance of the elevated blood pressure?
4. Explain the differences between a TIA and a CVA.
5. In what area of the brain would the diminished circulation and subsequent reduced oxygenation be anticipated?
6. Why would anticoagulant therapy be prescribed?
7. Research the importance of the ECG results indicating atrial fibrillation.

Internet Assignments

1. Go to the National Spinal Cord Injury Association to research advances in the treatment of spinal cord injuries.
2. Go to the National Parkinson's Foundation to research the latest developments in treatment interventions for Parkinson disease.
3. Research the diagnostic tests used by neurosurgeons at the American Association of Neurological Surgeons. What other procedures are used to treat head trauma and CVAs?

Critical Thinking

1. According to the Glasgow coma scale in Fig. 13.1, what would you consider a severe coma?
2. According to the figure shown in the Neurologic Assessment Enrichment box at the beginning of the chapter, what test is used to evaluate ocular movement?
3. Undetected cerebral bleeding and refusal of treatment often have what kind of outcome?
4. Identify some of the incidents where individuals may have a sudden onset of life-threatening occurrences.
5. A 74-year-old male has been diagnosed with a CVA. Although his speech is not affected, he has trouble with the use of nouns in sentences. Most of the time, he is able to groom and feed himself. He has difficulty making decisions and following complex commands. What would you recommend that his wife, the caretaker, do about obtaining help in his care? What kind of home health care might be available?
6. A 17-year-old male recently was involved in a motorcycle crash. He was not wearing a helmet and sustained a head injury and fractured lumbar vertebrae. As a result, he is a paraplegic and is unable to move his legs and control elimination. What type of care will this young male require? How will this affect his education? How

will his family find assistance for care and for financial needs?

7. A 78-year-old female has been diagnosed with Parkinson disease. She does not exhibit the usual symptoms of hand tremors with "pill-rolling" activity. Her mental status has been compromised, and she requires constant watching for her instability and her inability to perform activities of daily living. Her husband is her caretaker. What type of teaching will you provide to assist the family in the care of the patient? What can they expect in the future?

8. A 50-year-old female has been diagnosed with peripheral neuropathy. What kind of teaching would you provide to encourage her to get her diabetes under control? How would you assist her with dietary management? What resources would you encourage her to seek to get assistance?

9. What type of patient teaching would you provide to parents about the importance of childhood immunizations?

Prepare to discuss Critical Thinking case study exercises for this chapter that are posted on Evolve.

Credentialing Examination Questions

1. Which organs or structures are located in the CNS division of the nervous system?
   A. Brain
   B. Spinal nerves
   C. Spinal cord
   D. Brain and spinal cord

2. Which organs or structures are located in the PNS division of the nervous system?
   A. Brain
   B. Spinal nerves
   C. Spinal cord
   D. Brain and spinal cord

3. A patient experiences a cerebrovascular accident. Which side of the body will be affected?
   A. Same side as the cerebral insult
   B. Opposite side of the body
   C. Both sides if the stroke is a temporal stroke
   D. It depends on how quickly the patient receives medical intervention

4. Which arrhythmia is known to cause patients to be at a higher risk for stroke?
   A. Ventricular bradycardia
   B. Atrial bradycardia
   C. Atrial fibrillation
   D. Premature ventricular contraction

5. A "bubble test" can help diagnose which anomaly?
   A. Epilepsy
   B. Transichemic attack
   C. Brain tumor
   D. Patent foramen ovale

6. Which events may lead to a traumatic brain injury?
   A. Motor vehicle accident
   B. Fall
   C. Contact sports
   D. All of the above

7. Which condition occurs when the patient has a loss of nerve function at the cervical region resulting in paralysis of the arms, hands, trunk, and legs?
   A. Quadriplegia
   B. Paraplegia
   C. Hemiplegia
   D. Cardioplegia

8. Which type of seizure causes the patient to have short periods of staring or unconsciousness while their eyes are still open?
   A. Absence
   B. Tonic
   C. Atonic
   D. Myoclonic

9. Which disease causes symptoms of "dance-like" movements?
   A. Parkinson
   B. Huntington
   C. Epilepsy
   D. Amyotrophic lateral sclerosis

10. Which 5-year survival rate is most accurate for glioblastoma?
    A. Over 50%
    B. Over 75%
    C. 25% to 70%
    D. Less than 25%

14

Mental Disorders

CHAPTER OUTLINE

LEARNING OBJECTIVES

After studying this chapter, you should be able to:

1. Name some contributing factors to mental disorders.
2. List some of the many causes of intellectual developmental disorder.
3. Describe the characteristic manifestations of pervasive development disorders, including autism.
4. List criteria for diagnosis of attention-deficit/hyperactivity disorder.
5. List some examples of tic disorders.
6. Describe the progressive degenerative changes in an individual with Alzheimer disease.
7. Explain important factors in the treatment of Alzheimer disease.
8. Explain the cause of vascular dementia.
9. Relate treatment options for alcohol abuse.
10. Name the classic signs and symptoms of schizophrenia. Explain what is included in the multidimensional treatment plan.
11. Explain why bipolar disorder is considered a major affective disorder. Describe the treatment approach.
12. Discuss normal grieving process phases.
13. Discuss how each type of anxiety disorder prevents a person from leading a normal life.
14. Explain how posttraumatic stress disorder differs from other anxiety disorders.
15. Explain how a somatization disorder is diagnosed.
16. Discuss the relationship between anxiety and conversion disorder.
17. Describe factitious syndrome.
18. Contrast insomnia to narcolepsy.
19. List and discuss personality disorders, including their distinguishing characteristics.
20. Discuss the predisposing factor(s) of PANDAS (pediatric autoimmune neuropsychiatric disorders associated with streptococcal infections) syndrome.
21. Discuss options for animal therapy.

KEY TERMS

affect (AF-feckt)
amyloid (AM-ih-loyd)
anhedonia (an-hee-DOH-nee-ah)
autism (AW-tism)
catatonic (kat-ah-TOH-nic)
circadian (sir-KAY-dee-an)
cognitive (KOG-nih-tive)
deficit (DEAF-ih-sit)
delusion (dee-LOO-zhun)

endarterectomy (end-ar-ter-EK-toh-me)
hallucination (ha-loo-sih-NAY-shun)
hypoxia (hi-POX-ee-ah)
ischemia (is-KEY-me-ah)
mutism (MYOO-tizm)
narcissistic (nar-sis-SIST-ik)
paranoid (PAR-ah-noid)
psychotic (sigh-KOT-ik)
schizoid (SKIZ-oyd)

Mental Wellness and Mental Illness

At some time in life, almost everyone is affected by mental disorders, either personally or by the involvement of a family member or friend. Stress is considered a contributing factor that causes exacerbation of mental disorders. Other factors are hereditary or congenital, accidental, traumatic, psychosocial, socioeconomic, or related to drug toxicity. Chemical imbalances in the brain and its neurotransmitters also are factors. The specific causes of mental illness remain unclear in many cases. Power and control, along with bullying, contribute to many forms of mental illnesses.

Mental illness has been linked to the patient's inability to cope with stress imposed by modern society. Pressures imposed by life circumstances can be a source of personal pain and distress. The definition of mental wellness, or being in a good state of mental health, varies and is a relative state of mind. When healthy people have the capacity to cope and adjust in a reasonable manner to the ongoing stresses of everyday life, they are considered to be in a state of equilibrium, known as *mental wellness.*

Psychological pain is real, is intense, and can affect physical health. Subsequently, impaired or pathologic coping skills emerge in people's behavior. Some coping behaviors are conscious, and some are not easily controlled because they are unconscious. Certain disorders in thinking, perceiving, and behaving can be organized into clusters of signs and symptoms. These clusters become diagnostic criteria and a part of a total physical and psychological evaluation.

The American Psychiatric Association's *Diagnostic and Statistical Manual of Mental Disorders, Fifth Edition, Text Revision* (DSM-5-TR) was updated in 2022 and is the accepted reference that offers guidelines for criteria to be used in the clinical setting when diagnosing a mental disorder. In addition to diagnostic criteria, the DSM-5-TR gives the practitioner a standardized diagnostic code, similar to the *International Classification of Diseases,* tenth revisions, Clinical Modification (ICD-10-CM) coding systems.

Mental disorders include those of congenital and hereditary origins. Other categories, such as maladaptive disorders, phobias, anxiety, depression, addiction, and psychotic disorders, have uncertain or unknown causes and possibly more than one contributing factor. Psychosis, a symptom of a mental disorder, may be indicative of a severe mental disorder where the individual loses touch with reality. The individual may experience verbal or visual hallucinations, irrational thoughts, delusions, regressive behavior, and degeneration of personality.

Mental disorders cause mild to severe disruption in a person's ability to function in interpersonal relationships, self-care, and occupational settings. In some disorders, the person may experience incapacitating psychotic symptoms. The DSM-5-TR also includes substance use–related, eating, and sleep disorders. In some mental disorders, oxygen and nutrient deprivation with necrosis result in the death of brain cells; these are known as *organic disorders* and are permanent and cannot be reversed.

Modern therapeutic approaches include control of symptoms with psychotropic drugs, including antipsychotic drugs, antidepressants, anxiolytics (antianxiety agents), central nervous system (CNS) stimulants, and mood stabilizing medications. Hospitalization is necessary in some treatment cases and outpatient treatment is available and preferred in many cases. Play therapy is included in counseling sessions for some children. Patients with mental illnesses and conditions need established routines and consistency in treatment and daily living activities.

Pet therapy and service animals are also used as options in the treatment of various disorders. As defined and explained by the US Department of Justice, Civil Rights Division *Disability Rights Section,* "Service animals are defined as dogs that are individually trained to do work or perform tasks for people with disabilities. Examples of such work or tasks include guiding people who are blind, alerting people who are deaf, pulling a wheelchair, alerting and protecting a person who is having a seizure, reminding a person with mental illness to take prescribed medications, calming a person with posttraumatic stress disorder (PTSD) during an anxiety attack, or performing other duties. Service animals

The Child, the Therapist, and Play Therapy

Play is a natural means of expression for a child and a way for children to learn and develop a variety of skills. Therapists working with children use play therapy in assessment and treatment interventions, assisting the child to cope with emotional stress and trauma. Children often cannot verbalize their thoughts and feelings, and play therapy becomes a nonverbal avenue for them to communicate with the therapist. Play therapy may be employed on a one-to-one basis or in a group setting. During play therapy sessions, the therapist establishes rapport with the child and encourages the child to act out any feelings of anxiety and tension he or she may be experiencing. The therapist's goals are to give the child an opportunity to reveal feelings that he or she cannot verbalize, to understand the child's interactions and relationships with the important people in his or her life, and to teach the child appropriate coping mechanisms and adaptive socialization skills.

Therapists may use objects and toys during play therapy. All kinds of dolls, doll houses, stuffed animals, puppets, soft balls and foam bats, toy vehicles, punching toys, a sand tray, and paper and markers or crayons may be used during play therapy. During these play sessions, family interactions and dynamics may become apparent. Children who have suffered abuse may use dolls and "mimic" what took place. Sand therapy may include small plastic animals or people and allows the child to act out feelings (Fig. 14.1).

• **Fig. 14.1** Play therapy sessions with children. (Courtesy David L. Frazier, 2003.)

are working animals, not pets. The work or task a dog has been trained to provide must be directly related to the person's disability. Dogs whose sole function is to provide comfort or emotional support do not qualify as service animals under the Americans with Disability Act (ADA)."

Service animals require intensive training to provide their handler with assistance for the specific disability. Emotional support and therapy animals provide support are important, just have a different role in that they do not perform "specific" tasks to assist with a disability.

Traumatic events, including mass shootings, can cause anxiety and fear in many members of society. Children are being taught in schools how to protect themselves with books and backpacks in the event of an active shooter in the room. Students and school personnel are trained in school lockdowns. Parents recognize school lockdowns as safety measures for their children. Numerous individuals have expressed apprehension about being in crowded places or at overcrowded events to the point of avoiding occasions where they might feel they are in danger. Mass shootings at schools, public events, churches, and even rural areas can cause fear. Schools for prekindergarten to 12th grade are hiring resource officers to provide security in case of such events. Bomb threats are another concern facing schools because each one must be taken seriously, even though at times they are hoaxes. The children, however, are still affected by this type of threat.

Intellectual Developmental Disorder

Description

Intellectual developmental disorder is not a disease but a wide range of conditions with many causes. A causative factor interferes with the developmental processes, resulting in changes in the acquisition of intellectual skills and adaptive functioning in a variety of areas, including social and interpersonal skills, self-care, communication, self-direction, health, and safety. In addition, the level of behavioral performance is reduced. General intellectual functioning is subaverage, and the individual has noticeable **deficits** in adaptive behavior. This condition is manifested during the developmental period and before the age of 18 years.

ICD-10- CM Code	F70 *(Mild intellectual disabilities)*
	F71 *(Moderate intellectual disabilities)*
	F72 *(Severe intellectual disabilities)*
	F73 *(Profound intellectual disabilities)*
	F79 *(Unspecified intellectual disabilities)*

Symptoms and Signs

Intellectual disability disorder is identified by impairments that have an impact on a person's adaptation or function in three domains of their life. These domains include practical, social, and conceptual. The conceptual domain includes skills in reading, writing, language, math, and reasoning, as well as memory and knowledge. The social domain includes interpersonal communication skills with others, being able to make friends and keep them, and an ability to exhibit empathy to others and use good social judgment. The practical domain includes being able to take care of oneself and use good hygiene, manage money, participate in life activities or recreation, and being able to organize tasks associated with school or work.

Patient Screening

Signs of intellectual developmental disorder may appear on well-baby examinations or during preschool routine checkups. The first significant indications of intellectual developmental disorder sometimes appear when the child begins school or preschool. An appointment should be made for the earliest possible date when schedules will allow sufficient time for the physician to conduct a thorough assessment.

Etiology

Intellectual developmental disorder has a variety of causes, many of which are unidentifiable. The predisposing factors include heredity (inborn errors of metabolism, genetic disorders, or chromosomal abnormalities); early alterations of embryonic development (Down syndrome or damage from toxins); prenatal, perinatal, or postnatal conditions (prematurity, hypoxia, viral infections, or trauma); general medical conditions (infections, trauma, or poisoning); and environmental influences. Hypoxic-ischemic encephalopathy is a type of brain damage that may result in developmental or neurological abnormalities if the oxygen supply to the brain is compromised. It can occur before or shortly after birth. Fetal alcohol syndrome also may result in intellectual developmental disorder. Pregnant females should be told that all alcohol ingestion during pregnancy is to be avoided.

Diagnosis

Diagnosis requires observation and confirmation of the intellectual capabilities and adaptive behavior of the child. The individual must have symptoms that begin during the developmental period, but there is not a specific age requirement for making a diagnosis.

Standardized testing of intelligence in the conceptual, social, and practical domains will help ensure the health care provider makes a decision on diagnosis determined by the functioning needed for everyday life.

Treatment

Brain cells die and cannot be restored however the child can be taught to perform tasks at various levels. Underlying causes should be treated and intervention may prevent or delay progression. The full treatment plan is based on the areas of deficit, once identified.

Prognosis

The prognosis varies, depending on identifiable etiology and adaptive skills.

Prevention

Preventing all intellectual developmental disorders might not be possible, but early and good prenatal care and nutrition are encouraged for all pregnant females to reduce the occurrence. Fetal monitoring during labor may alert the labor and delivery staff when the fetus is deprived of adequate oxygen. In such a case, immediate intervention is necessary. Prompt attention to head injuries in children may prevent the onset of intellectual developmental disorder during childhood. Genetic counseling may be desirable before pregnancy for parents with a family history of intellectual developmental disorder.

Patient Teaching

Parents require encouragement to recognize that there is no cure. Some individuals with intellectual developmental disorders may be educated or trainable. Routines and consistency are important in enabling the individual to function at the highest possible level. Provide parents and caregivers with resources related to the diagnosis.

Learning Disorders

Description

Learning disorders, sometimes referred to as *learning differences* or *specific learning disabilities*, are conditions that cause children to learn in a manner that is not normal. The medical community may use the term learning disorder, and the educational community may use the term specific learning disability. Performance on standardized tests is lower than expected for age, schooling, and intelligence level. The brain's ability to receive and process information is affected.

ICD-10-CM Code	F81.81 *(Disorder of written expression)*
	F81.89 *(Other developmental disorders of scholastic skills)*

Symptoms and Signs

A person with a learning disorder exhibits difficulty in acquiring a skill in a specific area of learning, such as reading, writing, or mathematics. This lower level of achievement occurs despite the child's normal (sometimes above-normal) intelligence and adequate schooling. Many of these individuals become school dropouts, have low self-esteem, and feel demoralized. They also may exhibit deficits in social skills. Individuals with learning disabilities may have problems listening or paying attention, reading or writing, speaking, and/or performing arithmetic problems. The disability is no indication of intelligence level.

Patient Screening

Most learning disorders are noted as the child begins the formal education process. A teacher may notice that the child is not learning at the standard pace, or family members may be concerned about a child's grades at school. At this time, the child is tested by the school system to evaluate for any discrepancy between ability and performance. The school system develops an individualized education plan for teachers to adhere to when providing instruction to the student. The parents or guardians are involved in the process, too; and if a learning disability is identified, the child receives reasonable accommodations to enable their to achieve the highest potential.

Etiology

The etiology of this condition is uncertain, but there may be underlying abnormalities in cognitive processing. Deficits in visual perception, language processes, attention, or memory may contribute to the problem.

Diagnosis

When the school, after intensive testing, notifies parents of their findings, the physician will establish that the child has met all the diagnostic criteria listed in the DSM-5-TR, and further evaluation may be performed. In addition to ruling out normal variations in academic attainment, the physician eliminates inadequate schooling, language barriers, lack of opportunity, and poor teaching as causes. Hearing and vision must be tested. Other mental disorders are ruled out.

Treatment

Some children who have learning disabilities also may be diagnosed with hyperactivity and therefore may respond to drug therapy, usually with stimulants. Other children may respond favorably to special instructional techniques such as tutoring (Fig. 14.2). Research continues on how to find effective treatments for different types of problems.

Prognosis

The prognosis varies, depending on the etiology and support from the family, school system, and community.

Prevention

There is no known prevention, but good prenatal care and close monitoring during labor and birth may prevent hypoxia.

• **Fig. 14.2** Tutoring session in progress. (Courtesy Mark Boswell, 2003.)

Patient Teaching

Parents are encouraged to seek out community and educational resources and support groups in the community.

Communication Disorders

Children often exhibit difficulties in communication. These disorders may be psychologically based and are listed in the DSM-5-TR. There are a variety of expressive language disorders, including mixed receptive or expressive language disorders.

Stuttering

Description

Stuttering, a phonological or communication disorder, is defined as frequent repetitions or prolongations of sounds or syllables. Stuttering is considered a speech disorder.

ICD-10-CM Code	F98.5 *(Adult onset fluency disorder)*

Symptoms and Signs

The frequent repetition or prolongation of sounds or syllables constitutes a disturbance of the pattern and fluency of speech, a disturbance that is inappropriate for the child's age. There may also be broken words, filled or unfilled pauses in speech, word substitutions, or word repetitions. The onset usually occurs between ages 2 and 6 years. When stuttering occurs suddenly in a teenager or an adult, a thorough physical examination should be performed to rule out neurologic causes.

Patient Screening

When a parent or caregiver calls for an appointment for a child who is stuttering, the next available regular appointment should be given.

Etiology

No single cause has been identified as causing a person to stutter. Genetic factors have been identified in individuals who stutter with familial instances where one member of the family stutters as do other members of a family. Also, people who stutter may have minuscule changes in the way their brain processes language and speech when compared to those who do not stutter.

Diagnosis

Observation of the speech pattern usually is all that is needed for the diagnosis. Hearing should be assessed to identify potential hearing issues which can also affect speech.

Treatment

Speech therapy with a speech-language pathologist helps in the treatment. The condition may resolve spontaneously. Eliminating stressful situations and lowering anxiety may be of benefit since these seem to make stuttering worse.

Prognosis

Although there is no cure for stuttering, the prognosis is good with intervention.

Prevention

No prevention is known.

Patient Teaching

Parents and caregivers should take the child to all recommended appointments as instructed and help the child practice speech exercises at home. They should also provide positive reinforcement and exhibit patience.

Pervasive Development Disorders

Children diagnosed with pervasive development disorders (PDDs) differ widely in abilities, intelligence, and behaviors. The principal characteristics of PDDs are severe impairments in several areas of development, including communication and social interaction skills. The disorders can include particular behaviors that cause the failure to develop peer relationships and interactions with others, including lack of nonverbal communication and lack of reciprocation of emotions. This impairment is related directly to the person's developmental level or mental age. A category of disorders is referred to as *autism* spectrum, encompassing the broad group of developmental delays and disorders having an effect on social communication skills and possibly, to a larger or smaller degree, motor and language skills. The disorders listed as pervasive development type disorders are as follows: autistic disorder; pervasive development disorder, not otherwise specified (PDD-NOS) including atypical autism; Rett disorder; childhood disintegrative disorder (CDD); and Asperger disorder. Specific criteria are used when diagnosing PDDs.

Autism Spectrum Disorder (Autism)
Description

Autism spectrum disorder (autism) is a syndrome in which individuals have deficits in communication including social communication and interaction.

ICD-10-CM Code   F84.0 *(Autistic disorder)*
Autism is coded by active or residual status. When the activity status of the autism has been determined by diagnosis, refer to the physician's diagnosis and then to the current edition of the ICD-10-CM coding manual to ensure the greatest specificity of pathology.

Symptoms and Signs

The DSM-5-TR criteria include symptoms of problems with social-emotional reciprocity, nonverbal communication and both developing and maintaining relationships. Failure to maintain eye contact with the parent or caregiver may be one of the earliest symptoms identified. The child fails to establish normal peer relationships and to seek shared enjoyment. Communication impairments include delayed or absent verbal communication, inability to initiate a conversation, and repetitive use of inappropriate language. The child does not initiate age-appropriate play activities. Repetitive motions are noted along with inflexibility toward change and a compulsion for sameness. These children may have a memory for certain lists or facts.

Patient Screening

The parent of the child with autistic behavior is often aware of problems that are developing, but they do not know exactly why their child seems "different" than children of the same age. Often this issue is discussed on regular well-child (toddler) visits. When the parents first become aware of a problem, an appointment should be scheduled as soon as possible for an extensive examination and history.

Etiology

The etiology is uncertain, with no single cause identified. It is believed to be caused by a combination of genetic and nongenetic factors. Studies show that there is a familial tendency. The occurrence is four times more common in males than in females. Studies show that there is no link between childhood immunizations and autism.

Diagnosis

There is no specific test to determine if a child has autism. Developmental screenings at well-baby checkups are helpful in determining if a child is at the same milestones in development as other children the same age. Caregivers provide information and physicians observe behavior of the child. Tests may be performed to rule out other causes of communication barriers and to eliminate potential physical problems that could cause these communication delays.

Treatment

Applied behavior analysis (ABA) is one method for treating autism. According to the CDC website accessed October 2023, "ABA encourages desired behaviors and discourages undesired behaviors to improve a variety of skills. Progress is tracked and measured. Medications such as risperidone and aripiprazole have been approved by the US Food and Drug Administration (FDA) to treat irritability and aggressive behavior. Other medications may also be used as part of a treatment plan. These medications have not been

Asperger Syndrome, Childhood Disintegrative Disorder, Rett Syndrome, and Pervasive Development Disorder, Not Otherwise Specified

Asperger Syndrome

Similar to children with autism, children with Asperger syndrome experience problems with social interaction and communication. Additionally, they usually have a narrow range of interests. Usually, children experiencing Asperger syndrome tend to have average or above-average intelligence. They also appear to develop normally in the spheres of language and cognition. Many times, those with Asperger syndrome may have difficulty concentrating and may experience poor coordination. Children with Asperger syndrome seem to adjust better as they get older.

Childhood Disintegrative Disorder

A rare condition, childhood disintegrative disorder (CDD) allows children to start developing normally in all areas, both physical and mental. Typically between ages 2 and 10 years, the child may lose many of the skills he or she has acquired. Additionally, the child tends to lose language and social skills and may lose control of body functions, including bowel and bladder control. The long period of normal development before regression helps differentiate CDD from Rett syndrome.

Rett Syndrome

A very rare disorder, Rett syndrome, causes the child to experience symptoms associated with a pervasive development disorder (PDD). Additionally, the child also experiences problems with physical development. The child who commonly suffers the loss of many motor or movement skills, including ambulation and use of hands, along with the development of poor coordination, is placed in this category. The condition, usually affecting only girls, appears to be associated with a defect on the X chromosome.

Pervasive Development Disorder, Not Otherwise Specified

The child who does not meet all of the criteria for autism or Asperger's but demonstrates several of the traits or symptoms is considered to have a pervasive developmental disorder, not otherwise specified (PDD-NOS).

As previously mentioned, similar to autistic disorder, there is no known cure for PDD. Drug therapy may be used as a symptomatic treatment for irritability, aggression, serious behavioral problems, obsessive-compulsive behavior, anxiety, depression, seizure activity, inattention, and hyperactivity. Behavioral therapy is beneficial but should be specialized to the child's needs. Specialized classrooms with a small class size and one-on-one instruction are sometimes helpful to certain children, whereas regular classroom education serves others.

FDA approved specifically for autism but may be utilized to manage symptoms. These medications include selective serotonin reuptake inhibitor (SSRI) antidepressants, anticonvulsants, and stimulants. SSRI antidepressants are believed to decrease repetitive thoughts and behaviors. Anticonvulsants may help treat impulsivity and decrease aggression. Stimulants are useful for the treatment of attention-deficit/hyperactivity disorder (ADHD), which is often a comorbid condition with autism spectrum disorders.

Prognosis

The prognosis depends on the severity of the disorder. Greater public awareness is being generated to support additional research to cure the disorder. Children can learn adaptive behaviors. Early intervention is essential to prognosis. Some children with autism have normal to gifted intelligence. They can attend college and seek jobs where they are most suited for their abilities and personal level of comfort, with the support of their employers and communities.

Prevention

No prevention for this disorder currently is known.

Patient Teaching

Encourage parents to investigate community and educational resources and to seek out support groups. Consistency in routine and following the provider's instructions in regard to responding to the child's behaviors in a positive way.

Attention-Deficit/Hyperactivity Disorder

Description

ADHD is a condition of persistent inattention leading to hyperactivity and impulsivity. ADHD is traditionally considered a hyperactivity issue, but many children and adults simply have difficulty maintaining attention and have no hyperactivity problems. Therefore ADHD has been classified into subtypes: ADHD, predominately inattentive type; ADHD, predominately hyperactive-impulsive type; and ADHD, combined type.

ICD-10-CM Code	
F90.0	(Attention-deficit/hyperactivity disorder, predominantly inattentive type)
F90.1	(Attention-deficit/hyperactivity disorder, predominantly hyperactive type)
F90.2	(Attention-deficit/hyperactivity disorder, combined type)
F90.8	(Attention-deficit/hyperactivity disorder, other type)
F90.9	(Attention-deficit/hyperactivity disorder, unspecified type)

Symptoms and Signs

Typical ADHD behavior can be observed at any age, but symptoms are usually present before 12 years of age. Failure to pay close attention to details; careless mistakes; messy work, and difficulty sustaining attention and completing tasks are manifestations of the condition. The child avoids activities that require sustained attention, effort, concentration, and organization. The inability to sit quietly without fidgeting or squirming, or even to remain seated, denotes hyperactivity. Inappropriate running and climbing, difficulty in playing, and excessive talking are other signs of the condition. The American Psychological Association has established criteria for each of these disorders.

Displays of impatience, difficulty waiting for one's turn, frequent interruptions, and failure to listen to directions are manifestations of impulsivity. When someone asks a question, the child with ADHD may blurt out the answer before the question is finished. The inability to organize activities and define goals creates difficulty in performing simple tasks, such as picking up toys. Sexual and relationship problems may occur as the child grows older.

Any aspect of this behavior may be displayed at home, school, work, or social occasions. The behavior seems to be exaggerated in group situations.

The three subtypes are listed as follows:
- ADHD, predominantly inattentive type: This subtype is used if six (or more) symptoms of inattention have persisted for at least 6 months but no impulsiveness or hyperactivity is observed in a child who is under 16 years old. Five symptoms can be used for diagnosing those over 16 years old.
- ADHD, predominantly hyperactive-impulsive type: This subtype should be used if six (or more) symptoms of hyperactivity-impulsivity have persisted for at least 6 months in a child under 16 years old. Five symptoms can be used for diagnosis if the child is over 16 years old.
- ADHD, combined type: This subtype should be used if a child has symptoms of inattention and hyperactivity-impulsivity, which have persisted for at least 6 months in both areas.

Patient Screening
Similar to learning disorders, most ADHDs are first noted as the child begins the formal education process. The next available appointment should be scheduled.

Etiology
The cause is uncertain, but research indicates there may be a genetic link or familial pattern. Researchers are also trying to learn more about risk factors as well as other potential causes of the disorder.

Diagnosis
The diagnosis is based on observation of behavior and an evaluation concluding that the inattention is not age appropriate. The behavior severely impairs functioning.

According to the DSM-5-TR criteria above, symptoms and behaviors have been included to illustrate the types of behaviors that children, older adolescents, and adults with ADHD might exhibit. The descriptions will help clinicians

better identify typical ADHD symptoms at each stage of the patients' lives. Medical providers may also rule out physical conditions that could cause an individual to display those behaviors or symptoms. A questionnaire may also be administered for those who are around the child to fill out.

Treatment
An effective treatment for some children is the use of stimulants, such as dextroamphetamine (Dexedrine), methylphenidate (Ritalin), and mixed salts of a single-entity amphetamine and dextroamphetamine product (Adderall). Among the most commonly used stimulant medications are extended-release methylphenidate (Concerta), extended-release amphetamine and dextroamphetamine salts (Adderall XR), and lisdexamfetamine (Vyvanse). An alternative to stimulant therapy is the noncontrolled agent atomoxetine (Strattera). Atomoxetine provides similar results to stimulant therapy without many of the unwanted side effects. Guanfacine is a nonstimulant medication that may be used as a supplemental therapy, along with stimulant medications.

Behavior therapy is also helpful for some children in learning to change impulsiveness and other symptoms. Any over-the-counter drugs or supplements should be discussed with the provider.

Prognosis
Prompt diagnosis with appropriate management via medication and behavior therapy if indicated, leads to an excellent prognosis. Compliance with the medication dosage and frequency, however, is imperative.

Prevention
ADHD is genetic and therefore has no prevention.

Patient Teaching
Effective discipline and consistent routines are most successful in managing the condition. In addition, when medical treatment calls for drug therapy to treat the disorder, compliance is imperative. For children, regular weight monitoring is essential, because many psychostimulants decrease appetite.

Oppositional Defiant Disorder

Description
Oppositional defiant disorder (ODD) is a behavior disorder in which children demonstrate behaviors that are oppositional toward adults. This is the most common referral complaint to counselors and a major source of family stress, as ODD behaviors occur hundreds of times per week. Comorbid conditions include ADHD (incidence increases with age), conduct disorder, PTSD, learning disabilities, school underperformance, poor social skills, dysthymia, and

major depression. ODD is a strong predictor of poor outcomes (i.e., school underachievement, poor peer relations, delinquency, major depression, early substance initiation and abuse, and school expulsion and dropout).

| ICD-10-CM Code | F91.3 *(Oppositional defiant disorder)* (F91.0–F91.9 = 6 codes of specificity) |

Symptoms and Signs

Children with ODD often demonstrate behaviors, such as losing their tempers, arguing with adults, defying or refusing to comply with the adult's requests or rules, deliberately annoying others, and blaming others for mistakes and behaviors. In addition, they are irritable and easily annoyed. They are angry, resentful, spiteful, and vindictive. Additionally, these children may be involved in theft, vandalism, and bullying. They exhibit a negative attitude and are defiant.

Patient Screening

The appointment should be made as soon as schedules allow time for a thorough assessment by the physician. The parents may be experiencing great anxiety, and the child should be assessed as soon as possible.

Etiology

ODD has no identified single cause; however, there appears to be a combination of genetic and environmental factors.

Diagnosis

Some symptoms may appear as early as age 3 years or occur when a child is older. In most cases, the problem is discovered before the child becomes a teenager. For a diagnosis of ODD to be determined the behaviors have to be exhibited with a person other than a sibling. If a child is under the age of 5, the behaviors have to be exhibited on most days for a 6-month duration. If the patient is 5 years old or older, one incidence must occur per week for 6 months. A psychiatrist or mental health specialist is a provider who is specially trained to make a diagnosis of this condition, and the severity is designated according to the symptoms and exhibited behaviors. Other mental health conditions may be present too, which can make the diagnosis more difficult to determine.

Treatment

Mood stabilizers, such as risperidone (Risperdal) and olanzapine (Zyprexa), are often prescribed and are helpful for these patients. The most effective form of treatment is behavior and family therapy incorporating parent training and psychotherapy for the child.

Prognosis

Treatment is effective for children who demonstrate behaviors of ODD. If the child begins to demonstrate conduct disorder (a more severe disorder), the outcome is poor.

Prevention

There is no way to prevent ODD. Seeking medical advice when concerned about the behavior of a child may lead to an earlier diagnosis.

Patient Teaching

Encourage parent training courses and education. The child's lack of acceptance of responsibility for behaviors is somewhat indicative of this disorder. Use customized electronically generated educational materials to reinforce the treatment plan.

Tic Disorders

Tic disorders appear as sudden, rapid, recurrent motor movement or vocalization that is nonrhythmic. Resistance against tics is not possible, but they may be suppressed for varying lengths of time and diminish during sleep. Eye blinking, facial grimacing, coughing, and neck jerking are examples of simple motor tics. Making facial gestures, jumping, touching, and stamping are examples of complex motor tics. Simple vocal tics include throat clearing, sniffing, snorting, and grunting. The repetition of words out of context, the use of socially unacceptable words, and the repetition of one's own words or of the last sound heard are examples of complex vocal tics. Tic disorders may be motor or vocal and may be chronic.

Tourette Disorder

Description

Tourette disorder, also known as *Gilles de la Tourette syndrome*, is a syndrome of multiple motor tics coupled with one or more vocal tics, which may appear simultaneously or at different times.

| ICD-10-CM Code | F95.2 *(Tourette disorder)* (F95.0–F95.9 = 5 codes of specificity) |

Symptoms and Signs

The location, nature, and number of tics tend to change over time. The head typically is involved. Other body parts, such as the torso or the upper and lower limbs, may be involved. Clicks, grunts, yelps, barks, sniffing, and snorts are examples of vocal tics. The vocal tics also may include the uttering of obscenities. The patient has significant impairment in functioning at work and in socialization, and the condition is not the result of substance use or a general medical condition.

Patient Screening

The appointment should be made for the earliest date when schedules will allow sufficient time for the physician to conduct a thorough assessment.

Etiology

There is no specific cause identified; however, it is observed in families. Chemicals in the brain (neurotransmitters) that are responsible for movement and a person's behavior are also involved. Some research has associated the onset of Tourette syndrome with streptococcal infections caused by a reaction of antibodies to group A beta-hemolytic *Streptococcus* and nerve tissue. The incidence is higher in those assigned male at birth.

Diagnosis

There is no specific test to diagnose Tourette disorder. The observation of symptoms leads to the diagnosis. According to the CDC, to meet the diagnostic criteria, both at least two or more motor tics and at least one vocal tics must occur, although not necessarily at the same time. They occur several times a day over a period of a year or off and on. The patient has significant impairment in functioning at work and in socialization, and the condition is not the result of substance use or a general medical condition.

Treatment

Pharmacologic treatment is the only proven effective treatment for tics. Some patients with Tourette disorder have improved with the administration of haloperidol (Haldol). Other treatment options include clonidine and clonazepam for their calming effects. Additionally, fluoxetine (Prozac) may be helpful in treating repetitive and obsessive behaviors that occur with Tourette syndrome.

Prognosis

Although there is no cure for Tourette disorder, some patients experience a lessening of symptoms as they reach maturity. However, this usually is a lifelong, chronic condition.

Prevention

No prevention is known for this disorder.

Patient Teaching

Encourage the patient and the family to seek out credible support groups and access information from community health organizations. All those involved should work with the educational system to help the young person exhibiting Tourette syndrome obtain all possible educational assistance.

Dementia

Description

Dementia causes progressive, general deterioration of mental faculties, including a decline in perceiving, thinking, remembering, and cognitive functioning. Dementia, which is *not* a part of normal aging, represents a pathologic development. The irreversible brain damage may be the result of compromised blood flow to the brain resulting from atherosclerosis, thrombi, or trauma. In addition, toxins, metabolic conditions, organic disorders, infections, tumors, Parkinson disease, or Alzheimer disease may be responsible for the deterioration. The onset may be slow and insidious or may be sudden, depending on the cause.

Alzheimer Disease

Description

Alzheimer disease, a progressive degenerative disease of the brain, produces a typical profile of lost mental and physical functioning. It is the most common cause of deterioration in intellectual capacity, or dementia. It is most common in people older than 65 years of age, and its incidence increases in people older than 80 years of age.

ICD-10-CM Code	G30.9 *(Alzheimer disease, unspecified)* (G30.0–G30.9 = 4 codes of specificity)

Symptoms and Signs

The onset of Alzheimer disease is gradual and insidious, with early signs including loss of short-term memory, inability to concentrate, incapacity to learn new information, impairment of reasoning, and subtle changes in personality. Progression of symptoms corresponds with stages ranging from very mild decline (patients note memory lapses) to severe decline (patients frequently lose their capacity for recognizable speech and/or lose the ability to walk without assistance or sit without support). Staging provides useful frames of reference for making future plans of care. As the disease course continues, communication skills decline, and the patient struggles to find the right words, uses meaningless words, or interjects nonsensical phrases. Over a span of 5 to 10 years, there is profound deterioration of intellectual and physical ability. The patient becomes increasingly dependent on a caregiver. Response to stimuli from the outside world diminishes, and the patient seems emotionally detached. The patient may exhibit restlessness, sleep disturbances, disorientation, hostility, or combativeness. The patient eventually becomes bedridden and ultimately dies as a result of undercurrent infection or other complications.

Patient Screening

The onset is insidious, and symptoms may be uncovered during routine office visits. When a family member notices obvious signs and calls for an appointment, the appointment should be scheduled as soon as schedules will allow for a thorough assessment. Anxiety levels will be high, so the next available appointment should be provided.

Etiology

The cause of Alzheimer disease is not known, but the disease is age-related and may have a genetic basis in some families. Research has focused on an abnormality found on chromosome 21 as a genetic link. Patients with Down syndrome (a syndrome also linked to an abnormality on chromosome 21) show the same brain changes as do patients with Alzheimer disease. In later life, people with Down syndrome have the clinical symptoms of Alzheimer disease. Other theories for the cause of Alzheimer disease include biochemical changes in brain growth, an autoimmune reaction, infection by a slow virus, toxic chemical excess, chemical deficiency, blood vessel defects, and a deficiency

• **Fig. 14.3** Alzheimer disease. The diseased brain tissue *(H)* shows loss of cortex and white matter. (From Stevens A, et al: *Core pathology*, ed 3, St. Louis, 2010, Mosby/Elsevier.)

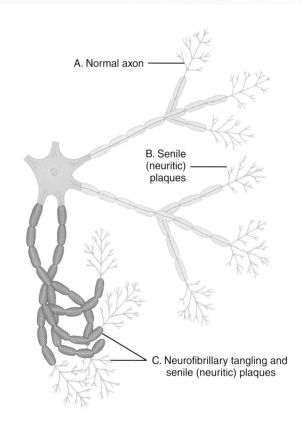

• **Fig. 14.4** Neurofibrillary tangles and senile plaques found in patient with Alzheimer disease. (From Black JM, Matassarin-Jacobs E: *Medical-surgical nursing*, ed 7, Philadelphia, 2004, Saunders.)

of neurochemical factors in the brain. Research has shown a higher rate of occurrence in people with a history of head trauma.

Diagnosis

Obtaining direct evidence of Alzheimer disease is difficult. When other causes of organic brain disease have been ruled out, the diagnostic criteria for Alzheimer disease include evidence of memory and cognitive disturbances. As the disease progresses, neurologic examination reveals sensory and motor deficits. In later stages, diagnostic studies include brain scans, which may detect brain atrophy, widened sulci, and enlarged cerebral ventricles. A positive diagnosis is possible after death, when evidence of brain atrophy and characteristic lesions in the cerebral cortex can be found on pathologic examination of the brain (Fig. 14.3).

The brain shows loss of neurons and the presence of senile plaques, which include microscopic deposits of amyloid material. Neurofibrillary tangles are also evident (Fig. 14.4).

Treatment

No cure is known for Alzheimer disease, so treatment is supportive and is geared toward helping alleviate symptoms.

Drug therapy to alleviate cognitive symptoms includes the use of cholinesterase inhibitors such as donepezil (Aricept) and rivastigmine (Exelon). Memantine (Namenda) is an *N*-methyl-D-aspartate inhibitor that regulates glutamate levels in the brain to help improve memory. Antipsychotic medications such as haloperidol; antianxiety agents, including buspirone; and SSRI antidepressants may be used to manage behavioral symptoms.

Other drugs used to treat the agitation associated with Alzheimer disease are risperidone and olanzapine in those who start to have delusional symptoms caused by

Alzheimer progression. Trazodone is sometimes used for "sundowning," a condition associated with Alzheimer disease, in which patients become confused and disoriented after dark.

In addition to reducing symptoms and suffering, treatment aims to increase the patient's ability to cope and reduce the patient's frustration level.

Research continues to delve into the etiology of Alzheimer disease. Researchers hope that identifying the cause may lead to prevention, because currently there is no way to reverse the neurologic damage caused by the disease. Early diagnosis and drug therapy may help slow the course of the disease. Some classes of and types of medications should be avoided, and a list should be provided to the patient and caregiver.

Prognosis

No cure is known for Alzheimer disease. Drug therapy may help delay the progression of the disorder. The advanced status of the disease usually indicates the need for custodial care.

Prevention

No prevention for Alzheimer disease is currently known. Continued research has identified that living a healthy lifestyle does put some people at lower risk.

Patient Teaching

Advise the caregiver to be consistent in planning daily activities for the patient and to keep the activities simple. Emphasize the importance of complying with the prescribed drug therapy regimen. Encourage the family to use community resources, trained individuals, and local groups for assistance in keeping the patient safe and functioning at the highest level possible. Memory Care facility information should be shared when appropriate.

Vascular Dementia

Description

A reduction in blood flow to the brain can result from narrowed and stenosed arteries. The functional areas of the cerebrum are shown in Fig. 14.5. The resulting hypoxia and reduced nourishment to the brain cells cause a general loss of intellectual abilities (Figs. 14.6 and 14.7 and Box. 14.1).

ICD-10-CM Code	F01.50 *(Vascular dementia without behavioral disturbance)*
	(F01.50–F03 = 6 codes of specificity)
	I67.2 *(Cerebral atherosclerosis)*
	F03 *(Unspecified dementia)*

Refer to the physician's diagnosis and then to the current edition of the ICD-10-CM coding manual to ensure the greatest specificity of pathology.

Symptoms and Signs

Along with the general loss of intellectual abilities in the patient, changes in memory, judgment, abstract thinking, and personality can be noted. A change in personal hygiene is observed. For example, one may not bathe or change clothes. Depression, anxiety, irritability, restlessness, sleeplessness, hallucinations, and psychotic tendencies can occur as the condition advances.

Patient Screening

Similar to the onset of Alzheimer disease, the onset of vascular dementia is insidious, and symptoms may be uncovered during routine office visits. When a family member notices obvious signs and calls for an appointment, enough

• **Fig. 14.6** Contusion. Contrecoup lesions in the frontal and temporal poles *(arrows)* are located opposite to a small coup lesion over the cerebellum *(bottom right arrow)*. (From Damjanov I, Linder J: *Pathology: a color atlas*, St. Louis, 1999, Mosby.)

• **Fig. 14.5** Map of the lateral surface of the cerebral cortex showing some of the functional areas. Areas 4, 6, and 8 are motor areas; areas 1, 2, 3, 41, 42, and 43 are primary sensory areas; and areas 9, 10, 11, 18, 19, 22, 38, 39, and 40 are association areas. (From Solomon EP: *Introduction to human anatomy and physiology*, ed 3, St. Louis, 2009, Saunders/Elsevier.)

• **Fig. 14.7** (A) Subdural hematoma. (B) Epidural hematoma. (From Vincent JL, et al: *Textbook of critical care*, ed 7, St. Louis, 2017, Elsevier.)

• BOX 14.1   **Drugs To Avoid In Patients With Dementia**

The following abbreviated list includes some of the medications that should be avoided in patients with Alzheimer disease and patients with other types of dementia. When selecting medications for this patient group, the following medications should be avoided or at least used in a limited manner. Generally, these medications may worsen cognitive function in patients with dementia.

Narcotic Analgesics

Meperidine, pentazocine, propoxyphene

Antiarrhythmics

Disopyramide

Tricyclic Antidepressants

Amitriptyline, clomipramine, doxepin, imipramine, protriptyline

Antiemetics

Cyclizine, dimenhydrinate, meclizine, promethazine, trimethobenzamide

Antipsychotics

Chlorpromazine, clozapine, pimozide, promazine, thioridazine, triflupromazine

Antihistamines

Azatadine, brompheniramine, chlorpheniramine, clemastine, cyproheptadine, diphenhydramine, hydroxyzine, promethazine

Benzodiazepines

Alprazolam, chlordiazepoxide, diazepam, lorazepam, triazolam

Gastrointestinal/Urinary Antispasmodics

Belladonna alkaloids, atropine, hyoscyamine, scopolamine, dicyclomine, flavoxate, oxybutynin, tolterodine

Muscle Relaxants

Carisoprodol, chlorzoxazone, cyclobenzaprine, metaxalone, methocarbamol, orphenadrine

---

time should be allowed for a thorough assessment. The next available appointment should be provided.

Etiology

Atherosclerotic plaque, as well as other conditions that affect blood vessels, may compromise blood flow to the brain, resulting in hypoxia and ischemia. When an embolism is the cause of the blockage, the hypoxia is sudden and complete. Small aneurysms may be responsible for smaller cerebral bleeds.

Diagnosis

Because symptoms may have an insidious onset, the family often does not notice the subtle changes taking place. When the patient's personal hygiene deteriorates, along with memory and judgment, family members may notice a problem prompting a visit to the health care provider. A thorough history, with physical and neurologic examinations, is necessary to rule out other causes of altered behavior. Vascular assessment of the carotid and cerebral arteries and cerebral or MRI arteriography confirm the condition or other physical conditions.

Treatment

To increase the blood supply to the brain, low-dose aspirin, clopidogrel (Plavix), prasugrel (Effient), and cilostazol (Pletal), are all used for their antiplatelet effect in preventing stroke or its recurrence, especially in patients who have hypertension or have had a myocardial infarction. When the carotid arteries are compromised, surgical intervention in the form of carotid **endarterectomy** may limit the progress of the condition. When the condition progresses, the patient may need to be at an inpatient care facility to ensure safety and care.

Prognosis

The prognosis depends on the extent of the cerebral insult.

Prevention

Very little is known about preventing this condition. Healthy lifestyles are recommended for all individuals. Early diagnosis and treatment may slow the progress of the dementia.

Patient Teaching

Caregivers should encourage patients to do what they can do for themselves. Advise the family that improvement is not likely and that they should prepare themselves and the patient for that possibility.

Substance Use–Related Disorders

ICD-10-CM Code   F10.10 *(Alcohol abuse, uncomplicated)*
(F10.1–F10.99 = 47 codes of specificity)
F19.20 *(Other psychoactive substance dependence, uncomplicated)*
(F19.20–F19.99 = 41 codes of specificity)

Alcohol Use Disorder

Description

Alcohol use disorder (alcoholism) is a disorder of physical and psychological dependence on daily or regular excessive intake of alcoholic beverages. The onset of this chemical dependency can be insidious or can be accelerated by an acute traumatic event.

ICD-10-CM Code   F10.20 *(Alcohol dependence, uncomplicated)*
(F10.1–F10.99 = 47 codes of specificity)

Symptoms and Signs

Alcohol acts on the CNS as a depressant. Individuals under the influence of alcohol may experience a decrease in activity, tension, and normal inhibitions. Ingestion of a few drinks of alcohol may change behavior, decrease the ability to think clearly, slow motor skills, and impair judgment and concentration. Excessive use of alcohol often is associated with anxiety, depression, insomnia, impotence, and behavioral disorders both before and during intoxication. Amnesia often occurs after intoxication. Repeated or prolonged heavy drinking of alcohol produces symptoms and signs in nearly every organ system. Examples include cirrhosis of the liver, pancreatitis, and peripheral neuropathy, resulting in muscle weakness and paresthesia. Chronic alcoholism causes pathologic changes in the nervous system (Fig. 14.8). The risk of cancer of the esophagus, stomach, and other parts of the GI system also is increased. The consequences of chronic alcohol abuse include dysfunction within family and social relationships and disruption in occupational responsibilities. Some people are prone to aggressive or violent behavior, accidents, and threatened

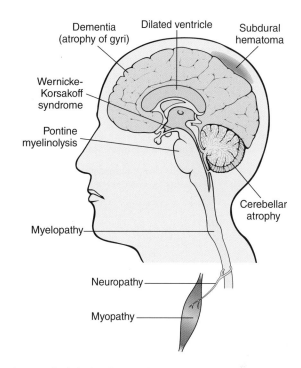

• **Fig. 14.8** Pathologic changes in the nervous system caused by chronic alcoholism. (From Damjanov I: *Pathology for the health-related professions*, ed 4, St. Louis, 2011, Saunders.)

or attempted suicide. The patient often denies his or her inability to control or discontinue alcohol abuse.

Patient Screening

When patients themselves call for an appointment, they require prompt assessment and intervention. When they state that they are in a crisis but cannot be seen in the office right away, they should be referred to an emergency facility.

Etiology

Alcohol abuse has no single cause but a cluster of possible causative factors. The origin may include genetic or biologic factors, depression, emotional conflict, social factors, and cultural attitudes. Because the patient history frequently includes a familial pattern of alcohol abuse, genetic factors pose a recognized statistical risk.

Diagnosis

Screening tests for alcohol use disorder include questionnaires that attempt to identify the behavior. Social history forms completed at a physical examination are designed to have patients answer questions about the use of alcohol and other substances, and the frequency and duration of use. Blood alcohol and toxicology tests can screen for misuse. Table 14.1 lists the effects of various levels of blood alcohol on the brain. Other laboratory tests may also be performed since increased alcohol ingestion can affect various organ systems, such as the gastrointestinal system.

TABLE 14.1	Effects of Rising Blood Alcohol Levels
Blood Alcohol Level	**Effects**
0.02	Mild euphoria, reduced inhibitions, slight body warmth, talkativeness
0.05	Noticeable relaxation, reduced alertness, increased self-confidence
0.08	**Legally drunk in 45 states;** impairment in coordination, judgment, memory, and comprehension
0.10	**Legally drunk in remaining states;** behavior becomes loud or embarrassing; mood swings are noticeable, and reaction time is reduced
0.15	Impaired balance and coordination; appears intoxicated
0.20	Disorientation, mental confusion, dizziness, lethargy, exaggerated emotional states
0.30	Staggering gait, slurred speech, visual disturbances, possible loss of consciousness
0.40	Inability to walk or stand, reduced response to stimuli, vomiting, incontinence, loss of consciousness, possible death ("dead drunk")
0.50	Respiratory effort depressed to point of ceasing, lack of reflexes, body temperature drops, impairment of circulation, possible death; immediate intervention and intense life-support measures required to sustain life
0.60	Death usually occurs or has occurred

ᵃBlood alcohol level (BAL) is measured in milligrams of alcohol per 100 mL of blood and reported as a percentage. An individual with a BAL of 0.10 has one-tenth of 1% (1/1000) of total blood volume as alcohol. BAL depends on the blood volume (blood volume increases with weight) and the amount of alcohol consumed over a given time.

Treatment

Rehabilitation consists of a specialized treatment plan that meets the patient's physical and psychological needs. Substance use disorder counseling and behavior modification techniques are just a couple of examples. There are also 12-step treatment programs and group therapy programs. Disulfiram, acamprosate, and naltrexone are the three FDA-approved medications for the treatment of alcohol use disorder. These medications may be used in conjunction with other therapies to treat this disorder.

Prognosis

The prognosis varies, depending on the duration of the alcoholism and the motivation of the person to work a program of recovery.

Prevention

No prevention is known for alcoholism. Educational programs in regard to avoidance of binge drinking and ingesting alcohol in excess may be beneficial.

Patient Teaching

Encourage patients and family members to be aware of the dangers related to excessive ingestion of alcohol. The provider will make referrals for support based on individual patient needs.

Drugs of Abuse

The misuse of various drugs that modify mood or behavior is called *drug abuse*. Many types of drugs may be suspected in abuse and dependence.

Peer pressure, a chaotic home environment, and poor coping skills can lead to drug abuse by individuals. The use of a prescription drug to treat illness and mental disorders often introduces the individual to the drug of abuse.

Table 14.1 presents popular drugs of abuse, their common names, and their many potential adverse effects. Suboxone is the combination of buprenorphine (a narcotic used for pain relief) and naloxone (an opioid antagonist). This combination decreases the symptoms of opioid withdrawal and reduces the cravings for the opioid high.

Steps have been taken to reduce the amount of opioids that are being prescribed. Patients with chronic or severe pain are often referred to a pain specialist for long-term relief from pain with the use of an opioid-containing medication.

Schizophrenia

Description

Schizophrenia, a major psychiatric disturbance, is a group of disorders that may result in chronic mental dysfunction, producing varying degrees of impairment.

ICD-10-CM Code	F20.9 *(Schizophrenia, unspecified)*

Symptoms and Signs

Schizophrenia is a mental disorder characterized by the presence of either positive manifestations (an excess or distortion of normal functions) or negative manifestations (a loss of normal functions). Positive symptoms include delusions

Substance Use Disorder

Substance use disorder is a significant social and medical concern. Altered behavior and medical complications of substance use disorder are found in all social, economic, ethnic, racial, educational, and professional groups. Some substances that are abused on a regular but episodic basis are alcohol, sedatives, stimulants, opioids, cannabis (marijuana), synthetic cannabis (spice), hallucinogens (including bath salts), inhalants, caffeine, nicotine, illicit synthetic (designer) drugs, and other chemical substances. These substances, prescribed or illegal, give the user a stimulant or depressant effect. The overindulgence in or dependence on chemical substances often produces a detrimental effect on the user's physical and psychological well-being and on the welfare of others.

During substance use disorder, tolerance to the chemical or drug often develops, necessitating increased amounts of the substance to achieve the desired effect. In addition to tolerance, both physical and psychological dependence can develop. Rapid withdrawal from certain drugs can cause life-threatening and even fatal reactions.

The individual under the influence of drugs often exhibits inappropriate behavior, while others may exhibit fairly normal behavior. Users are at risk for injury to themselves or others when driving or operating machinery while under the influence. They experience multiple social and interpersonal problems. Over an extended period, performance and relationships deteriorate. Dependability decreases, and desperation for more of the desired substance may lead to criminal behavior.

Many employers require applicants and employees to undergo drug screening prior to employment, at random, or after an accident or incident. Urine, saliva, and blood can be used for substance screening. Another method is an analysis of a hair sample (Fig. 14.9). Evidence of drug use stays in the hair shaft for about 90 days and is the only drug test that gives this length of drug use history. Drugs are absorbed into the bloodstream and circulated in blood, which nourishes the hair follicle, leaving trace amounts of residue entrapped in the core of the hair shaft.

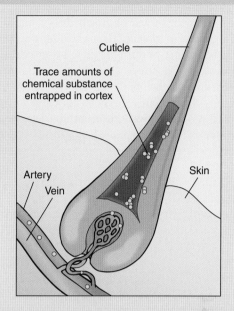

• **Fig. 14.9** The scientific principle behind hair analysis is that as drugs are ingested, they enter the bloodstream, which nourishes the hair follicles. In this way, trace amounts of drugs are deposited in the hair shaft, and, when analyzed, they can reveal a person's drug history. (With permission from Psychemedics Corporation, www.phychemedics.com.)

Law enforcement officers use a breath analyzer to measure blood alcohol levels quickly. Qualitative or quantitative drug assay tests (blood tests to detect the presence or level of specific drugs) also are performed. General toxicology drug screening determines only the presence or absence of a drug. Any identified drugs should be confirmed, and their levels determined through a test specific to that drug. Blood screening for nonspecific drugs usually is accompanied by urine drug screening.

(fixed, false beliefs), hallucinations, disorganized speech, and grossly disorganized or **catatonic** behavior. Negative symptoms are affective flattening, alogia, and avolition.

Schizophrenia is very disabling for the affected individual. In most cases, a person with schizophrenia will have difficulty finishing their education, maintaining employment, and participating in relationships. Many experience trouble with activities of daily living. Schizophrenia is rarely seen in children. Most symptoms begin to manifest in the mid to late 20s. Careful consideration must go into the diagnosis of schizophrenia, because some cultures and religions may regard some symptoms as normal. The onset of schizophrenia is usually insidious during adolescence or young adulthood.

Prodromal signs, such as withdrawal, odd behavior, disheveled appearance, and loss of interest in school or work may be noted. The patient may report feeling confused, isolated, anxious, and afraid. In the active phase of schizophrenia, a vast range of severe behavioral and perceptual manifestations is present, with notable social and occupational dysfunction.

One important feature is disorganized thinking, which is usually reflected in the patient's speech and disturbances in language and communication. For example, the patient may switch from one topic to another, speak incoherently, give an unrelated answer to a question, or experience difficulty speaking at all.

Distortions in perception called *hallucinations* are a common characteristic of schizophrenia. Hallucinations may be auditory, visual, olfactory, or sensory. The patient with auditory hallucinations acknowledges hearing voices that may be threatening, instructive, or conversational. Delusions, which are erroneous beliefs, represent exaggerations or distortions of perceptions or experiences. In persecutory delusion, for instance, people may believe that they are being mistreated, deceived, or stalked. More bizarre delusions may include the belief that one's thoughts are controlled by an "alien."

Inappropriate **affect** (feeling) is another identifying characteristic of schizophrenia. Lack of emotional expression (flat affect) or unreasonable outbursts of emotions may be noted. Eye contact is minimal.

Behavior may be bizarre or grossly disorganized, unpredictable, agitated, or violent. The patient may assume rigid posturing (catatonic posturing), dress in an odd manner, and neglect self-care. Any of these behaviors can stem from the patient's delusional thinking. As the symptoms and signs persist, the patient's ability to function in interpersonal, social, or occupational relationships deteriorates.

Schizophrenia has subtypes, which are determined by a clustering of characteristics, as shown in the table below.

ICD-10-CM Code   F20.0 *(Paranoid schizophrenia)*
Paranoid schizophrenia features anger, hostility, violence, grandiose or persecutory delusions, or hallucinations. The patient may be intelligent and well informed.

ICD-10-CM Code   F20.1 *(Disorganized schizophrenia)*
The patient is blatantly incoherent, with delusions that are not systematized into a theme. The patient's feelings are dull, inappropriate, or greatly exaggerated. Behavior may be odd or regressive. The patient has a history of extreme social impairment, poor functioning, and poor adaptation. The condition has a chronic course.

ICD-10-CM Code   F20.2 *(Catatonic schizophrenia)*
Catatonic schizophrenia features either excitement or stupor with mutism, negativism, rigidity, and posturing.

ICD-10-CM Code   F20.9 *(Schizophrenia, unspecified)*
The behavior is grossly disorganized, and the patient is obviously incoherent, grossly delusional, and hallucinatory. Prominent symptoms of psychosis may fit more than one subtype.

ICD-10-CM Code   F20.5 *(Residual schizophrenia)*
(F20.0–F20.9 = 8 codes of specificity)
The patient has experienced at least one episode of schizophrenia but is currently without prominent symptoms. Continuing evidence of illness, such as illogical thinking and odd behavior, may prevent the patient from functioning in the workplace.

Patient Screening

Scheduling of the appointment for the patient with schizophrenia varies, depending on the situation. When the patient or family member reports a crisis, they should be asked to report to an emergency facility.

Etiology

The cause of schizophrenia is unknown, but evidence suggests that genetic factors play a substantial role. Close biological relatives of patients with schizophrenia have a greater risk of schizophrenia.

Diagnosis

The diagnosis of schizophrenia requires recognizing a group of psychotic signs and symptoms, including delusions, hallucinations, disorganized speech, grossly disorganized behavior, affective flattening, alogia, and avolition. The DSM-5-TR includes the following information in regard to the diagnostic criteria for a determination of whether or not a person has schizophrenia.

The person must exhibit the presence of at least one positive and one negative symptom. The symptoms must interfere with the work or social life. The symptoms must be experienced for most days of at least 1 month over a 6-month period of time. In addition, other medical conditions have been excluded (ruled out).

There are no specific laboratory tests to diagnose this condition, but laboratory tests can be used to rule out other conditions. Recent advances in medical imaging of the brain now provide images of brain activity. These include positron emission tomography (PET), functional magnetic resonance, and magnetic encephalography. These tests, applied to patients with schizophrenia by researchers, have produced an insight into brain activity in these patients and in those without the disease.

Psychological tests that may help in diagnosis include the Rorschach (inkblot) test, the Thematic Apperception Test, and the Minnesota Multiphasic Personality Inventory. Organic causes, such as toxic psychosis associated with substance use disorder, cerebral arteriosclerosis, and hyperthyroidism, should be ruled out.

Treatment

During the acute phase of schizophrenia, antipsychotic drugs are used to control symptoms and to allow early release from the hospital. The minimal dose that produces remission of symptoms without troublesome side effects associated with antipsychotic medications is desirable. Subsequent long-term multidimensional treatment combines supportive psychotherapy, drugs, and family involvement. After the patient is stabilized, the goal of treatment is to help the patient to establish a better sense of self through personal, social, and vocational achievements.

Atypical antipsychotics are first-line therapy and include risperidone, olanzapine, asenapine (Saphris), clozapine (Clozaril), ziprasidone (Geodon), quetiapine (Seroquel), and lurasidone (Latuda). Some of these medications are supplied as injectable long-acting preparations. Atypical antipsychotics have less chance of causing extrapyramidal side effects compared with older drug therapies, although most atypical antipsychotics carry a black box warning regarding mortality risk in dementia-related psychosis and suicidal tendencies. Older antipsychotic drugs are used for those who do not respond well to atypical drugs and in cases where the patient has been on the older drugs for an extended period of time and reports no unmanageable side effects. These drugs include chlorpromazine, haloperidol, and fluphenazine. Intramuscular injections increase compliance because the medication can last for a month.

Potential side effects of the neuroleptic agents used to treat schizophrenia are known as *extrapyramidal side effects (EPSs)*, which are manifested as involuntary motor movements. Tardive dyskinesia is a type of EPS characterized by repetitive, involuntary, purposeless movements. Features may include grimacing, tongue protrusion, lip smacking, puckering and pursing of the lips, and rapid eye blinking. Weekly laboratory tests should be ordered and performed.

Prognosis

The prognosis is moderate if the patient takes prescription drugs regularly and if the family is supportive and willing to participate in treatment. Treatment in a community support program also is beneficial. Responses to treatment vary, and relapses may occur.

Prevention

Schizophrenia is genetic, so no prevention is known. Compliance with taking medications reduces psychotic breaks, helping to prevent the illness from worsening. Each time a patient has a psychotic break, baseline functioning is reduced.

Patient Teaching

Instruct patients to comply with the medication regimen despite the frequent unpleasant side effects. Because noncompliance can be an issue, involving the family is helpful. Advise family members and support persons that patients with schizophrenia are not bad people but are simply people with a bad illness. In addition, encourage family members to help the patient with activities of daily living.

Patients, families, and caretakers should be alert for side effects caused by risperidone. The physician should be notified if any of the following are noted in the individual taking risperidone: fever, confusion, rapid or irregular pulse, seizures, fainting, difficulty swallowing or breathing, or unusual, uncontrollable movements of the mouth or body. Refer to the Enrichment box about Neuroleptic Malignant Syndrome.

❖ ENRICHMENT

Neuroleptic Malignant Syndrome

Neuroleptic malignant syndrome (NMS), a unique life-threatening reaction to antipsychotic drugs, is suspected when patients suddenly develop a fever, muscle rigidity, altered mental status, and autonomic dysfunction. This is a danger that may accompany all neuroleptics, such as newer atypical antipsychotics and a range of other medications that have an effect on central dopaminergic neurotransmission. NMS is an important factor in the diagnosis of patients who suddenly experience fever, muscle rigidity and mental status changes. NMS needs prompt identification to prevent significant morbidity and death. Recommended treatment is to immediately stop the offending drug and to begin supportive measures. Additionally, drug interventions may be required in more severe cases.

Mood Disorders

Patients who are diagnosed with mood disorders experience a pathologic disturbance in mood that affects all aspects of his or her life. The terms *affect* and *mood* are used interchangeably to refer to the outward manifestation of a person's feeling or tone.

Bipolar Disorder

Description

Bipolar disorder is a major affective disorder with abnormally intense mood swings from a hyperactive, or manic, state to a depressive syndrome (Fig. 14.10). In some cases, symptoms of hyperactivity and depression may coexist. This is known as a "mixed" episode. The patient may remain manic for days, weeks, or months before experiencing depression. Assessment findings vary with the type of episode (manic, depressive, or mixed) that the patient is experiencing at the time of medical evaluation.

ICD-10-CM Code	F31.9 *(Bipolar disorder, unspecified)* (F31.0–F31.9 = 28 codes of specificity)

Symptoms and Signs

During a manic episode, the patient is excited, euphoric, and expansive. The person speaks rapidly with great certitude and conviction. Evidence of thought disorders, such as frequent changes of topic or flight of ideas, may be noted. Patients sleep little and seem to have excessive energy, which leads to overinvolvement in activities. Judgment is impaired, and they may spend money extravagantly. Behavior may

• **Fig. 14.10** Representation of bipolar disorder. (Courtesy David L. Frazier, 2003.)

appear bizarre, grandiose, or promiscuous. The patient may be delusional or experience auditory hallucinations.

During an episode of depression, the patient's mood becomes lowered, sad, or notably indifferent (flat affect). Thoughts and speech are slow, and the patient may avoid communication. The patient becomes withdrawn and demonstrates a loss of interest in life. Reports of sleep disturbance, loss of appetite, and feelings of guilt are common. The patient experiences a substantial decrease in physical activity. Suicide may be threatened or attempted.

Patient Screening

Most often, help will be sought during the depressive portion of the illness. Depressed individuals require immediate assessment.

Etiology

Bipolar disorder has no clear cause. Biochemical factors, such as alterations of neurotransmitter levels in the brain, endocrine disorders, and electrolyte imbalances, may play a role. The risk of mood disorders is higher among close relatives of the patient. Emotional or physical trauma may precipitate the onset of bipolar disorder in a predisposed person.

Diagnosis

A thorough family history and patient history of symptoms is obtained. The patient may appear to be experiencing only depression.

Bipolar disorder is identified when certain prescribed diagnostic criteria can be documented during physical and psychological evaluations. The mood disturbance must be pervasive and persistent and cause substantial impairment over a distinct period. Other medical causes, such as organic diseases, thyroid disorders, and psychiatric conditions, must be ruled out.

Treatment

After diagnosis, therapeutic treatment is dictated by the specific form of behavior the patient exhibits. Lithium carbonate is the drug of choice during an acute manic phase of bipolar disease. Valproate sodium and carbamazepine (Tegretol) are good drugs for supplemental therapy in stabilizing manic episodes. Antidepressant medications are best used in conjunction with anticonvulsants for optimal mood stabilization. Many of the drugs that fall into the category of anticonvulsant also function well to provide mood stabilization. Examples include lamotrigine (Lamictal) and gabapentin (Neurontin), as well as valproate sodium and carbamazepine. Atypical antipsychotics are often used for mood stabilization, such as lurasidone (Latuda), which is approved by the US Food and Drug Administration (FDA) for the treatment of bipolar disorder. Treatment includes a therapeutic environment, that meets the patient's physical needs, encourages personal responsibility, and sets reasonable limits and goals for behavior. During this time, the patient may need to be protected from self-injury.

Prognosis

The prognosis is good with treatment and drug therapy. Compliance is the key to successful treatment.

Prevention

No prevention is known.

Patient Teaching

Encourage patients to take medications and keep appointments with their therapist. Depending on the medications prescribed and taken, blood studies may be necessary. When available, use customized electronically generated educational materials to reinforce the treatment plan.

Major Depressive Disorder

Description

Major depressive disorder is a mood disorder characterized by one or more major depressive episodes. Persons with major depressive disorders have no history of manic or hypomanic episodes.

ICD-10-CM Code	F32.9 *(Major depressive disorder, single episode, unspecified)* (F32.0–F33.9 = 17 codes of specificity)

Symptoms and Signs

Major depressive disorder is a serious alteration in mood that may be described as deep and persistent sadness, despair, and hopelessness (Fig. 14.11). Symptoms develop gradually over several days, during which an anxious or brooding appearance may be noted. The person may experience an empty or heavy feeling inside accompanied by a vague sense of loss. The person also may have an attitude of self-blame, remorse, guilt, or loss of self-esteem. Other

• **Fig. 14.11** Depression. (Courtesy David L. Frazier, 2003.)

symptoms include sleep disturbance (insomnia or hyper-somnia), physical sluggishness or fatigue, loss of concentration, and inability to experience pleasure. In addition, a depressed person may have a variety of physical symptoms. Appetite disturbance results in a change in weight. The patient withdraws socially and may admit to having suicidal thoughts; suicidal behavior is common in major depression (Table 14.2).

TABLE 14.2	Depression on a Continuum	
Mild to Moderate		**Severe**

Communication

Mild to Moderate	Severe
• Slow speech • Long pauses before answering • Monotone	• Slow in extreme • May be mute and not talk at all

Affect

Mild to Moderate	Severe
• Crying and weeping, slumping in chair, drooping shoulders, look of gloom and pessimism • Anxiety may or may not be manifested • Anhedonia (inability to experience pleasure)	• May appear without affect • May be experiencing "nothingness" • Can sit for hours staring into space • Anhedonia

Thinking

Mild to Moderate	Severe
• No impairment in reality testing • Thinking is slow; concentration and memory are poor; interest narrows; perspective in situations is lost: • "Everyone always lets me down." • "No one cares." • Thoughts reflect doubts and indecisions; thinking is often repetitive in negative cycle: • "Why was I born?" • "What's life all about?" • Mild feelings of guilt and worthlessness • *May have suicidal ideation*	• Grasp of reality may be tenuous • Thoughts may indicate delusional thinking, reflecting feelings of: • Low self-esteem • Worthlessness • Helplessness • "I'm no good." • "God is punishing me for my terrible sins." • "My insides are rotting." • "My heart has stopped beating." • Concentration is extremely poor • Preoccupation with bodily symptoms • *May have suicidal ideation*

Physical Behavior

Mild to Moderate	Severe
• Fatigue and lethargy are hallmark symptoms; they do not prevent the person from working, but the person often works below potential; initiative and creativity are impaired • Grooming and hygiene usually are neglected	• Severe and extreme chronic fatigue and lethargy greatly interfere with occupational functioning, social activities, or relationships with others • Client may show extreme neglect of personal grooming and hygiene

Vegetative Signs

Mild to Moderate	Severe
• Sleep: Middle or late insomnia, hypersomnia; EEG studies show shortened REM latency • Energy is often highest in the morning, lowest in the evening • Eating: May have anorexia or overeat • Sexual appetite is diminished • Bowels: Constipation if psychomotor impairment is present; may have diarrhea if psychomotor agitation is present • Psychomotor impairment (slow motor movements): Everything is an effort	• Sleep: Usually insomnia; early-morning waking at 3:00 or 4:00 a.m. • Energy is often lowest in the morning, highest in the evening • Eating: Usually has anorexia; weight loss of more than 5% in 1 month • Loss of libido • Bowels: Usually constipation • Psychomotor impairment (most common)
Or	*Or*
• Psychomotor agitation (agitated depression); pacing up and down halls, wringing hands	• Psychomotor agitation

(From Varcarolis EM: *Foundations of psychiatric mental health nursing*, ed 3, Philadelphia, 1998, WB Saunders.)
EEG, Electroencephalogram; *REM*, rapid eye movement.

Patient Screening

People experiencing symptoms of depression require immediate assessment. The risk of suicide requires immediate assessment and intervention.

Etiology

No single cause has been identified for major depressive disorder. It is believed to result, though, from a variety of factors, which may include genes, hormones, chemistry of the brain, and biological differences.

Diagnosis

Major depressive disorder must be differentiated from a reactive type of depression that results from a difficult or stressful life circumstance, such as grief syndrome. Diagnostic criteria used in psychiatric evaluation include a prominent and persistent depressed mood lasting at least 2 weeks, with at least five or more depressive symptoms documented. A family history of depression is included in the assessment.

Treatment

The most effective treatment is a combination of medication and psychotherapy. Most patients have relief of symptoms and a good prognosis if they respond favorably to antidepressant therapy. SSRIs, including fluoxetine, are the first-line agents, but many patients with major depression also might be prescribed the tricyclics amitriptyline/nortriptyline along with the SSRI. Atypical antipsychotics may be used in severe cases of major depressive disorder. Depression may occur as a single episode or may be recurrent. Electroconvulsive therapy helps when a patient is severely incapacitated, has psychotic features, or does not respond to other therapeutic measures. Family support and education are considered important in the recovery process.

Patients who commit suicide have a high incidence of hopelessness or acute depression. The suicidal patient often wishes to discuss suicidal fears and does not want to die but sees suicide as the only escape from an intolerable situation. A reluctance to discuss suicidal thoughts makes it important for the examiner to explore the patient's preoccupation with death or such comments as "People would be better off without me" or "I am better off dead."

Suicide intervention is an attempt by medical, mental health, and community organizations to help the depressed individual through the crisis situation. Most telephone directories list crisis intervention centers. Hospital emergency departments and law enforcement agencies have professionals immediately available to offer support and personal contact to this individual. Mental health agencies routinely offer their clients a 24-hour "hotline" number for contacting a counselor. Structures that are often used as jumping points, such as bridges, have strategically placed signs that offer crisis intervention telephone numbers (Fig. 14.12). The increase in suicide rates continues to rise.

Anxiety Disorders

Description

Anxiety is a common form of psychological disorder. For most people, anxiety is just a temporary response to stress. For some people, however, anxiety becomes a chronic problem, and they regularly experience excessive levels of anxiety. They often exhibit anxiety that is inappropriate to the circumstance. Only when anxiety persists and prevents the person from leading a normal life does it become an illness. As a group, anxiety disorders represent the single largest mental health problem in the United States. They can lead to more severe disorders, such as depression and alcoholism.

Anxiety disorders, previously known as *neuroses*, include four specific disorders or syndromes that are different in behavioral manifestations but share the fact that the person's behavior is dominated by anxiety. The four disorders are generalized anxiety disorder, panic disorder, phobic disorder, and obsessive-compulsive disorder (OCD).

PUBLIC TELEPHONE

CRISIS CONTROL CENTER

• **Fig. 14.12** The Golden Gate Bridge, where many suicide jumps have been made. (Courtesy David L. Frazier, 1999.)

❖ ENRICHMENT

Grief Response

The grief response is initiated primarily by the death of a loved one, but grieving is also a normal sequela to any loss, including the loss of a function, body part, employment, or other important entity. The patient with a terminal illness faces the prospect of total separation and also must work through the various stages of grief.

The normal grieving process passes through several phases. The most recognized stages are those identified by Elisabeth Kübler-Ross. The first is denial: "No, I don't believe it." Second is anger: "Why did he or she do this to me?" or "Why is God letting this happen?" The third stage is bargaining: "If only this task can be accomplished or I can achieve this goal (live long enough), I will do this." Fourth is depression, in which people retreat within themselves and have little or no involvement with their environment. Finally, in the fifth stage, acceptance comes. Not everyone is able to move through these steps, and not everyone moves through them at the same pace or in the same order. Some people cannot express anger at the dead person or at God and do not move on. Many people never complete the grieving process, so they remain in a depressed state and have reduced coping mechanisms. Medical intervention may help during depression, but most people recover with minimal treatment.

Different cultures grieve in different ways. Many groups grieve quietly and privately, whereas others cry, moan, rant, and even throw themselves on the funeral pyre. The important goal of funerals and the viewing of the remains is to allow closure of the relationship and to allow loved ones to say goodbye (Table 14.3 and Fig. 14.13).

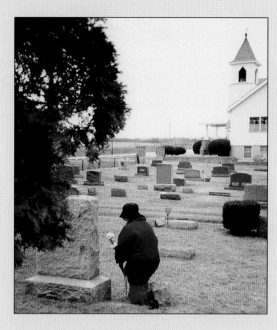

• **Fig. 14.13** Grief response. (Courtesy David L. Frazier, 1999.)

| TABLE 14.3 | **Phenomena Experienced During Mourning** |

Symptoms	Examples
Sensation of Somatic Distress	
• Tightness in throat, shortness of breath, sighing, "mental pain," exhaustion. • Food tastes like sand; things feel unreal. • Pain or discomfort may be identical to the symptoms experienced by the dead person. • Symptoms normally are brief.	A female whose husband died of a stroke complains of weakness and numbness on her left side.
Preoccupation With the Image of the Deceased	
• The bereaved brings up, thinks, and talks about many memories of the deceased. • The memories are positive. • This process goes on with great sadness. • The idealization of the deceased lets the bereaved relive the gratifications associated with the deceased and helps resolve any guilt the bereaved has toward the deceased. • The bereaved also may take on many of the mannerisms of the deceased through identification. • Identification serves the purpose of holding onto the deceased. • Preoccupation with the dead person takes many months before it lessens.	A male whose wife just died states, "I just can't stop thinking about my wife. Everything I see reminds me of her. We picked up this seashell on our honeymoon. I remember every wonderful moment we had together. The pain is so great, but the memories just keep coming." His friends notice that when he talks, his hand gestures and expressions are very like those of his recently deceased wife.
Guilt	
The bereaved reproaches himself or herself for real or fancied acts of negligence or omissions in the relationship with the deceased.	"I should have made him go to the doctor sooner." "I should have paid more attention to her, been more thoughtful."

Grief Response

Symptoms	Examples
Anger	
• The anger the bereaved experiences may not be toward the object that gives rise to it.	"The doctor didn't operate in time. If he had, Mary would be alive today."
• The anger often is displaced onto the medical or nursing staff. It is often directed toward the deceased.	"How could he leave me like this …? How could he?"
• The anger is at its height during the first month but is often intermittent throughout the first year.	
• The overflow of hostility disturbs the bereaved, resulting in the feeling that he or she is going "insane."	
Change in Behavior (Depression, Disorganization, Restlessness)	
• A person may exhibit substantial restlessness and an inability to organize his or her behavior.	Six months after her husband died, Mrs. Faye stated, "I just can't seem to function. I have a hard time doing the simplest tasks. I can't be bothered with socializing."
• Routine activities take a long time to perform.	"I feel so down … so, so empty."
• Depressive mood is common as the year passes and as the intensity of the grief declines.	
• The absence of depression is more abnormal than its presence.	
• Loneliness and aimlessness are most pronounced 6 to 9 months after the death.	
Reorganization of Behavior Directed Toward a New Object or Activity	
• The person gradually renews his or her interest in people and activities.	• Twenty months after her husband's death, Mrs. Faye tells a friend, "I'll be away this weekend. I am going fishing with my brother and his friend. This is the first time I've felt like doing anything since Harry died."
• The grieving thus releases the bereaved from one interpersonal relationship, and new ones are free to take its place.	

(From Varcarolis EM: *Foundations of psychiatric mental health nursing*, ed 6, St. Louis, 2010, Saunders.)

◆ **ENRICHMENT**

Postpartum Depression

Postpartum depression (PPD), often labeled "baby blues," ranges from mild depression to moderate depressive mood to severe postpartum psychosis. Depressive symptoms after the birth of a baby have been recorded for centuries. Although no specific cause has been identified, abrupt changes in the levels of hormones, including estrogen and progesterone, have been proposed as the cause of this condition. In addition, changes in thyroid status may play a role in some cases. A previous history of depression or other mental health conditions may increase the risk of PPD.

Symptoms usually begin within 24 to 48 hours after birth or during the first 6 weeks after giving birth. The symptoms may subside in a few days or a few weeks or may last for several months. The new mother experiences fatigue, changes in normal appetite and sleep patterns, feelings of worthlessness and despair, crying episodes, poor personal hygiene, despair about her ability as a mother, feelings of anger, and recurrent thoughts of suicide. Bonding with the baby may not take place. She also feels sad, has a flat affect, appears excessively angry, lacks interest in normal daily events, and experiences difficulty in concentrating and making decisions. She may express the desire to run away from everything, fears of being alone, and concern about potentially harming the baby. In the more severe cases of PPD, the mother may have thoughts of homicide, especially of killing the infant.

Maternal-child health care providers must be alert for any symptoms of PPD. Prenatal teaching of both parents should include the typical symptoms of PPD and instructions to seek prompt medical intervention if and when they occur. Early intervention with medication and therapy helps to reduce symptoms and prevent harm to the mother or child. The teaching also should urge parents not to feel any stigma for experiencing the condition, because it is a very common occurrence in many postpartum periods. Postpartum psychosis is considered a rare outcome, and when it does occur, it may bring about serious events.

Symptoms and Signs

Symptoms can range from worry and stress to extreme panic, depending on which anxiety disorder the patient is experiencing. Mild to moderate levels of anxiety can easily be mistaken for depression because of the similarity in symptoms, such as irritability, difficulty concentrating, and disturbance in sleep patterns.

Some symptoms of anxiety disorders are observed behaviors (e.g., nail biting), compulsive rituals (e.g., hand washing and checking), and other nervous movements.

Generalized Anxiety Disorder and Panic Disorder

ICD-10-CM Code	F41.0 (Panic disorder [episodic paroxysmal anxiety] without agoraphobia)
	F41.1 (Generalized anxiety disorder)
	(F41.0–F41.9 = 5 codes of specificity)

Patients with generalized anxiety disorder have a condition known as *free-floating anxiety* and live in a constant state of apparently causeless anxiety. They constantly worry about previous mistakes and future problems. These individuals dislike making decisions and worry about the decisions they have made. Their constant worrying often is accompanied by physiologic symptoms, such as diarrhea, elevated blood pressure, and sustained muscular tension. An inability to sleep and nightmares are common. Some patients are even prone to panic attacks.

In panic disorder, the anxiety also is unfocused. With a panic attack, the anxiety begins suddenly and unexpectedly, reaching a peak within 10 minutes. The attack often is accompanied by a sense of impending doom and a feeling that the person is "going crazy," losing control, or dying. The world may seem unreal (derealization), or patients may seem unreal to themselves (depersonalization). In addition, these patients may experience palpitations, rapid pulse, pounding heart, sweating, trembling, shortness of breath, chest pain, nausea, paresthesia, dizziness, and chills or hot flashes.

The anxiety characteristic of a panic disorder can be differentiated from generalized anxiety by its sudden, intermittent nature and greater severity. A person is said to have panic disorder if he or she has four panic attacks within a month's time or if one or more attacks have been followed by a persistent fear of having another attack.

Phobic Disorder

Description

A phobic disorder is marked by excessive, persistent, and irrational fear and the avoidance of the phobic stimulus. In phobic disorders, the person's excessive anxiety has a specific focus (Fig. 14.14), some object or a situation that presents no real danger. Many people with phobias realize that their fears are irrational but feel powerless to control or prevent them. Individuals with phobias must design their lives to avoid the things that they fear. When they confront

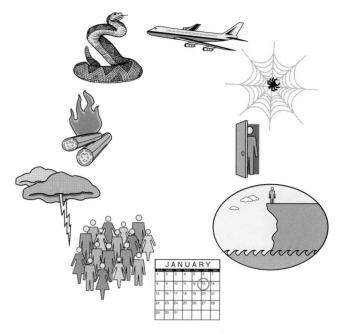

• **Fig. 14.14** Phobias.

an object or situation that causes them anxiety, they often have a severe attack of anxiety. Phobias can develop from or against almost anything (Table 14.4).

ICD-10-CM Code	F40.9 (Phobic anxiety disorder, unspecified)
	(F40.00–F40.9 = 23 codes of specificity)

Obsessive-Compulsive Disorder

Description

OCD is marked by the presence of obsessions (persistent unwanted thoughts) and compulsions (persistent urges to carry out specific actions).

ICD-10-CM Code	F42 (Obsessive-compulsive disorder)

Symptoms and Signs

Obsessions are persistent intrusions of unwanted thoughts, and compulsions are uncontrollable urges to carry out certain actions. The two features of this disorder usually, but not always, occur together. People with obsessions often have thoughts of harming others, committing suicide, or performing sexual acts considered immoral. These people feel as though they have lost control of their minds, which causes them great anxiety. People with compulsions develop senseless actions or rituals that relieve their anxiety temporarily (e.g., excessive hand washing). Examples include an obsession with germs that results in a compulsion to clean or wash one's hands and an obsession with fire or theft that results in a compulsion to check doors, appliances, and outlets.

TABLE 14.4 Phobias

Name	Description	Name	Description
Acrophobia	Fear of high places	Olfactophobia	Fear of odor
Agoraphobia	Fear of open spaces	Ombrophobia	Fear of rain
Algophobia	Fear of pain	Ophidiophobia	Fear of snakes
Androphobia	Fear of males	Pathophobia	Fear of disease
Arachnophobia	Fear of spiders	Pharmacophobia	Fear of drugs
Astrophobia	Fear of storms, thunder, and lightning	Phasmophobia	Fear of ghosts
Aviophobia	Fear of flying	Phobophobia	Fear of fear
Claustrophobia	Fear of closed or narrow spaces	Ponophobia	Fear of work
Hematophobia	Fear of blood	Pyrophobia	Fear of fire
Hodophobia	Fear of travel	Sitophobia	Fear of food
Hydrophobia	Fear of water	Thanatophobia	Fear of death
Iatrophobia	Fear of physicians	Toxiphobia	Fear of being poisoned
Kainophobia	Fear of change	Traumatophobia	Fear of injury
Kakorrhaphiophobia	Fear of failure	Triskaidekaphobia	Fear of the number 13
Lalophobia	Fear of speaking in public	Xenophobia	Fear of strangers
Monophobia	Fear of being alone	Zoophobia	Fear of animals
Ochlophobia	Fear of crowds		

Patient Screening

Patients with complaints of persistent intrusion of unwanted thoughts, compulsions, and uncontrollable urges to carry out certain actions require prompt assessment.

Etiology

Many theories attempt to explain the causes of anxiety disorders. Some anxiety disorders are caused by severe stress. In people who are anxiety prone, only slight stress, or none at all, can be a cause. A physical condition, such as hyperthyroidism (overactive thyroid gland) or a cerebrovascular disorder, also can produce the symptoms of anxiety. The role of neurotransmitters and genetic factors has been studied. OCD also may be related to dysfunction in the frontal lobe of the brain.

Diagnosis

Anxiety disorders are diagnosed after much investigation into the patient's symptoms and history, family history, and level of stress. In some cases, metabolic testing indicates abnormalities. PET to detect chemical activity or metabolism of the brain and biochemical studies also have been used. Using the DSM-5-TR criteria during assessment is important in arriving at a diagnosis; one must ask whether the individual meets the requirements for the diagnosis.

Treatment

If the anxiety prevents the person from living a normal life, a psychiatrist or a practitioner trained in treating psychological problems (e.g., psychologist or psychoanalyst) should be consulted. These therapists use many forms of treatment, depending on their perspective. Hypnosis is sometimes used to help the patient and the therapist to gain access to the subconscious mind. If the anxiety is caused by a specific stress (e.g., job related), steps should be taken to minimize or eliminate the problem.

Various methods of relaxation (e.g., systematic desensitization, progressive relaxation, breathing exercises, and guided imagery) can lessen the symptoms. Relaxation exercises (e.g., biofeedback) to relax tense muscles or physical activity (e.g., brisk walking, jogging, or swimming) may be beneficial. In addition, or as an alternative, the physician may prescribe an anxiolytic drug. SSRIs are a first-line therapy; fluvoxamine (Luvox) is FDA approved for the treatment of OCD. Benzodiazepines are also frequently prescribed. Examples are lorazepam (Ativan), clonazepam (Klonopin), and alprazolam (Xanax). These medications should be prescribed on an "as needed," short-term basis for severe anxiety because dependence can occur. In severe cases of anxiety, a period of hospitalization also may be necessary. If severe anxiety is not treated, psychotic depression may develop.

Prognosis

The prognosis is proportional to the patient's compliance with recommended medications and therapy interventions.

Prevention

No prevention is known.

Patient Teaching

Encourage patients to attempt relaxation techniques. When drug therapy is prescribed, encourage compliance and follow-up with therapy as recommended. Use customized electronically generated educational materials, when available, to reinforce the treatment plan.

Pediatric Autoimmune Neuropsychiatric Disorders Associated With Streptococcal Infections

Description

PANDAS (Pediatric autoimmune neuropsychiatric disorders associated with streptococcal infections), a form of obsessive-compulsive disorder with abrupt onset, follows the occurrence of a group A beta-hemolytic streptococcal infection.

ICD-10-CM Code	D89.89 *(Other specified disorders involving the immune mechanism, not elsewhere classified)*

Symptoms and Signs

An abrupt emotional personality change appears in 3-year-olds to prepubertal children, They may experience severe mood swings, separation anxiety, and abrupt, obsessive, and unusual behavior. Some may show signs of detachment from parents or caregivers, hyperactivity, or uncontrollable ADHD symptoms. They may encounter sleep disturbances, motor or vocal tics, and nighttime fears.

Patient Screening

The patient experiencing PANDAS suffers acute emotional pain and anxiety and requires prompt medical attention.

Etiology

The condition usually occurs after a bacterial streptococcal infection.

Diagnosis

Diagnosis is confirmed through the patient's history of a previous streptococcal infection and physical examination.

Treatment

Treatment with antibiotics to eliminate the streptococcal infection is primary. Short-term cognitive behavioral therapy may help deal with current behavioral changes. Medical intervention may involve managing OCD symptoms by prescribing the use of SSRIs. Additional options may include steroids.

Prognosis

The prognosis is good with therapy and medications; however, the reoccurrence of a streptococcal infection may trigger another episode.

Prevention

Prevention is to complete the course of prescribed antibiotics.

Patient Teaching

Parents should be instructed to make sure the child takes all of the antibiotics prescribed as treatment for any streptococcal infection.

Posttraumatic Stress Disorder

Description

PTSD is a delayed response to an external traumatic event that produces signs and symptoms of extreme distress.

ICD-10-CM Code	F43.0 *(Acute stress reaction)*
	F43.10 *(Posttraumatic stress disorder, unspecified)*
	F43.12 *(Posttraumatic stress disorder, chronic)*
	(F43.10–F43.12 = 3 codes of specificity)

Symptoms and Signs

PTSDs are different from other anxiety disorders because the cause of the stress is an external event of an overwhelmingly painful nature (Fig. 14.15). The person may experience this disorder for weeks, months, or even years (transitory episodes) after the event through painful recollections or nightmares. People with PTSD go out of their way to avoid being reminded of the painful event. They may be unable to respond to affection and have insomnia and irritability. These individuals also may exhibit strong physiologic responses to any reminder of the event. PTSDs can also be experienced by adults who were victims of child abuse and repress those memories until something triggers them during adulthood.

Symptoms of PTSD usually appear within a short time of the event. In some cases, however, the person has a delayed response (onset). The person may be symptom free for days or months after the event before signs of response to the painful event begin to appear. Not all people exposed to severely traumatic events have such symptoms.

Patient Screening

The patient experiencing PTSD suffers acute emotional pain and anxiety and requires prompt medical attention.

Etiology

PTSD caused by human actions (e.g., rape, acts of war, and continued abuse) tends to precipitate more severe reactions compared with PTSD caused by natural disasters (e.g.,

• **Fig. 14.15** Posttraumatic stress disorder (PTSD) sources. (A) Overwhelming numbers of violent deaths, as in wars. (B) Destruction of one's environment by fire, as by forest fires encroaching on communities. (C) Brush fires suddenly erupting on community property. (D) Fire destroying shelters and property. (Courtesy David L. Frazier, 1999.)

hurricanes, earthquakes, and floods). In the case of natural disasters, the greater the threat of death and the greater the number of people affected, the greater the likelihood of severe PTSD. The overwhelming experience of a threat to the individual's life is a causative factor.

Children also may be affected by experiencing or observing horrific events in their lives. Traumatic events include acts of war, in which they have observed family members being killed or being separated from the family unit. In addition, catastrophic events of nature, in which the children have witnessed violent destruction of homes and surroundings, may make them fearful and withdrawn. Abuse also is known to cause PTSD, especially sexual abuse. Recognizing traumatic events in children's lives is essential, as is involving them in therapy decisions.

Diagnosis

The provider will perform a physical and psychological examination to see if there are physical medical problems contributing to symptoms and to discuss what "led up" to the event. The provider will also use criteria in the DSM-5 TR to see which are met in regard to the individual.

PTSD diagnosis is also made based on a recent event in which the patient felt threatened with the possibility of dying, violence, or serious injury. The individual may witness the event, or be directly involved. Car crashes can also cause of trigger PTSD.

Often, children suffering from PTSD will reenact the event, have recurrent dreams or nightmares of the event, or have repetitive patterns of the event in their play. They may also have sadness and become withdrawn in addition to other symptoms that are not typical for a child.

Treatment

The goal of treatment of PTSD is to restore the individual's sense of control. Counseling and drug therapy are used in the treatment. Counseling therapy helps those with PTSD to accept the overwhelming memories without rearranging their lives to avoid the memories. They work to develop a sense of safety and control. Feelings of guilt and self-blame need to be addressed. Cognitive behavior training to increase self-esteem and self-control is employed.

Sleep disturbances must be recognized and treated. Benzodiazepines may be prescribed to help the patient regain normal sleep patterns. In addition, antianxiety agents or SSRIs may be used as drug therapy. Recovery may be complete in some individuals in a short time, whereas others may never recover completely.

Psychiatric service dogs may also be used to assist in the treatment of PTSD. These dogs are trained to perform tasks that can assist the person with PTSD. It should be understood that an emotional support animal is not considered a *service dog*.

Prognosis

The prognosis is good with therapy and medications; however, some patients with PTSD never fully recover. The treatment does help with day to day living and functioning in society.

Prevention

Seeking medical help from a physician or mental health therapist after an extremely violent or life-threatening event may help in preventing PTSD.

Patient Teaching

Encourage compliance with therapy and medication.

Somatoform Disorders

Somatoform disorders are a group of mental disorders in which the person experiences physical symptoms without the underlying organic cause. These symptoms are not under voluntary control and are real to the affected person. The opposite is true of factitious disorders (Munchausen syndrome) or malingering, in which the patient presents with feigned symptoms for personal or emotional gain. There is no confirmed, diagnosable, general medical condition that accounts for the symptoms of somatoform disorders.

Somatic System Disorder

Description

Somatic system disorder is multisymptomatic and typically occurs before age 30. The patient has symptoms that may or may not be associated with another diagnosis.

ICD-10-CM Code	F45.0 (Somatization disorder) (F45.0–F45.1 = 2 codes of specificity)

Symptoms and Signs

The patient experiences multiple recurring symptoms that may include nausea, vomiting, blood in the stool, pain, reproductive and neurologic system problems without a clinical basis. The patient will experience anxiety in regard to their symptoms and spend great amounts of time and resources in regard to the symptoms. Excessive thoughts and fears may also be experienced by the patient.

Patient Screening

Patients with initial complaints of severe pain and symptoms should be given the next available appointment. Patients demanding to be seen immediately should be referred to an emergency facility.

Etiology

The etiology is uncertain.

Diagnosis

The diagnosis is made after medical conditions are ruled out. The presence of pain is real, even though there may or may not be physical conditions that are diagnosed. This is a chronic condition without a symptom-free period of longer than 1 year. Clinically, there is no pathologic change, and no laboratory findings support the symptoms.

Treatment

Treatment includes investigating symptoms and ruling out any underlying general medical condition. Psychotherapy, including behavior modification, is a helpful treatment option.

Prognosis

The prognosis for cure is very poor.

Prevention

Because the etiology is unknown and a familial tendency for the disorder exists, no prevention is known. Encourage the patient to develop skills for dealing with stress.

Patient Teaching

Encourage patients to keep their regularly scheduled appointments. Using one health care provider may eliminate unnecessary tests and repeated procedures. Support the patient through the condition. Explain any diagnostic test results.

Functional Neurological Disorder (Conversion Disorder)

Description

Functional Neurological Disorder causes neurological symptoms that cannot be explained by a medical condition or neurological disease. These symptoms cause problems with functioning in daily life.

ICD-10-CM Code	F44.4 (Conversion disorder with motor symptom or deficit) F44.6 (Conversion disorder with sensory symptom or deficit)

Symptoms and Signs

Symptoms include deficits in voluntary motor or sensory functions (paralysis) that are unintentional and preceded by conflicts or other stressors. Clinically significant social and occupational functioning is present. The patient may not be able to walk or lose some of their "senses ability." Signs and symptoms vary, depending on the type of functional neurologic disorder, and may include specific patterns. Typically, this disorder affects your movement or your senses, such as the ability to walk, swallow, see or hear. Symptoms can vary in severity and may come and go or be persistent. However, you can't intentionally produce or control your symptoms.

Sensory symptoms may include anesthesia, hyperesthesia, analgesia, and paresthesia. Motor symptoms may include paralysis, tremors, tics, contractures, and ambulation disturbances. Speech disturbances may include aphonia and mutism, and visceral symptoms may include headaches, difficulty with swallowing and breathing, choking, coughing, nausea, vomiting, belching, cold and clammy extremities, weight loss, and pseudocyesis. Blindness and seizures also may be noted.

Patient Screening
Patients with initial symptomology, as previously described, require prompt attention. Many of the complaints warrant referral to an emergency facility. Careful neurologic and psychological screening will reveal the diagnosis of conversion disorder.

Etiology
The cause of this psychiatric syndrome is usually a highly stressful situation.

Diagnosis
The diagnosis is based on a history of the preceding event and the classic pattern of acute onset of symptoms. A complete physical examination rules out underlying pathologic conditions.

Treatment
Treatment is supportive and symptomatic. The course of this disorder is usually short, with many cases resolving in a few weeks, especially when the stressful situation is eliminated. Recurrence is common. Psychotherapy and hypnosis are treatment options.

Prognosis
The prognosis varies, depending on the intensity of the stress. Most cases do resolve within a few weeks, but recurrence is common.

Prevention
Avoiding extremely stressful situations may prevent the condition.

Patient Teaching
Encourage patients and families to find ways to reduce stressful situations. Help them find support groups, and encourage them to become involved in them.

Pain Disorder

Description
Pain disorder manifests as pain that causes significant distress and physical and social impairment. This pain is very real to the patient and takes control of the patient's activities.

ICD-10-CM Code F45.41 *(Pain disorder exclusively related to psychological factors)*
(F45.41–F45.42 = 2 codes of specificity)

Symptoms and Signs
Pain disorders include the subtypes that are associated with psychological factors, those associated with both psychological factors and general medical conditions, and those associated with only general medical conditions. The pain is severe and lasting and may have a clinical basis. The response to pain depends on the patient's interpretation, but this type of pain interferes with life activities (e.g., occupational, social, and other areas of functioning). The pain may be associated with musculoskeletal disorders (herniated disk, osteoporosis, and arthritis), neuropathies, and malignancies. Chronic pain often causes depression.

Patient Screening
Pain is very real in these patients, and underlying clinical factors should be assessed. These patients require prompt attention.

Etiology
The pain may be related to underlying clinical pathologic conditions. Psychological factors may play a role in the onset and severity of the pain. Occasionally, both clinical pathologic and psychological factors contribute to the manifestation of the condition. This condition is not intentionally produced, as is malingering.

Diagnosis
Diagnostic studies may reveal pathologic change. Because pain is subjective and pain disorder may or may not have a clinical basis, determining the extent of the pain and psychological involvement is difficult. Longstanding pain may cause depression and even lead to suicide.

Treatment
Any underlying identifiable pathologic change is treated. Patients with terminal disease may be given narcotics to relieve intractable pain. Psychotherapy may be of some help. The patient may be referred to a pain management specialist for evaluation and long-term treatment. This may include physical therapy, acupuncture, exercise regimens, meditation and or yoga, massage, dietary changes and weight loss. Weight loss physicians may also prescribe pain medications and recommend joint or epidural steroid injections, nerve blocks, spinal cord stimulation, radiofrequency ablation, or neuromodulation.

Prognosis
The prognosis varies, depending on the underlying pathology and the cause of pain.

Prevention
Because this condition is not intentionally produced, prevention depends on the underlying pathology.

Patient Teaching

Patient teaching includes information about their treatment plan and following all the physician's recommendations as directed.

Factitious Disorder

Description

Factitious disorder, formerly called *Munchausen syndrome*, is a serious mental illness in which the patient simulates symptoms of illness and presents for no apparent reason other than to get special attention and empathy given to those who are truly ill.

ICD-10-CM Code	F68.12 *(Factitious disorder with predominantly physical signs and symptoms)*
	(F68.10–F69 = 6 codes of specificity)

Symptoms and Signs

Patients with factitious disorder seek medical attention so that they can draw attention to themselves. If they are truly sick, they exaggerate their symptoms to appear sicker than they really are. Some individuals make themselves ill by injecting foreign material to cause a fever or doing other things to cause illness. They make up medical histories and may also tamper with instruments or results. These patients generally have extensive knowledge of medical terminology, medical diagnosis, and how the medical community functions.

Factitious disorder imposed on another occurs when someone, usually a parent, projects the symptoms to the child, usually a preschooler. This parent often stimulates or causes the illness in the child and then presents the child for treatment. The parent denies any knowledge of the actual cause and relates the symptoms to be GI, genitourinary, or CNS in nature. As in factitious disorder, the degree of the complaint is limited only by the caregiver or parent's medical knowledge.

Patient Screening

Until underlying clinical causes are eliminated, these patients require prompt attention.

Etiology

The cause of this behavior is uncertain. Some researchers believe it results from some type of trauma during childhood.

Diagnosis

These patients present at a hospital or physician's office with reports of fever, anemia, dermatitis, or seizure activity expecting to receive medical attention. The symptoms have an atypical clinical course with laboratory findings that are inconsistent with the symptoms. They have a dramatic flair but give vague answers when questioned closely. When the initial workup indicates no particular disease entity, symptoms change. The patient eagerly undergoes multiple invasive procedures. The patient has a history of repeated hospitalizations with no firm evidence of an underlying disease process. In addition, the patient has no motive for financial gain, only that of attention. Physicians may use the criteria in the Diagnostic and Statistical Manual of Mental Disorders (DSM-5 TR), published by the American Psychiatric Association to diagnose the condition.

Treatment

Eventually, the behavior is revealed, and when these patients are confronted with this fact, they seek attention at another facility. The patient may be coaxed to see a mental health expert for treatment in some cases.

Prognosis

The prognosis varies, depending on the duration of the condition. Intervention is necessary in a factitious disorder imposed on another. This is a severe form of child abuse and the authorities must be notified.

Prevention

There is no known prevention.

Patient Teaching

A nonjudgmental attitude by the health care provider may help reduce the severity of the condition. All instructions given by the provider should be followed.

◆ ENRICHMENT

Malingering

Malingering is the feigning of symptoms for financial or personal gain. The action is deliberate and fraudulent, and the symptoms are usually exaggerated. The patient may report these symptoms to avoid or delay various undesirable events. The diagnosis is difficult because the symptoms often are subjective and cannot be disproved.

Gender Dysphoria

Description

Gender dysphoria, according to the Diagnostic and Statistical Manual of Mental Disorders, is defined as a "marked incongruence between their experienced or expressed gender and the one they were assigned at birth."

ICD-10-CM Code	F64.2 *(Gender dysphoria of childhood)* F64.1 *(Gender dysphoria in adolescence and adulthood)*
	(F64.1–F64.9 = 4 codes of specificity)

Symptoms and Signs

Gender identity is a person's inner sense of maleness or femaleness. In this disorder, the person feels as if she or he really should be the opposite sex. Evidence of strong cross-gender identification is present, and the person has a discomfort about the assigned sex at birth.

Those assigned male at birth have a substantial preoccupation with feminine activities, including dressing in feminine clothing and playing with traditionally girl toys. Competitive sports and typical boy activities and play are avoided. Some people assigned male at birth indicate that they do not want their penis and would prefer to have a vagina.

Those assigned female at birth display a dislike for feminine attire and prefer male type of clothing. They prefer boys as playmates and engage in typical boy sports and games. Many claim that they will grow a penis and do not want breast growth or menses.

During adulthood, these persons have a strong desire to adopt the role of the opposite sex and to seek out physical change through hormonal or surgical intervention. They are not comfortable in the gender role defined by society. They take on the characteristics of the other sex and dress accordingly.

Regardless of age, many of these patients experience social isolation and ostracism. They frequently have anxiety, eating disorders, low self-esteem, and may have problems with substance use disorder. There are also individuals who have suicidal thoughts and may have attempted or died due to suicide.

Patient Screening
Gender dysphoria becomes a very important issue in the individual's and his or her parents' lives. When any patient or caregiver calls with a medical issue needing to be addressed, one should offer understanding and validation of the issue by scheduling an appointment at the earliest available time.

Etiology
The etiology of the syndrome is uncertain.

Diagnosis
Observation of the behavioral patterns leads to suspicion of gender dysphoria, but there is no known diagnostic test for this syndrome.

Treatment
Psychological counseling to recognize and acknowledge the feelings may be of value. Sex reassignment through hormone treatment and surgical intervention often helps these patients. Unisex bathrooms make such individuals feel more at ease in the office setting.

Prognosis
The prognosis varies, depending on the extent of the feeling and the extent of the action taken. Many sex change surgical procedures are successful when accompanied by intense psychotherapy. Family and employment relationships may affect the success of treatment.

Prevention
No prevention is known.

Patient Teaching
Patients should follow prescribed treatments, and postoperative care instructions if applicable.

Sleep Disorders

The "*The International Classification of Sleep Disorders (ICSD-3-TR)* divides sleep disorders into six major categories: Insomnia disorders, sleep-related breathing disorder, central disorders of hypersomnolence, circadian rhythm sleep-wake disorders, parasomnias, and sleep-related movement disorders.

Sleep disorders are assessed through polysomnography, which measures four rapid eye movement (REM) and the four nonrapid eye movement (NREM) sleep stages: stages 1, 2, 3, and 4. It takes approximately 90 minutes to go through one cycle of REM and NREM sleep.

The disorders can be caused by functional or organic disorders, so underlying pathologic conditions must be ruled out or treated.

Insomnia

Description
The individual experiencing insomnia has difficulty in falling asleep and/or staying asleep.

ICD-10-CM Code	G47.00 *(Insomnia, unspecified)* (G47.00–G47.09 = 3 codes of specificity)

Symptoms and Signs
Difficulty falling asleep, returning to sleep if awakened in the middle of the night, or staying asleep, are symptoms of insomnia. Those with insomnia feel physically and mentally tired, groggy, tense, irritable, and anxious on awakening. In addition, some people experience extreme early-morning awakening and report that their sleep was not restorative.

Patient Screening
Chronic insomnia becomes a very important issue in the individual's life. Schedule the first available appointment.

Etiology
The cause may be related to a situation, a medical problem, or time zone changes (e.g., jet lag), or the cause may be a change to high altitudes. Additional causes are pain, cardiovascular problems, thyroid conditions, and fever. Stimulants, including caffeine, amphetamines, steroids, alcohol, nicotine, and bronchodilators, tend to cause drug-related insomnia. Psychological causes include anxiety, stress, and even the fear of sleeplessness itself.

Other causative factors may be environmentally related and include room temperature that is too hot or too cold, noise, brightness, or light, an uncomfortable bed, or a sleep partner who snores, is restless, or has restless legs syndrome.

Diagnosis

To be diagnosed with insomnia, the sleeplessness must have been present for 3 nights per week for a period of 3 months. According to the DSM-5-TR, "The condition has three primary symptoms. 1. Challenges falling asleep (onset insomnia). 2. Inability to maintain sleep. (middle insomnia). 3. Early-morning wakefulness (late insomnia). The symptoms must be present for 3 nights per week for a minimum of 3 months. The individual must have enough or ample opportunity to sleep and cannot have another sleep-wake diagnosis or disorder, or another physical or mental condition to explain the insomnia experience." Sleep studies may also be performed to confirm the diagnosis and to rule out other causes.

Treatment

The first step in treatment is to identify and remove the cause; this is followed by an attempt to improve sleep. Patients are counseled to change their lifestyle to relieve tension and reduce stress. They are encouraged to keep a regular sleep schedule, to consider the bedroom only for sleep, and not to worry about stressful situations. Noise and disruptions during normal sleep time should be eliminated, and daily activities should be increased. Caffeine, nicotine, and stimulants should be avoided in the late afternoon and evening. Strenuous physical exercise also should be avoided in the few hours before retiring. A darkened and quiet environment would help. The patient should keep a regular bedtime and a regular time for arising. Psychotherapy may be indicated to help relieve anxiety and stress. Hypnotic medications such as zolpidem (Ambien), zaleplon (Sonata), eszopiclone (Lunesta), and ramelteon (Rozerem) are used to induce restful sleep. Benzodiazepines may be prescribed in some instances. Other therapies include the use of melatonin, trazodone, or diphenhydramine. When these therapies are ineffective, patients usually are referred to sleep disorder clinics.

Prognosis

The prognosis varies, depending on the cause.

Prevention

Eliminating caffeine, nicotine, and other stimulants during late afternoon and evening hours helps prevent insomnia. Developing good sleep habits, such as keeping regular hours of retiring, also helps prevent insomnia. Avoiding the use of electronic technology such as a cellphone, tablet, or computer can also help prevent insomnia, as these devices suppress the production of melatonin.

Patient Teaching

Instruct patients about normal sleep patterns and about avoiding caffeine, nicotine, and other stimulants in the late afternoon and evening hours. As previously mentioned, patients should be encouraged to avoid the habit of using digital technology and watching television or reading in bed. Help them to identify environmental changes they could make to improve the sleep environment.

Sleep-Related Breathing Disorder

Sleep-related breathing disorders include obstructive sleep apnea, parasomnias, narcolepsy, and restless leg syndrome. These disorders can contribute to insomnia. Sleep difficulties are linked to both physical and emotional or mental problems. Parasomnias, sleep-related disorders, and narcolepsy are explored more in-depth.

Parasomnias

Description

Parasomnias are a group of sleep disorders that involve strange or abnormal behaviors during sleep such as sleepwalking, night terrors, and nightmares. Parasomnias may also be termed *sleep arousal disorders* and often include dreams.

ICD-10-CM Code	G47.9 *(Sleep disorder, unspecified)* (G47.50–G47.9 = 12 codes of specificity)

Symptoms and Signs

Parasomnias are more common in children but can also affect adults. People who sleepwalk generally have no memory of the event; however, they are able to perform things they would normally do when awake, such as fix food or attempt to drive a car. They awake confused, with blank expressions on their faces, and are unaware of the environment. Those experiencing nightmares often have vivid recall and remember dreams of fear of attack, falling, and death. These dreams occur late at night.

Patient Screening

Although usually not an emergency, parasomnia becomes a very important issue in the individual's life. Schedule an appointment at the earliest available time. When safety is an issue, an appointment should be scheduled on the same day.

Etiology

Several elements, including possible genetic, developmental, psychological, and organic factors, may precipitate the incidents. Febrile episodes or brain tumors may be the causes. Lithium and certain drugs precipitate the condition. There is evidence that certain medications cause increased REM sleep periods and rebound REM sleep. Stress, anxiety, trauma, drug use, and other factors can result in nightmares.

Diagnosis

Reports of the episodes lead to further investigation. A thorough history should include any drug consumption. Any underlying cause in older adults and mature adults should be investigated and diagnosed.

Treatment

Protection from injury is primary for the sleepwalking person. Leading the person who is sleepwalking back to their bed is the best course of action. It is not dangerous to wake someone who is sleepwalking, but sometimes their reaction cannot be anticipated and could be aggressive, which is why the recommendation is to lead them to bed rather than wake them up. Minimizing exposure to terror, especially from movies, videos, and television programs, reduces the occurrence of night terrors. Children usually outgrow these conditions. Adults often are treated initially with zolpidem or zaleplon, because these drugs do not leave patients feeling drugged when they wake up in the morning. When drugs are suspected as a contributing factor, alternative drug therapy is considered.

Prognosis

The prognosis varies, depending on the cause. Many children will outgrow parasomnia. When the etiology is drug related, eliminating the causative drug helps.

Prevention

Minimizing stimulating factors, such as exposure to frightening movies, helps prevent this condition. Additionally, having a regular bedtime and a comfortable environment conducive to sleep and avoiding caffeine, electronics at bedtime, and other stimulants is helpful in prevention.

Patient Teaching

Family members should be advised not to interrupt or attempt to awaken the person who is sleepwalking unless there is an imminent danger. Parents are advised to use caution when discussing stressful events that may cause a child to become anxious.

Narcolepsy

Description

Narcolepsy, irresistible daytime sleep episodes, can have a duration of a few seconds to hours.

ICD-10-CM Code	G47.419 *(Narcolepsy without cataplexy)* (G47.411–G47.429 = 4 codes of specificity)

Symptoms and Signs

Narcolepsy, a chronic neurologic condition, is an overwhelming recurring compulsion to fall asleep. Usually precipitated by sedentary, monotonous activity, narcolepsy attacks occur while driving, sitting in a lecture, or even eating. The onset normally is before age 25 years but can happen at any time. A period of sleep paralysis may occur. Sleep paralysis may also be accompanied by hallucinations, however hallucinations can also occur as the person falls asleep. Those hallucinations are referred to as *hypnagogic*. Hallucinations are referred to as *hypnopompic* if they happen on waking. The person is unable to move, but breathing continues. There are two types of narcolepsy. People with type 1 narcolepsy may also experience cataplexy and have muscle tone loss during an episode. Cataplexy is brought on by strong emotions such as laughing.

Patient Screening

The patient experiencing episodes of narcolepsy requires prompt attention.

Etiology

People with narcolepsy enter REM sleep quicker than individuals who do not have narcolepsy. Some cases are believed to result from a lack of a chemical in the brain hypocretin(orexin). This chemical helps regulate sleep. Research continues in determining the exact cause of narcolepsy.

Diagnosis

A history of repeated episodes suggests narcolepsy. Seizure activity and sleep apnea should be ruled out. Sleep studies help in confirming the diagnosis.

Treatment

The patient should take therapeutic naps and establish a normal night sleep pattern. Drug therapy helps. Stimulants, including methylphenidate and dextroamphetamine, are prescribed. Modafinil (Provigil) and armodafinil (Nuvigil) are nonamphetamine stimulants and wakefulness-promoting drugs and may be prescribed for excessive daytime sleepiness. These patients must be warned of the dangers of falling asleep while driving or operating machinery. This chronic disorder is not under voluntary control.

Prognosis

The prognosis varies depending on the adaptation techniques the patient develops. The patient's response and tolerance to drug therapy may also dictate the outcome of this condition.

Prevention

No prevention is known.

Patient Teaching

Patients should follow the provider's recommendations and also understand that narcolepsy that occurs while driving or operating machinery is potentially dangerous. Assistance with accommodations may be available with medical documentation in the education and work setting. Workers should look for jobs that will keep them active and allow for interaction with others. Patients should avoid jobs that require them to make long drives or operate dangerous equipment.

Sleep-Related Breathing Disorders

Description

Sleep apnea is intermittent short periods of breathing cessation during sleep.

ICD-10-CM Code	G47.30 *(Sleep apnea, unspecified)* (G47.30–G47.39 = 9 codes of specificity)

Symptoms and Signs

Sleep apnea is considered a potentially life-threatening condition. During normal nocturnal sleep, the patient has periods in which breathing ceases, followed by snorting and gasping. The patient may snore loudly, sound like they are choking, or gasp for air during sleep. This condition occurs more often in males than in females and may be associated with obesity, hypertension, or an airway obstructive condition. The patient does not feel rested even after several hours of sleep.

Sleep apnea may be categorized as obstructive, central, or complex. The more common type is obstructive, in which air is unable to flow in or out of the upper airway. Attempts to breathe continue. During central episodes, the brain does not send appropriate messages to the intercostal muscles and the diaphragm to initiate the breathing process. The patient can experience many more periods of apnea in 1 hour. Complex sleep apnea is the term used when someone who is being treated for obstructive sleep apnea converts to central sleep apnea. This may also be referred to as *treatment-emergent central sleep apnea.*

Patient Screening

The patient experiencing episodes of sleep apnea requires prompt attention.

Etiology

Patients appear to have an inherent predisposition to this condition. Nasal obstruction often is the cause. Alcohol ingestion, smoking-related bronchitis, and sleep deprivation are other causes. Obesity can cause extra tissue to develop in the throat, creating a mechanical obstruction. As levels of oxygen (O_2) drop and levels of carbon dioxide (CO_2) increase, the brain is alerted to stimulate the breathing process, and the individual usually gasps for air.

Diagnosis

The diagnosis begins with a sleep history. The onset usually occurs in middle age. Daytime sleepiness, sleep attacks, and snoring and snorting episodes also suggest sleep apnea. Sleep laboratory studies and polysomnography confirm the diagnosis by observing periods of breathing cessation while the patient is sleeping.

Treatment

Weight loss is encouraged. Research indicates that if an individual is obese, weight loss of 10% can minimize symptoms.

• **Fig. 14.16** Adult using a continuous positive air pressure machine. (From Niedzwiecki B, Pepper J: *Kinn's the medical assistant: an applied learning approach*, ed 15, 2023, Elsevier.)

Protriptyline is prescribed. Continuous positive air pressure (CPAP) or dental appliances may be tried (Fig. 14.16). Any underlying pathologic condition should be diagnosed and corrected. The patient is advised to avoid the use of any drugs that depress the CNS. Uvulopalatopharyngoplasty, a surgical procedure to remove portions of the uvula, soft palate, and posterior pharyngeal mucosa, is attempted as a last resort. Alcohol, tobacco, and sedatives tend to cause a collapse of the upper airway passages during sleep and, therefore, should be avoided.

Prognosis

The prognosis varies depending on the cause. When overweight patients lose weight, they often experience significant improvement. Use of CPAP usually relieves symptoms and reduces the danger of respiratory arrest.

Prevention

No prevention is known.

Patient Teaching

Patients using CPAP will need instructions on how to use the equipment. They will also need patient education on healthy nutrition plans and surgery, if applicable.

Personality Disorders

Description

A personality disorder is a pattern of behavior that deviates from society's norms. In addition, a person with a personality disorder typically has thoughts about the self and the world that cause inappropriate behavior. Signs of a personality disorder become evident in adolescence. There are several named personality disorders, categorized into three clusters.

ICD-10-
CM
Code

Cluster A
F60.0 *(Paranoid personality disorder)*
F60.1 *(Schizoid personality disorder)*
F21 *(Schizotypal disorder)*
Cluster B
F60.2 *(Antisocial personality disorder)*
F60.3 *(Borderline personality disorder)*
F60.4 *(Histrionic personality disorder)*
F60.81 *(Narcissistic personality disorder)*
Cluster C
F60.6 *(Avoidant personality disorder)*
F60.7 *(Dependent personality disorder)*
F60.5 *(Obsessive-compulsive personality
         disorder)*
F60.9 *(Personality disorder, unspecified)*

Symptoms and Signs

Personality disorders influence the mental affect of a person and produce chronic, ingrained, maladaptive behavior. Disordered patterns of relating, thinking, and perceiving impair social and occupational performance. Personality disorders typically begin to appear in adolescence but should not be diagnosed until adulthood. A history of longstanding problems in interpersonal relationships and occupational difficulties is likely. Personality traits may give the person a reputation of arrogance or painful shyness and for rejecting responsibility for his or her behavior. The person tends to project negative feelings and blame others. Many types of personality disorders are recognized, each with unique distinguishing characteristics. Examples of personality disorders include paranoid, schizoid, antisocial, histrionic, and narcissistic disorders.

Cluster A

Cluster A personality disorders should be assessed and distinguished from delusional disorders and psychotic disorders.

Paranoid Personality Disorder
Those with paranoid personality disorder do not trust others and are suspicious of others. They assume others will exploit, harm, or deceive them. Individuals with paranoid personality disorder often misinterpret the meaning behind others' behaviors by thinking others are deliberately trying to exploit them.

Schizoid Personality Disorder
Individuals with schizoid personality disorder (SPD) appear to lack or show emotions of pleasure or pain. They tend to be loners and do not enjoy relationships with others. They appear to be indifferent, flattened, or detached.

Schizotypal Personality Disorder
Persons with schizotypal personality disorder are similar to those with SPD in that they have difficulty with social relationships. Individuals with schizotypal personality disorder, however, typically have ideas of reference; they may

be superstitious or preoccupied with paranoid phenomena. In addition, they may believe they have magical control over others. More often, they seek treatment for associated symptoms of anxiety or depression.

Cluster B

Antisocial Personality Disorder
Individuals with antisocial personality disorder have a disregard for and tend to violate the rights of others. They fail to conform to societal norms and often engage in behavior that could be grounds for arrest. These individuals are aggressive, manipulative, and reckless. They generally do not show remorse or make amends for their behavior.

Borderline Personality Disorder
A person with borderline personality disorder (BPD) has a pattern of unstable interpersonal relationships, self-image, and affects (feelings). Impending separation or rejection are central concerns for individuals with BPD. When those with BPD believe they are being rejected or abandoned, they often react with extreme emotions, such as anger, panic, or despair. They may display extreme sarcasm and verbal outbursts. They are impulsive and manipulative in their behavior.

Histrionic Disorder
Individuals with histrionic disorder display overly dramatic and theatrical mannerisms. They have a conscious or unconscious pervasive need to be the center of attention. People with this disorder are immature and dependent, constantly seeking approval and reassurance. Behavior or appearance may be inappropriately seductive.

Narcissistic Disorder
The narcissistic personality demonstrates pathologic self-love or grandiose self-admiration. When criticized, the person reacts with rage or humiliation, based on an exaggerated sense of self-importance. These individuals lack empathy and tend to exploit others. They exhibit a preoccupation with fantasies of unlimited success.

Antisocial disorder

Behavior patterns of the antisocial personality cause frequent conflicts with societal values. Troublesome conduct usually emerges before age 15 years, with truancy, fighting, stealing, a history of running away, or cruel behavior. Antisocial persons do not express guilt or learn from their mistakes. Other traits include a propensity for irresponsible and impulsive actions.

Cluster C

Avoidant Personality Disorder
The person with avoidant personality disorder avoids any social situation because of fears of criticism, disapproval, or rejection. Individuals with avoidant personality disorder view themselves as socially inept, personally unappealing, and inferior to others. They are preoccupied with being judged or criticized by their peers.

Dependent Personality Disorder

Individuals with dependent personality disorder have a pattern of excessively relying on others to make decisions for them. They are passive and have trouble disagreeing with others because they fear losing support or approval.

Obsessive-Compulsive Personality Disorder

Individuals with obsessive-compulsive personality disorder have an extreme pattern of preoccupation with orderliness, perfection, and mental and interpersonal control. They are preoccupied with details or lists to the point that they never finish a task.

Patient Screening

Individuals displaying these behaviors or family members reporting the behavior and requesting an appointment should be given an appointment as soon as convenient.

Etiology

The cause of personality disorders has not been identified. Various theories include possible biological, social, or psychodynamic origins.

Diagnosis

The diagnosis of personality disorders is based on the documentation of diagnostic criteria defined in DSM-5-TR.

Treatment

The treatment of personality disorders depends on the symptoms and includes psychotherapy and, in some cases, drug therapy. Pharmacologic treatments are often prescribed to address specific symptoms demonstrated by the individual. Improved coping mechanisms and control of symptoms are the goals of therapy. A trusting relationship between patient and therapist is advantageous because some people with these disorders tend to be noncompliant and resist therapy. Specialized psychotherapy incorporating specific limits and boundaries (dialectical behavioral training) has been shown to be effective in helping these clients feel more secure and in control. Hospitalization may be required during acute episodes that incapacitate the person. Family involvement in group therapy has proved beneficial for some patients. Treatment of comorbid conditions, such as anxiety and depression, with medications, is essential. Personality disorders themselves do not respond to drug therapy.

Prognosis

The prognosis for cure is very poor. Treatment of comorbid conditions improves outcomes. Long-term treatment is necessary.

Prevention

Treatment in adolescence when symptoms first appear, and ongoing treatment into adulthood, seems to lessen the frequency of behaviors. No prevention is known.

Patient Teaching

It is important to encourage the patient to comply with continued treatment and drug therapy.

Review Challenge

Answer the following questions:
1. What are the contributing factors to mental disorders?
2. What observations may indicate intellectual developmental disorder??
3. What variants are considered in the diagnosis of a learning disorder?
4. What are the characteristics of a child with autism?
5. What are the diagnostic criteria for attention-deficit/hyperactivity disorder?
6. What are the diagnostic criteria for a tic disorder?
7. Under what conditions may dementia occur?
8. Why is Alzheimer disease so difficult to diagnose?
9. How may vascular dementia be related to atherosclerosis?
10. How might head trauma cause dementia?
11. How does repeated heavy alcohol abuse harm the body?
12. What are some effects of a rising blood alcohol level on the brain?
13. Why is schizophrenia considered a major psychiatric disturbance?
14. How do bipolar disorders affect an individual?
15. What is thought to cause a major depressive disorder?
16. What are the phases of the grief process?
17. What are some of the longstanding problems typical of personality disorders?
18. How are the major anxiety disorders classified? How do they differ from each other?
19. What condition may result as a delayed response to an external painful event?
20. What is a somatization disorder?
21. How is anxiety related to a conversion disorder?
22. What condition results from preoccupation with illness and abnormal fear of disease?
23. Can severe pain cause illness?
24. How is factitious disorder diagnosed?
25. What is the typical pattern of sleep disorder in (1) insomnia, (2) narcolepsy, and (3) sleep apnea?
26. What are the three clusters of the 10 personality disorders?

Real-Life Challenge: Alzheimer Disease

A 75-year-old male is diagnosed with Alzheimer disease. The retired businessman noticed many memory lapses, primarily in the area of short-term memory and the inability to concentrate. His family states that his verbalization appears somewhat diminished in that he has difficulty expressing his thoughts in an appropriate manner and interjects nonsensical phrases. He becomes agitated quite easily and has very

little interest in grooming and self-appearance. The family has been advised that they may need help in the future to care for the patient and that he probably will have to be institutionalized.

Because the patient has exhibited both cognitive and behavioral symptoms of Alzheimer disease, he is treated with donepezil (Aricept) and alprazolam (Xanax).

Questions

1. Who is most likely to exhibit symptoms of Alzheimer disease?
2. List the typical symptoms.
3. What interventions may be taken?
4. What are some of the theories that have been advanced regarding the cause of Alzheimer disease?

5. How is Alzheimer disease diagnosed?
6. What is the anticipated prognosis for this patient?
7. What differentiates Alzheimer disease from senile dementia?
8. To what class of drugs does Xanax belong and what is the expected outcome of its administration?

Real-Life Challenge: Sleep Apnea

The wife of a 48-year-old male complains that she cannot sleep because of her husband's loud snoring. Questioning reveals she has noticed that he appears to stop breathing for periods of about 30 seconds when sleeping. The patient has a history of mild alcohol consumption

and also of smoking. He is approximately 30 pounds overweight.

Sleep studies are ordered because sleep apnea is suspected. He also says he does not feel rested after sleeping 8 to 9 hours a night.

Questions

1. What is the significance of the loud snoring?
2. Why is a history of social habits (smoking and alcohol consumption) important?
3. What are sleep studies?

4. What may happen if sleep apnea is not diagnosed?
5. Which treatment may be prescribed?
6. What is the anticipated outcome of the treatment?

Internet Assignments

Ascertain what services are available at the Alzheimer Association for families of individuals diagnosed with Alzheimer disease. Write a report listing and explaining these services and how the family may obtain the services.

Locate meeting sites for Alcoholics Anonymous in your community and the regular meeting times and days.

Critical Thinking

1. List some of the methods of play that a therapist might use with children who have been abused.
2. List some of the causes of intellectual developmental disorder.
3. What are some of the suggested ways to prevent intellectual developmental disorders?
4. Learning disorders affect performance on standardized tests, causing lower-than-expected scores for age, schooling, and intelligence level, as a result of the brain's ability to receive and process information. List and define some of the learning disorders.
5. What might be some of the psychological effects on the individual with learning disorders even after childhood? How may the diagnosis of learning disorders

affect the family? How does this diagnosis affect the educational system?
6. Children often exhibit difficulties in communication. These disorders may be psychologically based and are a variety of expressive language disorders, including mixed receptive or expressive language disorders. List some of the disorders along with how they may affect the child, the parents, the rest of the family, and the educational system
7. The individual who experiences stuttering may be made fun of in school. What might the school do about this form of "bullying"?
8. What is the prognosis for the autistic individual in society?

9. Research gender dysphoria, and create an informational handout for patients to share with their family members and friends.

10. List some of the symptoms of attention-deficit/hyperactivity disorder (ADHD). How may this disorder affect individuals in adult life?

11. Oppositional defiant disorder is a strong predictor of poor outcomes in children. List some of the possible poor outcomes.

12. List and describe some of the tic disorders.

13. An older individual has been diagnosed with early-onset dementia. The person's judgment and reaction times are slightly reduced. How would you approach the topic of cessation of driving?

14. List possible causes of dementia.

15. Alcoholism contributes to many crises in life. List some of the problems. How does alcoholism affect your community?

16. The misuse of various drugs that modify mood or behavior is called *drug abuse*. List various drugs that are commonly abused. How are these drugs obtained? What is the effect of drug abuse on your community?

17. What are some of the effects of drug abuse on the individual and the family?

18. How does schizophrenia affect the individual? What is the prognosis for the individual who has been diagnosed with schizophrenia?

19. In a mood disorder, a person experiences a pathologic disturbance in mood that affects all aspects of his or her life. List the mood disorders.

20. What is meant by a manic episode? List some of the activities an individual experiencing a manic episode may do.

21. What is the opposite of a manic episode? How does this affect the individual's life?

22. What is a major concern for the individual experiencing major depressive disorder?

23. How does depression affect the individual's family? How does it affect his or her employment?

24. What are the causes of major depression disorder?

25. List types of depression, their causes, and possible outcomes of the disorders.

26. What may be the cause of panic disorder?

27. List phobias, and describe how they are treated.

28. Posttraumatic stress disorders (PTSDs) are different from other anxiety disorders because the cause of the stress is an external event of an overwhelmingly painful nature. List some of the reactions of individuals experiencing PTSD.

29. How is PTSD treated? How does this disorder affect your community?

30. What are somatoform disorders? List the types and describe their symptoms,

31. How does factitious disorder affect the family?

32. How are individuals experiencing gender identity difficulties accepted in their families and their communities?

33. List the types of parasomnias.

34. What are treatment options for sleep apnea?

35. List the three clusters of personality disorders and each disorder within the cluster.

Prepare to discuss Critical Thinking case study exercises for this chapter that are posted on Evolve.

Credentialing Examination Questions

1. Which type of disorder is stuttering?
   A. Central nervous system
   B. Peripheral nervous system
   C. Speech
   D. Maxillofacial

2. Which statement best describes intellectual development disorder?
   A. Physical appearance is only noted abnormality
   B. Interferes with acquisition of intellectual skills
   C. Treated with medications
   D. Diagnosed after age 40

3. An individual has problems communicating but is able to memorize certain lists or cite facts. Which disorder do these characteristics describe?
   A. Autism spectrum
   B. Attention-deficit hyperactive
   C. Oppositional defiant
   D. Tourette

4. Which disorder involves symptoms of motor tics?
   A. Autism spectrum
   B. Attention-deficit hyperactive
   C. Oppositional defiant
   D. Tourette

5. Losing weight can have an effect on the symptoms of which sleep disorder?
   A. Nonobstructive sleep apnea
   B. Obstructive sleep apnea
   C. Parasomnias
   D. Narcolepsy

6. As a group, which disorders represent the single largest mental health problem in the United States?
   A. Anxiety
   B. Communication
   C. Phobias
   D. Bipolar

7. A patient feels uncomfortable with the gender they were assigned at birth and seeks medical help. Which term is accurate when discussing this diagnosis?
   A. Gender confusion
   B. Gender dysphoria
   C. Genetic gender disorder
   D. Nongenetic gender disorder
8. The patient experiences pain and medical conditions are ruled out. Which condition are they most likely experiencing?
   A. Functional neurological pain
   B. Obsessive-compulsive disorder
   C. Phobic disorder
   D. Somatic system disorder
9. A patient is diagnosed with factitious disorder. What symptoms are classic with this diagnosis?
   A. Atypical clinical course with laboratory findings that are not consistent with the symptoms
   B. Typical clinical course with consistent laboratory findings
   C. Symptoms consistent with metastatic cancer
   D. Abdominal pain with gastrointestinal ulcers confirmed by endoscopy
10. How many nights per week must a person have sleeplessness for a period of 3 months to be diagnosed with insomnia?
    A. One
    B. Two
    C. Three
    D. Four

15

Disorders and Conditions Resulting From Trauma

CHAPTER OUTLINE

LEARNING OBJECTIVES

After studying this chapter, you should be able to:

1. List the major types of trauma.
2. List the environmental factors that may result in trauma or other conditions.
3. Distinguish between an abrasion and an avulsion injury.
4. Describe conditions that require prophylaxis with tetanus toxoid.
5. Name three factors that generally need to be addressed in open trauma.
6. Explain the risk of puncture wounds to health care workers.
7. Describe the management of foreign bodies in the ear, eye, and nose.
8. Name the conditions classified as thermal insults.
9. Explain the "rule of nines" in adults with burns and how it is used.
10. Describe the possible injuries caused by (1) electrical shock and (2) lightning.
11. Define *hypothermia* and list those most at risk.
12. Describe the guidelines for treating (1) frostbite, (2) insect bites, and (3) snakebites.
13. Discuss various conditions resulting from cumulative trauma.
14. Explain the pathology that results in the pain and numbness of carpal tunnel syndrome.
15. Explain the importance of immediate intervention in shaken infant (baby) syndrome.
16. Name the best management strategies for child abuse and neglect and elder abuse and neglect.
17. Discuss special concerns in the diagnosis of (1) intimate partner violence, (2) sexual abuse, and (3) rape/sexual assault.
18. Discuss the signs of impending suicide and possible interventions.

KEY TERMS

abrasion (ah-BRAY-shun)
analgesic (an-ahl-GEE-sik)
antipyretic (an-tee-pye-RET-tic)
antiseptic (an-tih-SEP-tic)
avulsion (ah-VUL-shun)
biodefense (BY-O-DE-fens)
cautery (KAW-ter-ee)
débride (day-BREED)

ergonomic (er-go-NOM-ic)
hyperabduction (high-per-ab-DUCK-shun)
hyperthermia (high-per-THERM-ee-ah)
hypothermia (high-poh-THERM-ee-ah)
laceration (lass-er-AY-shun)
prophylaxis (proh-fih-LACK-sis)
tendinitis (ten-deh-NYE-tis)
vector (VECK-tor)

Trauma

Traumatic occurrences include physical and psychological injuries that are derived from external force or violence. Trauma may be self-inflicted, accidental, or the result of an act of violence and can interfere with body functions or the homeostatic status of the body. Trauma can result in a permanent disability, or it may be life threatening. Major types are open trauma, assault trauma, thermal trauma, and psychological trauma. Whether physical or emotional, trauma (including abuse and sexual attack) is prevalent in every society. Physical trauma is a leading cause of death in the United States among people ages 1 to approximately 44 years.

Environmental factors sometimes result in traumatic circumstances. Weather-related conditions are often contributing factors in the occurrence of thermal insults and motor vehicle accidents (MVAs), along with accidents involving other types of machinery or accidents caused by natural elements (e.g., lightning strikes or tornadoes). Severe wind and changes in barometric pressure are responsible for trauma to the tissues and to the respiratory system in those exposed to these elements. Poisons may come from contaminated groundwater, toxins in the air, ingestion of seafood gathered from contaminated locations, or chemical spills. Bites from animals, insects, reptiles, or humans may occur under particular environmental circumstances. High altitudes also can affect body functions. Precaution and prevention are of primary concern whenever people are subjected to potentially traumatic circumstances.

Triage means "to sort or pick" and is a process used to determine the severity of injury or illness in each patient who enters any medical facility. The goal of an effective triage system is the rapid identification of a patient's needs and the ability to identify urgent and life-threatening conditions. Placing a patient in the right place at the right time to use the proper resources and appropriate level of health care to meet the patient's medical needs is mandatory. A system should be in place in every medical facility to provide a communication system and support team to facilitate the needs of the patient. Trauma centers can provide specialized critical care on a 24-hour basis for those seriously injured. Services include a specially trained medical team, medical devices to provide intensive care measures, and a facility equipped for surgical intervention, if needed.

Open Trauma

Open trauma may involve only the skin surface, or it may extend to the soft tissue and structures far below the skin surface. It may be in the form of an abrasion, in which the skin surface is scraped away, or it may be an avulsion, in which the tissue or an appendage is torn away. The injury can involve only a small area of the skin, as with a puncture wound, a slightly larger area as in an injury caused by a missile, or encompass substantially larger areas, as with crushing injuries. All incidents of open trauma have a commonality: the risk of infection if the wound is not appropriately cleansed and dressed. Pain also is usually involved in most open trauma.

Open wounds can be the source of tetanus infection; therefore tetanus prophylaxis must be provided. Those who have completed the initial inoculation series for tetanus require a booster dose every 10 years. Those with no previous inoculation history are given tetanus immune globulin (human) and referred to a physician for the complete series of tetanus toxoid inoculations. When the patient has not had a booster injection within the past 10-year period, the booster injection of tetanus, diphtheria, and pertussis (Tdap) is recommended and/or administered.

Bleeding can be a factor in open trauma and must be addressed at once. Some injuries need only basic first aid, whereas others require medical intervention and surgical repair. Regardless of the severity of the injury, appropriate treatment aids healing and lessens scarring.

Abrasions

Description
Abrasions occur when the outer layers of the skin are scraped away or roughed up and the deeper layers are exposed.

ICD-9-CM Code	919.0 *(Abrasion or friction burn without mention of infection)*
ICD-10-CM Code	T07 *(Unspecified multiple injuries)*

Open wounds are coded by site and type. Once the diagnosis has been confirmed, refer to the current editions of the ICD-9-CM and ICD-10-CM coding manuals for the appropriate code.

Symptoms and Signs
The injured area appears raw and reddened, is painful, and has a small amount of bleeding (Fig. 15.1). The exposure of sensitive nerve endings causes a burning type of pain in the injured area; small foreign particles may be embedded in it.

Patient Screening
Abrasions require prompt cleansing. Current tetanus prophylaxis should be confirmed.

Etiology
Abrasions are caused by friction created when a rough, hard surface comes in contact with skin as a consequence of a scraping or sliding type of motion, often the result of a fall or scrape. An example is when a child falls off a bicycle and "skins" the knee. Such injuries are often referred to as *friction burns, floor burns, rug burns, strawberries or road rash.*

Diagnosis
Diagnosis is made on the basis of subjective information (what the patient says), history, and visual inspection.

Treatment
Treatment consists of gentle washing and irrigation of the area with a germicidal soap and water to remove any bacteria and contamination. Any foreign particles, such as gravel and dirt, which have not been removed by cleansing should be removed carefully with forceps. Failure to remove foreign particles left in the skin can stain the epidermis and cause scars or

• **Fig. 15.1** Abrasion. (A) Outer layers of the skin are scraped away. (B) Abrasion wounds of the elbow. (From Browner BD, Fuller RP: *Musculoskeletal emergencies*, Philadelphia, 2012, Saunders.)

• **Fig. 15.2** Avulsion. (A) A flap of skin has been torn away. (B) Avulsions over the foot and ankle. (From Browner BD, Fuller RP: *Musculoskeletal emergencies*, Philadelphia, 2012, Saunders.)

discoloration. Next, an antibiotic ointment or cream may be applied. A dressing may be applied as well, depending on the size and location of the abrasion to help keep the wound clean and protected. The dressing should be changed each day or if there is drainage present more frequently. Prophylaxis with Tdap injection is confirmed or administered, if necessary. Topical anesthetic spray can be purchased over the counter (OTC) and used to lessen the pain when an abrasion or similar wound needs initial or continued cleaning.

Prognosis
The prognosis for healing is good once cleansing to remove any foreign bodies or bacteria is accomplished. The extent of scarring depends on the depth and extent of the insult.

Prevention
Prevention is difficult, especially in active individuals. Protective gear or leather clothing worn sometimes by cyclists helps prevent extensive "road rash" abrasions.

Patient Teaching
Instruct the patient on appropriate wound care, the importance of keeping the wound clean and dry, and not to "pick"

at the scab once formed. The patient should also be told to avoid direct sunlight and to protect the new fragile skin with sunscreen or clothing for 6 months to prevent pigment changes in the skin. Provide written instructions to the patient regarding signs and symptoms of infection and when to report concerns.

Avulsion

Description
With avulsion injuries, a portion of the skin and possibly underlying tissue is torn away, either completely or partially (Fig. 15.2). At times, the injury may include separation of the bone area, which is a more serious injury.

ICD-10-CM Code	S31.000A (*Unspecified open wound of lower back and pelvis without penetration into retroperitoneum, initial encounter*)

Open wounds are coded by site and type. Once the diagnosis has been confirmed, refer to the current edition of the ICD-10-CM coding manual for the appropriate code.

Symptoms and Signs

An avulsion injury can involve a limb, an appendage, or any soft tissue area anywhere on the surface of the body. The patient usually has severe pain in the area. Bleeding from the wound is common. When the avulsion is partial, the avulsed tissue is still partially attached to the injured area. Larger avulsed areas are considered a serious injury. One type of severe avulsion is a "degloving" injury, in which the full thickness of skin is peeled away from the body, such as the skin on the hand or foot.

Patient Screening

Avulsion injuries require immediate attention. Prompt cleansing and closure of the open wound are important. When the avulsed tissue is available (i.e., still partially attached to the body or retrieved from the accident site, as in the case of a severed fingertip) and reattachment is possible, the surgical procedure is performed as quickly as possible. Current tetanus prophylaxis should be confirmed. An appointment should be made as soon as possible, or the patient sent to an emergency facility for larger and deeper avulsion injuries.

Etiology

The mechanism of this kind of injury is usually one in which the affected body part becomes entangled in machinery, clothing, or some other means of entrapment, causing the skin, tissue, and possibly bone to be torn and pulled away from the body. If the limb or appendage is severed completely from the body, it is termed an *amputation*.

Diagnosis

The diagnosis is made by performing a visual inspection of the affected part and examining the history of the injury mechanism.

Treatment

Treatment consists of controlling the bleeding, cleansing the area, and surgically repairing the tissue. If an amputation has occurred, the stump or remaining area must be cleansed and surgically repaired. The patient will likely be treated prophylactically with antibiotics to prevent infection. A sterile dressing is applied to the repaired wound. Tetanus prophylaxis is confirmed, or Tdap injection is administered, if necessary. Pain medication is prescribed and administered, when necessary. Revascularization is needed for increased blood supply in some instances when repairing with a skin graft. Application of basic fibroblast growth factor is also used to promote epithelialization in severe cases. Immobilization followed by physical therapy after bone healing may be necessary in cases of open fractures and avulsion.

Prognosis

The prognosis depends on the extent of the insult. Prompt intervention helps promote the healing process.

Prevention

Prevention is difficult, and the likelihood of injury is unpredictable. Following safety guidelines when operating machinery, especially wearing fitted and not loose clothes, is important, as is confining long hair that could be pulled into equipment and cause a scalp or facial avulsion.

Patient Teaching

Reinforce the importance of following safety guidelines. Instruct the patient on wound care and the importance of keeping the wound clean and dry. Provide the patient with written instructions regarding the signs and symptoms of infection. Encourage patients to keep any follow-up appointments as scheduled. Written instructions for wound care and signs of infection should be shared.

Crushing injuries

Description

Crushing injuries occur when a part of the body is compressed with extreme force between two surfaces.

> ICD-10-CM Code   S77.20XA
> *(Crushing injury of unspecified hip with thigh, initial encounter)*
> (S77.00–S77.22 = 9 codes of specificity)

Symptoms and Signs

A crushing injury may involve any body part, but most often, a finger, hand, toe, or foot is the involved part. The patient experiences pain and may not be able to move the injured part. Soft tissue is compressed or crushed, and depending on the amount of pressure involved in the mechanism of injury, bone, nerves, and vessels may also be crushed.

Patient Screening

Crushing injuries require prompt assessment and intervention. Many individuals who sustain such an injury are transported to an emergency facility. If not, they should be seen as soon as possible on the day of the injury or referred to an emergency facility. When a crushing injury occurs at the workplace, workers' compensation forms and any mandatory drug and alcohol screening must be completed. Witnesses may be interviewed if the patient is unable to give details and as with any patient interaction, all documentation is important.

Etiology

The crushing injury occurs when the affected body part becomes pressed between two hard surfaces. Examples of such injuries are fingers shut in doors, hands or fingers caught in presses, heavy objects being dropped on feet or toes, and compression of any body part as a result of an MVA. Falling debris, such as building parts broken loose in a storm, tornado, earthquake, or other natural disaster, can also cause crushing injuries.

Diagnosis

The diagnosis is made on the basis of history, visual inspection of the body area, and physical examination. Radiographic studies, ultrasound, and MRI of the injured part also aid in the diagnosis.

Treatment

Treatment depends on the severity and location of the injury. When an open wound is present, the area is cleansed, irrigated, and débrided, if necessary. Immobilization of the affected limb or appendage follows any surgical repair that is indicated. Sterile dressings will likely be applied to any open wound or surgical area to help prevent bacterial infection. If the crushing injury involves the head or trunk of the body, appropriate triage of the patient, monitoring of vital signs, and surgical intervention is undertaken. Tetanus prophylaxis is confirmed, or Tdap injection is administered, if necessary, and oral antibiotics may be prescribed as an additional prophylactic measure.

Prognosis

The prognosis depends on the extent of the insult. Prompt intervention and treatment help hasten the healing process.

Prevention

Prevention is difficult in some cases; however, there are things that can lessen the risk of crush injuries. Wearing a seatbelt at all times can help prevent crush injuries from MVAs. Following US Occupational Safety and Health Administration (OSHA) safety guidelines at work can also aid in prevention.

Patient Teaching

Reinforce safety guidelines to prevent further injury. Instruct the patient on wound care and the importance of keeping the wound clean and dry. Reinforce the value of being up to date with tetanus prophylaxis. Encourage patients to keep any follow-up appointments as scheduled.

❖ ENRICHMENT

Needlesticks

Health care providers are at risk for puncture wounds from contaminated needlesticks. US Occupational Safety and Health Administration (OSHA) guidelines and facility guidelines must be followed to lessen the risk of occurrence. This also reduces the likelihood of transmitting acquired immunodeficiency syndrome, hepatitis B, hepatitis C, and any other bloodborne diseases. Safety devices should be used for insertion of IV, performing phlebotomy and capillary punctures and administering injections, in addition to disposal of all sharps according to OSHA guidelines. Surgical instruments should also be handled with care to avoid puncture wounds.

❖ ENRICHMENT

Trauma and Compassion

MVAs occur throughout the world on a daily basis. Physical trauma resulting from an MVA or an accident can result in life-altering changes both physically and mentally. Stress, anxiety, and fear of driving or riding as a passenger in a car can result. Health care personnel should be aware that most patients involved in any type of accident or trauma will not understand the medical language being used or why they are being examined so extensively to check for neurological reflexes. Compassion is always important, especially when providing emergency care.

Images of injuries sustained by a 22-year-old female, front seat passenger, after a car turned directly in the path of a vehicle she was inside. The patient was treated at a trauma center for femur, left radius and ulna, and right metacarpal fractures. (A) Surgical site for femur repair. (B) Right metacarpals, lateral view. (C) Metacarpals were repaired with plates and pins. (Courtesy Kaitlynn Sue Fuqua.)

• **Fig. 15.4** Impaled object. A nail is impaled in the skin.

• **Fig. 15.3** Puncture wound. (A) A pointed object has punctured the skin. (B) Puncture wound of the foot. (From Browner BD, Fuller RP: *Musculoskeletal emergencies*, Philadelphia, 2012, Saunders.)

Puncture Wounds

Description

Puncture wounds result when a pointed or sharp foreign object penetrates the soft tissue (Fig. 15.3). Animal bites, discussed later in this chapter, also may be considered puncture wounds.

ICD-10-CM Code	S31.000A *(Unspecified open wound of lower back and pelvis without penetration into retroperitoneum, initial encounter)*

Open wounds are coded by site and type. Once the diagnosis has been confirmed, refer to the current edition of the ICD-10-CM coding manual for the appropriate code and modifier.

Symptoms and Signs

Puncture wounds cause pain and usually very little bleeding. Redness at the site may be noted, or there may be no indication of the wound other than the pain. A puncture wound may not have a dramatic appearance; therefore meticulous

inspection of the area and underlying structures should be carefully performed. If the foreign body that caused the injury is protruding out of the wound, it is described as an *impaled object* (Fig. 15.4).

Patient Screening

Puncture wounds require prompt assessment and cleansing. Tetanus prophylaxis needs to be confirmed. Impaled objects require stabilization to keep the object in the same position until assessment and treatment are accomplished. Removing an impaled object may cause more damage to tissues, nerves, and vessels.

Etiology

A puncture wound occurs when a sharp, pointed object penetrates the skin and underlying soft tissue. The offending object may be a needle, a nail, a splinter of glass, wood, or metal, a knife, or even a bullet. The object first penetrates the skin, and then the skin closes around the object or point of entry. As a result, bleeding is minimal. In some situations, bleeding will occur as the penetrating object is removed. Puncture wounds near joints are at risk for bacterial infection, and wounds on the bottom of the foot are at risk for cellulitis but any puncture wound can get infected and have complications. Some animal bites cause puncture wounds.

Diagnosis

Diagnosis is made by visual examination, history, and sometimes radiographic studies (if the object can be visualized by imaging). Some embedded objects can be visualized only by using magnetic resonance imaging (MRI). An impaled object is easily observed because it protrudes from the injured site.

Treatment

Treatment involves the removal of the foreign body, along with copious irrigation of the wound with sterile fluid. A sterile dressing is applied. Tetanus prophylaxis is confirmed or

Tdap injection is recommended and/or administered, if necessary. Antibiotics may be prescribed as an additional prophylactic measure. Impaled objects are stabilized until they can be removed by the physician. As with other work-related injuries, workers' compensation forms and any required drug or alcohol screening testing must be completed. Some puncture wounds are allowed to heal from the inside out to prevent infection. Once closed, if bacteria are inside the wound, the infection will typically worsen. If bacteria are present in the wound, the wound may become infected after it is closed with sutures, complicating the healing process.

Prognosis

The prognosis varies, depending on the extent and depth of the puncture wound.

Prevention

Prevention is difficult in some cases. All employees should follow OSHA-recommended safety device use and wear protective clothing such as steel-toed safety shoes, hard hats, and safety goggles.

Patient Teaching

Instruct the patient on wound care and on keeping the wound clean and dry. Provide the patient with instructions on the signs and symptoms of infection. Reinforce the importance of tetanus prophylaxis.

Lacerations

Description

Lacerations result when a sharp object cuts the skin and possibly underlying soft tissue.

> ICD-10-CM Code   S31.000A *(Unspecified open wound of lower back and pelvis without penetration into retroperitoneum, initial encounter)*
>
> *Open wounds are coded by site and type. Once the diagnosis has been confirmed, refer to the current edition of the ICD-10-CM coding manual for the appropriate code.*

◆ ENRICHMENT

Penetrating Injuries

Violence in today's society results in various forms of penetrating injuries. These injuries may be the result of knife wounds (stabbings), gunshot wounds, explosions, and intentional impaling of a pointed or sharp object or instrument.

Although the victims are not usually seen in an office setting, families often seek appointments to speak with the physician about the injury and prognosis. Some victims may be seen in the office after release from emergency care and/or during rehabilitation for treatment.

Symptoms and Signs

Lacerations result when a sharp object cuts the skin and possibly the underlying soft tissue. Lacerations cause pain and moderate to severe bleeding. The edges of the cut may be smooth or jagged depending on what object did the cutting. The bleeding is generally proportionate to the depth and length of the laceration.

Patient Screening

Lacerations require prompt cleansing and repair.

Etiology

Lacerations occur when a sharp instrument, such as a knife or sharp piece of glass or metal, cuts the skin and underlying soft tissue (Fig. 15.5).

Diagnosis

Diagnosis is made on the basis of visual examination. History may reveal the type of sharp object that caused the injury. A laceration with smooth edges that can be approximated cleanly is termed an *incision* (Fig. 15.6).

• **Fig. 15.5** Laceration. Skin is cut by a sharp object.

• **Fig. 15.6** Incision. A laceration with smooth edges.

Treatment

Lacerations should be cleansed gently with germicidal soap and water. If the laceration is not too deep and bleeding is controlled, approximating and securing the edges with tape, a butterfly dressing, or sterile adhesive strips (Steri-Strips) may be the only intervention necessary other than a sterile dressing application. In some cases a medical adhesive such as Dermabond may used to hold the edges together, thereby eliminating the need for sutures. Lacerations that are deep, have jagged edges, or continue to bleed need to be débrided and have the edges trimmed to facilitate good approximation. Bleeding should be controlled by either coagulation or suture. Suturing of the wound will probably be necessary. If the laceration is over a movable joint, immobilization of the area is indicated. A sterile dressing should be applied. Tetanus prophylaxis is confirmed, and Tdap injection is recommended and/or administered, if necessary, and antibiotics may be prescribed as an additional prophylactic measure.

If the laceration results from a work-related injury, workers' compensation forms and any required drug or alcohol screening testing must be completed.

Prognosis

The prognosis varies, depending on the location, length, depth, and condition of the laceration. The degree of approximation of the edges of the wound may determine the extent of the scarring.

Prevention

Prevention is difficult. Care when using knives should be stressed. Following OSHA guidelines when working can prevent some accidents.

Patient Teaching

Instruct the patient on wound care and the importance of tetanus prophylaxis. When sutures have been used for closure, instruct the patient regarding when to return for suture removal and that signs and symptoms of infection should be reported promptly. All medications should be taken as prescribed.

Foreign Bodies

Anything that enters a portion of the body where it does not belong is considered a foreign body. Common sites for entrapped foreign bodies include the ears, the eyes, and the nose, but any surface area of the body can be involved.

Foreign Bodies in the Ear

Description

Foreign bodies in the ear typically range from bugs, pebbles, and bits of cotton to anything small enough to fit in the ear canal.

ICD-10-CM Code	T16.1XXA *(Foreign body in right ear, initial encounter)*
	T16.2XXA *(Foreign body in left ear, initial encounter)*
	T16.9XXA *(Foreign body in ear, unspecified ear, initial encounter)*

Symptoms and Signs

The patient complains of feeling stuffiness and something in the ear. If the foreign object is a bug, the patient may also complain of a buzzing sound in the ear. Complaints of pain in the ear canal and decreased hearing capability may be expressed. Anything small enough to fit in the ear could be the offending foreign body. Visualization of the ear canal usually shows an apparent object.

Patient Screening

Although not a life-threatening condition, individuals with foreign bodies in the ear require prompt assessment and intervention.

Etiology

Flying insects may enter the ear canal accidentally in the course of flight, and instances of a bug crawling into the ear when an individual is lying down have been reported. Children have a tendency to place small objects in their ear canals. Small toys, beads, buttons, cereal, grapes, peas, beans, and pebbles are examples of some of the objects commonly found in the ear canals of children. Vegetative foreign bodies, such as wood splinters or thorns, may lead to infection. Foreign bodies in the ear should be removed as quickly as possible. Cotton from cotton-tipped applicators also may be the offending object; the cotton inadvertently comes off of the applicator stick during a cleaning process. Anything small enough to be placed into the ear canal could be a problem, especially in the case of children.

Diagnosis

Diagnosis is made on the basis of history and visual and/or otoscopic inspection of the ear canal (Fig. 15.7A).

Treatment

The goal of treatment is the removal of the offending object without damaging the ear canal or the tympanic membrane. Many times, the object simply may be grasped by forceps and removed. Food and cereal can absorb moisture from the ear canal and swell to the point of being compressed against the walls of the ear canal. Such objects may require removal by a physician with the use of gentle, controlled suctioning. The individual with a live bug in the ear should be placed in a dark room and have a flashlight shined in the ear. Bugs that are alive should crawl out of the ear toward the light. Bugs that are not responsive to the light technique may have to be washed out of the ear. In that case, the ear canal is

• **Fig. 15.7** (A) Foreign body in the ear. (B) Eye irrigation. (A, From Swartz MH: *Textbook of physical diagnosis*, ed 5, Philadelphia, 2006, Saunders; B, From Eagling and Roper-Hall: *Eye injuries: an illustrated guide*, 1986, Butterworth-Heinemann.)

gently irrigated. If this is not successful, then gentle suction may be necessary to remove the foreign body.

Prognosis

The prognosis is good with prompt removal of the foreign body, with no consequential damage to the ear canal or the tympanic membrane.

Prevention

Prevention includes educating children about not putting anything in their ears. Cotton-tipped applicators should be kept out of the reach of children and extreme caution used when attempting to cleanse the ears with them.

Patient Teaching

Stress the dangers of putting small objects in the ears and encourage parents to seek medical intervention when a child has a foreign body in the ear canal.

Foreign Bodies in the Eye

Description

Foreign bodies in the eye are objects that would not normally be found in the eye. Common offenders are bugs, rust, dust, sand, hair, small pieces of metal, or small pieces of brush or tree branches. Chemicals may be accidentally splashed in the eye.

ICD-10-CM Code	T15.90XA (Foreign body on external eye, part unspecified, unspecified eye, initial encounter)
	T15.91XA (Foreign body on external eye, part unspecified, right eye, initial encounter)
	T15.92XA (Foreign body on external eye, part unspecified, left eye, initial encounter)
	(T15.00 [7th digit]–T15.92 [7th digit] = 12 codes of specificity)

Foreign bodies in the eye are coded by site. Once the diagnosis has been confirmed, refer to the current edition of the ICD-10-CM coding manual for the appropriate code.

Symptoms and Signs

The individual complains of pain and a scratching sensation or irritation of the eye. The patient may report blurred or compromised vision. Tearing is usually present.

Patient Screening

Foreign objects in the eye require prompt evaluation and intervention. If the injury involves splashed chemicals, immediate irrigation of the eye is advised. If an immediate appointment is not available, the individual should be referred to an emergency facility. Patients should be encouraged to have someone else provide their transportation; they should not attempt to drive. If the object is impaled and sticking out of the eye, the emergency medical service (EMS) is the recommended mode of transport to the hospital after stabilization of the impaled object has been accomplished.

Etiology

Foreign bodies in the eyes can result from a number of sources and routes of entry. A common source of rust and metal particles in the eye is the undercarriage of a car; the person working under a car may inadvertently knock loose rust particles or minute scraps of metal that then fall into the eye. Accidents involving objects that have been propelled through the air, possibly as the result of an explosion, also can result in a foreign body entering the unprotected eye. Grass particles, tree leaves, and shrubbery debris can also get into the eye when working in a yard. Foreign objects also may be propelled into the eye as a result of an MVA or sports injury. A bug flying into the eye is a common occurrence. Occasionally just rubbing the eyes with dirty hands can be the source of entry for dirt or a chemical. Dust trapped under a contact lens are other sources of foreign substances in the eye.

Diagnosis

The diagnosis is made from visual and ophthalmoscopic examinations of the eye. A history of feeling something in the eye combined with the circumstance of possible exposure to foreign bodies is helpful. Staining the eye with fluorescein to visualize a corneal abrasion confirms the presence or previous presence of a foreign body.

Treatment

Treatment involves removing the offending material. Many times, gentle irrigation of the eye with normal saline will flush dust, bugs, or debris out of the eye (see Fig. 15.7B). Tears also help with the natural removal of a foreign body.

When the foreign body is embedded in the eye, the physician may attempt removal with surgical instruments. The eye may be numbed by using anesthetic eye drops such as proparacaine. If these procedures are unsuccessful, an immediate referral to an ophthalmologist or emergency department is made. Ophthalmic antibacterial drops or ointments may be placed in the eye, and the eye is usually covered with a patch. Because eyes have sympathetic movement, it is the usual procedure to bandage both eyes. Metal pieces or rust fragments falling from the undercarriage of a motor vehicle may result in eventual rust rings forming in the eye. These may have to be removed by an ophthalmologist to prevent staining.

Prognosis

The prognosis varies, depending on the offending material and the depth and involvement of the eye structures. Many injuries caused by bugs and dust will resolve after cleansing irrigation. Extensive corneal abrasions may result in residual scarring and compromised vision. Chemical burns may result in blindness. If the patient rubs the eyes while the foreign body is still in the eye, this can lead to more eye insult.

Prevention

Wearing approved eye protection is the best prevention for occupational and other possible insults by foreign objects to the eye. Protective eyewear while mowing grass, using a weed eater, and trimming shrubbery is also recommended.

Patient Teaching

Encourage the use of eye protection whenever any possible hazard to the eye is anticipated. When a foreign object other than minute dust particles enters the eye and is not removed successfully by gentle irrigation, encourage the individual to seek professional treatment. When one eye is patched or covered with a bandage, make the patient aware that depth perception will be absent, and encourage care in navigating steps.

Patients who have experienced metal in their eyes will need to be advised that if they require an MRI in the future, the radiology technician must be informed that the metal was in their eye as a foreign body.

❖ ENRICHMENT

Emergency Medical Service

The emergency medical service (EMS) provides prehospital care in emergency situations. Those responding may be paramedics, emergency medical technicians (EMTs), or first responders. This system is designed to provide early or lifesaving medical intervention for those who have a need for urgent and immediate medical care. This emergency care is followed by rapid transport to an emergency facility usually by ground or air transfer for further evaluation or advanced medical care.

Initially, the person experiencing a medical problem, or someone else at the scene, can quickly survey the situation and determine whether entry into the EMS system is warranted. Access to the EMS system is achieved by telephone and dialing 911.

It is important to realize that once an individual is entered into the system, emergency care will be provided until a physician orders it to cease. When a valid *Do Not Resuscitate* order exists for an individual, medical care is managed accordingly.

Illnesses for which the system may be called include chest pain; shortness of breath; unconsciousness; possible stroke; accidental injuries, including possible poisoning; possible suicide or accidental overdose; severe falls with neck, back, or leg injuries; serious motor vehicle crashes with serious injuries; burns; lightning injuries; electrocutions; possible or near-drownings; impaled objects; and gunshot wounds. Impending precipitous childbirth, severe bleeding, near-choking, and asthma attacks may require immediate emergency care provided by the EMS.

The caller will be asked to supply the phone number from which the call is being made, the location of the individual requiring the emergency treatment, and the nature of the emergency. Additionally, the caller will be instructed to remain on the line until help arrives. This is to maintain contact for updates on the individual's status, to provide instructions for treatment that can be rendered until help arrives, and for additional location information. In cases of cardiac arrest or cessation of breathing, the caller will be provided with instructions on beginning and performing cardiopulmonary resuscitation (CPR).

❖ ENRICHMENT

Mock Disaster Drills

Emergency medical management, emergency departments, police departments, fire departments, and emergency medical transport services conduct mock disaster drills. Hospitals, medical facilities and health educational institutions may also conduct mock drills. During these drills, mock disasters or accidents are orchestrated to provide as realistically as possible incidents for simulated events and health care professionals' training. Mock patients are transported to emergency facilities, and extra staff is called in to help provide service. Triage is practiced, and patients are assigned on the basis of their injuries or trauma to a health care provider.

Foreign Bodies in the Nose

Description

Any object or foreign material that is causing an obstruction in the nares should be considered a foreign body in the nose, and medical intervention for removal should be sought.

ICD-10-CM Code	T17.0XXA *(Foreign body in nasal sinus, initial encounter)*
	T17.1XXA *(Foreign body in nostril, initial encounter)*

Symptoms and Signs

Children have the most occurrences of foreign bodies wedged or stuck in the nares. Parents usually note mucus running from one of the nares, swelling near the bridge of the nose, and congested breathing. On investigation, they are able to confirm that one of the nares is constricted and that air is not moving through the affected side.

Patient Screening

Foreign bodies in the nose require prompt assessment and treatment.

Etiology

Children have a tendency to insert foreign objects into their noses. These foreign bodies include but are not limited to cereals, dried peas or beans, grapes, plastic, pebbles, toys or small doll shoes, and anything else small enough to fit in the nares. Dry materials, such as dried peas, beans, and cereal, have a tendency to absorb moisture from the mucous membrane and then swell, creating an obstruction.

Diagnosis

Ther diagnosis is made on the basis of history and visualization of the foreign body in the nares. Often mucus is dripping from the unobstructed nares and may be foul smelling.

Treatment

The child is encouraged to blow the nose in the hopes that the object will be expelled. Closing one side of the nare while blowing out the other side may provide a little more force when blowing. The child should be old enough to understand not to inhale, or the child may inhale the object. physician may need to grasp the object with forceps for removal or use a suction device if the forceps will not reach far enough.

Prognosis

The prognosis is good when the removal of the offending object is uncomplicated and complete.

Prevention

Prevention is difficult because children often have a tendency to insert small objects into their noses.

Patient Teaching

Counsel children not to place any objects in their noses. Emphasize that dried objects will swell and that medical intervention may be needed to correct the situation.

Thermal Insults

Thermal insults can be caused by either heat or cold, which includes burns or frostbite. Extreme temperatures cause conditions such as hypothermia, hyperthermia, heat stroke, and heat exhaustion. Regardless of the variance in temperature (hot or cold), most conditions resulting in a severely altered state can be life threatening if left untreated. However, hypothermia may be a protective factor in the case of a near-drowning in cold water.

Burns

Description

Burns are the result of thermal insults to tissue. The insults may be caused by heat, chemical sources, electrical sources, or radiation. Heat sources that cause injury may be in the form of dry heat, steam, or hot substances; sun rays are also capable of causing a burn.

ICD-10-CM Code	T30.0 *(Burn of unspecified body region, unspecified degree)*
	T30.4 *(Corrosion of unspecified body region, unspecified degree)*

Burns are coded by site, degree, and body surface involved. Once the diagnosis has been confirmed, refer to the current edition of the ICD-10-CM coding manual for the appropriate code.

Symptoms and Signs

The patient who has experienced a burn usually has pain. The extent of the burn, along with the percent of body surface involved, usually is related proportionately to the degree of pain. Depending on the depth and nature of the burn, the skin surface may be reddened, blistered, or charred (Fig. 15.8).

Patient Screening

Burns require prompt assessment and intervention. After evaluation and stabilization, patients with major burns are referred to burn centers for treatment. Knowing the mechanics of the injury is important in determining the type of treatment intervention required; this includes assessment of respiratory status, wound contamination, eye involvement, and fluid management. The emergency medical service (EMS) is appropriate for severe burns or those that cover large areas of the body.

Etiology

Burns can be caused by flame, dry heat, liquid scalds, radiation, chemicals, overexposure to the sun, or electricity. Exposure of the skin to any of these sources can cause

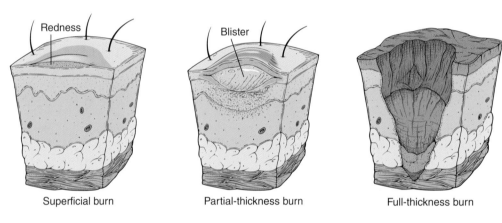

• **Fig. 15.8** (A) Examples of burns. Partial-thickness burn; note the blisters. (B) Full-thickness burn; note the dark color. (Courtesy Judy Knightton, Ross Tilley Burn Center, Sunnybrook and Women's College Health Center, Toronto, Ontario, Canada.)

Redness   Blister

Superficial burn   Partial-thickness burn   Full-thickness burn

• **Fig. 15.9** Depths of burns. The extent of involvement of layers of the skin.

destruction of the skin. Injury to the underlying soft tissue is proportionate to the duration of the exposure and the intensity of the thermal source.

Diagnosis

Diagnosis is made on the basis of visual examination and history. In the type of burn caused by flames, it is necessary to determine whether the burn occurred inside an enclosed space or out in the open. The respiratory state of any patient with this type of burn must be assessed. The status of the eyebrows, eyelashes, and nasal hair must be determined. Any singeing of these hairs indicates that the patient inhaled the flame or superheated air and that the respiratory status may be in grave danger.

Determination of the depth (Fig. 15.9) of burns is important. Pain intensity depends on the amount of nerve tissue that is involved or destroyed. Superficial burns involve only the outer layers of the skin, which usually appear only reddened, and yet these burns are painful. Partial-thickness

burns involve all layers of the skin; they produce blisters and are quite painful. Full-thickness burns involve both the skin and the underlying subcutaneous tissue. Resultant destruction of nerve endings often results in minimal pain in that particular area; however, pain may be reported in areas around the periphery of the burn site. Prompt assessment of the percent of skin surface area involved in the burn injury is achieved by applying the "rule of nines." The "rule of nines" provides a fast and fairly accurate calculation of the body surface involved. Percentages used to ascertain the burned tissue area in the adult are as follows: head, 9%; anterior trunk, 18%; posterior trunk, 18%; entire right arm, 9%; entire left arm, 9%; anterior surface right leg, 9%; posterior surface right leg, 9%; anterior surface left leg, 9%; posterior surface left leg, 9%; and perineum, 1%. (Fig.15.10) Percentages in children and infants are slightly different. The Lund & Browder and Palmer methods can also be used to estimate burn percentage based on different formulas. Another method of designating a percentage

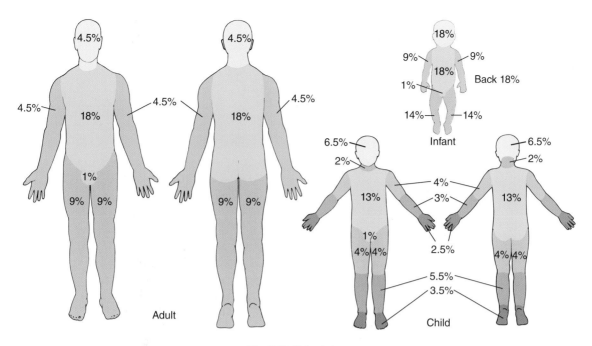

• **Fig. 15.10** Rule of nines.

of body surface involvement is used by the *International Classification of Diseases*, 10th revision, Clinical Modification (ICD-10-CM) code books. Refer to the current edition of the ICD-10-CM code books for these percentages.

Treatment

Treatment depends on the source of burns. Heat burns (from flames, liquid scalds, or superheated air) should be cooled with cool water and covered with dry sterile dressings until the patient can be seen by a physician. Sunburns should be treated with the application of cool water, and the damaged skin may be sprayed with **antiseptic** and **analgesic** sprays (Fig. 15.11). OTC medications such as ibuprofen or other nonsteroidal antiinflammatory drugs(NSAIDs) and or acetaminophen may be used for relief of sunburn pain. Cool compresses applied to the areas of sunburned skin may also provide pain relief.

Skin burned with chemicals other than lime must first be brushed away, should be flushed with cool water for at least 15 minutes, covered with a sterile dressing, and treated by a physician. The water can help reduce tissue damage if applied for an accurate amount of time. Electrical burns should be examined for points of entry (rings, belts, necklaces) and exit (knees, fingers, and toes) (Fig. 15.12A). These areas should be covered with dry sterile dressings and treated by a physician.

Minor burns are usually treated with an antibacterial cream or ointment. Severe burns require specialized treatment with surgical débridement of the burned tissue and skin grafts, if necessary.

Patients with severe large-area burns, older adults, the very young with burns, and those with severe burns to the face, hands, feet, or perineal area usually are admitted to a burn center, where they receive specialized burn care.

• **Fig. 15.11** Sunburn. (From Weston WL, et al: *Color textbook of pediatric dermatology*, ed 4, St. Louis, 2008, Mosby.)

Respiratory status (if the respiratory tract is involved), fluid and electrolyte balance, and vital signs are monitored. Pain control is accomplished with the use of narcotic analgesics. Tetanus prophylaxis is confirmed or administered, if necessary, and antibiotics may be prescribed as an additional prophylactic measure. A list of the patient's medicine allergies should be obtained. Skin grafting, including the use of cloned skin and the use of autografts, and adjacent tissue grafts, is used for the treatment of extensive destruction of tissue. There are newer methods of skin substitutes being used in burn treatment and studies continue to provide information regarding which type of substitute is best, and for which type of burn. These are divided into two classes of synthetic and biological skin substitutes.

Points of entry
• Necklace
• Belt
• Ring

Points of exit
• Knee
• Toes

A

• **Fig. 15.12** (A) Points of entry and exit for electrical burns. (B) Entry wound from electrocution on the palm of the hand. (C) Exit wound of the same injury on the dorsum of the hand. (B and C, From Klatt EC: *Robbins and Cotran atlas of pathology*, ed 2, Philadelphia, 2010, Saunders.)

The American Burn Association's National Burn Repository requests that forms be completed and submitted. These forms collect information for statistics about burns as well for research. The information submitted includes the name of the facility; admission year; patient age, sex, and race; admission type; discharge date; external causes; and total body surface area percentage.

Some communities request or require the completion and submission of a burn incident report, often to the fire department.

Work-related burns must be reported to state workers' compensation and, in some cases, OSHA. As with other work-related injuries, drug and alcohol testing may be required.

Prognosis

The prognosis varies, depending on the cause and extent of the burned tissue and other organ or system involvement. Prompt intervention helps promote a positive outcome. Scarring is typical.

Prevention

Safety guidelines at work should be followed. Prudent use of fire or combustible materials is helpful. It is wise to be proactive about avoiding situations where burns may occur. Applying sunscreen is strongly recommended when prolonged exposure to the sun is anticipated.

Patient Teaching

Stress the importance of keeping follow-up appointments and complying with prescribed therapy. Provide instruction on wound care and the signs and symptoms of infection. Provide patients information regarding medication use which are known to cause sun sensitivity.

Electrical Shock

Description

Electrical shock is an injury that occurs as the result of exposure to or contact with electricity.

Sunburn

Exposure to the ultraviolet alpha- and beta-rays from the sun can cause sunburn, ranging from mild to severe. A person who has experienced at least three severe sunburns with blistering is at risk for the development of skin cancer. Prevention of sunburn includes avoiding exposure from 10:00 a.m. to 2:00 p.m., which is when the sun's rays are the strongest, applying sunscreen to exposed skin areas, and wearing a hat to protect the scalp and eyes. Those at greatest risk have light or fair skin and freckles and blond or red hair. Acute injury results in hyperemia of the dermis and blister formation. Long-term exposure may stimulate pigmentation but may also promote carcinogenesis and aging of the epidermis and the dermis.

Sun protection factor (SPF) is the technical name for measurement of ultraviolet B (UVB; shortwave) protection provided by sunscreen. The numbers assigned to a product designate the length of time it takes to redden the skin compared with no protection. An SPF of at least 15 is recommended by the Skin Cancer Foundation as protection against the sun's harmful rays, or UVB.

Radiation Exposure

Exposure to radioactive material is another threat to society. "Dirty bombs," which are made of dynamite or other explosives, can have pellets or radioactive particles in their composition. These particles or pellets can be released into the environment by the explosion of the bomb. The three main types of exposure to ionizing radiation are slow, cumulative whole-body exposure; sudden whole-body exposure; and high-dose localized exposure. Sudden whole-body exposure is the most likely form of ionizing radiation exposure for the general public in a terrorist type of event. The body's exposure to radiation may be external irradiation of all or part of the body from an external source, including radiation therapy for cancer treatment, contamination by radioactive material in gases, liquids, or solids that have been released into the environment causing external, internal, or both types of contamination, or by incorporation of the radioactive material as a sequela to other contamination. Symptoms of radiation exposure include nausea, vomiting, and diarrhea; redness and blistering of skin burns; dehydration; weakness, fatigue, exhaustion, and fainting; hair loss, ulceration of oral mucosa, esophagus, and gastrointestinal (GI) tract; vomiting blood and experiencing bloody stools; bruising; sloughing of the skin; and bleeding from nose, mouth, and gums. The extent of the toxicity of ionizing radiation depends on the dose, the distance from the source of radiation, and the length of time of the exposure.

ICD-10-CM Code   T75.4XXA *(Electrocution, initial encounter)*
Burns are coded by site, degree, and body surface involved. Once the diagnosis of a burn has been confirmed, refer to the current edition of the ICD-10-CM coding manual for the appropriate code.

Symptoms and Signs

Patients who have experienced electrical shock may be in cardiac or respiratory failure. They have visible burns at the entrance wound and at the exit wound. If conscious, they experience pain at these sites. Charred tissue may be noted.

Patient Screening

Individuals who have suffered electrical shock constitute a life-threatening emergency. They need to be entered into the EMS for transport to an emergency care facility. Resuscitation and life support may be required during transport.

Etiology

The person who has sustained electrical shock experiences tissue damage from the point of entry of the electricity to the point of exit. The electrical current follows the path of least resistance through the body, usually along nerve routes. The current enters the body at the point of contact with the electrical source and exits at the point of grounding (see Fig. 15.12B and C). As the alternating current passes through the body, it may produce muscle contractions, causing the person to be thrown from the source. This can result in lacerations, fractures, or head trauma. One major concern with electrical shock injuries is the development of cardiac dysrhythmias.

Diagnosis

Diagnosis is made by visual examination and history. Radiographs, complete blood counts, urine and blood muscle enzyme tests, an ECG, and a CT scan may also aid in determining the severity of damage.

Treatment

Treatment consists of maintaining the cardiac and respiratory status. If indicated, cardiopulmonary resuscitation (CPR) must be administered after the patient has been removed from the electrical source. The patient must not be touched if he or she is still in contact with the electrical current. The patient's neurologic status and vascular status are assessed for the extent of tissue destruction. Any fractures, lacerations, and head injuries are treated. The burned areas are débrided and dressed with sterile dressings. Pain management is accomplished with the use of narcotic analgesics. Tetanus prophylaxis is confirmed or administered, if necessary, and antibiotics may be prescribed as an additional prophylactic measure.

Prognosis

The prognosis varies, depending on the extent of the insult and damage to organs and body systems. When a cardiac arrest has occurred, the prognosis may not be favorable, even with prompt resuscitative efforts. It is important to realize that electrical energy will follow nerves on its path through the body and therefore has the potential to cause damage to the peripheral nervous system.

Prevention

Extreme care should be taken in situations that involve repairing or being close to electrical power, and people should be alert for possible electrical accidents at all times. Electrical outlet covers should be used when the outlets are not in use. It is prudent to avoid standing in water when nearby electrical wires are at risk of coming in contact with the water.

Patient Teaching

Advise patients to follow the OSHA guidelines when working with electricity. Encourage them to be aware of potential sources of electrocution in the workplace and in the home environment. Wounds from electrical burns should be cared for as instructed to prevent infection.

Lightning injuries

Description

Lightning injuries occur when an individual is struck directly or indirectly (splash effect) by lightning.

ICD-10-CM Code	T75.00XA *(Unspecified effects of lightning, initial encounter)*
	T75.01XA *(Shock due to being struck by lightning, initial encounter)*
	(T75.00 [7th digit]–T75.09 [7th digit] = 3 codes of specificity)

Burns are coded by type and site. Once the diagnosis of a burn has been confirmed, refer to the current edition of the ICD-10-CM coding manual for additional burn codes.

Symptoms and Signs

Lightning injuries can be classified by the severity of the injury or by the type of strike the person receives. Usually the severity of the injury is in direct proportion to the intensity of the lightning strike.

The victim of a direct lightning strike is probably in a severely compromised state, unconscious, and not breathing. A heartbeat may be present if the apnea has not caused cardiac arrest. Clothing may be literally "blown off" the victim, and the victim may have been propelled through the air by the jolt. Burns usually are noted in areas of the skin where moisture is normally found, such as the axillae and groin or where metal was touching the body (see Fig. 15.12). Motor and sensory disturbances are noted, along with possible ruptured tympanic membranes. The patient who has experienced moderate contact will have less severe symptoms but with an altered level of consciousness and skin burns. The person with minor injuries exhibits fairly normal vital signs, some confusion, amnesia of preceding events, and some minor muscle or sensory nerve disturbances. All may experience some hearing or visual difficulties.

Patient Screening

Lightning strikes constitute a life-threatening situation. Respiratory efforts of the patient may be compromised; providing immediate rescue breathing is imperative. If apnea has caused cardiac arrest, CPR must be instituted immediately. An AED can be used to administer a shock if the patient is in cardiac arrest. It is important to call 911 promptly to enter the victim into the EMS.

Etiology

Lightning can strike a person in five different ways: (1) When the person is struck directly by a lightning discharge, it is termed a *direct strike*. (2) When lightning strikes an object that the person is touching, resulting in transference of the energy, it is termed a *contact strike*. (3) If lightning "jumps" from the primary object it strikes through the air and strikes the person, it is termed a *side splash*. (4) A *blunt injury strike* physically throws a person. (5) When the lightning bolt hits the ground and travels to the person by way of the ground, it is termed *ground strike. An upward streamer* occurs when electrical charges go upward to meet a downward charge.

Lightning tends to flow over the surface of the body, often sparing the deeper tissues.

Diagnosis

Diagnosis is made on the basis of visual examination and a history of the person having been outdoors when lightning occurred or inside a structure that was hit by lightning and in contact with a conductive or grounding source. A detailed neurologic assessment and a thorough examination of the surface of the body for burns should be completed. A classic fernlike pattern of burn may be noted on the skin. An eye examination should be conducted for retinal, optic nerve, or occipital lobe damage. Baseline visual acuity should be measured, because cataracts, corneal ulcers, or hemorrhage may occur. The ears should be examined for ruptured tympanic membranes. Vital signs should be assessed, including screening for hypertension. The cervical spine and the entire musculoskeletal system should be evaluated for injury.

Treatment

The patient should be entered into the EMS without delay. Treatment consists of restoring or maintaining the patient's respiratory effort. If the person is apneic, cardiac function ceases in a few minutes. If the person is in cardiac arrest, CPR must be initiated and continued for an extended period. An AED may be used if available. Cardiac monitoring is indicated, along with observation for cerebral edema and respiratory insult. Fractures, lacerations, burns, and other injuries need to be treated according to the facility protocol. Tetanus prophylaxis must be confirmed or administered, if necessary. Follow-up eye examinations should be conducted, because cataracts may develop in the year after the lightning strike. Treatment of ruptured tympanic membranes should be instituted.

Prognosis

The prognosis varies, depending on the extent of the insult. Cardiac dysrhythmias are a potentially lethal complication of lightning injuries. Prompt institution of CPR when respiratory efforts are found to be absent may also result in survival of the victim. According to the CDC, 90% of lightning victims survive but may have side effects. These individuals require follow-up examinations of the eyes and the ears for late-onset problems. Burn treatment of points of entry and exit and treatment of any other skin burns are required.

Prevention

Seeking shelter inside a building after hearing thunder is wise due to the fact that lightning can strike up to 25 miles from the storm. It is best to avoid seeking shelter under a tree. Getting into a car during a lightning storm is also a safe option if the car is metal on the top and sides; convertibles will not provide the same protection. When no shelter is available, positioning oneself as low as possible on the ground is a prudent action. Cancel outdoor activities if a storm occurs.

Patient Teaching

Provide patients and family members with safety information regarding lightning and thunderstorms. Emphasize the importance of having CPR training and of providing immediate intervention to a lightning strike victim when doing so is safe and possible. Teach the patient *"When thunder roars, go indoors"* which is a motto of the National Oceanic and Atmospheric Administration. Another motto *"See a flash, dash inside"* helps individuals who cannot hear know to take cover in a storm.

Extreme Heat (Hyperthermia)

Description

Hyperthermia occurs when an individual's core body temperature is much higher than the normal body temperature of 98.6°F.

ICD-10-CM Code	T67.9XXA *(Effect of heat and light, unspecified, initial encounter)* (T67.0 [7th digit]–T67.9 [7th digit] = 10 codes of specificity)

Effects of heat are coded by type. Once the diagnosis has been confirmed, refer to the current edition of the ICD-10-CM coding manual for the appropriate code.

Symptoms and Signs

The person with hyperthermia may be experiencing heat stroke or heat exhaustion as a result of prolonged exposure to extremely hot temperatures. The skin is hot, red, and usually dry. The patient may have a dry mouth, headache, nausea or vomiting, dizziness and weakness, and shortness of breath. The pulse is rapid and strong at the onset, gradually becoming weak, and blood pressure decreases. The pupils are constricted. Patients exhibit anxiety, mental confusion, irritability, aggression, and even hysterical behavior. In extreme cases, the person experiences altered levels of consciousness and may have seizure activity.

Heat exhaustion produces profuse sweating, fatigue, headache, weakness, nausea, dizziness, and possible heat or muscle cramps. The pulse is weak and rapid; the skin is pale and cool or hot and clammy or moist; and the body temperature is typically 101°F to 104°F if not cooled. The pupils are dilated.

Patient Screening

Hyperthermia is a life-threatening emergency. The individual should be entered into the EMS without delay. Until emergency care arrives to transport the person to an emergency facility, family, friends, or coworkers should move the individual from the extremely hot environment to a colder environment, loosen the victim's clothing, and place cool, moist cloths on the individual's face, neck, arms, and hands.

Etiology

Heat stroke results when the body's heat-regulating systems are unable to cope with the exposure to severe external heat sources. This can occur from exertion in the outdoors in extremely hot temperatures or from the body's failure to regulate heat due to another serious health problem, such as a stroke, which affects a large part of the brain. As the body overheats, its temperature rises from 105°F to 110°F. Because no effective cooling mechanism is functioning, the body stores the heat, eventually resulting in damage to the brain cells and, subsequently, permanent brain damage or death. Older adults, infants, children, and malnourished and debilitated people are the most susceptible to heat stroke. Others who experience heat stroke are those who work near furnaces and intense sources of heat and athletes who are exposed to the combination of high temperatures and high humidity.

Heat exhaustion is the result of salt or water depletion. Generally the person is involved in strenuous activity in a hot, humid environment. As a result, the person experiences prolonged and profuse sweating, causing the loss of excessive amounts of salt and water.

Diagnosis

The diagnosis of heat stroke is made by the presence of symptoms, especially the elevated body temperature. The history of exposure to high temperatures and humidity, along with the altered level of consciousness, aids in the diagnosis. In patients with a medical crisis, the diagnosis is made after tests are performed to confirm stroke or other brain injury.

The diagnosis of heat exhaustion is made from the history and clinical findings, specifically the moist, pale skin and normal or below-normal body temperature of the patient.

Treatment

Treatment of heat stroke, possibly a life-threatening condition, must be aggressive and instituted promptly. It consists of cooling the body down. The first step is to move the person to a cooler environment, to remove what clothing is possible, and to cool the body by pouring cool water over it or soaking it with a cool wet cloth. If the person begins to shiver, the cooling process should be slowed. It is imperative to bring the core temperature of the body below 100°F. The person should be transported to an emergency facility where vital signs can be monitored.

Treatment for heat exhaustion consists of moving the victim to a cool place and applying cool compresses. The individual should be made to lie down with the feet elevated. If the person is fully conscious, small sips of cool water should be given every 10 to 15 minutes. Once moved to the emergency department IV hydration is possible.

Many emergency departments are equipped with "Bair Huggers" used to cool or heat patients as indicated.

Prognosis

The prognosis varies, depending on the duration of the exposure and any underlying pathology. Heat stroke that is *nonexertional* resulting from a medical injury such as a stroke does not have a favorable outcome due to brain damage.

Prevention

All persons should be encouraged to avoid lengthy exposure to hot environments and advised of the importance of staying hydrated during hot weather or when working in hot environments. Employees who work in extreme temperatures should also rest in the shade or in an air-conditioned room and take breaks for hydration and cooling. Drinking fluids before going outside to work will help with hydration status. Older individuals and parents of young children should be provided education on the dangers of heat exposure. Employers can follow CDC recommendations in regard to "work and rest" schedules to prevent heat stroke.

Patient Teaching

Provide material to the patient or family on precautions to prevent hyperthermia from occurring.

Extreme Cold (Hypothermia)

Description

Hypothermia is generalized cooling of the body in which the core temperature of the body drops below 95°F (35°C).

ICD-10-CM Code	T68.XXXA *(Hypothermia, initial encounter)*

Symptoms and Signs

Hypothermia, which is generalized severe cooling of the body, causes the person to shiver and have a feeling of extreme cold or numbness. Fatigue is followed by loss of coordination, thick speech, and disorientation. The skin appears blue (in light-skinned people) or ash-colored (in dark-skinned people) and puffy, with the pulse being slow and weak. Core body temperature drops below 95°F. Breathing is slow and shallow, and the pupils are dilated. As the body temperature drops, the person experiences confusion, stupor, and unconsciousness.

Etiology

Hypothermia can occur when a person is exposed to cold wind, a cold environment, or cold water for prolonged periods. Older, very young, exhausted, and physically debilitated persons have the greatest risk of hypothermia. Lack of adequate clothing or becoming wet, as in a rainstorm, can add to the risk. Sudden immersion in cold water can cause hypothermia.

Diagnosis

The diagnosis is made on the basis of history, the clinical picture, blood tests, and the finding of severe abnormal low body temperature.

Treatment

Treatment of hypothermia, a life-threatening condition, must be aggressive and immediate. Any wet clothing must be removed, and gradual rewarming of the body is begun by wrapping the person in warm blankets and keeping the body dry. A barrier blanket should be placed between the person and the cold ground. Warm packs can be applied to the neck, chest, or groin but **not** to the extremities. If sources of heat such as warm packs or warm dry compresses are not available, the warmth from another person's body as he or she embraces the patient can also help warm the patient. If the person is conscious, warm liquids should be given orally in small quantities. Breathing should be monitored. The patient should be transported to an emergency facility where vital signs can be monitored.

Prognosis

The prognosis varies, depending on the duration of the exposure to cold and any underlying pathology.

Prevention

Prevention involves avoiding extremely cold temperatures. Packing an automobile with emergency supplies such as blankets and emergency warmers in the winter is a good idea for those who commute in extreme temperatures.

Patient Teaching

Encourage patients to avoid situations in which they may be exposed to extreme cold for long periods. Advise them to wear adequate layers of clothing when they must be in an extremely cold environment. Emphasize preparing for cold emergencies and power outages.

Frostbite

Description

Frozen or extremely cold tissue, usually on the face, ears, fingers, and toes, is termed *frostbite*.

ICD-10-CM Code   T33.90XA *(Superficial frostbite
of unspecified sites, initial
encounter)*
T33.99XA *(Superficial frostbite of
other sites, initial encounter)*
T34.90XA *(Frostbite with tissue
necrosis of unspecified sites,
initial encounter)*
T34.99XA *(Frostbite with tissue
necrosis of other sites, initial
encounter)*
*(T33.011 [7th digit]–T34.99 [7th
digit] = 74 codes of specificity)*
*Frostbite is coded by site. Once the diagnosis has been
confirmed, refer to the current edition of the ICD-10-CM
coding manual for the appropriate code.*

Symptoms and Signs

Frostbite, usually occurring on the face, fingers, toes, and ears, causes the skin in the affected area to become white in light-skinned people or ashen in dark-skinned people.

The person does not realize that the condition is occurring because little or no pain is felt as the tissue freezes. As the freezing deepens, the underlying tissue becomes firm, and the skin takes on a waxy appearance (Fig. 15.13).

Patient Screening

Frostbite requires prompt assessment and intervention. Most individuals will be seen in an emergency facility and assessed for additional hypothermal insults.

Etiology

Frostbite occurs when tissue is exposed to cold air, ice, snow, water, or freezing metal and objects. Ice crystals form between the cells of the skin. As the freezing continues, fluid that is drawn from the cells subsequently freezes. People who have undergone trauma, older adults, and newborns whose clothes are wet, or who are wearing tightly laced

• **Fig. 15.13** Frostbite. (From Elston J, Treat J, Rosenbach M: Andrews' diseases of the skin: clinical dermatology, ed 13, 2020, Elsevier.)

footwear, are at greatest risk when exposed to cold temperatures. Wearing clothes that are not protective against extremely cold temperatures and wind chill values also put one at higher risk.

Diagnosis

The diagnosis is made on the basis of visual examination and a history of exposure to cold. The depth or degree of the frostbite is determined by the color and appearance of the skin.

Treatment

Treatment consists of removing the patient from the cold environment. People suffering from superficial frostbite should be warmed with an external source of even heat. The temperature of the heat source should not be above 105°F. The affected skin area should *never* be rubbed. Patients suffering from frostbite should be treated by a physician, if possible. Rewarming of deep frostbite (frozen tissue) should not begin until professional medical care can be provided. The person should be kept warm, vital signs should be monitored, and alcohol should *never* be given. Pain medication may be administered. Additionally, dehydration may occur and require treatment with intravenous (IV) fluids.

Prognosis

The prognosis varies, depending on the length of exposure and the depth of the insult. Additional variables are the patient's age, general health status, and underlying pathology.

Prevention

Encourage patients to wear gloves, hats, scarves, and heavy socks when prolonged exposure to cold is anticipated. Advise them to replace any wet clothing with dry clothing to prevent additional trauma resulting from the cold temperature. Those playing in the snow should come inside, dry off, and get warm rather than staying out for long periods of time in wet snow. Children are very susceptible to frostbite due to their small size and losing body heat quicker than adults.

Patient Teaching

Provide patients with information concerning the prevention of frostbite. Advise parents to dress children in adequate gloves, hats, and scarves when they are engaged in outside winter activities and to come in periodically to warm up. Instruct patients to carry emergency blankets and supplies in extremely cold temperatures.

Bites

Bites can occur at any time and to any part of the body. They range from annoying insect bites to those by domestic animals, reptiles, or even other humans. Insect bites may be insignificant or life threatening. It has been

Rehabilitation

As recovery begins, many patients begin rehabilitation. The goal of rehabilitation is to help the patient regain some of the functions, both physical and mental, lost or diminished by the injury. The state of recovery depends on many things and often takes months or even years to regain most of the diminished functions. Factors involved include the mechanics of the injury, emotional challenges, family and social support, and complications from the injury. Before rehabilitation can begin, a thorough assessment of the physical state of the patient, along with identification of lost or diminished functions, must be made. The assessment is followed by the setting of obtainable and realistic goals. The sooner patients are entered into the rehabilitative stage, the more likely they are to succeed in returning to a near-preinjury state.

• **Fig. 15.14** Brown recluse spider bite after 48 hours of treatment. (From Miller JJ, Marks JG: Lookingbill and Marks' principles of dermatology, ed 6, Philadelphia, 2019, Elsevier.)

reported that insect bites are the most common cause of anaphylaxis in the United States. Mosquito bites can cause only itching, or they can cause encephalitis resulting from infection. An example is the West Nile virus, which is contracted through a bite from an infected mosquito. Additionally, tick bites can cause Rocky Mountain spotted fever, malaria, or Lyme disease. Animal bites range in severity from mere nips that do not break the skin and cause no serious disease to life-threatening bites that carry the risk of rabies and infection.

Some states require reportable incident forms. Medical professionals must recognize the reportable communicable diseases and conditions listed in the state board of health guidelines.

Insect Bites

Description
An insect bite, the puncture of the skin by the bite or sting of any insect or arthropod, may involve the injection of venom into the tissue of the individual.

> ICD-10-CM Code   T07 (Unspecified multiple injuries)
> Insect bites are coded by mention of infection. Once
> the diagnosis has been confirmed, refer to the current
> edition of the ICD-10-CM coding manual for the
> appropriate code.

Symptoms and Signs
The symptoms and signs of an insect bite or sting vary, depending on the type of insect that has bitten or stung the individual (Fig. 15.14). Usually a sharp, stinging pain is felt and may be followed by itching, redness, or swelling at the site. If the patient experiences a systemic reaction to the bite, he or she will have itching on the palms of the hands or soles of the feet, the neck, or the groin or may experience generalized itching, along with a rash over the entire body.

As the allergic reaction progresses, the patient experiences generalized edema, dyspnea, weakness, nausea, shock, and unconsciousness.

Patient Screening
Individuals reporting insect stings or bites require prompt assessment. Some bites or stings may precipitate an allergic reaction, often a very rapid and life-threatening reaction. Those with a known severe allergic response to certain types of bites or stings usually require emergency intervention as a lifesaving measure. Many such individuals and their families are aware of the potential danger and carry a "bee-sting" kit containing an epinephrine injection (EpiPen) with them at all times for emergency injection to reverse the allergic response. Follow-up appointments should be scheduled to educate the patient and the family about the dangers of insect stings and about taking preventive measures.

Etiology
The injury occurs when the insect either bites or stings the individual. Venom is injected into the tissue, resulting in the body's response to a foreign protein. Some of the more common types of bites or stings are those of mosquitoes, bees, wasps, hornets, spiders, fire ants, ticks, and fleas. Bites by black widow spiders, brown recluse spiders, and scorpions inject venom but do occur less often. Ocean animal bites cause pain and swelling and may be mild; however, sometimes they cause swelling of lymph nodes and difficulty breathing, depending on the type of bite.

Diagnosis
The diagnosis is made based on visual examination and patient history. It is hoped that the patient can identify or describe the offending insect. Some insect bites or stings leave characteristic signs.

Treatment

The first step in treating an insect sting is to determine whether the stinger is still present in the bite wound. If it is present, it must be removed to prevent further damage. The best method of removal is scraping across the site of the sting with a plastic card or a fingernail. (The use of forceps or tweezers squeezes more venom into the site.) The area is then cleansed with soap and water. The application of dry dressing, cold packs, or anesthetic sprays affords some comfort. The person should be observed for any signs of allergic reaction to the sting or bite.

People with black widow spider bites, brown recluse spider bites, or scorpion stings should be transported to an emergency facility. Aggressive treatment includes cleansing of the wound, administration of medication for pain relief, cold applications, and antivenin, and monitoring of vital signs. Antibiotics may be needed if the bite wound is open or if it becomes infected.

Prognosis

The prognosis varies, depending on the degree to which the person is sensitized to the offending foreign protein injected during the bite or sting. Many bites or stings resolve without treatment and no sensitization occurs. In those with moderate to severe reactions, recovery may be speedy or slow, depending on any underlying pathology.

Prevention

Prevention includes avoiding situations where exposure to the offending insect may occur. The use of insect repellant may be helpful. Education of family members and coworkers regarding possible severe reactions and the measures that are necessary to counteract a potentially life-threatening allergic response is beneficial. Pesticide services can help with elimination of spiders in homes and wasp nests ect.

Patient Teaching

Provide the patient with information on prevention of insect bites and stings. Instruct the family about procedures to follow in case of an emergency situation involving a severe reaction.

Rocky Mountain Spotted Fever/Tick Bite

Description. Rocky Mountain spotted fever, a tickborne disease, is a severe systemic infection. It is the most commonly reported rickettsial disease in the United States.

ICD-10-CM Code	A77.0 *(Spotted fever due to Rickettsia rickettsii)* (A77.0–A77.3 = 4 codes of specificity)

Symptoms and Signs. The patient may recall being bitten by a tick, typically during outdoor activity, such as camping and hiking. Patients are frequently unaware of the presence of the insects on their bodies because they are flat and small and may be hidden in an area covered by hair.

Several days to 2 weeks later, a sudden onset of fever, severe headache, vomiting, malaise, and myalgia occur. Four days after the onset of fever, a characteristic maculopapular rash is noted, and the rash spreads over the body. Small hemorrhages appear under the skin, the characteristic sign that gives the disease its name. Inflammation of blood vessels (vasculitis) affects the skin and other organs, leading to systemic manifestations in the heart, lungs, kidneys, and nervous system.

Patient Screening. Individuals reporting symptoms of fever, severe headache, vomiting, malaise, and myalgia require prompt assessment.

Etiology. The causative agent, *Rickettsia rickettsii*, is transmitted by the wood tick and carried in the feces of infected ticks. It is introduced into the bloodstream of a person during a prolonged tick bite (duration of 4–6 hours). Once it is in the bloodstream, the organism, an intracellular parasite, reproduces in certain cells and destroys them. The disease cannot be transmitted from person to person.

Diagnosis. Although Rocky Mountain spotted fever is difficult to diagnose, a history of a tick bite or recent outdoor activity in tick-infested areas and the onset of severe systemic symptoms, with the appearance of the characteristic rash, suggest the diagnosis (Fig. 15.15). Laboratory findings include a positive complement fixation reaction, which measures the antigen-antibody reaction occurring in the body, and thereby, the severity of infection. Changes in the clotting components in blood may be noted. Isolation of the organism in a blood culture confirms the diagnosis.

Treatment. The treatment of choice for Rocky Mountain spotted fever is antibiotic therapy with tetracycline or doxycycline and symptomatic relief with the administration of analgesics. Infection confers lifetime immunity.

Prognosis. The prognosis is good with rapid diagnosis and treatment with antibiotic regimen. The underlying pathology or concurrent health problems may complicate the outcome.

Prevention. Preventive measures include wearing protective clothing and applying insect repellent to clothing and exposed skin. Visual inspection of the skin for the presence of ticks should be made every few hours during and after outdoor activity in infested areas. If a tick is found, it should be removed carefully with tweezers, avoiding handling of the tick.

Patient Teaching. Encourage individuals to wear proper protective clothing and insect repellant when in environments where ticks may reside. Also instruct them to make a visual inspection of the skin for ticks or apparent tick bites every few hours and when they arrive home.

Malaria/Mosquito Bite

Description. Malaria is a severe generalized infection caused by the bite of an Anopheles mosquito that is infected by a Plasmodium type of protozoa.

ICD-10-CM Code	B54 *(Unspecified malaria)* (B50.0–B54 = 13 codes of specificity)

• **Fig. 15.15** Clinical signs identified in children with Rocky Mountain spotted fever. (A) Edema of the dorsum of the hand. (B) Periorbital edema. (C and D) Petechial rashes involving the palm and sole. (From Kimberlin D, Fischer M, Long S, Prober C: *Principles and practice of pediatric infectious diseases*, ed 6, 2023, Elsevier.)

Symptoms and Signs. Malaria is an acute, sometimes chronic, serious infectious illness. It is characterized by a classic cycle of chills, fever, and sweats, occurring in that order. The patient also may have headaches, nausea, fatigue, and myalgia. Although the course and severity of the disease can vary, bouts of malaria usually last from 1 to 4 weeks. Signs include an enlarged spleen, an enlarged liver, and anemia. The symptoms have a tendency to recur and may persist for years.

Patient Screening. An individual reporting symptoms of chills, fever, and sweats, possibly combined with headache, nausea, fatigue, and myalgia, requires prompt assessment.

Etiology. Malaria is caused by four species of the protozoan Plasmodium, which is transmitted from infected human to human by the bite of a mosquito vector or, less commonly, by blood transfusion or IV drug use. After they are introduced into the body, the protozoan parasites feed on hemoglobin and reproduce within red blood cells. Malaria is endemic in tropical and subtropical areas such as South and Central America, Asia, and Africa, and usually is brought to the United States by travelers returning from these areas. Cases have been reported in the United States recently but have been successfully treated with prompt medical care.

Diagnosis. Laboratory testing of infected individuals reveals decreased hemoglobin levels, decreased platelet count, prolonged prothrombin time (PT), and a positive serum antibody test result. Diagnosis is confirmed by identifying the Plasmodium organism in a blood smear.

Treatment. Malaria is treated with chloroquine, an antimalarial drug, given orally. Other drugs may include mefloquine, atovaquone-proguanil (Malarone), artemether-lumefantrine (Coartem), quinine, and artesunate. Tetracycline, doxycycline, and clindamycin may be used in conjunction with quinine. Antipyretics are given for fever. Infusion of packed RBCs may be required to treat anemia. Each new case of malaria must be reported to the local board of health.

Prognosis. The prognosis varies, depending on the response to treatment and any underlying pathology.

Prevention. Prophylactic medications may be administered before travel to known endemic areas. The choice of medication utilized depends on the country or region being visited. Recommendations for choosing medications are available from the CDC. A number of medications may be used for chemoprophylaxis, although some of these medications may cause serious or fatal side effects. Medications such as atovaquone/proguanil (Malarone), chloroquine, tafenoquine, primaquine, and doxycycline are among the most commonly used prophylactic treatments. Current CDC guidelines should be checked for dosage and duration of therapy instructions. An Environmental Protection Agency-registered insect repellent is recommended.

Altitude Sickness

Altitude sickness, or acute mountain sickness, is a disorder associated with the low oxygen content of the atmosphere at high altitudes. It occurs when individuals make a rapid ascent into high altitudes, usually greater than 8000 feet. Symptoms include loss of appetite, nausea and vomiting, headache, dizziness, rapid pulse, fatigue, difficulty sleeping, shortness of breath on exertion, and air hunger. Mild symptoms that mimic jet lag or the flu can subside as the body adjusts to the higher altitude. More severe symptoms include cough, chest tightness or congestion, confusion, cyanosis, decreased level of consciousness, pale or grayish skin, difficulty walking, and shortness of breath at rest. Life-threatening altitude sickness can cause prostration, cardiac disturbances, and cerebral edema, with possible seizures and death. Pulmonary edema is another severe state of altitude sickness. It is possible for those with heart problems to experience angina and subsequent myocardial infarction triggered by high-altitude conditions. In addition, dehydration is a contributing factor. Those who experience symptoms should descend to a lower altitude and drink plenty of water. Rest and curtailing stressful activities help relieve symptoms and are necessary interventions for shortness of breath and increased heart rate.

Prevention includes slowly acclimating to the higher altitudes over a few days, drinking extra fluids, and avoiding alcohol and smoking. When at elevations greater than 9000 feet, it is best not to climb more than 3300 feet a day. Increase altitude where sleeping by no more than 1,600 feet per day.

Patient Teaching. Provide patients who may be traveling to endemic areas with information on prophylactic medications. Also, instruct them regarding possible symptoms of malaria and encourage them to seek medical treatment at the onset of any such symptoms.

Animal Bites/Human Bites

Description

An animal bite is any bite inflicted on an individual by another animal. The source may be another human, a domestic pet, or any wild animal.

> ICD-10-CM Code   S codes by site
> *Refer to the current edition of the ICD-10-CM coding
>   manual for additional information and appropriate
>   codes according to site.*

Symptoms and Signs

Broken skin with evidence of teeth marks is the usual clinical finding related to an animal bite. Puncture wounds are present, with possible tearing of the skin. Bleeding is usually evident, and the flesh may actually be bitten away. Discoloration of the surrounding skin indicates bruising to the area. The patient usually reports pain at the site and swelling may be present.

Patient Screening

Individuals reporting animal bites require prompt assessment. The extent of the bite requires evaluation so that prompt treatment can begin. It is also important that information about the animal be obtained for animal control to confine the animal until possible rabies infection is ruled out. The patient should be given the next available same-day appointment. If this is not possible, the patient should be sent to an outpatient clinic or to an emergency department.

Etiology

Typically the bite occurs when the offending animal is agitated, frightened, threatened, or angry. Bites can be from domestic animals, such as cats and dogs; farm animals; or wild animals, such as skunks, bats, raccoons, and foxes. Human bites have been recorded. Shark bites are also a potential source of injury in some areas with an increase in shark presence.

Diagnosis

The diagnosis is made on the basis of history and physical examination. The pattern of the teeth marks is helpful in determining the type of bite, whether human or animal, and the type of animal that bit the patient.

Treatment

Treatment begins with cleansing of the wound with copious amounts of water and antibacterial soap to remove bacteria and contamination. If bleeding cannot be controlled, hemostasis is achieved with cautery or suturing. Depending on the site and severity of the wound, plastic surgery may be indicated for optimal repair.

Rabies is transmitted through the saliva of infected animals. If the offending animal is a domestic pet, it usually is not too difficult to confirm the most recent date of rabies inoculation or to quarantine the animal for the time necessary to rule out rabies infection. Most communities require reporting animal bites to the local animal control agency or a local law enforcement agency that will follow through on determining the rabies inoculation status of the animal. If it is not possible to determine if the animal is rabid, the injured person probably will have to undergo a series of injections to confer immunity against rabies.

Capnocytophaga bacteria, which lives in the mouths of animals such as dogs and cats, is known to cause very serious infections in humans. Animals should never be allowed to lick an open sore on a human under any circumstance, as the normal bacterial flora in their mouth can prove deadly to humans.

Human and animal bites are dangerous because of the organisms that may contaminate the wound. In addition, animal bites, such as the dog bite shown in Fig. 15.16, cause emotional trauma as well as physical trauma.

As with most invasive trauma, a sterile dressing should be applied. Tetanus prophylaxis is confirmed or administered, if necessary, and antibiotics may be prescribed as an additional prophylactic measure.

• **Fig. 15.16** Complex facial lacerations caused by a dog bite. (A) Initial injury. (B) Final result after repair and scar maturation. (From Nerad J: *Techniques in ophthalmic plastic surgery: a personal tutorial*, ed 2, 2022, Elsevier.)

Prognosis

The prognosis varies, depending on the extent of the damage to the tissue and on any underlying pathology. If the animal is rabid, the prognosis is guarded. There are cases where animals (packs) attack humans and cause trauma, which results in death.

Prevention

Be aware of surroundings at all times. Do not approach wild animals or any domestic animal who has never been around you despite an owner saying their pet "does not bite." Never leave small children unattended near an animal since any animal, even the family pet, can be unpredictable.

Patient Teaching

Encourage children not to approach or touch animals unfamiliar to them, even if the owner says the animal "does not bite," as animals are unpredictable. Advise individuals with pets to keep the animal's inoculations, especially for rabies, current. Instruct the patient or their family members on wound care and the importance of completing any antibiotic therapy that has been prescribed.

Snakebites

Description

A snakebite is a penetrating tissue wound made by the fangs or teeth of a snake.

ICD-10-CM Code	(T63.001A–T63.94XA = 152 codes of specificity)

Refer to the current edition of the ICD-10-CM coding manual for additional information and appropriate codes according to site.

Symptoms and Signs

The patient may have actually seen the snake that gave the bite or may not have been aware of the snake at the time the bite happened. In either event, the patient will have a noticeable bite to the skin or possibly only a slight skin discoloration at the site of injury. Burning pain is present, and swelling begins around the bite; however, this reaction may be delayed, developing slowly over time. The pulse rate becomes rapid, and the patient begins to experience weakness, visual difficulties, nausea, and vomiting. Signs and symptoms of the poisoning may take 30 minutes to several hours to develop. Coral snakes are extremely venomous and leave small chew types of teeth marks rather than the two distinct fang marks made by other venomous snakes. All snakebites should be treated as soon as possible.

Patient Screening

Complaints reporting a possible snakebite require prompt assessment and intervention. The EMS should be activated for transportation of the victim to the nearest emergency care facility.

Etiology

The poisoning from the snakebite usually takes 1 to 2 days to develop unless the person is allergic to the foreign protein

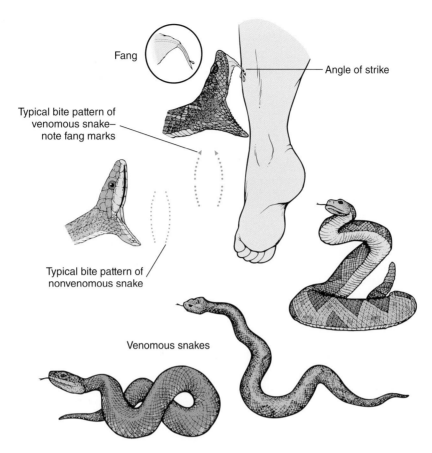

Fang

Angle of strike

Typical bite pattern of venomous snake–note fang marks

Typical bite pattern of nonvenomous snake

Venomous snakes

• **Fig. 15.17** Snakebite. (Redrawn with permission from *Patient Care Magazine*, Montvale, New Jersy, 1976, Patient Care Publications.)

of the venom, which will speed up the reaction time. Four kinds of venomous snakes are known to inhabit the United States: rattlesnakes, copperheads, water moccasins, and coral snakes. There are different species within each type. Rattlesnakes account for the greatest number of venomous snakebites. Some bites are the work of nonvenomous snakes, but all snakebites should be treated as venomous by the first aid provider.

Diagnosis

Diagnosis is made by history and visual examination of the affected area. Typically, two fang marks in the skin are indicative of venomous snakebites; the exception is the bite of a coral snake, which appears as a chew type of bite that leaves teeth marks (see Fig. 15.17).

The victim or other witness should not attempt to retrieve the head of any snake, as this can be extremely dangerous. Any rescuer must always remember that their own safety is a priority, and they *must never* jeopardize their own safety in a rescue.

Treatment

First aid and intervention at the scene consists of removing the person from the injury site to prevent further risk and keeping her or him calm and quiet. The EMS system should be activated. The bitten area is cleansed with soap and water. Any jewelry, including rings or other constricting objects, should be removed from the affected limb. The extremity should be immobilized, kept still, and positioned below the level of the heart if possible. Transport to the nearest emergency facility should be initiated as soon as possible so that aggressive treatment can begin immediately. Antivenin may be given to the patient and vital functions supported, as needed. The protocol for snakebite treatment indicates the following should *not* be applied after a snakebite: cold, tourniquet, suction, electrical shock. Cutting the skin and tissue where the bite occurred is *not* recommended.

Prognosis

The prognosis varies, depending on how venomous the snake is. Bites from nonvenomous snakes usually resolve and heal with few complications. Recovery from bites of venomous snakes depends on the availability of antivenin, the promptness of the treatment, and the location of the bite on the body. Preexisting pathology of the patient may dictate the outcome.

Prevention

Using caution in areas known to be inhabited by snakes is prudent. When in an area where snakes are likely to be present, heavy "snake" boots should be worn to prevent possible bites from penetrating tissue. Grassy, wet areas should be avoided, if possible.

Patient Teaching

Encourage individuals to regard all snakes as being potentially venomous. Provide information about areas in the community that snakes are likely to inhabit, and recommend avoidance of these areas. If travel within or occupation of these areas is necessary, encourage wearing of heavy boots to prevent bites around feet and lower legs.

❖ ENRICHMENT

Poisoning

Poisons are any substances that, when introduced into the body, cause illness or injury; many cause death. Poisoning can be accidental or intentional. Poisons can be introduced into the body by absorption through the skin, ingestion through the GI tract, inhalation through the respiratory system, and injection through a sting, bite, or hypodermic needle. The signs and symptoms vary according to the poison and the method of introduction into the body. Many poisons are found in the domestic setting and often are the cause of exposure. Many household cleaning products, laundry detergents, car cleaning and maintenance products, and air fresheners have the potential to become deadly if ingested. Most have warning labels. Ingested or swallowed poisons can include food, alcohol, chemicals, medications, and plants.

Inhaled poisons include gases, such as carbon monoxide, carbon dioxide, nitrous oxide, chlorine, and fumes from chemicals or drugs. Absorbed poisons include chemicals or oils from certain plants. Injected poisons include venom injected by bites from insects, spiders, ticks, snakes, or drugs given via a hypodermic needle.

Because of the vast number of poisons and methods of introduction into the body, it is impossible to identify symptoms, etiology, diagnosis, and treatment for each toxic substance. General guidelines include (1) identification of the toxic substance and (2) contacting a poison control center or emergency facility for assistance. Of utmost importance is that the rescuer or care provider not compromise their own safety, especially when inhalation of toxic fumes could be involved.

Poison control centers are available by phone and on the Internet. Hotlines are available 24 hours a day, 7 days a week. Many facilities contact poison control centers for recommended tests and management.

Cumulative Trauma (Repetitive Motion Trauma, Overuse Syndrome)

Cumulative trauma disorders, or repetitive motion injuries, are common in numerous occupations. They account for more time lost from work than any other single factor. At risk are those working in industries where repetitive tasks have to be performed, including those who work on computers on a regular and continuous basis, cashiers who scan products on conveyor belts, and those who engage in target practice and in certain other sports.

Cumulative trauma disorders are muscular conditions that result from repeated motions performed in the course of daily activities. These conditions are caused by repetitive movement that is unnatural or awkward, such as overexertion, twisting, or muscle fatigue. Soft tissue injuries that develop over time as a result of repetitive activities cause continuing stress on specific muscles or nerves. These injuries can result from improper posture of the wrist, arm, back, shoulder, or legs. Many occur because of pressure centered on the hand or the wrist, with frequent repetitive motions for an extended period. In the industrial setting, improper use of handheld tools, especially with excessive or improper grip, can cause cumulative trauma disorders. Additionally, continuous vibration contributes to the increased occurrence of trauma. The characteristics of cumulative trauma disorders are pain, tingling, numbness, swelling, redness, and loss of flexibility and strength. These disorders include but are not limited to white finger (Raynaud phenomenon), trigger finger, carpal tunnel syndrome, tennis elbow, thoracic outlet syndrome, de Quervain disease, synovitis, tenosynovitis, and nonspecific tendinitis. Cumulative trauma develops over an extended period, so the onset of symptoms is insidious. Much investigation may be necessary to pinpoint the repetitive task that has caused the trauma. Ergonomics is an assessment of how a person performs tasks. During the assessment, the individual is observed in a work situation or other action where a repetitive task is performed. An attempt is made to determine whether a subtle or other change in the way the task is done may help relieve symptoms or prevent an injury from occurring.

As with other work-related injuries, workers' compensation forms must be completed.

Carpal Tunnel Syndrome

Description

Entrapment and compression of the median nerve in the carpal tunnel causes pain and numbness in the wrist, hands, and fingers.

ICD-10-CM Code   G56.00 (Carpal tunnel syndrome, unspecified upper limb) (G56.00–G56.02 = 3 codes of specificity)

Symptoms and Signs

The patient experiences numbness of hands and fingers, with pain more pronounced at night. Swelling of the wrist or hand and "fluttering" of the fingers are additional symptoms. The patient often is observed cradling the arm or rubbing the hand or arm. Temporary relief is sometimes obtained by shaking or moving the wrist.

Patient Screening

Although not an emergency, assessment of this painful condition should be accomplished at the earliest available and convenient time.

Etiology

Tendons, blood vessels, and the median nerve pass through a narrow fibrous tunnel that extends from the wrist to the hand. Carpal tunnel syndrome results when the tendons within the tunnel become inflamed from repetitive overuse of the hand, wrist, or fingers, thereby causing entrapment of the median nerve as it passes through the wrist, which results in the pinching of the median nerve. Any condition that exerts pressure on the median nerve can cause carpal tunnel syndrome.

Diagnosis

The clinical findings, along with the history of repetitive motion activities, suggest carpal tunnel syndrome. Patients with carpal tunnel syndrome typically feel symptoms of numbness and tingling of the hand in the area of the thumb, index finger, middle finger, and part of the fourth finger. The carpal compression test or Durkan's test can be performed during the physical examination by compressing the median nerve to elicit a response. Another test is the Phalen wrist flexor test, in which the patient presses the backs of the hands together to bend the wrists as far downward as possible, without applying force, and holds them together for 60 seconds. The fingers should be kept pointing toward the floor. In a patient with a positive test result, numbness and tingling of the hand or fingers is present. Ultrasound, x-ray (to rule out other causes of pain), electromyography, and a nerve conduction test may be performed to aid in diagnosis.

Treatment

Treatment consists of physical therapy and identification and cessation of the repetitive motion to rest the wrist and the hand. Antiinflammatory drugs are prescribed; ice packs and a splint may be applied to maintain the wrist in a neutral position. Oral corticosteroids or a local injection into the affected area by an experienced clinician may quickly relieve symptoms. As a final resort, surgery to divide the carpal ligament is performed in an attempt to relieve pressure on the nerve.

Prognosis

The prognosis is usually favorable. If conservative measures are not successful, surgical intervention may be indicated. Compliance with the suggested or prescribed therapy is helpful in achieving a positive outcome.

Prevention

Prevention is important, so ergonomic studies and correction of improper repetitive activities should be implemented. Prevention involves using ergonomically correct devices and positions when engaging in activities such as typing, which tend to cause repetitive motion injuries.

Patient Teaching

Encourage patients to avoid repetitive motion that places the arm, hand, and wrist in compromised positions.

◆ ENRICHMENT

De Quervain Disease

De Quervain disease is an inflammation of the tendons of the thumb. It is caused by irritation of the long abductor and short extensor tendons. Repetitive motion such as those when playing online games, causes edema and tenderness in the thumb and its base.

Tennis Elbow

Description

Tennis elbow, technically known as *lateral humeral epicondylitis*, is the result of repetitive movement involving flexion of the wrist against resistance. The result of this repetitive action is an inflammatory condition of the tissue at the distal portion of the humerus.

ICD-10-CM Code	M77.10 *(Lateral epicondylitis, unspecified elbow)*
	(M77.00–M77.12 = 6 codes of specificity)

Symptoms and Signs

The patient has pain in the outer (lateral) aspect of the elbow and lower arm. Weakness is exhibited in the affected extremity.

Patient Screening

Tennis elbow is not an emergency but can be quite painful. Schedule the patient to be seen at the next available appointment.

Etiology

The extensor attachment to the lateral humeral condyle becomes inflamed. Repetitive motion in the elbow, usually with accompanying stress to the joint, causes this inflammatory condition.

Diagnosis

Diagnosis is made by evaluating the clinical findings and by physical examination. Doppler ultrasound, EMG, and MRI may be indicated. Radiographs may be used to rule out other causes.

Treatment

Treatment consists of stopping the repetitive task and resting the affected arm. An elastic brace can be placed distal to the elbow to alter the fulcrum of the activity. Physical therapy may be ordered. NSAIDs and ice packs to the area are also helpful in decreasing inflammation. Corticosteroids and plasma rich in platelets may be injected. Other types of injections include botulinum toxin A (Botox) or an alternative treatment such as prolotherapy, which, as of the authoring of this text has not been FDA approved. Needling, needle fenestration, ultrasonic tenotomy, extracorporal shock wave therapy are also potential treatments. Either laparoscopic or open surgery may be performed if other treatments are not successful in controlling pain.

Prognosis
The prognosis is good with treatment.

Prevention
Proper body mechanics when engaging in activities involving the shoulder and arm are helpful preventive measures. Recognition of stressful activities and modification of the activity may also be helpful. If the condition is the result of an occupational task, explore ergonomically correct methods for performing the task.

Patient Teaching
Provide the patient with information and suggestions regarding ergonomically correct methods of performing activities that place stress on the elbow joint. When physical therapy is prescribed, encourage compliance with the recommended exercises.

Trigger finger

Description
The technical term for trigger finger is *stenosing tenosynovitis*. The index finger has a lump or knot that appears on the flexor tendon. Flexion or extension of the finger may be interrupted and then begin again in a jerking or snapping type of motion when the hand is opened and closed.

ICD-10-CM Code   M65.30 *(Trigger finger,*
                        unspecified finger)
                        (M65.30–M65.35 = 16 codes of
                        specificity)

Symptoms and Signs
A lump or knot appears on the flexor tendon of the affected index finger. Movement of the finger may be temporarily interrupted and then continues with a jerking type of motion. Trigger finger can also affect the thumb or another finger. Closing the hand often causes pain at the base of the finger on the palm of the hand.

Patient Screening
The next available appointment should be given to the patient.

Etiology
The cause of trigger finger is excessive use of the finger or thumb resulting from difficult, repetitive finger movement or trauma to the tendon sheath. Trigger finger is caused by local swelling from inflammation or scarring around the tendons that provide the flexion motion of the finger.

Diagnosis
The diagnosis is made by evaluating the clinical findings, history, and physical examination results.

Treatment
As with other cumulative trauma, the prescribed course of treatment is cessation of repetitive activity and rest of the affected part. Ice packs on the inflamed area, stretching exercises, NSAIDs, and injecting cortisone into the inflamed tendon are effective treatments. Surgical intervention may be considered if all other conservative treatments fail.

Prognosis
The prognosis is good when the repetitive motion is halted.

Prevention
No method of prevention, other than avoiding the repetitive activity, is known.

Patient Teaching
Encourage the patient to allow the finger to rest and take medications as prescribed.

Neurogenic Thoracic Outlet Syndrome (Brachial Plexus Injury)

Description
Neurogenic thoracic outlet syndrome is the compression of the brachial plexus nerves.

ICD-10-CM Code   G54.0 *(Brachial plexus disorders)*

Symptoms and Signs
Neurogenic thoracic outlet syndrome is the most common type of thoracic outlet syndrome. The patient experiences pain in the arm of the affected side. The brachial plexus nerves are responsible for movement and feeling in the hand, arm, and shoulder. Paresthesia of the fingers also is experienced, along with weakness and diminished grasp capability in the fingers and the thumb. The patient may also experience shoulder and neck pain.

Patient Screening
Although not an emergency, the condition will cause the patient pain and possibly apprehension because of the numbness in the fingers and the continual dropping of items. Schedule the next available appointment for the patient.

Etiology
This syndrome is caused by the compression of nerves in the thoracic outlet which is the area between the shoulder and the neck. This can result from a continual dropping of the shoulder girdle, poor posture, trauma from an accident, having an extra "cervical" rib, or a fibrous band that causes compression. The performance of repetitive tasks that cause continual hyperabduction of the arm can also play a role in causing this condition

Diagnosis
The diagnosis is made by evaluating the clinical findings, history, and physical examination results. Electromyography

(EMG), ultrasound, and x-ray aid in confirming the diagnosis.

Treatment

Specific types of exercises or physical therapy may improve the condition. Antiinflammatory medications, analgesics, and muscle relaxers may help alleviate pain. Local injections of steroids, anesthetics, and onabotulinumtoxinA (Botox) may be injected. Surgical thoracic outlet decompression is also an option when other measures are not successful.

Prognosis

The prognosis is good with treatment.

Prevention

Avoid repetitive movements and lifting heavy objects. Avoiding carrying heavy bags over the shoulder may also prevent this type of compression injury. For a structural cause, there is no prevention but stretching to strengthen muscles may be of benefit.

Patient Teaching

If needed, follow all instructions for physical therapy and take medications as prescribed. If surgery is the chosen treatment, provide instructions for caring for the incision.

Tendinitis

Description

Tendinitis (tendonitis) is inflammation of a tendon that is usually caused by insult or injury to the tendon.

ICD-10-CM Code	M77.9 *(Enthesopathy, unspecified)* (M77.5–M77.9 = 5 codes of specificity)

Symptoms and Signs

The patient experiences nonspecific pain anywhere along the route of the tendon or its attachments. The most common symptom is acute pain. Swelling may occur and there may be tenderness in the affected area.

Patient Screening

The patient experiencing severe pain requires prompt assessment. Schedule an appointment as soon as possible.

Etiology

Tendinitis is inflammation of a tendon. It is caused by an insult to the tendon resulting from prolonged or improper activity of the affected part. Repeating the same action over and over can lead to overuse and inflammation.

Diagnosis

Nonspecific tendinitis is difficult to diagnose. A careful history indicates the event or events that caused the stress to the involved area. Movement into certain positions causes pain during the physical exam. An MRI and ultrasound may be ordered.

Treatment

Treatment is aimed at reducing pain, decreasing inflammation, and preserving the integrity of the joint involved. Resting the involved area is important, as is administering oral antiinflammatory drugs and applying ice. Steroids may be injected into the joint space. If the joint (e.g., the shoulder) becomes fixed (frozen shoulder), the adhesions that have formed may need to be released surgically to allow full range of motion of the joint.

Prognosis

The prognosis is good when the treatment plan is followed.

Prevention

Prevention involves avoiding the strenuous activity that initiates and subsequently aggravates the condition.

Patient Teaching

Encourage patients to be compliant with the prescribed drug therapy, physical therapy, and resting of the affected part.

Physical and Psychological Assault Trauma

Violence inflicted on a victim by others takes many forms, including child abuse, IPV, elder abuse, psychological abuse, sexual abuse, and rape. Victimization of individuals has become so prevalent that health care providers are now trained to identify people who have been victimized, to treat their physical and emotional trauma, and to report incidents or suspicion of abuse, as required by law.

Violence occurs in all areas of society, affecting both sexes, occurring at all socioeconomic levels, and including the entire age spectrum. The number of occurrences continues to increase, even though societal and cultural values typically expressed in the United States do not condone such behavior. Health care providers are encouraged to provide unconditional support to victims and to direct them to support groups or counseling for appropriate therapy.

Child Abuse/Neglect

Description

Physical, psychological, or sexual injury to a child is considered child abuse. The most commonly observed form is physical abuse because the resulting injuries are usually apparent. Signs of psychological abuse may be evidenced in the actions of the child. Sexual abuse may be discovered incidentally and investigated when the child complains of discomfort in the genital region or if the child reports

Bioterrorism

Bioterrorism is a source of great public concern. There are many different types of microorganisms and toxins that could cause diseases in humans and animals if used as a weapon. Anthrax, plague, botulism, smallpox, and radiation exposure are a few biological agents that could be used in terrorist attacks.

Biodefense is a measure to help prepare for such biological agents which could impact the world. Silent and deliberate attacks can seriously threaten life and cause social disruption. Awareness of the likelihood of the threats and knowledge of these conditions and possible intervention measures may prevent a potentially catastrophic final outcome. Updates about these conditions will be provided by the health care communities and government agencies should an attack of this type occur.

Similarly, data was provided during the COVID-19 pandemic in regard to reported cases and deaths in counties, states, and countries. This information was updated each day throughout the world in all news outlets. There has been debate as to whether this virus was initially an act of bioterrorism. All the answers are not clear, but one thing is certain. The pandemic provided a clearer picture of what can happen from a single virus, in a short period of time. This virus overwhelmed the medical communities with very sick patients who needed critical care. Ventilators were built by car manufacturers due to the need for patient care.

The world's response to the COVID-19 pandemic has opened the conversation for how to best respond to similar situations and keep people safe if biological terrorism occurs. Individuals who work in health care have seen just how important the balance is between life and death and how pivotal their role will continue to be in caring for patients.

the abuse. Neglect also may be considered a form of child abuse.

ICD-10-CM Code   T74.92XA *(Unspecified child maltreatment, confirmed, initial encounter)*
                        T76.92XA *(Unspecified child maltreatment, suspected, initial encounter)*

Additional codes may be required to identify any injury, the nature of the abuser or perpetrator, or the type of abuse. Once the diagnosis has been confirmed, refer to the current edition of the ICD-10-CM coding manual for additional appropriate codes.

Symptoms and Signs

Often, children who are victims of child abuse are identified as such by teachers, daycare providers, or health care providers. The injuries to the child encompass many forms, including bruises, fractures, burns, bites, and welts. The injuries can even be fatal (Fig. 15.18).

Bruising can have many telltale appearances, such as finger marks, which wrap around the child's limb and may show evidence of rings worn by the perpetrator; loop imprints of electrical cords or hangers; and horizontal wrap-around marks left by belts or straps, and possibly buckle marks. These bruises appear on soft tissue and not over bony prominences where normal falls would have caused them to be. The bruising is often in areas normally covered by clothing and in various stages of healing.

Burns from cigarettes appear as small circles (the diameter of a cigarette), often on hands, feet, buttocks, or genitals. Another form of burn is the scald burn with the pattern of "dipping," straight lines with no splash marks, a result of the child's body or part of the body being held in scalding water (Fig. 15.19).

Other observable injuries include teeth marks, bruising caused by human bites, and raised areas or welts caused by spankings with sticks, paddles, or belts on the buttocks or legs. A fracture, usually greenstick in nature, of a long bone may be noted.

Often the child is withdrawn, avoids eye contact, and does not respond appropriately to painful stimuli. When asked how the injury happened, the child denies any abuse and protects the abuser out of fear. In other cases, the child exhibits unusually aggressive behavior and has a neglected appearance. Emotional abuse also causes trauma to the child, many times through their adult life.

Neglect often is also considered a form of child abuse. When children are not provided with food or shelter, the caregiver is considered to be neglectful. Leaving young children unattended, thus endangering their well-being, is also a form of neglect. Child abuse or neglect is a reportable crime in all states, and the health care giver caring for the child victim can be found liable if the case is not reported to the appropriate agency. It is important to remember that when the abuser is a parent or family member, the child still has love for the person who inflicts harm.

Patient Screening

Any reports of child abuse require immediate investigation. An appointment is an urgent matter and should be scheduled as soon as possible, and if none is immediately available, a referral to an emergency facility should be made. Follow-up to verify treatment is necessary.

Etiology

Child abuse has many causes. These include emotional immaturity of the abuser; stress caused by economic or financial problems, social, or employment difficulties; poor parenting skills; drug or alcohol abuse; the abuser having a history of child abuse himself or herself; unrealistic expectations of the child; and the limitations of a physically or mentally challenged child. PTSD and stress have also been linked to child abuse.

Diagnosis

The diagnosis is made on the basis of history and clinical findings. Many times, health care providers are often the first professionals who are aware of child abuse or neglect; therefore careful documentation is critical if the case goes

• **Fig. 15.18** Imprint marks reflecting the weapons used to inflict them. (A and B) Fresh looped cord marks (A) and hypopigmented and hyperpigmented scars (B) that were the result of beatings with a looped electrical cord. (C) The characteristic pattern of parallel lines that results from blows with a belt. (D) This contusion in the configuration of a closed horseshoe with a central linear abrasion was inflicted with a belt buckle. (E) The red linear contusions on this child's thigh were the result of repeated blows with a switch. (F) These acute linear contusions over the back and buttocks were inflicted with a belt and a switch. (G) This boy was hit with a slipper with such force that imprints of the heel are evident. (H) The heel prints of a running shoe left on this boy's arm and thigh were distinct enough to enable identification of his abuser. (I) This girl was hit forcefully with a spatula. (J) This boy was struck with a chain, leaving a clear imprint of the links. (K) Child disclosed being hit with a phone charger, which caused this looped scar. (L) Severe bruising with underlying muscle damage. This toddler was covered from head to toe with severe looped cord contusions and lacerations. He had secondary myoglobinuria necessitating intensive care management to prevent renal failure. (From Zitelli B, McIntire S, Nowalk A, Garrison J: *Zitelli and Davis' atlas of pediatric physical diagnosis*, ed 8, 2023, Elsevier.)

• **Fig. 15.19** Child abuse. Well-demarcated burn caused by dipping the extremity in hot water. (From Schachner L, Hansen R: *Pediatric dermatology*, ed 4, 2011, Elsevier.)

to court. If the medical assistant suspects that child abuse or neglect is involved, further evaluation by an appropriate health care provider is necessary. Child abuse is not easy to diagnose; nevertheless, health care providers, teachers, and daycare providers are required, by law in most states in the United States, to report suspected child abuse to the local or state law enforcement agency or child protective agency. Health care workers should also be aware that there are certain medical conditions that may appear to be child abuse, such as making the skin appear to have bruising when there is none present.

Treatment

Any injuries must be treated in an appropriate manner. Documentation of the injuries is necessary, and the health care provider must remain alert for patterns of injuries. Radiographic studies of the long bones and the skulls of infants and toddlers should be performed to investigate the extent of abuse. Emotional support for the child should be given unconditionally. The child abuse hotline, the hospital protection team or the local or state protection service, and the local police department should be contacted, as indicated.

Prognosis

The prognosis varies, depending on the duration and extent of the abuse and the identity of the perpetrator of the abuse, that is, whether the abuser has custody of or easy access to the child. Removal of the child from the abusive environment by appropriate social service agencies usually is helpful. The emotional attachment of the child to the abuser may play a role in the resolution of this action. This is a difficult and sensitive issue that requires multiprofessional interaction.

Prevention

Prevention is the best treatment. Parents need to be taught good parenting skills and made aware of resources for crisis intervention. They need parenting skill classes to learn about alternatives to striking a child and methods of controlling their abusive reactions to the child's behavior (e.g., counting to 10). Abuse can also be prevented by teaching your child about online safety and monitoring their activities, putting on parental filters, and having conversations about the dangers of the internet. In addition, parents and caregivers should really know who they are leaving the child with at all times. There are times children are left with other adults who the parent met online and this person is left to care for the child while the parent is working or out of the house. Child predators use this to meet parents and have access to their children, and sexual predators fake their identity and use the internet to groom children and meet them away from the home to intentionally inflict harm.

Patient Teaching

Provide written information about the prevention of child abuse. Assist the family in locating and contacting community resources. Encourage family and community awareness of signs of child abuse and appropriate interventions. Teach parents to tell the child what to do if someone touches them, and to tell the parent immediately and assure them they are not "in trouble."

Shaken Infant (Baby) Syndrome

Description

Shaken infant syndrome (SIS), or *shaken baby syndrome (SBS)*, refers to the injuries incurred by the infant or toddler who has been shaken forcibly enough to cause intracerebral bleeding, resulting in a closed head injury.

ICD-10-CM Code   T74.4XXA (Shaken infant
                                            syndrome, initial encounter)
Once diagnosis of the injuries has been confirmed, referral to the current edition of the ICD-10-CM coding manual for appropriate codes is recommended.

Symptoms and Signs

The shaken baby may experience altered levels of consciousness to complete loss of consciousness. Irritability, changes in skin color to paleness or cyanosis, vomiting, lethargy, and convulsions are additional symptoms. Most of the time, there is no outward indication of physical trauma, but there may be hand marks on the infant's chest or abdomen made by fingers. Fractured or dislocated bones and neck or spinal injuries may be found. Examination of the eyes may reveal retinal hemorrhages (Fig. 15.20). Babies shaken into unconsciousness are often put to bed in the hope that the injury will resolve, and thus the opportunity for lifesaving treatment is usually lost.

• **Fig. 15.20** Shaken baby syndrome: retinal hemorrhages. (From Zitelli BJ, Davis HW: *Atlas of pediatric physical diagnosis*, ed 5, Philadelphia, 2008, Mosby; Courtesy Dr. Stephen Ludwig, Children's Hospital of Philadelphia, Pennsylvania.)

Patient Screening

SBS is a life-threatening emergency. These infants require prompt medical intervention. Contacting EMS for immediate transport to an emergency care facility is a prudent action. For a parent asking to speak with the physician after the diagnosis about treatment for their child, an appointment should be scheduled as soon as possible.

Etiology

The repeated rapid shaking of an infant results in the brain continually striking the inside of the cranial vault and then recoiling against the other side of the skull. As a result, tiny vessels rupture, causing minor or even major bleeds in and around the brain. The swelling and hemorrhage may lead to permanent severe cerebral (brain) damage or even death.

A form of child abuse, SIS usually occurs when the caregiver becomes irritated or upset and loses control, shaking the baby violently. Incidents of SIS resulting from tossing the baby into the air and catching him or her or even jostling the baby in a backpack as the caregiver jogs or runs, causing the baby to bounce up and down, have been documented. Young children have large heads and weak neck muscles and therefore are susceptible to intracerebral injury.

Diagnosis

The manifestation of three symptoms, subdural hematoma, cerebral edema, and retinal hemorrhage, leads to the diagnosis of SIS. CT and MRI should be performed to identify brain (bleeding) hemorrhages and radiographs can provide information regarding fractures. Blood tests should be performed to make sure there is no genetic reason, bleeding and clotting disorder, or other medical reason to explain the symptoms.

Treatment

Immediate and aggressive intervention, including life-sustaining measures, is necessary. Bleeding and cerebral edema must be controlled and intracranial pressure reduced. Nevertheless, damage may be permanent, even fatal. If the child survives, he or she may have visual deficits from retinal insults, including blindness, intellectual developmental disorder, or cerebral palsy. Trauma centers with traumatic brain injury programs are best prepared to handle these emergencies.

Prognosis

The prognosis varies, depending on the extent of the injury. Often the injuries to the brain are nonreversible or even fatal. Those children who do survive may be left with blindness, neurologic insults, and intellectual developmental disorders.

Prevention

SIS may be prevented by educating caregivers about the dangers of shaking a baby in anger and about methods of controlling their rage. Parents should be made aware of the importance of providing their children with competent caregivers. All caregivers, including parents, should develop a safe plan for dealing with and comforting a crying baby. When suspicions of nonaccidental injuries are raised, appropriate agencies must be notified.

ENRICHMENT

Family Violence

The incidence of family violence is increasing. All members of the family, regardless of age, sex, or place in the family line, are at risk for violence or abuse. Older adults and children are often targets of aggressive behavior from a stronger member of the family. Many members of dysfunctional families do not realize that abusive and violent behavior is not acceptable in today's society.

In family violence, one member of the family, either intentionally or unintentionally, causes physical or emotional harm to another member of the family. The core of the violence is the abuser's necessity to gain power and control over the victim. The individual perpetrating the abuse may use threats, isolation, verbal abuse, or intimidation to break down the victim's sense of their own power and security. The violent acts may be physical, including hitting, punching, slapping, kicking, or burning; emotional, including insults, threats, and harassment; or sexual, including incest or rape.

The cycle of abuse typically has three stages. Stage one is when tensions build. In stage two, the abuse actually takes place. During stage three, the abuser feels remorse. As the cycle repeats, the abuse has a tendency to become more severe. It is typical that the abuse is repeated, resulting in the victim realizing it is increasingly difficult to leave the relationship.

Patient Teaching

Provide all parents with infants or young children written information about SBS. Encourage all parents to have competent childcare for their children. Assist parents of shaken babies to locate and contact support groups in the community.

Elder Abuse/Neglect

Description

Elder abuse and neglect take on different forms: physical abuse, self-neglect, verbal abuse, psychological abuse, abandonment, violation of personal rights, and financial abuse. Withholding actions that result in harm or threatened harm to the health or welfare of older adults is considered abuse or neglect, depending on the extent of harm. The most commonly observed form is physical because the injuries are visually apparent. Psychological abuse may never be uncovered. Sexual abuse may be discovered incidentally with complaints of discomfort in the genital region or if reported by the older adult.

> ICD-10-CM Code   T74.91XA *(Unspecified adult maltreatment, confirmed, initial encounter)*
> T76.91XA *(Unspecified adult maltreatment, suspected, initial encounter)*
> *Once diagnosis of the injuries has been confirmed, referral to the current edition of the ICD-10-CM coding manual for appropriate codes is recommended. Additional codes are available for various forms of adult abuse.*

Symptoms and Signs

Elder abuse may never be reported to the authorities. Evidence of the abuse usually is discovered during examination for another purpose. Signs are similar to those of other forms of abuse, are varied, and are often hidden by clothing. Signs include bruising, fractures, malnutrition, skin breakdown (decubitus), poor hygiene, alopecia (hair loss) caused by repeated pulling or tugging of hair, and poor general health status. Other signs may include a series of missed appointments or frequently changing health care providers.

Similar to child abuse and domestic violence, victims often do not report or confirm the violence. One reason is that they love their abusers. Another is fear of losing a home and financial support. Additionally, they are afraid of more abuse from the abuser as a response to any complaint. Some older adults, as parents of the abuser, may feel that they have failed in raising their children. There are also older adults who cannot report the abuse due to a problem with communication or verbalizing what is occurring.

Neglect often is also considered a form of elder abuse. When these individuals are not provided with food or shelter, the caregiver is considered to be neglectful. Leaving the disabled older adult unattended, especially for long periods, thus endangering their well-being, is also a form of neglect.

Patient Screening

Reports of signs of elder abuse require prompt attention. Schedule an appointment for the patient to be seen as soon as possible.

Etiology

As with other forms of abuse, abuse of older adults is a complex situation. Often older adults may become more childlike or ill and dependent on their children for survival, including financial support and physical care. Society presumes that this group of people is protected by love, gentleness, and caring. Some of the older adults requiring care have diminished mental capacity and are confused. The care of these persons can be a source of stress to the caregiver, not only because of the physical care demands but also because of financial and emotional pressures. With the breakdown of the nuclear family structure and the stresses of being a single parent, the additional task of caring for an older person can become an overwhelming burden. Additionally, current society puts emphasis on youth. Other cases of elder abuse have a financial basis, either in the caregiver being unable to afford the necessities that the older person requires or in taking control of the older person's finances for the abuser's personal gain.

Diagnosis

The diagnosis is made on the basis of an evaluation of the situation and physical examination. Psychological abuse is difficult to diagnose. Many of the victims believe that revealing their child's abusive behavior toward them will suggest that they have failed as parents or that it will jeopardize their living arrangements.

Treatment

Treatment consists of treating any trauma with the appropriate care and determining the need for appropriate protective services. Counseling should be made available to all parties involved. If necessary, the victim should be removed from the abusive environment. Prevention is the best treatment; however, that is not always possible.

Prognosis

The prognosis varies, depending on the extent and duration of the abuse and the perpetrator of the abuse. Removal of the older individual from the abusive environment usually is helpful.

Prevention

The primary goal is to protect the patient from harm; however, prevention is not always possible. Close monitoring of situations in which an older person is dependent on others for care may be helpful. Suggestions of respite care may be helpful. Recognition of signs of extreme stress in the caregiver and suggestions of assistance for care provision may be helpful. Referrals for agencies that provide sitters may provide "help" for the primary caregiver, resulting in less stress for this person.

Patient Teaching
Assist family members in locating and contacting community resources that are available.

Psychological or Verbal Abuse
Description
Psychological or emotional abuse is the intentional and systematic diminishment of another's self-worth or self-esteem.

ICD-10-CM Code	T74.31XA (Adult psychological abuse, confirmed, initial encounter)
	T76.31XA (Adult psychological abuse, suspected, initial encounter)
	T74.32XA (Child psychological abuse, confirmed, initial encounter)
	T76.32XA (Child psychological abuse, suspected, initial encounter)

Symptoms and Signs
Symptoms of psychological or verbal abuse, the systematic diminishment of another, take on many forms. Often the abused person makes no complaints. Although emotional battering occurs in all age groups, children are the most frequent victims. The guilt that is imposed on these victims often leads to self-destructive behavior, including anorexia, bulimia, obesity, alcoholism, self-mutilation, drug addiction, depression, and suicide. Others manifest their guilt feelings by emotional guarding and turning their anger and rage inward against themselves. Abused individuals may display a lack of self-esteem and self-worth and find difficulty bonding with others.

Patient Screening
Psychologically or emotionally abused individuals usually do not have enough mental strength to seek help. Many of these individuals are unaware of the abusive actions directed toward them and feel that they deserve any abusive psychological behavior directed at them. Many are often referred from emergency care facilities and require an immediate appointment. The situations often are discovered on a visit to the physician for another reason.

Etiology
The cause of this form of abuse is unknown. Often a parent, partner, or caregiver is the abuser, denying the victim (child or partner) love and protection. The abuse can be active, with words such as "You're stupid," "I'm ashamed of you,"

or "You'll never amount to anything." It can be passive in the form of intentional neglect. Often it is a combination of the two. The abuse can take on the verbal form, or it may be shown by the abuser's actions. Most verbal abuse is done in secret; usually only the victim hears it. Emotional abuse becomes more intense over time; the victim begins to adapt to it. Verbal abuse consistently discounts the victim's perception of the abuse.

Diagnosis
Emotional abuse is difficult to diagnose because no physical contact occurs. The comments usually are made to the victim in private or in the home environment and rarely in a public setting. The abusive behavior takes place over time. The victim believes that he or she is responsible for the behavior of the abuser and does not realize that it is a form of abuse. The victims often defend the abusive behavior, believing that they deserve it. Victims feel lost, not knowing where to turn. These relationships are filled with inequity, competition, manipulation, hostility, control, and negation and create feelings of inadequacy, frustration, rejection, disappointment, sadness, fear, and confusion. In the medical office setting, many patient information forms now include questions about whether or not a person feels "safe" in their own home, if they are depressed, etc., which may lead to conversations about living conditions and emotional abuse.

Treatment
The best treatment is prevention. Education of the population as to what constitutes emotional abuse and ways to prevent the many forms is important. A building of self-esteem and self-worth is necessary to begin the healing process. Because of the varied forms of emotional abuse, each individual must believe in himself or herself and address the specific guilt felt, possibly with the help of a therapist.

Prognosis
The prognosis varies, depending on the duration of the abusive relationship. Psychological therapy may be helpful; however, many of these abused individuals are unable to accept the diagnosis of abuse and resist treatment. Some individuals enter into emotionally abusive relationships with other people willingly because they are victims who do not know how to avoid those relationships as adults.

Prevention
Prevention relies on the education of society as to what constitutes psychological or emotional abuse and how society can be helpful.

Patient Teaching
Help victims to build self-esteem and realize their self-worth. Assist them in locating and contacting community

resources that have programs to help individuals learn to avoid getting into relationships with emotionally abusive people.

Intimate Partner Violence

Description

Intimate partner violence (IPV) is the result of threatened or actual physical abuse, a pattern of behavior in which the victim is repeatedly physically assaulted by her or his partner. Other terms for IPV include domestic violence, spouse abuse, and battered spouse syndrome. Stalking is another form of IPV.

ICD-10-CM Code   T74.11XA *(Adult physical abuse, confirmed, initial encounter)*
T76.11XA *(Adult physical abuse, suspected, initial encounter)*

Symptoms and Signs

Victims of IPV in heterosexual and homosexual relationships can be either sex. The victim has evidence of bruising in various stages of healing, usually in an area of the body that is concealed by clothing, and has a tendency to avoid making eye contact with the examiner. Types of IVP include physical violence, sexual violence, stalking, and psychological aggression, but there are also other types of violence that can be attributed to IPV and have an impact on victims.

Patient Screening

An individual reporting a physical assault by a spouse or partner requires prompt attention and should be reported to the police according to state guidelines. Victims may also indicate their spouse or partner will not let them contact their family and that they feel "isolated and alone."

Etiology

IPV is a complex issue. There are many different factors that may play a part, some of which are societal, individual, relational, from the community where one lives. No one specific cause is known. Stress is suggested as an important factor, along with alcohol ingestion and possible intoxication. Many victims have low self-esteem, adding to their inability to escape the victimization. Both sexes can be abusers capable of inflicting physical and emotional harm.

Diagnosis

The diagnosis is made on the basis of the information provided by the victim or by others. Physical examination indicates physical injuries. As with child abuse and sexual abuse, the injuries are varied and often occur on areas of the body that normally are covered by clothing. Assessment of the emotional state is difficult but necessary. Proper evaluation and direct, appropriate questions should be a part of the examination. For example, "You have a bruise on your face. Did someone hit you?" Often intervention results from law enforcement involvement; other times, the abusive trauma is discovered by the physician and other health care staff when the victim is seen for another reason in the office or health care facility. Information obtained and physical findings should be carefully documented; photographs of the injuries should be included in the documentation. It should also be understood that, at times, the abuser is physically with the victim at the health care facility, which requires separating the two to question the victim about injuries.

Treatment

Treatment involves the normal protocol for treating physical injuries. Discussing the situation in a nonjudgmental way is imperative. Referral to the appropriate agencies for counseling is indicated; nevertheless, the health care provider must recognize that the victim may not want or seek counseling and may elect to stay in the abusive situation. Mandated reporting may be required by the state after probable cause is determined.

Prognosis

The prognosis varies, depending on the duration and extent of the battering. Additionally, the circumstances of the relationship in which the battering has taken place will affect the long-term outcome of any intervention. Moreover, the willingness of the battered individual to leave the situation and to report the battering to law enforcement also will affect the outcome. Murder and suicide can result.

Prevention

Prevention is difficult because many abused partners feel that they deserve the battering and that it is accepted behavior in society as they know it. Raising awareness of the issue in the community and in the educational system and teaching that battering is not acceptable behavior may prevent battering and acceptance of battering occurring in future generations. In some states, the individual committing the violence also faces additional charges if a minor child witnesses the violent act. The state, not the victim, is the complainant, removing the responsibility of filing a charge from the victim. Additionally, intervention programs for the batterer are becoming part of the sentencing protocols in domestic violence cases.

Patient Teaching

Reinforcing to the victim that no one deserves to be treated in such a manner may be helpful. Acceptance of the victim as an individual with inherent self-worth is a valuable tool in establishing rapport and in building trust between the caregiver and the individual. Provide the victim with local telephone contact numbers to be used in an emergency situation to obtain help. Additionally, assist them in locating and contacting community resources. Local IPV organizations are well-informed regarding the process of providing protection and can assist the victim with civil protective orders, shelters, and information regarding protective laws.

Sexual Abuse

Description

Any form of nonconsensual sexual contact or activity is considered sexual abuse. Sexual abuse may involve either sex and may be perpetrated by either sex. Another important factor is that the victim of sexual abuse may be of any age, from an infant to an older adult.

> ICD-10-CM Code T74.21XA *(Adult sexual abuse, confirmed, initial encounter)*
> T76.21XA *(Adult sexual abuse, suspected, initial encounter)*
> T74.22XA *(Child sexual abuse, confirmed, initial encounter)*
> T76.22XA *(Child sexual abuse, suspected, initial encounter)*

Symptoms and Signs

Sexual abuse takes on many forms; thus symptoms and signs can be numerous and different from one patient to the next. Any form of nonconsensual sexual activity can be considered sexual abuse. Some examples of sexual abuse are fondling of the genitals or breasts, penetration of the vagina or rectum with fingers or other objects, and forcing the victim to touch the perpetrator on or around the sex organs. Exposing a child to pornography is also considered abuse, as is taking pornographic photos of a child. The victim often does not report unwanted advances or activity and usually appears subdued. Itching, burning and discharge may be present in the urethral and vaginal areas. Anal and vaginal tears and scars may be found on physical examination. Sexually abused children have an unusual obsession with the genital region and frequently touch themselves abnormally. They often exhibit aggressive behavior.

Patient Screening

Any individual reporting sexual abuse requires prompt attention. Refer the patient to a sexual abuse or emergency facility for immediate intervention if the provider does not offer those services in the facility as a sexual assault forensic exam "rape kit" requires a chain of custody. Some victims may be resistant to this option; if so, schedule an appointment as soon as possible.

Etiology

As with other forms of abuse, the cause of sexual abuse is a complicated matter. Domination, control, and power issues can be reasons for this unacceptable form of behavior. Many of the perpetrators were sexually abused as children, and they do not regard what they are doing as wrong. Some simply have a sociopathic approach to society and its norms. It is important to consider that victimization of both sexes occurs and that the abuser can be of either sex.

Diagnosis

The diagnosis is made on the basis of the history given by the victim and is confirmed on physical examination. Often the sexual abuse is combined with physical abuse, and treatment of that abuse may lead to the victim confiding in the caregiver or health care provider regarding the unwanted sexual activity. Many times, the removal of the victim from a physically abusive environment allows the victim to feel safe enough to discuss the sexual abuse. Perpetrators of sexual abuse of children or infants have been babysitters, relatives, domestic partners, boyfriends, girlfriends, or parents. Sexual abuse can affect a person of any age.

Treatment

Immediately after the assault, strict legal guidelines must be followed when performing a physical examination. Emergency treatment of a victim of sexual assault involves both medical and forensic examinations. Any trauma is treated according to the protocol of the facility. Law enforcement agencies should be notified, with the victim's consent, or according to local or state policy. Prophylactic sexually transmitted disease (STD) treatments and pregnancy prevention therapy may be offered. If possible, the victim is removed from the abusive situation. Emotional support is provided, and reinforcement is given to the victim that he or she is not responsible for the sexual abuse. If the victim is receptive to counseling, arrangements are made to assist the victim in dealing with the abuse. If the victim is a child, child protective services are usually involved, and when the situation warrants, the child is removed from the environment. The social services agencies involved usually determine when a child is to be removed from this type of environment.

Prognosis

The prognosis varies, depending on the form, duration, and extent of sexual abuse. The physical wounds may heal quickly, but the emotional wounds often leave permanent scars. When possible, direct the victim to follow-up counseling. A resulting pregnancy or STD will require additional intervention.

> **ENRICHMENT**
>
> **DNA Parentage Testing**
>
> Deoxyribonucleic acid (DNA) parentage testing is the most reliable and powerful method of providing proof of parentage for legal and medical reasons. It conclusively answers difficult questions, resolves disputes, and helps streamline court proceedings.
> Testing is based on a highly accurate analysis of the genetic profiles of the mother, the child, and the alleged

Continued

Prevention

Prevention is difficult. It is not often possible to predict who may be a sexual abuser; nor is it possible to predict where or when sexual abuse may take place. Individuals should be encouraged not to provide personal details when communicating online with other people they do not know.

Patient Teaching

Assist the victim in locating and contacting community resource agencies that can provide support and assistance. Reinforce that sexual abuse is not accepted behavior. The victim should not be judged.

Rape/Sexual Assault

Description

Intercourse forced on a person against her or his will is termed *rape* or *sexual assault*.

ICD-10-CM Code	T74.21XA *(Adult sexual abuse, confirmed, initial encounter)*
	T76.21XA *(Adult sexual abuse, suspected, initial encounter)*
	T74.22XA *(Child sexual abuse, confirmed, initial encounter)*
	T76.22XA *(Child sexual abuse, suspected, initial encounter)*

Symptoms and Signs

The symptoms and signs of rape/sexual assault vary with the degree of violence incurred by the victim. Many come to an emergency care facility, physician's office, clinic, or a law enforcement agency stating, "I've been raped." Some report having pain in the pelvic and perineal regions or being choked or restrained in some manner. Others report the threat of death. Bruising may be noted in any area of the body, not just the pelvic area. Signs of rape include torn clothing, dirt and debris ground into clothing or hair, disheveled appearance, withdrawal, anxiousness, avoidance of eye contact, and bruising, tears, or lacerations around or on the genitals, rectum, or mouth. Pelvic and rectal examination often reveals tenderness in those areas and evidence of trauma. If the victim has not bathed or douched, evidence of semen may be present on the inner aspects of the thighs, genital areas, mouth, nares, or pubic region. Any part of the body, including the may be traumatized. Bruising or lacerations in the anal region are indicative of sodomy.

Patient Screening

Many rape victims will go to or be transported to an emergency facility for a sexual assault examination, which includes the gathering of any evidence. However, some victims resist reporting the attack to authorities and request an appointment to see a physician. Other victims may seek anonymity and seek a physician with whom they have had no previous contact. It is important to remember that both sexes can be victims of sexual assault. For any individual reporting rape or sexual assault, an appointment should be scheduled as soon as possible.

Etiology

Rape is a crime of violence and domination, not a sexual act. It occurs when there is no mutual consent between both parties involved in the sexual act, and it is a forced act. Rape can be in the form of date rape, acquaintance rape, rape by the victim's spouse or partner, or a violent act perpetrated by an unknown assailant.

Diagnosis

The diagnosis is made by evaluating the findings from the history, clinical examination, physical examination, including pelvic examination, and sex crime evidence gathering. Samples of debris, clothing, saliva, hair, pubic hair, fingernails, and scrapings from under the nails are collected. A specimen for urinalysis is obtained, along with specimens for blood tests for STDs, acquired immunodeficiency syndrome (AIDS), and possible pregnancy. Photographs may be taken for documentation of injuries. It is recommended that this type of complete examination take place in a facility with staff professionally educated in treating sexual assault victims. Many communities offer sexual assault response teams (SARTs) that are called in to perform sexual assault medical and legal examinations. All personal belongings of the victim must be handled carefully, and all items must be marked as evidence. Rape examinations for most victims are performed at no cost.

Treatment

Any patient who has suffered trauma is treated in an appropriate manner. Sexual assault victims should receive an emergent priority and be placed in a safe and secure location. Counseling at a rape crisis center should be offered. Information concerning the risks of possible pregnancy, STDs, and AIDS is given, along with an explanation of the protocol for follow-up testing. If the patient has no religious objection, prophylaxis for pregnancy may be considered.

Reinforcement that the victim is a survivor of a violent crime and is not responsible for the incident is necessary. Everyone dealing with the victim and her or his family must be nonjudgmental and supportive. According to state laws, victims must be informed that law enforcement must be notified, when applicable.

Prognosis

The prognosis for victims of rape varies. Physical healing may take place without any complications. However, a resulting pregnancy or STDs will need to be addressed. Ongoing psychological counseling may be required for lengthy periods. Undoubtedly, the physical and psychological effects on the victims will be longstanding, if not lifelong.

Prevention

It is difficult to prevent rape because it is difficult to predict who might be a perpetrator or what place might be a potential location of a rape. On the one hand, social media has played a role in strangers meeting each other for various purposes, which can give perpetrators easy targets because some individuals post a lot of information about their routines and personal lives. On the other hand, social media has also been used to help solve cases. Security cameras may deter some from committing crimes in those locations.

Patient Teaching

Have a nonjudgmental approach to providing care for rape victims. Assist them in seeking counseling and in contacting the local rape crisis center; and encourage them to follow through with the contact.

Suicide

Description

Suicide is taking one's own life or intentionally causing one's own death.

ICD-10-CM Code   T14.91×A *(Suicide attempt, initial encounter)*

Symptoms and Signs

Individuals contemplating suicide may appear depressed or make remarks about how they look forward to dying. They may give away certain items. They may state that they want to die and are thinking about committing suicide. Some may say, "You would be better off without me." They may withdraw from the family or the situation. They may say they are just tired, their body is tired, their mind is tired, and they are just exhausted. They may have tried cutting themselves or may be ingesting different drugs. To them, life is hopeless, and there is no relief. They feel that the only relief they will get will be by dying. This individual believes death is their final escape.

Patient Screening

When a patient or a family member calls about impending suicide, it is best to offer them the next available appointment. Additionally, the health care provider should be alerted and their instructions followed.

Etiology

Many factors may cause depression. Personal relationships may go bad. Difficult money situations may trigger the thought of escape. Loss of employment is a discouraging factor. Not being able to meet parental or partner expectations often is difficult. Being bullied can also lead to suicide.

Diagnosis

Some clients may be placed on a suicide watch if they have expressed a desire to end their life. Text messages, written messages, or letters indicating that the world or specific people would be "better off if I were dead" should be taken seriously. A psychologist or a psychiatrist is helpful in screening for this type of ideation. Social media platforms are also used to post personal feelings of depression, anxiety, and despair, and these posts can sometimes alert a friend that someone is considering suicide.

Treatment

If the patient is seen in the office, treatment may include antidepressant medications. The prevention hotline telephone number is 1-800-273-(TALK)8255 and is answered 24 hours a day, 7 days a week. The number 988 can also be called and the person will be routed to telephone assistance and support in their local area code. If the suicidal individual will not call the number, the individual attempting to help could call the number for advice on what to say and what to do.

Prognosis

Once the individual has committed suicide, nothing more can be done. Their family should receive counseling to help them deal with the circumstance. Grief counseling is recommended and arranged, if desired.

Prevention

Suicide may be stopped by recognizing sadness, depression, and intent to commit suicide. Talking with the person contemplating suicide and allowing him or her to know you care and want to help may stop or delay an impending suicide.

Patient Teaching

When an individual has attempted suicide or has expressed suicidal thoughts, express your recognition of the feeling. Recommend counseling, and discuss contacting the suicide hotline. Inform family members about the suicide hotline and its telephone number. Encourage the individual contemplating suicide to talk about their feelings. Suicide is a fatal action.

Review Challenge

Answer the following questions:

1. What are the major types of trauma?
2. What are some ways in which environmental factors can result in trauma?
3. What is the difference between an abrasion and an avulsion?
4. When is it appropriate to use tetanus toxoid in prophylactic treatment?
5. When is debridement of a wound necessary?
6. How are the depth and extent of burns assessed?
7. What are the possible effects of an electrical shock?
8. What are the types of lightning strikes? Which treatments may be required?
9. How are the signs and symptoms of heat stroke and heat exhaustion different?
10. What is the treatment for heat stroke? For heat exhaustion?
11. What are some precautions in the treatment of frostbite?
12. Which spider bites require emergency care?
13. What is Rocky Mountain spotted fever, and how is it transmitted?
14. Why is an animal quarantined after biting a human?
15. What are the signs and symptoms of a poisonous snakebite?
16. What is the relationship between repetitive activities and carpal tunnel syndrome?
17. Which physical patterns may be observed in child abuse?
18. How may elder abuse and neglect, child abuse and neglect, sexual abuse, or intimate partner violence be noted during the history and physical examination?
19. What testing is available for the rape/sexual assault victim?
20. How can parentage be determined in the laboratory?

Real-Life Challenge: Heat Exhaustion

The mother of a 14-year-old girl called the office about her daughter, who had just come home from attending marching band practice for approximately 3 hours. The girl was complaining of nausea, weakness, and headache. On questioning, the mother revealed that her daughter's skin appeared pale, cool, and moist. The weather had been hot and humid, and the girl told her mother that she had been practicing the marching routines for about 2.5 hours before she felt ill. When the mother took the girl's temperature, it was 98.2°F, and the girl's pulse was faint and fast.

The mother was advised to have her daughter lie down in a cool environment, with feet slightly elevated; to loosen her clothing; and to place cool compresses on the girl's face, forehead, neck, chest, abdomen, arms, back, and legs. She also was instructed to give her daughter 4 ounces of cool water to drink every 15 minutes. The office advised that they would call back in 1 hour to get a progress report.

The diagnosis was heat exhaustion.

Questions

1. What is the significance of the cool, moist skin?
2. What measures could have been taken to prevent the onset of heat exhaustion?
3. Compare the moist, cool skin and sweating of heat exhaustion with the skin condition of heat stroke.
4. What could be the anticipated outcome of the treatment that was suggested to the mother?
5. If the girl's condition did not improve in 1 hour, what would you expect the next step in treatment to be?
6. What is the significance of loosening clothing and applying cool compresses?
7. Why would the mother be instructed to use cool compresses and not ice?
8. Why would the patient with heat stroke require treatment in an emergency facility versus the heat exhaustion victim, who can be treated at home?

Real-Life Challenge: Intimate Partner Violence

A 36-year-old female is in the office being treated for pain and reduced hearing in the left ear. She is very vague about any history, saying only that her left ear is painful; she has noted some blood coming out of the canal, and she has reduced hearing in her left ear. Bruising is noted around the ear on the left cheek, on the left side of the neck, and behind the left ear on the skull. These areas are tender to the touch. The patient is very quiet, at times is tearful, and is wearing a long-sleeved turtleneck shirt and long pants. She is hesitant to remove her shirt for blood pressure measurement or for any other examination.

Examination reveals recent trauma to the left ear, blood is visualized in the canal, and otoscopic examination confirms a ruptured tympanic membrane. Audiometry confirms reduced hearing capability in the left ear. Bruises in various stages of healing are noted on the arms, neck, and chest. Further examination discloses similar bruising to the legs. The patient denies any abusive trauma and says she incurred the injuries in a fall. She avoids eye contact, tending to keep her eyes downward. Her demeanor is subdued, and her posture also appears subdued, with the shoulders slumped.

Gentle questioning eventually reveals that her husband, a male of large stature, recently lost his job as a result of drinking and aggressive or near-violent behavior. She also admits that in the past 2 weeks since the loss of his job, her husband has been "slapping her around" and that last night he struck her on the left side of her face and across the ear with his open hand. The patient does not want to file a police report and says she cannot leave the abusive situation.

She is referred to an ear, nose, and throat (ENT) specialist for treatment of the ruptured tympanic membrane. An appointment for follow-up is made for 2 days later, at which time additional support for the psychosocial situation will be supplied. She is instructed to call immediately in case of any recurrence of the abusive behavior. She also is advised to see whether she can get her husband to make an appointment for an examination.

Questions

1. What is typical behavior for a "battered" spouse or victim of intimate partner violence?
2. What is the significance of alcohol consumption and the loss of employment at the onset of abuse?
3. Why did not the victim want the abuse reported?
4. What are the legal responsibilities of your office in this situation?
5. What might be the reasons that the victim feels she cannot leave the abusive situation?
6. Explain the mechanics of the impact of the slapping causing rupture of the tympanic membrane.
7. Discuss the implications of both the abusive husband and the battered wife being patients of the practice.

Internet Assignments

1. Research the support available to families of major trauma victims at the American Trauma Society. Check this same website for suggested preventive measures.
2. Research suggested measures available to the victim of domestic violence at the National Coalition Against Domestic Violence.
3. Research the Bair Hugger concept.
4. Research your state's guidelines for reportable incidents.
5. Research your state's required reporting for workers' compensation injuries.
6. Access the SART digital toolkit at https://www.nsvrc.org/sarts. What are some of the tools that can assist members of the SART team?

Critical Thinking

1. Working in a facility where you see many patients filling out worker's compensation forms, you recently have noted that several from the same facility have been experiencing the same type of injury. What do you feel your role is in making someone aware that there might be a problem at that facility? How do you make sure that reports concerning this condition exist?
2. What teaching techniques would you use to explain to parents the importance of training their children not to place any objects in their noses? How would you attempt to explain to children the reason that they should not put things in their ears or their noses? What happens to cereal when they put it in their nose?
3. Explain the "rule of nines" when it comes to assessing a burn patient and the percentage of burns on their bodies.
4. Why is it important to have an understanding of radiation effects and burns? Explain how you would protect yourself from radiation.
5. Explain the guidelines in your community about animal bites. Are the animals quarantined? What are the reportable guidelines for animal bites? Are animals held for a certain length of time before being put down?
6. Family violence is escalating. What is happening to the statistics in your community? Can you remain objective while dealing with all members of the family?

7. After and while working with victims of abuse, what explanation do you have for why older adults and children are reluctant to come forward about being abused? Discuss some of the reasons older adults are abused.

8. Research the Duluth Model Power and Control Wheel, and discuss why you think this has an effect on family violence, domestic violence, and even sexual abuse.

Credentialing Examination Questions

1. Which wound is an example of closed trauma?
  A. Bruise
  B. Avulsion
  C. Puncture
  D. Abrasion
2. A hand is trapped between two surfaces. Which will most likely result in a crushing injury?
  A. Two soft surfaces
  B. Two hard surfaces
  C. Hard and soft surface
  D. Any of the above can result in a crushing injury
3. A person is impaled with an object. Which action should be taken *first*, when providing care?
  A. Call the immediate family
  B. Remove the impaled object
  C. Leave the object where it is until arrival at the emergency facility
  D. Stabilize the object prior to moving the patient
4. Which characteristic describes a partial-thickness burn?
  A. Skin and subcutaneous tissue involved
  B. All layers of skin and no subcutaneous tissue involved
  C. Absence of blisters
  D. No pain
5. Which venomous snake is responsible for the most bites in the United States?
  A. Coral
  B. Water Moccasin
  C. Rattlesnake
  D. Copperhead
6. What is the etiology of stenosing tenosynovitis (*trigger finger*)?
  A. Repetitive finger movement
  B. Compound fracture
  C. Avulsion of finger tissue
  D. Puncture
7. What is the purpose of biodefense?
  A. Justify increased use of antibiotics
  B. Teach individuals how to protect their homes
  C. Prepare for biological agents that could be used by terrorist
  D. Respond to natural disasters
8. Which person may be a victim of intimate partner violence?
  A. Spouses
  B. Partners
  C. Children
  D. Both spouses and partners
9. Which three digits can be entered into a telephone to be connected to a suicide and crisis lifeline?
  A. 899
  B. 988
  C. 788
  D. 987
10. Animal bites are dangerous for which reason or reasons?
  A. Animals have many bacteria in their mouths.
  B. The animal may have rabies.
  C. Animals have been responsible for fatal injuries to adults and children.
  D. All of the above.

Common Laboratory and Diagnostic Tests

Values may vary depending on laboratory reference values for each test. These values are for reference only. Results of one test alone are usually not conclusive and should be considered with the results of other diagnostic procedures, the symptoms and signs, and the findings of physical examination to arrive at a diagnosis.

Blood Analysis

Complete Blood Count

A complete blood count (CBC) is the evaluation of cellular components of blood. It includes red blood cell (RBC) count, RBC indices, white blood cell (WBC) count, WBC differential, hemoglobin (Hgb), hematocrit (Hct), and platelet count. Sometimes it is referred to as *hemogram*. Often the differential must be ordered specifically as CBC with differential.

Red Blood Cell Count

RBC count is the count of erythrocytes in a specimen of whole blood.

Normal Levels
Adult males: 4.5–6.1 million/μL
Adult females: 4.0–5.5 million/μL
Infants and children: 3.8–5.5 million/μL
Newborns: 4.1–6.1 million/μL

An elevated RBC count is indicative of many disorders, including, but not limited to, erythremia, polycythemia, erythrocytosis, dehydration, burns, hypoxia, diarrhea, cardiovascular disease, poisoning, pulmonary disease, and smoking. A reduced RBC count also is indicative of many disorders, including, but not limited to, anemias, bone marrow suppression, hemorrhage, lead poisoning, liver diseases, thyroid disorders, cardiovascular disease, malnutrition, vitamin deficiency, and adverse effects of certain drugs. When the RBC count is abnormal, cell morphology should be examined. As with most blood tests, results should be

evaluated with those of other tests, along with symptoms and signs, to determine a diagnosis.

Hemoglobin Count

An Hgb count is the measurement of the oxygen (O_2)-carrying pigments of the RBCs.

Normal Levels
Adult males: 13.0–18.0
Adult females: 12.0–16.0
Infants and children: 9.5–15.5
Newborns: 14–24

An elevated Hgb count is indicative of many disorders, including, but not limited to, congestive heart failure (CHF), chronic obstructive pulmonary disease (COPD), dehydration, burns, diarrhea, erythrocytosis, polycythemia, high-altitude sickness, and thrombotic thrombocytopenia. A reduced Hgb count is also indicative of many disorders, including, but not limited to, iron deficiency anemia, hemorrhage, hemolytic reaction to drugs or chemicals, liver diseases, and systemic lupus erythematosus (SLE) and is indicative of pregnancy.

Hematocrit Count

Hct count is the measurement of the percentage of RBCs in a volume of whole blood.

Normal Levels
Adult males: 38%–49%
Adult females: 36%–45%
Infants and children: 28%–50%
Newborns: 45%–64%

An elevated Hct count is indicative of many disorders, including, but not limited to, dehydration, burns, diarrhea, eclampsia, pancreatitis, shock, and polycythemia. A reduced Hct count is also indicative of many disorders, including, but not limited to, anemia, bone marrow hyperplasia, CHF, fluid overload, burns, thyroid disorders, pancreatitis, pneumonia, malnutrition, and adverse effects of certain drugs and is indicative of pregnancy.

White Blood Cell Count

The WBC count is the count of WBCs in a whole blood specimen.

Normal Levels
Adult males: 4500–11,000/μL
Adult females: 4500–11,000/μL
Infants and children: 6000–17,500/μL
Newborns: 9000–35,000/μL

An elevated WBC count is indicative of many disorders, including, but not limited to, acquired hemolytic anemia, anorexia, abscess, appendicitis, bacterial infections, bronchitis, burns, biliary disorders, respiratory disorders, disorders of the gastrointestinal (GI) tract, renal disorders, blood disorders, lactic acidosis, SLE, poisoning, rheumatoid arthritis, sepsis, shock, tonsillitis, trauma, uremia, and adverse effects of certain drugs, and indicative of pregnancy. Similar to an abnormal RBC count, a differential should be evaluated, and as with most blood tests, results should be evaluated with those of other tests—along with symptoms and signs—to determine a diagnosis. A decreased WBC is indicative of many disorders, including, but not limited to, acquired immunodeficiency syndrome (AIDS), anemias, chemical toxicity, Hodgkin disease, influenza, legionnaires disease, radiation therapy, shock, septicemia, vitamin B_{12} deficiency, cirrhosis, hepatitis, hypothermia, leukopenia, tuberculosis (TB), and adverse effects of certain drugs.

Differential White Blood Cell (Leukocyte) Count

The differential WBC (leukocyte) count is an assessment by percentage of leukocyte distribution in a specimen of 100 WBCs.

Leukocyte Count

Normal Levels
Segmented neutrophils (SEGs; mature "fighter" cell),
  adults: 50%–62%
Band neutrophils (immature "fighter" cells), adults:
  3%–6%
Eosinophil granulocytes (eosinophils), adults: 0%–3%
Basophil granulocytes (basophils), adults: 0%–1%
Monocytes, adults: 3%–7%
Lymphocytes, adults: 24%–44%

Increased neutrophils are indicative of many disorders, including, but not limited to, allergies, asthma, acute infections, appendicitis, burns, diabetic acidosis, cardiovascular

disorders, disorders of the GI tract, leukemia, respiratory disorders, poisoning, pyelonephritis, septicemia, tonsillitis, and adverse effects of certain drugs. A decrease in neutrophils is indicative of many disorders, including, but not limited to, endocrine disorders, anaphylactic shock, carcinoma, chemotherapy, anemias, pneumonia, influenza, septicemia, radiation therapy, and adverse effects of certain drugs.

An increase in eosinophils is indicative of many disorders, including, but not limited to, allergies, asthma, cancer, dermatitis, diverticulitis, eczema, Hodgkin disease, leukemia, parasitic infection, pernicious anemia, radiation therapy, sickle cell anemia, TB, and adverse effects of certain drugs. A reduction in eosinophils also is indicative of many disorders, including, but not limited to, aplastic anemia, CHF, eclampsia, infections, stress, and adverse effects of certain drugs.

An increase in basophils is indicative of many disorders, including, but not limited to, allergic reactions, Hodgkin disease, hypothyroidism, radiation therapy, sinusitis, urticaria, and adverse effects of certain drugs. A decrease in basophils is also indicative of many disorders, including, but not limited to, acute infections, anaphylactic shock, endocrine disorders, cancer, radiation therapy, stress, adverse effects of certain drugs, and pregnancy.

An increase in lymphocytes is indicative of many disorders, including, but not limited to, endocarditis, infectious mononucleosis, leukocytosis, lymphocytic leukemia, syphilis, toxoplasmosis chronic bacterial infection, viral infections, and adverse effects of certain drugs. A decrease in lymphocytes also is indicative of many disorders, including, but not limited to, aplastic anemia, Hodgkin disease, immunoglobulin deficiencies, leukemia, renal failure, SLE, uremia, sepsis, and adverse effects of certain drugs.

An increase in monocytes is indicative of many disorders, including, but not limited to, Epstein-Barr virus, Hodgkin disease, leukemia, rheumatoid arthritis, syphilis, SLE, TB, chronic inflammatory disease, and adverse effects of certain drugs. A decrease in monocytes is primarily indicative of aplastic anemia and hairy-cell leukemia.

Platelet (Thrombocyte) Count

The platelet (thrombocyte) count is the count of platelets in a whole blood specimen. Platelets help the blood clot.

Normal Adult Levels
150,000–450,000/μL

An increase in the platelet count (thrombocytosis) is indicative of many disorders, including, but not limited to, anemias, carcinoma, fractures, liver disorders, heart disease, hemorrhage, acute infection, inflammation, leukemia, pancreatitis, rheumatoid arthritis, surgery, adverse effects of certain drugs, and pregnancy. A decrease in platelet count (thrombocytopenia) is indicative of many disorders, including, but not limited to, anemias, bone marrow disorders, autoimmune disorders, severe burns, carcinoma, liver disorders, disseminated intravascular coagulation (DIC), hemolytic disease of the newborn, infections, radiation therapy, leukemia, celiac disease, vitamin K deficiency, and adverse effects of certain drugs.

Blood Chemistries

Chemistries

A normal chemistry profile may contain blood serum levels for albumin, alkaline phosphatase, aspartate aminotransferase (AST), bilirubin, calcium, creatinine, lactate dehydrogenase (LDH), phosphorus, total protein, urea nitrogen, and uric acid. Blood chemistries are often ordered in a panel of tests, which gives a profile of a certain organ or a number of organs. Chem7 is a basic metabolic panel consisting of seven tests: blood urea nitrogen (BUN), carbon dioxide (CO_2), creatinine, glucose, serum potassium, and serum sodium levels. A comprehensive metabolic panel generally consists of albumin, alkaline phosphatase, alanine aminotransferase (ALT), AST, BUN, calcium, chloride, CO_2, creatinine, LDH, glucose, potassium, sodium, total bilirubin, and total protein. These tests provide the health care provider with information regarding how the patient's liver and kidneys are working, blood sugar and calcium levels, electrolyte levels (sodium, potassium, chloride), and protein levels.

Albumin

Serum albumin is the measurement of one of the two major protein fractions in the blood.

Normal Adult Levels
3.5–5.0 g/dL

Increased levels of serum albumin are indicative of many disorders, including, but not limited to, dehydration, diarrhea, hepatitis, meningitis, carcinoma, myeloma, nephrosis, nephrotic syndrome, peptic ulcers, pneumonia, rheumatic fever, SLE, uremia, vomiting, and adverse effects of certain drugs. Below-normal levels of serum albumin are indicative of many disorders, including, but not limited to, ascites, alcoholism, burns, CHF, Crohn's disease, cystic fibrosis, diabetes mellitus, edema, hypertension, kidney disorders, malnutrition, GI disorders, trauma, stress, and adverse effects of certain drugs.

Alanine Transaminase

ALT is the measurement of the enzyme found in the liver.

Normal Adult Levels
4–36 units/L

ALT is released into blood when the liver is damaged. Elevated levels are indicative of cirrhosis of the liver, hepatitis, liver ischemia, mononucleosis, or inflammation of the pancreas.

Alkaline Phosphatase

Alkaline phosphatase level is the measurement of the enzyme found in bones, the liver, intestines, and the placenta.

Normal Adult Levels
25–100 units/L

Elevated alkaline phosphatase levels are indicative of many disorders, including, but not limited to, alcoholism, liver disorders, diabetes mellitus, fractures, GI disorders, endocrine disorders, hepatitis, Hodgkin disease, leukemia, neoplasms, myocardial infarction (MI), bone disorders, disorders of the pancreas, kidney disorders, and adverse effects of certain drugs. Below-normal levels of alkaline phosphatase are indicative of many disorders, including, but not limited to, pernicious anemia, cretinism, hypothyroidism, malnutrition, nephritis, and adverse effects of certain drugs.

Aspartate Aminotransferase (Serum Glutamic Oxaloacetic Transaminase)

AST (serum glutamic oxaloacetic transaminase [SGOT]) is the measurement of enzymes found primarily in the heart, liver, and muscles.

Normal Adult Levels
Females: 10–36 units/L
Males: 14–20 units/L

Elevated AST levels are indicative of many disorders, including, but not limited to, acute MI, alcoholism, liver disorders, mononucleosis, insult and injury to tissue (including trauma), cerebral and pulmonary infarctions, and adverse effects of certain drugs. Reduced AST levels are indicative of many disorders, including, but not limited to, diabetic ketoacidosis, liver disease, uremia, vitamin B_6 deficiency, and adverse effects of certain drugs.

Bilirubin

Bilirubin is a by-product of Hgb breakdown. Bilirubin is produced in the liver, spleen, and bone marrow.

Normal Adult Levels
Total: <1.5 mg/dL
Direct: 0.0–0.3 mg/dL
Indirect: 0.1–1.0 mg/dL

Total bilirubin is divided into direct bilirubin, primarily secreted by the intestinal tract, and indirect bilirubin, primarily circulating in the bloodstream. Obstructive or hepatic jaundice results in an increased amount of direct bilirubin entering the bloodstream rather than entering the GI tract and being filtered and eliminated by the kidneys. Conditions that cause an increase in direct bilirubin include, but are not limited to, biliary obstruction, pancreatic cancer (head of the pancreas), cirrhosis, hepatitis, and adverse effects of certain drugs. Hemolytic jaundice causes indirect bilirubin to accumulate in the blood because of the increased breakdown of Hgb. Conditions that cause an increase in direct bilirubin levels include, but are not limited to, pernicious and sickle cell anemias, autoimmune hemolysis, cirrhosis, hepatitis, intracavity and soft tissue hemorrhage, MI, septicemia, hemolytic transfusion reactions, and adverse effects of certain drugs.

Creatinine

Creatinine level is a measurement of an indicator of renal function.

Normal Adult Levels
Females: 0.5–1.1 mg/dL
Males: 0.6–1.2 mg/dL

Serum creatinine is continually excreted by the renal system, and elevated levels are indicative of slowing of glomerular filtration. Other conditions that may contribute to elevation of serum creatinine include, but are not limited to, CHF, diabetes mellitus, kidney disorders, hypovolemia, metal poisoning, endocrine disorders, subacute bacterial endocarditis, SLE, and adverse effects of certain drugs. Decreased serum creatinine levels are indicative of diabetic ketoacidosis and muscular dystrophy.

Lactate Dehydrogenase

LDH level is the measurement of body tissue intracellular enzyme released after tissue damage.

Normal Adult Levels
100–250 units/L

Elevated LDH levels are indicative of many disorders, including, but not limited to, alcoholism, anoxia, burns, cardiomyopathy, cerebrovascular accident (CVA), cirrhosis, CHF and MI, neoplasms, anemias, leukemia, renal disorders, pancreatitis, mononucleosis, muscle and bone pain, respiratory disorders, shock, trauma, and adverse effects of certain drugs. The levels of LDH decrease after radiation and after adverse effects of oxalates.

Total Protein

Total protein is the measurement of the total amounts of albumin and globulins in serum.

Normal Adult Levels
6.0–8.0 g/dL

Increased total protein is indicative of many disorders, including, but not limited to, Addison disease, dehydration, diarrhea, renal disease, vomiting, protozoal diseases, chronic inflammation or infections (including human immunodeficiency virus [HIV] infection and hepatitis B or C virus), and adverse effects of certain drugs. Decreased total protein is indicative of many disorders, including, but not limited to, autoimmune diseases, burns, cholecystitis, cirrhosis, CHF, Crohn's disease, diarrhea, hyperthyroidism, edema, leukemia, peptic ulcer, nephrosis, malnutrition, ulcerative colitis, and adverse effects of certain drugs.

Urea Nitrogen/Blood Urea Nitrogen

Urea nitrogen/BUN is an assessment of the urea content in the blood and gives an indication of the functioning of the renal glomeruli.

Normal Adult Levels
5–20 mg/dL

An elevated urea nitrogen level can be indicative of many disorders, including, but not limited to, kidney disease, CHF, shock, dehydration, burns, urinary tract blockage, and a high-protein diet. A decreased urea nitrogen level can be indicative of many disorders, including but not limited to malnutrition, overhydration, and liver damage.

Uric Acid

Uric acid is an end product of the metabolism of purines.

Normal Adult Levels
Females: 2.4–6.0 mg/dL
Males: 3.4–7.0 mg/dL

Elevated uric acid levels are indicative of many disorders, including, but not limited to, gout, hyperuricemia, hemolytic and sickle cell anemias, hypothyroidism, acute infections, lead poisoning, leukemia, neoplasms, nephritis, kidney stones and polycystic kidney disease, renal failure, malnutrition, psoriasis, uremia, urinary obstruction, and adverse effects of certain drugs. Reduced uric acid levels are indicative of many disorders, including, but not limited to, acromegaly, carcinomas, Hodgkin disease, pernicious anemia, and adverse effects of certain drugs.

Thyroid Function Tests

An evaluation of the levels of all three thyroid hormones is important in diagnosing thyroid disorders.

Thyroxine

The hormone thyroxine (T_4) is produced in the thyroid gland from iodide and thyroglobulin in response to stimulation by thyroid-stimulating hormone (TSH) produced by the pituitary gland. T_4 stimulates triiodothyronine (T_3) to be produced. It also stimulates basal metabolism. In the process of negative feedback, circulating levels of T_4 influence the levels of TSH.

Normal Adult Levels
5.0–12.0 mcg/dL

Increased levels of T_4 usually indicate the presence of hyperfunctioning thyroid disorders, including Graves disease, hyperthyroidism, thyrotoxicosis, and the adverse effects of certain drugs. Decreased levels of T_4 are indicative of hypothyroid disorders, including acromegaly, cretinism, and goiter, as well as hypothyroidism, liver disease, endocrine disorders, GI tract disorders, pituitary tumors, and adverse effects of certain drugs.

Triiodothyronine

T_3 stimulates the basal metabolic rate for the metabolism of carbohydrates and lipids, protein synthesis, vitamin metabolism, and bone calcium release. T_3 is the most active thyroid hormone and affects all body processes, including gene expression.

Normal Adult Levels
80–230 ng/dL

An increase in T_3 levels is indicative of many disorders, including, but not limited to, Graves disease, hyperthyroidism, thyrotoxicosis, and adverse effects of certain drugs. Decreased levels of T_3 are indicative of many disorders, including, but not limited to, iodine and thyroid deficiency disorders, such as goiter and myxedema; renal failure; starvation; thyroidectomy; and adverse effects of certain drugs.

Thyroid-Stimulating Hormone

TSH, produced in the anterior lobe of the pituitary gland, stimulates the production and release of T_3 and T_4 by the thyroid gland.

Normal Adult Levels
0.4–4.2 units/L

An increase in TSH levels may be indicative of many disorders, including, but not limited to, Addison disease, goiter, hyperpituitarism, hypothyroidism, thyroiditis, and adverse effects of certain drugs. A decrease in TSH may be indicative of many disorders, including, but not limited to, Hashimoto thyroiditis, hyperthyroidism, and hypothyroidism.

Lipid Profile

A lipid profile consists of a comparison of the results of four serum lipids: total cholesterol, triglycerides, high-density lipoproteins (HDLs), and low-density lipoproteins (LDLs). One consideration is the ratio of HDL:LDL; the recommended ratio is 3.4:5.0.

Total Cholesterol

Total cholesterol measures a widely distributed sterol that facilitates the absorption and transport of fatty acids. Cholesterol helps build cells and produce hormones.

Normal Adult Levels
Desirable: <200 mg/dL
Borderline: 200–240 mg/dL
High risk: >240 mg/dL

Elevated serum cholesterol levels are indicative of many disorders, including, but not limited to, atherosclerosis, CHF, biliary disorders, kidney disorders, lipid disorders, and adverse effects of certain drugs. Decreased levels of serum cholesterol are indicative of many disorders, including, but not limited to, anemias, carcinoma, cirrhosis, liver disease, hepatitis, endocrine disorders, GI tract disorders, and adverse effects of certain drugs.

Triglycerides

Triglycerides, the principal lipids in blood, are simple fat compounds of three molecules of fatty acid: oleic, palmitic, or stearic. Triglycerides give energy to muscles and store energy.

Normal Adult Levels
Normal: Below 150 mg/dL
Borderline: 150–199 mg/dL
High: 200–499 mg/dL
Very high: Above 500 mg/dL

Elevated triglyceride levels are indicative of many disorders, including, but not limited to, arteriosclerosis, MI, aortic aneurysm, hypercholesterolemia, hyperlipoproteinemia, alcoholism, diabetes mellitus, gout, renal disease, and malnutrition. Decreased triglyceride levels are indicative of many disorders, including, but not limited to, cirrhosis, malabsorption, hyperalimentation, and adverse effects of certain drugs.

High-Density Lipoprotein Cholesterol

HDL transports cholesterol and other lipids to the liver for excretion. HDL is believed to reduce the risk of coronary artery disease. It is often referred to as *good cholesterol*.

Normal Adult Levels
Desirable: 60 mg/dL or higher
Acceptable: 40–59 mg/dL
Undesirable: Less than 40 mg/dL

Increased levels of HDL are indicative of many disorders, including, but not limited to, alcoholism, hepatic disorders, cirrhosis, and adverse effects of certain drugs. Reduced levels of HDL are indicative of many disorders, including, but not limited to, arteriosclerosis, hypercholesterolemia, hyperlipoproteinemia, CHD, diabetes mellitus, liver disease, kidney disease, bacterial infections, and adverse effects of certain drugs.

Low-Density Lipoprotein Cholesterol

LDL has high cholesterol content, and it delivers lipids to body tissues. It is often referred to as *bad cholesterol*.

Normal Adult Levels
Optimal: Less than 100 mg/dL
Near optimal: 100–129 mg/dL
Borderline: 130–159 mg/dL
High: 160–189 mg/dL
Very high: 190 and above

Elevated levels of LDL are indicative of many disorders, including, but not limited to, diabetes mellitus, anorexia nervosa, renal failure, hepatic disease, and adverse effects of certain drugs. Decreased levels of LDL are indicative of many disorders, including, but not limited to, hyperlipoproteinemia, arteriosclerosis, pulmonary disease, stress, and adverse effects of certain drugs.

Electrolytes

Electrolytes are examined in serum to test for chloride, potassium, sodium, and carbon dioxide levels. Other electrolytes that may be included or can be tested individually are calcium, magnesium, and phosphorus.

Chloride

Chloride is an anion found predominantly in extracellular spaces. It helps maintain the balance of fluid inside and outside cells.

Normal Adult Levels
98–107 mEq/L

Increased blood serum levels of chloride may be the result of several disorders, including, but not limited to, metabolic disorders, dehydration, diabetes insipidus, hyperventilation, hyperparathyroidism, acidosis, respiratory alkalosis, CHF, Cushing disease, nephritis, renal failure, and adverse effects of certain drugs. Reduced blood serum levels of chloride may be the result of several disorders, including, but not limited to, metabolic alkalosis, diabetes, severe vomiting, burns, overhydration, salt-losing diseases, some diuretic therapies, central nervous system (CNS) disorders, diaphoresis, fasting, fever, heat exhaustion, acute infections, gastric obstructions, uremia, and adverse effects of certain drugs.

Potassium

Potassium is the major positive ion found inside the cells. Potassium is important in nerve conduction, muscle function, osmotic pressure, acid-base balance, and myocardial activity.

Normal Adult Levels
3.6–5.2 mEq/L

Increased blood serum levels of potassium may be the result of several disorders, including, but not limited to, renal failure, dehydration, burns, trauma, chemotherapy, metabolic acidosis, Addison disease, uncontrolled diabetes, dialysis, hemolysis, intestinal obstruction, sepsis, shock, pneumonia, uremia, and adverse effects of certain drugs. Reduced blood serum levels of potassium may be the result of several disorders, including, but not limited to, alkalosis, anorexia, vomiting, diarrhea, malabsorption, starvation, diuresis, excessive sweating, draining wounds, severe burns, endocrine disorders, pancreatitis, cystic fibrosis, GI stress, and adverse effects of certain drugs. Abnormally elevated or decreased potassium levels can cause life-threatening cardiac arrhythmias.

Sodium

Sodium is the major positive ion found outside the cell and is the main base in blood. Its functions include chemical maintenance of osmotic pressure, acid-base balance, and nerve transmission.

Normal Adult Levels
135–145 mEq/L

Increased blood serum levels of sodium may be the result of several disorders, including, but not limited to, dehydration, excessive fluid loss caused by vomiting, diarrhea, sweating, Cushing disease, kidney disease, diabetic ketoacidosis, diabetes insipidus, hyperaldosteronism, hypertension, hypovolemia, edema, and adverse effects of certain drugs. Decreased blood serum levels of sodium may be the result of several disorders, including, but not limited to, CHF, cirrhosis, cystic fibrosis, hypothyroidism, poor nutrition, psychogenic polydipsia, syndrome of inappropriate antidiuretic hormone secretion, severe burns, sweating, vomiting, diarrhea, and adverse effects of certain drugs.

Carbon Dioxide

CO_2 in normal blood plasma comes from bicarbonate. CO_2 levels in the blood affect abnormal kidney and lung functions.

Normal Adult Levels
23–30 mEq/L

Increased blood serum levels of CO_2 may be the result of several disorders, including, but not limited to, emphysema, aldosteronism, severe vomiting, dehydration, COPD, Cushing disease, bradycardia, cardiac disorders, renal disorders, and adverse effects of certain drugs. Decreased blood serum levels of CO_2 may be the result of several disorders, including kidney failure, alcoholic ketosis, dehydration, high fever, head trauma, malabsorption syndrome, uremia, and adverse effects of certain drugs.

Calcium

Calcium studies include the measurement of calcium levels in the blood.

Normal Adult Levels
8.5–10.2 mg/dL

Ionized Calcium

Ionized calcium is the amount of calcium that is not attached to the protein in the blood. It is also called *free calcium*.

Normal Adult Levels
4.4–5.3 mg/dL

Calcium is the most abundant mineral found in the human body. Calcium acts in bone formation, impulse conduction, myocardial and skeletal muscle contractions, and the blood-clotting process. Elevated serum calcium levels are indicative of many disorders, including, but not limited to, endocrine disorders, hepatic disease, respiratory acidosis, leukemia, neoplasms, blood disorders, respiratory disorders, and adverse effects of certain drugs. Reduced serum calcium levels are indicative of many disorders, including, but not limited to, alkalosis, bacteremia, burns, chronic renal disease and other renal disorders, endocrine disorders, osteomalacia, rickets, vitamin D deficiency, and adverse effects of certain drugs.

Magnesium

Magnesium studies include the measurement of magnesium levels in the blood.

Normal Adult Levels
1.7–2.3 mg/dL

Magnesium is an important mineral found in bones and inside cells. It is needed for proper nerve function, muscle maintenance, and bone strength. Elevated levels of magnesium are indicative of many disorders, including, but not limited to, chronic renal failure, dehydration, Addison disease, and diabetic ketoacidosis. Decreased levels of magnesium are indicative of many disorders, including, but not limited to, pancreatitis, alcoholism, cirrhosis of liver, chronic diarrhea, preeclampsia, malabsorption disorders, and ventricular arrythmias.

Phosphorus

Phosphorus studies include the measurement of phosphorus in the blood.

Normal Adult Levels
2.5–4.5 mg/dL

Phosphorus is the second-most abundant mineral found in the human body. It is needed in the building of bones and teeth, contraction of muscles, and nerve function. Elevated levels of phosphorus may be indicative of many disorders, including, but not limited to, renal disease, diabetic ketoacidosis, liver disease, and hypoparathyroidism. Decreased levels of phosphorus may be indicative of many disorders, including, but not limited to alcoholism, malnutrition, hypercalcemia, and hyperparathyroidism.

Clotting and Coagulation Studies

Activated Partial Thromboplastin Time

The activated partial thromboplastin time test is an evaluation of the time necessary to generate fibrin through the intrinsic pathway of coagulation. This test is a screening process used to detect coagulation factor deficiencies and to monitor the effectiveness of heparin therapy.

Normal values or standardized times used by the laboratory must be checked because various processes may be used.

Increased standardized times may be indicative of many disorders, including, but not limited to, hemophilia A or B, SLE, cardiac surgery, DIC, abruptio placentae, factor defects, hemodialysis, obstructive jaundice, vitamin K deficiency, presence of circulating anticoagulants, and adverse effects of certain drugs. Decreased standardized times are indicative of acute early hemorrhage and cancer spread.

Prothrombin Time

Prothrombin time (PT, also called *Pro Time*) is a measurement of the time taken for clot formation after the addition of reagent tissue thromboplastin and calcium to citrated plasma. In the clotting process, prothrombin converts to thrombin. Adequate vitamin K is necessary for adequate prothrombin production. This test helps in the evaluation of the extrinsic and common coagulation pathways and in monitoring oral anticoagulant therapy.

Normal Adult Levels
International normalized ratio (INR) ≤ 0.9–1.1
INR 2.0–3.0 is an effective standard therapeutic range
INR 2.5–3.5 is a high-intensity warfarin therapeutic range
9.4 to 12.5 seconds may vary from laboratory to laboratory

PT test results are generally reported as an **international normalized ratio (INR)**, which is a standardized result used with anticoagulation therapy. PT can also be reported in seconds.

Critical value: An INR of 5.0 or higher is considered a critical or panic value.

An increase in PT may be indicative of several disorders, including, but not limited to, vitamin K deficiency, liver disorders, adverse effects of anticoagulant therapy, prothrombin deficiency, salicylate intoxication, DIC, SLE, clotting disorders, biliary obstruction, CHF, pancreatitis, snakebite, vomiting, toxic shock syndrome, and adverse effects of certain drugs. A reduced PT may be indicative of certain disorders, including, but not limited to, deep vein thrombosis, MI, peripheral vascular disease, spinal cord injury, pulmonary embolism, and adverse effects of large amounts of foods rich in vitamin K or certain drugs.

Bleeding Time

Bleeding time is a screening test for coagulation disorders, a measurement of the time required for the platelet clot to form. It is often measured by using the Ivy method. The Ivy method involves placing a blood pressure cuff on the patient's arm, inflating the cuff to 40 mm Hg, and using a lancet or scalpel to make an incision on the underside of the forearm. The incision is to be shallow at 1 mm depth and about 10 mm long. Filter paper is used to "wick" blood from the cut every 30 seconds until bleeding ceases.

Normal time at most laboratories is between 1 and 9 minutes.

Increased bleeding times are indicative of several disorders, including, but not limited to, thrombocytopenia, DIC, aplastic anemia, platelet dysfunction, vascular disease, leukemias, liver disorders, aspirin ingestion, and adverse effects of certain drugs. Decreased bleeding time is clinically insignificant.

Erythrocyte Sedimentation Rate

Erythrocyte sedimentation rate (ESR) is the rate at which RBCs (erythrocytes) fall out of well-mixed whole blood to the bottom of the test tube. An alteration in blood proteins occurs during inflammatory and necrotic processes, causing aggregation of RBCs, thereby making them heavier and thus causing them to fall rapidly when placed in a special vertical test tube. A higher ESR is the result of faster settling of RBCs. Although not diagnostic of any particular disease process, an elevated ESR gives an indication of an ongoing disease process.

Normal Values by Westergren Method (most labs use this method, which is more accurate)

Adult males: 0–15 mm/h
Adult females: 0–20 mm/h
Children: 0–10 mm/h

Increased ESRs may be indicative of many disease processes, including, but not necessarily limited to, collagen diseases, infectious processes, inflammatory disorders, cancer, heavy metal poisoning, toxemia, pelvic inflammatory disease (PID), anemia, pain, pulmonary embolism, renal disorders, arthritis, subacute bacterial endocarditis, adverse effects of certain drugs, and pregnancy. Decreased levels may be found in CHF, sickle cell anemia, polycythemia, and as adverse effects of certain drugs.

Glucose Monitoring

Glucose Tolerance Test

Glucose tolerance test is a test that evaluates patients who have symptoms of diabetes mellitus or diabetic complications and screens for gestational diabetes. The test measures blood glucose levels at the following intervals: fasting, 30 minutes, 1 hour, 2 hours, and 3 hours after ingestion of a dose of glucose. Urine samples also are taken at these intervals.

Normal Adult Levels

Fasting: 70–110 mg/dL
30 min: 110–170 mg/dL
1 h: 120–170 mg/dL
2 h: 70–120 mg/dL
3 h: 70–120 mg/dL

All urine samples should test negative for glucose.

Increased glucose values or decreased glucose tolerance are indicative of certain disorders, including, but not limited to, diabetes mellitus, excessive glucose ingestion, certain endocrine disorders, hepatic damage, CNS lesions, pancreatitis, pheochromocytoma, and adverse effects of certain drugs. Decreased glucose values or increased glucose tolerance may be indicative of certain disorders, including, but not limited to, Addison disease, hypoglycemia, malabsorption, pancreatic disease, liver disease, hypoparathyroidism, hypopituitarism, and adverse effects of certain drugs.

Fasting Blood Glucose Levels

Fasting blood glucose levels are measured by the amount of glucose found in blood after 8 hours of fasting.

Normal Adult Levels

Serum: 70–99 mg/dL

Increased levels of blood glucose are indicative of several disorders, including, but not limited to, diabetes mellitus, excessive glucose ingestion, certain endocrine disorders, hepatic damage, status postgastrectomy, CNS lesions, pancreatitis, pheochromocytoma, and adverse effects of certain drugs. Decreased glucose values may be indicative of certain disorders, including, but not limited to, Addison disease, hypoglycemia, malabsorption, pancreatic disease, liver disease, hypoparathyroidism, hypopituitarism, and adverse effects of certain drugs.

Two-Hour Postprandial

Two-hour postprandial levels indicate blood glucose levels after fasting for 10 to 12 hours and then again 2 hours after consuming a normal meal.

Normal Adult Levels
Less than 140 mg/dL

Increased postprandial levels of blood glucose are indicative of several disorders, including, but not limited to, diabetes mellitus, excessive glucose ingestion, certain endocrine disorders, hepatic damage, status post gastrectomy, CNS lesions, pancreatitis, pheochromocytoma, and adverse effects of certain drugs. Decreased postprandial glucose values may be indicative of certain disorders, including, but not limited to, Addison disease, hypoglycemia, malabsorption, pancreatic disease, liver disease, hypoparathyroidism, hypopituitarism, and adverse effects of certain drugs.

Glycosylated Hemoglobin/Glycohemoglobin

Glycohemoglobin (HgbA1c) is the measurement of the blood glucose bound to Hgb and gives an overall view of the past 3 months of glucose saturation.

Normal Adult Levels
Normal: <5.7%
Prediabetic: 5.7%–6.4%
Diabetic: 6.5% and higher

Increased glycohemoglobin levels are indicative of several disorders, including, but not limited to, poorly controlled diabetes mellitus, iron deficiency anemia, splenectomy, alcohol or lead toxicity, and hyperglycemia. Decreased levels of glycohemoglobin may be indicative of certain diseases, including, but not limited to, hemolytic anemia, chronic blood loss, and chronic renal failure, and indicative of pregnancy.

Toxicology Studies and Drug Screens

Toxicology studies are conducted on blood, primarily serum, and on urine. Blood levels of various medications are checked by toxicology levels to determine whether a medication is at the therapeutic level or is approaching or at a toxic level. Blood alcohol levels are the preferred method of screening for blood alcohol content to provide the required qualitative information. Urine drug screens are used to detect the presence of various drugs or substances, primarily drugs of common abuse and/or of illegal origin and blood alcohol. Drugs detected by urine screening include depressants, hallucinogens, sedatives, and stimulants.

Blood Screening Tests

Drug Levels

Common blood serum testing for therapeutic drugs includes, but is not limited to, digoxin, digitoxin, theophylline, lidocaine, lithium, and various drugs for therapeutic or toxic levels.

Digoxin

Digoxin is a cardiac glycoside used to treat CHF and cardiac arrhythmias. Blood level studies produce information about therapeutic or toxic levels.

Normal Therapeutic Level
0.6–1.2 ng/mL

Therapeutic levels of digoxin vary according to each specific individual. Levels should be maintained according to the provider's specifications. The toxicity of the drug, which can occur at 4.0 ng/mL or higher, must be managed by medical intervention and is necessary to return to therapeutic levels.

Theophylline

Theophylline, a bronchodilator, is used to treat asthma and obstructive respiratory disorders. Blood level studies give information about therapeutic or toxic levels.

Normal Therapeutic Level
8–20 mcg/mL

Levels above 20 mcg/mL can indicate the toxicity of the drug. Medical intervention is necessary to return to therapeutic levels. Levels below 8 mcg/mL indicate that more theophylline is necessary to achieve the expected therapeutic effect.

Lidocaine

Lidocaine is used to treat acute ventricular arrhythmias resulting from MI or cardiac surgery. Blood level studies give information about therapeutic or toxic levels.

Normal Therapeutic Level
1.5–5 mcg/mL

Levels above 6 mcg/mL indicate potential toxicity of the drug, and levels greater than 9 mcg/mL are definitely toxic. Medical intervention is necessary to return to therapeutic levels. Levels below 1.5 mcg/mL indicate that more lidocaine is necessary to achieve the expected therapeutic effect.

Lithium

Lithium is used to treat bipolar disorder.

Normal Therapeutic Level
0.5–1.2 mEq/L

Levels above 1.6 mEq/L indicate toxicity of the drug. Medical intervention is necessary to return to therapeutic levels. Levels below 0.5 mEq/L indicate that more lithium is necessary to achieve the expected therapeutic effect.

Prograf (Tacrolimus)/FK-506

Prograf (Tacrolimus)/FK-506 is an immunosuppressive medication used in patients who have received organ transplants. It is used prophylactically to prevent organ rejection.

Normal Therapeutic Level
5–20 ng/mL

Therapeutic levels vary depending on other factors, such as the organ of transplant, the length of time with the transplant, the patient's race, and other medication therapies.

Phenytoin (Dilantin)

Phenytoin (Dilantin) is an anticonvulsant medication used to control seizures.

Normal Therapeutic Level
10–20 mcg/mL

Levels above 30 mcg/mL indicate toxicity of the drug. Medical intervention is necessary to return to therapeutic levels. Levels below 10 mcg/mL indicate more phenytoin is needed to achieve the expected therapeutic effect.

Alcohol Levels

Normal Level
0%

States have established blood levels or content of alcohol that are considered *legally drunk or intoxicated*. Refer to state guidelines for these levels.

Cardiac Enzymes/Cardiac Isoenzymes

Cardiac enzymes and isoenzymes are released by the myocardium as a result of an MI. Monitoring the levels of these enzymes helps evaluate the extent of the insult to the myocardium and the progress of the healing process.

Cross-Reactive Protein

The tissues of the body release cross-reactive (C-reactive) protein, a protein that can be detected and helps evaluate the general amount of inflammation in the body

Normal Adult Levels
<0.5 mg/dL

Baseline studies are recommended as a reference for future measurement of arterial conditions. An elevation may be indicative of rheumatic fever, rheumatoid arthritis, TB, cancer, pneumococcal pneumonia, SLE, or use of oral contraceptives. This protein is normally elevated in the last half of pregnancy. Inflammation in the body's tissues also

must be considered a source of the elevation. A high-sensitivity C-reactive protein test measures the risk for coronary artery disease and, thus, potential heart problems.

Creatine Kinase and Troponin

Creatine kinase (CK), an enzyme found in certain body tissues, becomes elevated with damage to cardiac and skeletal muscles.

Normal Adult Levels
Females: 30–145 units/L
Males: 55–170 units/L
Troponin: 0–0.04 ng/mL
Values may vary from laboratory to laboratory.

In MI, levels begin to rise in 4 to 6 hours, peak at 12 to 24 hours, and return to baseline 3 to 5 days after the onset of MI. The increased levels should be part of the total evaluation to confirm MI.

Creatine Kinase Isoenzymes (Creatine Phosphokinase Isoenzymes)

Isoenzymes increase during MI and are more specific in the diagnosis of MI.

Normal Values
MM-CK (muscle): 97%–100%
MB-CK (heart): 0%–4%
BB-CK (brain): 0%

MB-CK begins to rise within 2 to 6 hours after the myocardial insult; it usually peaks at 15 to 24 hours and then returns to normal within 72 hours. Troponin levels are drawn periodically after suspected MI. Small increases indicate some muscle damage and large increases in results are indicative of MI.

Lactate Dehydrogenase

LDH, an enzyme found in the tissues of the kidneys, heart, skeleton, brain, liver, and lungs, is released from cells, increasing serum levels and indicating cellular necrosis.

Normal Values
100–250 units/L
Values may vary among laboratories.

LDH levels begin to rise at 12 hours after the insult, reach a peak at 24 hours, and return to normal later than CK levels.

Lactate Dehydrogenase Isoenzymes

Lactate dehydrogenase (LDH) isoenzymes are found in many body tissues and are released when tissue necrosis occurs. There are five different LDH isoenzymes, and elevation of LDH-1 and LDH-II usually points to cardiac involvement and subsequent necrosis of myocardial tissue.

Normal Values: Percentage of Total
LDH-I: 17%–32%
LDH-II: 25%–40%
LDH-III: 19%–27%
LDH-IV: 5%–13%
LDH-V: 4%–20%

LDH-I and LDH-II are usually increased in myocardial insult and necrosis. Normally LDH-II is greater than LDH-I. When these values "flip," it is indicative of MI; however, troponin levels are used most frequently to diagnose MI. The ratio will return to normal within 48 hours. When LDH-V values are greater than those of LDH-IV, liver damage or disease is indicated.

Aspartate Aminotransferase (Serum Glutamic Oxaloacetic Transaminase)

AST (SGOT) is a measurement of enzymes found primarily in the heart, liver, and muscles.

Normal Adult Levels
Females over age 14: 8–43 units/L
Males: 8–48 units/L

Elevated AST levels are indicative of insult and injury to tissue. Low levels of AST in the blood are considered normal.

Alanine Aminotransferase (Serum Glutamic Pyruvate Transaminase)

ALT (serum glutamic pyruvate transaminase) evaluates liver insult and measures an enzyme product found primarily in the liver.

Normal Adult Levels
Females: 7–35 units/L
Males: 10–40 units/L

Elevated ALT levels are indicative of certain disorders, including, but not limited to, liver insult and liver disease, CHF, muscle injury, MI, pancreatitis, nonalcoholic fatty liver disease, mononucleosis, severe burns, trauma, shock, and adverse effects of certain drugs. Decreased levels of ALT are never found.

Urine Studies

Urinalysis/Clean Catch Urinalysis

Urinalysis/clean catch urinalysis is a physical, chemical, or microscopic analysis of a urine specimen. Clean catch is the method of collection used. Measurements include pH and specific gravity of urine and the presence of ketones, protein, sugars, bilirubin, and urobilinogen. Color and odor are noted, as is the presence of abnormal blood cells, casts, bacteria, other cells, and crystals.

Routine Urinalysis
Normal Characteristics
Color and clarity: Pale to darker yellow and clear
Odor: Aromatic
Chemical nature: pH is generally slightly acidic, 6.5
Specific gravity: 1.003–1.030; reflects the amount of
    waste, minerals, and solids in urine (concentration)
Normal Constituent Compounds
Protein: None or small amount
Glucose: None
Ketone bodies: None
Urobilinogen: −0.2 to 1 mg/dL
Bilirubin: None
Casts: None or small amount of hyaline casts
Nitrogenous wastes: Ammonia, creatinine, nitrites, urea,
    and uric acid
Crystals: None to trace
Fat droplets: None

Refer to Table 11.1 for abnormal findings and related pathology.

Culture and Sensitivity of Urine

Culture

The urine specimen is placed in/on a culture medium to see whether microbial growth occurs. If growth occurs, the pathogenic microbe is identified. Growth indicates pathogens residing in the urinary tract.

Normal Result
No growth

Sensitivity

Once the pathogen has been isolated, it is plated on the culture medium, and disks impregnated with specific antibiotics in specific concentrations are placed on top. Zones of inhibition of growth are measured around each disk to identify antimicrobials to which pathogens are sensitive.

Urinalysis (UA) with microscopy: Provides information regarding the sediment that may be present in urine. Sediment may include cells, casts, bacteria, yeasts, and crystals. Contaminants such as hair and fiber may also be recognized.

24-Hour urine collection: Urine is collected over a 24-hour period of time and is used to measure overall kidney function.

Estimated glomerular filtration rate: A calculation that is used to determine an estimate of the filtering capacity of the kidneys. This test is determined using blood, rather than urine.

Cardiology Tests

Electrocardiography (12-Lead)

Electrocardiography (ECG) is the recording of electrical activity of the myocardium used to diagnose ischemia, arrhythmias, conduction difficulties, and activity of cardiac medications.

Normal Result

No dysrhythmias/arrhythmias

The 12-lead ECG consists of three limb leads: I, II, and III; three augmented limb leads: aV_R, aV_L, and aV_F; and six precordial chest leads: V_1, V_2, V_3, V_4, V_5, and V_6. The conduction of an impulse through the myocardium is traced by three specific areas of the systolic and diastolic complex. The P wave represents atrial depolarization, the conduction of the stimulus from the sinoatrial node through the atrium to the atrioventricular (AV) node. The QRS complex represents ventricular depolarization, that is, the conduction of the stimulus from the upper portion of the ventricle and below the AV node through the AV bundle, through the right and left bundle branches, and through the Purkinje fibers, followed by its relay throughout the ventricular myocardium. The T wave represents the repolarization of the ventricular myocardium. The 12-lead ECG is used to detect conduction abnormalities, dysrhythmias, myocardial ischemia, and myocardial damage; to monitor recovery from an MI; and to assist in evaluation of the effectiveness of cardiac medications. Lead II normally is used to evaluate cardiac rhythm. Refer to Table 10.1 for an explanation of cardiac arrhythmias/dysrhythmias.

Echocardiography

Echocardiography is the ultrasound (acoustic imaging) examination of the cardiac structure to define the size, shape, thickness, position, and movements of cardiac structures, including valves, walls, and chambers.

Normal Result

Shows no abnormalities

This noninvasive procedure assists in diagnosing cardiac diseases and disorders, including structural abnormalities, congenital defects, myocardial damage, and blood flow through all structures of the heart.

Cardiac Stress Echocardiography

A cardiac stress echocardiography uses ultrasound imaging at rest and then during stress to evaluate the heart's walls, valves, and pumping action. The stress part of this examination can be accomplished in two different ways: (1) by walking on a treadmill or using a stationary bike or (2) by using the chemically induced method. The chemical agent that can be used to simulate exercise in the body is dobutamine, which is given intravenously. This test is performed in a safe environment, and a physician or cardiologist is present, along with specially trained staff.

Normal Result

Negative
Low risk of cardiac disease
Normal appearance of heart chambers and valves
No significant changes on ECG

Holter Monitor

A Holter monitor is a miniature electrocardiograph that records the electrical activity of the heart for an extended period, usually 24 to 48 hours. The patient may be asked to document all activities during the period to allow the examiner to correlate activity with cardiac abnormalities. The data may be transmitted to a programmed cellular phone the patient wears or another monitor where cardiac activity is downloaded and then assessed when the device is returned.

Cardiac Event Recorders

Cardiac event recorders are battery-powered, portable devices that record the electrical activity of the heart while the patient goes about his or her everyday activities. The monitors record the heart's rate and rhythm. Some monitors are attached to the chest with electrodes, whereas others are placed on the wrist. There are two types of monitors: (1) the loop memory recorder and (2) the symptom event monitor. The *loop memory recorder* records the ECG reading for a short period. The person must push a button when symptoms (e.g., feeling faint, dizziness, or feeling of irregular heartbeat) occur, and the monitor records the readings for the period before and after the event. The *symptom event monitor* is similar to the loop memory recorder in that one must place or activate the recorder during a symptom or event. But unlike the loop recorder, it is unable to record an ECG reading prior to the event. Both recorders have the capability to have their records transmitted over the phone to the physician's office. They may be worn for several days to several weeks, depending on what the physician deems necessary.

Normal Result

No dysrhythmias
Refer to ECG

Multigated Acquisition Scan

Multigated acquisition scan (MUGA) scanning is a nuclear medicine scanning method that assesses the function of the heart and identifies abnormalities of the myocardial walls. An MUGA scan may also be referred to as equilibrium radionuclide angiocardiography or radionuclide ventriculography.

<u>Normal Result</u>
55%–70% ejection fraction
Symmetric contraction of the left ventricle

A radioactive isotope "tracer" is injected, which attaches to RBCs to show all four chambers and the great vessels simultaneously. Technetium-99m is frequently used as the tracer; however, other pharmaceutical tracers may be used. A series of images are taken during both systole and diastole and then shown as a movie (or superimposed) to relate ventricular function and to allow the ejection fraction to be calculated. This test may be performed with or without the stress factor. The test demonstrates the percentage of blood that is pumped from the ventricles to the body with each beat and is reported as the patient's ejection fraction.

Doppler ultrasound:

A noninvasive procedure that bounces high-frequency sound waves from red blood cells that are circulating in blood vessels. Used to estimate the blood flow through blood vessels. It is helpful in diagnosing if valves in vessels are working, narrowing of vessels, blood clots, obstructed arteries, heart valve defects, and other blood vessel abnormalities.

Cardiac Stress Test (Cardiac Perfusion Scanning)

A cardiac stress test called *cardiac perfusion scanning* is used to detect and evaluate coronary artery disease. This test measures blood flow to the heart during stress and rest. The stress part of this examination can be accomplished in two different ways: (1) by walking on a treadmill or (2) by using a chemically induced method. Chemical agents that can be used to simulate exercise in the body are dobutamine, dipyridamole (Persantine), adenosine, or regadenoson (Lexiscan). Myoview, Cardiolite, and thallium are all radioactive agents used, and this test may be referred to accordingly. This test is performed in a safe environment, and a physician or a cardiologist is present, along with a specially trained staff.

<u>Normal Result</u>
Good blood flow during both the resting and exercise
  portions of test
No coronary blockage

Exercise Tolerance Test

The exercise tolerance test is an assessment of cardiac function during moderate exercise on a treadmill or stationary bicycle after a 12-lead ECG. No chemical agent is used to stress the heart during exercise.

<u>Normal Result</u>
Negative

The stress test measures the effects of exercise on myocardial output and O_2 consumption by the concurrent evaluation of the monitored ECG readings and O_2 consumption.

This test is performed in a safe environment to identify individuals who are prone to myocardial ischemia during activity.

Hepatobiliary (Gallbladder) Scanning With Ejection Fraction

Hepatobiliary iminodiacetic acid or gallbladder scanning with ejection fraction is a nuclear imaging scanning method used to evaluate the gallbladder and the ducts leading into and out of the gallbladder. It is also known as *cholescintigraphy* and *hepatobiliary scintigraphy*.

<u>Normal Results</u>
Negative scan
Ejection fraction: 30%–50%

Cardiac Catheterization

Cardiac catheterization is the fluoroscopic visualization of the right or left side of the heart by passing a catheter into the right or left chambers and injecting dye. In angiography, the catheter is passed into the coronary vessels, where the dye is injected and fluoroscopic images are recorded.

<u>Normal Results</u>
Varies with the area being assessed
Indicates normal anatomy and physiology, normal chamber
  volumes and pressures, normal wall and valve motion,
  and normal patent coronary arteries
<u>Normal Value for Cardiac Output</u>
5–6 L/min

Imaging Studies

Radiography

Radiography helps visualize internal organs and structures with electromagnetic radiation. Radiography of bone, the abdomen, the chest, paranasal sinuses, kidneys, ureters, and bladder, and mammography do not require contrast medium. A contrast medium is used to distinguish soft tissues and some organs (e.g., the gallbladder, esophagus, stomach, and small and large intestines). Normal results vary depending on the area being studied with the imaging process. The images are interpreted by the radiologist, and a report is then dictated and transcribed for the ordering physician. The ordering physician often visually inspects the films or images to evaluate the area himself or herself.

Magnetic Resonance Imaging/Magnetic Resonance Angiography

Magnetic resonance imaging (MRI)/magnetic resonance angiography (MRA) uses a magnetic field, instead of radiation, to visualize internal tissues. It is possible to view tissues and organs in three dimensions with MRI. MRA is used to examine major blood vessels in the body and to study the condition of blood vessels to detect tumors, differentiate healthy and diseased tissues, and detect sites of infection. It helps determine blood flow to tissues and organs. The patient is not exposed to ionizing radiation during MRI. Gadolinium-based contrast agents may be required for some examinations. Gadolinium does not contain iodine and is given intravenously. It is important to screen patients before the procedure to determine if they have any metal implants or pacemakers, if they work with metal shavings, or if they are claustrophobic. Open MRIs are best for those patients who are claustrophobic.

Normal results vary depending on the area being studied on MRI. The MRI scan is interpreted by the radiologist, and a report is then dictated and transcribed for the ordering physician. The ordering physician may also view the images.

Computed Tomography

Computed tomography (CT) is a radiographic technique that uses a scanner system, which can provide images of the internal structure of tissue and organs both geographically and characteristically. Depending on the area to be scanned and the reason indicated for scanning, oral and/or intravenous (IV) contrast media may be required. Iodinated contrast media may result in nephrotoxicity and renal failure, and, therefore, it is important to screen patients before they receive IV contrast media. Any patient receiving IV contrast media should be screened for the following risks:
- History of kidney disease, including tumor, surgery on kidneys, or transplantation
- Myeloma
- Diabetes
- Potentially nephrotoxic medications (e.g., metformin, chemotherapy, and/or long-term use of nonsteroidal antiinflammatory drugs)
- 70 years of age and older

If any of these risk factors are present, serum creatinine level needs to be measured to determine the glomerular filtration rate (GFR). If the GFR is below 45 mn/min/1.73 m^2, intervention to protect the kidneys may be required before administration of contrast.

Normal results vary, depending on the area being studied on CT. The scan is interpreted by the radiologist, and a report is then dictated and transcribed for the ordering physician. The ordering physician often visually inspects the films or images to evaluate the area.

Fluoroscopy

A real-time imaging process, fluoroscopy provides continuous visualization of the area being imaged. Films of the process are made for more extensive examination. Fluoroscopy is used in certain procedures and to study the functioning of tissues and organs.

Normal results vary, depending on the area being studied on fluoroscopy. The film is interpreted by the radiologist, and a report is then dictated and transcribed for the ordering physician. The ordering physician often requests for fluoroscopy, which can be a diagnostic tool and also a guide for the treatment procedure.

Sonography, Ultrasonography, and Echography

Sonography, ultrasonography, and echography all use an imaging system that projects a beam of sound waves into target tissues or organs and receives waves as they bounce back off the target structure. An outline of the structure is produced and recorded on film for examination. Tissues, organs, and systems that may be studied by using ultrasonography include, but are not limited to, the abdominal aorta, brain, breasts, gallbladder, pelvis for gynecologic and obstetric diagnostic examinations, heart, kidneys, liver, lymph nodes, pancreas, prostate, spleen, thyroid, urinary bladder, and upper GI tract.

Normal Result
Varies, depending on the area being examined

The ultrasound scan is interpreted by the radiologist, and a report is then dictated and transcribed for the ordering physician. The ordering physician may request to visually inspect the films or images to evaluate the area himself or herself.

Myelography

Myelography is an imaging examination of the spinal cord and spinal nerve roots. A contrast medium (dye) is injected into the subarachnoid space and recorded on radiographic film. Fluoroscopy generally is used in this procedure.

Normal Result
No lesions or abnormalities

It is used to diagnose ruptured or bulging disks, spinal cord lesions and tumors, spinal cord and spinal nerve trauma and edema, and other conditions involving the spinal cord and spinal nerves. This technique is used for those individuals who cannot have an MRI.

Positron Emission Tomography

Positron emission tomography (PET), a molecular imaging study, indicates how organs and tissues are actually functioning. It measures blood flow, O_2 use, and sugar metabolism. It is used to diagnose a variety of diseases, including many types of cancer, heart disease, certain brain abnormalities, and other CNS disorders. It is also helpful in assessing the effectiveness of cancer therapy.

A radioactive material, called a *radiotracer*, is injected intravenously or sometimes is inhaled as a gas. The energy that the tracer gives off is then detected and recorded by the gamma camera and PET scanner, and three-dimensional images are created with the aid of a computer.

Results are interpreted by a nuclear radiologist with specialized training in nuclear medicine. The standardized uptake value (SUV) is the amount of chemical activity in a certain spot and assists the radiologist in interpretation. Generally, an SUV of 2.5 or higher indicates malignancy and creates what is known as a "hot spot" on the scan. There are many other factors and variables that are taken into consideration by the physician.

Stool Analysis

Hemoccult/Guaiac Test/Fecal Occult Blood Test

The hemoccult/guaiac test looks for hidden (occult) blood in a stool sample. It is a qualitative detection of RBCs in the stool.

Normal Result
Negative

The presence of blood in the stool specimen is indicative of trauma, lesion, or other insult to the GI mucosa, producing blood. Blood in the stool may also be a sign of colorectal cancer. Fecal occult blood testing is used as a screening test for early detection (and thus treatment) of colorectal cancer. There are also tests that patients can perform in the privacy of their homes to determine blood in the stool.

Cologuard

Cologuard is a screening test for colorectal cancer. It can be used in those who do not have any family history of colorectal cancer (those who do have a family history should undergo colonoscopy). Cologuard detects certain altered deoxyribonucleic acid (DNA) in cancer cells. Abnormal cells or blood in the stool could indicate cancer, precancerous tumors, or polyps.

Normal Result
Negative

The Cologuard test is not definitive for cancer diagnosis. If the test shows a positive result, further testing (colonoscopy) must be performed.

Tests for Ova, Larvae, and Parasites

These tests are microscopic examinations of the stool to detect the presence of parasites at various stages of development.

Normal Result
None detected

A positive examination result indicates a parasitic infection of the GI tract.

Stool Culture

The test used to detect the presence of pathological bacteria that are not usually found in the stool.

Normal Result
Negative

Endoscopy Tests

Endoscopy

Endoscopy is the visual inspection of internal organs or body cavities through the use of a fiberoptic instrument with the appropriate scope. In addition, pathology may be removed, and insult to the tissue may be repaired during the diagnostic procedure.

Esophagogastroduodenoscopy/Upper Endoscopy

Esophagogastroduodenoscopy/upper endoscopy helps visualize the esophagus, stomach, and duodenum in a single procedure by using an endoscope. Biopsy and endoscopic therapies, such as esophageal dilation, may be performed.

Normal Result
Appearance of esophagus, stomach, and duodenum within normal limits

Abnormal findings may include, but are not limited to, hiatal hernia, Barrett esophagus, gastroesophageal reflux disease, esophagitis, and ulcers.

Esophagoscopy

Esophagoscopy is the visualization of the esophagus by using an esophagoscope.

Normal Result
The appearance of the esophagus mucosa is normal.

Foreign bodies may be visualized and removed. Inflammation may be noted, and biopsy specimens can be taken.

Gastroscopy

Gastroscopy is the visualization of the stomach by using a gastroscope.

Normal Result
Appearance of upper GI tract within normal limits

Hemorrhagic areas or erosion of a vessel may be revealed. Additional abnormal findings may include neoplasms, gastric ulcers, hiatal hernia, gastritis, and esophagitis.

Colonoscopy

Colonoscopy is the visualization of the colon by using a colonoscope.

Normal Result

Appearance of large intestinal mucosa is normal.

Inflammation, areas of ulceration, bleeding areas, strictures, polyps, colitis, diverticula, benign or malignant tumors, or foreign bodies may be observed in abnormal findings.

Sigmoidoscopy

Sigmoidoscopy is the visualization of the sigmoid portion of the colon and the rectum by using a sigmoidoscope.

Normal Result

Normal appearance of mucosa of sigmoid colon

Inflammatory bowel disease, polyps, benign and cancerous tumors, diverticula, and foreign bodies may be some of the abnormal findings during a sigmoidoscopic examination.

Proctoscopy

Proctoscopy is the visualization of the rectum by using a proctoscope.

Normal Result

Normal appearance of rectal mucosa and anal canal

Rectal prolapse, hemorrhoids, rectal strictures, fissures, abscesses, and fistulas are some of the abnormal findings during a proctoscopic examination of the rectum.

Cystoscopy

Cystoscopy is the visualization of the structures of the urinary tract by using a cystoscope.

Normal Result

Urethra, urethral orifices, urinary bladder interior, and male prostatic urethra appear normal.

Cancer of the bladder, benign prostatic hyperplasia, bladder calculi, prostatitis, ureteral strictures, urinary fistulas, vesicle neck stenosis, ureterocele, polyps, and abnormal bladder capacity are some of the abnormal findings during a cystoscopic examination of the urinary bladder.

Colposcopy

Visualization of the cervical epithelium, vagina, and vulvar epithelium with a colposcope

Normal Result

Normal appearance of mucosa of cervix

Lesions of the cervix are considered abnormal findings.

Ureteroscopy

Ureteroscopy is the visualization of the ureters and pelvis of the kidney.

Normal Result

Normal appearance of the ureters and pelvis of the kidney and its structures

Renal or ureteral stones, inflammation or bleeding of the urethral mucosa, and lesions or abnormal structures of the renal pelvis are some of the abnormal findings in a ureteroscopic examination.

Bronchoscopy

Bronchoscopy is the visualization of the trachea and bronchi using a bronchoscope.

Normal Result

Nasopharynx, larynx, trachea, and bronchi are normal in appearance.

Abnormalities revealed in a bronchoscopic examination include, but are not limited to, bronchitis, carcinoma and other tumors, inflammatory processes, TB, abnormal structures and disorders of the larynx and trachea, foreign bodies, and various pulmonary infections.

Laparoscopy

Visualization of abdominal or pelvic organs with a laparascope. A biopsy may be obtained, or procedures may be performed. Minimally invasive. A small incision is used to insert the laparascope, which enables faster recovery.

Technological advances have also opened the door for robotic-assisted surgeries. Robotic surgeries involve robotic arms that hold a camera and medical instruments to perform the surgery. The surgeon is able to maneuver the arms to perform the surgery and see the operative field, which is magnified on the computer screen.

Normal Result

Organ or body system examined appears as expected.

Arthroscopy

Arthroscopy is the visualization or inspection of the inner aspect of a joint by using an endoscope called an *arthroscope*. Biopsy specimens may be obtained.

Normal Result

Normal appearance of the inner aspect of the joint

Abnormal findings in the knee may include tears of meniscus, bone or cartilage fragments, and damage to other structures within the joint. Surgical repair may be attempted. Refer to Chapter 7 for additional information on arthroscopy.

Arterial Blood Gases

Arterial Blood Gas Analysis

Arterial blood gas (ABG) analysis is the measurement of dissolved O_2 and CO_2 in arterial blood. It is also a measurement of pH and O_2 saturation of the arterial blood. ABGs are used to assess oxygenation and ventilation, along with acid-base balance. In addition, they produce information about the effectiveness of therapy and the status of critical patients and are used in conjunction with pulmonary function studies.

Normal values are listed; however, these studies are complex and require interpretation by a physician, along with the results of other diagnostic studies, and consideration of symptoms and signs to arrive at a diagnosis or an evaluation.

Normal Adult Values
Acidity (pH): 7.35–7.45
CO_2 tension ($PaCO_2$): 35–45 mm Hg
Arterial O_2 tension (PaO_2): 75–100 mm Hg
Amount of bicarbonate (HCO_3) in the blood: 22–26 mEq/L
O_2 saturation: 95%–100%

Increased pH is indicative of several disorders, including, but not limited to, alkali ingestion, diarrhea, vomiting, hyperventilation, high-altitude sickness, metabolic acidosis, fever, and adverse effects of certain drugs. Decreased pH is indicative of several disorders, including, but not limited to, asthma, COPD, cardiac disease, MI, renal disorders, pulmonary disorders, respiratory acidosis, sepsis, shock, and malignant hyperthermia.

Increased $PaCO_2$ is indicative of several disorders, including, but not limited to, late-stage asthma, brain death, CHF, respiratory disorders, hypoventilation, renal disorders, poisoning, pneumothorax, respiratory acidosis, near-drowning, and adverse effects of certain drugs. Decreased $PaCO_2$ is indicative of several disorders, including, but not limited to, early-stage asthma, hyperventilation, dysrhythmias, respiratory alkalosis, metabolic acidosis, and adverse effects of certain drugs.

Increased PaO_2 is indicative of several conditions, including, but not limited to, hyperventilation and hyperbaric O_2 exposure. Decreased PaO_2 is indicative of several disorders, including, but not limited to, acute respiratory distress syndrome (ARDS), asthma, cardiac disorders, head injury, anoxia, hypoventilation, respiratory disorders, pneumothorax, respiratory failure, shock, smoke inhalation, and CVA.

Increased O_2 saturation is indicative of hyperbaric oxygenation. Decreased O_2 saturation is indicative of several disorders, including, but not limited to, anoxia, cardiac anomalies and disorders, carbon monoxide poisoning, ARDS, CVA, hypoventilation, respiratory disorders, pneumothorax, shock, smoke inhalation, and near-drowning.

Pulmonary Function Studies

Pulmonary function studies are complex and include evaluation of results from several tests. Most tests are performed by respiratory therapists and can be done with or without the use of bronchodilators. Results usually are reported to a pulmonologist for evaluation and correlation with symptoms and signs. Normal values are reported; however, the significance of these values is incomplete without the review and opinion of the pulmonologist, who is often assisted by the respiratory therapist.

Pulse Oximeter

A pulse oximeter is an instrument (spectrophotometer) that produces a noninvasive measurement of the O_2 saturation of peripheral blood.

Normal Result
Peripheral blood O_2 saturation $\geq$95%

Peak Flow

Peak flow is a measurement of inspiratory effort.

Normal Results
Calculations based on sex, height, and age

Spirometry

Spirometry is a measurement of lung capacity, volume, and flow rates used in the evaluation of asthma, bronchitis, COPD, and emphysema.

Methacholine Challenge

Methacholine challenge (also known as *bronchoprovocation test*) is a measurement of lung volumes before and after inhalation of methacholine chloride, which is used for the diagnosis of asthma.

Normal Result
Negative

The challenge is considered positive if there is a 20% or *greater* reduction in breathing compared with *baseline values*. A positive test indicates *that the* airways are "reactive," and an asthma diagnosis should be considered.

Sputum Studies

Sputum studies are analyses and cultures of sputum (material expelled from the respiratory tract) to detect the presence of pathogens. Common studies on sputum that are ordered include cytology testing, Gram staining, and culture and sensitivity (C&S).

Normal Result
Negative

Positive results might include respiratory disorders, such as fungal infections, mycobacterial infections (e.g., TB), or carcinoma.

Pulmonary Function Test

Normal findings are reported in percentages of observed values and by expected values calculated to include allowances for age, sex, weight, and height. Abnormal results are considered to be less than 80% of calculated values. A respiratory therapist or pulmonologist should be consulted for interpretation of values.

Normal Values
Tidal volume: 500 mL
Expiratory reserve volume: 1500 mL
Residual volume: 1500 mL
Inspiratory reserve volume: 2000 mL

Miscellaneous Tests

Culture and Sensitivity Studies

For wound, drainage, and blood C&S studies, specimens are obtained from various tissues and fluids of the body, placed on or in a medium to grow, and then studied for the presence of microbes. The specimens are placed on Mueller Hinton agar, and a variety of antibiotic disks are added on top of the specimen. Zones of growth inhibition determine which antibiotic will be effective in destroying or curbing the reproduction of the microbe.

Tissues and fluids that are sampled include blood, sputum, cerebrospinal fluid (CSF), urine, exudates from lesions, nasal secretions, stool, wound drainage, and any excised tissue.

Culture: A sample of a specimen is placed in/on culture medium to see whether microbial growth occurs; if growth occurs, identification of the pathogenic microbe is determined by sensitivity testing.

Sensitivity: Sensitivity disks (which are impregnated with specific antibiotics) are placed on the culture media to determine which antibiotic is most appropriate to use in treating the pathogen. The bacteria will grow up next to the round antibiotic disk if the antibiotic in the disc does not kill or destroy the bacteria. The bacteria will not grow up next to the antibiotic-impregnated disks if the antibiotic is one which will destroy or kill the bacteria. This method is used to determine which antibiotics will destroy or kill the pathogen.

Normal Result
No growth

The growth of any microbes requires microscopic identification. The antibiotic-impregnated disk requires inspection and identification of antibiotics showing effectiveness against the microbes.

- *Genetic tests*: Performed to assist a physician with a definitive diagnosis. Single-gene tests help identify specific syndromes or conditions. When there is a known genetic mutation present in a family, single-gene testing is beneficial. Panel genetic tests provide information for more than one gene. These tests can be categorized into groups that provide information regarding different medical concerns. In addition, these panel tests can provide information regarding the likelihood of developing different types of cancer, such as colorectal and breast cancers. https://www.cdc.gov/genomics-and-health/about/genetic-testing.html? CDC_AAref_Val=https://www.cdc.gov/genomics/gtesting/genetic_testing.htm

- *DNA testing*: Utilized in certain courtroom cases, or paternity genetic testing for proving or disproving paternity.

Bone Marrow Studies

For bone marrow studies, aspiration of bone marrow is obtained with a needle from the sternum, the posterior superior iliac spine, or the anterior iliac crest for the diagnosis of neoplasms, metastases, and blood disorders. Bone marrow studies provide a basis for the evaluation of hematologic disorders and infectious diseases.

Serologic testing: Analysis of blood specimens for antigen-antibody reactions. Used to detect bacterial infections, including syphilis, Lyme disease, chlamydia, and streptococcal infections; antibodies from viral sources, including infectious mononucleosis, rubella, hepatitis, rabies, human immunodeficiency virus (HIV), herpes, and cytomegalovirus; antibodies from fungal sources, such as histoplasmosis and Candida; and antibodies from the parasitic source toxoplasmosis.

Immune and Immunoglobulin Studies

Immune and immunoglobulin studies examine the functioning and malfunctioning of the immune system.

Normal Adult Levels
Immunoglobulin A (IgA): 60–400 mg/dL
Immunoglobulin G (IgG): 700–1600 mg/dL
Immunoglobulin M (IgM): 40–230 mg/dL
Immunoglobulin D (IgD): 0.13–15.27 mg/dL
Immunoglobulin E (IgE): 3–42 units/mL

Increased levels of immunoglobulins are indicative of many disorders, and the results need to be evaluated by a physician. Some disorders include arthritis, cancer, chronic infections, sinusitis, asthma, food and drug allergies, liver disease, SLE, and adverse effects of certain drugs. Decreased levels of immunoglobulins are indicative of many disorders, including, but not limited to, AIDS, bacterial infection, advanced cancer, hypogammaglobulinemia, and adverse effects of certain drugs.

Biopsy

A biopsy is the excision of tissue from the living body, followed by microscopic examination, for the purpose of arriving at an exact diagnosis.

Normal Result
No abnormal cells seen

Abnormal findings depend on cell structure discovered during microscopic examination.

Lumbar Puncture

Lumbar puncture is a surgical procedure to withdraw spinal fluid for analysis. It involves measurement and analysis of the chemical components of CSF and is used in the diagnosis of CNS diseases and disorders.

Normal Adult Results
Appearance: Clear, colorless
Specific gravity: 1.006–1.009
Pressure: 90–180 mm H_2O
AST: 05–35 units
Bicarbonate: 22.9 mEq/L
WBC count: 0.0–0.8 mm^3
RBC count: None
Glucose: 40–80 mg/dL
Total protein: 15–45 mg/dL
Lactic acid: 10–24 mg/dL
Venereal Disease Research Laboratory: Negative titer for syphilis
Bacteria or viruses: None present

Pressure depends on height and whether the patient is positioned in a sitting or horizontal position.

Abnormal findings are indicative of disorders or insults to the CNS.

Electroencephalography

Electroencephalography is the recording of the electrical activity of the brain. A neurologist interprets the brain wave activity to determine the presence of a neurologic disorder or any other medical condition.

Normal Result
Symmetric patterns of electrical brain activity

Abnormal findings include information indicative of CNS or brain insults, hematomas, CVAs, epilepsy, brain tumors, and seizure activity. Lack of any activity is an indication of brain death.

Electromyography

Electromyography (EMG) is the electrodiagnostic assessment and recording of the electrical activity of skeletal muscle at rest and in contraction. It is a nerve conduction study used to differentiate between muscle weakness caused by nerve injury and weakness caused by muscle diseases. EMG tests and nerve conduction tests are often done in combination.

Normal Results
Nerve conduction normal
Muscle action potential normal

Abnormal findings help identify the site and cause of muscle disorders and neuronal lesions, particularly those involving the anterior horn of the spinal cord.

Gastric Analysis

Gastric analysis is used in the diagnosis of pernicious anemia and peptic ulcers. The contents of the stomach are analyzed for acidity, appearance, and volume.

Normal Adult Levels
Bile: 0 or minimal
Mucus: Evenly mixed
Blood: 0 or scant
Fasting acidity: 2.5 mEq/L
Quantity: 62 mL/h
pH: 1.5–3.5

Increased levels of gastric acid are indicative of certain disorders, including, but not limited to, status post small-intestinal resection, gastric or duodenal ulcer, hyperplasia, Zollinger-Ellison syndrome, and hyperfunction of gastric cells. Reduced gastric acid levels are indicative of several disorders, including, but not limited to, pernicious anemia, status post vagotomy, renal failure, rheumatoid arthritis, gastric cancer, and atrophic gastritis.

Human Chorionic Gonadotropin

Human chorionic gonadotropin is measured for diagnosis of pregnancy, abortion, ectopic pregnancy, and uterine pathology.

Normal Result
Negative

A positive result is indicative of pregnancy, either intrauterine or ectopic. A positive result can also occur with testicular cancer in males, a trophoblastic tumor, hydatidiform moles, and ovarian cancer.

Gram staining: Used to identify gram-positive or gram-negative microorganisms of an infectious process.

Polysomnography: Sleep studies are indicated for excessive snoring, excessive daytime sleeping or drowsiness, insomnia or sleep-time cardiac rhythm disturbances.

Screening

Tuberculosis Screening (Mantoux Test)

An intradermal injection of tuberculin is given, usually on the inner aspect of the lower arm. Results are read between 48 and 72 hours. A two-step TB test may be indicated for certain populations.

Normal Result

Negative

Positive Result

Red, raised, hardened area at injection site; induration measures ≥5 mm for those who are immune compromised. 10 mm in populations at high risk, and 15 mm for those who have no identified risk factors.

Positive reaction requires further investigation, usually including chest radiography. Tuberculin blood test may also be performed.

Cancer/Tumor Markers as Screening Tools

Certain substances, including enzymes, antigens, and hormones, are produced by some tumors or cancers. These substances may be present in blood at higher-than-normal levels, indicating the presence of a tumor. Cancer/tumor markers cannot be used alone to diagnose cancer or a tumor. Some benign tumors may stimulate the production of these markers. In addition, elevated cancer markers are not always present, especially in the early stages of the disease process. Some physicians use these markers to track the progress of tumor growth, measure the effectiveness of treatment, and detect possible recurrence of the tumor. There are several markers, and many are specific in nature. The most widely used screening tool of this nature is the prostate-specific antigen (PSA) test. Other markers include CA 125, carcinoembryonic antigen, alpha-fetoprotein (AFP), CA 19-9, CA 15-3, and Papanicolaou (Pap) smear.

Prostate-Specific Antigen

The PSA test is a blood test used to determine the level of PSA in serum. This is a screening test that should be followed by a digital rectal examination (DRE) of the prostate gland to identify any abnormalities. Additional diagnostic studies are often indicated.

PSA blood test results are reported in nanograms per milliliter (ng/mL).

PSA is considered a marker in the screening for prostatic cancer; however, many other factors can cause an increase in PSA levels, when there is no cancer. Usually, 0 to 4 ng/mL is considered to be in the normal range. PSA levels increase with age.

PSA screening should be completed before DRE. A constant increase in the PSA level leads to suspicion of prostate cancer. The PSA test is a screening tool and must be combined with DRE for more accurate screening.

CA 125 Test

The CA 125 test measures the production of the protein marker CA 125. Increases in levels of CA 125 may be indicative of cancer of the ovaries.

Normal Levels

<35 units/mL (conventional units)

An elevation above normal may be indicative of cancer of the ovaries, pelvic organs (including the uterus and the cervix), pancreas, liver, breasts, colon, lungs, and digestive tract.

CA 19-9 Test

The CA 19-9 test measures the production of the protein marker CA 19-9. CA 19-9 levels may increase in the presence of pancreatic or colorectal cancer.

Normal Levels

<37 units/mL (conventional units)

An elevation may be indicative of the presence of colorectal, pancreatic, stomach, or bile duct cancer, infections, liver disease, and cystic fibrosis.

CA 15-3 Test

The CA 15-3 test measures the production of the protein marker CA 15-3. CA 15-3 levels may increase in the presence of breast cancer.

Normal Levels

<30 units/mL (conventional units)

An elevation may be indicative of the presence of breast cancer, benign conditions of the breast, ovarian disease, PID, endometriosis, and hepatitis, and indicative of pregnancy and lactation.

Carcinoembryonic Antigen

Carcinoembryonic antigen (CEA) is normally found in developing fetuses and decreases to very low levels after birth. CEA may be elevated in some individuals without any form of cancer. This test is not a screening test. It is used to monitor the recurrence or metastasis of colorectal cancer and other cancers after the disease has already been diagnosed.

Reference values vary depending on the health of the individual, smoking history, and the presence of existing intestinal or other disease processes. A baseline value should be established and monitored to determine effectiveness of treatment or exacerbation of the condition.

Alpha-Fetoprotein

Under normal circumstances, AFP is produced by the liver of a developing fetus and passes through the placenta to the mother's blood. Maternal levels decrease after birth. Certain conditions may cause an abnormal elevation of this protein as pregnancy progresses, suggesting a possible neural tube defect or other anomaly in the developing fetus(es). This test is not to be confused with the AFP tumor marker test, which is used in conjunction with other tests to diagnose liver, ovarian, or testicular cancer or to monitor the effectiveness of treatment of these cancers.

To compare or confirm normal values for amniotic fluid levels and serum AFP levels, their normal levels should be checked with a reference laboratory.

Elevations in maternal serum levels and amniotic fluid may be indicative of neural tube defects.

Papanicolaou Smear

A pap smear is the cytologic examination of cells that have been scraped or aspirated from the cervix and the cervical os. This screening test is recommended every 2 to 3 years, and yearly pelvic examinations are recommended.

The results of Pap smear are now reported to the physician in two different formats: (1) a system based on classes and (2) the Bethesda system, which uses descriptive diagnostic terms.

Class System May Need to Update This

The *class system*, based on classes, is used to report Pap smear results to the physician as follows:
- Negative: no abnormal or unusual cells seen
- Atypical: two types
  1. Atypical squamous cells, cannot exclude high-grade lesions.
  2. Atypical squamous cells of uncertain significance. A repeat Pap smear, other tests, and treatment of the underlying cause may be indicated.
- Low-grade squamous intraepithelial lesion: Abnormal cells are present. Mild dysplasia or the potential to become malignant. Further evaluation is indicated, possibly including colposcopy.
- High-grade squamous intraepithelial lesion: Indicates an increase in precancerous change. A complete evaluation with colposcopy is indicated, along with freezing or excision of the abnormality.
- Cancer: Very high likelihood of cancer. Complete evaluation with colposcopy and treatment. A plan of treatment is indicated for optimal results.

Bethesda System

When using the *Bethesda system*, the physician may relate the results as normal or abnormal because surface cervical cells may appear abnormal but are not always malignant. The six diagnostic categories are as follows:
- Nondiagnostic
- Benign
- Atypia of undetermined significance
- Follicular neoplasm
- Suspicious for malignancy
- Malignant

Mammography

Mammography is the radiographic examination of the soft tissues of the breast. This is a screening test performed on an annual basis in females 45 to 54 years of age to detect the presence of breast disease. Females aged 55 years or older should be screened every 2 years or can continue with annual screening. Screening should continue for those in good health and those expected to live 10 years or longer. Females should become familiar with their breasts and report any changes to their physician.

Normal Result
Negative for disease

Identification of abnormal conditions may indicate the need for further investigation. Various benign disorders, including fibrocystic disease of the breast, calcifications, and asymmetric densities, may be responsible for a positive result and require additional mammographic views with ultrasonography. It may also be recommended that in 6 months, repeat mammography and/or ultrasonography be done to follow up on any abnormality. Ultrasound-guided breast biopsy or stereotactic breast biopsy may be indicated to confirm the presence of a malignant neoplasm. Breast MRI may be indicated.

Testicular Self-Examination

Testicular self-examination is a screening test conducted monthly by the man himself at home for early detection of changes in testicular tissue.

Normal Result
No changes

If any changes are noted or a small hard lump is found, the physician should be contacted immediately. These findings could indicate testicular cancer and further testing is required.

BRCA1 and BRCA2 Gene Testing

BRCA1 and *BRCA2* are genes that suppress malignant tumors in humans. People with mutations in these genes are at higher risk of cancers.

Normal Result
Negative for mutation

Even if the test is negative for mutation, cancer development is still possible. A positive test indicates a higher risk for cervical, uterine, colon, pancreatic, biliary, testicular, prostate, or stomach cancer. The individual is also at higher risk for melanomas. *Note:* Approximately 5% to 10% of breast cancers and 10% to 15% of ovarian cancers are gene related or hereditary. *BRCA1* and *BRCA2* mutations also put males at higher risk for breast cancer.

Appendix II

Pharmacology

Pharmacology is defined as a branch of medicine concerned with the study of drug action. Drugs may be human-made, natural, or endogenous molecules and exert their effect on cells, tissues, organs, or organisms. Pharmacology is not only about how a drug works but, more importantly, why a drug works in the way it does.

Side effects are listed by various groups of medications and are not specific to any one drug in that group. Referral to the current edition of the *Physician's Desk Reference* (PDR) or other pharmacology reference is recommended to confirm the side effects of a specific drug.

This table presents the major drug groups, organized by the actions of medications. The examples are just that—examples—to represent the multiple medications found in each group. The example drugs are commonly prescribed and may be familiar in some way. Once again, refer to the current edition of the PDR or other pharmacology reference to locate additional drugs in the group.

Body System/ Drug Purpose	Drug Category	Drug Action	Examples	Side Effects	Comments
Chapters 1 and 2					
Drugs for pain and fever	Analgesics and/or opioids (narcotics)	Relieve pain	codeine, meperidine morphine, oxycodone hydrocodone, oxymorphone, hydromorphone, fentanyl	May cause drowsiness; blurred vision, dizziness, sedation; constipation can occur	May lead to physical and mental dependence. Patients should not drive or operate machinery while taking the drug.
	Nonopioids	Relieve pain and fever	acetaminophen (Tylenol), acetylsalicylic acid (aspirin), ibuprofen, naproxen, indomethacin	Aspirin and NSAIDs may cause GI irritation, anticoagulant effects, antiprostaglandin effects	Acetaminophen overdose has been linked to hepatic injury. The dose of acetaminophen-based products is limited to 4 g or less per day.
	Anesthetics[a]	Produce loss of sensation by interfering with nerve impulses			
	A. General		midazolam (Versed), propofol (Diprivan), etomidate (Amidate)	Versed: may cause amnesia, hypotension, headache	Versed is used for conscious sedation.
	B. Local		tetracaine, prilocaine, lidocaine	May cause skin rashes and/or edema	Lidocaine may be topical form; also used systemically as a cardiac drug.
Drugs for infectious diseases	Antibiotics	Destroy or inhibit the growth of bacterial strains of microorganisms.	penicillin, amoxicillin, amoxicillin/ clavulanic acid (Augmentin), tetracycline, doxycycline, minocycline, ciprofloxacin (Cipro), azithromycin (Zithromax)	Nausea, GI upset, urticaria	Caution must be used when administering IM penicillin and all antibiotics with regard to observation after injection for potential of anaphylaxis.
	A. Penicillins		penicillin V, amoxicillin/clavulanic acid (Augmentin), amoxicillin, piperacillin/ tazobactam	Stomach upset and diarrhea	Most contraindications involve hypersensitivity to the drug.
	B. Tetracyclines		minocycline, doxycycline, tetracycline	Stomach upset, diarrhea, vomiting	Should not be taken with dairy or antacids. Cause photosensitivity.

Category	Action	Drugs	Side effects	Notes
C. Cephalosporins[b]		cefazolin, cephalexin, cefaclor, cefdinir, cefepime	Nausea, vomiting, headache	Patients allergic to penicillin may also be allergic to cephalosporins.
D. Quinolone antibiotics		ciprofloxacin (Cipro), levofloxacin, moxifloxacin	Nausea, vomiting, dizziness	Cause photosensitivity. Are contraindicated during pregnancy.
E. Macrolide antibiotics		erythromycin, clarithromycin, azithromycin (Zithromax)	Stomach upset, nausea, vomiting	Should be taken with food.
F. Miscellaneous antibiotics		vancomycin (Vancocin), clindamycin, metronidazole (Flagyl), sulfamethoxazole/trimethoprim (Bactrim)		Vancocin: Used primarily for methicillin-resistant *Staphylococcus aureus*. Flagyl: Patients should avoid alcohol. Bactrim: Patients should drink 6–8 glasses of water daily to avoid renal crystallization of the drug.
Antifungals	Inhibit and kill fungal growth		Systemically administered antifungals may be nephrotoxic and hepatotoxic	Some are available in oral form for systemic treatment; others are available in topical form.
A. Polyene antifungals		amphotericin B, natamycin, nystatin		
B. Imidazole antifungals		clotrimazole, econazole, ketoconazole, miconazole, tioconazole		
C. Triazole antifungals		fluconazole, itraconazole, terconazole, voriconazole		
D. Allylamine antifungals		butenafine, terbinafine		
E. Echinocandin antifungals		anidulafungin, caspofungin, micafungin		
Antivirals	Inhibit viral growth	acyclovir, valacyclovir, zidovudine, amantadine	GI disturbances, headache, malaise, insomnia, dizziness	Should be taken at first sign of onset of viral attack for best relief of symptoms.
Antiprotozoals	Inhibit protozoal infections	artemether/lumefantrine (Coartem)	Headache, pruritus, GI disturbances, tinnitus	Also known as *antimalarials*.

Continued

Body System/ Drug Purpose	Drug Category	Drug Action	Examples	Side Effects	Comments
	Antitubercular agents	Suppress *Mycobacterium* causing tuberculosis	isoniazid, ethambutol (Myambutol), rifapentine (Priftin)	GI disturbances, hepatic disturbances	These drugs usually are given in combination.
Drugs used to treat cancer	Antineoplastics	Used as chemotherapy to inhibit the growth of neoplasms	cyclophosphamide (Cytoxan), methotrexate, fluorouracil, ofatumumab (Arzerra), pazopanib (Votrient)	Nausea; vomiting; hair loss; interference with blood cell production, resulting in anemia and suppression of the immune system	Historically used in combination to treat cancer. May be used in conjunction with radiation or surgery. Arzerra is a monoclonal antibody used for the treatment of chronic lymphocytic leukemia. Fluorouracil is used topically to treat actinic keratosis and basal cell carcinoma.
	Kinase inhibitors	Treat renal cell carcinoma	sorafenib (Nexavar) lenvatinib (Lenvima)	Hypothyroidism, GI disturbances, fatigue	
	CDK 4/6 inhibitors	HR-positive HER2-negative breast cancer	palbociclib (Ibrance) Abemaciclib (Verzenio) Ribociclib (Kisqali)	Neutropenia, respiratory issues, GI disturbances, hair loss	
	Angiogenesis inhibitors	Treat colon, lung, kidney, cervical cancers	bevacizumab (Avastin) ramucirumab (Cyramza)	Hemorrhage, blood clots, hypertension, GI issues	
	Checkpoint inhibitors	Treat melanoma, lung cancer, Hodgkin lymphoma	pembrolizumab (Keytruda) nivolumab (Opdivo)	Rash, fever, cough, GI disturbances, respiratory issues, hormonal issues	
	Antimetabolites	Treat carcinomas and sarcomas	methotrexate mercaptopurine (Purinethol), pazopanib (Votrient)	Bone marrow depression, stomatitis, mouth ulcers, GI upset, loss of hair, fever, chills	
	Estrogen receptor blockers	Used to treat breast cancer	tamoxifen (Nolvadex), anastrozole (Arimidex)	Reduce platelet count; may cause hot flashes, night sweats, insomnia	Side effects are relatively mild. Blood counts and liver studies are recommended.

Drugs used as nutritional supplements and alternative medicine	Electrolytes	Replace electrolytes	potassium chloride (K-Tab), 0.9% sodium chloride (normal saline), sodium polystyrene sulfonate (Kayexalate)	Rapid heart rate when levels are abnormally high	Potassium replacement therapy in use of diuretics. Potassium levels should be monitored.
	Vitamin/mineral supplements	Supplement or replace essential vitamins and minerals	cyanocobalamin (vitamin B_{12}), multiple vitamins, vitamins with minerals, carbonyl iron (Feosol)	Oral iron supplements may cause constipation; excessive oral iron intake may cause GI bleeding; caution must be used to avoid excessive ingestion of fat-soluble vitamins and iron to prevent toxicity	Vitamin B_{12} for treatment of pernicious anemia is by injection. Folic acid supplements are encouraged for females of childbearing capability to reduce incidence of neural tube deficits in the developing fetus.

Chapter 3

Drugs used to treat disorders of the immune system, immunizations	Immunizations	Provide artificially acquired active immunity to diseases; produce an antigen-antibody reaction	diphtheria, tetanus, and acellular pertussis vaccine, measles, mumps, rubella vaccine, oral poliovirus vaccine (Sabin vaccine), inactivated poliovirus vaccine (Salk vaccine)	Redness may develop at injection site, generalized malaise, fever	Follow the American Academy of Pediatrics' schedule recommendation.
	Immune globulins and antitoxins	Provide artificially acquired passive immunity	Rho(D) immune globulin (RhoGAM), immune globulin (GamaSTAN), tetanus antitoxin	Local inflammation at the injection site, slight fever	RhoGAM is given prenatally and postnatally to Rh-negative mothers to prevent Rh incompatibility in the infant and in subsequent pregnancies.
	Immunosuppressants	Reduce the body's autoimmune response to its own tissues	methotrexate, cyclosporine, azathioprine, mycophenolate, tacrolimus, adalimumab (Humira), abatacept (Orencia), etanercept (Enbrel), tocilizumab (Actemra), golimumab (Simponi), interferon, teriflunomide (Aubagio)	Imuran: Lower white blood cell count, upper GI symptoms, fatigue, alopecia, diarrhea, joint pain	Used to prevent rejection in transplant recipients and to treat rheumatoid arthritis. Increases risk of cancer in long-term use.

Continued

Body System/Drug Purpose	Drug Category	Drug Action	Examples	Side Effects	Comments
	Drug therapy for HIV infection	Prevent and reduce viral reproduction	efavirenz, tenofovir (Viread), emtricitabine (Emtriva), atazanavir (Reyataz), raltegravir (Isentress), darunavir (Prezista)	Various	Therapy is given per various protocols using combinations of antivirals.
Chapter 4 <u>Drugs for the endocrine system</u>	Hypoglycemics				
	A. Insulin and insulin analogs	Rapid acting: onset of action varies from 10 to 30min	Insulin lispro (Humalog), insulin aspart (NovoLog), insulin glulisine (Apidra), insulin regular (Humulin R, Novolin R)	Hypoglycemia, insulin shock	Glucophage reduces absorption of glucose from the intestine, helps prevent gluconeogenesis, and increases insulin use. Long-acting basal insulin. Once daily dosing.
		Intermediate acting	insulin isophane (Humulin N, Novolin N)		
		Long acting	insulin glargine (Lantus), insulin detemir (Levemir)		
		Other analogs	exenatide (Bydureon, Byetta Prefilled Pen), liraglutide (Victoza), pramlintide (Symlin)		
	B. Oral hypoglycemics	Stimulate insulin release	glipizide, glimepiride (Amaryl), glyburide	Sulfonylureas also may cause hypoglycemia	Patients taking Glucophage should be warned about the danger of iodine medium-based contrast imaging studies and the importance of advising any imaging technicians that they are taking Glucophage.
	Biguanides	Enhance insulin sensitivity in muscle and fat	metformin (Glucophage)	Stomach upset, gas	

Glitazones	Stimulate peroxisome proliferator–activated receptors	pioglitazone (Actos)	Reports of acute pancreatitis. Have a boxed warning regarding potential cardiovascular issues.	
DPP-4 inhibitors	Inhibit degradation of incretins and increase insulin secretion	sitagliptin (Januvia), saxagliptin (Onglyza), alogliptin (Nesina), linagliptin (Tradjenta)	Headache, respiratory tract infection	
SGLT-2 inhibitors	Cause kidneys to remove sugar in the body through urine	canagliflozin (Invokana) dapagliflozin (Farxiga)	Dehydration, ketoacidosis, kidney problems	
Alpha-glucosidase inhibitors	Slow the breakdown of carbohydrates to glucose	acarbose, miglitol (Glyset)	Gas, bloating, diarrhea	
Insulin antagonists or hyperglycemic agents	Elevate blood sugars	glucagon	Increase in blood glucose	Glucose tablets and gels are effective in emergency situations of low blood glucose levels.
Corticosteroids	Regulate immune response system and control of artificial immune response	hydrocortisone (Cortef), dexamethasone, prednisone, methylprednisolone (Medrol)	Nervousness; sleepiness; hypertension; muscle weakness; dry, itching, burning skin; depression	Treatment should not be stopped abruptly. Dosages should be tapered off. Long-term use may cause severe effects.
Thyroid replacements	Treat hypothyroidism	desiccated thyroid, levothyroxine, liothyronine,	Increased or irregular heartbeat, shortness of breath, headache, nervousness, irritability, sleeplessness, tremors, heat intolerance, weight changes, vomiting, diarrhea	Should be taken 30 min before breakfast on empty stomach. Once diagnosed with hypothyroidism, patient must take replacement therapy for life.
Antithyroid preparations	Inhibit the production of thyroid hormone	methimazole, propylthiouracil	Blood dyscrasias	Medication should be taken around the clock. Used to treat Graves disease.

Continued

Body System/ Drug Purpose	Drug Category	Drug Action	Examples	Side Effects	Comments
Chapter 5 Drugs for the sensory system					
A. Eyes	Mydriatics	Dilate the pupil of the eye	epinephrine, phenylephrine ophthalmic	Systemically cause increased heart rate, increased BP	Adrenergic drugs
	Miotics	Constrict pupil of the eye	pilocarpine (Isopto Carpine)	May slow heart rate and cause drop in BP	Cholinergic agonist
	Prostaglandin analogs	Decrease eye pressure from glaucoma	latanoprost ophthalmic (Xalatan), travoprost ophthalmic, bimatoprost ophthalmic (Lumigan),		Mast cell stabilizers
	Alpha-adrenergic receptor agonists	Decrease eye pressure from glaucoma	brimonidine ophthalmic (Alphagan P)		
	Ophthalmics	Treat allergic conjunctivitis, topical antibiotics	gatifloxacin (Zymaxid), alcaftadine (Lastacaft), bepotastine (Bepreve), besifloxacin (Besivance), neomycin/polymyxin B		
B. Ears	Cerumenolytics	Soften and emulsify ear wax	carbamide peroxide (Debrox)		Should not be used if tympanic membrane is ruptured or there is a discharge from ear.
	Antiinfectives	Inhibit growth of bacteria, as in swimmer's ear	hydrogen peroxide/ethyl alcohol, ciprofloxacin	Rash	Used routinely after swimming.
Chapter 6 Drugs for the integumentary system	Anesthetics	Produce lack of sensation to pain or abolish sensation to pain	lidocaine (Xylocaine), bupivacaine (Marcaine HCl)	Neurotoxicity, local reaction	May be mixed with epinephrine, causing vasoconstriction and extending duration of anesthesia.

Antiparasitics	Rid body of parasites (e.g., lice)	lindane, ivermectin (Sklice), pyrethrins/piperonyl, permethrin topical (Elimite), spinosad topical (Natroba)	Possibly carcinogenic	May be a blood toxin; must be used with care; all directions should be followed completely.
Antipruritics	Stop itching	calamine lotion, diphenhydramine cream, corticosteroid creams	Skin rash may rarely occur	Provide topical relief for dermatitis type of irritation.
Antiseptics	Inhibit bacterial growth, usually used on living tissue	hexachlorophene (pHisoHex), silver sulfadiazine topical (Silvadene), hydrogen peroxide, povidone/iodine (Betadine), isopropyl alcohol	pHisoHex: dermatitis, may be toxic when absorbed systemically Silvadene: Has a sulfa base; may cause reactions in those allergic to sulfa-based products Betadine: may cause skin rash when applied to those who have allergic reactions to topical iodine	Used as preoperative scrubs and cleansing. Silvadene is used on burn patients.
Disinfectants	Kill or inhibit bacterial growth; usually used on inanimate objects	formaldehyde, glutaraldehyde, phenol	Not for use on humans; may cause skin rash	Effective as disinfectant on inanimate objects.
Emollients/demulcents	Soothe and/or protect irritated tissue	A + D Cream, Eucerin, Lubriderm, many variants	vitamin E ointment, Desitin, Sween Cream	None likely	Frequently used to treat diaper rash or other localized skin irritation.
Keratolytics	Control abnormal skin scaling or promote peeling of overgrowths/ neoplasms of skin	coal tar topical (Tegrin Dandruff Shampoo, Neutrogena T/ Gel), salicylic acid, benzoyl peroxide (Clearasil), fluorouracil topical (Efudex), tretinoin (Retin A)	Retin A: Erythema, crusting lesions on skin; itching, burning, dryness of skin	Efudex is used to treat actinic keratosis and basal cell carcinoma.

Continued

Body System/ Drug Purpose	Drug Category	Drug Action	Examples	Side Effects	Comments
Chapter 7 Drugs for the musculoskeletal system	Antigout agents	Treat chronic gout	colchicine, allopurinol (Zyloprim), probenecid, febuxostat (Uloric)	Rash, headache, GI disorders, blood dyscrasias	Helpful in reducing excessive amounts of uric acid produced by the body.
	Antiinflammatories	Reduce inflammation in joints and muscles			
	A. Steroidal (see Drugs for the endocrine system, Corticosteroids)		prednisone, dexamethasone, methylprednisolone	GI upsets and bleeds, renal disturbances; steroids may mask infections	Patients usually are instructed to follow directions carefully and report any side effects as soon as possible.
	B. NSAIDs		ibuprofen (Motrin, Advil), naproxen (Aleve, Naprosyn), indomethacin (Indocin), celecoxib (Celebrex), meloxicam (Mobic)	GI symptoms, bleeding tendencies, changes in liver enzymes	Celebrex is a COX-2 inhibitor reported to have fewer gastric side effects.
	Bone replacement therapeutics	Treat and prevent osteoporosis	alendronate, ibandronate, risedronate, calcitonin-salmon (Miacalcin Nasal Spray)	Abdominal pain, muscle pain, constipation or diarrhea, nausea, flatulence	Instruct patients to take drug on an empty stomach with a glass of water and not to eat for at least 30 min.
	Muscle relaxants	Relax skeletal muscles	methocarbamol, cyclobenzaprine, baclofen, metaxalone, carisoprodol	GI upset, miosis, increased bronchial secretions, muscle cramps, tachycardia, elevated liver enzymes	May make patients drowsy; advise against driving or operating machinery.
Chapter 8 Drugs used for the gastrointestinal system	Antacids	Neutralize stomach acid	calcium carbonate (Tums)	Heartburn, indigestion, stomach upset	Chronic use of antacids may cause acid rebound effect.
	Antidiarrheals	Control diarrhea	bismuth subsalicylate (Pepto-Bismol), loperamide (Imodium), diphenoxylate hydrochloride (HCl)/atropine (Lomotil)	Constipation, abdominal cramping, diarrhea	Prolonged uncontrolled diarrhea should be reported to a physician.

		nitazoxanide (Alinia) aluminum hydroxide/magnesium hydroxide		
	Used as antiprotozoal/ infant use Used as antiprotozoal for diarrhea caused by *Cryptosporidium parvum* or *Giardia lamblia* in pediatric patients			
Antidotes	Neutralize toxins and poisons	syrup of ipecac, activated charcoal	Charcoal causes stool to be black	Syrup of ipecac is never given if the ingested substance is corrosive (e.g., lye, Drano) or is petroleum based, or if patient is lethargic or unconscious. Syrup of ipecac: Administration is followed by drinking a minimum of 4-6 glasses of water (adults). Vomiting should be expected and be prepared for. Activated charcoal is given after the vomiting has ceased; clothing should be protected; drug is given with a straw to get medication to back of mouth and prevent charcoal staining teeth.
Antiemetics	Prevent and treat nausea and vomiting	prochlorperazine (Compazine), metoclopramide (Reglan), dimenhydrinate (Dramamine), ondansetron (Zofran)	Drowsiness, dizziness, blurred vision, anticholinergic effects, hypotension, skin reactions	Slow peristalsis, may cause abdominal cramping and related constipation. Zofran may be given to patients with cancer on chemotherapy to treat nausea and vomiting.

Continued

Body System/Drug Purpose	Drug Category	Drug Action	Examples	Side Effects	Comments
	Antiflatulents	Provide symptomatic relief of gastric bloating and intestinal gas	simethicone (Mylicon, Phazyme)	None noted	Also used to treat colic in infants.
	Anthelmintics	Eradicate helminths (worms)	mebendazole (Vermox),	Abdominal pain, diarrhea	Treatment of entire family is recommended.
	Antispasmodics	Relieve smooth-muscle spasms of the stomach and intestines	hyoscyamine (Levsin), belladonna alkaloids/phenobarbital (Donnatal), hyoscyamine, dicyclomine (Bentyl)	Decreased peristalsis, dry mouth, headache, dizziness, palpitations, fatigue	Used to treat irritable bowel syndrome and similar intestinal disorders.
	Antiulcer agents	Reduce gastric acid secretions by acting as histamine-2 (H2)-receptor antagonists	cimetidine (Tagamet), ranitidine (Zantac), nizatidine (Axid), famotidine (Pepcid)	Headache, fatigue, myalgia, alopecia, diarrhea, rash, dizziness	Helpful in treatment of GERD.
		Act as proton pump inhibitors	omeprazole (Prilosec), pantoprazole (Protonix), esomeprazole (Nexium), lansoprazole (Prevacid)		More effective than H2-receptor antagonists.
	Digestants	Assist with digestion of food by replacing pancreatic enzymes	pancrelipase (Creon)	GI upset, rashes	Patient should be instructed not to chew or crush capsules.
	Emetics	Induce vomiting	syrup of ipecac		Syrup of ipecac is never given if the ingested substance is corrosive (e.g., lye, Drano) or is petroleum based, or if patient is lethargic or unconscious. Syrup of ipecac administration is followed by drinking a minimum of 4–6 glasses of water (adults). One should be prepared for vomiting.
	Laxatives/cathartics	Induce defecation and relieve constipation	bisacodyl (Dulcolax), sennoside alkaloids (Senna), mineral oil, psyllium (Metamucil)	Cramping, diarrhea	Patients should be cautioned about excessive continued use, which may cause a reverse reaction.

Chapter 9

Drugs used for the respiratory system				
Stool softeners	Soften feces	docusate sodium (Colace), docusate calcium (Surfak), polyethylene glycol (MiraLAX)	Leakage of oil-like substances from rectum, increased peristalsis, cramping	Used to ease evacuation of bowel contents.
Asthma prophylactics	Prevent exercise-induced asthma	cromolyn sodium (Intal), montelukast (Singulair)	Bronchospasm, cough, wheezing, nasal congestion	Have best action when used before exposure.
Leukotriene receptor antagonists		roflumilast (Daliresp)		
Antihistamines	Inhibit histamine to relieve allergy symptoms	diphenhydramine (Benadryl), clemastine (Tavist), chlorpheniramine (Chlor-Trimeton), fexofenadine (Allegra), cetirizine (Zyrtec), loratadine (Claritin), desloratadine (Clarinex), levocetirizine	Drowsiness, dry eyes, dry mouth, hypotension constipation, anorexia, palpitations	May cause drowsiness. Patient should be advised not to drive or operate machinery while taking medication. Contraindicated in patients with glaucoma.
Antitussives	Suppress cough	dextromethorphan, codeine, hydrocodone, benzonatate	CNS stimulation, blurred vision, palpitations, anxiety, weakness, insomnia	Patients should be instructed to follow directions. Hydrocodone and codeine may be habit forming.
Bronchodilators	Relax smooth muscle of bronchial tree; relieve bronchospasm	albuterol sulfate (Proventil), levalbuterol (Xopenex), epinephrine (Primatene), theophylline (Theo-Dur), ipratropium (Atrovent), tiotropium (Spiriva)	Hyperactivity, excitement, tremor, nervousness, insomnia, tachycardia	Routine theophylline blood level studies are recommended.
Decongestants	Shrink nasal mucous membranes	oxymetazoline (Afrin), pseudoephedrine HCl (Sudafed),	Nasal sprays may cause irritation to nasal membrane Constrict vessels; cause hypertension	Prolonged use of sprays may cause rebound effects. Should not be used by pregnant females because of possible constriction of vessels.

Continued

Body System/ Drug Purpose	Drug Category	Drug Action	Examples	Side Effects	Comments
	Expectorants	Increase respiratory secretions and reduce viscosity to allow for the expulsion of sputum	guaifenesin (Robitussin, Mucinex)	Excitability, constipation, nausea, vomiting, drowsiness	May cause drowsiness. Patient should be advised not to drive or operate machinery while taking medication.
	Mucolytics	Liquefy respiratory secretions	acetylcysteine	Runny nose, throat irritation, nausea	Used to treat asthma and cystic fibrosis. Also used as antidote in acetaminophen overdose.
	Smoking-cessation aids	Reduce nicotine levels while assisting with smoking-cessation programs	nicotine (Nicorette, NicoDerm), bupropion (Zyban),varenicline	Tobacco withdrawal symptoms, local effects from patches or sprays, dry mouth, insomnia	Patient may require emotional support while using these products. Chantix may elicit vivid dreams.
Chapter 10					
Drugs used for the cardiovascular system and for hematology	Antianginals	Used for prophylactic treatment of angina; dilate coronary arteries	nitroglycerin (Nitrostat, Transderm-Nitro), isosorbide monohydrate, isosorbide dinitrate	Lightheadedness, headache	Nitrostat sublingual tablets should be placed under the tongue to treat angina. May be repeated every 5 min, three times, to relieve angina. If no relief, entry into the emergency medical system is advised.
	Antiarrhythmics	Suppress cardiac arrhythmias	propranolol, verapamil, dronedarone (Multaq), dofetilide (Tikosyn)	Hypotension, GI upset, headache, fatigue	Regular monitoring of arrhythmias is recommended.
	Anticoagulants	Prevent formation of clots	warfarin (Coumadin), heparin sodium, ticagrelor (Brilinta), prasugrel (Effient), rivaroxaban (Xarelto)	Tissue or organ hemorrhage, rash, abdominal pain, headache	Blood coagulation studies are performed on a regular basis.
	Antihypertensives	Treatment and management of hypertension			
	A. Calcium channel blockers		amlodipine, diltiazem, verapamil	Constipation, dizziness	

Category	Action	Examples	Side effects	Notes
B. Beta-blockers		atenolol, carvedilol, metoprolol, propranolol, labetalol	Hypotension, lethargy, GI symptoms, slow heart rate, dizziness	
C. ACE inhibitors		enalapril, benazepril, lisinopril, fosinopril, ramipril, quinapril, trandolapril	Dizziness, hypotension, dry cough	
D. Angiotensin receptor blockers		candesartan, irbesartan, losartan, valsartan		
E. Diuretics		hydrochlorothiazide, furosemide, torsemide, bumetanide, spironolactone		
Antihyperlipidemics	Reduce serum cholesterol and low-density lipoproteins	gemfibrozil, fenofibrate, cholestyramine (Questran), niacin, fish oil, simvastatin (Zocor), atorvastatin (Lipitor), pravastatin (Pravachol), rosuvastatin (Crestor), ezetimibe (Zetia), pitavastatin (Livalo)	Myalgia, GI upset, headache, rash, dizziness, elevated liver enzymes. Zetia: Stomach pain, tiredness	Statin drugs are reported to reduce existing arterial plaque. Zetia is a cholesterol-lowering drug with less myalgia reported.
Cardiotonics/cardiac glycosides	Strengthen heartbeat	digoxin (Lanoxin), digitoxin	Irregular heartbeat, palpitations, loss of appetite, nausea, vomiting, diarrhea, visual changes	Patient should be instructed to take the drug in the morning, record daily weights, and take apical pulse before taking medication. If pulse rate is lower than 60 bpm, dose should be withheld and pulse recounted in 1 h. If pulse rate is still less than 60 bpm, medication should be withheld and the physician contacted. Patient may be prone to digitalis toxicity.
Coagulants/hemostatics	Control or stop bleeding by promoting coagulation	phytonadione, menadiol sodium, vitamin K	Normal aspirin side effects. Persantine: dizziness, headache, rash, GI upset	Administered to newborns to prevent hemorrhagic disease.

Continued

Body System/ Drug Purpose	Drug Category	Drug Action	Examples	Side Effects	Comments
	Platelet inhibitors	Inhibit platelet clumping	aspirin, dipyridamole (Persantine), prasugrel (Effient), dabigatran (Pradaxa), clopidogrel (Plavix), rivaroxaban (Xarelto), ticagrelor (Brilinta)	Normal aspirin side effects Aspirin side effects may include GI distress, ulceration, increased bleeding time (international normalized ratio). Persantine: dizziness, headache, rash, GI upset	
	Thrombolytics	Dissolve blood clots	streptokinase (Streptase), alteplase (Activase)	GI bleeds, bleeding in other sites	Best if administration begins within 2–3 h after onset of chest pain in MI.
	Vasoconstrictors	Constrict blood vessels	metaraminol, norepinephrine, epinephrine	Nausea and vomiting, cardiac arrhythmias, decreased urine output	Used to treat shock.
	Vasodilators	Dilate blood vessels	nitroglycerin, isosorbide dinitrate (Isordil), isosorbide mononitrate	Lightheadedness, headache	Nitrostat sublingual tablets should be placed under the tongue to treat angina. May be repeated every 5 min, three times, to relieve angina. If no relief, entry into the emergency medical system is advised.
Chapter 11					
Drugs used for the urinary system	Urinary analgesics	Lessen pain and burning of urinary tract infection	phenazopyridine HCl (Pyridium)	Produces orange- to red-colored urine that may stain clothing	Patients should be advised about possibility of stains to clothing from the orange- or red-colored urine.
	Urinary antiseptics	Used as specific antibacterials to treat urinary tract infections	nitrofurantoin (Furadantin), nitrofurantoin monohydrate/ macrocrystals (Macrobid), sulfamethoxazole/ trimethoprim (Bactrim)	GI disturbances, orange-colored urine	Patients should be informed about possibility of orange-colored urine.

	Action/Purpose	Examples	Side effects	Notes
Urinary antispasmodics	Relieve urgency, frequency, and incontinence	Oxybutynin HCl, flavoxate, darifenacin, fesoterodine (Toviaz), solifenacin (Vesicare), trospium	Dry mouth, constipation, somnolence, tachycardia	Relax bladder muscles and help to reduce incontinence.
Diuretics	Remove excessive fluid from body tissues; increase urinary output	Furosemide (Lasix), hydrochlorothiazide, bumetanide (Bumex), torsemide, spironolactone, metolazone	Hypokalemia, excessive diuresis, GI upset, dizziness, vertigo	Characterized by site of action. Many require monitoring of potassium levels and require daily potassium replacement. Patients should be instructed to take medication in morning to ensure restful nights. Recording of daily weights should be encouraged.
Enuretic agents	Control enuresis	Desmopressin	Dry mouth, constipation, somnolence, tachycardia	Relax bladder muscles and help reduce incontinence.
Chapter 12				
Drugs used for the reproductive system				
Contraceptives	Prevent conception/pregnancy		Thromboembolism associated with MI and CVA. Elevated blood pressure and blood glucose levels, acne, hair loss, gallbladder disease, hirsutism	A missed pill may result in pregnancy. Antibiotic therapy may render contraceptive ineffective. Now available in an intradermal patch form.
A. Low-dose monophasic birth control pills	Estrogen: ethinyl estradiol (EE) Progestins: Levonorgestrel, norethindrone, desogestrel, drospirenone, or ethynodiol diacetate.	EE/levonorgestrel (Aviane, Lessina, Lutera, Nordette, Orsythia), levonorgestrel/EE (Falmina), EE/norethindrone (Gildess Fe 1/20, Junel Fe 1/20, Loestrin Fe 1/20, Microgestin 1/20), EE/norgestrel (Cryselle, Lo/Ovral), EE/desogestrel (Apri)		
B. High-dose monophasic birth control pills		EE/norethindrone (Ovcon-50), EE/norgestrel (Ogestrel 0.5/50), Zovia (EE/ethynodiol diacetate)		

Continued

Body System/ Drug Purpose	Drug Category	Drug Action	Examples	Side Effects	Comments
	C. Biphasic birth control pills		EE/desogestrel (Kariva, Mircette), EE/norethindrone (Necon 10/11)		
	D. Triphasic birth control pills		EE/norethindrone (Estrostep Fe), EE/norgestimate (Ortho Tri-Cyclen, TriNessa, Tri-Previfem, Tri-Sprintec), EE/desogestrel (Cyclessa, Velivet), EE/levonorgestrel (Enpresse, Trivora)		
	E. Four-phase birth control pills		dienogest/estradiol (Natazia)		
	F. Extended-cycle birth control pills		EE/norethindrone/ferrous fumarate tablets (Lo Loestrin Fe), EE/levonorgestrel (Amethia Lo, Amethia, Seasonique), drospirenone/EE/levomefolate (Beyaz), drospirenone/EE (Gianvi, Loryna, Yaz)		
	G. Progestin-only pills (mini-pill)		norethindrone (Camilla, Errin, Nor-QD, Ortho Micronor)		
	Emergency contraception		ulipristal (Ella), levonorgestrel (Plan-B, Next Choice)		
	Alternative methods		medroxyprogesterone acetate (Depo-Provera), levonorgestrel intrauterine system (Mirena), etonogestrel (Nexplanon), EE/etonogestrel (NuvaRing)		Depo-Provera requires an injection every 3 months. Nexplanon implantation must be performed by a physician every 3 years. NuvaRing is a vaginal ring insert that is inserted/ removed by the patient. Mirena releases levonorgestrel. Included in grouping as a nonpill-related method.
	Fertility enhancers	Induce ovulation	clomiphene citrate	GI symptoms, CNS symptoms, acne, ovarian enlargement, ectopic pregnancies	Occurrence of multiple pregnancies is possible.
	Hormone replacements	Replace reproductive hormones			

	Action/Use	Drugs	Side Effects	Comments
A. Androgens	Stimulate the development of male sexual characteristics	testosterone cypionate (Depo-Testosterone), methyltestosterone	Urinary urgency, breast tenderness, priapism	Supplement low levels of testosterone
B. Estrogens	Stimulate the development of female sexual characteristics	estradiol (Estrace), conjugated estrogens (Premarin),	Anorexia, nausea, headaches, edema of lower extremities, hypercalcemia, thrombophlebitis	Used to treat symptoms of menopause; increases risk of breast and cervical cancers. Caution must be used in females who smoke; may cause deep vein thrombosis.
C. Progestins	Treat amenorrhea and abnormal uterine bleeding	medroxyprogesterone (Provera), medroxyprogesterone acetate (Depo-Provera)	Weight gain, stomach disturbances, edema, headaches, breakthrough bleeding	May be used for contraception, used in combination with estrogen for postmenopausal hormone replacement therapy.
Drugs used to treat prostatic conditions	Treats BPH and urinary retention	doxazosin, tamsulosin (Flomax), terazosin (Hytrin), finasteride	Hypotension, fatigue, edema, dyspnea	Used to relieve urinary retention and nocturia caused by enlarged prostate.
Drugs used to treat erectile dysfunction		sildenafil citrate (Viagra), tadalafil (Cialis), vardenafil	Nasal congestion, blurred vision, hypertension, dizziness, rash	Patients who have cardiac disease should be cautioned not to take Viagra. Drug should be taken on an empty stomach an hour before eating.

Chapter 13

	Action/Use	Drugs	Side Effects	Comments
Drugs used for the neurologic system — Adrenergic drugs	Mimic sympathetic nervous system	epinephrine, dopamine	Increased blood pressure, rapid heart rate	Initiate "fight or flight" system.
Adrenergic blockers	Block the action of sympathetic nervous system	Propranolol (Inderal), methyldopa	Hypotension, bradycardia, constricted bronchioles	Used to treat hypertension; Inderal also used for migraine headaches.
Analgesics	Relieve pain			

Continued

Body System/Drug Purpose	Drug Category	Drug Action	Examples	Side Effects	Comments
	A. Opioids (narcotics)		Codeine, meperidine, hydrocodone, hydromorphone, oxycodone, oxymorphone, fentanyl, morphine	May cause drowsiness; constipation can occur	May become addictive. Patients should not drive or operate machinery while taking the drug.
	B. Nonopioids		Acetaminophen (Tylenol), acetylsalicylic acid (aspirin), NSAIDs	Aspirin: may cause stomach upset and tinnitus	Aspirin also has anticoagulant, antiprostaglandin effects. All are antipyretic medications.
	Anesthetics	Produce loss of sensation by blocking nerve impulses			
	A. General		Thiopental sodium (Pentothal), midazolam (Versed)	Versed: may cause amnesia, hypotension, headache	Versed is used for conscious sedation.
	B. Local		Lidocaine (Xylocaine), procaine (Novocain)		Xylocaine may be topical form; also is used systemically as a cardiac drug.
	Anticholinergics	Block parasympathetic nervous system	Atropine, scopolamine	Dry mouth, increased heart rate, constipation, urinary retention, dilated pupils	May be used in treatment of Parkinson disease.

Classification	Action	Examples	Side Effects	Notes
Antiepileptics	Reduce the number and/or severity of seizures caused by epilepsy	Phenytoin (Dilantin), phenobarbital, clonazepam (Klonopin), gabapentin (Neurontin), vigabatrin (Sabril),	Reduced coordination, involuntary eye movement, slurred speech	Encourage good mouth care because Dilantin may cause gingival hyperplasia. Neurontin may be prescribed to treat post-therapy neuralgia. These medications should not be stopped abruptly.
Antiparkinsonism medications	Relieve symptoms and increase mobility of patients with Parkinson disease	Carbidopa-levodopa, amantadine (Symmetrel)	Dystonia, GI symptoms, dry mouth, increased hand tremors	Used to increase levels of dopamine in the brain.
Cholinergics	Mimic parasympathetic nervous system by liberating acetylcholine	Neostigmine (Prostigmin), pilocarpine	Increased peristalsis	
Hypnotics/Sedatives	Produce sedation or sleep			
Nonbarbiturates		Zolpidem (Ambien), eszopiclone (Lunesta)		May be habit forming. May cause confusion, sleep walking.
Stimulants	Increase the activity of brain/spinal cord	Caffeine, methylphenidate (Ritalin), modafinil (Provigil), armodafinil (Nuvigil)	Anorexia, euphoria, sleeplessness, dry mouth, GI disturbances, insomnia, weight loss	May be addictive. Ritalin is used to treat hyperactivity in children.
Drugs used in the treatment of Alzheimer disease — Alzheimer disease medications	Enhance transmission of cholinergic neurons to improve thought processes	Donepezil (Aricept), memantine (Namenda)	GI disturbances, insomnia, vomiting, anorexia	Help with memory and thinking processes; improve everyday activities; improve behavior.
Drugs used in the treatment of multiple sclerosis — Multiple sclerosis drugs	Used for relapsing forms of multiple sclerosis	Interferon beta-1b (Betaseron), interferon beta-1a (Avonex, Rebif, glatiramer (Copaxone), natalizumab (Tysabri), fingolimod (Gilenya), teriflunomide (Aubagio), dimethyl fumarate (Tecfidera)		Gilenya, Aubagio, and Tecfidera are oral agents. The remaining agents are given by injection.

Continued

Body System/ Drug Purpose

Chapter 14

Body System/ Drug Purpose	Drug Category	Drug Action	Examples	Side Effects	Comments
Drugs used for mental disorders	Antianxiety/anxiolytics/ minor tranquilizers	Used for short-term treatment of anxiety disorders, some psychosomatic disorders, and nausea and vomiting	diazepam (Valium), lorazepam (Ativan), clorazepate (Tranxene), alprazolam (Xanax), vigabatrin (Sabril), asenapine (Saphris), milnacipran (Savella), iloperidone (Fanapt)	CNS symptoms, GI disturbances, skin rash, nasal congestion. May be habit forming	May cause drowsiness; use caution when driving or operating machinery. Patient should not stop medication abruptly. Dosages should be tapered.
	Antidepressants/mood elevators	Treat depression	amitriptyline (Elavil), phenelzine (Nardil)	CNS symptoms, GI disturbances, weight gain, somnolence	May take 2–4 weeks for effects to be realized. Consumption of alcohol should be avoided.
			sertraline (Zoloft), fluoxetine (Prozac), venlafaxine (Effexor), paroxetine (Paxil), fluvoxamine (Luvox), milnacipran (Savella), vilazodone (Viibryd)	SSRIs have a lower incidence of side effects	
	Antimanics	Treat manic disorders	lithium (Lithobid)	Dry mouth, excessive thirst, weight gain, GI disturbances, tremors, cardiac arrhythmias, visual impairment, unsteady gait	Used to treat bipolar disorders. Blood level should be monitored on a regular basis.
	Antipsychotics	Relieve symptoms of psychosis and severe neurosis	haloperidol (Haldol), asenapine (Saphris), iloperidone (Fanapt)	Tachycardia or bradycardia, vertigo, postural hypotension, dry mouth, constipation, urinary retention, anorexia, blurred vision, fever, CNS system reactions	May cause drowsiness; caution should be exercised when driving or operating machinery.

Category	Use	Drugs	Adverse effects	Comments
A. Atypical antipsychotics		aripiprazole (Abilify), clozapine (Clozaril), olanzapine (Zyprexa), paliperidone (Invega), quetiapine (Seroquel), risperidone (Risperdal), ziprasidone (Geodon)		May cause significant drowsiness. Various agents may cause significant weight gain. Some may be weight neutral or produce weight loss.
B. Neuroleptics/major tranquilizers		fluphenazine HCl (Prolixin), chlorpromazine, imipramine (Tofranil), quetiapine (Seroquel)		May cause drowsiness; caution should be exercised when driving or operating machinery.

Chapter 15

Category	Use	Drugs	Adverse effects	Comments
Drugs used for first aid, emergency situations				
Sulfonamides	Treat burns topically	silver sulfadiazine (Silvadene), mafenide acetate (Sulfamylon)	Rash, redness	Helpful in treating infections; broad-spectrum agents effective against both gram-positive and gram-negative organisms.
Antivenoms	Counteract toxins, such as those from snakebites, spider bites	crotaline polyvalent immune Fab (rattlesnake), black widow spider antivenom	Made from sheep serum; less likely to produce severe reaction than antivenom from horse serum. Compartment syndrome may occur in affected limb	Often preceded by administration of antihistamine to lessen any allergic effects. Observation of individual for a minimum of 24 h is usual protocol.

aAnesthetics may be used alone or in combination to produce effects.

bDifferent generations of cephalosporins are effective against different strains of bacteria.

ACE, Angiotensin-converting enzyme; *BP,* blood pressure; *BPH,* benign prostatic hyperplasia; *bpm,* beats per minute; *CNS,* central nervous system; *COX-2,* cyclooxygenase-2; *CVA,* cerebrovascular accident; *DPP-4,* dipeptidyl peptidase-4; *GERD,* gastroesophageal reflux disease; *GI,* gastrointestinal; *HIV,* human immunodeficiency virus; *IM,* intramuscular; *MI,* myocardial infarction; *NSAIDs,* nonsteroidal antiinflammatory drugs; *SSRI,* selective serotonin reuptake inhibitor.

Glossary

Note: The Glossary contains the chapter Key Terms (unless they are defined in the text) and other important terms in the text. *Sp.*, Spanish

A

abduct (Sp. abducción, separar) move an arm or leg away from the body

ablation (Sp. ablación) excision or removal

abruptio placentae (Sp. desprendimiento de la placenta) detachment of the placenta from the uterus before birth; often results in severe bleeding

abscess (Sp. absceso) a localized collection of pus surrounded by swollen tissue

acetabulum (Sp. acetábulo) the cup-shaped cavity in which the ball-shaped head of the femur articulates

achalasia (Sp. acalasia) failure of the esophagogastric sphincter to relax with swallowing

acholic (Sp. arcilla) pale or clay-colored. Acholic stool usually results from problems in the biliary system

acidemia (Sp. acidemia) a decreased pH of blood (increased hydrogen ion concentration)

acidosis (Sp. acidosis) a pathologic condition resulting from an abnormal increase in the level of hydrogen ions in the body (decrease in pH), resulting from the accumulation of acid or loss of the alkaline reserve

acute abdomen (Sp. abdomen agudo) an abdominal condition of sudden onset, accompanied by pain resulting from intraabdominal inflammation or infection

acyanotic (Sp. acianótico) absence of a bluish appearance of the skin and mucous membranes

adenocarcinoma (Sp. adenocarcinoma, carcinoma glandular) a cancerous tumor arising from glandular tissue

adenoma (Sp. adenoma) a benign neoplasm in which cells are derived from the glandular epithelium

adenosarcoma (Sp. adenosarcoma) a cancerous glandlike tumor, such as Wilms tumor

adenovirus (Sp. adenovirus) a virus pathogenic to humans that causes conjunctivitis, upper respiratory infection, cystitis, or gastrointestinal infection; may persist in lymphoid tissue in latent period of the infection

adnexal (Sp. de los anexos) pertaining to accessory organs or tissues; appendage(s)

adrenocorticotropic hormone (ACTH) (Sp. hormona adrenocorticotrópica [ACTH]) a hormone secreted by the anterior lobe of the pituitary; also known as *corticotropin*

aerodigestive (Sp. aerodigestivo) pertaining to the respiratory and digestive tract considered together

agglutination (Sp. aglutinación) the clumping of antigens with antibodies or of the red blood cells from one type of blood with the red blood cells of another type

aggregation (Sp. agregación) the coming together of entities, such as platelets, blood cells, or diseases

agranulocytosis (Sp. agranulocitosis) a condition of the blood marked by a sudden decrease in the number of granulocytes (a type of white blood cell); occurs in lesions of the throat or other mucous membranes or as a side effect of the administration of certain drugs or radiation

alkalosis (Sp. alcalosis) excessive alkalinity of body fluids

allergen (Sp. alérgeno) an antigenic substance capable of producing an allergic response in the body

allograft (Sp. injerto alogénico) a graft of tissue between genetically different individuals of the same species

amblyopia (Sp. ambioplía) reduced vision in an eye without a detectable organic lesion

amnesia (Sp. amnesia) a loss of memory; inability to recall past experiences

amniogram, amniography (Sp. amniografía) radiography (after injection of radiopaque contrast medium into the amniotic fluid) of the pregnant uterus to detect placement of the placenta, the amniotic cavity, and the fetus

amniotic fluid (Sp. líquido amniótico) a transparent albuminous liquid made by the amnion and the fetus; surrounds and protects the fetus during pregnancy

amylase (Sp. amilasa) an enzyme produced in the salivary glands and pancreas that helps in digestion of starches

amyloid (Sp. amiloide) a waxy, starch-like protein that tends to build up in tissues and organs in certain pathologic conditions

analgesia, analgesic (Sp. analgesia, analgésico) relief of pain

analog (Sp. análogo) a drug that resembles another but has different effects

anaphylaxis (Sp. anafilaxia) a severe systemic allergic response characterized by redness, itching, swelling, and water buildup (angioedema); in severe cases, life-threatening respiratory distress occurs, and blood pressure drops rapidly (anaphylactic shock)

anaplastic (Sp. anaplástico) a change in the orientation and structure of cells; a loss of differentiation that is characteristic of malignancy

anastomosis (anastomoses) (Sp. anastomosis) the surgical or pathologic connection between two vessels or tubular structures

anesthesia, anesthetic (Sp. anestesia, anestésico) partial or complete loss of sensation caused by injury, diseases, or the administration of an anesthetic agent

angina pectoris (Sp. angina de pecho) paroxysmal chest pain, which often radiates to the arms and may be accompanied by a feeling of suffocation and impending death; the most common cause is a shortage of oxygen to the cardiac muscle linked with coronary artery disease

angioplasty (Sp. angioplastia) repair of a narrowed blood vessel through surgery or other angiographic procedures

angiotensin-converting enzyme (ACE) (Sp. enzima de conversión de la angiotensina [ECA]) an enzyme found on the surface of blood vessels in the lungs and other tissues with vasopressive action

angiotensin-converting enzyme (ACE) inhibitors (Sp. inhibidores de la enzima de conversión de la angiotensina) agents that inhibit angiotensin-converting enzyme (a potent vasoconstrictor) and promote relaxation of blood vessels

ankylosis (Sp. anquilosis) immobility of a joint

anorexia, anorectic (Sp. anorexia, anoréxico) loss of appetite for food

anosmia (Sp. anosmia) impairment or loss of smell

antibody (antibodies) (Sp. anticuerpo) an immunoglobulin that may combine with a specific antigen to destroy or control it

anticholinergic (Sp. anticolinérgico) a drug used to block the transmission of parasympathetic nerve impulses

anticholinesterase (Sp. anticolina esterasa) any enzyme that counteracts the action of the choline esters

anticoagulant (Sp. anticoagulante) any substance that delays or prevents blood clotting

antiemetic (Sp. antiemético) a medication that prevents or relieves nausea and vomiting

antigen (Sp. antígeno) any substance that stimulates the immune system to produce antibodies

antimicrobial (Sp. antimicrobiano) a substance that kills microorganisms or suppresses their growth

antipyretic (Sp. antipirético) a drug or treatment that reduces or relieves fever

antiseptic (Sp. antiséptico) a substance that inhibits the growth of microorganisms

antitrypsin (Sp. antitripsina) a substance that inhibits trypsin, an enzyme that hastens the hydrolysis of protein

anxiolytic (Sp. ansiolítico) a substance that diminishes anxiety

aphasia (Sp. afasia) a nerve defect that results in loss of speech

aphonia (Sp. afonía) inability to produce normal speech sounds or loss of voice

aphthous ulcers (Sp. úlceras aftosas) recurrent painful canker sores in the mouth

apicectomy (Sp. apicetomy) surgical removal of the apex of an infected or damaged tooth root

apnea, apneic (Sp. apnea, apneico) the temporary cessation of breathing

apoptosis (Sp. apoptosis) a pattern of cell death affecting single cells; refers to programmed cell death

arrhythmia (Sp. arritmia) variation or loss of normal rhythm of the heartbeat

arthrodesis (Sp. artrodesis) the immobilization of a joint accomplished surgically

arthroplasty (Sp. artroplastia) surgical reconstruction or replacement of a diseased joint

ascites (Sp. ascitis) abnormal intraperitoneal accumulation of serous fluid

aspiration (Sp. aspiración) drawing in or out by suction

assay (Sp. ensayar) the analysis of biologic substances, including laboratory and clinical evaluations

asymptomatic (Sp. asintomático) without symptoms

asystole (Sp. asístole) the absence of contractions of the heart; cardiac standstill

ataxia (Sp. ataxia) an uncoordinated gait associated with pathology of the central nervous system; an individual with this gait may be described as being *ataxic*

atrophy (Sp. atrofia) a wasting away; a degeneration of a cell, tissue, organ, or muscle because of disease or other influences

audiogram (Sp. audiograma) the record of a hearing test

aura (Sp. aura) a sensation or phenomenon that signals the onset of an epileptic seizure or a migraine

auscultation (Sp. auscultación) a diagnostic technique of listening for sounds within the body, particularly the lungs, heart, or abdominal viscera

autoantibody (Sp. autoanticuerpo) an antibody that attacks and destroys the body's own cells

autoimmunity, autoimmune (Sp. auto-inmunidad, auto-inmune) an immune response resulting in the presence of self-antigens or autoantigens on the surface of certain body cells; may result in allergy or autoimmune disease

autoinoculation (Sp. autoinoculación) refers to spreading a microorganism by contact with a lesion on one's own body

autonomic (Sp. autónomo) refers to the autonomic nervous system, which has two divisions (i.e., sympathetic and parasympathetic)

autosome, autosomal (Sp. autosoma, autosómico) any of the 22 ordinary paired chromosomes in humans, distinguished from the sex (X and Y) chromosomes

avulsion (Sp. separación) separation of a body part by tearing

azoospermia (Sp. azoospermia) an absence of spermatozoa in semen

azotemia (Sp. azotemia) an excess of urea or other nitrogenous bodies in blood

B

barium (Sp. bario) a pale, soft, alkaline metallic element; radiopaque barium (barium sulfate) compound commonly used in radiographic studies of the gastrointestinal tract

Battle sign (Sp. signo de Battle) bogginess of the temporal region of the head that may indicate fracture at the base of the skull

bicornuate uterus (Sp. útero bicorne) a uterus having two horns or horn-shaped branches

bifurcate (Sp. bifurcado) split into two branches

bilirubinemia (Sp. bilirrubinemia) the presence of bilirubin in blood

bilirubinuria (Sp. bilirrubinuria) the presence of bilirubin (a yellow- or orange-tinged pigment in the bile) in urine

biopsy (Sp. biopsia) the excision of tissue from the living body, followed by microscopic examination, for the purpose of exact diagnosis

biologic medications that are made from living organisms such as bacteria, animal cells or yeasts

biodefense measure to help prepare for such biological agents which could impact the world

biosimilar a biologic that can provide treatment benefits as an original biologic which already has FDA approval

blood gases (Sp. gases sanguíneos) the gases present in blood as a result of the use of oxygen and the production of carbon dioxide during metabolism; the blood is analyzed for evidence of deviations (acidosis or alkalosis) from normal levels

blood urea nitrogen (BUN) (Sp. nitrógeno ureico en sangre [NUS]) a measurement of urea nitrogen (a substance formed during protein breakdown) in the serum or plasma; an elevated BUN level may indicate impaired renal function

breech (Sp. nalgas) a presentation during an infants delivery where the buttocks or feet are positioned near the cervix

bronchoscopy (Sp. broncoscopía) examination of the bronchial tree with a bronchoscope to obtain a biopsy specimen, remove an obstruction, or diagnose a disease

bruit (Sp. ruido) an abnormal sound heard in auscultation

C

cachexia (Sp. caquexia) a profound and marked wasting disorder, usually associated with malnutrition and diseases, such as cancer and tuberculosis

calculus (calculi) (Sp. cálculo) a stone usually composed of mineral salts (e.g., kidney stones and gallstones) or calcified deposits on teeth

carcinogen, carcinogenic (Sp. carcinógeno) a substance that produces cancer or that causes transformation of a normal cell into a cancerous one

cardiac sphincter (Sp. esfínter cardiaco) the circular muscle at the opening of the esophagus into the stomach

cardiomegaly (Sp. cardiomegalia) enlargement of the heart

cardiomyopathy (Sp. cardiomiopatía) a defect of the heart muscle

cast (Sp. impresión) a negative mold or copy formed in a hollow organ or part (e.g., kidney or bronchi); a urinary cast is a small structure formed within the urinary system from mineral or protein matter and extruded from the body in urine

cataract (Sp. cataratas) a progressive disease in which the lens of the eye becomes cloudy, impairing vision or causing blindness

catatonic posturing (Sp. estado catatónico) a state of not being able to move, with the assumption of a rigid, often bizarre posture

cautery (Sp. cauterio) an instrument or chemical that destroys tissue as a therapeutic measure

cellulitis (Sp. celulitis) an acute, diffuse, spreading infection of the skin and subcutaneous tissue

centromere (Sp. centrómero) the constricted area of a chromosome

cephalgia, cephalalgia (Sp. cefalea) pain in the head; headache

cephalic (Sp. cefálico) referring to the head; cranial

cerclage (Sp. cerclaje) encircling of the cervix with a metal ring or suture ring to treat cervical incompetence during pregnancy to help prevent spontaneous abortion

chancre (Sp. chancro) a type of skin lesion usually associated with primary syphilis

cheilectomy (Sp. queilotomía) surgical removal of abnormal bone around a joint; also refers to the surgical removal of a lip

cholangiogram, cholangiography (Sp. colangiograma) a diagnostic radiographic study of the gallbladder and bile ducts

cholecystogram, cholecystography (Sp. colecistografía) a diagnostic radiographic study of the gallbladder

cholinergic (Sp. colinérgico) an agent that produces the effect of acetylcholine at the connections of muscles and nerves

chorea (Sp. corea) the ceaseless occurrence of involuntary muscular movements of the limbs or facial muscles

chromosome (Sp. cromosoma) structures in the nucleus of a cell that function in the transmission of genetic information

cicatricial (Sp. cicatriz) refers to a scar or the nature of a scar

circadian rhythm (Sp. ritmo circadiano) the biologic clock in humans; the rhythmic repetition of certain phenomena, such as hunger, fatigue, and changes in blood pressure, that tend to fluctuate within a 24-hour period

circumoral cyanosis (Sp. cianosis circumoral) a bluish discoloration around the mouth

clean-catch urine specimen (Sp. espécimen de orina limpia) a urine specimen obtained by cleaning the genitalia and then capturing a midstream urine sample for laboratory analysis

clonic (Sp. clónico) pertaining to increased reflex activity

closed reduction (Sp. reducción cerrada) the nonsurgical manipulative reduction of a dislocation or fracture

coagulation (Sp. coagulación) the process of clot formation

cognitive (Sp. cognitivo) pertaining to the mental processes of thinking, knowing, remembering, and perceiving

collateral (Sp. colateral) a small side branch of a blood vessel or nerve

colporrhaphy (Sp. colporrafia) suturing of the vagina

colposcopy (Sp. colcospia) examination of the vagina and cervix with an optical magnifying instrument frequently associated with biopsy of the cervix

comedo (comedones) (Sp. comedón) a blackhead, as seen in acne

commissurotomy (Sp. comisurotomía) surgical incision of component parts at the sites of junction between adjacent cusps of the heart valves to increase the size of the opening

comorbid (Sp. comórbido) two or more existing medical conditions

computed tomography (CT) (Sp. tomografía asistida por computadora [TAC]) a diagnostic technique using ionizing x-rays passed through a patient around specific sections of the body at multiple angles; useful in the detection of tumors

continuous positive airway pressure (CPAP) (Sp. presión positiva continua de las vías respiratorias [CPAP]) a form of respiratory therapy in which ventilation is assisted by a flow of oxygen delivered at a constant pressure throughout the respiratory cycle

contracture (Sp. contractura) immobility of muscles or a joint caused by shortening or wasting of tissue or muscle fibers

contrecoup a type of brain injury in which the tissue damage is on the opposite side of the trauma site controlled drug (Sp. drogas controladas) a drug regulated by the Federal Controlled Substance Act

corneal ulcer (Sp. úlcera de la córnea) ulcerative keratitis

corticotropin (Sp. corticotropina u hormona adrenocorticotrópica) a hormone secreted by the anterior lobe of the pituitary; also known as *adrenocorticotropic hormone (ACTH)*

cortisol (Sp. coritsol) major natural glucocorticoid synthesized in the adrenal cortex

craniotomy (Sp. craneotomía) incision into the skull—usually to relieve pressure, to remove a lesion, or to control bleeding

creatinine (Sp. creatinina) an important nitrogen compound that is a normal constituent of urine and blood; increased levels may indicate renal damage

Credé method (maneuver) (Sp. maniobra/ método de Credé) manual external compression of the bladder to aid in expulsion of urine

cryoablation (Sp. crioablación) the removal of tissue by destroying it with extreme cold

cryotherapy (Sp. crioterapia) the therapeutic use of cold

cryptorchidism (Sp. criptorquidismo) failure of one or both testicles to descend into the scrotum

cul-de-sac (Sp. fondo de saco) an area at the end of the abdominal cavity that is midway between the rectum and the uterus

curettage (Sp. curetaje/legrado) the removal of growths or other material from the wall of a cavity or other surface

cyanosis, cyanotic (Sp. cianosis, cianótico) bluish appearance of the skin and mucous membrane that usually indicates reduced hemoglobin levels in blood

cytology, cytologic (Sp. citología, citológico) the scientific study of cells

cytoreduction (Sp. citorreducción) a decrease in the number of cells (such as in a tumor)

D

débride (Sp. desbridar) remove foreign material or dead tissue in a wound

deficit (Sp. déficit) a deficiency from what is normal

delusion (Sp. falsa ilusión) a fixed false belief

demise (Sp. fallecimiento) destruction or death

demyelination (Sp. desmielinización) loss of the myelin sheath of a nerve

dermatome (Sp. dermatoma) a configured zone of skin innervated by a spinal cord segment

dialysate (Sp. dializado) the fluid that passes through a semipermeable membrane during dialysis

dialysis (dialyses) (Sp. diálisis) a procedure that filters out unwanted substances from the blood, usually in cases of renal failure

diaphoresis, diaphoretic (Sp. diaforesis, diaforético) profuse perspiration

diplopia (Sp. diplopía) double vision

discoid (Sp. discoide) shaped like a disk

diuresis, diuretic (Sp. diuresis, diurético) increased formation and excretion of urine

Doppler (Sp. Doppler) ultrasonogram, Doppler ultrasonography ultrasonographic technique used to evaluate blood flow velocity

dorsiflexion (Sp. dorsiflexión) to bend a joint toward the posterior aspect of the body; for example, the hand is dorsiflexed when it is extended or bent backward at the wrist

drusen (Sp. drusen) small yellowish deposits that develop beneath the retina; commonly associated with age-related macular degeneration

dyscrasia (Sp. discrasia) a pathologic condition; an abnormal condition of blood

dyspareunia (Sp. dispareunia) pain or discomfort in the pelvis or the vagina during or after sexual intercourse

dysphagia (Sp. disfagia) difficulty swallowing

dysphasia (Sp. disfasia) difficulty speaking, usually caused by a lesion in the central nervous system

dysphonia (Sp. disfonía) hoarseness; difficulty speaking

dysplastic, dysplasia (Sp. displástico) marked by abnormal adult cells

dyspnea (Sp. dispnea) labored or difficult breathing

dysrhythmia (Sp. disritmia) an abnormal cardiac rhythm

dysuria (Sp. disuria) painful or difficult urination

E

ecchymosis (Sp. equimosis) discoloration of the skin associated with a contusion

echocardiogram, echocardiography, echocardiographic (Sp. ecocardiograma, ecocardiografía, ecocar-diográfico) an ultrasonographic study of the motion of the walls or structures of the heart

ectopic (Sp. ectópico) out of normal position

effacement (Sp. borramiento) the thinning or obliteration of the cervix during labor

electrocardiogram (ECG), electrocardiography, electrocardiographic (Sp. electro-cardiograma, electrocardiografía, electro-cardiográfico) a record of the electrical activity of the heart

electromyogram (EMG), electromyography, electromyographic (Sp. electromiograma, electromiografía, electromiográfico) an electrodiagnostic assessment of the activity of skeletal muscles

embolization (Sp. embolismo) a treatment that blocks the flow of blood (i.e., to "starve" a tumor)

embolus (emboli), embolism (Sp. émbolo) a mass (e.g., foreign body, blood clot, or a piece of tumor) that breaks off and causes occlusion of an artery

emergency medical service (EMS) (Sp. servicios médicos de urgencia [SMU]) trained services provided on the scene

empyema (Sp. absceso) accumulation of pus in a hollow organ; abscess

encephalitis (Sp. encefalitis) inflammation of the brain

endarterectomy (Sp. endarterectomía) the surgical excision of the innermost lining of an artery to remove blockage

endemic (Sp. endémico) condition in which a disease is prevalent in a particular geographic area or in a population

endometriosis (Sp. endometriosis) a growth of endometrial tissue at various sites outside the uterus

endometrium (Sp. endometrio) the lining of the uterus that changes with the menstrual cycle; if the ovum is fertilized, the endometrium serves as the place where implantation occurs

endorphins (Sp. endorfina) one of the body's own morphine-like painkillers

endoscopy (Sp. endoscopia) examination of any cavity of the body with an endoscope

enzyme-linked immunosorbent assay (ELISA) (Sp. prueba de inmunoabsorción enzimática [prueba ELISA]) a test used to detect antibodies to the virus (human immunodeficiency virus) that causes acquired immunodeficiency syndrome in serum

epidural (Sp. epidural) an anesthetic injected into the epidural space around the spine, often used in labor and delivery

epigastric (Sp. epigástrico) refers to the upper middle region of the abdomen

epiphysis (epiphyses), epiphyseal (Sp. epifisis, epifiseal) the long end of a bone where bone growth occurs

epistaxis (Sp. epistaxis) bleeding from the nose

ergonomics (Sp. ergonomía) the science concerned with people and their work; it explores mechanical principles enhancing efficiency and well-being in the work environment

ergot (Sp. cornezuelo) a drug obtained from a fungus that grows on rye plants

erythema (Sp. eritema) redness or inflammation of the skin produced by capillary congestion

erythrocyte sedimentation rate (ESR) (Sp. tasa de sedimentación eritrocítica) a measurable reflection of the acute-phase reaction in inflammation and infection

esophagoscopy (Sp. esofagoscopia) examination of the esophagus with an esophagoscope

exacerbation (Sp. exacerbación) an increase in the severity of a disease or aggravation of its symptoms

exotoxin (Sp. exotoxina) bacterial toxins excreted outside of the bacterial cell

exsanguination (Sp. desangramiento) excessive loss of blood from a body part

exudate, exudative (Sp. exudado) fluid, cells, or cellular debris that has oozed into tissue because of injury or swelling

F

fascia (Sp. fascia) a fibrous membrane that covers, separates, and supports the muscles

fasciculation (Sp. fasciculación) involuntary contraction or twitching of muscles

fibrin (Sp. fibrina) a protein material produced by the action of thrombin on fibrinogen

fibrosis, fibrotic (Sp. fibrosis, fibrótico) the abnormal formation of fibrous tissue

fissure (Sp. fisura) a crack or groove on a surface

fistula (Sp. fístula) an abnormal tubelike passageway

fluorescein angiography (Sp. angiografía fluoresceínica) a procedure in which light-sensitive material is injected into a blood vessel

foramen (foramina) (Sp. foramen) an opening or hole in a bone, allowing the passage of nerves or blood vessels

foramen ovale (Sp. agujero ovale) an opening in the septum between the right and left atria of the fetal heart

Fowler position (Sp. posición de Fowler) a semisitting position, usually at 45 degrees, used to facilitate breathing and drainage

fulguration (Sp. fulguración) tissue destruction with high-frequency electrical sparks

fulminant (Sp. fulminante) occurring with great intensity; refers to severe pain with sudden onset

G

gamete (Sp. gameto) male or female sex cell

gangrene (Sp. gangrena) death of tissue caused by a decrease or absence of blood supply

gastrectomy (Sp. gastrectomía) surgical removal of the stomach

gastroscopy (Sp. gastroscopía) visual examination of the stomach using a gastroscope

genitourinary (Sp. genitourinario) referring to the genital and urinary systems of the body

Giemsa stain (Sp. tinción de Giemsa) a process of staining bacteria for identification

glenoid (Sp. glenoideo) having the semblance of a socket

glomerulosclerosis (Sp. glomerulo-esclerosis) hardening of the renal glomerulus

glomerulus (glomeruli) (Sp. glomérulo) a tiny ball of microscopic blood vessels on the end of the renal tubules

glucosteroid (Sp. glucosteroid) steroid produced by the adrenal cortex

goitrogenic (Sp. bociógeno) pertaining to substances causing goiters

gonadotropin (Sp. gonadotropina) a hormone that stimulates the testes and the ovaries to function

Gram staining (Sp. coloración de Gram) a process of staining bacteria for identification

Guthrie test (Sp. prueba de Guthrie) a test to detect phenylketonuria

gynecomastia (Sp. ginecomastia) abnormal enlargement of breast tissue in males

H

H2-receptor antagonist (Sp. antagonista del receptor H2) chemical agent that blocks the interaction of histamine or acetylcholine with receptors in stomach cells; drugs that inhibit secretion of gastric acid

hallucination (Sp. alucinación) a false perception of reality; may be visual, auditory, or olfactory

hallux (Sp. hallux) the great toe

hematemesis (Sp. hematemesis) vomiting of blood

hematocrit (Sp. hematocrito) the percentage of the total blood volume consisting of erythrocytes

hematoma (Sp. hematoma) localized swelling filled with blood as a result of a broken blood vessel

hematopoiesis, hematopoietic (Sp. hemato-poyesis, hematopoyético) pertaining to the production and development of blood cells or a substance that stimulates their production

hematuria (Sp. hematuria) blood in urine

hemiparesis (Sp. hemiparesia) paralysis affecting one side of the body

hemoccult (Sp. hemoccult) trademark for a guaiac reagent strip test for occult blood

hemochromatosis (Sp. hemochromatosis) a rare inherited disease of iron metabolism characterized by excess iron deposits in the body; a bronze color of the skin may be noticed

hemodynamic (Sp. hemodinámica) refers to forces involved in the circulation of blood within the body

hemolysis, hemolytic (Sp. hemólisis, hemo-lítico) the destruction of red blood cells with the release of hemoglobin

hemoptysis (Sp. hemoptisis) spitting up of blood

hemostasis (Sp. hemostasis) the condition of controlled bleeding

hepatomegaly (Sp. hepatomegalia) enlargement of the liver

histoplasmosis (Sp. histoplasmosis) a systemic respiratory disease caused by a fungus

homeostasis (Sp. homeostasis) a state of equilibrium within the body

human chorionic gonadotropin (hCG) (Sp. gonadotropina coriónica humana [GCH]) hormones produced by the placenta and detected in the urine and blood of a pregnant female

humoral (Sp. humoral) refers to body fluids or substances found in them

hyaline membrane (Sp. membrana hialina) a membrane that forms in the lung sacs of a developing fetus; a respiratory distress syndrome of the newborn

hydronephrosis (Sp. hidronefrosis) accumulation of urine in the renal pelvis caused by obstruction, forming a cyst

hymen (Sp. himen) the membrane partially covering the entrance to the vagina

hyperabduction (Sp. hyperabducción) abduction beyond normal limits

hyperalimentation (Sp. hiperalimentación) infusion of life-sustaining fluids, electrolytes, and elements of nutrition intravenously or via the gastrointestinal tract

hypercapnia (Sp. hipercapnia) increased carbon dioxide levels in blood

hypercoagulable (Sp. hipercoagulable) refers to the increased ability of any substance to coagulate, especially blood

hyperemic (Sp. hiperémico) refers to an excessive amount of blood in a body part or area

hyperesthesia (Sp. hiperestesia) increased sensitivity to pain

hyperglycemia (Sp. hiperglicemia) an increase in the normal blood glucose level

hyperkalemia (Sp. hipercalemia) a greater than normal amount of potassium in blood

hyperkeratosis (Sp. hyperqueratosis) results when an excess of proteins called *keratins* are produced, leading to thickening of the skin

hyperlipidemia (Sp. hiperlipemia) an increase of fat levels in blood

hyperparathyroidism (Sp. hiperpara-tiroidismo) a condition caused by overactive parathyroid glands

hyperplasia (Sp. hiperplasia) abnormal multiplication of the number of cells resulting from an increased rate of cellular division

hypertrophy, hypertrophic (Sp. hipertrofia, hipertrófico) enlargement of an organ or structure

hyperuricemia (Sp. hiperuricemia) excessive uric acid levels in blood

hypoalbuminemia (Sp. hipoalbuminemia) low albumin levels in blood

hypocalcemia (Sp. hipocalcemia) low calcium levels in blood

hypogammaglobulinemia (Sp. hypogamma-globulinemia) a below normal concentration of gamma globulin in blood associated with a decreased resistance to infection

hypogonadism (Sp. hipogonadismo) a condition resulting from a deficiency in the secretions of the ovary or the testis

hypokalemia (Sp. hipocalemia) low potassium levels in blood

hypoparathyroidism (Sp. hipopara-tiroidismo) a condition caused by greatly reduced function of the parathyroid glands

hypothalamus (Sp. hipotálamo) a portion of the diencephalon of the brain

hypovolemic shock (Sp. choque hipovolémico) a condition that occurs when blood in the circulatory system is decreased (e.g., as a result of hemorrhage)

hypoxia (Sp. hipoxia) low oxygen levels in tissues

hysterosalpingography (Sp. histerosalpingo-grafía) radiographic images of the uterus and the fallopian tubes

I

iatrogenic (Sp. iatrogénica) pathology inadvertently introduced by medical treatment or a diagnostic procedure

idiopathic (Sp. idiopático) refers to a disease without a known or recognizable cause

immunocompetent (Sp. inmunocompe-tente) the immune system has the ability to defend the body against disease

immunocompromised (Sp. con inmunidad comprometida) refers to an immune system incapable of fighting disease

immunodeficiency (Sp. inmuno-deficiencia) the diminished ability of the immune system to react with appropriate cellular immunity response; often the result of loss of immunoglobulins or aberrance of B- or T-cell lymphocytes

immunoelectrophoresis (Sp. inmuno-electroforesis) a technique used to separate and allow identification of complex proteins

immunogen (Sp. inmunógeno) an antigen (i.e., a substance capable of stimulating an immune response)

immunoglobulin (Sp. inmunoglobulina) a protein that can act as an antibody

immunoincompetence (Sp. inmuno-incompetencia) immunodeficiency

immunosenescence (Sp. inmunosenescencia) the gradual advanced age-related deterioration of the immune system that increases the risk for, and severity of, infection in the older adults

immunosuppressive (Sp. inmunosupresor) having the property of suppressing the body's immune response to antigens

incompetent cervix (Sp. cervix incompetente) premature painless dilation of the cervical os during pregnancy

infarct, infarction (Sp. infarto, infartado) an area of dead tissue caused by lack of blood supply

inguinal (Sp. inguinal) pertaining to the groin

insidious (Sp. insidioso) refers to the onset of a disease without symptoms

intractable (Sp. incurable) incurable or resistant to treatment

intravenous pyelogram, intravenous pyelography (Sp. pielograma intravenoso, pielografía intravenosa) radiographic study of the renal pelvis and ureter using injected dye

intravenous urogram, intravenous urography (Sp. urograma intravenoso, urografía intravenosa) radiographic study of the urinary tract using injected dye

intrinsic (Sp. intrínseco) refers to the essential nature of a substance or structure

intrinsic factor (Sp. factor intrínseco) a substance normally found in gastric juices; essential for the absorption of vitamin B$_{12}$

iontophoresis (Sp. iontoforesis) the therapeutic introduction of ions into the body tissues by direct current

ischemia, ischemic (Sp. isquemia, isquémico) holding back or obstructing the flow of blood

ischemic necrosis (Sp. necrosis isquémica) the death or sloughing off of small areas of tissue or bone, caused by insufficient circulation or lack of blood supply

J

jaundice (Sp. ictericia) yellowing of the skin

K

karyotype (Sp. cariotipo) a picture of chromosomes in the nucleus of a cell

Kegel exercises (Sp. ejercicios de Kegel) isometric pelvic exercises used by females to strengthen pelvic muscles and/or to improve retention of urine

keratin (Sp. queratina) a hard protein substance found in hair, nails, and skin

keratoconjunctivitis sicca (Sp. querato-conjuntivitis seca) dryness of the conjunctiva resulting from a decrease in lacrimal function

keratolytic (Sp. queratolítico) a substance that causes shedding of skin

keratosis (Sp. keratosis) a skin lesion where there is overgrowth and thickening of cornified epithelium

keratotomy (Sp. queratotomia) surgical incision of the cornea

kernicterus (Sp. kernicterus) a form of icterus (bile pigmentation of tissues and membranes) occurring in infants

ketone (Sp. cetona) acid chemical that builds up in blood when the body burns fats instead of glucose

L

laparoscopy (Sp. laparoscopia) a surgical procedure to examine the abdomen by using an endoscope called a *laparoscope*

laryngectomy (Sp. laringectomía) surgical removal of the organ of voice (larynx)

laryngoscopy (Sp. laringoscopia) visual examination of the larynx by using a laryngoscope

laser ablation (Sp. ablación por láser) separation, detachment, destruction, or removal of a part using laser surgery

laser photocoagulation (Sp. fotocoagulación por láser) coagulation of the blood vessels in the eye by using a laser

lavage (Sp. lavado) the cleaning out of a cavity by using liquid

leukocoria (Sp. leucocoria) the appearance of a whitish "reflection" or mass in the pupillary area behind the lens of the eye

leukocytosis (Sp. leucocitosis) a slight increase in the number of white blood cells

leukopenia (Sp. leucopenia) a decrease in the number of white blood cells

leukorrhea (Sp. leucorrea) a white or yellow mucous discharge from the vagina

lipase (Sp. lipasa) a fat-splitting enzyme produced by the pancreas

liposome (Sp. liposoma) a small, spherical particle in an aqueous solution, formed by a bilayer of phospholipid molecules

lithotripsy (Sp. litotripsia) crushing of stones (e.g., kidney stones and gallstones)

lumbar puncture (Sp. punción lumbar) a surgical procedure to withdraw spinal fluid for analysis or the injection of an anesthetic solution

lumpectomy (Sp. tumorectomia) removal of just the tumor from the breast

lymph (Sp. linfa) a mostly clear, colorless, transparent, alkaline fluid found within the lymphatic vessels; formed in tissues throughout the body

lymphadenitis (Sp. linfadenitis) inflammation of the lymph nodes

lymphadenopathy (Sp. linfadenopatía) disease of the lymph nodes

lymphocyte (Sp. linfocito) one of two types (B cells and T cells) of leukocytes (white blood cells) found in blood, lymph, and lymphoid tissue

lymphocytosis (Sp. linfocitosis) an excessive number of lymph cells

M

macrophage (Sp. macrófago) a monocyte blood cell

macula (Sp. mácula) a small spot or a colored area

maculopapular (Sp. maculopapular) pertaining to or consisting of macules and papules

magnetic resonance imaging (MRI) (Sp. formación de imágenes por resonancia magnética [RM]) a procedure similar to computed tomography that does not require radiation; a large magnetic field is applied and creates an image; useful in visualizing the cardiovascular system, brain, and soft tissues

malaise (Sp. malestar) a feeling of discomfort, illness, or uneasiness

malocclusion (Sp. maloclusión) improper positioning and faulty contact of teeth

mastectomy (Sp. mastectomía) surgical removal of breast tissue; can be partial or radical

McBurney point (Sp. punto de McBurney) the point of special tenderness in acute appendicitis; corresponds with the normal position of the base of the appendix

meconium (Sp. meconio) the first stool of a newborn, greenish black and with a tarry consistency

mediastinal shift (Sp. desplazamiento mediastinal) abnormal movement of the structures within the mediastinum to one side of the chest cavity

mediastinum (Sp. mediastino) the area in the chest between the lungs

megakaryocyte (Sp. megacariocito) a large bone marrow cell having large or many nuclei

megaloblastic (Sp. megaloblástico) pertaining to abnormally large red blood cells found in pernicious anemia

meibomian gland (Sp. glándula de chalazion) a sebaceous gland on the posterior margin of each eyelid

melanin (Sp. melanina) the black pigment found in the basal layer of the epidermis

melena (Sp. melena) the passage of very dark, tarry stools stained with digested blood

meningitis (Sp. meningitis) inflammation of the coverings around the brain and the spinal cord (meninges)

menorrhagia (Sp. menorragia) painful menstruation

metabolic acidosis (Sp. acidosis metabólica) excessive acid in body fluids, caused by dehydration, diarrhea, vomiting, renal disease, or hepatic impairment

metaplastic (Sp. metaplástico) characterized by metaplasia (a reversible change of cells usually caused by stress or injury); cancer formation can occur with chronic inducing stimulus by injury or irritation

metastasis (metastases), metastatic, metastasize (Sp. metástasis, metastásico, metastatizar) spreading of a malignant disease or pathogenic microorganisms from one organ or body part to another not directly connected with it

metatarsophalangeal (Sp. metatarsofalángico) pertaining to the metatarsus and phalanges of the toes

metrorrhagia (Sp. metrorragia) irregular menstruation

monoclonal antibodies (MAB) (Sp. anticuerpos monoclonales [MAB]) antibodies produced from a single clone of B lymphocytes

monocyte (Sp. monocito) a phagocytic white blood cell that engulfs and destroys cellular debris

multiparous (Sp. multiparos) having had multiple pregnancies

murine (Sp. roedor) pertaining to mice or rats

murmur (Sp. murmullo) a blowing sound heard when listening to the heart or vessels with a stethoscope

mutation (Sp. mutación) a variation or change in genetic structure

mutism (Sp. mutismo) the condition of being unable to speak

myalgia (Sp. mialgia) muscle pain

mycoplasma (Sp. micoplasma) microscopic organisms that lack a rigid cell wall; some species cause infections in humans

myelin (Sp. mielina) the protective fat and protein covering around the axons of many nerves

myelogram, myelography (Sp. mielograma, mielografía) radiographic study of the spinal cord after the injection of a dye

myringotomy (Sp. miringotomía) a surgical incision of the eardrum performed to release fluid or pus from the middle ear

N

necrosis, necrotic (Sp. necrosis, necrótico) death of tissue

neoadjuvant therapy (Sp. quimioterapia) a preliminary cancer treatment

neonate (Sp. neonato) a newborn baby

neoplasm, neoplasia, neoplastic (Sp. neoplasma, neoplasia, neoplástico) abnormal formation of new tissue; can be benign or malignant

neovascularization (Sp. neovascularización) the formation of new blood vessels

nephrectomy (Sp. nefrectomía) the surgical removal of a kidney

nephron (Sp. nefrona) the functioning unit of the kidney or renal tubule

nephropathy (Sp. nefropatía) any disease or damage of the kidney

nephrotoxic (Sp. nefrotóxico) a quality of being destructive to kidney tissue

neurotransmitter (Sp. neurotransmisor) a chemical released by the terminal end fibers of an axon

nociceptor (Sp. nociceptor) nerve that receives and transmits painful stimuli

normal flora (Sp. flora normal) the presence of normal bacteria and fungi adapted for living in, and characteristic of, the area considered (e.g., skin, intestine, or vagina)

nuchal rigidity (Sp. rigidez en la nuca) neck stiffness

nullipara (Sp. nulípara) a female who has never produced viable offspring

O

odynophagia (Sp. odinofagia) painful swallowing; a severe burning, squeezing pain while swallowing caused by irritation or muscular disorder of the esophagus

oligospermia (Sp. oligospermia) insufficient number of spermatozoa in semen

oliguria (Sp. oliguria) scanty urination

oncogene (Sp. oncógeno) a gene in a virus that can prompt a cell to become malignant

onycholysis (Sp. onicolisis) a spontaneous separation of the nail plate or supporting structures

oophorectomy (Sp. ovariotomía) the surgical removal of one or both ovaries

opacity (Sp. opacidad) the state of being opaque or not transparent

open reduction (Sp. reducción abierta) exposure of a fractured or dislocated bone through a surgical incision to realign the bone ends

ophthalmoscopy, ophthalmoscopic (Sp. oftalmoscopia, oftalmoscópico) an examination of the interior of the eye

opportunistic infection (Sp. infección oportunista) infection resulting from a defective immune system

orchiectomy (Sp. orquiectomía) the surgical removal of one or both testes; also called *orchidectomy*

orchiopexy (Sp. orquidopexia) surgical procedure to mobilize an undescended testis and bring it into the scrotum

orchitis (Sp. orquitis) inflammation of the testes

orthodontics (Sp. ortodoncia) branch of dentistry concerned with correction of dentofacial structures (e.g., teeth)

orthopnea (Sp. ortopnea) a condition in which breathing becomes easier in the upright standing position or in the sitting position

orthoptic training (Sp. entrenamiento ortóptico) eye muscle exercises

Ortolani sign (Sp. prueba de Ortolani) an assessment maneuver designed to detect a hip dislocation

ossification (Sp. osificación) the development of bone

osteogenesis (Sp. osteogénesis) the formation of bone tissue

osteophyte (Sp. osteofito) a bony outgrowth, usually branch shaped

ostomy (Sp. ostomía) a surgical opening of the bowel to the outside of the body

otitis media (Sp. otitis media) middle ear infection

otoscopy (Sp. otoscopia) visual examination of the ear by using an otoscope

oxygen saturation (Sp. saturación de oxígeno) refers to the oxygen content in blood, divided by oxygen capacity, and expressed in volume percent

P

palliative (Sp. paliativo) alleviating symptoms without curing the underlying cause

panhypopituitarism (Sp. panhipopituitarismo) a condition in which the entire pituitary gland ceases to function and is not producing any pituitary hormones

papule (Sp. pápula) a circular area on the skin that is reddened and elevated

parasympathetic (Sp. parasimpático) the division of the autonomic nervous system mediated by the release of acetylcholine, which has many effects on body functions, such as slowing heart rate and stimulating peristalsis

paresis (Sp. paresia) partial paralysis

paresthesia (Sp. parestesia) abnormal, usually increased, sensations

parietal (cells) (Sp. células parietales) the cells on the wall of a cavity, such as the stomach; pertaining to or located near the parietal bone (of the parietal lobe) of the skull

paronychia (Sp. paroniquia) inflammation of soft tissue surrounding the nail

partial thromboplastin time (PTT) (Sp. tiempo parcial de tromboplastina [TPT]) a measure of the coagulation sequence of plasma and screen for platelet abnormalities

patch test (Sp. prueba del parche) a screening test in which a small piece of material containing the allergy-causing substance is placed on the skin; redness or edema indicates a positive reaction

patent (Sp. de patente, accisible) open and unblocked

pathogenesis (Sp. patogénesis) the development of disease; pathologic mechanisms

pathologist (Sp. patologista) one who specializes in the study of disease

peau d'orange (Sp. piel de naranja) condition in which the skin is dimpled, resembling the skin of an orange

pelvic inflammatory disease (PID) (Sp. enfermedad inflamatoria pélvica [EIP]) inflammation of the female pelvic organs, usually caused by bacteria

perfusion (Sp. perfusión) delivery of oxygen and other nutrients to the tissue by blood

pericoronitis (Sp. pericoronitis) inflammation of gum around the crown of a tooth

periosteum (Sp. periostio) the fibrous covering of long bones

peritonitis (Sp. peritonitis) inflammation of the membrane that lines the abdominal cavity and covers the viscera

pessary (Sp. pesario) an object placed in the vagina to support the uterus

petechia (petechiae) (Sp. petequia) a tiny spiderlike hemorrhage under the skin

phagocyte, phagocytic, phagocytosis (Sp. fagocito, fagocítico, fagocitosis) the process by which cells surround and digest certain particles (e.g., bacteria, protozoa, debris)

phenotype (Sp. fenotipo) the entire physical appearance and biochemical and psychological makeup of an individual as determined by the interaction of genetic makeup and environmental factors

phlebotomy (Sp. flebotomía) surgical puncture of a vein to withdraw blood

phonologic (Sp. fonológico) refers to oral communication or vocal sounds

photocoagulation (Sp. fotocoagulación) the coagulation (clotting) of tissue by controlled use of a laser to seal off bleeding blood vessels

photon (Sp. foton) the smallest quantity of electromagnetic energy; a particle with no mass and no charge; may occur in the form of x-rays, gamma rays, or quanta of light

photophobia (Sp. fotofobia) unusual sensitivity to light

phototherapy (Sp. fototerapia) treatment of disease by exposure to light

plaque (Sp. placa) a deposit of hardened material lining a blood vessel; or a gummy accumulation of microorganisms that clings to teeth and is considered the forerunner of caries and periodontal disease

plasmapheresis (Sp. plasmaféresis) the process of separating blood into its components by centrifuging

polydipsia (Sp. polidipsia) excessive thirst

polyphagia (Sp. polfagia) excessive eating

polyposis (Sp. poliposis) a condition of multiple polyps

polyuria (Sp. poliuria) excretion of abnormally large amounts of urine

positive end-expiratory pressure (PEEP) (Sp. presión positiva al final de la expiración [PEEP]) mechanical ventilation with pressure maintained, thereby increasing the volume of gas remaining in the lungs at the end of expiration

positron emission tomography (PET) (Sp. tomografía por emisión de positrones [PET]) a noninvasive radiographic study of the blood flow in specific organs and body tissues

postprandial (Sp. posprandial) after meals

primipara (Sp. primípara) a female who has delivered one child of at least 20 weeks' gestational age

probiotic (Sp. probiotico) a substance that stimulates the growth of microorganisms with beneficial properties (such as those of the intestinal flora)

proctoscopy (Sp. proctoscopia) visual examination of the rectum by using a proctoscope

prodromal (Sp. prodrómico) refers to the initial stage of a disease before the onset of actual symptoms

prophylaxis, prophylactic (Sp. profilaxis, profiláctico) the prevention of disease

prostate-specific antigen (PSA) (Sp. antígeno específico de la próstata [APE]) an enzyme that is measured in a blood test to detect cancer of the prostate

proteinuria (Sp. proteinuria) the presence of protein in urine

prothrombin time (PT) (Sp. tiempo de protrombina [TP]) a measure of the time taken for clot formation

proton pump inhibitor (Sp. inhibidor de la bomba de pro-tones) a drug that blocks gastric acid secretion; used to treat ulcers of the gastrointestinal tract and gastroesophageal reflux disease

pruritus (Sp. prurito) itching

pseudomembranous (Sp. membrana pseudo) a false membrane

pseudoneurologic (Sp. pseudoneurológico) refers to a neurologic symptom that is without clinical basis

pseudopregnancy (Sp. pseudoembarazo) false pregnancy, also known as *pseudocyesis*

psychosexual (Sp. psicosexual) refers to the relationship between the psychological and emotional aspects of sex

psychosis, psychotic (Sp. psicosis, sicopático) a major mental disorder usually accompanied by perceptional distortion of reality, regressive behavior, and diminished impulse control

psychotropic drugs (Sp. erogas psicotrópicas) drugs that have an effect on the mind or that alter a person's state of mind

ptosis (Sp. ptosis) drooping of one or both eyelids

purpura (Sp. púrpura) a red-purple discoloration of the skin caused by multiple minute hemorrhages in the skin or mucous membrane

purulent (Sp. purulento) containing pus

pustule (Sp. pústula) a small elevation of the skin containing pus

putrefaction (Sp. putrefacción) decomposition of organic matter

pyelogram, pyelography (Sp. pielografía) radiography of the pelvis of the kidney and ureter by using a contrast solution

pyelonephritis (Sp. pielonefritis) a purulent infection of the kidney tissue and renal pelvis

pylorus (Sp. píloro) the narrow part of the stomach toward the duodenum

pyuria (Sp. piuria) pus in urine

R

raccoon eyes (Sp. ojos de mapache) dark discoloration (bruising) around the eyes; a sign of possible basilar skull fracture

radioimmunoassay (Sp. radioinmuno-análisis) radiology used to detect the concentration of an antigen or antibody or other protein in serum

rale (Sp. estertor) an abnormal crackling sound made by the lungs during inspiration; indicative of fluid in a bronchus

Raynaud phenomenon (Sp. fenómeno de Raynaud) a temporary constriction of arterioles in the skin causing short episodes of numbness and color changes in the fingers and toes; this condition is usually idiopathic

reflux (Sp. reflujo) a backward flow

regenerative medicine (Sp. medicina regeneradora) a field where stem cells are induced to differentiate into a specific cell type that can be used to repair damaged tissue

renal calculi (Sp. cálculo renal) kidney stones

reticuloendothelial (Sp. reticuloendotelial) refers to the system responsible for phagocytosis of cellular debris, pathogens, and foreign substances and for removing them from the circulation

retinopathy (Sp. retinopatía) refers to noninflammatory eye disorders

retrovirus (Sp. retrovirus) a family of viruses that contains ribonucleic acid (RNA) and reverse transcriptase; some retroviruses are oncogenic and can induce tumors

rheumatoid factor (Sp. factor reumatoide) a macroglobulin type of antibody; increased levels are found in the blood of persons with rheumatoid arthritis

rhonchus (rhonchi) (Sp. ronquido) dry rattling in the throat or bronchus caused by partial obstruction

ribonucleic acid (RNA) (Sp. ácido ribonucleico [ARN]) controls protein synthesis in cells and takes the place of deoxyribonucleic acid (DNA) in some viruses

S

salpingo-oophorectomy (Sp. anexectomía) the surgical removal of a fallopian tube and an ovary

Schick test (Sp. prueba de Schick) an intradermal skin test to detect immunity to diphtheria; a positive result indicates lack of immunity or negative immunity

Schilling test (Sp. prueba de Schilling) a 24-hour urine test for gastrointestinal absorption of vitamin B$_{12}$

sclerosis, sclerosing (Sp. esclerosis) hardening of a body part

sclerotherapy (Sp. escleroterapia) use of sclerosing chemicals to treat esophageal varices or hemorrhoids

seborrhea (Sp. seborrea) the excessive secretion of sebum from sebaceous glands

sebum (Sp. sebo) oily secretion of sebaceous glands

semi-Fowler position (Sp. posición semi-Fowler) position of lying on the back with the head elevated 8 to 10 inches and the knees flexed

senile (Sp. senil) refers to growing old with decreased physical and mental capacity

senile plaque (Sp. placa senil) microscopic patch of fragmented nerve around amyloid deposits found in the cerebral cortex of normal older people; found in larger amounts in people with Alzheimer disease

sensorineural (Sp. sensorineural) pertaining to a sensory nerve

septicemia (Sp. septicemia) a disease in which pathogenic microorganisms or toxins are present in blood

sequestrum (Sp. secuestro) a segment of dead bone; the result of an abscess from a bacterial infection in a bone and bone marrow

serology, serologic (Sp. serología, serológico) a study of blood serum to measure antibody titers

sigmoidoscopy (Sp. sigmoidoscopia) visual examination of the sigmoid colon by using a sigmoidoscope

sinopulmonary (Sp. sinopulmonar) pertaining to the paranasal sinuses and lungs

sinusotomy (Sp. sinusotomía) incision into the sinus

skeletal traction (Sp. tracción ósea) a method of immobilization and reduction of a long-bone fracture, in which traction is applied by means of pins and wires

somatoform (Sp. forma somática) psychogenic symptoms without an underlying disease process

somatotropin (Sp. somatotropina) growth hormone secreted by the anterior pituitary gland

spermicidal (Sp. espermicidal) destructive to sperm

splenomegaly (Sp. esplenomegalia) enlarged spleen

squamous cell (Sp. células escamosas) flat and scaly epithelial cell

status asthmaticus (Sp. estado asmático) severe asthmatic episode that does not respond to normal treatment

steatorrhea (Sp. esteatorrea) the presence of malabsorbed fat in feces

stenosis, stenosed (Sp. estenosis, estenosado) narrowing of an opening

stent (Sp. stent) a device used to hold tissue in place or provide support

Steri-Strips (Sp. Steri-Strips) trademarked brand name for sterile adhesive strips used to approximate and hold together the edges of a wound

stomatitis (Sp. estomatitis) an inflammatory condition of the mouth

stress incontinence (Sp. incontinencia por presión) leakage of urine when stress is placed on the perineum

stridor (Sp. estridor) a high-pitched respiratory sound caused by obstruction of air passageway

subluxation (Sp. subluxación) partial dislocation

substernal retraction (Sp. retracción del esternón) condition in which the chest wall under the sternum sinks in with each respiration

sulfonylurea (Sp. sulfonilurea) oral hypo-glycemic agent that stimulates the pancreas to produce insulin

supine (Sp. supino) lying on the back

surfactant (Sp. agente de superficie) an agent (normally present in the lungs as a phospholipid) that lowers surface tension; abnormal in the lungs of premature infants or in hyaline membrane disease

symptomatic (Sp. sintomático) concerning the nature of a symptom indicative of a disease

syncope (Sp. síncope) fainting, lightheadedness

syncytial virus (Sp. virus de síncytial) a type of minute parasitic microorganism

synovial (Sp. sinovial) pertaining to a lubrication fluid around a joint, bursa, and tendon sheath

synthesize (Sp. sintetizar) to produce a substance by combining two or more elements or chemicals

T

tachycardia, tachycardic (Sp. taquicardia, taquicár-dico) rapid heartbeat; greater than 100 beats per minute

tachypnea (Sp. taquipnea) rapid and shallow respirations

tamponade (Sp. tamponar) compression of a part by pressure or a collection of fluid

tendinitis (Sp. tendinitis) inflammation of a tendon

tenesmus (Sp. tenesmo) ineffectual spasms of the rectum accompanied by a desire to empty the bowel; sometimes mistaken as constipation

tetany (Sp. tetania) hyperexcitability of nerves and muscles resulting from low serum calcium

levels; a syndrome characterized by intermittent tonic spasms of the extremities, cramps, and convulsions

tetralogy of Fallot (Sp. tetralogía de Fallot) a congenital cardiac condition

tetraplegia (Sp. tetraplejia) another term for quadriplegia; the inability of a person to move the upper and lower extremities; impaired mobility includes the upper and lower extremities; the head, neck, and shoulders may or may not be affected, depending on the level of injury to the spine

thallium scan (Sp. escáner con talio) a cardiac stress test using intravenous thallium injection to diagnose ischemia and coronary artery disease

thoracentesis (Sp. toracentesis) surgical puncture into the parietal cavity for aspiration of fluids

thoracostomy (Sp. toracotomía) an incision in the chest wall for the purpose of drainage; a chest tube may be inserted for drainage of air or fluid from the pleural space

thrill (Sp. estremecimiento) vibration felt on palpation, especially over the heart

thrombocytopenia (Sp. trombocito-penia) reduced number of thrombocytes (platelets)

thrombus (Sp. trombo) a blood clot attached to the interior wall of a blood vessel, often causing vascular obstruction

thyroidectomy (Sp. tiroidectomía) surgical removal of the thyroid gland

thyrotoxicosis (Sp. thyrotoxicosis) a toxic condition caused by hyperactivity of the thyroid gland

thyrotropin (Sp. tirotropina) thyroid-stimulating hormone

tinnitus (Sp. tinnitus) ringing or buzzing in the ears

tonometry (Sp. tonometría) measurement of intraocular pressure

toxin, toxic (Sp. toxina, tóxico) poisonous substance

toxoplasmosis (Sp. toxoplasmosis) a disease caused by infection with protozoa found in many mammals and birds

transcutaneous electrical nerve stimulation (TENS) (Sp. estimulación nerviosa eléctrica transcutánea [ENET]) electrical stimulation of nerves for relief of pain

transferrin (Sp. transferrina) globulin in blood serum that transports iron

triiodothyronine (T3) (Sp. triyodotironina) a hormone that helps regulate growth and development, metabolism, and body temperature

trisomy (Sp. anormalidad chromosomal) one or more than the normal number of chromosomes

Trousseau phenomenon (Sp. fenómeno de Trousseau) sign in which pressure applied to the upper arm produces muscular spasms, indicating latent tetany

truss (Sp. braguero) a device that holds a reduced hernia in place

tumor necrosis factor (Sp. factor de necrosis de tumor) a natural body protein with anticancer effects; also produced in response to bacterial toxins (can be produced synthetically)

turgor (Sp. turgor) normal tension in a cell that results in normal strength and tension of the skin

tympanic membrane (Sp. membrana del tímpano) eardrum

Tzanck test (Sp. análisis de Tzanck) diagnostic test that examines the tissue of a lesion to determine the type of cell present

U

ulcer, ulceration (Sp. úlcera, ulceración) a craterlike sore on the skin or mucous membrane

ultrasonogram, ultrasonography (Sp. ultrasonografía) imaging deep structures of the body using high-frequency sound waves

ultrasound diathermy (Sp. diatermia por ultrasonidos) medical diathermy (heating of body tissue) by using ultrasound

uremia (Sp. uremia) toxic condition of excessive waste products, protein, and nitrogen in blood caused by renal insufficiency

urethritis (Sp. uretritis) inflammation of the urethra

urodynamics (Sp. urodinámica) study of the mechanics of urinary bladder, filling and emptying liquid

urothelium (Sp. urotelio) transitional epithelium in the wall of the bladder

V

vaginismus (Sp. vaginismo) a spasm of the muscles surrounding the vagina, causing painful contractions of the vagina

Valsalva maneuver (Sp. maniobra de Valsalva) forced exhalation with the mouth and nose closed, causing increased intrathoracic pressure, slowing of heart rate, increased venous pressure, and a reduced amount of return blood flow to the heart

varicocele (Sp. varicocele) a condition in which the veins in the scrotum near the testicles are swollen and enlarged

vector (Sp. vector) carrier of infectious agent of disease from one person to another (usually insects)

venom (Sp. veneno) poison secreted by an animal

ventricular shift (Sp. desplazamiento ventricular) lateral movement of one of the ventricles of the brain to one side caused by pressure on the other side

vertex (Sp. vertex) top of the head

vertigo (Sp. vértigo) loss of equilibrium or sensation of instability; dizziness

vesicle (Sp. vesícula) a small blister-like elevation of the skin containing clear fluid

vitrectomy (Sp. vitrectomía) a surgical procedure that removes the contents of the vitreous chamber of the eye

W

Western blot test (Sp. prueba Western blot) a laboratory blood test to identify and analyze specific protein antigens; sometimes used to confirm the validity of the ELISA test

wheal (Sp. ampolla) a smooth, round, elevated area of the skin with red edges and a white center, usually accompanied by itching; hives

white blood cell (WBC), WBC count (Sp. glóbulos blancos, conteo de glóbulos blancos) see Appendix I, Common Laboratory and Diagnostic Tests, under Blood Analysis

X

xerostomia (Sp. xerostomía) dry mouth; reduced amount of saliva

Z

zygote (Sp. zigoto) fertilized ovum

Index

Page numbers followed by *f* indicate figures, *t* indicate tables, and *b* indicate boxes.

Rosiglitazone maleate, 159
Rotator cuff tears, 288–289
Rotavirus, immunization schedule, 72*f*
Round window, 190*f*
RSV (respiratory syncytial virus) pneumonia, 373
Rubella (German measles), 77–79, 78*f*
Rubeola (measles), 76–77, 76*f*
Rule of nines, 625*f*
Ruptured disk, 553
Ruptured tympanic membrane
    etiology and diagnosis, 200, 200*f*
    symptoms and signs, 200
    treatment and prognosis, 200

S

Saccular aneurysm, 425*f*
Sacral nerves, 534*f*–535*f*
Sacral plexus (L5-S3), 538*f*–539*f*
Sacrum, 254*f*, 258*f*
Salivary glands, 293*f*
    in Sjögren syndrome, 124–125
Salpingo-oophorectomy, 502–503
Saphenous vein grafts, 397*f*
Sarcoidosis
    diagnosis and treatment, 386
    etiology, 386
    patient screening, 386
    patient teaching, 386
    prevention, 386
    prognosis, 386
    symptoms and signs, 385–386
Sartorius muscle, 253*f*
Scabies
    description, 229
    etiology and diagnosis, 229–230
    patient screening, 229
    patient teaching, 231
    prevention, 230–231
    symptoms and signs, 229
    treatment and prognosis, 230
Scalded child, 642
Scale
    in cradle cap, 210
    dermatologic, 211*f*–212*f*
    of dermatophytoses, 226
    of psoriasis, 217
Scaling and root planing (SRP), 299
Scapula, 254*f*
Scars, hypertrophic, 232, 232*f*
Scheuermann disease, kyphosis associated with, 259*f*
Schirmer tear test, 125*f*
Schizoid personality disorder, 608
Schizophrenia
    etiology and diagnosis, 590
    prognosis and prevention, 591
    symptoms and signs, 588–590
    treatment, 590–591
Schizotypal personality disorder, 608
Sciatic nerve injury, 554–555
SCID (severe combined immunodeficiency), 111–112
Sclera, 167, 168*f*, 169*t*
    rosacea involving, 218
Scleritis
    description, 180
    etiology and diagnosis, 180
    patient teaching, 181
    symptoms and signs, 180
Scleroderma
    chronic, progressive disease, 123

Scleroderma *(Continued)*
    etiology and diagnosis, 124
    skin involvement in, 123*f*
    symptoms and signs, 123
    treatment and prognosis, 124
Scleroplasty, 180–181
Sclerotic stage, 268
Scoliosis
    description, 260, 261*f*
    diagnosis, 260
    etiology, 260
    patient screening, 260
    patient teaching, 261
    prevention, 261
    prognosis, 261
    symptoms and signs, 260
    treatment, 260
Screening
    breast cancer, 525*t*
    drug, 589*b*
    tests, 12
Screening test
    alpha-fetoprotein, 674–675
    BRCA1 and *BRCA2* gene testing, 675
    cancer/tumor markers, 674
    carcinoembryonic antigen, 674
    CA 15-3 Test, 674
    CA 19-9 Test, 674
    CA 125 test, 674
    mammography, 675
    Mantoux test, 673–674
    Papanicolaou smear, 675
    prostate-specific antigen, 674
    testicular self-examination, 675
    tuberculosis screening, 673–674
Scrotal sac, 479*f*
    and abdominal hernia, 321*f*
Sea salt, in simple goiter, 147
Sebaceous cysts, 232, 233*f*
Sebaceous glands, 209
Seborrhea, 175
Seborrheic dermatitis
    description, 209
    etiology and diagnosis, 210
    patient teaching, 213
    prevention, 213
    prognosis, 212–213
    symptoms and signs, 209–210
    treatment, 210–212
Seborrheic keratosis, 231, 231*f*
Secondary hypopituitarism, 144
Secondary syphilis, 486*f*
Second-degree heart block, 414*t*–415*t*
Seizure disorder (epilepsy), 557–558
Seizures, first aid for, 559*f*
Selective IgA deficiency
    etiology and diagnosis, 110
    patient screening, 110
    patient teaching, 111
    symptoms and signs, 110
    treatment and prognosis, 110
Semicircular canals, 190, 190*f*, 199*f*
Sense of smell, loss of, 363
Sensitization, contact dermatitis developed via, 214
Sensorineural hearing loss, 190
    patient teaching, 203
    prevention, 203
    symptoms and signs, 202
Sensory cortex, 534*f*–535*f*
Septicemia, 483
Septum, deviated, 361–362, 362*f*

Serous otitis media, 194
Serum markers
    CA-125, 512
    in testicular cancer, 497
Service animals, 575–576
Sesamoid bones, 252
Severe combined immunodeficiency (SCID)
    diagnosis and treatment, 112
    etiology, 112
    patient screening, 112
    patient teaching, 112
    symptoms and signs, 112
Severed tendon, 283–284
Sex, as predisposing factor for disease, 3
Sex chromosome abnormalities, 69*f*
Sexual abuse
    diagnosis and treatment, 649
    symptoms and signs, 649
Sexual assault, 650–651
    response teams and evidence maintenance, 651*b*
Sexual dysfunction
    contraception/birth control, 490–491
    erectile dysfunction/impotence, 488–489
    male and female infertility, 489–490
Sexually transmitted diseases (STDs)
    chancroid, 487–488
    chlamydia, 481–482
    genital herpes, 484–485
    genital warts, 485–486
    gonorrhea, 482–483
    hepatitis B, 338
    risk factors for, 480*b*
    syphilis, 486–487
    transmission of, 481–488
    trichomoniasis, 483–484
Sexually transmitted infections (STIs), risk factors for, 480*b*
SGLT2 (sodium-glucose linked transporter 2) inhibitors, 159
Shaken baby syndrome
    etiology and diagnosis, 645
    prognosis and prevention, 645
    symptoms and signs, 644
Shiatsu, 24–25
Shingles, 220–221
Shin splints, 284–285
Shock
    cardiogenic, 419–420
    causes of, 419*f*
    diagnosis and treatment, 417–418
    spinal, 550*f*
    symptoms and signs, 417
Short bones, 252
Short bowel syndrome, 331–332
Shoulder, 255*f*
    bursae, 265*f*
    dislocation of, 282*f*
    major nerves of, 538*f*–539*f*
    structures, 288*f*
    tendonitis, cupping placement for, 24*f*
Shunting procedures, for hydrocephalus, 52*f*
Sickle cell anemia, 432, 433*t*
Side splash lightning strike, 628
SIDS (sudden infant death syndrome), 79
Sigmoid colostomy, 329*f*
Sigmoid diverticular disease, 327*f*
Sigmoidoscopy, 332
Sildenafil citrate, precautions, 489*b*
Silicosis, 379
Simple goiter, 147*f*
    etiology, 147